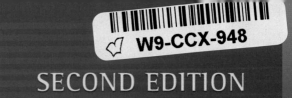

SECOND EDITION

PHARMACOLOGY
PRINCIPLES AND APPLICATIONS

Eugenia M. Fulcher, RN, BSN, EdD, CMA
Former Program Director, Medical Assisting
Swainsboro Technical College
Swainsboro, Georgia

Robert M. Fulcher, BS, BSPh, RPh
Pharmacist-in-Charge
CVS Pharmacy
Waynesboro, Georgia

Cathy Dubeansky Soto, PhD, MBA, CMA
Program Director, Medical Assisting
El Paso Community College
El Paso, Texas

SAUNDERS
ELSEVIER

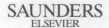

SAUNDERS
ELSEVIER

11830 Westline Industrial Drive
St. Louis, Missouri 63146

PHARMACOLOGY: PRINCIPLES AND APPLICATIONS

978-1-4160-2540-5

Notice

Knowledge and best practice in this field are constantly changing. As new research and experience broaden our knowledge, changes in practice, treatment and drug therapy may become necessary or appropriate. Readers are advised to check the most current information provided (i) on procedures featured or (ii) by the manufacturer of each product to be administered, to verify the recommended dose or formula, the method and duration of administration, and contraindications. It is the responsibility of the practitioner, relying on their own experience and knowledge of the patient, to make diagnoses, to determine dosages and the best treatment for each individual patient, and to take all appropriate safety precautions. To the fullest extent of the law, neither the Publisher nor the Authors assume any liability for any injury and/or damage to persons or property arising out of or related to any use of the material contained in this book.

The Publisher

Library of Congress Control Number 2007932285

Executive Editor: Susan Cole
Developmental Editors: Celeste Clingan, Jennifer Presley
Publishing Services Manager: Patricia Tannian
Senior Project Manager: Sarah Wunderly
Design Direction: Andrea Lutes

Printed in China

Last digit is the print number: 9 8 7 6 5 4 3 2 1

We dedicate this second edition to our parents,

Harold L. and Rosabel L. Mills and Robert M. and Lucy F. Fulcher,

who gave us dreams and the desire for and the means

to obtain professional educations, only wishing you were here to be proud.

To our children, Lee, Gene, and Kim, and grandchildren, Mac and Allie,

we know you have dreams and we hope you will succeed in reaching them.

We thank each of you for the love and support that you have provided during

the preparation of this text. To all allied health professionals

who will use this text, may you achieve your professional dreams—

they can come true. You are the reason this text has been written—

to provide the educational background for patient safety.

Bobby and Genie Fulcher

To my best friend, my husband, Jose Soto III, I dedicate this book—

thank you for your constant compassion and dedication

in seeing me through all my "special projects" during our 32 years of marriage.

To our daughters and their families:

Cathy June, Ed, Joshua, and Matthew; and Jenny, Fernando, and Victoria;

to my dad, Edward D. Dubeansky of Mentor, Ohio,

and to the memory of my mom, June E. Dubeansky;

to my siblings, Ed Jr., Steve, Clyde, Allan, and Bernadette Bileci;

and to the entire Dube' support group,

I thank each of you for your constant enthusiasm

and words of encouragement. I treasure our times together.

Cathy Dubeansky Soto

Reviewers

Vanessa Austin, RMA, CAHI
Clinical Education Specialist
Clarian Health Partners
Indianapolis, Indiana

David Frame, PharmD
Assistant Professor of Pharmacy, Clinical
    Hematology Oncology Specialist
University of Michigan
Ann Arbor, Michigan

Julie Golembiewski, PharmD
Clinical Associate Professor
Pharmacy Practice and Anesthesiology
University of Illinois
Chicago, Illinois

Kathy Gudgel, RN, MSN
Instructor, Nursing
School of Health Sciences
Pennsylvania College of Technology
Williamsport, Pennsylvania

Maureen Messier, CMA, RMA, AS, BA
Instructor, Medical Assisting/General Education
Branford Hall Career Institute
Southington, Connecticut

Joshua Neumiller, PharmD
Geriatric Resident/Clinical Research Associate
Elder Services
Washington State University
Spokane, Washington

Tami Remington, PharmD
Clinical Associate Professor
College of Pharmacy
University of Michigan,
Ann Arbor, Michigan

April Schroer, MSN, RN, CS
Southwest Region Nursing Director
Vocational Nursing
Kaplan Higher Education Corporation
San Antonio, Texas

Angela Taylor, RN, PhD, BC
Associate Professor
Department of Nursing
University of Virginia
Wise, Virginia

Marsha Lynn Wilson, BS
Health Careers Counselor/Educator
Educational Services
Clarian Health Partners
Indianapolis, Indiana

Preface

The goal of the second edition of *Pharmacology: Principles and Applications* is to help the student master not only the principles of pharmacology but also the skills to transfer this knowledge to a clinical setting for patient safety. We have sought to achieve this in various ways, some of which are found in other pharmacology texts and others of which are unique to this text.

The purpose of this text has remained constant—to provide an introduction to pharmacology that gives allied health professionals an in-depth knowledge about medications that are used on a day-to-day basis in the ambulatory and some inpatient care settings. Thus, the text includes information on medications used to stabilize a patient in outpatient emergency situations but not medications frequently used in inpatient emergency situations, such as intensive care units. Similarly, because medications that are used on a "stat," or immediate, basis in specialized intensive care units and in surgical areas typically are not used in ambulatory care settings, information about these drugs is not included.

As the world of medicine has evolved from a predominately inpatient setting for acute and chronic care to ambulatory care for many conditions previously seen on an inpatient basis, allied health professionals have integrated the skills needed to complete tasks ordered by the health care provider to provide safe, necessary patient care in the ambulatory setting. Because the tasks health professionals are legally permitted to perform vary from state to state, it is important for all health care personnel to understand state statutes in their particular employment setting. This text is designed to provide a solid background in pharmacology as well as the necessary skills to administer prescription and over-the-counter medications safely.

The organization of material by body system lends itself to the study of disease processes along with the study of medications used to therapeutically and prophylactically treat these diseases.

This comprehensive study helps students achieve additional competency and critical thinking skills and helps prepare them for examinations that are required for licensure or certification. The depth of material is sufficient for critical thinking skills that can be readily transferred to patient care and patient teaching.

Because pharmacology is a specific science associated with many distinct health care fields, interaction among the professionals who work in these various health care settings is essential to ensure patient safety and compliance with therapeutic care. This professional intercommunication creates safeguards for the patient as well as checks and balances among professionals. It is essential for each professional—health care provider, pharmacist, and allied health professional—to keep his or her medication knowledge as current as possible. In addition, communication among health care workers is important because of the multitudes of medications released each year and the increase in indications for usage of established medications. The allied health professional must also be careful to ensure that correct medications are being charted in the medical record and are being relayed to the pharmacist as allowed by state laws.

Organization of the Text

Pharmacology: Principles and Applications has been organized in a student-friendly manner intended to facilitate the study of pharmacology. Each chapter contains special elements that help make learning fun and easy.

Section I: General Aspects of Pharmacology

Section I, an introduction to pharmacology, gives a short history of the field and how it has changed our world. To ensure safety for both the student and patient, specific legislation and ethical issues related to pharmacology are stressed. The discussion also includes basic pharmacology terminology and provides an understanding of how drugs are used by the body and the skills needed to read and interpret medication orders and document medications appropriately.

Section II: Mathematics for Pharmacology and Dosage Calculations

Section II has a basic math review for the student who needs to practice rudimentary math skills and necessary content to calculate drug dosages so that medications are administered safely. The discussion covers the three systems of measurement used to prescribe medications and the conversions needed to change a medication order from one system to another. The calculation of dosages for adults and children and other special applications are also discussed. New to this edition is Chapter 11, *Principles and Calculations in Intravenous Therapy,* which provides an overview of basic intravenous therapy principles, techniques for administration, and the calculations specific to intravenous administration of medications.

Check Your Understanding math review boxes allow students to check the application and calculation concepts that they have learned as they work their way through each math module. (Answers to these sections are found in **Appendix B.**)

Pretests gauge students' knowledge *before* each math chapter material is covered, allowing both instructors and students to identify areas of weakness. Further review of the material can be accomplished by retaking the pretest before completing the review section. This will indicate areas that need extra attention prior to completing the chapter-ending **Review Questions** that cover chapter concepts related to the ambulatory care setting.

Section III: Medication Administration

Section III presents the general principles of medication administration. The discussions about routes of medication administration are organized according to the AAMA/CAAHEP and ABHES curriculums, starting with enteral (routes that begin with introduction into the gastrointestinal tract), followed by percutaneous (routes through the skin and mucous membranes), and ending with parenteral routes (by injection).

Procedures for drug calculation and administration are presented in storyboard format, displaying illustrations that present specific steps to assist

the visual learner. The Procedure Boxes include **icons** that represent OSHA-mandated and methodology-related protocols that should be followed prior to administering medications. The following icons are presented:

 Handwashing required

 Gloves required

 Sharps container required as indicated

 Use the 3 "befores" and 7 "rights" of medication administration.

Section IV: Pharmacology for Multisystem Application and Section V: Medications Related to Body Systems

Sections IV and V are directly related to medications. Section IV presents medications that affect multiple body systems, such as analgesics, immunizations, antimicrobials, and antineoplastics. The rapidly growing use of herbs and nutritional supplements and their interactions with other medications are also addressed. Section V discusses medications specific to body systems. Tables are included in these sections that present both generic and trade names for drugs, usual adult dosage, typical routes of administration, and drug interactions.

Each chapter in these sections lists the **Common Signs and Symptoms of Diseases** found in the applicable body system. These can be compared to the **Common Side Effects of Medications** commonly prescribed for these diseases, which are presented at the beginning of the chapters. Using these tools, the allied health professional can learn to assist in distinguishing between disease progression and medication reactions by asking pertinent questions for the health care professional to evaluate. This allows the allied health professional to teach patients which signs and symptoms must be reported to the health care provider and which they might expect as side effects—information that is critical for patient education. Medication safety is best reinforced when the patient becomes an active member of the medication administration process.

Easy Working Knowledge tables list medication classifications used with applicable body systems or systemic medications. This listing, which helps locate discussions of specific medication types, corresponds to the quick reference of drug classifications found inside the text's cover. The student can learn to group medications by systemic disease processes to help with correct documentation of medicines. When the student knows the medications used for specific body systems and specific disease process, the potential for drug errors is reduced.

Icons representing the body systems are located next to associated medication names. These icons, listed below, help students begin to identify drugs as they relate to particular body systems.

 Medications used for integumentary disorders

 Medications used for sensory system disorders

 Medications used for infectious diseases

 Medications used for immune system disorders

 Medications used for endocrine system disorders

 Medications used for musculoskeletal disorders

 Medications used for gastrointestinal system disorders

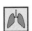 Medications used for respiratory tract disorders

 Medications used for circulatory disorders

 Medications used for blood disorders

 Medications used for urinary system disorders

 Medications used for reproductive system conditions

 Medications used for mental disorders

 Medications used for neurological conditions

 Medications used for pain management

 Medications used as antineoplastics

 Medications used as nutritional supplements

Workbook

The *Workbook* includes multiple review questions and practice problems that not only promote continued learning but also offer thought-provoking, critical thinking questions on how a variety of realistic situations would be handled safely by the allied health professional.

Instructor's Resource Manual with TEACH

The *Instructor's Resource Manual with TEACH* contains answer keys to the text and workbook, a test bank and answer key, as well as detailed lesson plans and lecture outlines. The lesson plans are linked to each chapter and are divided into 50-minute units in a three-column format. The lecture outlines in PowerPoint provide talking points, thought-provoking questions, and unique ideas for lectures. The electronic resource on CD includes all the instructor's resource manual assets plus the test bank in Examview, and PowerPoint slides to help the instructor save valuable preparation time and create a learning environment that fully engages the student.

Purpose of the Textbook

Our goal has been to provide a student-friendly pharmacology text that helps the allied health professional to administer medications safely and to teach patients to administer medications safely at home. The book's early introduction of drugs to their corresponding body systems is designed to help the student begin to recognize the drugs that are most often used with a specific body system. The introductory section on body system and systemic-related medications is designed to help the allied health professional accurately record information about the medication administered and to obtain information from the patient that will assist the health care provider in deciding on the needed medications for the specific patient. This multidisciplinary process must be directed to each individual patient, with the health care provider, pharmacist, and allied health professional providing a system of checks and balances for patient safety.

As authors, we hope that the second edition of *Pharmacology: Principles and Applications* provides students with an enjoyable and in-depth way to learn how to administer medications safely, document medications in the medical record, and relay needed information to other health care professionals and patients who are a part of the medication therapy process.

Acknowledgments

With both of us having worked in the medical field for over 40 years, we have seen the importance of having a strong background in pharmacology to ensure patient safety and education. As health professionals—an ambulatory care nurse and a pharmacist—we understand that safe patient care is only as strong as the individuals involved in medication administration. This book is intended to provide the foundation for that knowledge.

We give special thanks to some special people at Elsevier. To Celeste Clingan, our Developmental Editor, who has been our friend, confidante, and consultant, we give a big thanks for a job well done. To Susan Cole, Executive Editor, we acknowledge the time you have taken ensure the text is as it should be. To Michael Ledbetter, Publisher, for your faith in our abilities. We also thank you for being a friend to both of us throughout many text preparations. To Andrew Allen, Vice President and Publisher, your continuous support of our endeavors is so appreciated. You have been a guide that has produced a light for many years. To Sue Hontcharik, Administrative Assistant—you are friend in need and a friend indeed. Your encouraging words on so many occasions helped us complete this text. Finally, to Sarah Wunderly, Senior Project Manager, your desire for the best text is so apparent. We are so lucky and thankful for your guidance through the production process. We thank all of the Elsevier staff for being there for us when we needed assistance. You are the greatest!

We are also thankful to Carolyn Duplessis for giving us so many great ideas that were incorporated into the first edition and have been continued in this one. Your initial efforts helped bring the book into logical order for student learning and thus patient safety.

To our reviewers, we say a big thank you for providing guidance throughout the publication of this text. To those who reviewed the first edition and gave suggestions for the new edition—from what materials could be excluded to those that needed inclusion—know that your ideas have been incorporated. To those who reviewed the chapters during the production of this second edition for providing many ideas and guidance for this text. You are special people to take time to give us the needed assistance.

We also must thank some special individuals who have provided background materials and direction as well as moral support when needed. To Don Balasa at the American Association for Medical Assistants, we owe our thanks for providing information about the medical practice acts of the states. To Judy Jondahl at the AAMA, thanks for being a friend who gave us moral support during this busy time. To my dear friend, Gail Voyles, thanks for being my friend—a friend for life. To all who have provided encouragement, but a special thanks to our sons, Lee and Gene, we offer our gratitude for their patience and support throughout the entire project. To our grandchildren (and they are really grand) Mac and Allie, you have been the light that made the long days seem shorter. Thanks for being such great children during the times that we were busy writing. Through the love, understanding, and patience of all who have helped with this book, a dream continues to be a reality that will assist allied health students in the future.

Genie and Bobby Fulcher

I wish to acknowledge Man Tai Lam, MD, El Paso, TX, in Private Practice for Internal Medicine and Infectious Diseases (and EPCC Medical Assiting Program Medical Advisor); Panagiotis Valilis, MD, with the El Paso Cancer Treatment Center, and Amir Sajadian, MD, Medical Assisting faculty at El Paso Community College. I want to recognize and thank each of you for your professional support and continued words of encouragement!

I would like to thank my co-authors Genie and Bobby Fulcher for their input and patience in creating this second edition. I also appreciate and want to send a BIG "thank you" to the entire Elsevier staff who worked so diligently on this project, especially Susan Cole, Executive Editor, and Senior Project Manager Sarah Wunderly.

Cathy D. Soto

Critical Thinking Scenario. These scenarios stimulate class discussion by introducing the real-world aspect of pharmacology to students.

End of chapter **Critical Thinking Exercises** and **Review Questions** offer challenging, thought-provoking questions on how a variety of realistic situations would be handled by the allied health professional.

The **Top 100 Drugs** are shaded in the tables and indicate the most popular medications prescribed by health care providers throughout the United States.

Did You Know? boxes provide enrichment facts about relevant topics of interest, such as new medical trends, history, diagnostics, treatments, and diseases.

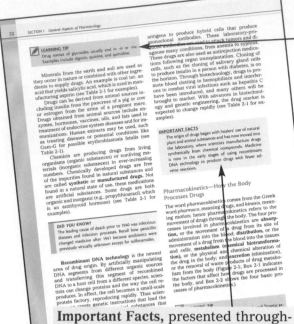

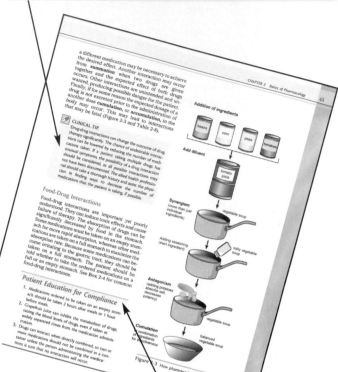

Learning Tips and **Clinical Tips** give helpful hints about medications and their clinical administration and about studying pharmacology.

Important Facts, presented throughout each chapter, contain bulleted summations of previously learned material that provide an at-a-glance resource for students to consult in reviewing important points.

Patient Education for Compliance boxes contain information pertinent to instructing patients on medication administration and about possible side effects or adverse reactions. It is crucial for the allied health professional to take special care in instructing patients about these important issues.

Extensive math review. All math chapters begin with a pretest that highlights material covered within the chapter. If a student masters the pretest with a 90% or better, the student should then move on to the review questions. If the student can score 90% on both, he or she is ready to move to the next chapter. Students are encouraged to go back to the pretest when studying the chapter to check for mastery of the chapter's concepts.

Contents

Section I: General Aspects of Pharmacology

Introduction, 2
1   Legal and Ethical Aspects of Pharmacology, 12
2   Basics of Pharmacology, 29
3   Drug Information and Drug Forms, 48
4   Understanding Drug Dosages for Special Populations, 64
5   Reading and Interpreting Medication Labels and Orders and Documenting Appropriately, 80

Section II: Mathematics for Pharmacology and Dosage Calculations

6   Math Review, 98
7   Measurement Systems and Their Equivalents, 128
8   Converting Between Measurement Systems, 145
9   Calculating Doses of Nonparenteral Medications, 164
10 Calculating Doses of Parenteral Medications, 189
11 Principles and Calculations in Intravenous Therapy, 205

Section III: Medication Administration

12 Safety and Quality Assurance, 226
13 Enteral Routes, 237
14 Percutaneous Routes, 247
15 Parenteral Routes, 261

Section IV: Pharmacology for Multisystem Application

16 Analgesics and Antipyretics, 288
17 Immunizations and the Immune System, 305

18 Anitmicrobials, Antifungals, and Antivirals, 331
19 Antineoplastic Agents, 365
20 Nutritional Supplements and Alternative Medicines, 382

Section V: Medications Related to Body Systems

21 Endocrine System Disorders, 404
22 Eye and Ear Disorders, 435
23 Skin Conditions, 455
24 Musculoskeletal System Disorders, 475
25 Gastrointestinal System Disorders, 493
26 Respiratory System Disorders, 523
27 Circulatory System Disorders, 546
28 Urinary System Disorders, 583
29 Reproductive System Disorders, 593
30 Neurologic System Disorders, 620
31 Drugs for Mental Health and Behavioral Disorders, 656
32 Drugs of Abuse and Misuse, 680

Appendixes

A   Basic Intravenous Therapy Medications, 698
B   Check Your Understanding Answers, 705
C   Drug-Food and Drug-Drug Interactions, 711

Glossary, 712
Index, 723

General Aspects of Pharmacology

Introduction, 2

CHAPTER 1
Legal and Ethical Aspects of Pharmacology, 12

CHAPTER 2
Basics of Pharmacology, 29

CHAPTER 3
Drug Information and Drug Forms, 48

CHAPTER 4
Understanding Drug Dosages for Special Populations, 64

CHAPTER 5
Reading and Interpreting Medication Labels and
Orders and Documenting Appropriately, 80

Introduction

OBJECTIVES

After studying this chapter, you should be capable of doing the following:

- Explaining the differences among the terms *drugs, pharmacology, clinical pharmacology,* and *therapeutics.*
- Describing the role of the allied health professional in pharmacology and the role of each participant in medication delivery.
- Explaining the allied health professional's knowledge base as a safeguard for the medication team.
- Describing why patient education is important for safe medication delivery.

Judy, a new allied health professional, has little background in pharmacology. Sara, a young mother of a 2-year-old, calls and states that her child has a cold with fever. She asks Judy to call in a prescription to the local pharmacy for the child. Judy does not think that it is necessary to ask any further questions about the child's condition because "a cold is a cold." Judy does pull the medical record and sees that the child is allergic to penicillin but has been given Augmentin in the past. So, without consulting the physician, Judy orders the same antibiotic for the child. The next day Sara calls to say the child has a rash covering the entire body and cannot breathe properly. Judy tells Sara to continue the medicine because it sounds like the child has measles and will be fine. Later that day Judy learns that the child is in intensive care at the local hospital with an adverse reaction.

- What are some of the implications for Judy?
- What has she done that could be grounds for litigation?
- Should she have called in the prescription without consulting the physician?
- What is the physician's responsibility?
- What is the pharmacist's responsibility?

KEY TERMS

Administer	Dose	Medication
Adverse reaction	Drug	Over-the-counter (OTC) drug
Anatomy	Food and Drug Administration	Pathology
Bioequivalency	(FDA)	Pharmacology
Brand-name drug	Generic drug	Prescribe
Clinical pharmacology	Homeostasis	Prescription
Dispense	Legend drug	Side effect
Dosage	Managed health care	

An important responsibility of the allied health professional is understanding drugs, drug interactions, and routes of administration. All health care professionals should know the answers to questions about medications such as these: What is the correct **dose** to be given? Is the **dosage** within normal limits? What are the signs of drug overdose? How do various drugs interact? What **adverse reactions** can occur when drugs are given singly? What adverse reactions and **side effects** can occur when drugs are given in combination? How do routes of administration affect the drug's effectiveness and the body's response to the medication?

With knowledge of medications, the health care professional can prepare the patient for a realistic expectation and safe outcome. As a team member, the allied health professional is responsible for obtaining the medical background of patients, both new patients and established patients, especially those seen in more than one medical setting. The health team member must have basic knowledge of pharmacology to document current prescription and over-the-counter medications in medical records and to ensure accuracy with medications that sound alike or are spelled similarly (Figure I-1). This action alone can help prevent legal and ethical problems for the physician.

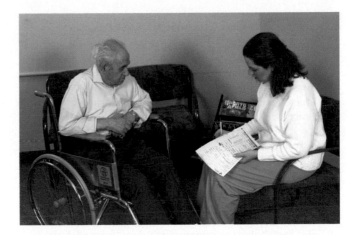

Figure I-1 The allied health professional plays a major role by taking the patient's complete medicinal health history.

DID YOU KNOW?

The word *pharmacology* comes from the Greek *pharmagon*, which has three related meanings: claim, poison, and remedy.

Understanding pharmacology is important in providing good patient care. Pharmacology has changed immensely in the last half of the twentieth century. Many medications used today were not available as recently as 10 years ago. New medicines and new uses of older medicines are constantly being researched and approved for use by the **Food and Drug Administration.** The developments in pharmacology require constant and diligent study, even as the health care professional remembers and uses the medical essentials of the basic health sciences.

IMPORTANT FACTS

- A complete medication profile, including both prescription and over-the-counter drugs, must be documented for all patients.
- Allied health professionals must continue to learn about new medications as they are released and keep current on new uses for older drugs.

What Is Pharmacology?

Pharmacology is the study of drugs, their uses, and their interaction with living systems. The science of pharmacology draws on many disciplines including anatomy, physiology, chemistry, pathology, microbiology, and psychology. **Anatomy** and **physiology** provide essential information about body parts and normal physical function. **Pathology** describes changes from normal structure and function of cells, tissues, and organs and describes the function of medications when the body is out of **homeostasis**. *Psychology* guides the health care provider in understanding how a person's mental state and lifestyle influence medication compli-

ance. The allied health professional must be able to integrate established knowledge in the basic sciences with new information from the rapidly advancing field of pharmacology.

A **drug** is any chemical that can affect body functions. Drugs assist in maintaining homeostasis, or in restoring homeostasis following a decline in body functions caused by illness. Drugs can become dangerous if they are used to create unnecessary dependence, but when used intelligently, they provide a lifesaving benefit (if used unwisely, of course, they can cause irreversible harm). When patients and prescribers use medications appropriately, medications can restore health, prolong life, and increase the quality of life for patients with diseases and abnormal conditions.

Researchers today build on the accumulated knowledge of the past to produce major new advances. Through the years, the increasing knowledge about disease processes has led to the need for refined medications and to rapid changes in the field of pharmacology. Pharmacology will continue to change rapidly in the future as medical research makes innovative studies in the field. The allied health professional must remain current with these advances. However, the four basic terms used in pharmacology—*drug, pharmacology, clinical pharmacology,* and *therapeutics*—remain the same (Box I-1).

IMPORTANT FACTS

- Pharmacology is the study of drugs and their uses.
- Pharmacology draws information from many scientific disciplines including anatomy, physiology, chemistry, microbiology, psychology, and pathology.

1. **Drug**—Any chemical that can affect living processes. Under this broad definition, all chemicals are considered drugs when given in amounts large enough to alter or affect life.
2. **Pharmacology**—The study of drugs and their interactions with living systems. The definition includes the study of the physical and chemical properties of drugs, as well as their effects on the body. It also includes the history of drugs, their sources and uses, and how they are used by the body. This is a broad field, and this book will consider only those areas of pharmacology relevant to an ambulatory medical setting.
3. **Clinical pharmacology**—The study of drug absorption and metabolism in humans including those who are healthy, as well as those who are not, in homeostasis.
4. **Therapeutics**—The use of drugs to diagnose disease **(diagnostic agents),** prevent disease or a condition such as pregnancy **(prophylactic agents),** or treat disease **(therapeutic drugs).** This definition, simply stated, is the medical use of drugs, even though some may cause adverse reactions. (Adverse reactions are those effects that are undesirable or unintended.) The term *therapeutics* also encompasses the basic reasons for giving a particular drug to a particular patient, in a particular dosage, by a particular route, and on a particular schedule. Knowledge of pharmacology helps show what strategies will promote a beneficial drug effect for a patient while minimizing undesired effects.

IMPORTANT FACTS—*Cont'd*

- Medications aid in keeping the body in homeostasis and are of lifesaving benefit when used correctly and with discrimination. If used incorrectly, drugs can cause irreparable harm.

History of Pharmacology

Pharmacology is one of the oldest sciences, with roots in ancient cultures. Ancient civilizations recorded the use of drugs more than 2000 years ago. Through trial and error, humans discovered which plants might be used for food and which had medicinal value. Folk remedies largely did, and still do, make use of herbs and other plants. In previous generations, serious illnesses were considered to be of supernatural origin, the result of spells cast on the victim by an enemy, a demon, or an offended god. The ancient medicine men using frog bile, pig teeth, spider webs, and sour milk were actually witch doctors or sorcerers who treated the whole body. Herbal treatments for illnesses became a part of every cultural heritage, with many cultural communities choosing healers—

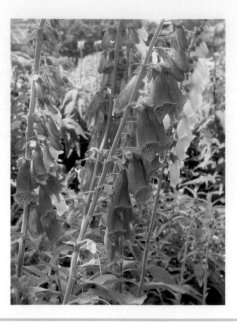

Figure I-2 Foxglove *(Digitalis purpurea),* used for cardiac disorders, is an example of plant materials that have been used as medications over many centuries.

wise men, witch doctors, "root doctors," *curanderos,* or shamans—whom culture members saw as having "cures" because of their special knowledge of plants. Some of these ancient forms of healing are still used today. Over the years, folk uses of plants and other natural remedies became the basis for certain modern medicines and for the current pharmacology field. For example, the digitalis plant, also called foxglove *(Digitalis purpurea),* is the basis of the commonly used cardiac medication digitalis (Figure I-2).

Many medications are related to times of war or to legislation that is discussed in Chapter 1. See the time line in Box I-2 for an annotated history of pharmacology.

In the early years of the twenty-first century, patches and small dots are being used for medication administration in increasing number because of their convenience for treating conditions from smoking cessation to hormone replacement therapy to contraception and even attention deficit hyperactivity disorder (ADHD). Pumps and nasal sprays to administer insulin are being used by people with type 1 diabetes mellitus. Solid-state silicon microchips containing microreservoirs filled with saline to which drugs and biomaterials can be added are in the near future. The wells will be individually sealed, and the dose will be dissolved by an electrical impulse passed through the metal coating. The chip can be programmed and reprogrammed to meet the needs of the patient.

BOX I-2   TIME LINE OF MEDICATIONS

Pre-Eighteenth Century	Prior to the sixteenth century, Egyptian Sumerians collected plants for treatment of specific diseases and used molded bread for treatment of infection. India's version of Materia Medica was written as a drug formulary of plants used for treating diseases. During the sixteenth century, the Chinese devised a 52-volume formulary of concoctions prepared to restore and maintain body harmony. Reserpine (rauwolfia) was prescribed for high blood pressure and ginseng as a diuretic. In the seventeenth century, Greek physicians, and especially Hippocrates, used opium for pain and herbal remedies such as belladonna (atropine) for nausea and vomiting and Jesuit's bark (quinine) for malaria. The Greeks also used natural cures for dieting. The Romans began the use of prescriptions for obtaining patient medications.
Eighteenth Century	Edward Jenner developed the first vaccine, which was used for immunity against cowpox (smallpox).
Nineteenth Century	Morphine (1806), strychnine (1817), quinine (1820), and nicotine (1828) were created.
1865	During the American Civil War, carbonic acid was used for surgical asepsis.
1895	Pierre and Marie Curie invented the technique of making x-rays.
1897	During the Spanish-American War, typhoid vaccines were administered to troops.
1898	Pierre and Marie Curie discovered radium.
Twentieth Century	
Early 1900s	Prontosil (1908—forerunner of sulfa drugs), salvarsan (1910—synthetic arsenic for syphilis), and phenobarbital (1912—drug used for epilepsy) were created.
1914-1918 (World War I)	Tetanus antitoxin was developed and used for military personnel
1920s	Diphtheria vaccine (1922)
1930s	Sulfa (antiinfective), phenytoin (Dilantin for epilepsy), and yellow fever vaccine were created.
1940s (World War II)	Penicillin (antiinfective), Benadryl (1945—antihistamine), cortisone (1948—immunosuppressant), antibiotics, chemotherapeutic agents, influenza vaccine
1950s (Korean War)	Oral contraceptives, and Salk vaccine (1954—polio vaccine) were created. Medications to treat mental illness were introduced.
1960s	Sabin oral polio vaccine was introduced. Vaccines for rubella, rubeola, and mumps were created, as were beta blockers to treat hypertension and clotting factors for hemophilia.
1970s	Cimetidine for treatment of peptic ulcers and ibuprofen for treatment of inflammation were introduced.
1980s	Vaccine for chickenpox, medications for cardiac arrhythmia, ACE inhibitors (angiotensin-converting enzyme), and medications for benign prostatic hypertrophy were developed. DNA-produced insulin (1980) was the first DNA medication.
1990s	AIDS medications and chemotherapy were developed at rapid pace to treat these devastating illnesses. Newer forms of medications were developed to treat peptic ulcers, impotence, and diabetes, especially newer forms of insulin that caused fewer reactions.
Twenty-first Century	New drug administration techniques are being developed, such as insulin delivered via nasal spray, continuous oral contraception, and inhaled antibiotics.

Inhalation medications using aerosol particles are another trend of the future. Gene therapy and the splicing of genes for medications are down the road in pharmacy practice.

Internet pharmacy has brought ethical and safety dilemmas of its own. New consumer safety regulations are being put into place to ensure safety for patients who use the Internet to fill medication prescriptions. The government is even looking into ways to ensure that Internet sites provide patient safety and that the medications are those specified and protected by regulations pertaining to the manufacture and distribution of the drugs.

IMPORTANT FACTS

- By trial and error, early civilizations found plant sources that could be used to treat disease processes. Folk medicine used herbs and other plant materials for medicinal purposes.
- In the sixteenth century the Chinese created the first pharmacopoeia, which listed drugs of animal,

vegetable, and mineral origin that were used to maintain body harmony.

- At the end of the nineteenth century and beginning of the twentieth century, many laws were enacted to protect the public in the field of pharmacy.
- Medications for previously fatal chronic illnesses were introduced during the first half of the twentieth century. Many of these medications arose out of the needs of uniformed military personnel, especially those serving in combat.
- The pharmaceutical field developed rapidly in the last half of the twentieth century. This period saw the introduction of oral contraceptives, medications for hypertension, insulin produced by recombinant DNA technology, drugs to treat impotence, and chemotherapeutic drugs, as well as new administration techniques.
- At the start of the twenty-first century, medication delivery systems that have a prolonged effect and do not require the frequent application of medications are available. Among these delivery systems are patches, insulin pumps, and silicon microchips.

Why Study Pharmacology?

Before administering medications safely, health professionals must know the forms of drugs available and what patient factors could affect the actions of the drugs. The knowledge includes the expected action of the drugs within the body, the correct dosage of the drugs, methods and routes of administration, symptoms of abnormal reactions, and appropriate patient education for the delivery of the medication.

The allied health professional functions as a link in the health care chain to ensure that the physician is aware of all medications, both prescription and over-the-counter, that the patient is taking. A complete history of medication use must be documented with each patient encounter to assist the physician in safely and effectively prescribing medications for the patient. The use of alcohol, recreational drugs, and alternative medications such as herbals and vitamins should also be recorded.

In many cases the allied health professional will reinforce patient teaching about a drug's purposes, its method and route of administration, and the regimen for medication efficacy. Therefore safe, effective drug therapy requires that the health care professional have a working knowledge of pharmacology so that critical decisions and medication administration can assure appropriate patient care.

For legal and educational purposes and to ensure patient safety the health professional must provide accurate documentation including the knowledge concerning medications that sound alike or are spelled similarly. This professional interaction is critical to the health professional–patient relationship, as well as to the employee-employer association.

With the growing number of **over-the-counter (OTC)** drugs, the need for information concerning their actions and interactions with **prescription** medications (or **legend drugs**) will prevent reactions detrimental to the patient. People today frequently use OTC drugs to treat themselves for common ailments or illnesses such as allergies, colds, arthritis, and gastric conditions without consulting a physician. Because many medications previously available on a prescription-only basis have become OTC items, these drugs must be noted in the medical record. The use of OTC drugs by the patient must be followed as the use of prescription medications would be followed, even if the drug seems insignificant.

Medication Administration and Professionals

According to guidelines of the Drug Enforcement Agency, a regulatory agency of the U.S. Department of Justice, each person in the medication pathway has a specific duty. A physician **prescribes** a drug when he or she gives an order including a prescription to be filled by the pharmacy in an outpatient setting. In **dispensing** a drug, a health care professional, usually a pharmacist, distributes the drug in a correctly labeled container with specific instructions for the patient on how and when to take the medication. To **administer** a drug means to give the medication by the route prescribed. Drug administration may be done by the patient personally or by a health care professional in a medical facility (Figures I-3 and I-4).

For the safety of the patient, a professional pathway of tracking medications from physician's prescription to the patient taking the medication must be done. Just as the U.S. government has a system of checks and balances, so there is a system of checks and balances in place for administering and prescribing medications. The potential for human error always exists when prescribing, administering, or dispensing medications, so health care providers take on interconnected roles to reduce the chance of error.

A triangular pathway among the physician, pharmacist, and allied health professional is essential for patient safety and compliance. The patient

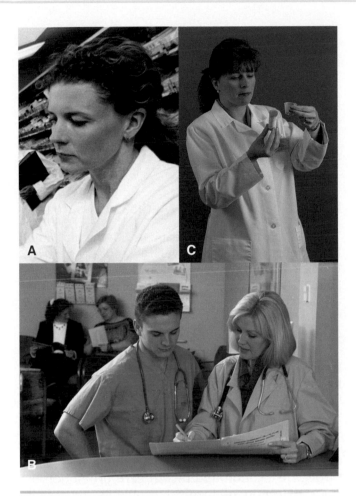

Figure I-3 The three members of the health care team with direct use of pharmacology for the safety of the patient. **A,** Pharmacist; **B,** physician; **C,** allied health professional.

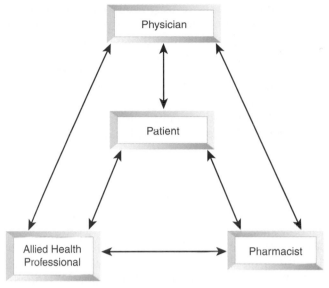

Figure I-4 Triangulation of health care professionals for the safety of medication use by the patient.

is always in the center of this pathway to ensure the highest level of safety in patient care (see Figure I-4). The patient who needs medication may begin at any point in the triangle of health care personnel to obtain the needed medication. Perhaps the office visit or discharge from a hospital stay begins the triangle, with the physician writing the prescription after checking for the possibility of adverse reactions. As a legal safeguard, the allied health professional should again check for errors and then be sure the chart has appropriate documentation. If the medication is appropriate, the patient then takes the prescription to the pharmacy, where it is dispensed. The pharmacist then uses checks and balances to ensure that unsafe drug interactions do not occur, as well as to check for the appropriateness of the drug, dose, and duration of the prescription prior to dispensing the medication. In modern pharmacies a complete drug profile is maintained, and a "red flag" appears if any possible danger is present after the pharmacist enters the prescription into the computer. In today's world, however, where patients go to multiple physicians, specialists, and pharmacies, patients may either not understand or forget the importance of having a total drug profile at one pharmacy. This one step could prevent severe, life-threatening drug interactions. Therefore patients should be encouraged to use the same pharmacy when filling prescriptions. The pharmacist may serve as a resource for possible interactions and also act as a gatekeeper to identify and prevent the use of similar drugs prescribed by more than one physician, thereby preventing overuse or abuse of medications.

In another case, a patient may go to a pharmacy to have a prescription refilled. The pharmacist then begins the cycle as needed by contacting either the medical office or the physician for refill or prescription authorization. The allied health professional in these cases must be aware of the medications taken by the patient by obtaining the medical record, checking prescriptions, and giving pertinent information to the physician, who makes the decision about prescribing medications. Depending on the laws of the state, the physician or the allied health professional may then telephone the pharmacy with refill instructions.

Similar to the phone call to the physician's office requesting a refill, the allied health professional obtains the information and asks the physician whether the patient needs to come to the office to be examined or whether the medication prescription is one that can be telephoned to the pharmacy. Variables in this triangulation for safety include the specific policies and procedures of each medical office and the laws governing the prescribing of medications in each state.

The physician is central to medication delivery when he or she determines the specific drug therapy required for a specific patient in a specific situation. Some physicians may also dispense sample medications or administer some drugs, such as antipyretics for fever or analgesics for pain, in their medical practice.

The pharmacist is primarily concerned with the use of drugs. Sixty percent of visits to a physician result in a prescription. Therefore pharmacists are involved not only in providing the correct drug product but also in helping to ensure its proper use. The pharmacist ensures that the course of therapy prescribed is safe, effective, and correct in every detail for the patient. If a question concerning the therapy is evident, the pharmacist will contact the physician for verification.

The allied health professional begins the education of the patient in proper drug use while also functioning as a liaison between the physician and pharmacist. The health care professional must have adequate knowledge to ensure accurate and timely transfer of information among all of the involved health professionals.

In other cases the allied health professional is the person who receives phone calls from patients with questions about their prescriptions. He or she is usually the first person on the professional team to hear that the medication has caused problems or has not had the expected results. Most patients do not feel comfortable discussing medications that have not had the desired effect with a physician. Rather, they turn to other health care professionals such as a pharmacist or office staff member to ask questions. It is an important role for allied health professionals to provide knowledgeable answers and to include other health care professionals such as physicians and pharmacists in safe patient care. The pathway of medication delivery requires that the entire team know medications, their uses and misuses, and the patient who will be using the drugs. And just as the physician and the office staff must know the patients and their medical needs, so the pharmacist must keep updated records of all medications being taken by a patient to ensure safety.

IMPORTANT FACTS

- Physicians *prescribe*, pharmacists *dispense*, and allied health professionals (depending on state law) may *administer* medications, as well as be a liaison to other health care professionals.

IMPORTANT FACTS—*Cont'd*

- Allied health professionals must have a working knowledge of all medications used at the site of employment, including new drugs and new applications of established drugs.
- The physician, pharmacist, and allied health professional must cooperate in a system of checks and balances to ensure safety for the patient.

Patient Education for Medication Safety

The health care worker must use diligent and intelligent observations, as well as moral integrity. Using common sense based on accurate pharmacology knowledge when administering medications will create a climate for understanding by the patient and help establish patient trust and cooperation.

Today's health care professional must counsel patients concerning medications and must help the patient understand how to follow the treatment for optimal therapeutic effect. This teaching role requires understanding of nonmedical uses of drugs and of the signs and symptoms of drug misuse, abuse, and addiction. The responsibility also includes preventing problems in healthy people through education and health care promotion by early detection of medical problems and when the possibility of drug side effects and adverse reactions exists. By imparting accurate and up-to-date knowledge of medications, the allied health professional can assist the patient in complying with therapy. The key to achieving safe, high-quality medical care is having knowledgeable answers that will clarify any misunderstandings about the patient's therapy and increase compliance by the patient.

With the medical field being influenced in so many ways by **managed health care** and other insurance company interests, as well as the current culture of pursuing legal actions with medical errors, the importance of educating patients cannot be emphasized enough. Most insurance companies look for a proactive stance with patient education and will reimburse for time spent in education in the medical office. This helps ensure patient compliance with a prescribed treatment and drug regimen. In the past, patients received only the information that the physician thought was necessary. Little literature was available that could be understood by the patient. The general consensus was that patients should be given only essential information, which did not include information

For faster refills, phone in 24 hours in advance

Rx/pharmacy #44 Ph:001-555-4444
505 South Bell St
Holly, GA
00111-0000
www.RX.com

05-23-2007
Prscbr: Lawrence, Merry
Refills: 12

PATIENT PRESCRIPTION INFORMATION
IF YOU HAVE ANY QUESTIONS ABOUT YOUR MEDICATION, PLEASE CONTACT YOUR PHARMACIST:
Foster, Richard

ZETIA 10 MG TABLET M/S
MERCK/SCHERING
TAKE 1 TABLET BY MOUTH EVERY DAY

This is a WHITE, OBLONG-shaped, TABLET imprinted with 414 on the front.
EZETIMIBE - ORAL (eh-ZET-ih-mibe)

COMMON BRAND NAME(S): Zetia

USES: This medication is used either alone or with other drugs (e.g., HMG-CoA reductase inhibitors or "statins"), along with a low cholesterol/low fat diet, to help lower cholesterol in the blood. Reducing cholesterol helps prevent strokes and heart attacks. Ezetimibe works by reducing the amount of cholesterol your body absorbs from your diet.

HOW TO USE: Read the Patient Information Leaflet provided by your pharmacist before you start taking this medication and each time you get a refill. If you have any questions regarding the information, consult your doctor or pharmacist. Take this medication by mouth usually once daily with or without food. If you are also taking a bile acid sequestrant (e.g., cholestyramine, colestipol), take ezetimibe at least 2 hours before or at least 4 hours after the bile acid sequestrant. It may take up to 2 weeks before the full benefit of this drug takes effect. Use this medication regularly in order to get the most benefit from it. Remember to use it at the same time each day. It is important to continue taking this medication even if you feel well. Most people with high cholesterol do not feel sick.

SIDE EFFECTS: Dizziness, headache, diarrhea, back pain may occur. If any of these effects persist or worsen, notify your doctor or pharmacist promptly. Remember that your doctor has prescribed this medication because the benefit to you is greater than the risk of side effects. Many people using this medication do not have serious side effects. Tell your doctor immediately if any of these serious side effects occur: chest pain, fatigue, stomach pain. This drug can very rarely cause muscle damage. Tell your doctor immediately if you experience the following: muscle pain/tenderness/weakness (especially with fever or unusual tiredness). A serious allergic reaction to this drug is unlikely, but seek immediate medical attention if it occurs. Symptoms of a serious allergic reaction include: rash, itching, swelling, dizziness, trouble breathing. If you notice other effects not listed above, contact your doctor or pharmacist.

PRECAUTIONS: Before taking ezetimibe, tell your doctor or pharmacist if you are allergic to it; or if you have any other allergies. This medication should not be used along with a statin agent if you have certain medical conditions. Before using this medicine, consult your doctor or pharmacist if you have: active liver disease. Before using this medication, tell your doctor or pharmacist your medical history, especially of: liver disease (moderate to severe). This medication should be used only when clearly needed during pregnancy. Discuss the risks and benefits with your doctor. It is not known whether this drug passes into breast milk. Consult your doctor before breast-feeding.

DRUG INTERACTIONS: Your doctor or pharmacist may already be aware of any possible drug interactions and may be monitoring you for them. Do not start, stop, or change the dosage of any medicine before checking with them first. Before using this medication, tell your doctor or pharmacist of all prescription and nonprescription products you may use, especially of: "blood thinners" (e.g., warfarin), cyclosporine, fibrates (e.g., fenofibrate, gemfibrozil).

OVERDOSE: If overdose is suspected, contact your local poison control center or emergency room immediately. US residents can call the US national poison hotline at 1-800-222-1222. Canadian residents should call their local poison control center directly.

NOTES: Do not share this medication with others. Laboratory and/or medical tests (e.g., cholesterol levels) should be performed periodically to monitor your progress. When ezetimibe is given with a statin agent, liver function tests should be performed to monitor for side effects. Consult your doctor for more details. For best results, this medication should be used along with exercise and a low cholesterol/low fat diet. Consult your doctor.

MISSED DOSE: If you miss a dose, use it as soon as you remember. If it is near the time of the next dose, skip the missed dose and resume your usual dosing schedule. Do not double the dose to catch up.

STORAGE: Store at room temperature at 77 degrees F (25 degrees C) away from light and moisture. Brief storage from 59-86 degrees F (15-30 degrees C) is permitted. Do not store in the bathroom. Keep all medicines away from children and pets. Properly discard this product when it is expired or no longer needed. Consult your pharmacist or local waste disposal company for more details about how to safely discard your product.

Information last revised April 2007
Copyright(c) 2007 First DataBank, Inc.

Keep Out of Reach of Children

Rx Item# 000000

IMPORTANT DISCLAIMER: The side effects listed above are not all of the possible risks that could be caused by this medication. For further information, please consult with your physician about the uses, precautions and risks of the medication specific to your health. This information is obtained from First DateBank for use as an educational aid.

Figure I-5 Handout typical of those given to patients with their prescriptions.

about possible adverse reactions and side effects. Patient education related to medication safety was not of primary concern, and patients often had detrimental effects, waiting until the effects were severe to contact a health care professional because of the lack of knowledge.

Today there are legal implications for the physician, pharmacist, and allied health professional who fail to provide and document education to the patient. Even the roles of medical and allied health professionals have changed because of the current need for patient education concerning medications. Because patients are ill and under stress, often the educational materials must be reviewed several times and provided in writing, and this repeated educational effort should be documented (Figure I-5). Medication errors can be avoided, prevented, or reduced with proper patient teaching so that patients are part of and knowledgeable about their medical and pharmaceutical treatment. Another means for the patient to maintain a full drug profile and to provide it to all health care providers would be to carry a pocket or wallet medication card listing all drugs, prescription and OTC, taken on a regular basis. The sooner a physician is aware of any medication-related problem, the sooner steps can be taken to correct the problem and improve patient care.

Patient Education for Compliance

Eight questions to which patients should know the answers follow:

1. What is the medication I have been prescribed?
2. What is this prescription for?
3. How long should I take this medicine?
4. What side effects can I expect while taking this medicine?
5. Do any special instructions apply to taking this medication?
6. Are there any foods, other prescription medications, or OTC medicines (including herbals, vitamins, and natural products) that I should not take with this medicine?
7. Is an equally effective generic form of this medication available at a lower price?
8. If I am taking several medicines, should I be aware of any potential interactions?

Summary

As partners with pharmacists and physicians, allied health professionals are one of the major links in the medication delivery pathway in today's health care environment. The administrative assistant must know medications in order to refer medication questions appropriately to other members of the health care team. Knowledge of drugs, their actions, their interactions, their side effects, and their adverse reactions is necessary for appropriate patient care. Depending on the laws of individual states, allied health professionals may administer medications, while physicians prescribe and pharmacists dispense. The ideal working relationship among all of these professionals provides a system of checks and balances for patient safety. All medications, whether prescription or OTC, should be documented in the medical record to prevent overdosing or adverse reactions from multiple medications from multiple providers. Through education about the importance of providing information to all physicians and taking medications as ordered, the patient becomes an active participant in pharmacologic therapy, and this role will only increase in the future.

With the rapid appearance of numerous new medications in the last half of the twentieth century, patients must take an active role in their own care. Health care providers must constantly update patients' basic understanding, and allied health professionals *must* keep current on all pharmaceutical products used in the medical practice where they work.

Critical Thinking Exercises

SCENARIO

Mary Ann, an administrative allied health professional, is manning the phone at Dr. Merry's office. Janelee calls to say that she has been to the pharmacy to get her medication and has read on the patient information sheet that the drug prescribed should not be taken with aspirin that she takes daily.

1. What should Mary Ann do first?
2. Should she make a decision or should she ask Dr. Merry?
3. The pharmacist had called earlier and asked to speak to Dr. Merry but Mary Ann took a message and did not give the message to Dr. Merry. Should she give the information to the physician as soon as possible—why or why not?
4. What should be provided to the physician at the time the message is relayed?

REVIEW QUESTIONS

1. Define:
   Pharmacology _____
   Drug _____
   Medication _____
   OTC _____
   Dispense _____
   Prescribe _____
   Administer _____
   Prescription drugs _____
   Legend drugs _____

2. The three health professionals in the medication pathway are _____, _____, and _____.

3. Describe the role of each health professional in the system of checks and balances to ensure the safe use of medicines. _____
   _____

4. Explain why allied health professionals, including those in administrative roles, must have a knowledge base of pharmacology and the medications prescribed in the medical office of employment. _____

_____

5. Patient teaching is an important element of health care. What are four areas of patient teaching that are important in pharmacology? How can patient teaching be used to lessen society's preconceived ideas about the use and abuse of drugs? _____

_____

_____

CHAPTER 1

Legal and Ethical Aspects of Pharmacology

OBJECTIVES

After studying this chapter, you should be capable of the following:

- Differentiating among the major governmental agencies and the role and regulations of each in medication development and delivery.
- Identifying the legal aspects of the 1970 Controlled Substances Act and describing regulations for the five schedules of controlled substances.
- Describing the registration and documentation process with the Drug Enforcement Administration for compliance with administering, dispensing, and prescribing controlled drugs.
- Differentiating among drug dependence, drug abuse, drug misuse, and habituation.
- Listing and describing the signs of drug abuse and the ethics involved in addressing these problems with patients and medical professionals.
- Identifying the ethical procedures regarding prescriptions and the use of protocol to ensure that ethical procedures are followed, including who may prescribe medications.

George, an allied health professional, is working in an outpatient setting when a new patient without an appointment visits the office. When Mr. James, the patient, is in the examination room, George asks him the reason for his visit. Mr. James replies that he wants a prescription for a controlled substance for pain and has no other reason to be in the office. When asked about the pain, the answers are vague and the level of pain cannot be described.

What are the implications for George regarding obtaining a medical history?

Why would the vagueness and the desire only for pain medication be a signal that needs to be relayed to the physician?

Why would it be important for George to be sure no prescription pads are available in the examination room?

Does the allied health professional have a responsibility other than to report the information to the physician? Why or why not?

KEY TERMS

Bioequivalency
Controlled substance
Dangerous drug
Diagnostic agent
Drug abuse
Drug addiction
Drug dependence
Drug efficacy
Drug Enforcement Administration (DEA)

Drug purity
Drug quality
Drug sample
Drug standardization
Drug standards
Drug strength or potency
Narcotic
National Formulary (NF)
Physical dependence
Placebo

Prophylactic agent
Psychologic drug dependence or habituation
Respondeat superior
Standardization
Therapeutic drug
United States Pharmacopoeia (USP)

Throughout history, some members of societies have chosen to misuse or even abuse medicinal substances such as herbs, chemicals, and drugs. As societies became more progressive, governing members saw the need to establish regulations to control the use of these substances by enacting laws and regulations.

Over the past 25 years the public has become more knowledgeable about medications as the number of over-the-counter (OTC) medications has increased, making patient education about drug interactions and adverse reactions an important public issue. The government has taken steps to ensure that the consumer has quality drugs that have the expected therapeutic properties. Prior to the twentieth century, drug legislation would have been almost impossible—detailed information about drugs was not available because there was no way to analyze drugs as they were developed. A **drug's strength,** or concentration of active ingredients, varied with the conditions under which the drug was prepared. The consistency of the drug might vary from one bottle of medication to the next, and patients' reactions to medication also varied. Since the beginning of the twentieth century, however, research methods mandated by legislation have resulted in the consistent manufacture of medications and thus safety in their preparation and effectiveness for patient treatment. Legislation now also requires that all new medications undergo stringent testing before release to assure **standardization** of these therapeutic agents and therefore consistency with the use.

Pharmaceutical companies spend vast amounts of money on drug development, advertising, and promotion. Therefore legislation is necessary to protect consumers and enforce quality control of the medication. Advertisements for medication stress their positive effects to increase sales. By law, adverse reactions, drug interactions, and other negative effects are required to be given equal coverage in the media so that people are given sufficient information to make informed choices about the value of the therapeutics. Because of today's information highways such as the Internet, the U.S. government is currently investigating ways to ensure that the information gathered from computer sources is accurate and complete.

Controls for ensuring safety and promoting informed choices have been a direct result of legislation at the federal, state, and local levels. State and local regulations, such as the classification of certain controlled drugs, are usually more stringent and precise than federal regulations because more exact details are added at each level of regulation. Restrictions found in the policy and procedures manual of individual offices or medical facilities may be even more stringent than government regulations. The allied health professional *must* have a working knowledge of regulations at all levels to comply with all restrictions.

International, Federal, and State Statutes for the Regulation of Medications

The international control of medications comes under the authority of the World Health Organization of the United Nations. This group provides technical assistance in the drug field and promotes research on drug abuse. Because no world judicial groups enforce laws concerning drugs, drug control varies from country to country. Some nations have stringent laws, even stricter than those of the United States.

DID YOU KNOW?
Harsh punishments including long prison sentences and even death are imposed for the possession of illegal drugs and for drug trafficking in some countries. Other countries have lenient laws concerning drug possession and lenient enforcement of those laws, even to the point of allowing the use of some drugs that are illegal in the United States.

Because of the strict regulation of standards and safety for new drugs in the market, drugs are often available in other countries before they are available in the United States. Before the turn of the twentieth century, detailed information such as content analysis, drug strength, and the consistency of medications during manufacture was lacking for most medications. Many drugs containing opium and the new miracle drug, morphine, did not require a prescription, and pharmacists and physicians were not required to hold a license. Labeling of ingredients on the bottles was not a requirement, nor was the potency of the medication consistent from bottle to bottle. The use of many addicting and **dangerous drugs** resulted in injury or death from their use, addiction, or inconsistency in the medications.

DID YOU KNOW?
Before 1906, patent medicines were sold by medicine men in traveling shows, by mail order, in stores, by trained physicians, and even by individuals who just called themselves "doctors." Medications with names like Dr. Smith's Miraculous Cough Medicine or

Federal Legislation Related to Drugs

The earliest federal regulation occurred with the *Pure Food and Drug Act of 1906* that included the following but still allowed the medicine man to flourish because of loopholes in the law and lack of enforcement:

- Drug manufacturers must label medication packages to indicate the presence of 11 specific dangerous or addictive ingredients.
- Drugs could not be labeled as curative if the claims were false and misleading, but advertisement by word of mouth, newspapers, almanacs, and the like was not covered and only drugs found in interstate commerce were included.
- The **United States Pharmacopoeia (USP)** and the **National Formulary (NF)** were created as the compendia containing the official standards for **strength** and **purity** by which a drug is to be manufactured, including an indication of the amounts of dangerous products present that may cause **drug addiction.**

In 1912, to tighten the law, Congress passed the *Shirley Amendment*, which prevented fraudulent therapeutic claims by drug manufacturers. This amendment was followed 2 years later by the *Harrison Narcotic Act* or *Federal Narcotic Drug Act* with provisions related to dangerous drugs:

- Established the word *narcotic* and required the use of a stamp on the containers of these drugs
- For patient safety, regulated the importation, manufacture, sale, and use of opium, codeine, and their derivatives and compounds

In the late 1930s sulfonamide was widely used as an antibacterial agent. The lethal elixir was in a raspberry-flavored base for flavor and fragrance but had not been tested for safety. With no need for approval of the chemicals used in manufacture, the company did not use an alcohol but made the drug using an industrial-strength liquid solvent, diethylene glycol—a major ingredient in antifreeze. More than 100 children died after ingesting less than an ounce of the medicine, and more than 350 were poisoned. In response to the public demand for drug safety, Congress passed the *Food, Drug and Cosmetic Act of 1938* to provide safety testing on all drugs. The **Food and Drug Administration** (FDA) was formed to enforce the laws, seize goods that were improperly manufactured or packaged, and undertake criminal prosecution of the responsible persons or firms. Furthermore, pharmaceutical firms were required to report all adverse effects associated with their drugs at regular intervals.

In 1951 the *Durham-Humphrey Amendment* to the Food, Drug and Cosmetic Act of 1938 placed in position further regulations:

- Stated how prescriptions could be ordered or dispensed by designating prescription and OTC medications
- Required that all prescriptions, or legend drugs, be labeled "Caution: Federal law prohibits dispensing without a prescription"
- Designated the OTC drugs that were considered sufficiently safe not to require a prescription

Drug companies in the mid–twentieth century made large profits and engaged in drug promotions that were misleading or even false. An example is thalidomide, a hypnotic that was taken by pregnant women early in pregnancy because the manufacturer claimed it was a miracle drug for the nausea of pregnancy and a sleeping aid without realizing the associated dangers. The drug caused severe deformities in fetuses, leading to a wave of "thalidomide babies." Because the medication was only on the market in the United States for a short period, most cases of adverse reactions occurred in Europe. Some pregnant women in the Northeast took the drug, but the tragedy was more a "might-have-been" catastrophe than a widespread, actual one. This opened eyes in Congress and led to the passage of more stringent legislation, the *Kefauver-Harris Amendment of 1962*, increasing drug safety and effectiveness to be enforced by the FDA.

After many confusing amendments to the Harrison Narcotic Act of 1914 (the initial laws concerning narcotic, or controlled, medications) and the possible tragedies that could have occurred, the *1970 Comprehensive Drug Abuse Prevention and Control Act* was passed to regulate the manufacture, distribution, and dispensing of potentially abusive drugs and to prevent indiscriminate use of controlled drugs. These acts of 1970 repealed the 50 laws passed between 1914 and 1970 concerning drug control and provided regulations for the therapeutic use of controlled substances as follows:

- Required proven effectiveness of a drug prior to marketing, with all drugs (old and new) requiring testing
- Indicated drugs that had potential for abuse and placed these medications in categories sorted by that potential
- Required security of controlled substances by anyone who dispenses, receives, sells, or destroys controlled substances by using special DEA forms to show current inventory
- Regulated the use of controlled substances to legitimate handlers only to help reduce the widespread illicit use of controlled drugs
- Provided for prevention of **drug abuse** and **drug dependence** and for the treatment and rehabilitation of abusers and drug-dependent persons
- Two important agencies came into being:
  - The **Bureau of Narcotics and Dangerous Drugs** (BNDD) was formed to register all persons who manufacture, dispense, prescribe, or administer any controlled substances and to provide for necessary revision of the categories of controlled drugs and their classes.
  - The **Drug Enforcement Administration** (DEA), an agency of the Department of Justice, was established to regulate and enforce the manufacturing and dispensing of dangerous and potentially abused drugs. Any-

one who handles **controlled substances** must follow the stringent requirements of the law. (See section on DEA that follows.)

The *Poisoning Prevention Packaging Act of 1970* created standards to ensure that both prescription and OTC medications were in child-resistant packages. The National Drug Code is used by the FDA to identify the manufacturer, including the drug formulation and the size of the packaging, by a unique and permanent code that was instituted with the *Drug Listing Act of 1972*.

In 1978 the *Drug Regulation and Reform Act* allowed for briefer investigation of new drugs to allow for faster access by the consumer. In response to the removal of drugs because of potential dangers or the lack of research for rare conditions, Congress passed the *Orphan Drug Act* in 1983 to fund research into drugs for the treatment of rare chronic illnesses. Historically this research had been unprofitable and therefore had been done on a limited basis. With the grant money available through the Orphan Drug Act, drug companies have found new drugs and new uses for older drugs.

DID YOU KNOW?

Thalidomide, which caused severe birth defects in the 1960s, has been found today to be effective for leprosy, acquired immunodeficiency syndrome, and other rare conditions because of the enactment of the Orphan Drug Act.

Several other acts of importance include the following:

- 1984—*Drug Price Competition and Patent Term Restoration Act* eased requirements for marketing generic drugs by allowing generic drug companies to prove bioequivalence without having to duplicate trials and extended the length of time of patents to compensate for the time lost in premarketing trials
- 1990—*Omnibus Budget Reconciliation Act of 1990 (OBRA-1990)* mandated that OTC drugs are considered an important part of the medical record and must be documented
- 1990—*Anabolic Steroids Control Act of 1990* placed anabolic steroids under the umbrella of the Controlled Substances Act of 1970
- 1992—*Amendment to Applications for FDA Approval to Market New Drugs* and in 1997,

Food and Drug Administration Modernization Act allowed rapid approval by the FDA for medications for life-threatening diseases and debilitating conditions.

Over the years, federal legislation has established standards for medicines that provide patient safety. Citizens of the United States can feel assured that their medications have been tested and found effective with minimal adverse reactions and that all prescriptions for the same medication will contain the same therapeutic ingredients. Box 1-1 provides a timeline of important federal drug legislation.

At the state level, almost all states have laws concerning the substitution of **generic drugs** for **brand-name drugs.** State laws are governed by the state boards of pharmacy. Some states and some insurance companies permit generic substitution by the pharmacist, although the person prescribing the medication, usually a physician, retains the right to require the dispensing of a brand-name drug by writing "brand necessary" on the prescription. If the state has mandatory substitution, the pharmacist is required to use less expensive generic drugs to dispense the prescription. If a generic name is used on the prescription, the pharmacist may use his or her discretion to select the drug with a **bioequivalency** that is identical to the brand-name medication. A generic medication must go through the same testing as a trademarked drug unless the active ingredients have not changed and the inert ingredients provide the same bioequivalency.

Drug Standards and Patient Safety

Drug standards are regulations to assure consumers that they are receiving safe medications. Legislation requires that *all* drugs with the same name and strength be of uniform strength, quality, and purity so that each prescription filled for a medication is the same in all pharmacies, no matter where they are in the United States. Drug manufacturers must meet the standards set in the USP/NF for quality, efficacy, strength or potency, and purity of a drug. **Drug purity** specifies the type and concentration of a chemical substance present in a drug. Most products are combinations of ingredients including fillers, buffers, solvents, and so on that are necessary to give form to tablets and capsules and to make the product more palatable or change the absorption

rate of the medication. Purity standards also ensure that excessive contaminants are not found in the medication. **Drug potency,** or strength, is the concentration of active ingredients in the preparation and is measured by chemical analysis. **Drug quality** ensures that consumers receive the same standard of medications that meet the federally approved requirements found in the NF. **Drug efficacy** refers to the ability of a drug to produce the desired chemical change in the body. Clinical trials are used to compare the response of individuals taking the drug with the response to a **placebo.**

Even OTC drugs are studied to make sure they are safe for administration without professional guidance if the manufacturer's directions are followed and to make sure that the labels bear sufficient warnings and instructions. By 1983, OTC medications were either found safe or were removed from sale except by prescription. One of the problems in medicine today is that vitamin and herbal supplement standards are not enforced by the FDA but are supervised as food products by the Department of Agriculture, the restrictions of which are not as strenuous. The supplements may not have the same purity and quality with each manufacturer or batch. Consumers must be careful to choose reputable companies and to carefully read labels to lower the risks of taking poor-quality supplements.

In the illicit drug market, the consumer does not enjoy the protection of these standards with the inherent dangers of using illicit drugs similar to those found in the time of the medicine man. The lack of control over illegal drugs has resulted in overdoses and death among those willing to take the risks involved.

IMPORTANT FACTS

- Drug standards ensure that consumers will receive safe medications and that the drugs are those expected.
- Drug purity specifies the type and concentration of a substance that is allowed to be present in a drug.
- Drug potency or strength is the concentration of active ingredient in a medication.
- Drug quality ensures that the consumer receives drugs meeting the standards published in the National Formulary.
- Drug efficacy is the ability of the drug to produce the desired chemical change in the body.
- OTC medications must meet the same standards as legend drugs.

BOX 1-1	TIME LINE OF DRUG LEGISLATION

Pre-1900s   Medicine men traveled throughout the United States, selling "drugs" and "potions" without regulation.

1906   **Federal Pure Food and Drug Act of 1906**

Established the *U.S. Pharmacopoeia* (USP) and *National Formulary* (NF) as compendia of officially approved drugs, thereby providing the first official written source for medication formulas.

First governmental attempt to protect consumers of foods and drugs by requiring minimal standards of strength, purity, and quality.

Drug preparations containing any of specified "dangerous" drugs had to have the ingredient labeled on the container.

No enforcement agency.

1914   **Harrison Narcotic Act or Federal Narcotic Drug Act**

Established the word *narcotic* and required a tax stamp on containers of narcotic drugs.

Regulated the importation, manufacture, sale, and use of opium, codeine, and their derivatives and compounds.

This law saw many revisions and was eventually replaced in its entirety by the Controlled Substances Act of 1970.

1938   **Federal Food, Drug and Cosmetic Act**

Response to use of toxic materials in new medications.

Established the responsibility of the Food and Drug Administration for supervising and regulating drug safety under the U.S. Department of Health and Human Services.

Specified that all new drugs must be tested for toxicity, with the test results reviewed by the FDA prior to approval for marketing.

Enforced by the FDA.

1951   **Durham-Humphrey Amendment**

Specified how prescription drugs could be ordered and dispensed.

Recognized OTC drugs that did not require a prescription.

Required warning labels concerning drowsiness, nervousness, habit-forming potential, and the like, to be placed on packaging.

Certain drugs are *legend* drugs, so called because they bear the label (legend), "Caution: Federal law prohibits dispensing without a prescription."

1962   **Kefauver-Harris Amendment**

Response to severe deformities in fetuses caused by thalidomide

Required proof of both safety and efficacy of a new drug before that drug can be approved by FDA for use.

Medications, both prescription and OTC, must be safe and effective.

Enforced by the FDA.

1970   **Comprehensive Drug Abuse Prevention and Control Act of 1970**

Established the Drug Enforcement Administration (DEA) as a division of the Department of Justice.

Drugs with potential for abuse by the public were indicated as substances needing to be controlled.

Isolated drugs with the potential for abuse and addiction were placed into one of five schedules (I through V).

Required security of controlled substances by anyone who dispenses, receives, sells, or destroys controlled substances.

Required reporting on special DEA forms to indicate current inventory.

Set limitations on the use of controlled medications. Guidelines were established for each schedule of controlled drugs.

Each prescriber, dispenser, or drug manufacturer must register and have a DEA number.

Enforced by DEA.

1978   **Drug Regulation and Reform Act of 1978**

Permitted briefer investigation of new drugs to allow earlier access by consumers.

Enforced by FDA.

1983   **Orphan Drug Act**

Gives pharmaceutical firms incentives to develop and manufacture medications for diseases affecting only a small number of people.

Enforced by FDA.

1984   **Drug Price Competition and Patent Term Restoration Act**

Eased requirements for marketing generic drugs.

Extended the length of some patents to compensate for the time lost in premarketing approval.

Allowed generic drug companies to prove bioequivalence without having to duplicate expensive clinical trials done for the original drug.

Enforced by FDA.

(continued)

BOX 1-1	TIME LINE OF DRUG LEGISLATION—*Cont'd*

1990	**Omnibus Budget Reconciliation Act of 1990 (OBRA-90)** Mandated that OTC drugs be considered an important part of an individual's medical record.	Changed FDA regulations to allow faster approval of drugs for life-threatening or severely debilitating diseases.
1992	**Amendment to Applications for FDA Approval to Market New Drug (CFR314)**	1997 **Food and Drug Administration Modernization Act** Granted the FDA authority to quickly approve drugs for life-threatening diseases.

FDA and the Introduction of New Drugs

As an agency of the U.S. Department of Health and Human Services, the FDA is responsible for testing all drugs before they are released to the public. The drugs go through several steps in development. The process is lengthy, taking 6 to 12 years, and expensive. At the end, only about 1 drug emerges for each 5000 to 10,000 different compounds tested. The two steps in testing new drugs are preclinical testing and clinical testing. (See Box 1-2 for the process.) At any time during the process or even after approval, the FDA advisory committee may ask for additional information from the manufacturer, for revisions in the trials, or for returning the medication to the company for further research or testing. Therefore manufacturers that develop a drug are given a 20-year patent on the medication to cover the time and expense of trials necessary to show that the drug is therapeutic in humans for the intended purpose. The process of FDA approval uses up to half of the patent time, leaving the company with about 10 years of marketability under the patent, or the trade, name. At the end of that time, another company may manufacture the drug under its own brand name or use the generic name that has been assigned by the USP.

DID YOU KNOW?

Many brand names may be available for the same generic drug. For example, ibuprofen is sold under the brand names of Motrin, Nuprin, and Advil, and naproxen is sold as Naprosyn by prescription and as Aleve as an OTC medication, although the strength is not the same.

The FDA also reviews proposals for new indications for already approved drugs—new uses for drugs on the market—with the clinical testing process being performed as for a new drug. Also,

if a manufacturer finds new indications for an already patented drug, the patent on the medication may be extended for a longer period of time. If a drug appears to be associated with too many adverse reactions, the FDA or manufacturer has the right to withdraw the drug from the market after approval has been granted. This is a means of protecting the public from unsafe medications, such as removal of most of the COX-2 inhibitors.

Many prescription medications are becoming OTC drugs at a strength decreased below the legend strength. An OTC drug has gone through the same rigorous evaluation as the prescription drug; it is a medication, and as such, the consumer must use it as the FDA has approved it for OTC use. Educating the patient to follow directions is an important element in the safe use of OTC drugs. For a review of the role of the FDA in drug regulations, see Table 1-1.

IMPORTANT FACTS

- The development of a new drug is a lengthy process, taking up to 12 years, and only one of up to 10,000 compounds tested may reach the stage of a new drug.
- A company introducing a new drug has approximately 10 years of exclusive use of the drug.
- Preclinical and clinical testing must be done on a new medication to ensure its safety. Any adverse reactions to medications, especially newly marketed drugs, should be reported to the FDA.
- The FDA regulates the manufacture of medications to ensure the safety of the public.

DEA and Controlled Substances

Controlled substances became regulated by the Controlled Substances Act, Title II of the Comprehensive Drug Abuse Prevention and Control Act of

| BOX 1-2 | STEPS IN THE DEVELOPMENT OF NEW DRUGS |

Development of a New Compound by a Pharmaceutical Company

Preclinical Testing in Animals

Drugs are tested for toxicity, pharmacokinetics (use of the drug in the body), and possible useful effects. Animal testing: range of 1-3 years, usually 18 months

FDA safety review

Investigational New Drug Status if Approved

(Go back to earliest research if not approved)

↓

Clinical Trials in Humans

Range of 2-7 years, usually 5 years

Testing for safety, effectiveness, dosage range, and therapeutic use

Phase I: Subjects are normally volunteers with a specific disease to be treated by the new drug. Trials test for the metabolism of the drug and its effects in humans.

Phase II: Subjects are patients.

Trials test for therapeutic use, dosage range, and safety.

Phase III: Subjects are patients.

Trials test for safety and effectiveness.

(Usually a sample size of 500-3000 subjects in phases II and III)

↓

New Drug Application (NDA) Sent to FDA

FDA review: Range of 2 months to 7 years, usually 24 months

↓

FDA Approval of NDA

(If not approved, return to manufacturer for further initial testing or further research)

↓

Postmarketing Surveillance

Drug is released for use, permitting observation in large numbers of patients

Surveys, sampling, and inspections by FDA and physicians using the medication are performed

Adverse reactions are reported to FDA

1970. The drugs covered under this act are those with the potential for abuse, addiction, or both, and are classified according to their abuse potential. This abuse potential applies not only to pain relievers but also to drugs with the potential to be addictive or habit forming such as steroids, depressants, and stimulants. Drugs cannot be placed on the controlled substances list unless the potential for abuse has been established. Criteria for placement on the list follow:

- Evidence that the substance is being used in sufficient amounts to pose a medical threat to individuals or a hazard to the community
- Significant diversion of the substance from legitimate use to illegal drug traffic and use
- Tendency of consumers to take the substance on their own initiative rather than on medical advice
- A new drug with an action related to the action of a drug already on the controlled substances list would be included until a decision could be made concerning its potential for abuse

The controlled substances are grouped into five categories, or schedules, each with its own prescription and dispensing restrictions (Table 1-2). Medications with the highest potential for abuse and with no accepted medical use are placed on Schedule I. Those with the least abuse potential are placed on Schedule V. A drug may be moved from one schedule to another or may be removed from the list as the abuse potential is reevaluated by the DEA. Any revision of the list is compiled and sent to practitioners by the DEA, and the health professional's knowledge of this information must be current.

Because the DEA strictly enforces the regulations pertaining to scheduled medications, precise and complete records are required for Schedule II medications (Figure 1-1). These records must indicate the flow of the medicines from the time of arrival until they are administered. The scheduled drugs must be stored in a secure manner in a locked cabinet.

IMPORTANT FACTS

- Controlled substances may be moved between schedules on the controlled substances list. Therefore a current list of all medications controlled by the DEA should be kept in the office. This list is available from the DEA.
- The controlled substances are placed in one of five groups, or categories, each with its own restrictions on prescribing and dispensing, on the basis of the danger of abuse or misuse.
- Controlled substances can be abused and misused with or without prescription use.

TABLE 1-1 *Agencies Responsible for Drug Surveillance*

AGENCY	CONCERN	RESPONSIBILITY	SUPERVISING DEPARTMENT OF U.S. GOVERNMENT
Food and Drug Administration (FDA)	General safety standards in the production of drugs, foods, and cosmetics	Approves and removes products on the market Regulates labeling and advertising of prescription drugs (cooperates with Federal Trade Commission on regulation of nonprescription drugs) Regulates drug manufacturing practices Engages in postmarketing surveillance to detect unanticipated adverse and therapeutic effects on drugs	Department of Health and Human Services
Drug Enforcement Administration (DEA)	Controlled substances only	Enforces laws against drug activities Assigns identification numbers (DEA numbers) for those entities that prescribe, dispense, and manufacture scheduled drugs Monitors scheduled drugs for the need to change the level of possible abuse	Department of Justice

The DEA and Controlled Substances in the Medical Office

Controlled substances are labeled in a specific way so that they can be easily identified. A large **C** shows that the drug is a controlled drug, with the Roman numeral of the class (I through V) appearing within the **C.** For example, a Schedule II medication would be shown as appears in Figure 1-2.

Physicians or other health professionals (such as dentists) who administer, dispense, or prescribe controlled substances must have a current state license, must register with and be assigned a DEA number, and in some states must have a state controlled-substance license. Exceptions to this ruling are physicians who are interns, residents, in the armed services, from a foreign country, or on the staff of a Veterans Administration facility, who dispense and prescribe using a special code under the registration of the hospital or institution. At the appropriate time for renewal (every 3 years), the DEA will automatically send a renewal form 45 days prior to the renewal date. If this form is not re-

ceived, it is the responsibility of the physician to notify the DEA that the form has not been received. The medical office should have a method of ensuring that renewal is returned in a timely manner.

Ordering and Securing Controlled Substances

A prescription may not be used to order the supplies of controlled substances that are for patient therapy in the medical office. Schedule II substances for use in the medical office or in the physician's medical bag must be ordered from suppliers using the Federal Triplicate Order (DEA Form 222). When scheduled medications are ordered, one copy of the form goes to the DEA, the second copy goes to the supplier, and the third copy is retained by the physician. On receipt of the drugs, the physician attaches the documentation showing the receipt of the medication. This necessary documentation could be a packing slip with the cash receipt showing payment for the medication or the

TABLE 1-2 *Drug Classifications According to the Controlled Substances Act of 1970*

DRUG SCHEDULE	CHARACTERISTICS	PRESCRIPTION REGULATIONS	EXAMPLES
Schedule I	High potential for abuse, severe physical or psychologic dependence No accepted medicinal use in United States For research use only	No accepted use in United States Marijuana may be used in cancer and glaucoma for research and may be obtained for patients in research situations	Narcotics—heroin Hallucinogens—peyote mescaline, PCP, hashish amphetamine variants, LSD Cannabis—marijuana, TCH
Schedule II	High potential for abuse, severe physical or psychologic dependence Accepted medicinal use with specific restrictions	Dispensed by prescription only Oral emergency orders for Schedule II drugs may be given, but physician must supply written prescription within 72 hr No refills without a new written prescription from the physician	Narcotics—opium, codeine morphine, methadone, hydromorphone (Dilaudid), meperidine (Demerol), oxycodone (Percodan), fentanyl (Duragesic) Stimulants—amphetamines, methylphenidate (Ritalin), amphetamine salts (Adderall)
Schedule III	Moderate potential for abuse, high psychologic dependence, low physical dependence Accepted medicinal uses	Dispensed by prescription only May be refilled 5 times in 6 mo with prescription authorization by physician Prescription may be phoned to pharmacy	Narcotics—paregoric (opium derivative), certain codeine or hydrocodeine combinations (with acetaminophen, aspirin, or ibuprofen) Depressants—glutethimide (Doriden), pentobarbital (Nembutal) Stimulants—benzphetamine
Schedule IV	Lower potential for abuse than Schedule III drugs Limited psychologic and physical dependence Accepted medicinal uses	Dispensed by prescription only May be refilled 5 times in 6 mo with physician authorization Prescription may be phoned to pharmacy	Narcotics—propoxyphene (Darvon), pentazocine (Talwin) Depressants—chloral hydrate (Noctec), phenobarbital, diazepam (Valium), Librium, Xanax, Tranxene, benzodiazepines (Ativan, Dalmane), Versed, Serax, Halcion, Valmid, meprobamate (Equanil), Restoril, paraldehyde Stimulants—Tenuate, phentermine
Schedule V	Low potential for abuse Abuse may lead to limited physical or psychologic dependence Accepted medicinal uses	OTC narcotic drugs sold by registered pharmacist Buyer must be 18 years of age, show ID, and sign for medications	Narcotic preparations containing limited quantities of narcotics, generally cough and antidiarrheal preparations—cough syrups with codeine, diphenoxylate HCl with atropine sulfate (Lomotil) and attapulgite (Parepectolin)

From the Drug Enforcement Administration, U.S. Department of Justice, Washington DC. Local DEA offices can provide current lists of medications on these schedules.

Registrant Name: Lawrence Merry, M.D.		DEA Reg #: AD0000000	
Address: 4th Street and Jones Ave.		Inventory of Schedule: II ✓ III,IV,V ____	
City/St. Zip: Holly, GA 00111		Inventory Date: 11/01/01	
		Inventory Time: Opening of business ✓ Close of business ____	

Drug/Preparation	# Containers	Contents*	CS Contents**
morphine sulfate	1 vial	100 tabs	gr 1/4 (16 mg)
Demerol HC1 ampule	10	1.0 mL	25 mg
Percocet	1 bottle	50 tabs	5/325 mg

The above stock controlled substances was inventoried by the person(s) signed below, who attest that the above inventory is maintained at the location appearing at the top of this inventory and has been maintained at the location appearing at the top of this inventory for at least two years.

June Smith, CMA
Inventoried by

Jane Joy, CMA
Inventoried by

* Number of grams, tables, ounces, or other units per container.
** Controlled substance content of each unit.

Drug Name	Patient	Dose	Date	Hour	MD	MA

Reviewed by   Reviewed by

_____, CMA   _____, MD

Figure 1-1 Typical inventory of controlled substances form.

C II

Figure 1-2 Symbol that indicates a drug is a controlled substance in Class II (Schedule II).

invoice and a copy of the check showing payment. Office personnel who keep good records are not only invaluable to the physician—they also assist the physician in following state and federal regulations related to controlled substances.

To purchase controlled substances on Schedules III through V, the physician does not use Form 222 but may purchase these medications through local pharmacies. However, the records of the suppliers' invoices and a logbook of the administration of the medication must be kept for 2 years. The date of receipt and the quantity of the drug received should be on the invoice and/or in the logbook.

Controlled substances must be kept separate from other drugs and must be placed in a securely locked area. Some states require a double lock on opioid products. The stock of controlled substances should be kept to a minimum. For the office needing large amounts of controlled substances, higher security measures, such as an alarm system, should be in place. The physician or his or her designee should keep the key. The statutes of each state provide guidelines on the allied health professional's role in the handling of controlled substances.

If a theft or loss of inventory occurs, the local DEA field office must be notified immediately. If theft has occurred, it is *required* that the local police department be notified, as well as the state bureau of narcotic enforcement. *Any* theft or loss is significant and must be reported, even if it is a single tablet or a single dose. If damage or contamination of significant amounts of controlled substances occurs, the local DEA office should be contacted for appropriate disposal instructions.

Record Keeping and Inventory Control

As controlled substances are received, the medication should be recorded on a special inventory form. The receipt should be signed by two employees and should show the exact amount of stock medication received. To take an inventory count, the allied health professional counts the amount of the medication on hand and compares this with the amount ordered and the amount either administered to or dispensed to patients. The total of the medications on hand plus the dispensed medications should equal the inventory received.

An inventory is required by the DEA every 2 years. This inventory includes the following information:

- The name and quantity of each controlled substance
- The name, address, and DEA registration number of the physician
- The date and time of the inventory process
- The signature of the person(s) taking the inventory; preferably two persons should take the inventory

Included with the inventory must be invoices or copies of invoices from the drug suppliers. Schedule II drug records must be kept separate from other records and must be readily available for inspection by DEA or government agencies interested in drug administration. Other scheduled drug records may either be kept separate or be easily retrievable from professional records. All of these records must be kept for at least 5 years.

If a medication for controlled substances is administered and none is dispensed, then the medical record of the patient must show the medication administration and must have ease of availability for DEA review. If controlled substances are administered and dispensed, the records must be maintained separate from the medical charts and must be readily available for inspection. States vary as to the exact requirements of record keeping, and allied health professionals should be aware of the state regulations where they practice.

Disposing of Scheduled and Nonscheduled Drugs

To dispose of controlled drugs, such as expired drugs, call the DEA office for instructions for disposal. If the drug must be mailed, the allied health professional should be sure that registered mail is used to ensure safe shipment. Once the drugs have been destroyed, the DEA will issue a receipt that the physician should place with the controlled substance records.

Outdated, noncontrolled medications do not come under these stringent regulations. Depending on the state law, they may be flushed down the toilet, washed down a sink, or placed in the trash. If placed in the trash, the physician should maintain security to ensure these medications do not fall into the hands of the public. Incineration may be necessary for medications such as topicals or injectables that are difficult to destroy.

IMPORTANT FACTS
- The DEA is an agency of the U.S. Department of Justice responsible for monitoring controlled substances. The FDA is an agency of the U.S. Department of Health and Human Services responsible for regulating the manufacture and safety of drugs.
- Controlled substances are marked with C, with the schedule number within the letter.

Role of Allied Health Professionals in Medication Administration

State governments must comply with federal regulations, and each state has legislation concerning the storage and dispensing of controlled drugs. The medical practice act of each state provides the guidelines for the prescribing and administration of medications by allied health professionals, who must be knowledgeable of the statutes in their locale. Because some allied health professionals perform tasks under the legal premise of **respondeat superior,** the physician needs a working understanding of the state and federal laws governing the legal job performances in his or her state of practice. Any legal interpretation of the law must come from the agency in each state that enforces the medical practice act. For example, in some states allied health professionals may administer parenteral medications, whereas in others that would be illegal; in some states allied health professionals may call prescription orders from the physician to the pharmacist, whereas in others it is not allowed. As an agent or representative of the physician, allied health professionals work under the laws of the state in which they practice their profession and have a legal and ethical responsibility to know what their state allows under that state's medical practice act.

When federal and state laws concerning medications differ, which law prevails? The stricter laws, whether they are federal or state, prevail. The policy and protocol concerning who may handle prescriptions and administer medicines in the medical office must be in compliance with state and national laws. Some states allow allied health professionals to write prescriptions for a physician's signature or allow a physician's agent, such as a nurse practitioner, to sign. In other states this practice is illegal. Some states allow medication administration by allied health workers; other states do not. Because many medications have similar names, health care professionals should be sure that their knowledge of medications is adequate to perform telephone transmittal of prescriptions with accuracy before doing so in the medical office. For commonly prescribed medications, health care professionals should know the indications, normal dosage, side effects, adverse reactions, and what patient education is necessary before handling telephone orders. New medications should be researched before the health care professional administers them or relays orders.

Other laws may come from regulatory agencies such as the Federal Trade Commission, which regulates business practices in the medical field, or the Consumer Products Safety Commission, which has a routine that must be followed, such as drug packaging to prevent poisoning in children.

Preventing Drug Dependence and Drug Abuse

Substance abuse is a national and international problem that affects all of us. Health care workers have a responsibility to patients and society to assess the chances for abuse or misuse of drugs. A patient's frequent request for a given medication and "doctor-hopping" may be signs of potential abuse or misuse of medications. A pharmacist may make the medical office aware of the patient's use of multiple medical offices and will provide the information to prevent further abuse. The medical office professional should be sure the physician is aware of any information provided by other health care professionals. Other signs that may indicate substance abuse include pinpoint pupils, lethargy, or a change in, or unusual, behavior.

Drug dependence includes both **psychologic drug dependence,** or **habituation,** and **physical dependence.** The physical dependence begins with the use of a medication over a prolonged period of time and is a normal adaptation to continued drug use. The medication may involve a drug used to relieve pain or to control physical or emotional problems, or it may be one used for such conditions as blood pressure or respiratory disease. Psychologic drug dependence is a craving to take a drug for pleasure or to relieve discomfort and a psychologic crutch used to relieve anxiety. However, drug addiction is the compulsive use of a drug despite physical harm and is therefore a dysfunctional behavior.

Drug abuse depends in part on why a drug is taken and what is culturally defined as acceptable. What is considered abuse in one culture may not be considered abuse in another culture. Drug abuse is the use of a drug in a way that is not consistent with medical or social reasoning. It is the administration of drugs in quantities over an excessive time that is inconsistent with accepted medical practice with resultant physical or psychologic dependence. (See Chapter 32 for a discussion of drug abuse and misuse.)

Some actions by patients may indicate possible abuse, as with the patient who asks for a particular medication and is not satisfied without that specific drug. Drug abusers, or those with drug-seeking behaviors, usually know which drugs they want and will continue to ask for a specific drug rather than accept the medical care offered by the physician. Many times drug-seeking persons will state they have lost a previously obtained prescription or lost the medication after the prescription was filled and therefore need a new prescription. The health care professional should follow office protocol exactly by pulling medical records and checking for signs of possible misuse of medications, such as repeated prescriptions for pain medications, sedatives, or behavior-altering medications. Documenting all prescriptions precisely is of utmost importance for all patients so that the physician can evaluate early signs of possible misuse.

Finally, the prescription pads should be safeguarded at all times. Prescription pads should never be used as note pads or for orders other than those for prescription medications. Signature lines may have the imprint of the health care professional's signature, and drug abusers may copy the imprint and forge a prescription. A prescription pad should never be left in an examining room unattended. The patient who abuses medications may be able to obtain the drugs more easily by stealing blanks from the prescription pad. Although all prescriptions should be documented in the medical record, another safeguard is to copy all prescriptions leaving the medical office and place copies in the medical records. The patient seeing this procedure would certainly be less likely to forge a prescription because the pharmacist could easily confirm whether the prescription had been written. Medical office personnel are an important link in preventing drug abuse and misuse by participating in the checks and balance system between the physician and the pharmacist. This system often is the first line of defense as early warning signs are observed and proper action is taken.

IMPORTANT FACTS

- Allied health professionals must have a working knowledge of all medications used in the office of employment. Health professionals with questions about a drug should investigate the drug.
- Health professionals should establish a working relationship with local retail pharmacists. Pharmacists are excellent sources of information about medications, legal responsibilities for drugs, and the uncertainties of drug therapy, as well as observing for early signs of drug abuse and misuse.

Ethics of the Health Professional in Pharmacology

Ethically, all members of the medical team must have a working knowledge not only of drugs with potential for abuse but of all medications that are used in their practice area. The physician or health care professional is responsible for writing the prescription or orders, but the person administering the medication must also have a working knowledge of the medication—its dosage, strength, physical appearance, side effects, and adverse reactions. If there is any doubt about the order, the person administering the medication should ask the physician or health care professional for clarification. With a written or phoned prescription, this accountability becomes a responsibility of the pharmacist. The ultimate goal in medication administration is the safety of the patient and the reduction of possible mistakes.

All health professionals must use confidentiality in all areas of medications and their administration. Some drugs indicate certain conditions such as HIV infection, and the health professional must carefully protect prescriptions from anyone who does not have a need to see them. If prescriptions are sent by facsimile equipment to pharmacies, a protocol must be in place to safeguard confidentiality. The procedure will vary among medical offices, but it must be in place to protect the provider against the possibility of legal actions.

Drug Samples and Ethics

Drug samples are a manufacturer's way of promoting sales by providing free supplies of medications to health care professionals. These samples may not be sold. The sample drug requiring a prescription is marked "sample," bears the federal legend ℞, and a prescription is recommended. These medications must be inventoried before being left with the physician. Manufacturers may also supply drug coupons for a discount on the price of the prescribed drugs. These coupons may not be sold or traded for use on a drug other than the one identified on the coupon.

Samples are distributed to health care professionals (prescribers) only when the physician provides a written request for any sample and identifies the desired quantity of the drug, the manufacturer's name, and the prescriber's name. Medical personnel in the physician's office may not sign for samples; the physician must sign the required form to receive samples. (Box 1-3 outlines the protocol for receiving drug samples and the DEA surveillance of controlled substances.)

Samples should be stored immediately in an area that is not accessible to patients and should be organized by indication of use or of disease process and expiration date. Samples approaching their expiration date should be placed toward the front of the storage area so that they are used first. Office personnel should assist the physician in being sure that only those medications that will be used are left by the sales representative. If the medications are not used or distributed before the expiration date, the drugs must be properly destroyed so that unauthorized persons cannot use them. Destruction may be accomplished by flushing the medication down the toilet, pouring liquid medications into sink drains (followed by flushing with water), or incinerating. Drug destruction requires time and effort and should be avoided (by not allowing medications to expire) if at all possible. Distributed drugs may *not* be returned to sales representatives.

Finally, drug samples may not be repackaged but must be provided to the patient in the package in which they came from the manufacturer.

Before taking any medicine samples for personal use, for use by family and friends, or for

---

BOX 1-3   DRUG SAMPLES AND DRUG ENFORCEMENT AGENCY (DEA) SURVEILLANCE

Responsibilities of Manufacturer
- Supply samples
- Provide documentation to DEA for scheduled medications

Responsibilities of Sales Representative
- Inventory drugs on receipt and yearly
- Show place for safe keeping
- Maintain records of distribution
- Report theft or loss
- Verify current valid DEA registration of health care professionals

Responsibilities of Physician's Office
- Provide prescription or representative's form signed by the health care professional
- Safeguard against theft and misuse
- Document that samples are supplied to patients
- Dispose of unused samples properly
- Retain samples at office once signed for; no return to manufacturer's representative
- Do not use outdated samples
- Obtain authorization by allied health professionals from health care professional to use prescription samples
- Do not repackage samples
- Do not charge for samples
- Keep samples in a secure area that is not accessible to patients

---

use by patients, medical personnel should always ask permission from the physician and office protocol should be followed.

Ethics of Medications with Medical Personnel

Because of the easy availability of medicines in the medical office, health care workers are at risk for drug abuse and misuse. Many medications, especially sample medications, are found in the outpatient setting, which can lead to the indiscriminate use of drugs. Career pressures, such as stress and lower back pain, place professionals at greater risk of drug abuse and misuse. Many people begin the road to drug abuse by having medications prescribed for legitimate health problems, only to find they have become chemically dependent health care workers.

The impaired health care professional is a danger not only to himself or herself but to the patient. The patient is in danger because of erratic behavior that causes errors in judgment and accidents. The impaired health care worker is also a problem for coworkers because they cannot depend on the person to do assigned duties. Tension in the workplace is increased, and financial implications such as embezzlement are possible.

How the problem is handled is an ethical matter (and in some states a legal issue) that must be faced with each situation. As suspicion increases a decision must be made concerning the need to tell someone in management of the concerns about the fellow professional. By confronting the problem head-on, patient safety is protected and the impaired worker has the opportunity to receive the needed care.

IMPORTANT FACTS

- Know the protocol of the health care facility where you work, as well as the abilities of your coworkers. Know the lines of authority—who is in charge of what, who supervises whom.
- Have a working knowledge of drug samples and their place in the medical office. Be sure to follow office protocol when distributing these samples.
- Know the signs of drug abuse and work within a legal framework to be sure you do not provide a way for drug abuse within the medical office or with patients.
- Work with pharmaceutical sales representatives to gain knowledge of new medications, new uses for medicines, and information on the drug samples left at the office.
- Drug samples should be suitable for the physician's practice and should be organized by their use for disease processes or categories of use. All similar drugs should be grouped together, with those with the nearest expiration date placed at the front. Because packaging varies with pharmaceutical companies, a storage container may be helpful in keeping drug samples together.
- Health care professionals are at risk for drug abuse or misuse because of the ready availability of the medicinal agents such as drug samples and the tensions of the profession.
- Drug abuse or misuse by health care professionals is a physical issue but more importantly an ethical problem because of the impact on patient care.

Summary

Today's health market has come a long way from the early twentieth century, when medicine men hawked their wares from wagons. Those wares were not subject to quality assurance oversight for ingredients or the manufacture of the drug.

One bottle of medication might do wonders, but the next might be ineffective or deadly. Today, with federal and state legislation, the public can be assured that the medication prescribed and dispensed will be of the same strength and purity every time they fill the prescription or receive the medicine in the physician's office. Through multiple statutes, the FDA continues to follow previously recognized drugs and studies proposing new uses of these medications while watching closely as new medications are developed. The process is long, time consuming, and expensive, but the public can feel assured that drugs are safe. If for any reason safety is questioned, drugs are recalled or taken off the market until their quality and safety can be established.

Controlled substances have the potential to be abused, and through stringent laws these drugs are watched closely by the drug enforcement agencies. Written prescriptions are required for drugs with the most potential for abuse, and it is unlawful for a person to possess a controlled substance without a valid prescription. The 1970 Controlled Substances Act was designed to provide increased research into the prevention of drug abuse and drug dependence. It also required labels for drugs with the potential for abuse, dependence, or both to ensure they would be administered or dispensed by legal drug handlers and not used illicitly. To avoid illegal use of these controlled substances, the public should be aware of potentially abusive or dependent drugs and the signs of abuse or dependency.

Health care workers must know the federal and state laws because ignorance of the law is not a defense in court if mishandling or poor administration of drugs occurs. The allied health professional must know the laws in the state of employment because the medical practice act varies from state to state. These laws concerning medications are specific and must be followed exactly. Allied health personnel often work under the doctrine of *respondeat superior,* with the physician assigning a protocol that is appropriate to a given situation.

Ethics in the medical office requires ensuring confidentiality for the patient, safeguarding prescription pads, and proper handling of drug samples. By working with other health care professionals such as physicians and pharmacists, the allied health professional can be effective in patient safety. Because medicines are readily available in the medical field, the allied professional should be extremely careful about drug misuse and drug abuse and be observant for the early signs and symptoms of misuse.

Critical Thinking Exercises

SCENARIO

Connie is a medical assistant in a family physician's office in a small city. Just after the office opens one morning, a well-dressed gentleman appears at the window, gives his name as John, and flashes his DEA badge. John says he is there to examine the records of the Class II controlled substances that have been administered in the office. John asks specifically for a certain patient's record.

1. Can John legally ask for this record?
2. What should be documented in the record if the patient has received Demerol on several occasions?

3. John also wants to see the records showing the ordering and receiving of the medications for administration. What records does Connie need to have available?
4. What forms does the physician need to be able to order controlled substances?
5. Are the same requirements necessary for Schedule III, IV, or V substances as for the Schedule II substances? Why or why not?
6. Can a drug representative leave samples of controlled substances? If yes, which classes? If no, why not?
7. Connie finds some Schedule II medications that are out of date. What procedure must be followed to dispose of these drugs?

REVIEW QUESTIONS

1. Define:
   Drug abuse _____
   Drug dependence _____
   Drug standards _____
   Drug Enforcement Administration (DEA) _____
   Food and Drug Administration (FDA) _____

2. Outline major drug legislation of the twentieth century pertaining to drug manufacturing, distribution, and advertising. _____
   _____
   _____

3. Name and define the five schedules found in the Controlled Substances Act. Place common medications that fall under this legislation in the correct schedule. _____
   _____
   _____

4. Describe the process of drug development. How does this process make medications expensive?
   _____
   _____
   _____

5. Drug abuse, drug dependence, and habituation are real problems in the medical office. Describe signs of patients who are abusers or are dependent on certain drugs. What measures can the medical office take to assist the patient yet ensure that the office does not aid in further abuse or dependency?_____
   _____
   _____

6. Why are the ethics in handling and dispensing of medication samples so important to health care workers? _____
   _____
   _____

CHAPTER 2

Basics of Pharmacology

OBJECTIVES

After studying this chapter, you should be capable of doing the following:

- Providing definitions of the keywords using the glossary or a medical dictionary.
- Stating health care workers' responsibility in regard to adverse reactions, side effects, and toxic reactions.
- Defining a drug and an ideal drug.
- Describing the five fundamental categories of pharmacology and how these factors influence medications in the body.
- Describing the indications for medicines.
- Knowing drug classifications and some commonly prescribed medications in each classification.

Joyce works in a physician's office that has several patients who do not think that going to a physician is necessary until an illness becomes life threatening. These patients often see folk healers and use herbal supplements and over-the-counter (OTC) preparations rather than prescription medications. Joyce does not think it is necessary to document the herbal supplements and OTC medications in the medical record.

What harm may Joyce cause these patients?

Thinking that the patient is taking medications as ordered, the physician cannot understand why the maintenance dose is not working and increases the dosage. What are the dangers of cumulation, polypharmacy, synergism, and antagonism?

KEY TERMS

Absorption	Distribution	Pharmacodynamics
Active ingredient	Drug blood level	Pharmacognosy
Agonist	Drug half-life	Pharmacokinetics
Alkaloid	Drug interaction	Pharmacotherapeutics
Allergic reaction	Excretion	Polypharmacy
Analgesic	First-pass effect	Potentiation
Anaphylaxis	Free or unbound drug	Receptor site
Antagonism	Glycoside	Recombinant DNA technology
Antagonist	Habituation	Replacement therapy
Antidote	Hypersensitivity reaction	Safe drug
Antiinflammatory	Ideal drug	Solubility
Antimetabolite	Idiosyncratic drug reaction	Stimulant
Antipyretic	Indication	Summation
Biotransformation	Inert ingredient	Supplemental medication
Chelator	Irritant	Supportive medication
Cumulation	Legend drug	Synergism
Curative (healing) medication	Local action	Synthetic or manufactured drug
Demulcent	Maintenance medication	Systemic action
Depressant	Metabolism	Toxic
Desired effect	Oil	Toxicology
Destructive agent	Palliative medication	Usage
Dispersion	Pharmacodynamic agent	Vehicle

With the possible exception of computers, in no area of life in the twentieth and twenty-first centuries has technology transformed everyday life more than in pharmacology. Drugs are not new; they have been used from prehistoric times through all eras of civilization (see Introduction chapter). Only in the twentieth century, however, have laws and regulations regularly been put in place to ensure quality in medications. The government has set standards for all drugs (see Chapter 1). The allied health professional is responsible for knowing the action of drugs within the body; the routes of administration; the forms of drugs for administration; and the symptoms, side effects, adverse reactions, and **toxic** effects of drugs on all patients including children and older adults. The allied health professional's understanding of pharmacology can be critical to the patient–health professional relationship, as well as to the employer-employee relationship. The allied health professional is responsible for having current knowledge of medications and their actions and reactions in the body.

What Is a Drug? What Is an Ideal Drug?

The word *drug* comes from the Dutch word *droog*, which means dry. The term is appropriate because for centuries most drugs that were used to treat people came from dried plants. Today a drug is considered to be any substance that causes chemical changes within the body. Virtually all chemicals including such substances as tea and coffee may be classified as drugs when given in large doses. In this book, a **drug** is any chemical used for a therapeutic application such as treating an illness, relieving a symptom, or for diagnostic testing. Drugs are chemical substances that can help or harm individuals, and therefore how drugs alter the biochemical function of the body must be studied and understood. Most drugs contain various components—active and inactive or inert ingredients. An **active ingredient** is the pure, undiluted form of the chemical or ingredient that produces an effect. An active ingredient is rarely given by itself. Usually it is combined with one or more **inert ingredients** that somehow affect or assist the drug's action by adding flavor, bulk, color, and so on. In most drugs the active ingredient is carried in an inert primary base or **vehicle,** which may contain ingredients such as preservatives, colorings, and flavorings.

An **ideal drug** is one that has only qualities of effectiveness and safety and produces no side effects or adverse reactions. An ideal drug is a theoretical construct only because there is no such drug as a perfect drug. However, some characteristics help a drug draw near to ideal such as the following:

- Predictability. The drug will produce the same effect each time the same dose is given.
- Ease of administration. The drug is simple to administer, convenient to use, and requires only one dose a day, to help the patient follow the directions for the medication.
- Inexpensive. Low cost will help lighten the financial burden of taking medications over prolonged periods. Because of ongoing expense, even moderately priced drugs can devastate the family budget.
- A name that is easy to pronounce and remember.

No drug is completely safe, no drug has all the properties of an ideal drug, and all drugs have side effects, but selectivity in prescribing is necessary to reduce the chance of side effects and possible injury. A **safe drug,** although not ideal, causes no harmful effects when taken over a long period of time. The drug should be selective: it should produce only the response for which it is given. The drug response may be difficult to predict from person to person and may change if the patient takes other medications. The health care team—the physician, pharmacist, and allied health professional—should work together to ensure that the medications are producing the desired or intended results to minimize the chance of a drug-induced injury.

IMPORTANT FACTS
- No ideal drug exists. All drugs cause some side effects or adverse reactions. The allied health professional must be aware of these effects and acquire an adequate knowledge of medications for safe administration.
- Safe drugs are those that can be taken in adequate doses over long periods of time with no harmful effects.

Five Basic Categories of Pharmacology

Medicines are foreign to the body and are capable of causing side effects, adverse reactions, and unexpected results, as well as the desired therapeutic effects. Medications do not necessarily achieve these effects by eliminating the cause of symptoms but rather by changing body chemistry or function to diminish the disease process causing the symptoms. Health care professionals must have a basic understanding of how drugs affect the body. Pharmacology terms are **pharmacognosy,** or the natural origins of drugs; **pharmacokinetics,** or how drugs are processed by the body; **pharmacodynamics,** or the actions of drugs in the body; **pharmacotherapeutics,** or the effects of drugs on the body; and **toxicology,** or the toxic or poisonous effects of drugs on the body.

IMPORTANT FACTS

The fundamental divisions in pharmacology follow:
- Pharmacognosy—The origin of drugs
- Pharmacokinetics—How the body processes drugs (what the body does to the drug)
- Pharmacodynamics—Drug actions on the body (what the drug does to the body)
- Pharmacotherapeutics—The effect of drugs in the treatment of disease
- Toxicology—The poisonous effects of drugs on the body

Pharmacognosy—Origins of Drugs

In the past, drugs came from basically four sources: (1) plants, (2) animals (including humans), (3) minerals or mineral products, and (4) synthetic or chemical substances. To this list we can now add the modern engineered drugs. No longer is the drug industry bound to natural substances in either crude or natural states. Today, chemicals and even human tissues, such as in stem-cell therapy, can be manipulated to increase drug sources.

The early drugs from plants (leaves, roots, bulbs, stems, seeds, buds, or blossoms) had an unknown purity and varying strength. Often materials not desired entered the plants and therefore produced toxic effects in the body. The dried parts of the plant were known as *crude drugs*. The active ingredient was later separated from the plant, and the substance became more reliable for administration.

Plant sources are grouped by their physical and chemical properties. **Alkaloids** are alkaline organic compounds that are combined with acids to make a salt to extract the chemical from its natural state. **Glycosides** are active plant substances that yield a sugar (glycose or glucose) plus an active ingredient. The sugar is thought to increase the absorption and metabolism of the drug. **Gums** are usually polysaccharides that produce thick substances and are sticky when wet and hard when dry. Gums can attract and hold water, causing swelling and the formation of gelatin-like masses. **Oils** are thick and sometimes greasy liquids that may cause an odor or bad taste. Volatile oils evaporate easily and are used as flavoring agents. Fixed oils do not evaporate easily and are greasy. (Table 2-1 shows examples of these plant sources.)

TABLE 2-1 *Drug Sources*

SOURCE	DRUG
PLANTS	
Purple foxglove (digitalis)	Digoxin (glycoside)
Rose hips	vitamin C
Cinchona bark	Quinidine (glycoside)
Opium poppy	morphine, codeine, paregoric (alkaloid)
Periwinkle (vinca)	Vincristine (alkaloid)
Snakeroot	reserpine
Grapefruit	methylcellulose
Belladonna	atropine, scopolamine (glycoside)
Willow bark	aspirin
Castor bean	castor oil (oil)
MINERALS	
Gold	Solganal, auranofin
Zinc	zinc oxide
Calcium	Os-Cal, Cal-Bid, Citracal, Rolaids, Tums
Magnesium	milk of magnesia, Mylanta, Maalox
Aluminum	Amphojel, Gelusil
ANIMALS	
Codfish	cod liver oil
Pancreas of cows and hogs	insulin
Stomachs of hogs	pepsin
Animal thyroid glands	thyroid hormone
Placenta	hair products
SYNTHETICS AND SEMISYNTHETICS	
Inorganic	sulfonamides, oral contraceptives, barbiturates meperidine (Demerol)
Organic	penicillin, cephalosporins
RECOMBINANT DNA TECHNOLOGY	
Insulin	Humulin
Erythropoietin	Epogen

Minerals from the earth and soil are used as they occur in nature or combined with other ingredients to supply drugs. An example is coal tar, an acid that yields salicylic acid, which is used in manufacturing aspirin (see Table 2-1 for examples).

Drugs can be derived from animal sources including insulin from the pancreas of a pig or cow or estrogen from the urine of a pregnant mare. Drugs obtained from animal sources include enzymes, hormones, vaccines, oils, and fats used in treatment of endocrine system diseases and for immunizations. Human extracts may be used, such as treating diseases or potential conditions like Gam-G for possible erythroblastosis fetalis (see Table 2-1).

Chemists are producing drugs from living organisms (organic substances) or nonliving materials (inorganic substances) in ever-increasing numbers. Chemically developed drugs are free of the impurities found in natural substances and are called **synthetic** or **manufactured drugs.** Not found in a natural state of use, these medications are artificial substances. Some drugs are both organic and inorganic (e.g., propylthiouracil, which is an antithyroid hormone) (see Table 2-1 for examples).

DID YOU KNOW?
The leading cause of death prior to 1940 was infectious diseases and infection processes. Recall how penicillin changed medicine after 1941 because antibiotics were previously virtually unknown except for sulfonamides.

Recombinant DNA technology is the newest area of drug origin. By artificially manipulating DNA segments from different organic sources and transferring this segment of recombined DNA to a host cell from a different species, scientists can change proteins and the way the cell reproduces. In effect, the cell becomes a small-scale protein factory, reproducing rapidly. Thus scientists can create genetic instructions that lead the organism to produce chemical substances that can be used as drugs. The newer forms of insulin for use in humans have been produced by this technique to prevent interactions from animal sources that may cause immune reactions.

Another biotechnological method of drug production is the use of cells from animals with antigens to produce hybrid cells that produce monoclonal antibodies. These laboratory-produced antibodies are used to attack tumors and diagnose many conditions, from anemia to syphilis. These drugs are also used as antirejection medications following organ transplantation. Cloning of cells, such as the cloning of salivary gland cells to produce insulin in a person with diabetes, is on the horizon. Through biotechnology, drugs to promote blood clotting in hemophiliacs and interferons to combat viral infections such as hepatitis C have been introduced, and many others will be brought to market. With advances in biotechnology and genetic engineering, the drug market is expected to change rapidly (see Table 2-1 for examples).

IMPORTANT FACTS
The origin of drugs began with healers' use of natural plant and animal substances and has now moved into the laboratory, where scientists manufacture drugs synthetically from chemical compounds. Medicine is now in the early stages of using recombinant DNA technology to produce drugs with fewer adverse reactions.

Pharmacokinetics—How the Body Processes Drugs

The word *pharmacokinetics* comes from the Greek word *pharmaco*, meaning drugs, and *kinesis*, meaning motion; hence pharmacokinetics refers to the movement of drugs through the body. The four processes involved in pharmacokinetics are **absorption,** or the movement of a drug from its site of administration into the blood; **distribution,** or the movement of a drug from the blood into the tissues and cells; **metabolism (chemical biotransformation),** or the physical and chemical alteration of the drug in the body; and **excretion** (elimination), or the removal of waste products of drug metabolism from the body (Figure 2-1; Box 2-1 indicates the factors that affect how drugs are processed in the body, and Box 2-2 shows the four basic processes of pharmacokinetics.)

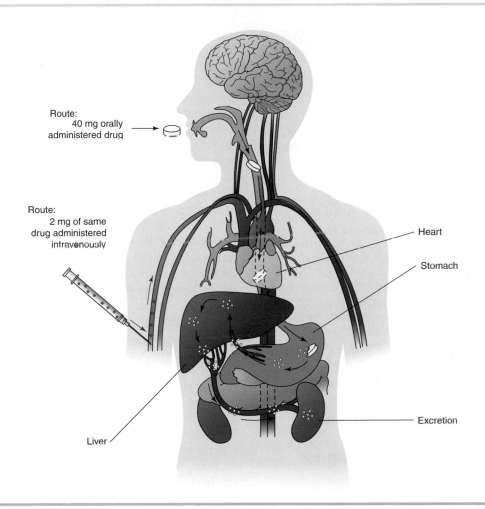

Figure 2-1 Pharmacokinesis is the movement of drugs through the body via absorption, distribution, metabolism, and excretion. (From Klieger DM: *Saunders textbook of medical assisting*, St Louis, 2005, Saunders.)

BOX 2-1	FACTORS THAT AFFECT DRUG ACTIVITY IN THE BODY

Drug Administration
- Patient compliance or medication errors

Disintegration/Dissolution of Drug
- Availability of drug for absorption

Pharmacokinetics
- Absorption
- Distribution
- Metabolism
- Excretion

Pharmacodynamics
- Drug-receptor cell interactions

Intensity of Responses
- Individual differences including: physiologic (e.g., age, gender); psychologic; genetics; diet; disease states; interactions from other drugs

Absorption

The rate of absorption of a medication is directly related to its route of administration. Medications may be administered by three routes: (1) enterally (directly into the gastrointestinal [GI] system by oral, rectal, or nasogastric tube); (2) parenterally (most often by intradermal, subcutaneous [SC], intramuscular [IM], or intravenous [IV] injections); and (3) percutaneously or through the mucosa (by inhalation, sublingually, transdermally, or topically). The rates of absorption for the various routes of administration vary according to the route of administration and drug **solubility** or its ability to dissolve (Tables 2-2 and 2-3). Absorption is affected by the rate that blood flows through the tissues with some medications dissolving rapidly, whereas others dissolve slowly, depending on the form of the drug and the amount of blood flow in the area. The primary sites of absorption are the mucosa of the mouth, stomach, small intestines, and rectum and the blood vessels in the muscles and subcutaneous tissues. Examples

BOX 2-2   FOUR BASIC PROCESSES OF PHARMACOKINETICS

Drug Administration
Routes: enteral, parenteral, percutaneous, or mucosal

Absorption
Active ingredients are absorbed and transported to sites of action. The amount of absorption depends on the drug's ability to cross cell membranes.

Distribution
Drug molecules are transported to various body areas via circulating body fluids (such as blood). The permeability of the capillaries to the drug determines the rate of distribution.

Metabolism (Biotransformation)
The drug is chemically altered by the action of enzyme in the blood, liver, lungs, kidneys, and intestines that convert drug molecules into water-soluble compounds or metabolites for the body's use or elimination.

Excretion
Unused drug molecules (intact, changed, or inactivated) are removed from their sites of action, usually through the urinary tract, respiratory tract, GI tract, or skin.

TABLE 2-2 *Rate of Drug Absorption by Route of Administration*

ROUTE	RATE OF ABSORPTION FROM FASTEST TO SLOWEST
Enteral	Rectal → Nasogastric → Oral
Parenteral	Intravenous → Intramuscular → Subcutaneous → Intradermal
Percutaneous/mucosal	Inhalation (lungs) → Sublingual (tongue) → Transdermal (through skin) → Topical (on skin)

The rate of absorption is specific to each route of administration.

TABLE 2-3 *Oral Preparations and Their Absorption Rates*

PREPARATION	RATE
Syrups, elixirs, liquids	Fastest
Suspensions	
Powders	
Capsules	
Tablets	
Coated tablets	
Enteric-coated tablets	
Timed-release capsules	Slowest

include nitroglycerin placed under the tongue next to blood vessels, albuterol (Ventolin) taken into the lungs by inhalation, or dextrose in water administered intravenously directly into the bloodstream (see Box 2-2). Once a drug has reached the bloodstream and is ready for use by the body, it is called a **free** or **unbound drug.** The drug binds to the proteins in cells and tissue to be called a "bound drug" that can now be metabolized and used. (Table 2-4 shows the route of administration versus the time for absorption of the medications.)

Factors that may cause variation in the absorption rate include the following:

Incorrect Administration Poor technique in giving a medication may destroy the drug before it reaches the bloodstream or its site of action. Specific directions must be given, when necessary, to enhance absorption of the drugs.

pH Drugs of an acidic pH such as aspirin are easily absorbed in the acid surroundings of the stomach, whereas alkaline medications are more readily absorbed in the alkaline environment of the small intestine.

Absence or Presence of Food in Stomach Food in the stomach slows the absorption rate and amount of irritation, whereas an empty stomach increases the rate of absorption and irritation in most medications, but some drugs do require food in the intestinal tract for absorption to take place.

Fat or Lipid Solubility Drugs that are highly soluble in fats or lipids, such as alcohol and alcohol-containing substances, are readily absorbed, whereas those with low lipid solubility are better absorbed by some means other than the GI tract.

Length of Contact The absorption of topical drugs is influenced by the length of time they are in contact with the skin, the size of the area, the skin thickness, and the hydration of the tissues at the site of application.

Inhalation Factors The depth of respirations, surface area of the mucous membranes, hydration of the patient, blood supply to the lungs, and concentration of the drug influence the rapidity of absorption. Inhalation is actually one of the most rapid forms of medication administration and absorption.

Drug Concentration High concentrations of drugs tend to be absorbed more rapidly; thus initial or first doses may be higher than maintenance or daily doses (see Box 2-2).

Distribution

Once a drug reaches the bloodstream it is ready to travel through body fluids to its site of action. Areas with an extensive blood supply receive a

TABLE 2-4 *Drug Administration Route and Rate of Absorption or Action*

ROUTE	TIME INVOLVED	WHEN USED	EXAMPLES
ENTERAL ROUTES			
Oral	30-60 min	As often as possible Safest and most convenient	Most medications Tablets, capsules
Sublingual	Several sec to several min	Rapid effect	Nitroglycerin for angina
Buccal	Several min	Rapid effect	Nitroglycerin for angina
Rectal	15-30 min, depending on contents of rectum	When oral medications cannot be used (i.e., with nausea/vomiting) and parenteral route is not indicated For local effect	Suppositories for nausea/vomiting or for constipation Preparation H for hemorrhoids
PARENTERAL ROUTES			
Subcutaneous (SC)	Several min; 20-30 min	Medications inactivated by gastrointestinal tract or when fast absorption is not indicated	Insulin, vaccines
Intramuscular (IM)	Several minutes, shorter than SC route; 15-25 min	Medications with poor absorption or when more rapid effects are desired—higher blood levels are obtained faster	Narcotics for pain, antibiotics, hormones
Intravenous (IV)	Approximately 1 min; administered directly into bloodstream	When immediate effects are necessary; when absorption in muscles is not adequate or is damaging to tissues	IV fluids, antibiotics, supplements, cytotoxics
Intraarterial	Approximately 1 min	Local effects within an internal organ	Cancer medications
PERCUTANEOUS/MUCOSAL ROUTES			
Transdermal	30-60 min	Convenient to provide continuous absorption and systemic effects over hours	Nitroglycerin and estrogen
Intrathecal	Several min	Local effects in the spinal cord	Spinal anesthesia, epidurals
Inhalation	Approximately 1 min	Local effects on respiratory tract	Medications for asthma, chronic obstructive pulmonary disease; oxygen
Topical	Approximately 1 hr	Local effects on skin, ears, eyes	Creams, ointments, drops
Vaginal	15-30 min	Local effects	Creams, foams, suppositories
Urethral	15-30 min	Local effects	Gels, jellies

drug rapidly, whereas areas with less blood supply have a delay in distribution. *Although a drug is delivered to the organ or tissues through blood vessels and capillaries, the effect of the drug is in the tissues, not the blood vessels.* The rate at which a drug enters different areas of the body depends on the permeability of the capillaries to the drug's molecules and to the chemical makeup of the drug, amount given, size of the person, and amount of protein in the blood. The amount of drug circulating in the bloodstream is called the **drug blood level.**

Two factors that influence drug distribution are fat solubility and protein binding. The body provides storage reservoirs in which the fat-soluble drug accumulates, resulting in a sustained pharmacologic effect on the body. Lipid- (fat-) soluble drugs are more readily absorbed by fat tissue for storage there. Because little blood flows through fat tissue, the storage site for the drug is established and a relatively stable reserve of the drug is maintained. Lipid-soluble drugs, such as hormones given by injection in an oil base, tend to have a longer-lasting effect.

The other means of storage is by plasma protein binding, whereby drugs in the circulatory system attach to proteins in the blood. Protein binding causes the storage of a drug in the blood as a bound drug and decreases the amount of free drug circulating in the body. This limits the amount of drug at the site of action. As the body uses the free drug, the protein-bound drug breaks down for use. Sulfa drugs are typical of this process: they remain in the body with antiinfective action for longer periods of time than other antibiotics.

Some drugs cannot pass through certain types of cell membranes such as in the blood-brain barrier. As an additional barrier, the brain is protected by restricting entry of water-soluble electrolytes, but lipid-soluble drugs are allowed distribution into the brain and cerebrospinal fluid because the brain is composed of many lipids. The placental barrier, another membrane, is less selective in the distribution of medications, allowing water- and lipid-soluble drugs to cross. Thus many medications given to a mother may also reach the fetus, producing either a therapeutic effect (such as cardiac drugs that may be necessary for the fetus) or harmful effects (such as anesthetics, alcohol, or narcotics). Other drugs may be selectively distributed to specific sites such as sending hCG to the ovaries to treat infertility (see Box 2-2).

Metabolism, or Biotransformation

Metabolism, or **biotransformation,** is a series of chemical reactions that alter and convert drugs into water-soluble compounds for excretion. The drug is detoxified, or turned into a relatively harmless substance, by enzymes that break down the medication and allow the body to rid itself of the drug. Without metabolism the drug would continue to have an effect on the body and would eventually cause harm to the person by cumulation to toxic levels.

Although other organs can contribute to metabolism of drugs, the liver is the primary site for drug metabolism. Orally administered drugs absorbed in the stomach or upper intestines enter the bloodstream and pass through portal circulation in the liver before reaching systemic circulation that takes the drug to the site of action in the intestinal tract. The amount of the drug that may be metabolized during this pass through the liver varies from a small amount to a substantial portion of the drug. This pass through the liver leaves only a limited amount of the medication to reach the site of action. This is called the **first-pass effect.** Drugs that are administered parenterally or sublingually do not undergo a first-pass effect. Therefore often medications administered parenterally require lower doses than those given by enteral routes (see Figure 2-1).

The rate of metabolism is an important issue in drug dosage. The **drug half-life** is the time the body takes to inactivate half of the available drug. Elderly adults or persons with impaired liver or renal function may have inefficient or insufficient metabolism of the drug and may be at risk for drug toxicity because the drug's half-life is prolonged (see Box 2-2).

Excretion or Elimination

The rate of **excretion** or **elimination** depends on the chemical composition of the drug, rate of metabolism, and route of administration (see Tables 2-2, 2-3, and 2-4). The conditions of the excreting organs such as the kidneys and lungs also determine how quickly and how completely excretion occurs.

IMPORTANT FACTS

- Absorption, distribution, metabolism, and excretion are steps used to process drugs. These processes are dependent on many factors including age, mental state, route of administration, gender, and the physical condition of the patient.
- The drug blood level is the amount of drug circulating in the bloodstream.
- The half-life of a drug is the time at which half of the initial dose has been metabolized. The half-life is different for different drugs and is essential in establishing the correct dosage.
- Drug excretion occurs most commonly via the kidneys; therefore adequate renal function must be present to remove the drug from the body.

Pharmacodynamics—Drugs and Their Actions in the Body

Pharmacodynamics, or drug action, is the term for how a drug works or its mechanism of action in the body. In pharmacodynamic terms, drugs produce chemical effects that affect biochemical or physiologic processes in the body or control changes in the body caused by disease. *Drug action* is the physiologic change in the body or the response to the pharmacologic effect. It is the chemical reaction of drugs in the body. *Drugs can modify the way the body acts, but they do not give body organs and tissues a new function.*

LEARNING TIP

Dynamite causes an explosion at the site that has been chosen for its use. Pharmacodynamics refers to drug action, as drugs "explode" into action in the body.

The effects of drugs usually either slow down or speed up ordinary cell processes and protect the body from the actions of foreign agents (Table 2-5).

No drug has a single action. When the drug enters the body, a predictable chemical reaction is expected. However, because there is no ideal drug and because individuals react to drugs differently, many unpredictable chemical reactions occur. The **desired effect** happens when the expected response occurs, such as Benadryl stopping the runny nose or watery eyes caused by allergies. However, when other effects are predictable but not the desired effects, a **side effect** has occurred. Because medications affect more than one body system, the action may not be specific and may cause undesired responses. The drowsiness that occurs with Benadryl is expected, and is sometimes a therapeutic use to assist with insomnia, but is not the desired effect. It is a side effect. Lowering the dosage of the medication will often reduce side effects, but in some cases the drug may have to be discontinued because of the side effects. (Adverse reactions that tend to be more severe are discussed later in the section on toxicology.)

The site of action for the drug may be either local or systemic. **Local action** is limited to the site of administration and the tissues immediately surrounding the application site; examples of medications with local action are nasal sprays and topical creams. When the drug effect is felt throughout the body, not just at the site of administration, the effect is considered **systemic.** Intravenous and intramuscular drugs always reach systemic circulation for their effect, whereas oral and subcutaneous drugs may produce systemic or local effects. The same drug may be manufactured for either systemic or local effect. An example is Benadryl, which is manufactured in capsules for systemic use and as a cream for topical or local use. A drug that has its effect on a part of the body that is distant from the site of administration is said to have a remote effect; an example is nitroglycerin placed under the tongue to treat the acute symptoms of angina pectoris. (Rather than having systemic action, some drugs have specific sites of action, such as thyroid hormone that has a primary site of action in the thyroid gland for hormone replacement in hypothyroidism.)

IMPORTANT FACTS

- Drug effects fall into four major categories:
  - *Depression*, or a lessening of some body function or activity
  - *Stimulation*, or an increase in some body function or activity
  - *Irritation*, or the production of inflammation, generally by drugs applied to mucous membranes or the skin
  - *Demulcence*, or a relief of irritation or the production of a soothing effect
- Drugs do not have a single action, although each drug has an expected action or desired effect. Because drugs may not be specific to a single body system, side effects may occur when another system is influenced.
- Drug action is also related to the site of action. A drug that is not absorbed into the bloodstream but works at the site of application is said to act *locally. Systemic action* refers to a total-body effect of a drug that is absorbed into the bloodstream. *Remote action* refers to the effect of a drug on the body at a site distant from the site of administration.

TABLE 2-5 *Four Major Drug Effects*

EFFECT	DEFINITION	EXAMPLE
Depressant	Reduces the activity of the body part	Detrol depresses the urge to void
		Dilantin depresses seizure activity
Stimulant	Increases body function or activity	Laxatives stimulate peristalsis
		Oral hypoglycemics stimulate the pancreas to release insulin
Irritants	Produce symptoms of inflammation at site of application	Efudex irritates skin lesions for destruction of the lesion
		Ichthammol increases the inflammation of boils
Demulcent	Soothing action for irritation, usually to skin or mucous membranes	Hydrocortisone cream soothes allergic skin reactions
		Solarcaine relieves pain of sunburn

Pharmacotherapeutics—Indications for or Effects of Medication Use

The effect of a drug differs from its action. The *action* of a drug refers to *how* and *where* a drug acts in various body systems. The *effect* of a drug is the sum of the biologic, physical, and psychologic changes that occur in the body or the result of the drug's action. Because a perfect drug does not exist, effects that are not part of the desired therapeutic response do occur. Moreover, drugs given systemically will usually affect more than one body tissue, not just the target receptor site.

   LEARNING TIP

If we have therapy of any kind, we expect it to affect or change our body in some way. Pharmacotherapeutics refers to how a drug affects our body—how it changes what is happening in our body or the therapeutic effect of the medication to treat symptoms or diseases such as a headache or cough.

Indications and Uses of Medications

Illnesses present with signs and symptoms, which may then become **indications** for treatment with certain medications, or pharmacotherapeutics. In-dications are the reason why medical treatment is instituted. **Usage** is the prescribing and application or administration of a medication for a given purpose (Table 2-6). Many drugs produce therapeutic effects in several ways while still having the same indications and usage. For example, aspirin is used as an **analgesic** and **antipyretic,** but it is also used to slow blood clotting and as an **antiinflammatory** agent. Diuretics may be used both to relieve edema and to lower blood pressure, in this way affecting both the urinary and circulatory systems. A final example is ibuprofen, which was first introduced for the relief of arthritic pain and is also used as an antipyretic and analgesic.

Drug therapy is an integral part of the physician's plan of treatment in patient care, but it does not stand on its own. It is merely one part of the total treatment of the medical condition.

Contemporary Medication Indications

As the field of pharmacology has evolved, a new classification of indications for drug use has come into being. The same uses are present, but the list is shorter because some categories have been combined from those found in the traditional indications. The terms *therapeutic, diagnostic, destructive, pharmacodynamic,* and *prophylactic*

TABLE 2-6 *Traditional Medication Indications*

INDICATION	EXPLANATION OF TERM	USAGE
Therapeutic	Relieve symptoms	Muscle relaxants for muscle spasms
		Diuretics for edema
Diagnostic	Diagnostic testing to pinpoint disease processes	Dyes for radiologic testing
		Allergens for allergy testing
Replacement therapy	Replace missing chemicals	Hormones for menopause
		Thyroid replacement in hypothyroidism
Supplemental	Avoidance of deficiencies or to reinforce existing body chemicals	Vitamins for pregnant women
		Calcium for prevention of osteoporosis
Preventive/prophylactic	Prevent or lessen the severity of disease	Influenza vaccine for prevention of influenza
		Contraceptive to prevent pregnancy
		Fluorides for prevention of tooth decay
Palliative	Reduce the symptoms of a disease but not necessarily treat the disease or condition	Narcotics for pain
		Decongestants for nasal congestion
		Antiinflammatories for arthritis
Curative/healing	Kill or remove the causative agent of disease	Antibiotics for infection
		Antivirals for viruses
Maintenance	Maintain a condition of health put at risk by chronic disease processes or surgical interventions	Insulin for diabetes mellitus
		Antihypertensives for elevated blood pressure
		Antihypercholesterolemics for elevated serum lipids
Supportive	Maintain the body in homeostasis until a disease process can be resolved	Corticosteroids for persons with allergic reactions such as asthma
		Oxygen therapy

represent broad drug uses and are in keeping with good pharmacologic terminology. This classification tends to avoid the overlap found with the older classifications and should also prevent confusion in using medications (Table 2-7).

When a drug enters the body, a predictable chemical reaction is expected. However, because each person is different, unpredictable chemical reactions may occur. Each patient must be monitored closely to determine the effects of the medication on that person. The expected response is called the **desired effect.** When the medication produces the effect the physician intended and the expected therapy occurs, the desired effect has been achieved.

Because a medication may influence more than one body system at a time, the action of the drug may not be specific and may produce side effects. **Side effects** are usually mild but sometimes annoying responses to a medication, although in some cases medications are used for the side effects such as minoxidil (Rogaine) with a side effect for hair growth. An example of a side effect is the drowsiness caused by antihistamines. Side effects may decrease when the medication is taken over a period of time. Lowering the dosage of the drug may reduce other side effects. In some instances the drug must be discontinued or stopped because of its side effects. (Adverse reactions are discussed under Toxicology because they tend to be more severe and less predictable.)

Toxicology—Poisonous Effects of Drugs on the Body

All drugs or chemicals have a toxic level or, if taken in excess, act as poisons. The dose of a medication can mean the difference between a therapeutic effect and a toxic effect. The goal of pharmacology is to select the medication in the dose that is therapeutic and to avoid medications and doses that produce toxic effects. The difference

TABLE 2-7 *Contemporary Medication Indications*

INDICATION	EXPLANATION OF TERM	USAGE
Therapeutic	To maintain homeostasis, to relieve symptoms, to fight illness, and to reverse disease processes	Promote normal growth and functioning Replacement of hormones Antiinfectives for infections Alleviation of pain Treatment of mental illness
Diagnostic	Aid in diagnosing diseases, aid in examination of the patient, and to discover the nature or extent of conditions	Barium for x-ray studies Dyes for diagnostic radiologic studies Acetic acid for use during colposcopy to detect abnormal cervical tissue
Destructive	Destroy cells and tissues	Radioisotopes to treat hyperactive glands Bactericidals and antiseptics to destroy bacteria Chemotherapeutics for destruction of malignant cells
Pharmacodynamic	Alter normal body function	Anesthetics for either sleep or numbness Contraceptives to alter hormone balance Aspirin for blood "thinning" Digitalis to increase heart muscle contractions
Prophylactic	Prevent occurrence of illnesses or diseases	Antihistamines for allergies Antivenoms

between a therapeutic dose and a toxic dose is considered the margin of safety. For some drugs, just a small increase in drug levels can cause toxic effects, whereas slightly lowering the blood levels of other drugs may cause the therapy to fail. When the toxicity level has been exceeded, an **antidote** is given to stop the toxic effect.

Adverse reactions usually imply problems or symptoms more severe than side effects. Adverse reactions are unintended, undesirable, and often unpredictable effects that cause unintentional pain or discomfort or unwanted symptoms for the patient. When Benadryl causes hyperactivity or a rash, the reaction is adverse versus the side effect of drowsiness and the relief of a rash. Because the U.S. Food and Drug Administration (FDA) requires substantial testing of drugs before allowing them to be marketed, common adverse reactions may be predictable. The allied health professional has a responsibility to monitor a patient for adverse reactions, and serious adverse reactions should be reported. The physician usually takes the necessary action for reporting adverse reactions to the appropriate authorities as designated by law.

CLINICAL TIP

All adverse reactions should be documented in red ink in the patient's record and should be noted in an obvious place such as the front of the chart so that the patient does not receive the same drugs again, either in the office or as a prescription.

Allergic reactions, or drug allergies, are a type of **hypersensitivity reaction** to drugs. Allergic reactions may occur after only one dose of a drug is taken either because the drug was taken many years before or the person is allergic to a similar antigenic substance. The person becomes sensitized to the drug by an antigen-antibody reaction following the administration of a single dose or multiple doses of a drug. The reaction appears with the next administration of the drug and may be mild to severe to life threatening. Mild reactions may have no immediate effect but may manifest with a rash for 3 to 4 days. These mild reactions must be recognized and reported before another dose of the drug is taken. Some reactions occur almost immediately, whereas others may be delayed for hours or days. Those that occur rapidly are usually more serious. Signs and symptoms of allergic reactions are itching, rashes, hives, difficulty breathing, wheezing, and swelling of the eyes, lips, or tongue. The patient should be educated to report all adverse reactions.

CLINICAL TIP

The allied health professional must use extreme caution when giving any medication for the first time to a person with known allergies to medications, foods, or other substances. People with other allergies are more susceptible to drug allergies.

Anaphylaxis, or anaphylactic shock, is a severe adverse reaction that is a potentially fatal, allergic response occurring a short time after drug administration to a person who is sensitive or allergic to the medication. The symptoms of anaphylaxis are hives, reddened skin, bronchospasm, elevated blood pressure followed by a drop in blood pressure, cyanosis, dyspnea, vascular collapse, loss of consciousness, cardiac arrhythmias, and cardiac arrest. The initial symptoms may be rapid swelling of the mouth and throat with difficulty breathing. Angioedema, or the accumulation of fluid in the subcutaneous tissues, may occur in the eyelids, lips, mouth, throat, hands, and feet. This is a medical emergency and must be treated immediately. Anaphylaxis has been noted most often after the administration of antibiotics, especially penicillin and its derivatives, and the dyes used in diagnostic studies, especially those containing iodine, but it could potentially occur with any medication at any time. Insect stings and some foods such as shellfish, peanuts, and eggs may also produce anaphylaxis.

Patient Education for Compliance

All patients who have had adverse reactions to medications should wear a medic-alert bracelet or tag to identify the substance of extreme allergy. All allergies should be listed on a card and placed in the wallet of a hypersensitive person. Some people allergic to insect stings or bites may even be prescribed a small kit of emergency medications to carry with them when they might be exposed to the significant allergen. An example is the stinging insect kit for persons allergic to bee stings and who work outdoors or engage in activities that might put them in contact with bees or other stinging insects.

IMPORTANT FACTS

- Toxic effects can occur with all drugs. A small change in a dose of a medication may separate a therapeutic effect from a toxic effect.
- Adverse reactions are indications of hypersensitivity to a drug in response to changes in the immune system. These reactions have unpredictable effects including allergic reactions and anaphylaxis.

Identifying Undesirable Effects of Drugs

Undesirable and sometimes unpredictable reactions can affect the body systems, causing side effects or toxic adverse reactions. The allied health professional should be aware that about 50 percent of adverse reactions occur in patients older than 60 years of age. Severe illness and polypharmacy (see Chapter 4), conditions often found in the elderly, increase the risk of these reactions. Deciding whether the patient is experiencing adverse reactions or some other symptom of an illness may be difficult. The questions found in Box 2-3 will assist in helping the professional make this decision. If the drug regimen has caused no problems in the past, then perhaps a new medication recently added could be the cause. Identifying unwanted reactions should be a part of the history taking for patient safety.

Drug manufacturers and health care professionals play complementary roles in minimizing unwanted reactions. The pharmaceutical industry strives to produce safe drugs. Health care providers in turn strive to select the least harmful medications for their patients. The allied health professional must assist in evaluating for possible adverse reactions and should educate the patient in ways to minimize or avoid harm from medicines. By teaching the possible unwanted reactions, the allied health professional can alert the patient for early identification of the signs and implement correction before

BOX 2-3	QUESTIONS FOR DETERMINING ADVERSE REACTIONS

- Did the patient follow the directions accurately?
- When did the symptoms first occur? How long after the first use of the drug?
- Has the patient started anything else new or changed something (such as adding herbals or vitamins)? Has a new household product, such as a new detergent, been used?
- If the drug was discontinued, did the signs and symptoms disappear?
- If the drug was restarted, did the same effects return?
- Could the illness cause the symptoms? Are the signs and symptoms consistent with the diagnosis?
- Could other drugs or products that are being used concurrently cause the reaction?
- Is there a possibility of a drug-drug or drug-food interaction?

the harm from the drugs is too great. Remember that idiosyncratic reactions—those unwanted reactions that occur with the first dose of the drug or when a subsequent dose is given—are unpredictable and may be from genetic predispositions.

By evaluating medications on an individualized basis, the health care professionals can reduce unwanted drug effects. The risks of the drugs and the probable benefits to the patient should be evaluated, and a balance sought during drug therapy.

Drugs and Their Receptor Sites

For drugs to be effective, the medication must attach to an appropriate **receptor site** in some manner. Free drug molecules, not yet bound to a site of action, travel in the blood until they are attracted to specific receptor sites. If the drug just continues to move about the body in the blood, the desired effect cannot take place. For a drug to be therapeutic, the chemicals found in that drug must be selective of the specific cell receptor site. The receptor site on the cell wall and the drug chemical fit together like pieces of a jigsaw puzzle. The better the fit of the drug and the receptor site, the better is the expected response to the medication. If the pieces do not fit together, the stimulation of the receptor sites may not occur and the drug may block another medication from being effective. Thus drugs at the receptor sites may either mimic or block the action of a medication when it mimics the body's physiologic actions. A drug's selectivity of a specific receptor site, however, does not guarantee its safe medicinal use (Figure 2-2).

Some medications may compete with previously bound drugs at receptor sites to form new

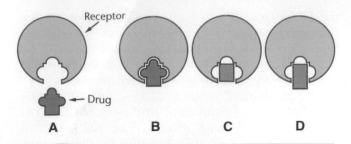

Figure 2-2 **A,** Drugs act by forming a chemical bond with specific receptor sites, similar to a key and lock. **B,** The better the "fit," the better the response. Those with complete attachment and response are called *agonists*. **C,** Drugs that attach but do not elicit a response are called *antagonists*. **D,** Drugs that attach, elicit a small response, and also block other responses are called partial agonists. (From Clayton BD, Stock YN: *Basic pharmacology for nurses,* ed 13, St Louis, 2004, Mosby.)

bonds. When the medication stimulates the receptor site, a chain of biochemical events is initiated and the response occurs. The drug works with the body to mimic its function and is called an **agonist.** Drugs may also compete with previously bound drugs at receptor sites. When drugs are attached strongly and do not produce a chemical reaction but do prevent agonists from binding at the receptor site, the medication is called an **antagonist.** The antagonist binds to the receptor site, does not activate it, and prevents it from being activated by the agonist drug. Antagonists thus counteract the expected effects of other drugs.

A weak bond that prevents other chemicals or drugs from binding to the receptor sites on the cell wall is called a *partial agonist*. Some drugs act by changing cell wall permeability, whereas others act as enzyme inhibitors. Examples are **antidotes,** used to neutralize toxic substances; **chelators,** used to treat metal poisonings; and **antimetabolites,** used with cancer to disrupt essential cell metabolic process, either by inhibiting enzymes or by interrupting DNA replication and function.

Mechanisms of Drug Interactions

Some medications are prescribed together to achieve the desired response. Other drugs may counteract or augment each other's effect if given together; other drugs may be wholly incompatible when given together and may interfere with the absorption, metabolism, or excretion of medications. Moreover, special precautions must be used with pregnant women, young children, and the elderly (see Chapter 4).

Drugs interact in various ways with other drugs and foods. These interactions must be addressed, or they may result in permanent bodily damage or even death. When multiple drugs are given together and induce simultaneous reactions, the combination of drugs may change the expected outcome of each drug, producing either better or worse results. Some of these actions are desirable, but others are undesirable.

Drug interactions, or the combined effect of drugs administered together, may take the form of **synergism, potentiation,** or **antagonism.** In addition to drug-drug interactions, there may also be drug-food interactions. For example, tetracyclines interact with milk, and antigout medications interact with cheese. Alcohol also interacts with many drugs, especially hypnotics, sedatives, and antianxiety medications. Another area of concern is the use of vitamins, minerals, and herbal supplements because these substances, too, can interact with prescribed medications.

Drug-Drug Interactions

When two or more medications are prescribed together, either (1) the drugs have no effect on each other's action, (2) the drugs increase each other's effect, or (3) the drugs decrease each other's effect. Any of these results may also be affected by the ingestion of food. Most drugs do not interact with other drugs or food, but when such interactions do occur, some may be life threatening. Because patients are taking more than one medication for more than one disorder, the potential for interactions increases. Patients may also be taking OTC drugs or herbal supplements that contain chemicals such as alcohol, nicotine, or caffeine for conditions that are not related to the illness being treated, but these have an effect on the body or the action of the prescribed drugs. All interactions are important in patient safety with medication administration.

If one drug potentiates another drug's effect such that the effect of the two drugs given together produce a stronger effect than if the two drugs are given individually, the action is referred to as **synergism.** The converse of synergism is **antagonism,** which occurs when two drugs cancel or decrease the effects of one another. Synergism and antagonism can be either desirable or undesirable. **Potentiation** occurs when one drug prolongs or augments the effects of another. The long-term use of some drugs may result in a lessening of the expected effect of the drug, a condition referred to as **tolerance.** The body simply gets used to the drug in the bloodstream, and a higher dose or a switch to a different medication may be necessary to achieve the desired effect. Another interaction may occur from **summation** when two drugs are given together and the expected effect of both drugs occurs. Other interactions are unintended and unwanted, producing possible danger for the patient. Finally, if for some reason the expected dosage of a drug is not excreted prior to the administration of another dose **cumulation,** or **accumulation,** in the body may occur. This may lead to interactions that may be fatal (Figure 2-3 and Table 2-8).

 CLINICAL TIP
Drug-drug interactions can change the outcome of drug therapy significantly. The chance of undesirable interactions can be lowered by reducing the number of medications taken. If a patient taking multiple drugs has unusual symptoms, the possibility of a drug interaction should be considered, as all possible interactions may not have been documented. The allied health professional should take a thorough history and assist the physician in finding ways to decrease the number of medications that the patient is taking, if possible.

Food-Drug Interactions

Food-drug interactions are important yet poorly understood. They can induce toxic effects and cause failure of therapy. The absorption of drugs can be significantly decreased by food in the stomach. Some medications must be taken on an empty stomach for more rapid absorption, whereas other medications are taken on a full stomach to maximize the absorption rate. Because some medications can become irritating to the gastric tract, they should be taken on a full stomach. The patient should be told whether to take the ordered medications on a full or an empty stomach. See Box 2-4 for common food-drug interactions.

Patient Education for Compliance

1. Medications ordered to be taken on an empty stomach should be taken 2 hours after meals or 1 hour before meals.
2. Grapefruit juice can inhibit the metabolism of drugs, raising the blood levels of drugs, even if taken at widely separated times from the medication administration.
3. Drugs can interact when directly combined, so two or more medications should not be combined in a container unless the person administering the medications is sure that no interaction will occur.

Addition of ingredients

beans   corn   peas   tomatoes

Add diluent

tomato juice

Synergism
(more than just individual ingredients)

vegetable soup

Adding seasoning
(inert ingredient)

salty vegetable soup

Antagonism
(adding potatoes absorbs salt, decreases potency)

vegetable soup

Cumulation
or combination of ingredients for effectiveness

balanced vegetable soup

Figure 2-3 How pharmacodynamics works.

TABLE 2-8 *Effects of Drugs in the Body*

EFFECT	REACTION IN BODY	EXAMPLES
Agonism (desired effect)	Drug stimulates the desired response at the receptor site	Penicillin to successfully treat infections
Synergism	One drug brings about a stronger effect of another drug when taken together	
Desirable synergism		meperidine (Demerol) for pain and promethazine (Phenergan) for nausea that prolong the effects of each
Undesirable synergism		warfarin sodium (Coumadin) and aspirin that increase bleeding tendencies
Potentiation	Drug increases the effect of another drug in the body	
Desirable potentiation		penicillin and probenecid (antigout medication) to prolong excretion time of penicillin
Undesirable potentiation		cimetidine (Tagamet) and theophylline where Tagamet increases the effects of theophylline
Antagonism	Drugs weaken or stop the effects of each drug when given together	
Desirable antagonism		vitamin K to decrease effects of Coumadin
Undesirable antagonism		aspirin and ibuprofen when given together decrease the action of both tetracyclines and antacids cause a decrease in absorption of tetracyclines
Summation or addition	Combining of two drugs and achieving the expected medicinal effects of each by adding the drugs together	Antihistamine plus antibiotic for sinus infection
Cumulation	Drug has stronger effect than expected because previous dose has not been metabolized or excreted from the body	Hyperactivity caused by excessive caffeine ingestion
Tolerance	Drug has less effect than expected; body gets used to drug (may be acquired or congenital)	Need for increased dosage of estrogen therapy for menopausal symptoms
Idiosyncrasy	Drug produces different effect than expected	Allergic reaction
Dependence/addiction/habituation	Body dependent on drug to function	Need for more and more pain medication to obtain the same result
Psychologic dependence	Emotional attachment to or craving for drug	Using sleep preparations without insomnia
Physical dependence	Physiologic dependence with possibility of withdrawal symptoms	Use of pain medications over a long period of time, especially scheduled drugs
Allergy	Hypersensitivity to drug; body develops antigen-antibody reaction	Most common is the allergic reaction to penicillin including rash, difficulty breathing, and possible anaphylaxis
Interference	One drug promotes the rapid excretion of another, reducing the activity of the first	Taking a laxative with an antacid

BOX 2-4	COMMON FOOD-DRUG INTERACTIONS

FOOD/DRUG	EFFECTS
Milk and calcium products/tetracycline	Tetracycline becomes insoluble, and antibacterial properties are ineffective with binding to calcium
High-fiber diets with wheat bran and oats	Reduce the absorption of many drugs
Grapefruit, grapefruit juice/"statin" drugs for hypercholesterolemia and sildenafil (Viagra)	Inhibit drug metabolism and raise blood levels of many medications; in other medications, stop the action of the drug; the juice seems to affect drug metabolism even if the medication and juice are taken at different times; the greater the amount of juice consumed, the greater the inhibition of medications.
Wine, yogurt, cheese/monoamine oxidase inhibitors (MAO inhibitors that act as antidepressants)	Cause potential toxic effects when used together
Caffeine or caffeine-containing foods/central nervous system stimulants	Toxic stimulation of the nervous system
Salt substitutes/potassium-sparing diuretics	Dangerously high potassium levels
Citrus juices (orange juice)/aluminum-based antacids	Excessive absorption of aluminum
Broccoli, brussels sprouts, cabbage/warfarin sodium (Coumadin)	Inactivate the medication because they contain vitamin K

IMPORTANT FACTS

- Medications may work together to either (1) increase the expected outcomes of each drug (synergism), (2) decrease the action of one or more of the drugs (antagonism), or (3) result in no change in the absorption and metabolism of each drug (agonism).
- Drugs bind to receptor sites on cell walls. The drug and the receptor site fit together like pieces of a puzzle.
- Drugs interact with other drugs for synergism, potentiation, or antagonistic action. These interactions may range from desirable to life threatening.
- Antagonism, synergism, and potentiation may be desirable or undesirable responses. Many times medications are given together for their synergistic or potentiating actions.
- Not all patients can tolerate all medications. Drug idiosyncrasies become evident when a patient does not respond to a drug in an expected way.
- Drugs accumulate in the body (a process called cumulation) if metabolism or excretion is not complete before another dose is given.
- Tolerance to a medication may occur if the patient receives the drug over a prolonged period of time. If tolerance occurs, the patient needs more medication to achieve the same effect as formerly.
- Foods (e.g., grapefruit juice) may have adverse effects on drugs and may potentiate the action of drugs or act as antagonists. Alcohol needs to be used with caution with medications. High-fiber diets can affect the metabolism of drugs.

Summary

A drug is a chemical compound used to prevent, cure, or treat disease or to diagnose abnormal conditions. No drug is ideal because chemicals interact differently in each person because of the distinct body functions of each person. In choosing medications, it is desirable to find a medication that is as close to ideal as possible—a drug with the fewest side effects and adverse reactions. Drugs may occur in natural substances such as plants, minerals, or animals or may be made in chemical laboratories. The study of the origins of medicines is pharmacognosy. The synthesis of new drugs including the manipulation of genes with recombinant DNA techniques is on the frontier of today's pharmacology.

The way drugs are processed by the body—through absorption, distribution, metabolism, and excretion—is the field of pharmacokinetics. Age, weight, gender, route of administration, and disease processes found in the patient will affect how a particular drug produces its effect. Pharmacodynamics refers to how and where drugs act in the body to produce a therapeutic or diagnostic action. The sites of action—local, systemic, selective, remote, and specific—are where drugs act on target cells or tissues. Pharmacotherapeutics refers to the physiologic changes brought about by the drug. Drugs are selected to cure a disease, palliate disease symptoms, prevent disease, or diagnose disease. Drugs may also produce toxic effects including adverse, allergic, idiosyncratic, and ana-phylactic reactions; serious reactions should be reported to the FDA. The potential side effects and adverse reactions are reported in drug inserts so that health care professionals are aware of these findings.

Medications are prescribed to aid in diagnosing disease, as well as to treat diseases after they have been identified. Medications may be used to replace missing substances in the body or to maintain the body as it adjusts to what is necessary. From therapeutic to curative to palliative to supportive indications, medications are an important part of medicine today.

No matter how careful the physician or how compliant the patient, undesirable reactions may occur. Deciding whether an adverse reaction or an undesirable effect is occurring may be difficult, but by eliminating possible causes of the reaction, health care professionals can recognize adverse reactions and stop the medication as needed. Undesired reactions include physical or psychologic dependence of the patient on the medicine. People may even take medicines out of habit rather than need, and these situations need to be addressed and the necessary changes made to the drug therapy.

Drug usage is complicated and varies because each patient is an individual with different needs and different physiologic and sometimes psychologic determinants. The allied health professional must be careful to see each patient as an individual and must take a detailed pharmacologic history to avoid detrimental side effects and adverse reactions.

When two or more medications are given together, they can increase each other's action, decrease each other's action, or have no effect on each other's action. These drug-drug interactions depend on how the receptor site on the cell and the drugs fit together. In some instances, medications are given to stop the actions of other drugs that might be detrimental to the body. In other cases, drugs are given to neutralize toxins. Some drugs work locally, whereas others work systemically, or throughout the body. Drug-drug interactions can be life threatening.

Also important are foods that can interfere with medicines. Some food-drug interactions can be dangerous to the patient, and these interactions should be fully discussed when drug therapy is prescribed.

Critical Thinking Exercises

SCENARIO

Mrs. Jones likes to take her medications each day with grapefruit juice. Since drinking the grapefruit juice and taking cholesterol-lowering medications, her cholesterol level has started to rise although her diet has not changed. A known effect of the juice is to inhibit the effects of the medications.

1. How would you determine that Mrs. Jones is drinking grapefruit juice? What questions would you ask?
2. Mrs. Jones asks if she can take her medicine 2 hours after drinking her juice because she thinks the grapefruit helps her arthritis. How would you respond?
3. When she asks about changing her medications to keep drinking the juice, what would be your response?

REVIEW QUESTIONS

1. Why is it impossible to have an ideal drug? _____
   _____
   _____
   _____

2. What is a drug? An active ingredient? A safe drug? _____
   _____
   _____
   _____

3. Drugs are excreted by four routes. What are they? What organs are involved in excretion? Which organ is most commonly involved? _____
   _____
   _____
   _____

4. What are the differences among a side effect, an adverse reaction, and an allergic reaction?_____
    _____
    _____
    _____

5. Drugs work at various receptor sites. How do agonists work at receptor sites? Antagonists? Partial agonists? Antidotes? Chelators? Antimetabolites?_____
    _____
    _____
    _____

6. Drug-drug interactions occur when medications are taken together. Some interactions are wanted; others are undesirable and even life threatening. Give two reasons for giving medications together, and cite two types of dangerous drug interactions._____
    _____
    _____
    _____

7. What role do OTC drugs play in drug-drug interactions? _____
    _____
    _____

8. Define *synergism, antagonism, potentiation, idiosyncratic drug reactions, cumulative effect,* and *drug tolerance.* _____
    _____
    _____
    _____

9. Describe what happens in drug-food interactions. Give two examples of drug-food interactions. ___
    _____
    _____
    _____

CHAPTER 3

Drug Information and Drug Forms

OBJECTIVES

After studying this chapter, you should be capable of doing the following:

- Determining the different means of classifying medications.
- Discussing what is meant by off-label medications.
- Contrasting drug names—generic, legend, over-the-counter, and chemical.
- Using the main sources of drug information.
- Using the *Physicians' Desk Reference* (PDR) or other drug reference guide to list brand and generic names, drug classifications, product identification by shape, identifying marks, and color, major precautions, available forms, dosage, and manufacturer.
- Identifying and describing drug forms.

Susan works in a local physician's office that specializes in gerontology. Mrs. Elder has come to see the physician for a small, painful wound on her leg that will not heal. Dr. Merry asks Susan to apply a dressing to Mrs. Elder's leg using an ointment. Unable to find an ointment in the medicine cabinet, Susan uses a cream. When Mrs. Elder tries to change the dressing, it has stuck to her leg.

What difference would an ointment make in this scenario?

Is it permissible for Susan to swap an ointment and cream? Why or why not?

Mrs. Elder has difficulty swallowing pain medication because her mouth is dry. Would you suggest that she take medications in a capsule or a tablet form? Why?

KEY TERMS

Aerosol	Emulsion	Nomenclature
Aerosol foam	Enteric-coated tablet	Ocular insert
Ampule	Extract and fluid extract	Off-label uses
Buccal tablet	Gel/jelly	Ointment
Buffered tablet	Gelcap	Package insert
Caplet	*GenRx*	Paste
Capsule	Gum	Pellet
Chewable tablet	Habituation	*Physicians' Desk Reference* (PDR)
Colloid suspension/solution	Implant	Plaster
Contraindication	Insulin pen	Powder
Cream	Liniment	Precaution
Delayed-release capsule/tablet	Lotion	Premeasured cartridge
Drug Facts and Comparisons	Lozenge	Reconstitution
Drug nomenclature	Magma	Solution
Effervescent powder	Metered dose inhaler	Spirits
Elixir	Nebulizer	Sublingual tablet

Suppository
Suspension
Sustained-release tablet
Sustained-release/time-release
  capsule
Syrup

Tablet
Tincture
Topical
Transdermal
Transdermal patch/disk
Troche

United States Pharmacopoeia/
  Dispensing Information
  (USP/DI)
Vial
Viscous suspension

Drugs can be named and classified in several ways. Several sources of information concerning medications, their names, and their classifications are available. These resources are important in providing safe dosages of medications for each patient and for providing information prior to the administration of drugs.

In this text drugs will be classified according to the body system where the therapeutic effect is expected. Icons for body systems will be used throughout the remainder of the book to assist in identifying medications with the receptor sites in the body's organ system. Other drugs such as antibiotics and analgesics that have systemic effect will be placed in chapters without relationship to a specific body system.

Medication forms vary according to the route of administration and the speed at which the body needs to absorb the drug for therapeutic effects. In this text the medication forms will be considered as enteral to include all routes involving the gastrointestinal (GI) tract, parenteral to include all medications injected into the bloodstream (IV), into the muscle (IM), or under the skin (subcutaneous [SC] or intradermal [ID]), or percutaneous for drugs that are absorbed through the skin. The rates of absorption for these routes are found in Tables 2-2, 2-3, and 2-4.

Drug Classifications

Drugs may be classified or grouped in several ways. Classifying drugs is complex and difficult because drugs may be indicated for use in treating conditions in several body systems. One classification is based on a drug's therapeutic action on body organs; examples are diuretics used to relieve edema and analgesics used to relieve pain. Drugs may also be classified according to their general use, in which case the classification is similar to their therapeutic action, producing such terms as *diuresis* or *analgesia*. Families of drugs may also be used to classify, such as penicillins used as antibiotics or thiazides for diuresis. Grouping drugs by the specific body system or organ on which they have their effect, as well as by their action on that system,

assists understanding. It should be remembered that some medications have more than one use and may have therapeutic effects on more than one body system. Some examples are diuretics, which are used for diuresis and to lower blood pressure, and aspirin, which is used for analgesia to reduce inflammation and as an antithrombotic (to prevent blood clots) in patients with coronary disease. The classification by therapeutic effect and drug families are usually found in the drug reference materials that are discussed later.

> **IMPORTANT FACTS**
> - Drugs are classified by their medicinal uses and their therapeutic actions, as well as by family. A single drug may have more than one classification, may affect more than one body system, and may be used in several ways in the treatment of illnesses and conditions.
> - Most drug classifications are based on medical terminology for the symptoms or disease processes for which they are used.

"Off-Label" Uses for Medications

Drugs are used for conditions found in the package insert for uses approved by the FDA. However, some medications have "off-label" uses, which means that the medication can be used for a condition other than that approved by the FDA. Off-label medication means that medications are being prescribed for an indication that has not been studied by the manufacturer and submitted to the FDA for approval. These drugs are routinely used but have never been officially approved for a specific use, although the desired use may be therapeutic. The "off-label" use of drugs is becoming more widespread as physicians use the medications and report their effects after the drugs have already received initial FDA approval and because of physicians reporting different, unrelated effects on patients who were using the drugs as prescribed. Some drugs have been used in the past but now have approval for "off-label" indications because of financial gain from further testing for FDA approval. Rogaine, which was originally developed as a blood pressure medication and is used to prevent or slow balding, and Viagra, which was originally used to stimulate the heart during heart surgery and is now prescribed for erectile dysfunction in men, are examples of the changes by manufacturers. However, some of the older generic medications are truly used as "off-label" situations because of the money necessary for the extra studies. An example is Periactin, which is an antihistamine used for weight gain, usually in geriatric patients.

Drug Nomenclature

Drugs are named in a variety of ways including using names that include the family of drugs. For example, the "cillin" in amoxicillin indicates the drug is a penicillin derivative. (Drugs that affect body systems are classified by mode of action in subsequent chapters in Sections IV and V.) Since 1962, legislation has required that the FDA assign an *official or generic name* to any drug approved for human use in the United States. With this nomenclature, any drug with the same generic or official name must have the same chemical name and structure, no matter who manufactures the drug. Listings of official drug names can be found in drug reference books such as the *United States Pharmacopoeia/National Formulary* (USP/NF). This system is called **drug nomenclature.** Each drug has several ways of being named, which can be confusing to health care professionals and patients. For proper prescription dispensing and medication administration, drug names must be spelled correctly.

CLINICAL TIP
Health professionals must check the exact spelling of all medications to be administered before giving the medication. Some drug names look and sound alike or are spelled similarly.

The *chemical name* of a drug identifies the exact chemical compound of a medication and its molecular structure. Any drug with the same generic or official name must have the same chemical name and structure, no matter who manufactures the drug.

The *generic*, or *nonproprietary*, name, also called the common name, is the one given a drug when a manufacturer first proposes it to the FDA for approval. The generic name is never capitalized, is easier to remember than the chemical name, and is not the property of the manufacturer. Generic drugs are often prescribed in preference to proprietary drugs because they tend to cost less, have the least potential for errors, and identify the drug no matter who manufactures it.

Several interchangeable terms for *trademarked* drugs exist. *Trade name, brand name,* and *proprietary name* all refer to a drug name owned by a specific manufacturer. After the drug has been introduced for clinical trials, the manufacturer has the right to the sole manufacturing for 20 years. After 20 years, other companies may make the drug, but they may not use the original trade name. The symbol® follows a trade name, indicating that the name is a registered trademark and is restricted to use by the owner of the name, usually the manufacturer who owns the patent of the drug. Trade names are designed to be easily remembered (e.g., Viagra, Claritin). The first letter of a trade name (proprietary name) is capitalized, and the name usually suggests some special feature of the drug. Confusion is possible when trade names are used because names for entirely different compounds may be pronounced or spelled similarly.

Examples of drug nomenclature follow:

Chemical name—
    2-(4-isobutylphenyl)propionic acid
Trade name—Motrin
Generic name—ibuprofen
Over-the-counter drug name—ibuprofen, Advil, Nuprin, Motrin IB (the last three are also proprietary names)

Chemical name—
    N-cyano-N'-methyl-N''-[2-[[5-methyl-1H-imidazol-4-yl]methyl]thio] ethyl] guanidine
Trade name—Tagamet
Generic name—cimetidine
Over-the-counter drug name—Tagamet HB (also a proprietary name)

Legend drug is another name for drugs sold only by prescription, such as Demerol (meperidine) and Valium (diazepam). These drugs are so named because they must bear the federally mandated warning or legend, "Caution: Federal law prohibits dispensing without a prescription."

OTC drugs do not require a prescription. They are found on the shelves of pharmacies, grocery stores, and the like and are sold in dosages that are considered safe if the directions of the manufacturer are followed. Usually the doses are lower than found with prescription strengths of the drug.

Patient Education for Compliance

1. Health care professionals should teach patients to read all ingredients and drug interactions listed on the packaging before they take OTC drugs.
2. Generic and trade named drugs contain the same formulation even if the drug is manufactured by different companies (e.g., Amoxil by Beecham is the same amoxicillin as Trimox by Apothecon).

CLINICAL TIP
OTC drugs are medications and should always be listed in the clinical record as drugs taken by the patient. These drugs can interact unfavorably with prescription medications.

IMPORTANT FACTS
- Drug nomenclature refers to all the names by which a drug can be identified—all drugs have a chemical name, an official or generic name, and a trade name, and may have an OTC name.
- The trade name belongs to the company that developed the drug. The company also owns the right to be the sole manufacturer of the new drug for 20 years after the drug is introduced to the FDA for clinical trials.

Sources of Drug Information

Many sources of drug information are on the market. Individuals who function in different roles in health care can find sources suitable to their needs. The USP/NF is the official drug list recognized by the U.S. government. The book is revised annually (the latest edition, USP 30/NF 25 in 2007), with supplements twice a year to keep it updated. Its primary purpose is to provide standards regarding the identity, quality, strength, and purity of substances used in health care. It contains the official standards adopted by the FDA for the manufacture and quality control of medications and nutritional supplements produced in the United States.

The *United States Pharmacopoeia/Dispensing Information* (USP/DI) comes in several volumes including one for health care professionals and another, *Advice for the Patient,* in lay language. Both are large volumes of practical information about drugs and highlight significant information that will reduce patient risks. The patient volume stresses tips for proper use of medications and the necessary precautions to ensure safety in their administration.

Before a new drug is marketed, the manufacturer develops **package inserts** (Figure 3-1 and Table 3-1). The inserts provide a comprehensive and concise description of the drug, its indications and precautions in clinical use, recommendations for dosage, known adverse reactions, contraindications, and all other pharmacologic information relating to the drug. The FDA must approve this material before the product is marketed to the public. The insert must accompany each package of the product for dispensing, whether in bottles for pharmacy use or on samples for the physician's office.

The *Physicians' Desk Reference* **(PDR)** is published yearly by Medical Economics Publishing and financed by the pharmaceutical industry. The publication includes information about approximately 2500 drugs in an easily accessible form, making it a frequently used reference in a physician's office. The company also provides several supplements per year with revised information or information on new products; in addition, another volume for OTC drugs is available. All drugs are cross-referenced by manufacturer, trade and generic names, and drug classification. Color photographs of many of the drugs are included to assist with product identification.

The PDR consists of seven sections, each separated by color for easy access:

- Section I (white), Manufacturer Index: This section includes an alphabetical listing of each manufacturer, the address, emergency phone number, and a partial list of available products.
- Section II (pink), Brand and Generic Name Index: This section is a comprehensive alphabetic listing of medications by generic and trade names. The drugs found in the Product Information Section (Section V, white) are referenced and indexed here.
- Section III (blue), Product Category Index: This section subdivides medications by therapeutic class (e.g., antibiotics, antiarthritics, analgesics)
- Section IV (gray), Product Identification Guide: Each manufacturer supplies full-color photographs of actual-size tablets, capsules, and other drug forms. This section is invaluable for identifying products in the office.
- Section V (white), Product Information Section: This section contains the information found

Rx only

WARNINGS:

1. ESTROGENS HAVE BEEN REPORTED TO INCREASE THE RISK OF ENDOMETRIAL CARCINOMA IN POSTMENOPAUSAL WOMEN.

Close clinical surveillance of all women taking estrogens is important. Adequate diagnostic measures, including endometrial sampling when indicated, should be undertaken to rule out malignancy in all cases of undiagnosed persistent or recurring abnormal vaginal bleeding. There is no evidence that "natural" estrogens are more or less hazardous than "synthetic" estrogens at equi-estrogenic doses.

2. ESTROGENS SHOULD NOT BE USE DURING PREGNANCY.

There is no indication for estrogen therapy during pregnancy or during the immediate postpartum period. Estrogens are ineffective for the prevention or treatment of threatened or habitual abortion. Estrogens are not indicated for the prevention of postpartum breast engorgement.

Estrogen therapy during pregnancy is associated with an increased risk of congenital defects in the reproductive organs of the fetus, and possibly other birth defects. Studies of women who received diethylstilbestrol (DES) during pregnancy have shown that female offspring have an increased risk of vaginal adenosis, squamous cell dysplasia of the uterine cervix, and clear cell vaginal cancer later in life; male offspring have an increased risk of urogenital abnormalities and possibly testicular cancer later in life. The 1985 DES Task Force concluded that use of DES during pregnancy is associated with a subsequent increased risk of breast cancer in the mothers, although a causal relationship remains unproven and the observed level of excess risk is similar to that for a number of other breast cancer risk factors.

DESCRIPTION:

Estropipate, (formerly piperazine estrone sulfate), is a natural estrogenic substance prepared from purified crystalline estrone, solubilized as the sulfate and stabilized with piperazine. It is appreciably soluble in water and has almost no odor or taste - properties which are ideally suited for oral administration. The amount of piperazine in Estropipate Tablets is not sufficient to exert a pharmacological action. Its addition ensures solubility, stability, and uniform potency of the estrone sulfate. Chemically estropipate is represented by estra-1,3,5(10)-trien-17-one, 3-(sulfooxy)-, compound with piperazine (1:1). The structural formula may be represented as follows:

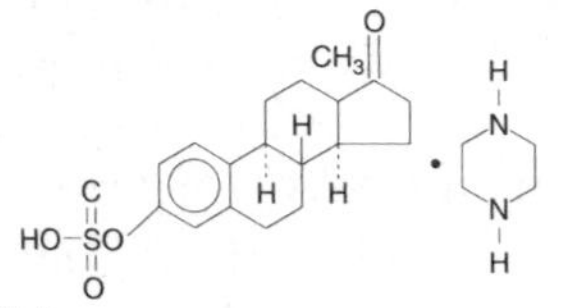

$C_{18}H_{22}O_5S.C_4H_{10}N_2$ **Molecular Weight: 436.58**

Estropipate Tablets are available for oral administration containing 0.75 mg, 1.5 mg or 3 mg estropipate (calculated as sodium estrone sulfate 0.625 mg, 1.25 mg and 2.5 mg, respectively).

Inactive Ingredients: Colloidal silicon dioxide, crospovidone, lactose monohydrate, magnesium stearate, and pregelatinized starch. The 0.75 mg also contains D&C yellow no. 10 aluminum lake and FD&C yellow no. 6 aluminum lake. The 1.5 mg also contains FD&C yellow no. 6 aluminum lake. The 3 mg also contains FD&C blue no. 2 aluminum lake.

CLINICAL PHARMACOLOGY:

Estrogen drug products act by regulating the transcription of a limited number of genes. Estrogens diffuse through cell membranes, distribute themselves throughout the cell, and bind to and activate the nuclear estrogen receptor, a DNA-binding protein which is found in estrogen-responsive tissues. The activated estrogen receptor binds to specific DNA sequences, or hormone-response elements, which enhance the transcription of adjacent genes and in turn lead to the observed effects. Estrogen receptors have been identified in tissues of the reproductive tract, breast, pituitary, hypothalamus, liver, and bone of women.

Estrogens are important in the development and maintenance of the female reproductive system and secondary sex characteristics. By a direct action, they cause growth and development of the uterus, Fallopian tubes, and vagina. With other hormones, such as pituitary hormones and progesterone, they cause enlargement of the breasts through promotion of ductal growth, stromal development, and the accretion of fat. Estrogens are intricately involved with other hormones, especially progesterone, in the processes of the ovulatory menstrual cycle and pregnancy, and affect the release of pituitary gonadotropins. They also contribute to the shaping of the skeleton, maintenance of tone and elasticity of urogenital structures, changes in the epiphyses of the long bones that allow for the pubertal growth spurt and its termination, and pigmentation of the nipples and genitals.

Estrogens occur naturally in several forms. The primary source of estrogen in normally cycling adult women is the ovarian follicle, which secretes 70 to 500 micrograms of estradiol daily, depending on the phase of the menstrual cycle. This is converted primarily to estrone, which circulates in roughly equal proportion to estradiol, and to small amounts of estriol. After menopause, most endogenous estrogen is produced by conversion of androstenedione, secreted by the adrenal cortex, to estrone by peripheral tissues. Thus, estrone—especially in its sulfate ester form—is the most abundant circulating estrogen in postmenopausal women. Although circulating estrogens exist in a dynamic equilibrium of metabolic interconversions, estradiol is the principal intracellular human estrogen and is substantially more potent than estrone or estriol at the receptor.

Estrogens used in therapy are well absorbed through the skin, mucous membranes, and gastrointestinal tract. When applied for a local action, absorption is usually sufficient to cause systemic effects. When conjugated with aryl and alkyl groups for parenteral administration, the rate of absorption of oily preparations is slowed with a prolonged duration of action, such that a single intramuscular injection of estradiol valerate or estradiol cypionate is absorbed over several weeks.

Administered estrogens and their esters are handled within the body essentially the same as the endogenous hormones. Metabolic conversion of estrogens occurs primarily in the liver (first pass effect), but also at local target tissue sites. Complex metabolic processes result in a dynamic equilibrium of circulating conjugated and unconjugated estrogenic forms which are continually interconverted, especially between estrone and estradiol and between esterified and non-esterified forms. Although naturally-occurring estrogens circulate in the blood largely bound to sex hormone-binding globulin and albumin, only unbound estrogens enter target tissue cells. A significant proportion of the circulating estrogen exists as sulfate conjugates, especially estrone sulfate, which serves as a circulating reservoir for the formation of more active estrogenic species. A certain proportion of the estrogen is excreted into the bile and then reabsorbed from the intestine. During this enterohepatic recirculation, estrogens are desulfated and resulfated and undergo degradation through conversion to less active estrogens (estriol and other estrogens), oxidation to nonestrogenic substances (catecholestrogens, which interact with catecholamine metabolism, especially in the central nervous system), and conjugation with glucuronic acids (which are then rapidly excreted in the urine).

When given orally, naturally-occurring estrogens and their esters are extensively metabolized (first pass effect) and circulate primarily as estrone sulfate, with smaller amounts of other conjugated and unconjugated estrogenic species. This results in limited oral potency. By contrast, synthetic estrogens, such as ethinyl estradiol and the nonsteroidal estrogens, are degraded very slowly in the liver and other tissues, which results in their high intrinsic potency. Estrogen drug products administered by non-oral routes are not subject to first-pass metabolism, but also undergo significant hepatic uptake, metabolism, and enterohepatic recycling.

INDICATIONS AND USAGE:

Estropipate tablets are indicated in the:

1. Treatment of moderate to severe vasomotor symptoms associated with menopause. There is no adequate evidence that estrogens are effective for nervous symptoms or depression which might occur during menopause and they should not be used to treat these conditions.
2. Treatment of vulval and vaginal atrophy.
3. Treatment of hypoestrogenism due to hypogonadism, castration or primary ovarian failure.
4. Prevention of osteoporosis.

Since estrogen administration is associated with risk, selection of patients should ideally be based on prospective identification of risk factors for developing osteoporosis. Unfortunately, there is no certain way to identify those women who will develop osteoporotic fractures. Most prospective studies of efficacy for this indication have been carried out in white menopausal women, without stratification by other risk factors, and tend to show a universally salutary effect on bone. Thus, patient selection must be individualized based on the balance of risks and benefits. A more favorable risk/benefit ratio exists in a hysterectomized woman because she has no risk of endometrial cancer (see Boxed **WARNINGS**).

Estrogen replacement therapy reduces bone resorption and retards or halts postmenopausal bone loss. Case-control studies have shown an approximately 60 percent reduction in hip and wrist fractures in women whose estrogen replacement was begun within a few years of menopause. Studies also suggest that estrogen reduces the rate of vertebral fractures. Even when started as late as 6 years after menopause, estrogen prevents further loss of bone mass for as long as the treatment is continued. The results of a double-blind, placebo-controlled two-year study have shown that treatment with one tablet of estropipate 0.75 mg daily for 25 days (of a 31-day cycle per month) prevents vertebral bone mass loss in postmenopausal women. When estrogen therapy is discontinued, bone mass declines at a rate comparable to the immediate postmenopausal period. There is no evidence that estrogen replacement therapy restores bone mass to premenopausal levels.

At skeletal maturity there are sex and race differences in both the total amount of bone present and its density, in favor of men and blacks. Thus, women are at higher risk than men because they start with less bone mass and, for several years following natural or induced menopause, the rate of bone mass decline is accelerated. White and Asian women are at higher risk than black women.

Early menopause is one of the strongest predictors for the development of osteoporosis. In addition, other factors affecting the skeleton which are associated with osteoporosis include genetic factors (small build, family history), endocrine factors (nulliparity, thyrotoxicosis, hyperparathyroidism, Cushing's syndrome, hyperprolactinemia, Type I diabetes), lifestyle (cigarette smoking, alcohol abuse, sedentary exercise habits) and nutrition (below average body weight, dietary calcium intake).

The mainstays of prevention and management of osteoporosis are estrogen, an adequate lifetime calcium intake, and exercise. Postmenopausal women absorb dietary calcium less efficiently than premenopausal women and require an average of 1500 mg/day of elemental calcium to remain in neutral calcium balance. By comparison, premenopausal women require about 1000 mg/day and the average calcium intake in the USA is 400-600 mg/day. Therefore, when not contraindicated, calcium supplementation may be helpful.

Weight-bearing exercise and nutrition may be important adjuncts to the prevention and management of osteoporosis. Immobilization and prolonged bed rest produce rapid bone loss, while weight-bearing exercise has been shown both to reduce bone loss and to increase bone mass. The optimal type and amount of physical activity that would prevent osteoporosis have not been established, however in two studies an hour of walking and running exercises twice or three times weekly significantly increased lumbar spine bone mass.

CONTRAINDICATIONS:

Estrogens should not be used in individuals with any of the following conditions:

1. Known or suspected pregnancy (see Boxed **WARNINGS**). Estrogens may cause fetal harm when administered to a pregnant woman.
2. Undiagnosed abnormal genital bleeding.
3. Known or suspected cancer of the breast except in appropriately selected patients being treated for metastatic disease.
4. Known or suspected estrogen-dependent neoplasia.
5. Active thrombophlebitis or thromboembolic disorders.

WARNINGS:

Induction of Malignant Neoplasms:

Endometrial Cancer: The reported endometrial cancer risk among unopposed estrogen users is about 2 to 12 fold greater than in non-users, and appears dependent on duration of treatment and on estrogen dose. Most studies show no significant increased risk associated with use of estrogens for less than one year. The greatest risk appears associated with prolonged use—with increased risks of 15 to 24-fold for five to ten years or more. In three studies, persistence of risk was demonstrated for 8 to over 15 years after cessation of estrogen treatment. In one study a significant decrease in the incidence of endometrial cancer occurred six months after estrogen withdrawal. Concurrent progestin therapy may offset this risk but the overall health impact in postmenopausal women is not known (see **PRECAUTIONS**).

Breast Cancer: While the majority of studies have not shown an increased risk of breast cancer in women who have ever used estrogen replacement therapy, some have reported a moderately increased risk (relative risks of 1.3 - 2.0) in those taking higher doses or those taking lower doses for prolonged periods of time, especially in excess of 10 years. Other studies have not shown this relationship.

Congenital Lesions with Malignant Potential: Estrogen therapy during pregnancy is associated with an increased risk of fetal congenital reproductive tract disorders, and possibly other birth defects. Studies of women who received DES during pregnancy have shown that female offspring have an increased risk of vaginal adenosis, squamous cell dysplasia of the uterine cervix, and clear cell vaginal cancer later in life; male offspring have an increased risk of urogenital abnormalities and possibly testicular cancer later in life. Although some of these changes are benign, others are precursors of malignancy.

Gallbladder Disease:

Two studies have reported a 2- to 4-fold increase in the risk of gallbladder disease requiring surgery in women receiving postmenopausal estrogens.

Cardiovascular Disease:

Large doses of estrogen (5 mg conjugated estrogens per day), comparable to those used to treat cancer of the prostate and breast, have been shown in a large prospective clinical trial in men to increase the risks of nonfatal myocardial infarction, pulmonary embolism, and thrombophlebitis. These risks cannot necessarily be extrapolated from men to women. However, to avoid the theoretical cardiovascular risk to women caused by high estrogen doses, the dose for estrogen replacement therapy should not exceed the lowest effective dose.

Elevated blood pressure:

Occasional blood pressure increases during estrogen replacement therapy have been attributed to idiosyncratic reactions to estrogens. More often, blood pressure has remained the same or has dropped. One study showed that postmenopausal estrogen users have higher blood pressure than nonusers. Two other studies showed slightly lower blood pressure among estrogen users compared to nonusers. Postmenopausal estrogen use does not increase the risk of stroke. Nonetheless, blood pressure should be monitored at regular intervals with estrogen use.

Hypercalcemia:

Administration of estrogens may lead to severe hypercalcemia in patients with breast cancer and bone metastases. If this occurs, the drug should be stopped and appropriate measures taken to reduce the serum calcium level.

PRECAUTIONS:

General:

Addition of a Progestin: Studies of the addition of a progestin for ten or more days of a cycle of estrogen administration have reported a lowered incidence of endometrial hyperplasia than would be induced by estrogen treatment alone. Morphological and biochemical studies of endometria suggest that 10 to 14 days of progestin are needed to provide maximal maturation of the endometrium and to reduce the likelihood of hyperplastic changes.

There are, however, possible risks which may be associated with the use of progestins in estrogen replacement regimens. These include: (1) adverse effects on lipoprotein metabolism (lowering HDL and raising LDL) which could diminish the purported cardioprotective effect of estrogen therapy (see **PRECAUTIONS** below); (2) impairment of glucose tolerance; and (3) possible enhancement of mitotic activity in breast epithelial tissue, although few epidemiological data are available to address this point (see **PRECAUTIONS** below).

The choice of progestin, its dose, and its regimen may be important in minimizing these adverse effects, but these issues remain to be clarified.

Cardiovascular Risk: A causal relationship between estrogen replacement therapy and reduction of cardiovascular disease in postmenopausal women has not been proven. Furthermore, the effect of added progestins on this putative benefit is not yet known.

In recent years many published studies have suggested that there may be a cause-effect relationship between postmenopausal oral estrogen replacement therapy without added progestins and a decrease in cardiovascular disease in women. Although most of the observational studies which assessed this statistical association have reported a 20% to 50% reduction in coronary heart disease risk and associated mortality in estrogen takers. the following should be considered when interpreting these reports:

(1) Because only one of these studies was randomized and it was too small to yield statistically significant results, all relevant studies were subject to selection bias. Thus, the apparently reduced risk of coronary artery disease cannot be attributed with certainty to estrogen replacement therapy. It may instead have been caused by life-style and medical characteristics of the women studied with the result that healthier women were selected for estrogen therapy. In general, treated women were of higher socioeconomic and educational status, more slender, more physically active, more likely to have undergone surgical menopause, and less likely to have diabetes than the untreated women. Although some studies attempted to control for these selection factors, it is common for properly designed randomized trials to fail to confirm benefits suggested by less rigorous study designs. Thus, ongoing and future large-scale randomized trials may fail to confirm this apparent benefit.

(2) Current medical practice often includes the use of concomitant progestin therapy in women with intact uteri (see **PRECAUTIONS** and **WARNINGS**). While the effects of added progestins on the risk of ischemic heart disease are not known, all available progestins reverse at least some of the favorable effects of estrogens on HDL and LDL levels.

(3) While the effects of added progestins on the risk of breast cancer are also unknown, available epidemiological evidence suggests that progestins do not reduce, and may enhance, the moderately increased breast cancer incidence that has been reported with prolonged estrogen replacement therapy (see **WARNINGS** above).

Because relatively long-term use of estrogens by a woman with a uterus has been shown to induce endometrial cancer, physicians often recommend that women who are deemed candidates for hormone replacement should take progestins as well as estrogens. When considering prescribing concomitant estrogens and progestins for hormone replacement therapy, physicians and patients are advised to carefully weigh the potential benefits and risks of the added progestin. Large-scale randomized, placebo-controlled, prospective clinical trials are required to clarify these issues.

Physical Examination: A complete medical and family history should be taken prior to the initiation of any estrogen therapy. The pretreatment and periodic physical examinations should include special reference to blood pressure, breasts, abdomen, and pelvic organs, and should include a Papanicolaou smear. As a general rule, estrogen should not be prescribed for longer than one year without reexamining the patient.

Hypercoagulability: Some studies have shown that women taking estrogen replacement therapy have hypercoagulability, primarily related to decreased antithrombin activity. This effect appears dose- and duration-dependent and is less pronounced than that associated with oral contraceptive use. Also, postmenopausal women tend to have increased coagulation parameters at baseline compared to premenopausal women. There is some suggestion that low dose postmenopausal mestranol may increase the risk of thromboembolism, although the majority of studies (of primarily conjugated estrogens users) report no such increase. There is insufficient information on hypercoagulability in women who have had previous thromboembolic disease.

Familial Hyperlipoproteinemia: Estrogen therapy may be associated with massive elevations of plasma triglycerides leading to pancreatitis and other complications in patients with familial defects of lipoprotein metabolism.

Fluid Retention: Because estrogens may cause some degree of fluid retention, conditions which might be exacerbated by this factor, such as asthma, epilepsy, migraine, and cardiac or renal dysfunction, require careful observation.

Uterine Bleeding and Mastodynia: Certain patients may develop undesirable manifestations of estrogenic stimulation, such as abnormal uterine bleeding and mastodynia.

Impaired Liver Function: Estrogens may be poorly metabolized in patients with impaired liver function and should be administered with caution.

Information for the Patient:

See text of Patient Package Leaflet below.

Laboratory Tests:

Estrogen administration should generally be guided by clinical response at the smallest dose, rather than laboratory monitoring, for relief of symptoms for those indications in which symptoms are observable. For prevention and treatment of osteoporosis, however, see **DOSAGE AND ADMINISTRATION** section.

Drug/Laboratory Test Interactions:

Accelerated prothrombin time, partial thromboplastin time, and platelet aggregation time; increased platelet count; increased factors II, VII antigen, VIII antigen, VIII coagulant activity, IX, X, XII, VII-X complex, II-VII-X complex, and beta-thromboglobulin; decreased levels of anti-factor Xa and antithrombin III, decreased antithrombin III activity; increased levels of fibrinogen and fibrinogen activity; increased plasminogen antigen and activity.

Increased thyroid-binding globulin (TBG) leading to increased circulating total thyroid hormone, as measured by protein-bound iodine (PBI), T4 levels (by column or by radioimmunoassay) or T3 levels by radioimmunoassay. T3 resin uptake is decreased, reflecting the elevated TBG. Free T4 and free T3 concentrations are unaltered.

Other binding proteins may be elevated in serum, i.e., corticosteroid binding globulin (CBG), sex hormone-binding globulin (SHBG), leading to increased circulating corticosteroids and sex steroids respectively. Free or biologically active hormone concentrations are unchanged. Other plasma proteins may be increased (angiotensinogen/renin substrate, alpha-1-antitrypsin, ceruloplasmin).

Increased plasma HDL and HDL-2 subfraction concentrations, reduced LDL cholesterol concentration, increased triglycerides levels.

Impaired glucose tolerance.

Reduced response to metyrapone test.

Reduced serum folate concentration.

Carcinogenesis, Mutagenesis, Impairment of Fertility:

Long term continuous administration of natural and synthetic estrogens in certain animal species increases the frequency of carcinomas of the breast, uterus, cervix, vagina, testis, and liver. See **CONTRAINDICATIONS** and **WARNINGS.**

Pregnancy:

Teratogenic Effects: Pregnancy Category X: Estrogens should not be used during pregnancy. See **CONTRAINDICATIONS** and Boxed **WARNINGS**.

Nursing Mothers:

As a general principle, the administration of any drug to nursing mothers should be done only when clearly necessary since many drugs are excreted in human milk. In addition, estrogen administration to nursing mothers has been shown to decrease the quantity and quality of the milk.

ADVERSE REACTIONS:

The following additional adverse reactions have been reported with estrogen therapy: (see **WARNINGS** regarding induction of neoplasia, adverse effects on the fetus, increased incidence of gallbladder disease, cardiovascular disease, elevated blood pressure, and hypercalcemia.)

Genitourinary System:

Changes in vaginal bleeding pattern and abnormal withdrawal bleeding or flow; breakthrough bleeding, spotting.

Increase in size of uterine leiomyomata.

Vaginal candidiasis.

Change in amount of cervical secretion.

Breasts:

Tenderness, enlargement.

Gastrointestinal:

Nausea, vomiting.

Abdominal cramps, bloating.

Cholestatic jaundice.

Figure 3-1 Typical drug insert showing a warning box (Reprinted with permission of Barr Laboratories, Inc., Pomona, NY).

TABLE 3-1   *Reading a Package Insert*

ITEM	MEANING
Drug form	Tablet, syrup, elixir, etc.
Drug trade name® (capitalized first letter)	Manufacturer's registered name for the drug
Drug generic name (lowercase first letter and in parentheses)	USP/NF official name
Chemical description and structural formula	Indicates chemical compound found in the drug
Clinical pharmacology	Purpose of the drug and expected effects on the body
Indications and usage	Therapeutic actions of the drug, conditions or disease processes for drug use
Contraindications	Conditions in which the drug should not be used
Warnings	General risks when taking the drug; include drug interactions, potential toxic effects, and possible diseases/conditions that might be potentiated
	Black box indicates possible life-threatening interactions
Precautions	Reasons to adjust dosage or to discontinue use of drug, and pregnancy category
Adverse reactions	Compilation of possible reactions to the drug
Drug abuse and dependence	Information present only for drugs with the potential for abuse or dependence
	DEA scheduled drug; if no "C," not scheduled
Overdosage	Effects and treatment of overdosage
Dosage and administration	Usual dosage and route of administration of drug
How supplied	Dosage of drug, description of its forms, and how they are supplied, with the NDC number for each supply source; how to store; also shows the marking on the drug for identification
Drug company	Name, address, and logo of the drug manufacturer
Date of package insert	Information on when insert was written or last revised

DEA, Drug Enforcement Administration; NDC, National Drug Classification; USP/NF, United States Pharmacopoeia/National Formulary.

on package inserts for the major products of manufacturers. The section is alphabetized by manufacturer and then by product.

- Section VI (white), Diagnostic Product Information: This section includes an alphabetic listing of many of the diagnostic test medications and products used in hospitals and physicians' offices.
- Section VII (white), Miscellaneous: This section assembles miscellaneous information including the following:
  - Key to controlled substances categories
  - Key to FDA use-in-pregnancy ratings
  - List of poison control centers
  - FDA telephone directory
  - Drug information centers
  - Look-alike, sound-alike drug names
  - Adverse event report forms

Elsevier publishes *GenRx,* a comprehensive compilation of drug information with drug product identification charts. It includes drug costs and comparisons among various similar medications and provides the equivalence of similar medications. *GenRx* is published annually. A companion volume for use by the general public is available.

Pharmacists use *Drug Facts and Comparisons,* a loose-leaf binder source for comparison of medications that is updated monthly. It contains information that allows for comparison and evaluation of medications. The manufacturer, the form of packaging, and comparison tables of medications are included along with a section on orphan drugs, diagnostic aids, and drugs in developmental stages that makes these easily found for comparisons and new uses.

Other references include books and electronic drug information sources such as Micromedix, Lexi-Comp Drug Information Handbook, and Lexi-Comp Pediatric Drug Information Handbook. Manufacturers also include information on their websites concerning the drugs they manufacture. Using such reliable medication sites as Rxlist.com and Drug Info Base will provide rapid information for the Internet user.

Pharmacists are another professional source of information on drugs. They keep current on medications and have access to the package inserts found on each bottle of medication. With each prescription, pharmacists give patients drug information sheets about their new or refilled prescriptions (Figure 3-2).

Allied health professionals should make drug cards for the medications used in their employment setting. It is vital that anyone giving medications

Rx/pharmacy®
505 South Bell St
Holly, GA
00111-0000

#44 Ph:001-555-4444
www.Rx.com

05-23-2007
Prscbr: Lawrence, Merry
Refills: 12

PATIENT PRESCRIPTION INFORMATION
IF YOU HAVE ANY QUESTIONS ABOUT YOUR
MEDICATION, PLEASE CONTACT YOUR PHARMACIST:
Foster, Richard

For faster refills, phone in 24 hours in advance

Keep Out of Reach of Children

Rx Item#
000000

ZETIA 10 MG TABLET M/S
MERCK/SCHERING
TAKE 1 TABLET BY MOUTH EVERY DAY

This is a WHITE, OBLONG-shaped, TABLET imprinted with 414 on the front.
EZETIMIBE · ORAL (eh-ZET-ih-mibe)

COMMON BRAND NAME(S): Zetia

USES: This medication is used either alone or with other drugs (e.g., HMG-CoA reductase inhibitors or "statins"), along with a low cholesterol/low fat diet, to help lower cholesterol in the blood. Reducing cholesterol helps prevent strokes and heart attacks. Ezetimibe works by reducing the amount of cholesterol your body absorbs from your diet.

HOW TO USE: Read the Patient Information Leaflet provided by your pharmacist before you start taking this medication and each time you get a refill. If you have any questions regarding the information, consult your doctor or pharmacist. Take this medication by mouth usually once daily with or without food. If you are also taking a bile acid sequestrant (e.g., cholestyramine, colestipol), take ezetimibe at least 2 hours before or at least 4 hours after the bile acid sequestrant. It may take up to 2 weeks before the full benefit of this drug takes effect. Use this medication regularly in order to get the most benefit from it. Remember to use it at the same time each day. It is important to continue taking this medication even if you feel well. Most people with high cholesterol do not feel sick.

SIDE EFFECTS: Dizziness, headache, diarrhea, back pain may occur. If any of these effects persist or worsen, notify your doctor or pharmacist promptly. Remember that your doctor has prescribed this medication because the benefit to you is greater than the risk of side effects. Many people using this medication do not have serious side effects. Tell your doctor immediately if any of these serious side effects occur: chest pain, fatigue, stomach pain. This drug can very rarely cause muscle damage. Tell your doctor immediately if you experience the following: muscle pain/tenderness/weakness (especially with fever or unusual tiredness). A serious allergic reaction to this drug is unlikely, but seek immediate medical attention if it occurs. Symptoms of a serious allergic reaction include: rash, itching, swelling, dizziness, trouble breathing. If you notice other effects not listed above, contact your doctor or pharmacist.

PRECAUTIONS: Before taking ezetimibe, tell your doctor or pharmacist if you are allergic to it; or if you have any other allergies. This medication should not be used along with a statin agent if you have certain medical conditions. Before using this medicine, consult your doctor or pharmacist if you have: active liver disease. Before using this medication, tell your doctor or pharmacist your medical history, especially of: liver disease (moderate to severe). This medication should be used only when clearly needed during pregnancy. Discuss the risks and benefits with your doctor. It is not known whether this drug passes into breast milk. Consult your doctor before breast-feeding.

DRUG INTERACTIONS: Your doctor or pharmacist may already be aware of any possible drug interactions and may be monitoring you for them. Do not start, stop, or change the dosage of any medicine before checking with them first. Before using this medication, tell your doctor or pharmacist of all prescription and nonprescription products you may use, especially of: "blood thinners" (e.g., warfarin), cyclosporine, fibrates (e.g., fenofibrate, gemfibrozil).

OVERDOSE: If overdose is suspected, contact your local poison control center or emergency room immediately. US residents can call the US national poison hotline at 1-800-222-1222. Canadian residents should call their local poison control center directly.

NOTES: Do not share this medication with others. Laboratory and/or medical tests (e.g., cholesterol levels) should be performed periodically to monitor your progress. When ezetimibe is given with a statin agent, liver function tests should be performed to monitor for side effects. Consult your doctor for more details. For best results, this medication should be used along with exercise and a low cholesterol/low fat diet. Consult your doctor.

MISSED DOSE: If you miss a dose, use it as soon as you remember. If it is near the time of the next dose, skip the missed dose and resume your usual dosing schedule. Do not double the dose to catch up.

STORAGE: Store at room temperature at 77 degrees F (25 degrees C) away from light and moisture. Brief storage from 59-86 degrees F (15-30 degrees C) is permitted. Do not store in the bathroom. Keep all medicines away from children and pets. Properly discard this product when it is expired or no longer needed. Consult your pharmacist or local waste disposal company for more details about how to safely discard your product.

Information last revised April 2007
Copyright(c) 2007 First DataBank, Inc.

IMPORTANT DISCLAIMER: The side effects listed above are not all of the possible risks that could be caused by this medication. For further information, please consult with your physician about the uses, precautions and risks of the medication specific to your health. This information is obtained from First DataBank for use as an educational aid.

Figure 3-2 Drug information sheet.

be knowledgeable about the drugs routinely being administered. Trade and generic names, as well as usual dosage, should be included, along with side effects and adverse reactions. These drug cards should be readily available for answering questions prior to the administration of medications. New drug cards should be prepared as new medications are introduced for clinical use.

Drug handbooks and textbooks with information on medications are available at different levels of detail. Because information in books may not be completely current, journal articles and news releases should be read to update the information. With the numerous journal articles posted on Internet sites, health professionals should be able to keep current without difficulty. Because some of the material that passes for information on Internet sites is not accurate, health professionals should be selective in the sites they review. Good sites are those associated with medical, nursing, and pharmacy schools, as well as the FDA, National Institutes of Health, American Heart Association, and similar associations making specialized and accurate information from manufacturers and government agencies only a click away.

Knowing all there is to know about drugs on the market is impossible, but the health care professional must know how and where to obtain the necessary information to ensure patient safety and compliance with medications. No single source can always provide all of the information needed.

IMPORTANT FACTS

- Drug references including drug package inserts, the USP/NF, the PDR, drug handbooks, and drug cards are important to ensure proper administration of medications and safety in drug usage.
- The allied health professional should be knowledgeable about all medications that he or she might administer.

Drug Forms and Drug Delivery Systems

Drugs come in many dosage forms. These forms differ in their rate of action, site of action, and amount of medication delivered at the site of action. The dosage forms may be a solid, semisolid, liquid, or gas. The route of delivery influences the efficiency and action of the drug. The drug may be given orally, or through the GI tract; parenterally, or through routes outside the enteral route (although this route is usually considered to be by injection); or percutaneously, by medications applied to the skin or mucous membranes (including instillations).

Oral Medications

The oral route, in which the medication is taken by mouth and swallowed, is the simplest way to administer medications because it is usually more convenient, economical, and safer than other routes. A drug taken by mouth is subject to the actions of the GI tract and may be affected by variations in peristalsis, gastric secretions, and other GI functions. Vomiting and diarrhea may alter medication availability for absorption and may even be reason to avoid the oral route for drug administration. The disadvantage of the oral route is that drugs administered orally are absorbed slowly and at an unpredictable rate because of patient-to-patient differences in gastric function. Some drugs, such as insulin, are destroyed by digestive fluids and must be administered by other routes.

Oral drug forms include solids, liquids, powders, and other miscellaneous forms. The terms *tablet* and *capsule* have replaced the term *pill* (a globular mass compounded by a pharmacist), and this term should not be used in medicine today.

Solid Oral Preparations

Tablets (Box 3-1) are dried powder forms of medication that have been compressed into a small disk or solid mass that come in many shapes, colors, and sizes (Table 3-2). In addition to active ingredients, tablets contain binders (adhesives to hold the substances together), disintegrators (substances that encourage dissolving in the body), lubricants (to give the tablet a sheen for ease in swallowing and to assist with the manufacturing process), and fillers (inert ingredients that make the tablet a convenient size). Some oral medications can be mixed with food to give the drug a more acceptable taste, whereas others must be taken on an empty stomach. The medication should never be mixed in a whole serving of food because the person may not eat all of it.

Capsules are cylindrical gelatin containers made of two pieces that fit together (Table 3-3

BOX 3-1   IMPORTANT FACTS ABOUT ADMINISTRATION OF TABLETS

1. Drugs that may discolor teeth should not be given orally. Oral iron preparations for children are given by dropper or straw to prevent staining of the teeth.
2. Oral medications should not be given to someone who is unconscious, vomiting, or unable to swallow.
3. Enteric-coated tablets should be swallowed whole, not crushed or chewed, because the desired place of absorption is in the intestines.
4. Sustained-release tablets should not be crushed because crushing changes the absorption rate of the drug and may result in an overdose.
5. Patients should not swallow or chew buccal or sublingual tablets, nor should the tablets be taken with water because water would dissolve the tablet too rapidly and prevent the desired absorption.
6. Oral dissolving tablets should be allowed to dissolve in the mouth and should not be swallowed whole. The mouth must have sufficient moisture to allow the tablet to disintegrate.

---

and Box 3-2). This form is a convenient way of giving medications with an unpleasant odor or taste. Capsules usually contain powder, granules, or a combination of the two and may have one or more active ingredients. In most cases the capsule also contains an inert filler substance and does not need flavorings because the medications are enclosed.

CLINICAL TIP
Except for sustained-release capsules, capsules may be pulled apart and the entire contents added as powder to foods for patients who have difficulty swallowing.

Troches or **lozenges** are hard medications in a candy or fruit base that are designed to dissolve in the mouth for local effect. Examples of lozenges are cough drops or lozenges for the relief of a sore throat.

Liquid Oral Preparations

Liquid oral preparations consist of one or more active ingredients placed in a liquid medium. **Gelcaps,** a cross between liquid medications and capsules, are soft gelatin shells made in one piece and filled with a liquid form of medication. Gelcaps should not be chewed because the gelatin shell is provided when the medication has an unpleasant taste. With some medications, the drugs may be squeezed into the oral cavity for patients who

TABLE 3-2 *Solid Oral Preparations—Tablets*

FORM	DESCRIPTION	EXAMPLE
Unscored tablet	Tablets that are intended to be swallowed whole	aspirin
Scored tablet	Tablets with indentions cut into the tablet to allow for partial doses by breaking the tablet on the line	furosemide (Lasix)
Enteric coated	Tablets that have a special coating so that the drug dissolves in the intestines rather than the stomach; may be coated with sugar for taste enhancement or with film-coating for ease of swallowing	enteric coated aspirin (Ecotrin)
Chewable tablets	Medications in a flavored or sugar base that are designed to be chewed	antacids (Tums), chewable vitamins
Sublingual tablets	Tablets designed to dissolve under the tongue for short-term release of medication	nitroglycerin
Buccal tablets	Tablets placed between the cheek and the gum to dissolve and be absorbed through the buccal membrane for short-term release of medication	nitroglycerin
Buffered tablets	Tablets with antacids added to the active ingredients to prevent irritation of the stomach and gastrointestinal tract	aspirin (Bufferin)
Sustained-release (controlled-release) tablets	Tablets that are layered to allow incompatible active ingredients to be given in one medication for release in stages over a period of time	chlorpheniramine/phenylpropanolamine (Allerest 12 Hour)
Caplets	Tablets in the shape of a capsule for ease of swallowing	acetaminophen (Tylenol)
Oral dissolving tablets	Tablets designed to dissolve in the mouth	desloratadine (Clarinex) soluble tablets

TABLE 3-3 *Solid Oral Preparations—Capsules*

FORM	DESCRIPTION	EXAMPLE
Capsules	Gelatinous containers that hold powdered medications	amoxicillin (Amoxil)
Sustained-release capsules	Capsules designed to deliver medications over a particular period of time	phenylpropanolamine/chlorpheniramine (Ornade Spansule)
Delayed-release capsules	Capsules prepared to release drugs at a particular site; some of these medications contain beads that are designed for release at different times or at a particular site to meet the metabolism of the body; these capsules provide a steady flow of medications over a period of time	theophylline (Theo-24)

have difficulty swallowing gelcaps; however, this should only be done on the advice of a physician because the exact amount of medication delivered may change. The patient's mouth needs to be moist for the patient to be able to swallow a gelcap, or the gelcap will adhere to the dry mucous membranes of the mouth.

BOX 3-2	IMPORTANT FACTS ABOUT ADMINISTERING CAPSULES

Timed-release products should never be opened; they should be swallowed whole because opening the capsule will alter the absorption rate and could result in an overdose of the medication.

TABLE 3-4 *Liquid Oral Medications—Solutions*

FORM AND BASE	DESCRIPTION	EXAMPLE
Syrups/aqueous (water-based)	Solutions that are sweetened with sugar or sugar substitute to disguise the medicinal taste; also contain flavorings, color, and aromatic agents	guaifenesin (Robitussin)
Elixirs (alcohol and water)	Sweetened, flavored medications that contain alcohol and water to improve solubility; if the solution is mainly water, the sweetener is natural sugar; if the solution is mainly alcohol, the sweetener is artificial	diphenhydramine (Benadryl)
Extracts and fluid extracts (water or alcohol, or both)	Highly concentrated preparations that move desired materials into a solution and then evaporate to leave a syrup, mass, solid, ointment-like substance, or dry powder; fluid extracts are from plant sources that are used in syrups; extracts are used in compounding medications.	vanilla extract, peppermint extract
Tinctures (alcohol or hydroalcohols)	Pure chemicals or extracts from plants that are potent medications	camphorated tincture of opium (Paregoric)
Spirits (alcohol or hydroalcohols)	Solution containing volatile aromatic ingredients that may be diluted with water prior to administration; aromatic spirits containing oils and other substances are easily released into the air to provide a pleasant smell and are therefore used in vaporizers and humidifiers	spirits of ammonia, peppermint spirit

Other oral liquids are divided into two major categories—solutions and dispersions. **Solutions** (Table 3-4 and Box 3-3) are medications in which the active ingredient has been dissolved in a liquid vehicle. In **dispersions,** the medication is not dissolved in a liquid but instead is distributed as particles throughout the liquid. Dispersions (Table 3-5 and Box 3-4) are classified by the size of the particles. The most common dispersion is a suspension.

Miscellaneous Oral Medications

Miscellaneous oral products include powders that contain finely ground particles or **granules,** which are larger and of irregular shape. Granules are better suited than powders for use in solutions because powders tend to float on the surface of a liquid. Laxative granules are used to relieve constipation; an example is Metamucil. **Effervescent powders** are coarsely ground medicinal agents that have been mixed with an effervescent salt that releases carbon dioxide when mixed with

| BOX 3-3 | IMPORTANT FACTS ABOUT SOLUTIONS |

1. If syrups are added to juice or milk, the person must drink the entire amount to receive the total dose. Be careful in using milk, because the medication may change the flavor of the milk and a child might refuse to drink it. Also, milk may change the property of the drug.
2. Because of the high sugar content of elixirs, care should be taken when used with people with diabetes. Because of the alcohol content, persons who are alcohol dependent should not take these medications, especially patients taking disulfiram (Antabuse).
3. Elixirs may have to be diluted for children. The medication should be diluted one dose at a time, because adding water to the entire bottle may cause the active ingredients to precipitate, or settle out of the solution.
4. Paregoric should always be diluted prior to administration.

water or another liquid. They typically give off a bubbling action. Examples are analgesics, such as B-C Powders or Alka Seltzer, and effervescent antacids or laxatives.

TABLE 3-5 *Liquid Oral Medications—Dispersions*

FORM	DESCRIPTION	EXAMPLE
Dispersion	Large, undissolved particles of medication are mixed with, but not dissolved in, a solvent; most are suspensions require reconstitution using purified or distilled water	amoxicillin suspension (Amoxil Oral Suspension)
Emulsion	A water-in-oil mixture in which one liquid is dispersed in another; the liquids do not mix readily	Fat emulsion used in total parenteral nutrition; whole milk with cream, oil in vinegar
Gel	A semisolid jelly-like product containing a large amount of water; thick viscous liquid that easily penetrates without a residue	Orajel
Magma	Viscous suspensions of medications that contain ultrafine particles blended in liquid	milk of magnesia, aluminum hydroxide (Aludrox)

BOX 3-4   IMPORTANT FACTS ABOUT DISPERSIONS

1. A suspension settles slowly but may be redispersed by shaking prior to pouring. A suspension should always be shaken prior to administration. If a suspension is not shaken, the active ingredient will settle to the bottom of the container and will not be administered.
2. After a suspension is reconstituted, it has a short shelf-life (usually 7 to 14 days) at room temperature. Some must be under refrigeration for a 14-day shelf-life. The label will specify whether the medication should be refrigerated and will indicate the shelf-life.
3. Because a residue is expected on the spoon, medicine cup, or other means used to administer the suspension, the container for the dose should be cleaned between doses to ensure that the proper dosage is given with each dose.
4. Emulsions to be taken orally may be diluted with water just prior to administration. Shaking well ensures that the medications are mixed just prior to dispensing.

CLINICAL TIP

- Eardrops should be warmed to body temperature to prevent vertigo (dizziness). Holding the bottle in the hand for a few minutes will do this.
- When otic preparations are applied, the head should be tilted away from the affected side to prevent drainage of the medication from the ear.
- Shake ear medication in a suspension for 10 seconds to place the active ingredient back into the suspension.

Percutaneous Medications

Percutaneous or topical medications (Table 3-6 and Box 3-5) are those applied to the skin and mucous membranes for local effect. Many are OTC drugs that are not absorbed systemically, but some preparations are absorbed into the bloodstream from the topical application. **Topical** refers to the application of medications directly to any body surface. **Transdermal** refers to absorption of a drug through the skin from a patch impregnated with a medication (Figures 3-3 to 3-5).

DID YOU KNOW?

Transdermal patches were used by astronauts on the space shuttle to prevent nausea. Patches have found a growing market that is expected to increase in the future for the treatment of such conditions as angina, smoking cessation, chronic pain, and estrogen replacement therapy and to perform allergy testing.

Parenteral Medications

Parenteral medications are those given by injection. Liquid preparations for injection must be sterile solutions or sterile reconstituted powders. They are stored in **vials, ampules,** or **premeasured cartridges** for ease of administration (Figure 3-6). All of these systems are small glass or plastic containers that hold drugs in powder or liquid form. If the drug is in powder form, it must be mixed with a sterile liquid, or **reconstituted,** before administration. Some drugs are unstable as liquids and are packaged in powder form to provide a longer shelf-life. After reconstitution, these medications have a limited shelf-life.

Water-Based Parenteral Medications

Sterile normal (isotonic) saline, a water-based solution of salt in water with approximately the same concentration as is normally found in body tissue, is used to reconstitute or dilute drugs for injection. It is also used to replace lost body fluids when given intravenously. Sterile distilled water is used similarly to saline but tends to be more irritating because it is not isotonic with the body fluids. In solutions in which the drug precipitates (settles

TABLE 3-6 *Percutaneous Medications*

FORM	DESCRIPTION	EXAMPLE
Liniments	Drugs containing oil, soap, water, or alcohol that are applied to the skin to produce heat for relief of muscular aches and pains	Ben-Gay
Colloids	A gluelike suspension or solution that contains particles dispersed in a solvent such as water, volatile ether, or alcohol and leaves a residue on the skin	Suspension—Aveeno oleated oatmeal bath; solution—Compound W and flexible collodion
Tinctures	Alcohol-based liquids that evaporate to disinfect the skin	Tincture of iodine
Lotions	Free-flowing liquids or suspended ingredients in water	Hand lotions, calamine lotion for itching
Creams	Semisolid preparations in a water base that are absorbed into the tissues for slow, sustained release of the drug	Bactroban cream (antiinfective) and corticosteroid cream; Solarcaine
Ointments (see Figure 3-3)	Semisolid greasy preparations in an oil base that are not absorbed into the skin; prevent adherence of bandages to the skin	Triple antibiotic ointment; Solarcaine; eye preparations
Pastes	Semisolid preparations that are stiffer than ointments because they contain more solid materials and apply more thickly	Toothpaste
Gels	Semisolid preparation with a high proportion of water with a drug plus a thickening agent; used to reduce friction and to provide lubrication	Antiseptic, antifungal, and contraceptive gels and lubricants; topical anesthetics
Plasters	Solid or semisolid medicated or nonmedicated preparations that adhere to the body by means of a backing	Salicylic acid spots for removal of corns or warts
Aerosol foams	A water-in-oil emulsion that disperses as a spray and slows vaporization in the air	Vaginal preparations, hair products
Transdermal patches and disks (see Figure 3-4)	Drug-containing reservoirs of medication that are applied to the skin for absorption of medication through the skin	Nicotine patches, fentanyl patches; estrogen patches for menopause and contraception
Suppositories (see Figure 3-5)	Medication placed in a base of cocoa butter, hydrogenated vegetable oil, or glycerinated gelatin to form a solid dosage for insertion into a body orifice; some have local action, whereas others have systemic action	Glycerin suppositories, vaginal suppositories
Sprays	Emit a fine dispersion of liquids, solids, or gaseous materials	
	Nasal—solutions designed for both local and systemic effects in alcohol or water pump-type dispenser	decongestants, fluticasone (Flonase)
	Translingual—used under the tongue	nitroglycerin
	Topical—applied to skin	Hormones to treat postmenopausal symptoms, sunscreens
Aerosols	Liquid in a pressurized can that releases a fine mist or a coarse liquid spray	Primatene mist aerosol
Metered dose inhalers	Fine mist of medications that are breath activated and are delivered into the respiratory tract to treat airway diseases	Albuterol MDI
Nebulizer	Small micronized powders, as well as liquids that deliver medications into a reservoir for inhalation into the respiratory tract	levalbuterol (Xopenex), albuterol (Ventolin), Advair Diskus
Ophthalmic/otic solutions and suspensions	Sterile solutions or suspensions for use in the eye and solutions or suspensions for use in the ear that are inserted using a dropper	Ophthalmic—Ocu-Sol, Vasocon-A Otic—Cortisporin
Ocular inserts	Small, transparent membranes containing medications that are placed between the eye and the lower conjunctiva; the medication is slowly released	pilocarpine (Ocusert)

BOX 3-5   IMPORTANT FACTS ABOUT PERCUTANEOUS MEDICATIONS

1. Liniments should not be used with heating pads or external heat because the patient may be burned by the combination.
2. The drug molecules in the transdermal patches and disks are present in different sizes and shapes for absorption through the skin over various time periods. The drug flow persists over a longer period of time and provides a more constant blood level than the up-and-down level found with oral and parenteral medications. Transdermal medications may be absorbed over days or hours.
3. The patch consists of a backing, a drug reservoir, a protective strip, and an adhesive layer. The drug moves by osmosis through the patch's controlled membranes to the skin for systemic absorption. In some patches the absorption rate is controlled by the size of the openings in the membrane; in others, control comes from the skin itself. Body temperature and climate affect the absorption rate. On a hot, sunny day, the skin's pores are open wider, which promotes faster absorption, whereas cold temperatures may slow the rate at which the medication enters the body.
4. Sites of application for patches or disks should be rotated with each application to ensure proper absorption and to prevent damage to the skin and blood vessels over a period of time.
5. Patches should be wrapped prior to disposal to prevent an accidental overdose by a child or pet that may come into contact with the discarded patch.
6. The person applying the patch should wear gloves or wash hands immediately after application to avoid unintended absorption of the medication while applying the patch.
7. Vaginal, rectal, and urethral suppositories are made to melt at body temperature for release of the medication and come in a variety of shapes, depending on the site of administration and the age and sex of the patient.
8. Because of the large number of blood vessels in the rectum, suppositories are often used in comatose patients or those with nausea and vomiting. Suppositories with a local effect in the rectum are used to stimulate defecation. Vaginal suppositories are used as antiinfectants and contraceptives.
9. If a suppository is wrapped, the patient should be educated to remove the outer wrapper prior to administration.
10. Handling of suppositories should be kept to a minimum to prevent melting prior to insertion into the body opening.
11. Suppositories may have to be stored in a refrigerator during warm weather so that the medication remains solid for insertion.
12. Inhalants are being increasingly used to treat systemic conditions, as well as for their local effects. Drugs such as penicillin are now in clinical trials for this manner of administration.
13. Ocular inserts are much like transdermal patches in that the medication is slowly released through the membrane of the eye over a period of time.
14. Placing pressure on the inner canthus of the eye for a few minutes after instilling eye drops can diminish the systemic absorption of eye preparations. This pressure blocks the ducts and reduces drainage of the medication.
15. Ophthalmic preparations must remain sterile and should be used by only one person. Care should be taken not to touch the body surfaces with the applicator's tip.
16. An ophthalmic preparation may be used in the ear in an emergency situation, but an otic preparation may never be used in the eye. The sterility of an ophthalmic preparation may be necessary with tubes inserted into the eardrum. The physician should prescribe when an ophthalmic preparation can be used in the ear.
17. Sports creams should be used only as recommended by the manufacturer. Overuse may lead to severe toxic effects, even death, as the active ingredient (salicylates) will be systemically absorbed.

out) of the solution, the solutions must be shaken until no sediment is seen.

CLINICAL TIP

When reconstituting powders or crystals in multidose vials, the health care professional should be sure to record the date and time of reconstitution and initial the entry.

Oil-Based Parenteral Medications

Some parenteral medications come in an oil base, which provides slow release and prolongs the absorption time and duration of action. Because of the oily nature of the medication, these drugs are thick, or viscous, in appearance and are given by IM injection for less irritation of body tissue. Oil bases are used for many of the hormones that are used in hormone replacement therapy and for the treatment of certain cancers.

Injectable Parenteral Suspension

Injectable suspensions such as insulin are small, undissolved particles in a liquid base. These suspensions need to be rotated by hand, not shaken, prior to administration to ensure the redistribution of the particles. As with all suspensions, the drug settles slowly but can be redispersed by gentle shaking or by rotating the container between the hands.

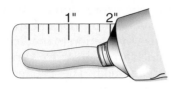

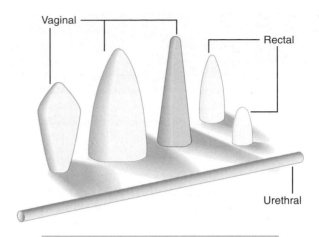

Figure 3-5 Typical shapes of suppositories.

Figure 3-3 Paper for measuring transdermal nitroglycerin ointment.

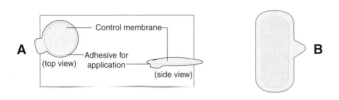

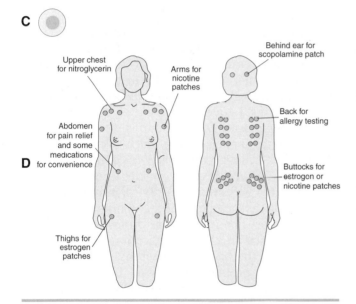

Figure 3-4 Transdermal applications of medications. **A,** Side view of a transdermal patch. **B,** Transdermal patch. **C,** Transdermal spot. **D,** Sites for transdermal medical applications and the medications typical for each site.

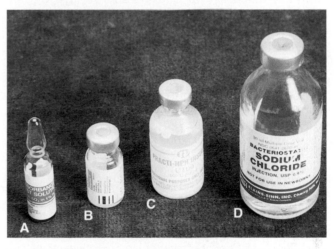

Figure 3-6 Typical containers for injectable medications. **A,** Ampule. **B,** Single-dose vial. **C** and **D,** Multidose vials.

Other Forms of Medications

Implants or **pellets** are dosage forms that are placed intradermally, or under the skin, by means of minor surgery or special injections. This drug form is used for the long-term, controlled release of medications, especially hormones. Radioactive isotopes, used in the treatment of cancer, may also be administered in the form of implants. **Tampons** are drug-impregnated packs, pads, or plugs made of cotton or sponge that are inserted for release of medication. **Douches** are water-based solutions used to irrigate any part of the body—topically, otically, ophthalmically, intracavitarily—or to cleanse surgical wounds. Many vaginal douches are available OTC. **Medicated enemas** may be ordered to administer a medication either locally or systemically. The medication is suspended in a solution for administration in the rectum and is often used with patients in whom oral consumption is restricted or who cannot swallow. Oil-retention enemas to soften feces are another type of medicated enema.

Packaging Medications for Patient Compliance

Some medications are packaged for easy use and compliance such as the compacts used for oral contraceptives. The medication container is designed to remind the user to take the medication daily.

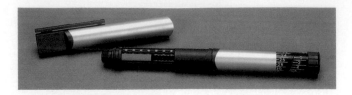

Figure 3-7 Pen for administration of insulin.

Automatic insulin delivery systems are a new system for administering insulin for easy compliance. An example is the Novolin Pen, by Squibb-Nova, which delivers either regular insulin, NPH insulin, or the combination Novolin 70/30, which is 70% NPH insulin and 30% regular insulin. (Types of insulin are discussed in Chapter 21.) A cartridge of insulin is attached to the pen and remains attached throughout the use of the container. The pen is disposed of along with the cartridge when it is empty. This method of administration has a mechanism for presetting the dose of insulin to reduce errors in dosage and contamination. This is especially helpful for patients with visual problems or arthritis (Figure 3-7).

IMPORTANT FACTS

- Drugs come in solids and liquids and are administered orally, parenterally, and topically.
- The rate of absorption of medications varies with the form and route of administration. Solid medications must be dissolved prior to absorption. Liquid medications given parenterally are absorbed faster. Inhalation and translingual sprays have fast absorption. Topical medications tend to have a longer absorption time but also a longer time of action.
- Topical medications can have systemic, as well as local effects, although most are applied for local action.
- Some medications are packaged for compliance, such as compacts for oral contraceptives and Novolin pens for insulin administration.
- Drug forms must be adjusted to a patient's lifestyle and physical condition.

Summary

Drugs are classified in several complex ways. In this book drugs are grouped by their effects on body systems, and icons are used to indicate the body systems where the drug has its usual effect.

The allied health professional should acquire general knowledge of drug classifications and their indications for use in relation to medical diagnoses.

Drug nomenclature refers to various ways in which drugs are named. The chemical name describes the chemicals involved in the production of the drug. For the allied health professional, the generic, or official, name and the trade name are the important names to know. When a new drug is proposed to the FDA, the manufacturer assigns it a trade name and has the right to sole production of the drug for 20 years after the beginning of clinical trials. Thereafter other companies may manufacture the drug and use either the generic name or a trade name of their own devising for the same compound. Other terms applied to medications are *over-the-counter*, *legend*, and *controlled substances*. The allied health professional *must* learn the drugs that are used routinely in the medical office of employment.

With so many medications used today, various drug references are used by health care workers, depending on their specialty, to distinguish among drugs and ensure accurate administration. The USF/NF is the official government source used to ensure that the drug meets FDA regulations. The drug inserts supplied with all marketed products are an excellent source of information on all aspects of the drug. The *Physician's Desk Reference* provides a compilation of drug inserts, with many cross-reference abilities. Other resources include *GenRx* and drug handbooks. Drug cards provide health care professionals with a quick reference on all the medications routinely administered in the health care setting. This helps ensure that the proper checks and balances are in place for accurate drug administration.

Medications come in many forms. Solid drugs, given orally or topically, come in tablet, capsule, and powder form. Liquids may be in a water base or in other bases such as alcohol. Liquids may be given either orally (enterally), by injection (parenterally), or topically (percutaneously). The health care professional should know the drug forms and how they affect administration techniques. Disease conditions of the patient such as alcoholism or diabetes mellitus are important factors in deciding the form of medication to use. More often the form of medication administered relies on the ability of the patient to take oral medications such as those with nausea and vomiting or children and older adults who require a liquid because of the inability to swallow solid drugs. When a severe illness occurs, oral medications may not be appropriate and intravenous medications may be administered because of the rapidity of medication absorption. Patient compliance may also be considered when the medication needs sustained periods of time for administration. Sustained release or transdermal patches may be used because daily administration is not necessary. Finally, topical preparations may be used when only local effects are required.

Before administering medications or performing patient education about prescribed medications, the allied health professional should be aware that many factors affect the choice of medication and should be sure that contraindications are discussed with the physician or patient as necessary.

Critical Thinking Exercises

SCENARIO

Mrs. Smith, 75, has difficulty swallowing an enteric-coated tablet. While you are taking Mrs. Smith's history, her daughter tells you that she has been crushing this tablet and mixing it with her food. The daughter is concerned that her mother may not be receiving all the medicine, as the food now tastes bitter (from the medication) and she may not be eating all of it.

1. What is your response to the daughter?
2. Is it safe to crush an enteric-coated tablet?

REVIEW QUESTIONS

1. What is the placebo effect? Does it work with all patients? What is necessary for a placebo to be effective? _____

2. Explain why oral medications are absorbed slower than injectables. Why are sublingual medications faster acting than swallowed oral medications? _____

3. What are the advantages of injectable medications when rapid action is desired? What are the dangers of giving medications by injection? Why do drugs take longer to be absorbed after oral administration? _____

4. If you wanted to find a medication for smoking cessation, in what part of the PDR would you look? A manufacturer's address? Identification of a medication brought to the office but not found in the medical record? A trade name for a generic drug? The telephone number of the local poison control center? _____

5. Why are oral medications more often prescribed? _____

6. What is meant by using a medication "off label"? _____

7. What is the difference between liquids that are solutions and those that are dispersions? What are the implications of each for the allied health professional? _____

8. What is the base of a cream? An ointment? Which would you suggest to keep a dressing from sticking to a wound? Which would you suggest if you wanted the medication to be absorbed into the skin?

CHAPTER 4

Understanding Drug Dosages for Special Populations

OBJECTIVES

After studying this chapter, you should be capable of doing the following:

- Discussing the variables that affect the dosages of medications.
- Providing general patient education about contraindications and precautions for medication use.
- Identifying populations in whom special understanding of medication administration may be required such as pregnant and lactating women, the elderly, and children.
- Identifying medication indications, dosage, and special precautions or contraindications with elderly, children, and pregnant or lactating women.
- Providing essential information about medications to promote patient compliance.

Mary, a-29-year old, has come to the gynecology office in November thinking that she may be 6 weeks' pregnant for the first time. She has been waiting to have a child because of employment opportunities. When she calls for an appointment, Mary says she has been taking herbal supplements and over-the-counter (OTC) medications for headaches during the past 4 months and wants to know if it will be safe to continue. She states that she has read of the dangers of herbal supplements and pregnancy. Her other concern is that she has allergic rhinitis during the spring for which she takes OTC antihistamines. Her concern is about what medications she can take at that time and when the greatest danger of medications is during pregnancy.

What answer would be appropriate for the allied health professional to make about the taking of herbal supplements?

Why is it important for her to not take medications prior to seeing the physician if she thinks she might be pregnant?

Why would it be safer for Mary to take OTC medications for allergic rhinitis in the spring rather than during the early months of pregnancy?

What advice should the allied health professional give Mary about medications for headaches?

KEY TERMS

Biotransformation

Body surface area (BSA)

Dentition

Precaution

Teratogen

The effects of medications on the body are related to the drug dosages and the forms of medications used for administration. No one method of determining dosages will guarantee safety because individual differences in drug effects and tolerances must be taken into account, especially in children. Variables in the person such as gender, age, weight, dose, genetics, and diseases affect how the patient responds to the medication. As patients are examined by more than one physician, the chances of polypharmacy and drug interactions increase. The system of checks and balances among the physician, pharmacist, and allied health professional become more important for patient safety.

In January 1997 the U.S. Food and Drug Administration (FDA) was concerned that the lack of information made available to patients concerning the possible reactions to prescription medications was leading to improper use of drugs. The FDA appropriations bill required the pharmaceutic industry to develop a plan to provide useful consumer medication information to 95% of the people receiving prescriptions by 2006. A plan that asked for voluntary compliance by health professionals, who would provide accurate, unbiased, understandable, timely, and useful information to the patient, was designed. It was determined that by empowering patients with the knowledge of how the drug works, when to take it, why they are taking it, what results they could expect, and what the risks or side effects might be, preventable drug-related illnesses could be drastically reduced. In response to this action plan the U.S. Pharmacopeial Convention, Inc., copyrighted 81 standardized pictograms in 1997, which are graphic images that show patients how the medication is intended to be taken, as well as any warnings or precautions the patient should know. The U.S. Pharmacopeia Pictogram Library is available for use free by any health care facility and can be downloaded from this Internet site: *www.usp.org*. In order to meet the goal of providing the needed consumer information to patients, the National Council on Patient Information and Education has developed a website, *http://www.talkaboutrx.org*, to provide patients with accurate information.

Today written patient instructions are provided by the pharmacy with each prescription dispensed. These printed materials include the common uses for the medication, when the medication should not be used, how the medication should be used, what to do if a dose is missed, how to store and dispense the medication, drug and food interactions, warnings, and possible side effects. Verbal instructions should be provided to the patient in the physician's office and then should be reinforced at the pharmacy.

Of importance to allied health professionals is the liability risk if a problem occurs with the medication and information provided was either incomplete or inaccurate. Information provided to the patient in the medical office when sample medications are distributed meets the same requirements as if a pharmacist is dispensing the medication. Labeling, record keeping, and providing written information to meet the FDA requirements is necessary.

Cultural influences on how medications are taken and the interactions of medications that are not prescribed, such as OTC herbal supplements, with prescription drugs influence the way the patient takes and responds to medications. The basic cultural and ethnic beliefs may even interfere with the prescribed care placing the patient in danger. The need to gain information concerning patient compliance is a necessity with each encounter for patient safety.

Variables Affecting Drug Dosage and Actions

No two persons respond exactly alike to drugs, which is why there is no ideal drug. Even the same person may not respond in the same way to the same dose of a drug given on different occasions. Responses to medication can be influenced by several factors (Figure 4-1):

Age

Dosages considered safe for infants, children, adults, and the elderly have been established for some drugs. However, many drugs do not have dosages established for all age groups because children are rarely studied and the differing dosages for the geriatric patient have only lately become an area of interest. An individual's metabolism can affect the appropriate dosage. The very young may be more sensitive to medications because of immature organs. The elderly are more sensitive than younger adults because of organ degeneration or increased sensitivity.

Weight

Whether the person is thin, "average," or obese will have a bearing on the drug effect. What is wanted in drug therapy is a certain concentration of a drug in the body that provides therapeutic effects. Adult doses are based on an average age and body weight (usually 18 to 65 years and weighing approximately 150 lb are considered average). Therefore doses may seem to need adjustment for patients who do not fall within the "normal" weight and age, but because the therapeutic effects may be adequate, these doses may not need to be adjusted. Heavier individuals may need higher doses, and those with little body fat may need lower doses. For example, highly fat-soluble medications that act on the central nervous system, such as fentanyl, require larger initial doses for obese adults, but maintenance doses may be that for "normal" adults. The dosage may be determined on the basis of body surface area (BSA) rather than just body size for medications with a

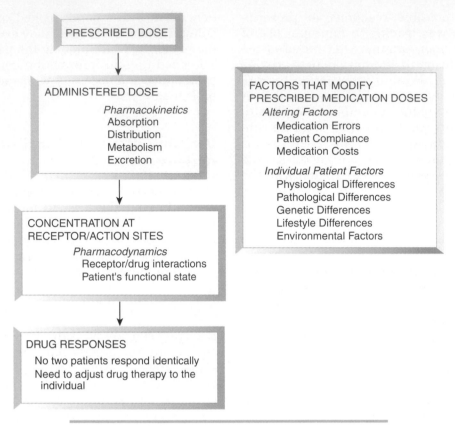

Figure 4-1 Factors that affect drug responses in the body.

high toxicity rate such as chemotherapeutics. This method accounts not only for the patient's weight but also for the relationship of weight to height (see Chapter 9).

 CLINICAL TIP

Because the correct drug dosage can vary on the basis of the weight of the patient, the allied health professional in inpatient and outpatient facilities should accurately measure weight and height, especially in children and the elderly, at each office visit.

Diet

The effects of certain drugs are altered by diet. Diets that promote health will help to elicit a therapeutic effect of a medication, whereas poor nutrition will promote adverse effects, such as the patient who eats a diet high in fat content slowing the metabolism of some drugs or the person who eats many milk products and needs to take certain antibiotics. Starvation produces a more intense response to medical therapy. Even the foods eaten in a therapeutic diet may affect the potency, availability, metabolism, absorption, and thera-

peutic effect of the medications. See Chapter 2 for drug-food interactions.

 CLINICAL TIP

The patient's diet should be investigated as part of the medical history to ascertain if dietary considerations are significant with drug selections. Diets that promote health will help elicit a therapeutic effect of a medication.

Gender

Women may react more strongly than men to some medications because of their smaller size and a higher proportion of body fat. Remember that body fat can be a reservoir for lipid-soluble medications, slowing the drug's excretion.

Genetics

The slight differences in body processes caused by genetic disposition make some people more sensitive or more resistant to certain medications. The metabolic rate of the individual, often a genetic factor, influences pharmacokinetics.

Diseases

Some diseases impair body functioning and the metabolism and excretion of medications. Renal and hepatic diseases are especially significant. Renal diseases reduce the excretion of some drugs, causing drugs to accumulate in the body. If the dosage is not lowered in a person with renal insufficiency, toxic levels may be reached even with low doses of the medication. The same is true of hepatic diseases because the liver is the major organ of metabolism for most drugs.

Mental State

The patient with a positive attitude is more likely to respond positively to medications. The patient who is depressed or despondent may not take medication and may not respond to some drugs. Strong emotions such as anger, fear, jealousy, or extreme worry will have an effect on drug actions because metabolism and other physiologic processes are affected.

Patients' investments in drugs and their desire for positive effects on the body can strongly influence and potentiate the effects of drugs. A strong belief that a drug will be helpful influences the potential for positive results. In patients with negative feelings and mistrust, any medication may have a diminished effect.

History of Previous Medications

Long-term use of a drug can result in increased effects because of accumulation of the drug in the body or, alternatively, can result in a reduced response because the individual has developed a tolerance to the drug. In either case the dosage may have to be adjusted for continuing effectiveness.

Time of Administration

Drugs should be taken at the time ordered by the physician. Some drugs need to be taken on an empty stomach to be effective, whereas others require food in the gastrointestinal tract. Drugs that stimulate the body should not be taken just before sleep. Body functions change with the time of day and as the body adjusts to periods of work and rest. Those who work at night and sleep in the day might take medications at different times than people with more routine work hours.

Route of Administration

The nearer the drug is administered to the blood supply or mucous membranes, the faster the drug is absorbed, distributed, and metabolized (see Table 2-4).

Environment

Because local weather conditions affect the blood supply, with heat causing dilation of the blood vessels and cold causing constriction of the vessels, drug effects are influenced by the environment. At high altitudes, less oxygen is available to the body, which also affects drug distribution in the blood. For the patient with respiratory disorders, a smoking environment at home may be of importance in the effectiveness of medications; the patient with employment requiring prolonged standing may have the need for increased medications for arthritis. Perhaps one of the greatest environmental factors is that related to patients living in poverty who cannot afford medications and must choose between medications and food. Also, many of these patients do not eat the food necessary for safety with medication administration.

Drug Dependence

Physical or psychologic dependence on drugs may lead to increased drug use because the patient needs to consume more of the medication for the same effects.

Patient Compliance

Patient compliance in taking medications as prescribed affects the response to the medication. Doses missed or extra doses taken result in variations in the intended response. Patient cooperation with medical therapy is desired, but such variables as manual dexterity, vision, intellectual capacity, mental state, attitude toward medications, and socioeconomic factors (such as ability to pay for the drugs) play a major role in compliance. Location—whether close to or far from pharmacies and public transportation—can be a major factor in compliance for people who lack private transportation or are dependent on other people to obtain medicines. Poor education or the inability to follow directions can result in life-threatening situations from underdosage or overdosage. In rural areas, where transportation problems, medical availability, and other socioeconomic issues can be exaggerated by great distances to travel for medical care, patient compliance may be a prominent reason for the success or failure of medicinal care.

Precautions and Contraindications to Medication Use in Certain Populations

The ideal drug does not exist. Any medication prescribed has an undesired effect on some person. "No two people are alike" is a familiar saying but one that is especially true with medications. Individual variations do occur, with one person exhibiting an intense response and another person exhibiting no response. Several factors might cause contraindications to medication in certain populations such as tetracyclines with pregnant women because of the teratogenicity in the fetus. A contraindication is a condition in which a medication should not be used. Manufacturers evaluate drugs for contraindications and provide this information to the Food and Drug Administration (FDA). A drug insert, the *PDR*, and various other drug compendia list contraindications. Precautions are specific warnings that should be considered when administering drugs to patients with specific conditions or diseases such as the use of cough syrup for the person with diabetes. With a warning, the medication may still be prescribed if the benefits of use outweigh the possible harm.

Certain groups of people must be monitored more closely than usual during medication use because of body size or its functional ability to metabolize or excrete drugs. Groups in which medications appropriate for "normal" adults may not be appropriate include pregnant women, children, and the elderly.

Medications During Pregnancy and Lactation

The use of any medication—prescription, OTC, or "natural"—during pregnancy or lactation could carry a risk for causing birth defects to the developing fetus or the risk that the drug will be transferred to the baby in breast milk. Such factors as drug route, dosage, and pharmacokinetic activities are important in determining the amount of drug that will circulate in the blood of the mother and its po-

tential effect on the baby or fetus. Many drugs cross the placental membrane, but the potential for adverse fetal effects depends on the drug type, its concentration, and fetal age. No drug can be considered totally safe because problems may arise later in life or in subsequent generations, as occurred with use of diethylstilbestrol (DES) in the 1930s and 1940s to prevent miscarriages, which was later linked to an increased risk for cervical and vaginal cancer in female offspring of DES users.

The first trimester is the time when the developing embryo and fetus are at greatest risk for fetal defects or abnormalities if exposed to **teratogens.** Medications should be avoided at this stage if at all possible and certainly limited to only those absolutely needed and approved by the physician.

In the 1950s and 1960s the teratogenic effects of thalidomide caused the Kefauver-Harris legislation to protect pregnant women from possible teratogens. Cocaine and other recreational drugs, alcohol, and smoking are causes for teratogenic effects today, and many states have passed legislation concerning the use of these substances during pregnancy and the effects found at birth. Because of its vasoconstrictive effects, cocaine can cause the placenta to malfunction and lead to intrauterine death. Excessive alcohol use can cause fetal alcohol syndrome. Smoking can cause pregnancy complications, preterm delivery, or a low infant birth weight in addition to serious chronic health problems for the baby. Certain drugs such as the measles-mumps-rubella (MMR) vaccine should not be given during the first trimester of pregnancy because of an association with fetal defects caused by the live virus in the vaccine. Even the use of tetracycline (an antibiotic) by a pregnant woman may cause stained teeth in her baby later.

As a precaution, in 1983 the FDA established a system for classifying drugs according to their potential for fetal risks. Drugs are now placed into one of five pregnancy categories (Box 4-1). Because the law does not require the manufacturer to classify drugs in use prior to 1983, many drugs have not been assigned to an FDA pregnancy category. For conditions that require medications, the physician will try to find the least toxic drug and will consider the fetal gestational age at the time of the drug's administration, how long the therapy is necessary, and what other medications are being taken at the same time.

During lactation, some drugs in the maternal circulation are readily transferred to the infant through diffusion of the drug to breast milk. Unlike medications that may cross the placenta to the fetus, drugs are not transferred directly to the breast-feeding infant because the mother has metabolized the drugs, so the dose has already been reduced prior to passage to the infant. The amount of a medication ingested by the baby includes the age of the infant, as well as how much and when the breast milk was consumed in relation to the drug's administration. Medications ordered for the lactating mother will be ordered with consideration for the possibility of transfer to the child, and at times breast-feeding may be temporarily interrupted while medicinal therapy is occurring. Changes in the activity level of the nursing infant may signal the effects of drugs, and mothers should be made aware of the signs of potential problems (Boxes 4-2 through 4-4).

BOX 4-1 FDA PREGNANCY CATEGORIES

CATEGORY	DESCRIPTION
A	Remote risk of fetal harm—Studies have not demonstrated risk to the fetus in the first trimester, and there is no risk in the second and third trimesters.
B	Slightly more risk than category A—Two distractions exist. One is that animal studies have not demonstrated risk to the fetus, but the studies are inadequate in the pregnant woman. The other is that animal studies have demonstrated adverse effects, but studies in pregnant women have not demonstrated a risk during any of the trimesters of pregnancy.
C	Greater risk than category B—One category is that animal studies have shown adverse effects in the fetus, but there are no adequate studies in pregnant women. The other is that there are no animal reproduction studies and no studies in humans.
D	Proven risk of fetal harm—Studies in women have shown proof of fetal damage, but the potential benefits of use during pregnancy may be acceptable despite the risk.
X	Proven fetal risk—One category is that studies show a definite risk of fetal abnormalities in either humans or animals. Another category is that adverse reaction reports indicate evidence of fetal risk. The risks clearly outweigh any possible benefit.

IMPORTANT FACTS
- Special medication precautions and contraindications exist for pregnant or lactating women, young children, and the elderly.
- Medications taken by pregnant women may be teratogenic, causing abnormalities in the embryo or fetus. The danger is directly related to the trimester of the pregnancy and the rate of fetal growth at the time of the drug administration. Therefore drugs should only be administered during the first trimester of pregnancy when absolutely necessary.
- Medications introduced after 1983 have been assigned to a pregnancy category by the FDA according to their potential for teratogenicity.

BOX 4-2	SELECTED DRUGS CONTRAINDICATED DURING PREGNANCY BECAUSE OF TERATOGENICITY

ACE inhibitors—all
   captopril (Capoten)
   enalapril (Vasotec)
   benazepril (Lotensin)

Anticancer agents/immunosuppressants
   busulfan (Myleran)
   cyclophosphamide (Cytoxan, Neosar)
   methotrexate (Folex, Mexate)
   thalidomide

Antiseizure drugs
   carbamazepine (Atretol, Carbatrol, Tegretol)
   phenytoin (Dilantin, De-Phen)
   trimethadione (Tridione)
   valproic acid (Depakene)

Vitamin A derivatives
   etretinate (Tegison)
   isotretinoin (Accutane)
   vitamin A (Aquasol A)

Sex hormones
   estrogens, progestins, androgens

lithium (Eskalith, Lithobid)

tetracycline (Vibramycin, Minocin, Achromycin, Panmycin, Sumycin)

warfarin (Coumadin, Panwarfin, Sofarin)
HMG CoA reductase inhibitors or statins (Lipitor, Zocor)

Live vaccines

Other drugs
   alcohol in large or continuous doses (exact amount not known)
   cocaine in large or continuous doses (exact amount not known)
   misoprostol (Cytotec)

BOX 4-3	SELECTED DRUGS CONTRAINDICATED DURING LACTATION

Controlled substances
   amphetamines and amphetamine-like drugs
   cocaine
   heroin
   marijuana
   phencyclidine
   nicotine

Anticancer agents/immunosuppressants
   cyclophosphamide (Cytoxan, Neosar)
   cyclosporine (Neoral, Sandimmune)
   doxorubicin (Adriamycin, Rubex)
   methotrexate (Folex, Mexate)

Other drugs
   bromocriptine (Parlodel)

   ergotamine (Ergomar)

   gold salts (Ridaura, Myochrysine, Solganal)

   lithium (Lithobid, Eskalith)

   ciprofloxacin (Cipro)
   sulfa preparations
   misoprostol (Cytotec)

Medications in Children

Children are not miniature adults. Their ability to absorb, metabolize, and excrete medications is very different from that of adults. These differences affect the amount of drug needed to produce a therapeutic effect and the amount that causes toxic effects. A standard medication dosage for children is nearly nonexistent, and drugs are ordered according to body weight or body surface area (BSA).

Age is no longer considered a reliable guide for administering medications to infants and small children because chronologic age correlates poorly with organ system development. Height is a better correlation in children with lean body mass, whereas larger, more obese children may need higher dosages or those calculated according to BSA. The dosage of medications supplied to children should be recalculated regularly. As children grow, physiologic changes in the fast-growing body affect pharmacodynamics or how the drug acts in the body. Other factors such as skin hydration in infants allow the absorption of water-soluble topical drugs. The ability to swallow medications and the size and form of the oral preparation must be considered when administering medications to young children. Gastric acidity and gastric motility in infants and children cause differences in absorption rates.

When working with pediatric patients (birth to 16 to 18 years), it is important to consider the height and weight of the child and the child's ability to swallow medications so that medicines are administered as safely as possible. Because children grow rapidly, accurate height and weight measurements at each office visit are important

BOX 4-4 MEDICATIONS CONSIDERED RELATIVELY SAFE DURING LACTATION*

Analgesics
  acetaminophen (Tylenol)
  codeine
  propoxyphene (Darvon)

Antiinfectives
  cephalosporins
    cefadroxil (Duricef)
    cefazolin (Ancef)
    cefoxitin (Mefoxin)
    ceftriaxone (Rocephin)
  erythromycin (E-Mycin)
  isoniazid (INAH)
  azithromycin (Z-Pak)

Cardiovascular drugs
  digoxin (Lanoxin) (must be monitored
    very closely)
  guanethidine (Ismelin)

Diuretics
  spironolactone (Aldactone)

Hypoglycemics
  insulin
  Thyroid preparations (must be monitored
    more closely)

Vaccine
  immune globulins (RhoGAM)

Gastrointestinal drugs
  antacids (Maalox, Mylanta)
  cisapride (Propulsid)
  laxatives (except cascara sagrada
    derivatives)

*All medications used during lactation have the potential for passing to the infant through breast milk. Most drugs are contraindicated during lactation and should be carefully evaluated by a health care professional prior to administration.

statistics that the physician uses in calculating appropriate medication doses.

Because pediatric patients are more sensitive to drugs and respond on an individual basis to medications, drug dosages are quantitative with the inherent risk for medication errors caused by the need to measure or dilute oral doses and the miscalculation of doses. These differences increase the chance of adverse reactions and heightened sensitivity. Premature infants and newborns have intense responses to some drugs. Because their organ systems are not developed, medications may remain in the body longer than in older children before being eliminated. Both prolonged drug time in the body and delayed responses may change the pharmacokinetics (absorption,

IMPORTANT FACTS FOR ADMINISTRATION OF PEDIATRIC MEDICATIONS

- The infant and the very young child have immature organ systems, making them highly sensitive to medications.
- In the infant and small child, medications may have a more intense effect for a prolonged period as a result of gastric motility and slow biotransformation by an immature liver.
- The use of intramuscular medications in infants and children is different from their use in adults because of faster absorption of the medication in the muscle tissue of the young.
- Pediatric doses are approximations of the needed medication and should be carefully calculated. The child should be watched closely for adverse reactions and adjustments made as needed.
- Pediatric dosing handbooks should be used or dosing with the calculation double-checked and compared with the available drug. Doses may be rounded to an easily administered amount.

distribution, metabolism, and excretion) in the body and their safety and effectiveness. Of most importance is that gastric emptying times vary, and thus the impact of a drug cannot be predicted. The thin skin of the premature or newborn infant allows more rapid absorption of topically used medications, and this faster absorption in turn increases the chance of toxic effects.

With the metabolic rate of drugs in infants up to 1 year old and the young child being low because of immaturity of the liver, the dosages of the drugs and their time between doses must be recalculated and often reduced because of the rapid metabolism of drugs. Healthy infants older than 1 to 2 weeks may be dosed on the milligram-per-kilogram basis, although the medications may need more frequent dosing because of increased metabolism. By 1 year of age, the liver and kidneys have matured to the point that they have the ability to metabolize drugs at the adult level, and the child's body can process drugs pharmacokinetically in much the same fashion as an adult's body. Children do metabolize drugs faster, especially after the second birthday and again at puberty.

Young children are more vulnerable to adverse reactions because of the immature state of the organs and ongoing growth and development. Effects such as suppression of growth and development by glucocorticosteroids and discoloration of teeth by tetracyclines may occur when medications are given during times of rapid growth and development. Table 4-1 lists medications that should be avoided or used with extreme caution in children.

IMPORTANT FACTS FOR PEDIATRIC PATIENTS
- Pediatric patients cannot be treated with medications used for adults unless some changes are made to the dosage. Children are not small adults; their metabolism and excretion are not well developed.
- Height and weight should be measured in children and elderly patients at each office visit to ensure correct dosing.

Medications in the Elderly

The geriatric population (those older than 65), which represents approximately 12% of the U.S. population, uses approximately 30% of all prescribed drugs and 50% of all OTC medications. Because of their high rate of medication use, the elderly experience more drug-related incidents than any other age group. Older people are more sensitive to drugs than younger adults and exhibit wider variation in how medications affect their bodies. This age group will be of increasing importance to health care professionals with the changing demographics of the U.S. population. Experts estimate that by the year 2030, at least 20% of the population will be more than 65 years old, making seniors the fastest-growing segment of the population.

As adults age, the normal changes in the body affect pharmacokinetics. Individuals with chronic disease processes are at greater risk for toxic effects, adverse reactions, or the lack of therapeutic effect than patients with acute diseases. Some older adults weigh no more than an average large child, and some weigh even less, yet often these people are prescribed the large "normal" adult dose, leading to toxic effects.

Factors Affecting Drugs in the Geriatric Patient

Factors leading to possible dangerous effects caused by the accumulation of drugs within the body include slower metabolism, poor circulation, and impaired function of the liver, lungs, kidneys, or central nervous system. Chronic or debilitating conditions that are accompanied by dehydration or electrolyte imbalance can affect how the aging body uses a drug and may interfere with the

TABLE 4-1 *Medications to Avoid or Use with Extreme Caution in Children*

MEDICATION	ADVERSE REACTION
salicylates/aspirin	Reye's syndrome following viral diseases, especially chickenpox and influenza
androgens	Premature closure of epiphyseal lines of bones
glucocorticoids	Suppress growth
hexachlorophene (Dial soap)	Central nervous system toxicity
nalidixic acid (NegGram)	Erodes cartilage
fluoroquinolones (Cipro, Floxin)	Weakens tendons and causes their rupture
phenothiazines (Thorazine, Mellaril)	Sudden infant death syndrome
sulfonamides	Kernicterus (jaundice and collection of bile in the spine and brain)
tetracyclines	Stain developing teeth

expected therapeutic effect. Estimates indicate that 70% to 80% of all adverse drug reactions in the elderly are related to drug dosage. Because the drug's pharmacokinetics are diminished, body tissues retain a higher level of the medication, resulting in an increase in adverse reactions. There may be a narrow separation between maximum drug effectiveness and drug toxicity in the elderly. The use of multiple drugs simultaneously and poor compliance by many elderly add to the problems associated with aging and medications.

With the gradual, progressive decline of organ function in the aging body, drug pharmacokinetics also decline. Older adults who are physically active will have minimal changes, whereas those who are inactive or bedridden will exhibit dramatic changes. Slowed gastric and intestinal emptying time allows medications to remain in the stomach, increasing absorption and therefore serum levels while simultaneously increasing the risk of stomach irritation because of the prolonged contact time. The amount of the drug's oral dose absorbed does not change with age, but delayed stomach emptying may cause another dose of drugs to be administered prior to the total absorption of the previous dose; distribution changes caused by changes in body fat and water ratio and less muscle mass; slowed metabolism caused by less blood flow to the liver and less enzymatic activity to metabolize a drug; and delayed excretion caused by less blood flow to kidneys and renal function. This decrease in the processing of a drug by the body can decrease the drug's half-life and cause drug accumulation in the body. The concentration of a drug rises to a higher level, and the drug effects are more intense. Because individuals respond at different rates, dosing and monitoring for effects must be individualized.

The dosages and effects of medications applied transdermally may also be difficult to predict in older patients. Although skin thickness decreases, drying, wrinkling, and decreased hair follicles may change the rate of absorption. Decreased cardiac output may also affect the rate at which medications are absorbed through the skin. Because of decreased salivary flow, sublingual tablets may not be properly dissolved and absorbed, nor may tablets be easily swallowed. **Dentition** should be evaluated prior to giving chewable tablets because many elderly adults have insufficient teeth to chew tablets. Many drugs can affect the mental status of older individuals, leading to confusion and unintentional overdosing of medications.

Polypharmacy and the Elderly

With the increasing numbers of geriatric patients and the increased medications found as OTC preparations, many older adults become caught in the vicious circle of polypharmacy. The era of medical specialization has only added to this problem because a person who sees multiple physicians for multiple problems is usually prescribed multiple medications without the discontinuance of any of the drugs the person was previously prescribed by someone else. The problem is increased by the patient's self-medication with OTC drugs. By taking accurate medical histories (Box 4-5) including full documentation of *all* medications being taken, the allied health professional assists in the elimination of inappropriate medications and thus improves the patient's quality of life and reduces the undesirable effects of polypharmacy (Box 4-6).

Some of the polypharmacy is apparent when the patient receives more than one drug in the same class of medications or several different medications from different medication classes to treat the same symptoms. More likely is the fact that medications are added to treat the side effects of another medication, leading to the use of more and more drugs and possible negative outcomes. The negative effects include adverse drug reactions, drug-drug interactions, medication errors, increased treatment costs, and increased risk of hospitalization. Because of these inherent problems, it is important to use the lowest effective dose in the geriatric patient.

BOX 4-5   QUESTIONS TO ASK TO PREVENT POLYPHARMACY

- What dietary supplements, vitamins, and OTC drugs do you take?
- What pharmacies have you used in the past 2 years to fill your prescriptions?
- Who are all of the physicians that you see and what medications has each prescribed for you?
- How would you describe your ability to read medication labels?
- When do you take your medications? Of those times, which are you most likely to forget to take the doses? How often do you forget your medications?
- Do you have any questions about your medications and how to take them?

BOX 4-6   CONDITIONS THAT MAY OCCUR WITH POLYPHARMACY

- Cardiac arrhythmias
- Disturbances in balance
- Cognition changes, confusion, depression, suicidal ideation
- Constipation
- Gastric ulcers
- Hypertension or hypotension
- Rash
- Unexpected failure of treatment

The elderly individual who responds in an expected way to a drug at a given time may experience toxic or adverse reactions in the future. The elderly person is in a constant state of physiologic change, and the medications ordered must change with the individual. The use of drugs may remain relatively safe as long as each physician maintains a total drug profile, and as long as the potential for drug interactions and the physiologic changes in the patient are evaluated each time medications are prescribed. For this reason, it is important for the geriatric patient to fill prescriptions at the same pharmacy each time so that the drug profile is current and accurate.

The allied health professional should be aware that 40% or more of elderly individuals do not take their medications correctly. Some fail to get prescriptions filled initially, whereas others never refill the prescription to continue the medicines. Yet others do not adhere to the prescribed dosage or follow the schedule for taking the medicines. These factors can lead to toxic effects from overdosing or nontreatment from underdosing. Underdosing and failure to respond to a medication are more common by far, accounting for approximately 90% of the problem. Unintentional

IMPORTANT FACTS ABOUT ELDERLY PATIENTS AND THEIR DRUGS

- Older people are usually more sensitive to medications than younger adults.
- Medications must be individualized for the older adult because of changes in the body organ systems and in drug pharmacokinetics associated with body changes.
- Adverse reactions are more common in older persons.
- Adverse reactions may be caused by polypharmacy, severe illness, the presence of multiple diseases, and the resultant use of multiple drugs.
- Noncompliance is common. About 90% of noncompliance is intentional and is caused by expense, side effects, or the patient feeling the medication is not necessary.
- Unintentional noncompliance is usually caused by forgetfulness or failure to understand the pharmaceutic treatment.
- After age of 50, only three medications should be taken at the same time. If more than three medications are necessary, the patient should be instructed to wait 10 minutes between each dosage of three or less to allow for absorption.

noncompliance may result from forgetfulness; from not understanding instructions because of poor vision, inadequate hearing, or decreased ability to understand; or from the complexity of remembering how to take multiple drugs. Sadly, however, 75% of noncompliance is intentional: The older person feels the medicine is not necessary or finds the side effects unpleasant. A major reason for noncompliance may be inability to pay for drugs by people on a fixed income. Because the medications are necessary for good treatment, the allied health professional needs to listen to the patient and ask sufficient questions to obtain a full history of the medicines being taken and to look for clues that may signal an unrecognized noncompliance problem.

Assisting the Elderly with Medication Compliance

To help elderly patients comply with medication orders, simplifying the instructions for taking medications and being sure the medication schedule is convenient for the patient is necessary. Encourage the patient to read all labels carefully and to use only one pharmacy. The patient should make a list of all medications taken, their strength, dose,

and length of time each has been taken. This list should be taken to each physician with each visit so that the medical record can be updated. The allied health professional should thoroughly explain the medication schedule, making the medication times fit as closely to the person's schedule as possible. The reason for administration should be explained clearly and concisely, followed with precise written instructions. Using a calendar or a weekly pill container will assist in reminding the patient to take the medicines as prescribed. Finally, providing sample medications to those who cannot afford the medicines may help with compliance and will provide small amounts of medications for trial before expensive prescriptions are dispensed and side effects prevent the use of the medicine.

IMPORTANT FACTS FOR GERIATRIC DOSAGES

- Elderly individuals have decreased metabolism and excretion compared with younger adults; therefore the danger of overdose is increased.
- Drugs tend to accumulate in the elderly and are more likely to have a cumulative effect in debilitated patients or those with chronic medical problems.
- Compliance with medicinal treatment declines as the elderly become more forgetful. Some 40% or more of elderly individuals do not comply with medical treatment.

Assisting Other Special Populations with Medications

The health care professional should spend time with each patient to ensure that he or she understands the condition, treatment prescribed, and reasons for and actions of the medication ordered. Providing this understanding increases the likelihood that the patient will take prescribed medications routinely. Some pharmaceutic companies provide audio, video, and written materials to assist with patient education for their new medications. Asking that the patient explain what he or she has heard and understood can reveal any information that has not been adequately covered. Patients with low incomes or fixed incomes such as retirees may have difficulty paying for their medications, and this may also be discussed with the patient. Compliance will be more easily accomplished if affordable methods of procuring the medications are discussed with the patient. If a trade-name medication is required, for example, the health care professional may be able to provide the patient with samples, and some pharmaceutical companies even have special programs for those who cannot afford their medications.

The medical office should keep a list of available local resources that can assist with medication compliance. In some communities pharmacies cooperate with other medical entities to provide low-cost prescription copayments. Some agencies will come to the home and prepare medications for the patient to take. Others will assist with transportation for the patient to obtain medicines. For some elderly patients, it may be the caregiver who needs to understand the medication administration. In these cases the caregiver should be present whenever medicines are discussed. Some patients such as the visually impaired may need special labels, whereas others may need to contact social agencies that can help defray the cost of prescription medications. Conditions that involve loss of memory, vision, hearing, or movement, as well as socioeconomic situations that result in inadequate transportation or financial resources, may cause real barriers for some patients. The health care professional's knowledge of available resources can play a major role in assisting with patient compliance.

A patient who is illiterate and who is embarrassed to ask for help in reading prescription labels or OTC labels is at risk for inadvertent double dosing, adverse reactions to medications, and dangerous drug interactions. The illiterate person may also have problems understanding the language of prescriptions. Because even most literate people are not medication literate, it is important to provide an increased knowledge base for reading drug ingredients. It is not commonly understood by most patients, for example, that medications such as OTC headache preparations with salicylates such as aspirin may cause bleeding in the person who is taking Coumadin and its derivatives or that ibuprofen and aspirin should not be taken together because ibuprofen is an aspirin-like compound.

Taking time to answer questions during an office visit will help the patient stay focused on the goals of the treatment. Taking 5 to 10 minutes to explain areas of concern can save the time that would be involved if a problem had to be corrected later after adverse effects have occurred. Compliance may entail making lifestyle changes to ensure therapeutic results. The health care team can improve compliance by helping patients integrate the medical treatments into their daily lives. Con-

venience in taking medications helps a person comply with treatment.

For patients who have difficulty with medication compliance, written instructions can help ensure accuracy of dosage. Some health care facilities have printed materials that provide checklists for the areas of compliance that need special attention. These checklists should also include areas where specific instructions about medications can be provided. Written instructions provide the patient with a guide that can be followed at home.

IMPORTANT FACTS ABOUT COMPLIANCE WITH SPECIAL POPULATIONS

- Because barriers such as language, hearing, vision, culture, and religion can cause noncompliance, they should be evaluated before any medications are prescribed.
- Written instructions should be provided for patients who have difficulty remembering desired schedules or who have disabilities that make compliance difficult.
- The allied health professional should be sure that patients who are illiterate or who have language barriers understand medication schedules before they leave the physician's office.
- If a patient requires a caregiver, the caregiver should be present when medication administration is discussed.

Medications and Cultural Differences

Perceptions about medications that influence the acceptance or refusal of medicinal treatment come from the cultural, social, and religious beliefs and convictions of people. A person's ideas become part of the reason for compliance or noncompliance with therapy. By understanding some of these cultural differences, the health care professional can assist with communication to improve patient care and compliance.

Ethnic and cultural differences seldom affect the action of medications in the body (even though some diseases occur only in certain racial or ethnic groups), but a patient's compliance with a physician's orders can be greatly affected by the patient's understanding of the therapy and by good communication between patient and provider concerning the need for medication therapy. People of some cultures may refrain from expressing views that conflict with the views of others, especially those in medical communities. Even nonverbal communication can hinder compliance. Through patient assessment and awareness of sociocultural differences, health care professionals can surmount certain obstacles to good health care.

The allied health professional must be aware of his or her attitudes because these attitudes are transmitted both verbally and nonverbally. Self-analysis of our own beliefs, expectations, attitudes, and practices establishes the way we accept differences. An open mind and a willingness to expand personal knowledge of diversity assists in establishing patient-caregiver interactions. Barriers to communication can be overcome through tone of voice, body language, and actions that convey reassurance. Patience with the patient and allowing time to be sure that the patient understands medication orders are important steps in promoting compliance with medical therapy.

In 1989 Albers Herberg noted that attitudes toward health and illness generally reflect one of three views: scientific-biomedical, holistic, and magicoreligious. Each perspective regards illness and health in different, culturally determined ways (Table 4-2). In the United States the scientific-biomedical paradigm predominates, with professionals undergoing extensive training in the biomedical sciences. In the scientific-biomedical domain, disease and illness have a cause and the goal of health care is to find a cure. Scientific research is based on finding cures for diseases and illnesses.

The holistic paradigm focuses on achieving harmony of body, mind, and spirit to prevent illness. Disharmony or imbalance among these natural components leads to disease or illness. Once the person is in harmony, health is restored. Thus health requires bringing the mind, body, and spirit into balance (Figure 4-2).

The magicoreligious paradigm regards humans as under the control of supernatural, mystical forces. Witchcraft, good and evil spirits, spells, voodoo, and other forces bring about illness and disease. Health is a blessing from God for being good, whereas illness is a sign that the individual has not carried out God's will. Illness may or may not be part of God's plan, but it comes from supernatural forces.

Culture must be considered in the use of medications for the treatment of illnesses. One third of the U.S. population consists of individuals from racial, ethnic, or cultural subgroups that are referred to as minorities. Beginning in the twenty-first century, however, persons from a minority background accounted for more than 50% of the total population, making the need to know and understand diversity a necessity to meet the health care needs of patients. For an accurate and meaningful gathering of data, care must be sensitive to differences and respect those ideas that are in conflict with the biomedical-scientific outlook prevalent in American medical institutions.

When making health care decisions, people draw on their cultural background and rely on various personal relationships in seeking assistance with those decisions. In some cultures, individuals

TABLE 4-2 Beliefs Concerning Health and Illness as Life Events

	SCIENTIFIC-BIOMEDICAL	HOLISTIC	MAGICORELIGIOUS
Health	Prevention activities and restorative therapy through exercise, medications, and treatment	Environment, behavior, and sociocultural factors influence and maintain health and the prevention of illness or disease; maintaining and restoring health are vital	A reward of God's blessings and good will
Illness and disease	Cause-effect relationship to life events; wear and tear happens to the body, as do accidents, injuries, diseases, and chemical imbalances; the body functions as a machine; mind and body are two distinct entities	Disease, chemical or physical imbalance, and chaos occur when the laws of harmony and natural balance have been disturbed; human life is only one part of the cosmos; everything has its place and role to maintain order	Cause of health and illness is not organic but mystical; evil spirits, sorcery, taboos, and supernatural forces cause illness; humans are at the mercy of good and evil forces, which may initiate diseases or illnesses with or without a reason
Societies in which belief predominates	White Americans Europeans	Native Americans Various Asian groups	African Americans Persons of Hispanic culture

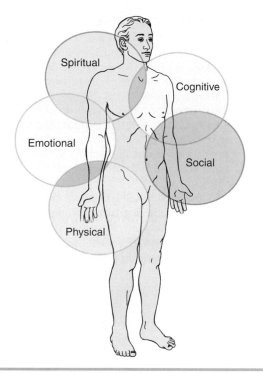

Figure 4-2 The individual in a holistic health perspective. The diagram shows the dynamic interactions among the physical, social, emotional, spiritual, and cognitive aspects of a person.

seek assistance from family members, and parents or grandparents may make decisions about health matters. In other groups the patient may make decisions while assessing how the decision will affect the entire group or family. In yet other groups the individual makes his or her own health care decisions. Although family members may participate to some degree, either through influence or through participation in the therapy, identifying the person who makes the decisions about the medical care and including that person in the teaching sessions will assist with providing successful therapy.

A number of people in the United States have as their primary language a language other than English. To comply with drug therapy, the patient must first understand the language of instruction. For the person who does not speak English, giving the directions in English will not lead to comprehension and compliance. Instruction sheets in the patient's language or pictographs will assist with comprehension. A person who can act as an interpreter and who will accompany the patient to the physician's office will further assist with compliance.

A person's feelings about medications and home or folk remedies that are considered important to health in that individual's culture may influ-

ence how he or she accepts medication therapy. Individuals from certain cultural backgrounds may consider home remedies such as roots, teas, and poultices to be more effective than prescription or nonprescription medications. (Home remedies and folk medicine are discussed in Chapter 20.) The allied health professional should attempt to discover the home remedies that the patient is using because these remedies could interfere with the prescribed medical care. Understanding cultural differences toward illness and treatment makes an important step toward gaining patient confidence and compliance with prescribed treatments.

Communication and Medication Compliance

Communication, both verbal and nonverbal, is vital to compliance with medication treatment. Nonverbal communication between persons of different cultures may enhance acceptance or inadvertently show disrespect for the patient. Even eye contact is interpreted differently by various cultures. Life experiences, historical and cultural backgrounds, and the patient's perception of the situation are social factors that the allied health professional must try to understand while remaining nonjudgmental and trying to clarify any information that could have been miscommunicated. In today's multicultural world, the allied health professional should adapt medical materials to meet a variety of cultural needs. Written materials may not suffice, for a patient who cannot read and write may lack understanding of why the prescribed medical therapy is important.

IMPORTANT FACTS
- Cultural differences in how people regard illness and health can affect compliance not only with medications but also with the total medical care of the patient.
- Problems in communication can lead to noncompliance with treatment.

Summary

Many patient variables must be considered when prescribing medications. Among these variables are the patient's age, weight, gender, diet, genetics, concurrent diseases, and mental state. Some people respond to placebos when the psychologic need is more intense than the physiologic response. How a medicine is given, what medicines have been previously prescribed, and the possibility of drug dependence are all important factors that the physician must consider when prescribing drug treatment. The elderly and children have different rates of metabolism than the average adult, the person for whom the average dosage is designed. Dosages must be adjusted in these individuals, and special precautions followed in drug use. Pregnancy and lactation may preclude the use of some drugs because of the danger to the fetus and infants.

People from different cultures have different perspectives on the role of medications in sickness and health, and their cooperation with medical treatment may be culturally based. The allied health professional must be sure that cultural differences do not interfere with therapy and that the patient complies with the course of treatment.

Critical Thinking Exercises

SCENARIO

Jane, age 23, thinks she may be pregnant because she has missed one menstrual period. It is spring, and she has a history of allergic rhinitis that causes sinus headaches. She asks you, the medical assistant, what medications she may take for her allergies. The physician has previously prescribed an antihistamine for the condition, and she wants you to call in the same prescription to the pharmacy.

1. What should you do?
2. What do you need to tell Jane about taking medicines during the first trimester of pregnancy?
3. If there were medications that could be safely given during the first trimester, in what pregnancy category would the medications be listed?

REVIEW QUESTIONS

1. What is polypharmacy? Who is at risk for polypharmacy? _____

2. What is the role of the allied health professional in polypharmacy? _____

3. How do variations in weight and the gradual decline in body functions affect dosages for the elderly? _____

4. Why is medication therapy potentially harmful in the first trimester of pregnancy? _____

5. Communication barriers and cultural differences may cause noncompliance with drug therapy. How can the allied health professional be sure that those from other cultures comply with medication therapy? _____

6. Compare the scientific-biomedical, holistic, and magicoreligious paradigms of health and illness. How can the allied health professional work with those of different cultures to promote understanding of the medicinal treatment? _____

7. What variables (weight, height, and so on) affect drug dosage and actions? What does the allied health professional need to do to ensure correct dosage? _____

   _____

   _____

   _____

8. What are three of the negative outcomes of polypharmacy? _____

   _____

   _____

   _____

9. Why is it important to obtain weight and height at each medical visit? _____

   _____

   _____

   _____

10. Why is age a variable in drug dosages? _____

    _____

    _____

    _____

CHAPTER 5

Reading and Interpreting Medication Labels and Orders and Documenting Appropriately

OBJECTIVES

After studying this chapter, you should be capable of doing the following:

- Explaining the parts of a National Drug Code (NDC).
- Listing warning and caution label information and its relevance.
- Identifying items to look for when inventorying medications.
- Distinguishing between a prescription and a medication order.
- Using correct abbreviations when assisting with prescription writing.
- Describing the parts of a prescription.
- Describing the steps necessary to prepare prescriptions for a physician's signature.
- Telephoning prescriptions to pharmacies and medication orders to health facilities.
- Documenting prescriptions and medical orders in patients' records.
- Safeguarding prescription pads.
- Recognizing when prescription refills might be necessary and transferring orders for refills accurately by telephone.
- Writing a prescription.
- Interpreting a physician's medication orders.

Tonya, an allied health professional, knows that Mrs. Kline likes to see several physicians at the same time. Tonya asks Mrs. Kline to give her a list of the medicines that she is taking on a regular basis so that she can enter this information into the medical record. Mrs. Kline tells Tonya that she can remember some of her medicines but not all of them.

  Does Tonya need to get the medicines from all of the physicians or just those prescribed by the internist? Why?
  If Mrs. Kline uses the same pharmacy to fill all prescriptions, can Tonya call that pharmacy to obtain the needed information?
  Is that ethical? Why or why not?
  Should Tonya tell Mrs. Kline to bring all of her medications each time she sees the physician? Why or why not?
  How can Tonya help Mrs. Kline remember the medications she is taking for inclusion in the medical record?
  If samples are given to Mrs. Kline, what steps does Tonya need to take to be sure patient safety is provided?

KEY TERMS

Auxiliary labels	Inscription	Standing order
Compounding	Medication order	Subscription
Concentration	National Drug Code (NDC)	Superscription
DEA number	Refill	Volume
Documentation	Signature (Sig or Signa)	Verbal order
Dosage strength (weight)	Standard protocol	

Medications may be prescribed, dispensed, or administered in a medical office. Sample medications or other medications supplied by the health care provider and given to the patient are considered dispensed, but a pharmacist in a pharmacy setting does most of the dispensing. Drugs are administered (given) in health care facilities by health care professionals. Being able to read the label on a medication, whether prescription or over the counter (OTC) is a necessity for allied health professionals. Forgetting to read the label or improperly identifying the information on a label may result in the wrong medication being given ("look-alike-sound-alike" medications), undermedication or overmedication, unwanted side effects, improper usage and storage, and improper preparation of the dose. Reading and understanding the medication label that contains both generic and trade names and strength and providing an understanding of the terms associated with the standardized format of labels for both prescription medications and OTC purchases is important to ensure correct administration and proper usage of medications by health professionals and patients.

Prescribing medications is a daily routine in physicians' offices. The allied health professional plays a role in prescription therapy by assisting the physician with samples, phoning prescriptions to pharmacies, and documenting the administration of medications to patients. This role varies with state laws and with the protocol of the specific health care setting.

Reading a Label for Stock Medications

The *manufacturer's label* found on stock medication bottles contains information about the size of the bottle, the strength of the medication, and other important facts that are necessary in providing the correct medication for patient safety. Some labels contain more detail than others, but reading the entire label is most important to ensure quality assurance in patient care. Reading all medication labels prior to dispensing or administering medications is important. If a patient is supplied with a new medication, counseling of the patient is required by law and pharmacies provide a patient education sheet about the drug for the patient to take home and read (Figure 5-1).

Parts of a Medication Label

In the following section the parts of the label are indicated by a letter of the alphabet with the figures showing the indication on the label.

A. Trade (or Proprietary or Brand) Name

This is the copyrighted name assigned to the medication after initial approval by the U.S. Food and Drug Administration that can only be used by the company that created the drug. Trade names are always capitalized and are usually seen first on the drug label in bold type. The symbols ® for registered or ™ for trademark will follow the name. ™ is used until the U.S. Patent and Trademark Office has registered the name, and then ® is the correct symbol. In Figures 5-2 and 5-3, Dilaudid is the trade name.

B. Generic Name

Also called the *official name*, the name given to the medication by the U.S. Pharmacopeia together with the manufacturer is indicated using lowercase letters. This is the name given the drug when it is first developed. After the patent rights have expired, the drug may be manufactured by other companies under the same generic name but with another trade name. In Figures 5-2 and 5-3, the generic name is hydromorphone HCL. In Figures 5-4 and 5-5, the drug does not have a trade name—phenobarbital is the generic name.

C. Drug Strength (Weight)

The drug strength or weight, such as milligrams, micrograms, milliequivalents, and grains, is the amount of active ingredient of a medication in dosage form. In tablets this is the amount of active ingredient in the tablet. In liquid form the medication is the weight of medication in a specified number of milliliters or other indication of the volume of medication. The dosage strength of a medication may come in various weights. The labels in Figures 5-2 and 5-3 indicate Dilaudid 2 mg per tablet and 4 mg per milliliter, respectively. Using Figures 5-4 and Figure 5-5, notice that the same medication may come in different strengths and often tablets may even be of different colors or shapes, or both, to prevent medicinal errors.

D. Form

Form indicates whether the medication is a solid (e.g., tablets, capsules, powders), liquid (e.g., solutions, dispersions, syrups), or semisolid (e.g., creams, ointments, suppositories). (See Chapter 3 for a review of this material.) Some medication labels have indications of specific dosage forms such as those seen in Box 5-1.

E. Route of Administration

The route of administration indicates the way the drug enters the body. Some labels, especially those for parenteral use, tell the routes that are acceptable for the medication on hand. Other labels do not provide the route to be used, but tablets, caplets, capsules, and other medications found in

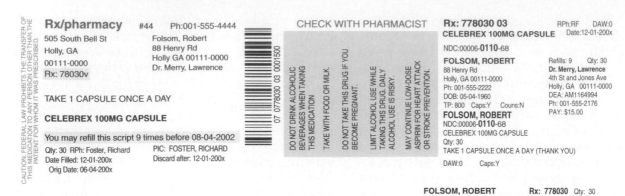

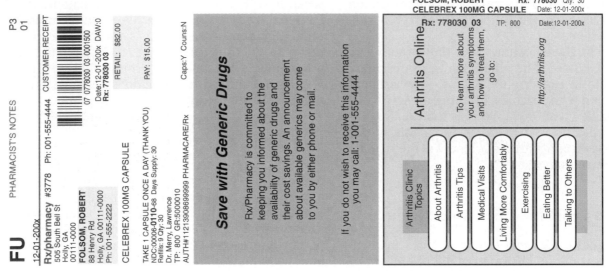

CELECOXIB-ORAL

USES: This medication is a nonsteroidal anti-inflammatory drug (NSAID) which relieves pain and swelling (inflammation). It is used to treat arthritis, menstrual pain or other acute pain.

HOW TO USE THIS MEDICATION: Take this drug by mouth, generally once daily as directed. To decrease the chance of stomach upset, this drug is best taken with food. Dosage is based on your medical condition and response to therapy. Take this medication with 6 to 8 ounces (180-240ml) of water. Do not lie down for at least 30 minutes after taking this drug.

SIDE EFFECTS: Stomach upset or tiredness may occur. If these effects persist or worsen, notify your doctor promptly. Unlikely but report promptly black or bloody stools, stomach pain, severe headache or a change in the amount of urine. Very unlikely but report promptly dark urine or yellowing eyes or skin. In the unlikely event you have an allergic reaction to this drug, seek immediate medical attention. Symptoms of an allergic reaction include rash, itching, swelling, dizziness or trouble breathing. If you notice other effects not listed above, contact your doctor or pharmacist.

PRECAUTIONS: Tell your doctor your medical history, including any allergies (especially to aspirin/other NSAIDs); liver, kidney, or heart disease; stomach/intestinal ulcers or bleeding; history of smoking, alcoholism, asthma, high blood pressure; growths in the nose (e.g., nasal polyps); serious infections, swelling (edema), blood disorders (anemia) or poorly controlled diabetes. This medicine may cause stomach bleeding. Daily use of alcohol, especially when combined with this medicine, may increase your risk for stomach bleeding. Check with your doctor or pharmacist for more information. Caution is advised when this drug is used in the elderly, as this group may be more sensitive to drug side effects. This medication should be used only when clearly needed during the first six months of pregnancy. It should not be used during the last three months of pregnancy. Discuss the risks and benefits with your doctor. it is not known whether this drug is excreted into breast milk. Because of the potential risk to the infant, breast-feeding while using this drug is not recommended. Consult your doctor before breast-feeding.

DRUG INTERACTIONS: Tell your doctor of all prescription and nonprescription medication you may use, especially medicines for high blood pressure (e.g., ACE inhibitors such as lisinopril); "water pills" (diuretics such as furosemide or thiazides); other NSAIDs or aspirin (e.g., ibuprofen); lithium, methotrexate; corticosteroids (e.g., prednisone); rifamycins (e.g., rifampin) or "blood thinners" (e.g., warfarin). Check all nonprescription medicine labels carefully, since many contain pain relievers/fever reducers (NSAIDs/aspirin) which are similar to this drug. Aspirin as prescribed by your doctor for reasons such as heart attack or stroke prevention (i.e., non-arthritis doses) should be continued. Consult your pharmacist. Do not start or stop any medicine without doctor or pharmacist approval.

OVERDOSE: If overdose is suspected, contact your local poison control center or emergency room immediately. Symptoms of overdose may include severe stomach pain, coffee ground-like vomit, dark stool, ringing in the ears, change in amount of urine, unusually fast or slow heartbeat, muscle weakness, slow or shallow breathing, confusion, severe headache or loss of consciousness.

NOTES: Do not share this medication with others. Laboratory or medical tests may be performed to monitor your progress.

MISSED DOSE: If you miss a dose, use it as soon as you remember. If it is near the time of the next dose, skip the missed dose and resume your usual dosing schedule. Do not double the dose to catch up.

STORAGE: Store at room temperature (77 degrees F or 25 degrees C) away from light and moisture.

For faster refills, phone in 24 hours in advance

Keep Out of Reach of Children

Figure 5-1 Handout typical of those given to patients with their prescriptions.

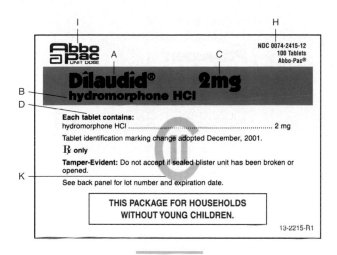

Figure 5-2

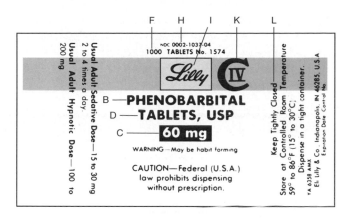

Figure 5-4

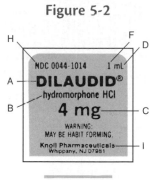

Figure 5-3

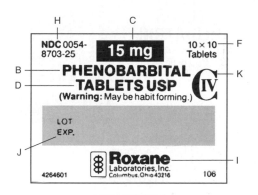

Figure 5-5

Table 2-4 are to be administered orally, as are the oral liquids found in Table 2-3. Notice that the label for phenobarbital in Figure 5-4 is for a tablet and does not give the route of administration, whereas atropine (Figure 5-6) is a parenteral that states the medication may be given SC, IM, and IV.

F. Total Amount of Medication in the Container

The amount of medication in the container will indicate the total number tablets, capsules, and the like of the solid oral forms of medication (see Figure 5-4). With oral liquid medications, the total volume of medication and the weight per volume of medication are included on the label (Figure 5-7). Medications that are found in powdered form for reconstitution (see Chapter 10) will provide the total weight of the medication, as well as the concentration following reconstitution in either injectable or oral medications (Figures 5-8 and 5-9).

G. Directions for Reconstitution

Medications that must be mixed with a diluent prior to administration will provide the directions for reconstitution (see Figures 5-8 and 5-9).

BOX 5-1	ABBREVIATIONS THAT MODIFY DRUG FORMS
ABBREVIATIONS	**EXAMPLE**
SR = Sustained Release	Pronestyl SR
CR = Controlled Release	Sinemet CR
LA or XL = Long Acting	Entex-LA, Procardia XL
DS = Double Strength	Septra-DS
TR = Time Release	Triaminic TR

H. National Drug Code

All medications are assigned an NDC to identify the manufacturer, product, and size of the container. This code number, containing 11 digits, is shown on the label preceded with the letters NDC at the front.

An example of the NDC code and its meaning (related to Figure 5-4) is 0002-1037-04.

The drug manufacturer number 0002 is assigned to Eli Lilly, Inc.

The product, phenobarbital, is coded 1037.

The size of the container is designated as 04 for 1000 tablets.

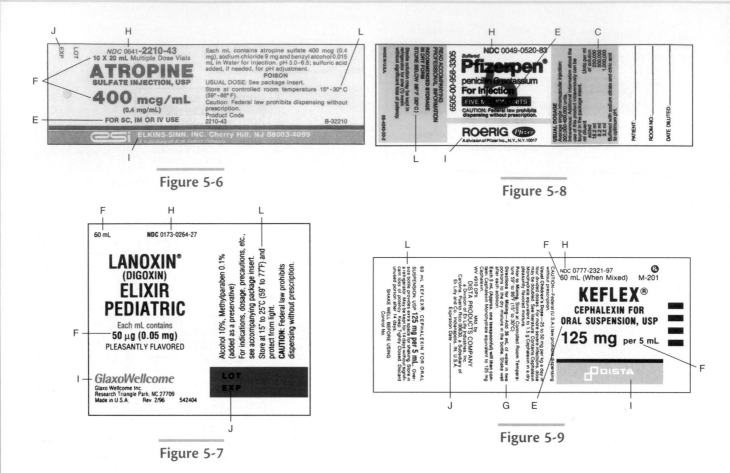

Figure 5-6

Figure 5-8

Figure 5-7

Figure 5-9

I. Manufacturer's Name

The name of the manufacturer, and sometimes the address, is found on the label (see Figure 5-7).

J. Expiration Date

The expiration date is the last date for safe use of the medication. After this date, the drug should be discarded (see Figure 5-6). Lot numbers are also included with the expiration date so that if a product is recalled, the patient can be notified and the medication either discarded or returned to the manufacturer.

K. Labels for Controlled Drugs

The symbol for controlled drugs, as well as the warning that the medication may be habit forming, is found on medications that are listed in the Controlled Drug Schedules (see Figures 5-2 and 5-4).

L. Auxiliary Labeling

This labeling placed by the pharmacy gives specific additional information and advice to the patient about use of or special handling of the med-

ication (see Figure 5-9). These labels include storage labels stating that the medication must be stored at a certain temperature and conditions with more than one direction found on a single label, instructions for patients, and precautions and cautions for use. All auxiliary labels are not seen on all containers, but those needed for patient safety with the specific medication are found.

> **DID YOU KNOW?**
> A study on medications concluded that only 8% of drugs shipped were arriving within the temperature and humidity limits developed by manufacturers. More than 26% were subjected to excessive heat, and 65% of the drugs were subjected to temperatures between 86° F and 104° F, making the drug use less than optimum and in some cases dangerous. The health care professional should always check the condition of drugs on arrival.

Labeling of OTC Medications

Not only can OTC medications be bought by anyone, but many people do not bother to read the directions on the label and falsely believe that because the

BOX 5-2	FDA LABELING GUIDELINES FOR OVER-THE-COUNTER MEDICATIONS

This information must appear on the product packaging, in a standard format.
- Brand name of the drug
- Active and inactive ingredients (and amounts of each in a single dose)
- Drug's purpose
- The type of treatment for which the drug is designed (the use)
- A section on warnings, precautions
- Possible adverse reactions
- When to stop using the drug
- When to consult a physician
- Directions and dosage chart
- Lot or batch number
- Quantity of contents

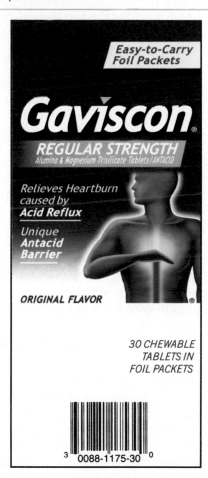

Figure 5-10

medication is available without a prescription, the ingredients are not harmful. Because the Federal Trade Commission recognized that many OTC medications were being misused, new label guidelines with more specific information are now in place. The information must be in a recognizable and standardized format in a language that is understandable by most

TABLE 5-1 *TJC Official "Do Not Use" List*

DO NOT USE (OLD ABBREVIATION)	USE INSTEAD (NEW TERMINOLOGY)
U (unit)	Unit
IU (International Unit)	International Unit
Q.D., QD, q.d., qd (daily)	Daily
Q.O.D., QOD, q.o.d., qod (every other day)	Every other day
Trailing zero (X.0 mg)	X mg
Lack of leading zero (.X mg)	0.X mg
μg	mcg or micrograms

people. For the information found on labels of OTC medications, refer to Box 5-2 and Figure 5-10.

Ordering Medications

Medications may be ordered for the patient using either a prescription or a medication order to provide drugs deemed needed by the physician. Orders may be written orders as on a prescription or medication order, verbal orders, or standing orders. The safest and preferable means of ordering medications is written, but in some instances a verbal order is necessary with standard medical abbreviations often being used as a means of medical shorthand.

Common Abbreviations Used in Prescriptions and Medication Orders

The allied health professional must be familiar with terms and abbreviations used in writing prescriptions or medication orders. These abbreviations come from Latin or Greek words, are shorthand for directions, and are used daily in the medical field. The list of commonly used standard abbreviations such as qid, tid, q4h and the like for writing prescriptions or orders is found inside the back cover of this text. Recently The Joint Committee (TJC) has made recommendations of an official "Do Not Use List." However, these abbreviations are included in the abbreviation list of this text because the use is still seen in some medical settings and the meaning must be known (Table 5-1).

> **IMPORTANT FACTS ABOUT ABBREVIATIONS**
> - Only standard, commonly used abbreviations should be used so that the abbreviation is understood by other health care professionals.
> - The prescription is a legal document, and "local" abbreviations, or those not universally accepted, should not be included because the prescription could be misinterpreted.

Verbal Orders

When the physician tells an allied health professional which drug or drugs to administer to a patient, the physician is giving a **verbal (oral) medication order.** The order is for a specific patient and designates the medication to be given, the dose, the form of the medication, the time, and the route of administration. Orders should not be routinely given verbally because of the possibility of error and confusion. However, if an order is given verbally, the person receiving the order should read back the order to the person who gave it. If there is a possibility of confusion, especially if the drug name sounds like other drug names, the medication name should be spelled to reduce the chance of error. All verbal orders should be documented, using V/O (verbal order) prior to writing the order, as soon as possible to prevent errors in administration of the medication. *Legally, any order not documented has not been performed.* This order should be countersigned by the person giving the order as soon as possible.

Standing Orders

Physicians may have **standing orders** that are assigned for use in specific instances. An example of a standing order might be to give a specific antipyretic, such as acetaminophen, to children with a high fever while they are waiting to see the physician. Physicians may also use a **standard protocol,** which is a signed set of orders to be used with specific procedures; an example is the use of a suppository, a laxative, and an enema prior to a colonoscopy. "Standard protocol" may be the order written in the medical record; the allied health professional knows what the physician expects and performs the specific tasks exactly as they are documented in the office manuals. The health care worker should ascertain the appropriateness, dose, allergy, and weight information before administering medications to standing orders or standard protocol and should ascertain that the patient has no condition that would cause adverse reactions. Standard protocol and standing orders should be kept in a designated place in the office, and the documents should be signed by a physician. Following drug administration or procedures, documentation in the medical record should be performed immediately.

Medication Orders

A **medication order,** telling the allied health professional which drug or drugs to administer, should be written but may also be given verbally. It is not given to the patient for filling at a pharmacy, but rather is used for administration of drugs in hospitals and ambulatory facilities. In the physician's office, medication orders may be called *standing orders* or *standard protocol,* as discussed earlier. The allied health professional has the responsibility to follow these orders within his or her legal scope of practice, which varies by state law. The six components of medication orders listed in Box 5-3 are again discussed in Chapter 12.

| BOX 5-3 | SIX COMPONENTS OF MEDICATION ORDERS |

1. Date
2. Patient's name
3. Medication name
4. Dosage or amount of medication
5. Route of administration. (If no route is given, oral administration is appropriate. If there is doubt as to the route of administration, the allied health professional should *always* ask the physician.)
6. Time or frequency of administration

Prescriptions

A **prescription,** a legal document, indicates the medication needed and the directions for use to meet the health needs of the patient for whom it was prescribed. Medicines are prescribed after the physician has evaluated the patient's symptoms and has made a diagnosis of the disease or condition that requires medication. The word *prescription* commonly refers to a slip of paper on which the physician's orders are written for the **compounding**, dispensing, or administering of medicines to a particular patient. Prescriptions may be written by health care providers such as physicians, nurse practitioners, and physician's assistants, who are licensed to do so by the medical practice act of their state of practice. The order should always be recorded in the patient's medical record. Although only licensed health care professionals may sign prescriptions, often the allied health professional may be delegated the responsibility of completing the prescription form for signature. The physician ultimately has the responsibility of checking the information for accuracy prior to signing.

Prescription Preparation

Prescription orders should be written on a prescription blank for a pharmacist to fill. Any drug not available as an OTC drug requires a prescription.

The prescription has several parts—four that are required, with other optional information—and should always be written in permanent blue or black ink. Some physicians are now using computer-generated prescription forms for refills, and the physician need only sign these computer-printed blanks. Some physicians prefer blanks that have space for one medication per sheet, whereas others may prefer to use multiple-line prescription blanks (if allowed by state medical practices act) for patients whose conditions require the prescribing of several

medicines at the same time. These blanks eliminate the need to write the patient's name, address, and so forth on more than one order and also save the physician from having to sign each blank. If not all prescription lines on a multiple-line form are used, the unused lines should be crossed through. Physicians should never leave signed prescription blanks that are not prepared for a specific patient.

Some states require a multiple-copy prescription program (MCPP) to deter illegal diversion of drugs. In those states the physician is required to write prescriptions for Schedule II controlled substances in triplicate—one copy for the pharmacist, one for the state drug agency, and one for the physician's records. If multiple-copy prescriptions are not used, many offices make a practice of copying all prescriptions for the medical record for tracing the source of possible errors if needed.

Parts of a Prescription

The following description should be read against the sample prescriptions shown in Figure 5-11, *A* and *B*. The four required components of a prescription are the superscription; inscription; signa, or signature; and subscription.

Line A

Prescriptions are preprinted with the physician's name, address, and phone number.

Line B

The patient heading includes the patient's name and address, the date the prescription was written, and the patient's age, if a child. The date is important because prescriptions must be filled within 12 months of writing, and some prescriptions may be refilled for 12 months after initial filling. Variations of this may occur with individual pharmacies and with state regulations. Prescriptions for Schedule III, IV, and V controlled substances must be filled within 6 months of the original date of the prescription.

Line C

The **superscription** contains the symbol ℞ meaning "take thou" or "recipe."

Line D

The **inscription** specifies the name and strength of the drug or the ingredients and the quantity to be included in each dose. The amount (weight) of

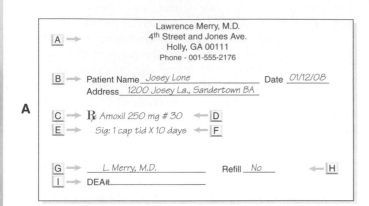

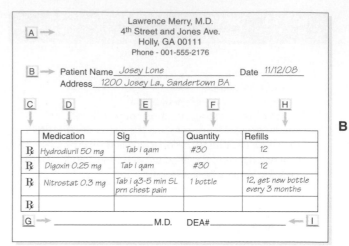

Figure 5-11 Examples of prescription blanks and their components. **A,** Single-line prescription; **B,** multiple-line prescription. The four major components of a prescription are the superscription *(Line C)*; the inscription *(Line D)*; the signa, or signature *(Line E)*; and the subscription *(Line F)*.

the active ingredient shown is in milligrams, grains, or other pharmacologic weight found in each tablet, capsule, or other dosage forms. Weight usually indicates the strength of a medication, whereas a fluid measurement indicates the volume (e.g., milliliters, teaspoons, ounces) of the medication to be taken, administered, or dispensed. If the medicine is an oral liquid, this will be stated as the concentration or weight per fluid volume such as milligrams per milliliter. If it is a topical medication, the strength is indicated by the percentage of the medication in the base.

Line E

The **signa or signature (Sig)** gives the directions to the patient, usually in abbreviations, for taking the medications. The directions should include when the patient is to start and stop the medication and the route of administration.

Line F

The **subscription** designates the number of doses, the quantity to be dispensed, and the form of the drug.

Line G

The physician's signature line is for the signature of the physician. The prescription is not a legal document until the signature has been affixed. If the physician wants the patient to receive a brand-name drug, he or she must write on the prescription, "Dispense as Written," "Brand Necessary," or "Medically Necessary." The permissibility of

substituting generic drugs for brand-name drugs depends on the laws of each state. Many third-party insurers require the use of generic medications if no medical reason is documented for the need of brand-name drugs, and the copay for using brand-name medications is often greater than with a generic drug.

Line H

The **refill** line designates the number of refills permitted. This line should never be left blank. If no refills are designated, either "none" or "0" should be inserted. The use of "12" will allow the prescription to be filled as needed for up to a year. If the permitted refills have not been used within a year of initial filling, any remaining refills are not permitted.

Line I

A line for the Drug Enforcement Administration **(DEA) number** may be found on prescription blanks. This number is required for prescribing controlled substances. To prevent the abuse of controlled drugs, the DEA number should be written only on those prescriptions that require its use and these numbers should not be preprinted. The health professional's state license number is required on the prescription pad for third-party payments in some states.

Prescriptions may also be telephoned or faxed to the pharmacist if the physician requests that the allied health professional do so and if state laws allow. The information provided to the pharmacist over the phone is the same that would be given if the prescription were written. Schedule II medications cannot be phoned in except in certain emergency situations and then only the amount needed for 72 hours can be dispensed. (The phoned-in prescription must be followed with a written prescription within 72 hours.) Before prescriptions are phoned in to the pharmacy, the patient's record should be reviewed by the physician and the refill order or new medication order should be documented in the record. If the physician refuses to prescribe for the patient, this too should be documented, either by the physician or by the allied health professional, showing that the physician refused the request. When phoning in prescriptions, the allied health professional should ask the pharmacist to read back the prescription and confirm that the pharmacist has the correct medication and dosage before concluding the conversation. If there is a chance of misinterpretation or confusion with other medications, the pharmacist should spell the name of the drug.

The allied health professional should maintain patient confidentiality by being sure that any faxed prescription is either placed in the medical record or destroyed. This prevents its improper use or the chance that it will be dispensed twice by mistake. The fax machine should be located in an area accessible only by medical personnel.

IMPORTANT FACTS ABOUT PRESCRIPTIONS

- Prescribing medications and refilling prescriptions are major tasks in a medical office. The role of the allied health professional in the prescription process depends on the legal statutes of the state in which he or she practices.
- Prescriptions are written orders for a drug or treatment that are usually dispensed by a pharmacist. Medication orders may be either written or verbal. They are commonly used in the clinical setting.
- New and refill prescriptions are legal documents and should be recorded in the medical record. Prescriptions may be written by the allied health professional but must be signed by a practitioner licensed to prescribe in the state of practice. All Schedule II medications require a physician's signature.
- Some states allow the allied health professional to relay prescription orders verbally to other health professionals such as pharmacists; other states do not. The law of the state where the person is employed applies.
- The components of a prescription include the superscription, subscription, inscription, signa, physician's signature, refill information, and certain other information such as the need for brand name medication, if applicable.

IMPORTANT FACTS ABOUT PRESCRIPTIONS—*Cont'd*

- A prescription may designate single drug orders or multiple orders on a single sheet. The physician's preference is the determining factor. Some prescriptions are computer generated.
- No lines for writing a prescription should be left blank. If necessary, a line should be drawn through the area not needed for the prescription.

Prescription Refills

Prescription refills may be conveyed to the pharmacy either in writing, such as by a new prescription or by fax, or verbally over the phone. Schedule II medications cannot be refilled but require a new written and signed prescription. For convenience, patients may phone in a request for a prescription to the allied health professional for medications other than Schedule II medications (Box 5-4). A phoned request requires the physician to make decisions about refills on the basis of information obtained during the phone conversation. Pharmacists may also call with requests for refills. In either circumstance, the allied health professional should obtain the patient's medical record for the physician to use in evaluating the medication need. Verbal orders for refills should be written into the medical record immediately, and the physician should confirm all prescriptions prior to phoning in refills.

Often a physician prefers to have patient messages taken and left in a designated place for evaluation at certain times of the day. Many physicians do not want to be disturbed while examining a patient but prefer to review requests for refills either at the end of the morning or the end of the day depending on the office protocol.

To decrease the confusion for patients and pharmacists who call for a prescription, the allied health professional should give an approximate time that

---

BOX 5-4   INFORMATION NEEDED FOR REFILLS

- The date and time of the call
- The pharmacy to be called and its phone number (be sure to obtain the correct location and number for a chain pharmacy)
- The medication desired, its strength, and the last time the prescription was refilled
- How the patient is taking the medication
- A telephone number where the patient can be reached if questions should arise
- Signature of person receiving the request

the person can expect the prescription to be phoned to the pharmacy for dispensing. To ensure the refill will be available when needed, patients should be instructed to call 1 or 2 days before the refill is actually needed. Forty-eight-hour notice of the need for a refill allows time for the office to notify the patient concerning the status of the request.

IMPORTANT INFORMATION ABOUT PRESCRIPTION REFILLS

- Documentation of refills and medication orders must be done in a timely manner as soon as the orders are given.
- Documentation is essential. An undocumented order is legally a nonentity. Remember, "Not charted, not done."
- If samples are given to the patient, these also should be documented in the medical record including the lot number and expiration date and with the directions in case a refill or a prescription is necessary.
- A stenographer's pad for prescription refills near the phone will assist with compliance. One column may be used to take the patient's request in either blue or black ink, and the other column may be used for the physician's response, preferably in another color ink. Using this system, the refill verification is easily viewed.

When the physician reviews the request, he or she may note approval on the request form or may document the refill in the medical record. If the physician has not documented the refill, the allied health professional who calls in the refill should document it immediately. The documentation shows that the order has been conveyed to the pharmacist. The allied health professional should also be sure that all orders have been called in to the pharmacy before the medical record is filed and that all orders have been conveyed before the end of the work day.

If a refill request is denied, the patient should be notified and given instructions for follow-up visits or informed of the physician's concerns. If the physician wants to see the patient, the allied health professional should call the patient, make an appointment for the patient to be seen, and explain why the prescription request was denied.

If the patient uses mail order for prescriptions, two prescriptions will be necessary for new prescriptions—one to be filled at a local pharmacy for use until the mail order prescription can arrive and the other to be sent to the mail order pharmacy for long-term drug dosages. If the prescription is for refills, the patient should allow sufficient time

for the shipment of the medications. Patients who wait until the last minute for obtaining refills of prescriptions may find that doses are missed because of lack of medicine and the therapeutic effect of the medications is diminished. For the patient who consistently waits too long for approval of medication refills, the allied health professional should educate the patient about the timing needed for the entire process.

IMPORTANT DOCUMENTATION ABOUT PRESCRIPTION REFILLS

1. The physician, or in some states nurse practitioners and physician's assistants, are the only persons who may approve a refill request.
2. A refilled prescription is like a new prescription.
3. The physician should indicate the number of allowable refills.
4. The pharmacist, physician, and the allied health professional work as partners to meet the prescription needs of the patient. This triangular process provides checks and balances in prescribing medications.
5. The allied health professional should always check for allergies and adverse reactions of the patient before relaying refill requests, as well as monitoring for therapeutic effects as appropriate.

DID YOU KNOW?

The U. S. Department of Health and Human Services is currently moving full steam ahead to adopt electronic means of prescribing medications (e-prescribing) and keeping electronic health records (EHRs). One of the first steps to be accepted is e-prescribing using databases between health professionals and pharmacies to provide a higher level of patient safety.

Safeguarding Prescription Pads

Prescription pads should be handled carefully and should be safeguarded to prevent unauthorized use. The prescription blank should be designed so that any erasure is immediately apparent. It should also be designed so that it cannot be counterfeited or duplicated by photocopying. Counterfeit proofing may be accomplished by using colored paper, colored ink, or a watermark. Another way to safeguard prescription pads is to use carbonless duplicates. The original copy of the prescription is given to the patient, and the duplicate is placed in the patient's record. Finally, prescription pads should have preprinted numbers so that theft of the contents of a prescription pad can be easily detected and reported. It is good practice to keep all prescription pads locked in a safe place, with only a single pad kept on the physician's person or in a safe place that can only be accessed by office personnel.

Prescription pads should not be left unguarded at any time. Experienced drug abusers and drug seekers can take entire pads or sheets from the pad without being seen. Drug seekers forge prescriptions and take the prescriptions to areas where the physician's handwriting and signature are not readily identified. If the pharmacist becomes suspicious of a forged prescription, he or she will phone the physician's office for verification. The allied health professional should check the medical record to verify any prescription, but he or she should also inform the physician and verify the prescription with the physician if a copy is not in the medical record.

IMPORTANT FACTS ABOUT SAFEGUARDING PRESCRIPTION PADS

- A safe practice for legal protection is to add a copy of all prescriptions to the medical record. If carbonless prescription pads are not used, the allied health professional should photocopy the written prescription. If a multiple-line prescription pad is used, the health professional obliterates the unused lines to prevent alteration of prescriptions.
- Prescription blanks are never to be used as notepads but are used only for writing medication prescriptions. Orders for laboratory tests should be on a laboratory request form, and instructions should be written on memo pads, not prescription pads.
- Prescription pads must be safeguarded against theft and misuse and should be printed to prevent counterfeiting or photocopying of blank sheets.

Prescription blanks should only be used to write prescriptions. They should not be used as notepaper. Orders for anything other than medications should be written on notepaper or memo pads, and laboratory tests should be written on a laboratory request form.

Prescriptions should not be used for ordering stock medicines for the office. Stock bottles should be ordered on a pharmacy order form. On delivery of these medications, the invoice should be checked against the medications received, and the invoice should be filed with the records of the office.

Summary

Allied health professionals have professional responsibilities in reading, interpreting, and documenting medication orders. Their expectations may include writing prescriptions and preparing them for a physician's signature. In some states allied health professionals may be allowed to relay prescriptions verbally to a pharmacist, depending on the medical practices act of that state. To relay medication orders or prescriptions correctly, the allied health professional must know the medications prescribed by the physician. If additional knowledge is necessary, the professional should use reference materials to research drugs. Medication errors can occur because of similarities in drug names; therefore the allied health professional should be careful to repeat all verbal orders to the physician as he or she gives them. In relaying the information, the health professional should ask the pharmacist or nurse (e.g., in an inpatient facility) to repeat the orders.

The allied health professional needs a working knowledge of the parts of a prescription and the abbreviations used in writing a prescription. Refills of prescriptions are a major task in the medical office. Before the physician can evaluate the appropriateness of refill requests, the allied health professional needs to obtain information from the patient concerning any adverse reactions that might have occurred and whether the medications prescribed were taken properly. Proper documentation of refills is an important task of the allied health professional. The allied health professional should also ascertain whether the patient understands the prescribed treatment. This information was covered in previous chapters.

Critical Thinking Exercises

SCENARIO

Dr. Merry asks you to write prescriptions for J. Rex for medications for her arthritis. She takes ibuprofen 600 mg three times a day, at breakfast, in the midafternoon, and at bedtime. The ibuprofen needs to be taken with food, which may be a snack. Dr. Merry wants J. to have a 1-month supply at a time; the prescription may be refilled three times. Also needed is Extra-Strength Tylenol one caplet every 4 to 6 hours as needed for pain. Finally, one Norflex 100 mg tablet to be taken twice a day, at breakfast and bedtime, is prescribed. This should also be for a 1-month supply.

1. What prescriptions need to be written?
2. What documentation should be included in the medical record for these medications?

REVIEW EXERCISES

Using the label shown, answer the following:

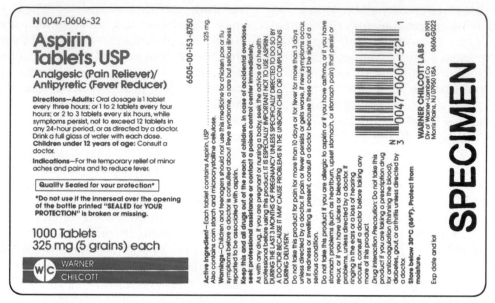

1. What is the generic name? _____

2. What is the trade name? _____

3. What are the storage requirements? _____

4. Who is the manufacturer? _____

5. What cautions are given? _____

6. What is the recommended dosage in a 24-hour period? _____

7. What is the dosage strength? _____

8. What is the manufacturer's NDC code? _____

9. What is the storage container size? _____

10. What is the usual dose? _____

11. What are the warnings given? _____

Reading and Writing Prescriptions

In the following exercises, interpret the order of the physician.

12. Keflex 250 mg #20, Sig: cap i po qid with food

_____

_____

13. Brethine 5 mg #30, Sig: tab i po tid

_____

_____

14. Restoril 15 mg # 30, Sig: cap i hs prn sleep

_____

_____

15. naproxen sodium 275 mg #60, Sig: tab i tid

_____

_____

16. furosemide 20 mg tabs #90, Sig: 40 mg qam and 20 mg @ 1 pm

_____

_____

In the following exercises, write the prescription for signature by the physician. Check a drug reference to be sure the dosage is appropriate. If the dosage is incorrect, make note of that fact.

17. Dr. Merry wants Arthur Rice to have ibuprofen 600 mg tablets four times a day for 10 days for his arthritis. Ibuprofen should be taken after meals and at bedtime with a snack. Decide on the number of tablets needed for compliance. The prescription may be refilled three times.

> Lawrence Merry, M.D.
> 4th Street and Jones Ave.
> Holly, GA 00111
> Phone - 001-555-2176
>
> Patient Name_____   Date _____
> Address_____
>
> R℞
>
>
> _____   Refill _____
> DEA#_____

18. Sara Hurt fell and fractured her leg. Dr. Merry wants her to have a prescription for Tylenol No. 3 for pain. He wants the prescription to allow her 30 tablets, and she may take one or two tablets every 4 to 6 hours as needed for pain. Tylenol No. 3 is a controlled substance.
Dr. Merry's DEA number is AM0000000.

a. Can the prescription be refilled?   Yes   No
b. Can a generic substitute be used?   Yes   No

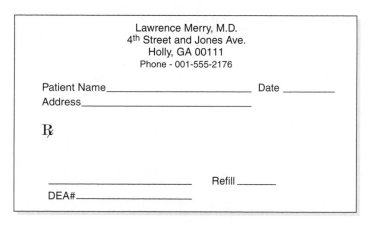

> Lawrence Merry, M.D.
> 4th Street and Jones Ave.
> Holly, GA 00111
> Phone - 001-555-2176
>
> Patient Name_____   Date _____
> Address_____
>
> R℞
>
>
> _____   Refill _____
> DEA#_____

19. Dr. Merry has seen Susie Illy, age 3, for a bacterial upper respiratory tract infection. He wants her to have a prescription for 5 oz of amoxicillin suspension. (Write in the apothecary measure.) She is to be given one teaspoonful three times a day for 10 days, or until all the medication has been taken. No refills are allowed.

```
Lawrence Merry, M.D.
4th Street and Jones Ave.
Holly, GA 00111
Phone - 001-555-2176

Patient Name_____    Date _____
Address_____

Rx


_____    Refill _____
DEA#_____
```

20. Dr. Merry also wants Susie to have some Benadryl for her allergic rhinitis. He orders a bottle of Benadryl elixir for Susie, with orders for her to take half a teaspoonful every 4 to 6 hours for runny nose.

```
Lawrence Merry, M.D.
4th Street and Jones Ave.
Holly, GA 00111
Phone - 001-555-2176

Patient Name_____    Date _____
Address_____

Rx


_____    Refill _____
DEA#_____
```

21. Dr. Merry wants Hy Tension to take Lopressor 50 mg tablets at breakfast and supper for his high blood pressure. Dr. Merry wants 60 tablets dispensed now, with refills for 3 months, but he wants the label to remind Hy to get his blood pressure checked once a week and to call the office if it drops below 130/70 mm Hg.

```
Lawrence Merry, M.D.
4th Street and Jones Ave.
Holly, GA 00111
Phone - 001-555-2176

Patient Name_____    Date _____
Address_____

Rx


_____    Refill _____
DEA#_____
```

Documentation

Document the following exercises as they would appear in a medical record.

22. J. Smith brings the following medicines from other physicians to the office to be included in her medical record:

    a. digoxin 250 micrograms, taken daily at breakfast

    b. indomethacin 25 milligrams, taken three times daily with meals

    c. nifedipine-XL 30 milligrams, taken daily

    d. Lopressor 50 milligrams, one tablet taken at breakfast and again at bedtime

    e. acetaminophen 325 milligrams, one to two tablets taken every 4 to 6 hours as needed for pain.

Mathematics for Pharmacology and Dosage Calculations

CHAPTER 6
Math Review, 98

CHAPTER 7
Measurement Systems and Their Equivalents, 128

CHAPTER 8
Converting Between Measurement Systems, 145

CHAPTER 9
Calculating Doses of Nonparenteral Medications, 164

CHAPTER 10
Calculating Doses of Parenteral Medications, 189

CHAPTER 11
Principles and Calculations in Intravenous Therapy, 205

Math Review

OBJECTIVES

After studying this chapter, you should be capable of doing the following:

- Identifying proper, improper, and equivalent fractions.
- Changing improper fractions to mixed numbers.
- Reducing fractions to lowest terms.
- Finding the lowest common denominator for fractions.
- Adding, subtracting, multiplying, and dividing fractions and mixed numbers.
- Rounding decimals to whole numbers, tenths, hundredths, and thousandths.
- Converting fractions and mixed numbers to decimals.
- Adding, subtracting, multiplying, and dividing decimals.
- Changing percents to decimals.
- Changing decimals to percents.
- Multiplying and dividing percents.
- Using fractions to figure percentages.
- Using proportions to figure percents.

KEY TERMS

Decimal	Lowest common denominator (LCD)	Proper fraction
Denominator	Lowest common multiple (LCM)	Proportion
Dividend	Mixed number	Proportional method
Divisor	Numerator	Quotient
Equivalent fraction	Percent	Ratio
Improper fraction	Product	Reciprocal

CHAPTER 6 PRETEST

FRACTIONS AND MIXED NUMBERS

Write the following as an improper fraction.

1. $4\frac{3}{4} =$ _____

2. $6\frac{1}{2} =$ _____

3. $1\frac{5}{8} =$ _____

4. $2\frac{7}{12} =$ _____

5. $3\frac{2}{3} =$ _____

Convert the following to a mixed number.

6. $\frac{11}{3} =$ _____

7. $\frac{51}{5} =$ _____

8. $\frac{35}{6} =$ _____

9. $\frac{37}{4} =$ _____

10. $\frac{73}{9} =$ _____

CHAPTER 6 PRETEST—cont'd

Simplify the fraction to the lowest terms. The answer will be a whole number.

11. $\dfrac{81}{9} =$ _____

12. $\dfrac{36}{18} =$ _____

13. $\dfrac{27}{3} =$ _____

14. $\dfrac{144}{72} =$ _____

15. $\dfrac{32}{8} =$ _____

Solve by adding or subtracting fractions. Simplify to the lowest terms.

16. $\dfrac{1}{2} + \dfrac{3}{4} + 2\dfrac{5}{6} =$ _____

17. $6 + 3\dfrac{1}{3} - 7 =$ _____

18. $8 - 2\dfrac{3}{4} + 4\dfrac{1}{7} =$ _____

19. $1 + 5\dfrac{1}{6} - 2\dfrac{2}{3} =$ _____

20. $3\dfrac{2}{3} + \dfrac{1}{6} + 4 - \dfrac{2}{5} =$ _____

Solve by multiplying fractions. Simplify to the lowest terms.

21. $4\dfrac{1}{2} \times 6\dfrac{1}{3} =$ _____

22. $3\dfrac{2}{5} \times 7\dfrac{1}{5} =$ _____

23. $5\dfrac{1}{4} \times 2 \times 4 =$ _____

24. $3\dfrac{1}{6} \times \dfrac{1}{7} =$ _____

25. $2\dfrac{1}{3} \times 4\dfrac{2}{3} \times 3 =$ _____

Solve by dividing fractions. Simplify to lowest terms.

26. $\dfrac{4}{5} \div \dfrac{1}{3} =$ _____

27. $6\dfrac{1}{2} \div 5\dfrac{1}{4} =$ _____

28. $7 \div \dfrac{7}{8} =$ _____

29. $3\dfrac{1}{8} \div 2 =$ _____

30. $4\dfrac{1}{3} \div 2\dfrac{1}{5} =$ _____

DECIMALS

Round the decimal to the nearest whole number.

31. $537.64 =$ _____

32. $0.972 =$ _____

33. $1.65 =$ _____

34. $99.25 =$ _____

35. $4.5 =$ _____

Round the decimal to the nearest hundredth.

36. $674.3333 =$ _____

37. $4.790 =$ _____

38. $88.010 =$ _____

39. $1.0010 =$ _____

40. $5000.0016 =$ _____

Convert the fraction to a decimal.

41. $4\dfrac{3}{4} =$ _____

42. $\dfrac{21}{2} =$ _____

43. $6\dfrac{1}{3} =$ _____

44. $8\dfrac{5}{8} =$ _____

45. $\dfrac{25}{4} =$ _____

Solve by adding or subtracting decimals. Round to the nearest tenth.

46. $34.5 + 27 + 15.801 =$ _____

47. $80 - 54.33 + 17.21 =$ _____

48. $72.5 - 66.409 =$ _____

49. $66 + 34.667 + 91.3 =$ _____

50. $54.33 - 16.008 =$ _____

(continued)

CHAPTER 6 PRETEST—cont'd

Solve by multiplying decimals. Round to the nearest thousandth.

51. $7.234 \times 124.35 =$ _____

52. $27 \times .0001 =$ _____

53. $3 \times 2.4501 =$ _____

54. $61.0001 \times 34.75 =$ _____

55. $32.1 \times 64.25 =$ _____

Solve by dividing decimals. Round to the nearest hundredth.

56. $46.35 \div 3 =$ _____

57. $18 \div 5.5 =$ _____

58. $98.5514 \div 88.58 =$ _____

59. $47.5 \div 22 =$ _____

60. $74.25 \div 5.001 =$ _____

PERCENT

Change the decimal to a percent.

61. $0.0157 =$ _____

62. $3.651 =$ _____

63. $4.4 =$ _____

64. $0.050 =$ _____

65. $0.172 =$ _____

Change the percent to a decimal.

66. $1.10\% =$ _____

67. $47.55\% =$ _____

68. $3\% =$ _____

69. $99\% =$ _____

70. $14.88\% =$ _____

Multiply Percents

71. Find 6% of 17 = _____

72. Find 25% of 34 = _____

73. Find 3% of 80 = _____

74. Find 55% of 75 = _____

75. Find 40% of 40 = _____

Divide percents. Round your answer to two decimal places.

76. 3 is what percent of 70? _____

77. 12 is what percent of 60? _____

78. 25 is what percent of 175? _____

79. 4 is what percent of 9? _____

80. 6 is what percent of 40? _____

Solve for the unknown percent.

81. What number is 25% of 84? _____

82. What number is 14% of 50? _____

83. What number is 60% of 70? _____

84. What number is 15% of 500? _____

85. What number is 90% of 90? _____

Solve for the unknown number using proportions.

86. 20 is 60% of what number? _____

87. 45 is 25% of what number? _____

88. 3 is 15% of what number? _____

89. 30 is 40% of what number? _____

90. 48 is 30% of what number? _____

RATIO AND PROPORTION

Solve for x using proportion.

91. $2 : x :: 100 : 300$ _____

92. $1 : 15 :: x : 45$ _____

93. $5 : 100 :: 20 : x$ _____

94. $x : 30 :: 2 : 5$ _____

95. $4 : x :: 8 : 32$ _____

96. $2\frac{1}{2} : 250 :: x : 750$ _____

97. $1 : 320 :: x : 480$ _____

98. $\frac{1}{4} : 500 :: \frac{1}{2} : x$ _____

99. $x : \frac{1}{3} :: 2 : \frac{2}{3}$ _____

100. $1\frac{1}{2} : x :: \frac{1}{2} : 200$ _____

Fractions

Fractions, used in the apothecary system, are a method of writing a whole number that has been divided into parts (e.g., $\frac{1}{2}$, $3\frac{2}{5}$). Fractions are written with a *numerator* (number on the top), a *line* (meaning "divided by"), and a *denominator* (number on the bottom). When a number in the numerator is divided by the same number in the denominator, the equivalent is 1.

> **EXAMPLE 1:** $\frac{2}{2} = 1$; $\frac{3}{3} = 1$; $\frac{12}{12} = 1$, and so forth.

Proper Fractions

With *proper fractions*, the numerator is always a lower number than the denominator.

> **EXAMPLE 2:** $\frac{1}{2}$ **1** is the numerator. **2** is the denominator. Using a pizza as an example, the numerator states how many pieces of pizza have been taken, or a numerator of **1**. The denominator of **2** states how many equal pieces the whole pizza has been divided into, or 2 equal pieces.

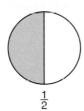

$$\frac{1}{2}$$

> **EXAMPLE 3:** $\frac{5}{6}$ **5** is the numerator and states how many equal pieces of the pizza have been taken. The denominator of **6** states there are six equal pieces to make one whole pizza. So $\frac{5}{6}$ of pizza has been taken.

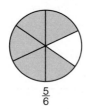

$$\frac{5}{6}$$

Improper Fractions

Improper fractions are fractions in which the numerator is equal to or greater than the denominator.

A whole number is formed when the numerator and denominator are the same or the numerator can be divided evenly by the denominator. A whole number plus a fraction occurs when the numerator is not divided evenly by the denominator and a fractional portion is a remainder.

> **EXAMPLE 4:** If a pizza is cut into 8 equal pieces and we take all 8 pieces, the improper fraction to express this is $\frac{8}{8}$. The whole number would be 1.

Two pizzas would be needed to increase the numerator to a number larger than 8. With two pizzas, each being equally cut into 8 pieces, there are now 16 possible numerators (eight pieces from one pizza and eight pieces from the second pizza).

> **EXAMPLE 5:** Two pizzas cut into 8 pieces are available, and you take 11 pieces. The improper fraction to describe the pizza taken would be $\frac{11}{8}$.

Equivalent Fractions

Equivalent fractions show two or more different fractions that have the same portion of the whole. The fractions have different numerical values but are equivalents, such as $\frac{1}{2}$ and $\frac{2}{4}$.

> **EXAMPLE 6:** One pizza can be divided into any number of equal pieces, such as 6 pieces, 8 pieces, or even 12 pieces.

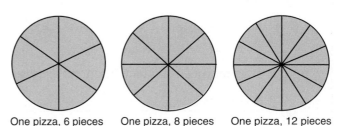

One pizza, 6 pieces   One pizza, 8 pieces   One pizza, 12 pieces

The equivalent fractions in this example are $\frac{6}{6}$, $\frac{8}{8}$, and $\frac{12}{12}$. If each pizza is divided into two equal halves, the equivalent fractions would now be shown as $\frac{3}{6}$, $\frac{4}{8}$, and $\frac{6}{12}$.

Simplifying Fractions to the Lowest Term

Fractions should be reduced to the lowest terms, or simplified. To simplify a fraction, divide the numerator and denominator by the largest number that divides evenly into both.

> **EXAMPLE 7:** The fraction $\frac{3}{6}$ can be simplified to its lowest terms by dividing the numerator and denominator by 3:

$$\frac{3}{6} \div \frac{3}{3} = \frac{1}{2}$$

And the largest number that will equally divide into $\frac{4}{8}$ is 4:

$$\frac{4}{8} \div \frac{4}{4} = \frac{1}{2}$$

Finally, to simplify $\frac{6}{12}$, the largest number to divide by is 6:

$$\frac{6}{12} \div \frac{6}{6} = \frac{1}{2}$$

Equivalent fractions (equal fractions) can be simplified to the same fraction.

In this example, the fractions $\frac{3}{6}, \frac{4}{8}$, and $\frac{6}{12}$ are called equivalent (or *equal*) fractions because when divided by the largest number possible, they are all simplified to the same final fraction of $\frac{1}{2}$. Therefore it can be stated that $\frac{3}{6} = \frac{4}{8} = \frac{6}{12} = \frac{1}{2}$.

> **EXAMPLE 8:**

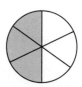

$\frac{3}{6} = \frac{1}{2}$ of the pizza

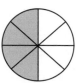

$\frac{4}{8} = \frac{1}{2}$ of the pizza

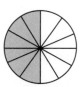

$\frac{6}{12} = \frac{1}{2}$ of the pizza

CHECK YOUR UNDERSTANDING—FRACTIONS   6-1

Identify each fraction; write (P) for a proper fraction, (I) for an improper fraction, or (E) for an equivalent fraction.

1. $\frac{4}{4} = $ _____

2. $\frac{12}{10} = $ _____

3. $\frac{6}{5} = $ _____

4. $\frac{1}{2} = $ _____

5. $\frac{3}{3} = $ _____

6. $\frac{11}{5} = $ _____

7. $\frac{3}{4} = $ _____

8. $\frac{20}{30} = $ _____

9. $\frac{1}{1} = $ _____

10. $\frac{2}{1} = $ _____

Change to as many equivalent fractions as possible.

11. $\frac{30}{90} = $ _____

12. $\frac{6}{24} = $ _____

13. $\frac{15}{60} = $ _____

14. $\frac{8}{32} = $ _____

15. $\frac{10}{40} = $ _____

Improper Fractions and Mixed Numbers

Improper fractions are those in which the numerator is greater than the denominator, or if two or more whole pizzas are equally divided and a portion is taken, an improper fraction can be formed. Improper fractions can be simplified to show how many whole pizzas + partial pizzas (pieces of pizza) exist. When this is simplified and written with a whole number and a fraction, the result is called a *mixed number*.

EXAMPLE **9:** In Example 4 there are two pizzas that were each cut into 8 pieces, and 11 pieces were already taken.

The improper fraction of $\frac{11}{8}$ can be simplified to $1\frac{3}{8}$, meaning one whole pizza plus three pieces of the second pizza were gone.

Remember to keep the 8 as the denominator because both pizzas are cut into 8 pieces.

Therefore the improper fraction is $\frac{11}{8}$, and the mixed number is $1\frac{3}{8}$.

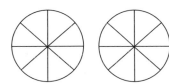

2 pizzas, each cut into 8 equal pieces

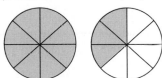

8 pieces + 3 pieces = 11 pieces

EXAMPLE **10:** Always simplify the fraction to its lowest possible term. If we had taken 12 pieces of pizza from Example 4, the improper fraction would be $\frac{12}{8}$ and the mixed number would be $1\frac{4}{8}$, which can be simplified to $1\frac{1}{2}$.

The mixed number for $\frac{12}{8} = 1\frac{1}{2}$ (one whole pizza and $\frac{1}{2}$ of the second pizza).

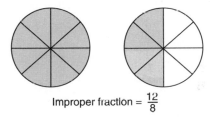

Improper fraction = $\frac{12}{8}$

Adding Fractions and Mixed Numbers with the Same Denominator

To add fractions with the same denominator, add all the numerators of the fraction, then carry forward the denominator. Be sure to simplify improper fractions and mixed numbers to their lowest terms.

EXAMPLE **11:** Solve $\frac{1}{4} + \frac{2}{4} = ?$

The denominators are the same, so

$$\frac{1}{4} + \frac{2}{4} = \frac{3}{4}.$$

CHECK YOUR UNDERSTANDING—MIXED NUMBERS   6-2

Change the improper fraction to a mixed number.

1. $\frac{14}{3} =$ _____

2. $\frac{19}{2} =$ _____

3. $\frac{31}{5} =$ _____

4. $\frac{72}{4} =$ _____

5. $\frac{55}{7} =$ _____

6. $\frac{69}{8} =$ _____

(continued)

CHECK YOUR UNDERSTANDING—MIXED NUMBERS (cont'd)   6-2

7. $\dfrac{25}{6} =$ _____

8. $\dfrac{74}{9} =$ _____

9. $\dfrac{19}{3} =$ _____

10. $\dfrac{23}{8} =$ _____

Change the mixed number into an improper fraction.

11. $1\dfrac{2}{5} =$ _____

12. $13\dfrac{3}{4} =$ _____

13. $6\dfrac{1}{2} =$ _____

14. $2\dfrac{5}{6} =$ _____

15. $4\dfrac{5}{6} =$ _____

16. $2\dfrac{3}{11} =$ _____

17. $17\dfrac{1}{4} =$ _____

18. $16\dfrac{3}{5} =$ _____

19. $5\dfrac{7}{10} =$ _____

20. $70\dfrac{1}{3} =$ _____

Simplify to lowest terms and show as a mixed number.

21. $\dfrac{70}{8} =$ _____

22. $\dfrac{50}{24} =$ _____

23. $\dfrac{26}{6} =$ _____

24. $\dfrac{30}{4} =$ _____

25. $\dfrac{35}{10} =$ _____

26. $\dfrac{75}{9} =$ _____

27. $\dfrac{30}{20} =$ _____

28. $\dfrac{10}{4} =$ _____

29. $\dfrac{70}{16} =$ _____

30. $\dfrac{52}{14} =$ _____

Before a mixed number can be used, it often has to be changed into an improper fraction. To do this, you need to know how to add fractions.

Recall that any number divided by itself is equal to 1 ($\dfrac{8}{8} = 1$).

EXAMPLE 12: Change $3\dfrac{1}{4}$ into an improper fraction.

STEP 1: Change the whole number into equivalent fractions:

$$3 = \dfrac{4}{4} + \dfrac{4}{4} + \dfrac{4}{4} \text{ (same as saying}$$
$$3 = 1 + 1 + 1, \text{ because } \dfrac{4}{4} = 1)$$

STEP 2: Add the numerators of the fractions and carry forward the denominator.

$$\dfrac{4}{4} + \dfrac{4}{4} + \dfrac{4}{4} + \dfrac{1}{4} = \dfrac{13}{4} \ (4 + 4 + 4 + 1 = 13)$$

Therefore $3\dfrac{1}{4}$ is equivalent to the improper fraction $\dfrac{13}{4}$.

Adding Fractions and Mixed Numbers with Different Denominators

Often the denominators are not the same, so additional steps are necessary because the lowest common denominator must be found before solving. For example, suppose there are two pizzas. The first pizza is cut into five equal pieces, and the second pizza is cut into eight pieces.

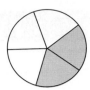 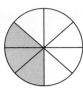

1 pizza, 5 pieces   1 pizza, 8 pieces

If two pieces are taken from the first pizza, the fraction is $\frac{2}{5}$. If three pieces are taken from the second pizza, the fraction is $\frac{3}{8}$. The total amount taken from the two pizzas can be determined by adding $\frac{2}{5} + \frac{3}{8}$.

EXAMPLE 13: Solve: $\frac{2}{5} + \frac{3}{8} = ?$

> STEP 1: Make both denominators the same.

Do this by finding the smallest number that each denominator will divide into without leaving any remainder. This is called finding the lowest common denominator (LCD). The number must be the same for both fractions and must be a multiple of the original denominator. Because $5 \times 8 = 40$, see if any number smaller than 40 can be divided by both 5 and 8 (the denominators). This method is also called finding the least common multiple (LCM).

Do the math:

$5 \times 1 = 5$	$8 \times 1 = 8$
$5 \times 2 = 10$	$8 \times 2 = 16$
$5 \times 3 = 15$	$8 \times 3 = 24$
$5 \times 4 = 20$	$8 \times 4 = 32$
$5 \times 5 = 25$	$8 \times 5 = 40$
$5 \times 6 = 30$	
$5 \times 7 = 35$	
$5 \times 8 = 40$	

By doing the math, we can verify that no number smaller than 40 divides equally into both denominators (5 and 8); therefore 40 is the LCD.
Replace each denominator with the number 40.

$$\frac{2}{5} = \frac{?}{40} \quad \text{and} \quad \frac{3}{8} = \frac{?}{40}$$

> STEP 1a: Write the first fraction: $\frac{2}{5} = \frac{?}{40}$

> STEP 1b: Solve for ? by dividing the denominator into 40.

Do the math: $40 \div 5 = 8$

> STEP 1c: Take the answer from step 1b and multiply it by the numerator.

Do the math: $8 \times 2 = 16$

The first new equivalent fraction is $\frac{2}{5} = \frac{16}{40}$.

Recall in Example 3, that $\frac{8}{8}$ is the same as 1. Here is another way to do the math:

$$\frac{2}{5} \times \frac{8}{8} = \frac{16}{40}$$

Continue this step by taking the second fraction and repeating steps 1a, 1b, and 1c.

> STEP 1a: Write the second fraction:
> $$\frac{3}{8} = \frac{?}{40}$$

> STEP 1b: Solve for ? by dividing the denominator into 40: $40 \div 8 = 5$

> STEP 1c: Take the answer from step 1b and multiply it by the numerator.

Do the math: $3 \times 5 = 15$

The second new equivalent fraction is

$$\frac{3}{8} = \frac{15}{40}.$$

> STEP 2: Add the numerators, and carry forward the like denominators.
> $$\frac{16}{40} + \frac{15}{40} = \frac{31}{40}$$
> Therefore :
> $$\frac{2}{5} + \frac{3}{8} = \frac{31}{40}$$

> STEP 3: Simplify your final answer if possible. In this example, the answer $\frac{31}{40}$ cannot be further simplified.

EXAMPLE 14: Simplify the fraction to the lowest form in the following problem:

$$\frac{1}{5} + \frac{3}{10}$$

$$\frac{1}{5} + \frac{3}{10} = \frac{2}{10} + \frac{3}{10} = \frac{5}{10} \div \frac{5}{5} = \frac{1}{2}$$

Subtracting Fractions

Subtracting fractions uses the same steps to find the LCD as adding fractions.

CHECK YOUR UNDERSTANDING—ADDING FRACTIONS   6-3

Find the lowest common denominator for the two fractions.

1. $\frac{2}{5}, \frac{3}{8} = $ _____

2. $\frac{1}{2}, \frac{3}{7} = $ _____

3. $\frac{3}{4}, \frac{1}{6} = $ _____

4. $\frac{1}{5}, \frac{2}{3} = $ _____

5. $\frac{5}{6}, \frac{4}{7} = $ _____

6. $\frac{1}{4}, \frac{1}{5} = $ _____

7. $\frac{2}{3}, \frac{1}{6} = $ _____

8. $\frac{1}{9}, \frac{1}{10} = $ _____

9. $\frac{2}{5}, \frac{5}{7} = $ _____

10. $\frac{1}{2}, \frac{3}{4} = $ _____

Add the fractions. Simplify your answer if possible.

11. $\frac{1}{2} + \frac{3}{4} = $ _____

12. $\frac{5}{6} + \frac{1}{4} = $ _____

13. $\frac{1}{8} + \frac{1}{4} = $ _____

14. $\frac{2}{3} + \frac{5}{8} = $ _____

15. $\frac{1}{7} + \frac{1}{5} = $ _____

16. $\frac{2}{5} + \frac{5}{6} = $ _____

17. $\frac{1}{4} + \frac{2}{7} = $ _____

18. $\frac{4}{5} + \frac{1}{6} = $ _____

19. $\frac{1}{3} + \frac{4}{7} = $ _____

20. $\frac{6}{7} + \frac{3}{5} = $ _____

EXAMPLE 15: Solve $\frac{5}{6} - \frac{1}{2} = ?$

STEP 1: Make both denominators the same. The LCD for the denominators of 6 and 2 is 6. $\frac{5}{6}$ does not change; $\frac{1}{2}$ becomes $\frac{3}{6}$.

STEP 2: Subtract the numerators and carry forward the like denominators:

$$\frac{5}{6} - \frac{3}{6} = \frac{2}{6}$$

STEP 3: Simplify the final fraction if possible. $\frac{2}{6}$ can be simplified to $\frac{1}{3}$.

STEP 1: Change $1\frac{1}{2}$ to an improper fraction (see Example 13):

$$1\frac{1}{2} = \frac{3}{2}$$

STEP 2: Make the denominators the same LCD (4 in this case):

$$\frac{3}{2} = \frac{6}{4} \text{ and } \frac{3}{4}$$

STEP 3: Subtract the numerators and simplify the answer if possible:

$$\frac{6}{4} - \frac{3}{4} = \frac{3}{4}$$

Subtracting Fractions and Mixed Numbers

Subtracting fractions that use mixed numbers requires you to first change the mixed number into an improper fraction.

EXAMPLE 16: Solve $1\frac{1}{2} - \frac{3}{4} = ?$

Multiplying Fractions

To multiply two fractions, first multiply the two numerators, then multiply the two denominators. Simplify your answer if possible.

EXAMPLE 17: Solve $\frac{1}{4} \times \frac{2}{5}$

CHECK YOUR UNDERSTANDING—SUBTRACTING FRACTIONS AND MIXED NUMBERS

6-4

Find the LCD, then subtract. Simplify answer if possible.

1. $\dfrac{4}{7} - \dfrac{1}{4} =$ _____

2. $\dfrac{5}{6} - \dfrac{1}{3} =$ _____

3. $\dfrac{7}{8} - \dfrac{1}{4} =$ _____

4. $\dfrac{9}{10} - \dfrac{1}{3} =$ _____

5. $\dfrac{5}{9} - \dfrac{2}{7} =$ _____

6. $\dfrac{3}{4} - \dfrac{1}{8} =$ _____

7. $\dfrac{5}{8} - \dfrac{3}{16} =$ _____

8. $\dfrac{5}{7} - \dfrac{1}{12} =$ _____

9. $\dfrac{2}{3} - \dfrac{1}{6} =$ _____

10. $\dfrac{7}{8} - \dfrac{3}{5} =$ _____

Change the mixed numbers into improper fractions, then subtract. Simplify answer to lowest terms if necessary.

11. $16\dfrac{1}{2} - 4\dfrac{1}{3} =$ _____

12. $1\dfrac{3}{8} - \dfrac{1}{2} =$ _____

13. $12\dfrac{1}{4} - 6\dfrac{5}{7}$ _____

14. $5\dfrac{1}{5} - 4\dfrac{1}{4} =$ _____

15. $9\dfrac{1}{8} - 7\dfrac{2}{3} =$ _____

16. $3\dfrac{3}{8} - 1\dfrac{5}{16} =$ _____

17. $4\dfrac{1}{4} - 2\dfrac{1}{2} =$ _____

18. $10\dfrac{7}{8} - 8\dfrac{5}{6} =$ _____

19. $6\dfrac{1}{6} - 5\dfrac{4}{5} =$ _____

20. $14\dfrac{1}{3} - 12\dfrac{3}{4} -$ _____

STEP 1: Rewrite as $\dfrac{1 \times 2}{4 \times 5} =$

STEP 2: Multiply the numerators, then the denominators

$1 \times 2 = \mathbf{2}$ and $4 \times 5 = \mathbf{20,}$

so the fraction is written as: $\dfrac{2}{20}$

STEP 3: Simplify answer if possible.

$\dfrac{2}{20} = \dfrac{1}{10}$

Use the following shortcuts to save time in obtaining the answer.

Shortcut: When changing a mixed number to an improper fraction, multiply the whole number and denominator, then add the numerator to obtain the improper fraction.

Shortcut: Cancel any numerator and denominator that can be divided equally by the same number. In the above problem, the canceling would be as follows: $\dfrac{1}{\cancel{4}} \times \dfrac{\cancel{2}^{1}}{5}$. Therefore the answer will be $\dfrac{1}{2} \times \dfrac{1}{5}$ or $\dfrac{1}{10}$.

Multiplying Mixed Numbers

EXAMPLE 18: Solve $4\dfrac{1}{10} \times 5 = ?$

STEP 1: Change $4\dfrac{1}{10}$ to an improper fraction and 5 to an improper fraction:

$4\dfrac{1}{10} = \dfrac{41}{10}$

(instead of $\dfrac{10}{10} + \dfrac{10}{10} + \dfrac{10}{10} + \dfrac{10}{10} + \dfrac{1}{10} = \dfrac{41}{10}$, multiply $4 \times 10 + 1 = \dfrac{41}{10}$)

Then change 5 to an improper fraction, by placing the 5 over the 1 or $\dfrac{5}{1}$.

STEP 2: Cancel (if possible) any numerators with denominators:

$\dfrac{41}{10} \times \dfrac{5}{1} = \dfrac{41}{\underset{2}{\cancel{10}}} \times \dfrac{\cancel{5}^{1}}{1} = \dfrac{41}{2} \times \dfrac{1}{1}$

CHECK YOUR UNDERSTANDING—MULTIPLYING FRACTIONS AND MIXED NUMBERS

6-5

Cancel the numerator and denominator that can be divided equally by the same number, then multiply.

1. $\dfrac{2}{3} \times \dfrac{3}{4} =$ _____

2. $\dfrac{5}{6} \times \dfrac{8}{8} =$ _____

3. $\dfrac{1}{5} \times \dfrac{5}{8} =$ _____

4. $\dfrac{10}{12} \times \dfrac{1}{2} =$ _____

5. $\dfrac{1}{4} \times \dfrac{2}{7} =$ _____

Change the whole number into a fraction.

6. $17 =$ _____

7. $6 =$ _____

8. $4 =$ _____

9. $12 =$ _____

10. $3 =$ _____

Multiply, then simplify the answer if possible.

11. $\dfrac{1}{3} \times 2 \times \dfrac{5}{8} =$ _____

12. $2\dfrac{1}{2} \times 3\dfrac{1}{2} \times 6 =$ _____

13. $4 \times 1\dfrac{3}{4} \times \dfrac{1}{9} =$ _____

14. $1\dfrac{5}{16} \times 3 \times 4 =$ _____

15. $\dfrac{2}{5} \times 3\dfrac{3}{4} \times 8 =$ _____

16. $2\dfrac{5}{7} \times 1 \times 3\dfrac{3}{7} =$ _____

17. $\dfrac{1}{4} \times \dfrac{2}{3} \times \dfrac{1}{2} =$ _____

18. $3\dfrac{1}{3} \times 11 \times 2\dfrac{1}{4} =$ _____

19. $2\dfrac{1}{5} \times 2\dfrac{1}{4} \times 2\dfrac{2}{3} =$ _____

20. $4 \times \dfrac{11}{12} \times 3 =$ _____

STEP 3: Multiply across the numerator line and denominator line to solve:

$$\frac{41 \times 1}{2 \times 1} = \frac{41}{2}$$

STEP 4: Simplify the fraction, and change it into a mixed number if possible:

$$\frac{41}{2} = 20\frac{1}{2}$$

EXAMPLE 19: Solve: $\dfrac{2}{3} \times 3 \times 2\dfrac{3}{4} = ?$

STEP 1: Change to improper fractions:

$$\frac{2}{3} \times \frac{3}{1} \times \frac{11}{4} =$$

STEP 2: Simplify numerators with denominators:

$$\frac{\overset{1}{\cancel{2}}}{\underset{1}{\cancel{3}}} \times \frac{\overset{1}{\cancel{3}}}{1} \times \frac{11}{\underset{2}{\cancel{4}}} = \frac{1}{1} \times \frac{1}{1} \times \frac{11}{2}$$

STEP 3: Multiply across to solve:

$$\frac{1 \times 1 \times 11}{1 \times 1 \times 2} = \frac{11}{2}$$

STEP 4: Change to a mixed number and simplify if possible:

$$\frac{11}{2} = 5\frac{1}{2}$$

Dividing Fractions

When dividing fractions, invert the second fraction (use the reciprocal) and then multiply the two fractions. The *reciprocal* of a fraction is the inversion of a fraction, or the fraction "flipped" or inverted. The reciprocal of $\dfrac{1}{2} = \dfrac{2}{1}$, the reciprocal of $\dfrac{3}{4} = \dfrac{4}{3}$, the reciprocal of $\dfrac{11}{20} = \dfrac{20}{11}$, and so forth. Simplify your answer after multiplication if possible, and write answer as a mixed number.

EXAMPLE 20: Solve: $\frac{3}{4} \div \frac{1}{2} = ?$

STEP 1: Find the reciprocal of the second fraction and change division sign to multiplication sign:

$$\frac{3}{4} \div \frac{1}{2} \text{ becomes } \frac{3}{4} \times \frac{2}{1}$$

STEP 2: Cancel the numerators and denominators that divide evenly

$$\frac{3}{\cancel{4}_2} \times \frac{\cancel{2}^1}{1}$$

STEP 3: Multiply across to solve:

$$\frac{3}{2} \times \frac{1}{1} = \frac{3}{2}$$

STEP 4: Simplify the fraction if possible, then change it to a mixed number.

$$\frac{3}{2} = 1\frac{1}{2}$$

Dividing Mixed Numbers

To divide fractions that include mixed numbers, the mixed number must first be changed to an improper fraction. Next, write whole numbers as a fraction, and solve by inverting the second fraction and multiplying. Simplify if necessary.

EXAMPLE 21: Solve: $3\frac{5}{8} \div 2\frac{1}{2} = ?$

STEP 1: Change to improper fractions:

$$3\frac{5}{8} = \frac{29}{8} \text{ and } 2\frac{1}{2} = \frac{5}{2}$$

The problem now looks like this:

$$\frac{29}{8} \div \frac{5}{2} =$$

STEP 2: Invert the second fraction, and change the sign from division to multiplication.

$$\frac{29}{8} \times \frac{2}{5} = ?$$

STEP 3: Cancel the numerators and denominators that divide evenly:

$$\frac{29}{\cancel{8}_4} \times \frac{\cancel{2}^1}{5} = \frac{29}{4} \times \frac{1}{5}$$

STEP 4: Multiply across to solve:

$$\frac{29}{4} \times \frac{1}{5} = \frac{29}{20}$$

STEP 5: Simplify the fraction if possible, then change it to a mixed number:

$$\frac{29}{20} = 1\frac{9}{20}$$

CHECK YOUR UNDERSTANDING—DIVIDING FRACTIONS AND MIXED NUMBERS

6-6

Change the mixed number to an improper fraction.

1. $3\frac{4}{5} = $ _____

2. $7\frac{1}{8} = $ _____

3. $1\frac{1}{4} = $ _____

4. $4\frac{1}{2} = $ _____

5. $10\frac{1}{5} = $ _____

Divide, then simplify the answer if possible.

6. $4\frac{2}{5} \div \frac{1}{3} = $ _____

7. $3\frac{2}{3} \div \frac{1}{3} = $ _____

8. $7 \div 2\frac{5}{8} = $ _____

9. $5\frac{4}{9} \div 2\frac{1}{3} = $ _____

10. $2\frac{1}{2} \div 4 = $ _____

11. $4 \div \frac{5}{6} = $ _____

12. $6\frac{1}{2} \div 2\frac{3}{4} = $ _____

13. $8\frac{5}{9} \div 6\frac{1}{3} = $ _____

14. $1\frac{1}{36} \div \frac{5}{8} = $ _____

15. $10\frac{1}{5} \div 1\frac{1}{4} = $ _____

CHECK YOUR UNDERSTANDING—FRACTION REVIEW   6-7

Change to improper fractions.

1. $3\frac{1}{2} =$ _____

2. $2\frac{1}{4} =$ _____

3. $1 =$ _____

4. $1\frac{2}{5} =$ _____

5. $2\frac{1}{3} =$ _____

Change to as many equivalent fractions as possible.

6. $\frac{4}{8} =$ _____

7. $\frac{6}{12} =$ _____

8. $\frac{10}{25} =$ _____

9. $\frac{8}{24} =$ _____

10. $\frac{17}{51} =$ _____

Change to mixed numbers.

11. $\frac{11}{8} =$ _____

12. $\frac{14}{3} =$ _____

13. $\frac{9}{5} =$ _____

14. $\frac{7}{2} =$ _____

15. $\frac{7}{4} =$ _____

Simplify to the lowest terms.

16. $\frac{15}{6} =$ _____

17. $\frac{20}{6} =$ _____

18. $\frac{27}{4} =$ _____

19. $\frac{18}{12} =$ _____

20. $\frac{12}{9} =$ _____

Add; then simplify to lowest possible term.

21. $2\frac{1}{2} + \frac{1}{4} =$ _____

22. $\frac{5}{8} + \frac{2}{3} =$ _____

23. $\frac{1}{3} + 1\frac{1}{2} =$ _____

24. $2\frac{1}{2} + \frac{1}{4} =$ _____

25. $6 + 1\frac{3}{8} =$ _____

Subtract; then simplify to lowest possible term.

26. $7 - 2\frac{1}{3} =$ _____

27. $2\frac{1}{2} - \frac{1}{8} =$ _____

28. $4\frac{1}{2} - 3\frac{2}{3} =$ _____

29. $2\frac{5}{8} - \frac{3}{4} =$ _____

30. $\frac{2}{3} - \frac{1}{4} =$ _____

Multiply; then simplify to lowest possible term.

31. $2 \times \frac{1}{8} \times \frac{3}{4} =$ _____

32. $5 \times \frac{1}{2} \times 7 =$ _____

33. $2\frac{5}{8} \times 4 \times \frac{1}{3} =$ _____

34. $3\frac{2}{5} \times \frac{4}{7} \times \frac{1}{2} =$ _____

35. $\frac{2}{3} \times \frac{1}{2} \times \frac{3}{8} =$ _____

Divide; then simplify to lowest possible term.

36. $4\frac{1}{3} \div 3 =$ _____

37. $6\frac{2}{5} \div 4\frac{1}{2} =$ _____

38. $4\frac{3}{4} \div 1\frac{1}{2} =$ _____

39. $5 \div \frac{1}{2} =$ _____

40. $4 \div 2\frac{1}{2} =$ _____

Decimals

Decimals are used to show a fractional part of a number. Metric measurements are expressed as decimals.

Decimal places appear to the right of a whole number that is followed by a decimal point to indicate a number less than 1. If no digit is to the left of the decimal point, a zero must be inserted in the medical field to prevent errors (e.g., 0.5).

EXAMPLE **22:** 432.1568

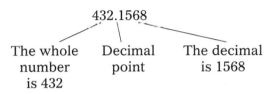

The whole   Decimal   The decimal
number   point   is 1568
is 432

A decimal can be converted to a mixed number or fraction by dropping the decimal point, using the following rules:

The digits to the left of the decimal point remain a whole number.

The digits to the right of the decimal point become the numerator of the fraction.

The denominator, when using decimals, becomes a power of 10, with one zero for each number or decimal place to the right of the decimal point.

EXAMPLE **23:** Convert 66.78 to a mixed number. 66 is the whole number.

78 becomes the numerator.

100 is the denominator because 78 is two places to the right of the decimal point, indicating hundredths.

The mixed number is $66\frac{78}{100}$.

 LEARNING TIP
The decimal point acts as one place in the decimal.

Rounding Decimals

Decimals can be rounded to the nearest whole number or multiples of 10, usually in 10ths, 100ths, or 1000ths. Rounding shortens a decimal by dropping one or more digits after the decimal point (e.g., 0.76 = 0.8 when rounding to tenths).

When rounding to a whole number, the digit 5 will determine how rounding will occur. If the last digit to the right of the decimal is less than 5, the whole number does not change and the digits after the decimal point are dropped. For example, to round 76.4 to a whole number, the whole number would remain 76. To round to places in the decimal, choose the place, such as tenth or hundredth, and follow the rule of rounding using 5 as the decision point. To round to hundredths, 16.444 would be rounded to 16.44.

When the decimal is 5 or larger, drop the decimal but increase the whole number to the next whole number. For example, to round 76.5 to a whole number, the whole number would be 77 and the .5 is dropped. If rounding to hundredths, 88.876 would be rounded to 88.88.

EXAMPLE **24:** Round the following decimals to thousandths:

942.0099 ⟶ 942.010 (in this case, the final zero would be dropped, and the answer would be 942.01)

3.6666 ⟶ 3.667

0.9875 ⟶ 0.988

EXAMPLE **25:** Round the following decimals to hundredths:

78.754 ⟶ 78.75

9.553 ⟶ 9.55

100.4893 ⟶ 100.49

EXAMPLE **26:** Round the following decimals to tenths:

88.569 ⟶ 88.6

12.69 ⟶ 12.7

92.385 ⟶ 92.4

Converting Fractions to Decimals

To convert a proper fraction to a decimal, divide the numerator by the denominator. The answer will be a fraction of a whole number, or a decimal.

EXAMPLE **27:** Convert the fraction $\frac{4}{5}$ to a decimal.

CHECK YOUR UNDERSTANDING—ROUNDING DECIMALS   6-8

Round the decimal to the nearest whole number.

1. 0.8 = _____

2. 42.35 = _____

3. 0.95 = _____

4. 100.41 = _____

5. 67.6 = _____

Round the decimal to the nearest tenth.

6. 33.67 = _____

7. 56.78 = _____

8. 54.11 = _____

9. 121.334 = _____

10. 600.707= _____

Round the decimal to the nearest hundredth.

11. 233.332 = _____

12. 19.5726 = _____

13. 88.8883 = _____

14. 78.654 = _____

15. 100.0593 = _____

Round the decimal to the nearest thousandth.

16. 400.0099 = _____

17. 234.5574 = _____

18. 1616.1616 = _____

19. 357.9753 = _____

20. 357.9758 = _____

STEP 1: Divide the numerator by the denominator. Add the number 0 as many times as necessary. (In the example, 5 will not divide into 4, but 5 will divide into 40, so one 0 is added). Before adding a 0 in the numerator, place a decimal point behind the numerator number. Then move the decimal point to the same place on the equivalent (answer) line.

$$5 \overline{)\begin{array}{c} 0. \\ 4. \end{array}} = 0 \quad \text{(5 does not go into 4, so add a zero)}$$

$$5 \overline{)\begin{array}{c} 0.8 \\ 4.0 \\ \underline{4.0} \\ 0 \end{array}} = 0 \quad \text{(Because a zero was added, the answer will have a decimal point)}$$

For each 0 added, the decimal point is moved to the **left** one space past the decimal point.

So the answer is not 8, it is 0.8. Remember any number that is a decimal should show 0 before the decimal point if a whole number is not present in that place.

Therefore, $\frac{4}{5} = 0.8$ (not .8)

When an improper fraction is converted to a decimal, the answer will contain a whole number and a remainder (the remainder is shown as a decimal).

EXAMPLE **28:** Convert the improper fraction $\frac{21}{5}$ to a decimal.

STEP 1: The number 5 will go into 21 four times with a remainder of 1. Be sure the decimal is in the correct place.

$$5 \overline{)\begin{array}{c} 4. \\ 21.0 \\ \underline{-20} \\ 1 \end{array}} \quad \text{(5 will not go into 1, so add a zero)}$$

$$5 \overline{)\begin{array}{c} 4.2 \\ 21.0 \\ \underline{-20} \\ 10 \\ \underline{-10} \\ 0 \end{array}} \quad \text{(Because a zero was added, the answer will have a decimal point)}$$

$$\frac{21}{5} \text{ or } 5 \overline{)21} = 4.2$$

To convert a mixed number to a decimal, first change the mixed number to an improper fraction. Repeat the math in example 27 to convert the answer to a decimal.

CHECK YOUR UNDERSTANDING—CONVERTING FRACTIONS TO DECIMALS
6-9

Convert the proper fraction to a decimal.
Round your answer to the nearest thousandth.

1. $\dfrac{5}{8} =$ _____

2. $\dfrac{3}{4} =$ _____

3. $\dfrac{1}{6} =$ _____

4. $\dfrac{2}{3} =$ _____

5. $\dfrac{3}{8} =$ _____

Convert the improper fraction to a decimal,
round answer to the nearest tenth.

6. $\dfrac{21}{2} =$ _____

7. $\dfrac{17}{9} =$ _____

8. $\dfrac{14}{5} =$ _____

9. $\dfrac{8}{3} =$ _____

10. $\dfrac{10}{7} =$ _____

Convert the mixed number to a decimal,
round to the nearest hundredth.

11. $3\dfrac{1}{2} =$ _____

12. $6\dfrac{2}{5} =$ _____

13. $4\dfrac{3}{4} =$ _____

14. $5\dfrac{7}{9} =$ _____

15. $2\dfrac{7}{11} =$ _____

Adding and Subtracting Decimals

To add or subtract numbers with decimals, the problem must be set up as a list of numbers with the decimal point of each number of the list being written directly below the decimal point in the previous number. After aligning the decimals, do the math calculation.

Place a decimal point after any whole numbers that are not followed by decimals.

Insert a decimal point and sufficient zeros after whole numbers to make all the decimals the same length as the decimal with the greatest number of places following the decimal point.

EXAMPLE 29: Find the sum of $64.3 + 18 + 0.33$

$$\begin{array}{r} 64.30 \\ 18.00 \\ 0.33 \\ \hline 82.63 \end{array}$$

EXAMPLE 30: Find the difference of $69.3 - 5.94$

$$\begin{array}{r} 69.30 \\ -5.94 \\ \hline 63.36 \end{array}$$

Multiplying Decimals

When multiplying decimals, align the numbers without regard to the decimal points and complete the regular multiplication.

To insert the decimal point after multiplication, count the number of decimal places in each line of the multiplication problem.

In the answer, place the decimal point at the sum of the decimal places from each line. Be sure to count from right to left when placing the decimal point.

EXAMPLE 31: Determine the product of 92.3×4.66

STEP 1: Multiply without considering the decimal places.

$$\begin{array}{r} 92.3 \\ \times\, 4.66 \\ \hline 5538 \\ 5538 \\ 3692 \\ \hline 430118 \end{array}$$

STEP 2: After finding an answer, find the number of decimal places in the answer by counting the one decimal place in 92.3 and two decimal places in 4.66. There

CHECK YOUR UNDERSTANDING—ADDING AND SUBTRACTING DECIMALS
6-10

Add the following decimals.

1. $71.4 + 16.32 + 38 =$ _____

2. $53 + 14.762 + 9.3 =$ _____

3. $33.33 + 66.7 + 1245.121 =$ _____

4. $54.01 + 21.5 + 78.667 =$ _____

5. $0.001 + 1.34 + 654.2 =$ _____

6. $40.267 + 17.6 + 0.003 =$ _____

7. $123.5 + 688.8 + 99.99 =$ _____

8. $26.83 + 45.761 + 0.9 =$ _____

9. $9.1 + 8.23 + 765.124 =$ _____

10. $32 + 67.84 + 0.1 =$ _____

Subtract the following decimals.

11. $38.672 - 32.43 =$ _____

12. $142.637 - 14.263 =$ _____

13. $77.4 - 37.46 =$ _____

14. $44.62 - 14.01 =$ _____

15. $5.04 - 1.67 =$ _____

16. $374.5 - 98.44 =$ _____

17. $98.7 - 8.662 =$ _____

18. $0.4 - 0.016 =$ _____

19. $1.06 - 0.92 =$ _____

20. $246 - 0.91 =$ _____

CHECK YOUR UNDERSTANDING—MULTIPLYING DECIMALS
6-11

Multiply the following decimals, round answer to nearest hundredth.

1. $6.34 \times 42.44 =$ _____

2. $34.33 \times 16 =$ _____

3. $43.011 \times 17.92 =$ _____

4. $0.988 \times 942.01 =$ _____

5. $31.97 \times 16.3 =$ _____

6. $0.41 \times 2.34 =$ _____

7. $1.01 \times 0.011 =$ _____

8. $4.012 \times 77 =$ _____

9. $89.98 \times 76.4 =$ _____

10. $22.73 \times 15.5 =$ _____

are three decimal places total. Show the answer with three decimal places: 430.118

Drop zeros from the answer when they are to the right of the decimal place if they are not followed by any other digit. Remember to count decimal places from right to left of the total.

Dividing Decimals

To divide decimals, the divisor must first be changed to a whole number by moving the decimal point. For each place that a decimal point is moved to the right in the divisor, the decimal point in the dividend is moved to the right the same number of places. Add zeros if necessary in the divisor to handle movement if decimal places are not sufficient for the number of places needed.

EXAMPLE 32: Determine the quotient: $\frac{5.32}{8}$

$$
\begin{array}{r}
0.665 \\
8\overline{)5.320} \\
-4\,8 \\
\hline
52 \\
-48 \\
\hline
40 \\
-40 \\
\hline
0
\end{array}
$$

EXAMPLE 33: Determine the quotient of $48.2 \div 0.68$ to the hundredth.

$0.68\overline{)48.2}$ First, move two decimal places in the divisor.

68 $\overline{)4820.}$ Now move two decimal places in the dividend, add a zero to accommodate the decimal move, and drop the decimal point in the divisor and place a decimal point after the "0" in the dividend.

Do the math: The quotient is 70.88. This can be rounded to 70.9 or, if a whole number is desired, 71.

```
        70.88
0.68 )48.20.00
      -47 6
         600   (68 will not go into 60,
       - 544    so add zero)
         560   (68 will not go into 56,
       - 544    so add zero)
          16
```

CHECK YOUR UNDERSTANDING—DIVIDING DECIMALS   6-12

Divide the following decimals, round answer to nearest tenth.

1. $72.6 \div 31.5 =$ _____

2. $0.63 \div 3.11 =$ _____

3. $41.37 \div 6.777 =$ _____

4. $27.9 \div 3.33 =$ _____

5. $2.3 \div 0.76 =$ _____

6. $76.5 \div 41.5 =$ _____

7. $39.7 \div 18.4 =$ _____

8. $40.6 \div 5.12 =$ _____

9. $99.8 \div 16.22 =$ _____

10. $73.2 \div 37.8 =$ _____

CHECK YOUR UNDERSTANDING—DECIMAL REVIEW   6-13

Convert to mixed numbers. Do not simplify answer.

1. $98.6 =$ _____

2. $32.84 =$ _____

3. $432.67 =$ _____

4. $17.666 =$ _____

5. $27.3 =$ _____

Round to the nearest whole number.

6. $33.333 =$ _____

7. $674.75 =$ _____

8. $34.5 =$ _____

9. $18.99 =$ _____

10. $0.88 =$ _____

Round to the nearest tenth.

11. $99.109 =$ _____

12. $0.476 =$ _____

13. $123.456 =$ _____

14. $66.666 =$ _____

15. $3.717 =$ _____

Round to the nearest hundredth.

16. $99.8599 =$ _____

17. $0.3826 =$ _____

18. $345.678 =$ _____

19. $2.653 =$ _____

20. $33.456 =$ _____

Round to the nearest thousandth.

21. $68.2467 =$ _____

22. $987.6543 =$ _____

23. $4.2468 =$ _____

24. $98.9372 =$ _____

25. $1047.3218 =$ _____

(continued)

CHECK YOUR UNDERSTANDING—DECIMAL REVIEW (cont'd)   6-13

Convert to decimals.

26. $\dfrac{7}{8} = $ _____

27. $3\dfrac{1}{2} = $ _____

28. $44\dfrac{3}{4} = $ _____

29. $\dfrac{11}{8} = $ _____

30. $17\dfrac{2}{5} = $ _____

Add; then round to the nearest hundredth.

31. $46.38 + 27.4 + 0.44 + 17 = $ _____

32. $34.75 + 16.333 + 8 + 16.479 = $ _____

33. $16.334 + 31.6 + 34.567 + 17.889 = $ _____

34. $64.5 + 88.92 + 14 + 81.267 + 544.445 = $ _____

35. $91.25 + 44.337 + 16.4 + 88 + 391.24 = $ _____

Subtract; then round to the nearest tenth.

36. $47.314 - 16 = $ _____

37. $598.7 - 394.621 = $ _____

38. $33 - 16.2 = $ _____

39. $274.651 - 35.7 = $ _____

40. $34.5 - 1.047 = $ _____

Multiply; then simplify to the nearest whole number.

41. $91.47 \times 16.3 = $ _____

42. $37.1 \times 4.333 = $ _____

43. $31.456 \times 18 = $ _____

44. $19 \times 18.2 \times 66.234 = $ _____

45. $3 \times 17.2 \times 0.47 = $ _____

Divide. Then simplify to the nearest thousandth.

46. $7.49 \div 6.33 = $ _____

47. $77.99 \div 7.99 = $ _____

48. $35.92 \div 14.64 = $ _____

49. $44.333 \div 16.333 = $ _____

50. $97 \div 33.66 = $ _____

Percents

Percent (%) means "hundredths" or "parts per 100." Percents may be seen as a fraction (such as $\dfrac{1}{4}\%$), a decimal (such as 0.25%), a whole number (such as 25%), or a mixed number (such as $1\dfrac{1}{4}\%$).

Important step: When changing a percent that is expressed as a fraction to a percent that is expressed as a decimal, remember that the result or number is still a percentage that must be changed to a decimal number for further calculations.

 LEARNING TIP

Remember to change a fraction to a decimal by dividing the numerator by the denominator.

EXAMPLE 34: $\dfrac{1}{4}\% = 0.25\%$

and $1\dfrac{1}{4}\% = 1.25\%$

Changing Percents to Decimals

Drop the % sign. Then divide by 100 because the word "percent" means part of a hundred. The division causes the decimal to move two places to the *left*.

EXAMPLE 35: 4% becomes $\dfrac{4}{100}$ or 0.04

1.8% becomes $\dfrac{1.8}{100}$ or 0.018

Hint: Remember to carry over the decimal point from the percent problem to the fractional problem.

Percents that contain a fraction must first be changed to decimal percents before dividing by 100.

EXAMPLE 36: $\dfrac{1}{4}\% = 0.25\%$ then divide by 100, so

$\dfrac{25}{100} = 0.0025,$

$2\dfrac{1}{2}\% = 2.5\%$, then divide by 100, so

$\dfrac{2.5}{100} = 0.025$

Hint: Be sure to keep the decimal point in the numerator when dividing by 100.

Changing Decimals to Percents

First, multiply the decimal by 100. This causes the decimal to be moved two places to the *right*. Second, add a % sign.

> **EXAMPLE 37:** 2.64 becomes 264%
>
> $$2.64 \times 100 = 264.$$
>
> 264 becomes 264%

> **EXAMPLE 38:** 0.022 becomes 2.2%
>
> $$0.022 \times 100 = 2.2$$
>
> 2.2 becomes 2.2%.

Multiplying Percents

In the statement "Find 5% of 20," the term "of" means to multiply a number by a percent. The first step is to change the percent to a decimal, 5% becomes 0.05. Next, multiply the number found in the problem by the decimal, $20 \times 0.05 = 100$ (before correct decimal placement). The final step is to input the correct number of decimal places. In the example, 0.05 has two decimal places, so the answer, 100, would need two decimal places. The answer is 1 (1.00).

Hint: Remember to move decimal places from right to left, and always drop zeros that appear after the decimal point as trailing zeros.

> **EXAMPLE 39:** Find 3% of 42.
>
> STEP 1: Change % to a decimal: 3% = 0.03
>
> STEP 2: Multiply: $42 \times 0.03 = 126$
>
> STEP 3: Input decimal places as needed. Two decimals in step 1 (0.03) means the answer has two decimal places. Answer = 1.26

In the next example, an additional step must be performed because the mixed number must be changed to decimal form. As in Example 28, change the mixed number to an improper fraction,

---

CHECK YOUR UNDERSTANDING—CHANGING PERCENTS TO DECIMALS 6-14

Change the percent to a decimal. Round your answer to nearest hundredth.

1. $\frac{2}{3}\%$ = _____

2. 8% = _____

3. $4\frac{1}{2}\%$ = _____

4. $64\frac{3}{4}\%$ = _____

5. 31% = _____

6. 5.5% = _____

7. $7\frac{7}{8}\%$ = _____

8. $3\frac{1}{3}\%$ = _____

9. $17\frac{7}{10}\%$ = _____

10. $98\frac{7}{10}\%$ = _____

CHECK YOUR UNDERSTANDING—CHANGING DECIMALS TO PERCENTS 6-15

Change the decimal to a percent, simplify answer to nearest tenth.

1. 3.59 = _____

2. 44.2 = _____

3. 0.06 = _____

4. 7.34 = _____

5. 0.047 = _____

6. 0.0352 = _____

7. 1.17 = _____

8. 78.421 = _____

9. 0.055 = _____

10. 3.672 = _____

then convert the improper fraction to a decimal before attempting to find the percent.

EXAMPLE 40: Find: $3\frac{1}{2}\%$ of 90

STEP 1: $3\frac{1}{2}$ is the same as $\frac{7}{2}$, which in decimal form is 3.5 ($\frac{1}{2}$ can be changed to 0.5% by dividing 2 into 1 to obtain 3.5%)

STEP 2: Change % to a decimal: 3.5% = 0.035

STEP 3: Multiply 90 × 0.035 = 3150

STEP 4: Input decimal places as needed. Three decimals in step 2 (0.035) means the answer has three decimal places. Answer = 3.150 (same as 3.15 because the last zero should be deleted because it is not necessary as fifteen hundredths is equivalent to 150 thousandths, or it is a trailing zero).

Dividing Percents

Dividing percents answers the question of "what." To find "what" percentage one number is of another number, use these steps:

STEP 1: Set up the problem as a fraction.

STEP 2: Simplify the fraction (if possible).

STEP 3: Divide the fraction's denominator into its numerator to obtain a decimal.

STEP 4: Change the decimal to a percent.

EXAMPLE 41: 15 is what percent of 45?

STEP 1: Write as a fraction: $\frac{15}{45}$

STEP 2: Simplify the fraction: $\frac{15}{45} = \frac{1}{3}$

STEP 3: Divide: $3\overline{)1.00} = 0.33$

STEP 4: Change step 3 answer to a percent: 0.33 = 33%

Using Fractions to Figure Percentages

With this method, two fractions will be determined. The first fraction will show the numbers given in the problem. The second fraction will show a number as a percentage of 100. The unknown number in either fraction is labeled x. Set up the two fractions as shown in the following example. Then solve for x that is identified by "what." Use an equals sign (=), identified by "is," to indicate equality when showing the relationship between two equal fractions. Always round the answer to the nearest whole number.

Formula for Fractions

$$\frac{a}{b} = \frac{c}{d}$$

a = numerator for fraction one is the amount or part of a whole being compared to the base. May be a number found in the problem, or may be the unknown

b = denominator for fraction one is the base or the whole in the problem or standard used for comparison. The base often follows the word "of." This may be a number found in the problem, or may be the unknown

c = numerator for fraction two will be a percent of 100 (the number or unknown followed by %), and may be the unknown

d = denominator for fraction two will always be 100 when solving for percents

---

CHECK YOUR UNDERSTANDING—MULTIPLYING PERCENTS   6-16

Multiply by a percent, round answer to nearest hundredth.

1. Find 14% of 28 = _____

2. Find $3\frac{1}{2}\%$ of 17 = _____

3. Find $6\frac{2}{3}\%$ of 80 = _____

4. Find $5\frac{1}{4}\%$ of 14 = _____

5. Find 19% of 75 = _____

6. Find 27% of 10 = _____

7. Find 48% of 100 = _____

8. Find 11% of 20 = _____

9. Find 82% of 19 = _____

10. Find $\frac{41}{2}\%$ of 11 = _____

CHECK YOUR UNDERSTANDING—DIVIDING PERCENTS   6-17

Divide by a percent. Round your answer to tenths.

1. 70 is what percent of 84? _____

2. 32 is what percent of 50? _____

3. 14 is what percent of 77? _____

4. 11 is what percent of 15? _____

5. 3 is what percent of 7? _____

6. 15 is what percent of 19? _____

7. 2 is what percent of 13? _____

8. 44 is what percent of 63? _____

9. 7 is what percent of 77? _____

10. 4 is what percent of 9? _____

The letters of a, b, or c can be the unknown, so any one of these letters can be labeled "*x*" in a given problem. When finding percents, the letter d is always 100 because it signifies 100%.

For example: What is 20% of 200?

$$a \quad = \quad c \quad \times \quad b$$

Note: The 20% is "c" because the "%" sign is attached; d is always 100; what is unknown; 200 is base.

$$\frac{x\,(a)}{200\,(b)} = \frac{20\,(c)}{100\,(d)}$$

A problem can be stated three different ways when using fractions. The following three examples show each way the question can be asked, followed by the solution. The most difficult part of the problem is understanding what is unknown and then correctly placing the known "*x*" into either the a, b, or c part of the fraction.

EXAMPLE 42: 15 is what percent of 45?

When a problem is asked like Example 42, the unknown "what" is the percentage. The number beside the word "is" becomes the numerator of fraction one. The number beside the word "of" becomes the denominator of fraction one. In the second fraction, *x* is used for the percentage over 100. Using the formula shown earlier, the letter a = 15, b = 45, c = *x*, and d = 100.

STEP 1: Set up the problem as two equivalent fractions.

$$\frac{15 \text{ (part of whole)}}{45 \text{ (base)}} = \frac{x \text{ (percent)}}{100}$$

STEP 2: Cross-multiply.

$$45 \times (x) = 15 \times 100$$
$$45x = 1500$$

STEP 3: Isolate the *x* so that it is by itself (by dividing both sides by 45).

$$x = 45\overline{)1500}$$
$$x = 3333$$

STEP 4: Remember that you must still move the decimal two places to the left and add a percent sign to obtain an answer shown in percent. Show final answer in whole percentage number only.

$$x = 33.33 \text{ will be written as } 33\%$$

The fractions in this problem could have been simplified. $\frac{15}{45}$ is the same as $\frac{1}{3}$. The answer would still be the same, $x = 33\%$.

EXAMPLE 43: 15 is 33% of what number?

In Example 42, the unknown "what" is a number. Therefore the unknown "*x*" is in the first fraction, and the second fraction is $\frac{33}{100}$. The number beside the word "is" becomes the numerator of fraction one. The denominator of fraction one is the unknown.

STEP 1: Set up the problem as two equivalent fractions.

$$\frac{15 \text{ (portion of base)}}{x \text{ (base)}} = \frac{33 \text{ (percent)}}{100}$$

STEP 2: Cross-multiply:

$$33x = 1500$$

STEP 3: Isolate x:

$$x = \frac{1500}{33}$$

$$x = 45.45$$

STEP 4: Show the answer in a whole number only. *Hint*: Always remember what you are solving for. You may be solving for a percent or a number. In this problem, you are looking for a number so:

$$x = 45$$

EXAMPLE 44: What number is 33% of 45?

In Example 43, the unknown "what" is a number, therefore the unknown "x" is in the first fraction, and the second fraction is $\frac{33}{100}$. Since there is no number beside the word "is," the numerator in fraction one is "x." The denominator in fraction one is 45. Use the formula shown previously.

STEP 1: Set up the problem as two equivalent fractions.

$$\frac{x \text{ (portion of base)}}{45 \text{ (base)}} = \frac{33 \text{ (percent)}}{100}$$

STEP 2: Cross-multiply.

$$100x = 1485$$

STEP 3: Isolate x

$$\frac{100x}{100} = \frac{1485}{100}$$

$$x = 14.85$$

STEP 4: Show the answer as a whole number.

So $x = 15$

Using an Equation to Figure Percentage

To solve percentage problems using an equation, the parts of the problem are translated to the equivalent parts. "Of" translates to "times"; "what" translates to the unknown or "x"; "is" translates to "=."

For example What (x) is (=) 20% of ($\times$) 200?

$$x = 0.2 \times 200$$

Note: 20% has been changed to a decimal for calculation.

$$x = 40$$

The following are the same as examples 41 to 43 that have been placed in the equation method.

EXAMPLE 45: 15 is what percent of 45?

$$15 = \quad x \qquad \times \ 45$$
$$45x = 15$$
$$x = 33.33\% \text{ or } 33\%$$

EXAMPLE 46: 15 is 33% of what number?

$$15 = 33 \quad \times \quad x$$
$$33x = 15$$
$$x = 45.45\% \text{ or } 45\%$$

EXAMPLE 47: What number is 33% of 45?

$$x \qquad\qquad = 33 \quad \times \ 45$$
$$x = 14.85\% \text{ or } 15\%$$

CHECK YOUR UNDERSTANDING 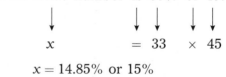   6-18

Using the equation method, translate the following and solve. Round to whole numbers.

1. What number is 25% of 40? _____

2. 16 is what % of 64? _____

3. 15 is 60% of what number? _____

4. 30 is what % of 90? _____

5. 5 is 10% of what number? _____

6. What number is 3% of 90? _____

7. What number is 25% of 500? _____

8. 4 is what % of 80? _____

9. 12 is 40% of what number? _____

10. 13 is 5% of what number? _____

CHECK YOUR UNDERSTANDING—PERCENT REVIEW   6-19

Change to decimals.

1. $\frac{1}{2}\% = $ _____

2. $3\frac{1}{4}\% = $ _____

3. $1.44\% = $ _____

4. $7.25\% = $ _____

5. $33\frac{1}{3}\% = $ _____

Change to percents.

6. $1.89 = $ _____

7. $72.34 = $ _____

8. $0.0631 = $ _____

9. $0.05 = $ _____

10. $0.11 = $ _____

Solve, rounding to the nearest tenth.

11. 27% of 2 = _____

12. 70% of 44 = _____

13. 66.67% of 49 = _____

14. $84\frac{1}{2}\%$ of 99 = _____

15. $33\frac{1}{2}\%$ of 50 = _____

Solve, writing as a percent.

16. 20 is what percent of 80? _____

17. 67 is what percent of 200? _____

18. $\frac{1}{2}$ is what percent of 2? _____

19. 30 is what percent of 45? _____

20. $4\frac{3}{4}$ is what percent of 19? _____

Solve for the number. Round to the whole number

21. 6 is 10% of what number? _____

22. 20 is 25% of what number? _____

23. 25 is 50% of what number? _____

24. 30 is 70% of what number? _____

25. 2 is 60% of what number? _____

Solve for the number and round to whole number.

26. What number is 15% of 45?

27. What number is 40% of 80?

28. What number is 5% of 55?

29. What number is 80% of 60?

30. What number is 25% of 16?

Ratio and Proportion

A *ratio* shows a relationship between two numbers by using a colon to separate the numbers.

A *proportion* shows the relationship between two equal ratios or fractions.

The *proportional method* is used to find the relationships between ratios, including finding unknowns and dosage calculations.

Use two colons (::) to show a relationship between two ratios.

EXAMPLE **48:** This is a ratio **1 : 3**

This is a ratio **2 : 6**

This is a proportion: **1 : 3 :: 2 : 6**

Notice that if you divide the second ratio by 2, the two ratios are identical.

Solving for *x* in a Proportion

In a proportion the product of the means must equal the product of the extremes. In the following proportion multiply the extremes together **1 × 8** and then the means together **4 × 2**. Therefore $1 \times 8 = 4 \times 2$

extremes
1 : 4   ::   2 : 8
means

Knowing that proportions must be equal makes it easy to solve for an unknown part of the equation. Let *x* stand for the unknown.

If the problem is *x* : 3 :: 2 : 6, solve for the unknown *x* by multiplying.

STEP 1: Multiply the extremes together.
$x \times 6 = 6x$

STEP 2: Multiply the means together.
$3 \times 2 = 6$

STEP 3: The problem would now be $6x = 6$. Isolate x by dividing each side by the number that is in front of x. In this problem, divide by 6. This will allow x to be equal to 1.

STEP 4: Prove the computation by replacing x in the original problem with your answer. The answers of the means and extremes should be equal.

EXAMPLE 49: Solve for x in this proportion: $1 : x :: 2 : 8$

STEP 1: Multiply extremes: $1 \times 8 = 8$

STEP 2: Multiply means: $2 \times x = 2x$

STEP 3: Isolate x:
$$\frac{2x}{2} = \frac{8}{2}$$
$$x = 4$$

STEP 4: Prove answer: $1 : 4 :: 2 : 8$ The means and extremes are equal therefore this is a true proportion.

Using Ratios and Proportions to Figure Percents

The method of using ratios and proportions to figure the percent is similar to the fractional method once you have determined "x." The first ratio will show the numbers in the problem, and the second ratio will show a number as a percentage of 100. The unknown number in either ratio is labeled "x." Set up the two ratios as a proportion (as shown in the following example). Remember to use two colons (::) to show a relationship between the two ratios. Always round the answer to the nearest whole number.

Formula for Ratios and Proportions

a : b :: c : d

a = one of the extremes is the amount or part of the whole being compared to the base, always a number or the unknown variable in the first ratio

b = one of the means or the whole number in the problem or the standard used for comparison, always a number or the unknown variable in the first ratio

c = one of the means; when figuring percents, "c" will always be a percent of 100. In practical applications, this number is a portion of the total of an item.

d = one of the extremes; when figuring percents, this will always be 100. When using practical applications this number is the "total" amount of an item.

CHECK YOUR UNDERSTANDING—RATIO AND PROPORTION 6-20

Solve for x in the proportion.

1. $5 : x :: 4 : 20$ $x = $ _____
2. $1 : 3 :: 3 : x$ $x = $ _____
3. $11 : 22 :: x : 44$ $x = $ _____
4. $16 : 20 :: 4 : x$ $x = $ _____
5. $50 : x :: 3 : 9$ $x = $ _____
6. $4 : x :: 32 : 16$ $x = $ _____
7. $x : 14 :: 12 : 24$ $x = $ _____
8. $6 : 24 :: 1 : x$ $x = $ _____
9. $8 : 2 :: x : 4$ $x = $ _____
10. $x : 30 :: 5 : 6$ $x = $ _____
11. $x : 5 :: 12 : 10$ $x = $ _____
12. $64 : 2 :: 32 : x$ $x = $ _____
13. $1 : 9 : x : 81$ $x = $ _____
14. $8 : 250 :: x : 125$ $x = $ _____
15. $6 : x :: 3 : 1$ $x = $ _____
16. $x : 9 :: 3 : 1$ $x = $ _____
17. $2 : x :: 4 : 250$ $x = $ _____
18. $x : 325 :: 1 : 650$ $x = $ _____
19. $3 : 600 :: 2 : x$ $x = $ _____
20. $10 : 100 :: 25 : x$ $x = $ _____

The following three examples show each way a ratio and proportion question can be asked using percents, followed by the solution.

The letters a, b, or c can be the unknown, so any one of these letters can be labeled "x" in a given problem. In the following examples, letter d is always 100 for 100%.

EXAMPLE **50:** 15 is what % of 45?

In this example the two numbers being compared are 15 and 45. Set the first ratio up to express this comparison. The second ratio is asking "what" percent 15 is to 45, so the "unknown" is a percent. *Hint:* Recall that a proportion is a comparison between two equivalent ratios. Using the formula shown earlier, the letter a = 15, b = 45, c = x, and d = 100.

STEP 1: Write as a ratio and proportion

$$15 : 45 :: x\% : 100$$

STEP 2: Multiply the means and the extremes

$$45 \times x = 15 \times 100$$
$$45x = 1500$$

STEP 3: Isolate the x so that it is by itself (by dividing both sides by 45).

$$\frac{45x}{45} = \frac{1500}{45}$$
$$x = 33.33$$

STEP 4: Since the question is asking for a percent, move the decimal two places to the left, add a percent sign, and write as a whole number.

$x = 33.33$ will be written as 33%

If you wish to prove your answer, replace the x with 33 in the original problem.

15 : 45 :: 33 : 100

The answer is correct because 1500 is approximately equal to 1485. Remember that you rounded from 33.33% to 33%.

The problem can be asked three different ways depending on what is known or given, as well as where the "x" is placed in the proportion. In Examples 50-52, the same numbers as found in previous examples are used to show

how to set up the problem using ratios and proportion.

EXAMPLE **51:** 21 is what percent of 35?

STEP 1: Set up the two ratios. The numbers in the first ratio are given. The "what" is the percent.

$$21 : 35 :: x : 100$$

STEP 2: Multiply the means and the extremes.

$$21 \times 100 = 35 \times x$$
$$2100 = 35x$$

STEP 3: Isolate the x.

$$x = 60$$

STEP 4: The problem is asking for a percent, so the answer will be 60%.

EXAMPLE **52:** 21 is 60% of what number?

STEP 1: Set up the two ratios. Only one number in the first ratio is given. The "what" is the second number. The percents are given.

$$21 : x :: 60 : 100$$

STEP 2: Multiply the means and the extremes.

$$21 \times 100 = 60 \times x$$
$$2100 = 60x$$

STEP 3: Isolate the x.

$$x = 35$$

STEP 4: The problem is asking for a number, so the answer will be 35.

EXAMPLE **53:** What number is 60% of 35?

STEP 1: Set up the two ratios. Only one number in the first ratio is given. The "what" is the first number. The percents are given.

$$x : 35 :: 60 : 100$$

STEP 2: Multiply the means and the extremes.

$$x \times 100 = 35 \times 60$$
$$100x = 2100$$

STEP 3: Isolate the x.

$$x = 21$$

STEP 4: The problem is asking for a number, so the answer will be 21.

CHECK YOUR UNDERSTANDING—USING PROPORTIONS TO FIGURE PERCENTS

6-21

Solve for the unknown percent using the proportional method. Round answer to the nearest whole number.

1. What number is 12% of 500? _____
2. What number is 70% of 250? _____
3. What number is 81% of 11? _____
4. What number is 66% of 75? _____
5. What number is 34% of 60? _____
6. What number is 22% of 21? _____
7. What number is 47% of 400? _____
8. What number is 53% of 19? _____
9. What number is 38% of 70? _____
10. What number is 85% of 90? _____

Solve for the unknown number using the proportional method. Round answer to the nearest whole number.

11. 16 is 25% of what number? _____
12. 32 is 10% of what number? _____
13. 50 is 40% of what number? _____
14. 5 is $33\frac{1}{3}$% of what number? _____
15. 14 is 75% of what number? _____
16. 3 is 20% of what number? _____
17. 7 is 15% of what number? _____
18. 11 is 5% of what number? _____
19. 72 is 90% of what number? _____
20. 60 is 80% of what number? _____

Practical Applications

Many applications in a medical facility require the practical use of basic math calculations. The math problems will not be set up for you, and oftentimes setting up the problem correctly is the most difficult part of finding a solution. Always check your solution by placing your answer into the original math problem for *x*. The following section shows a math calculation used in inventory replacement and in determining medication administration.

EXAMPLE 54: There are 24 ampules of Xylocaine in one box of medication. How many ampules of Xylocaine are in two boxes?

STEP 1: Set up the equation:

$$\frac{24 \text{ ampules}}{1 \text{ box}} = \frac{x \text{ ampules}}{2 \text{ boxes}} \text{ or}$$

24 ampules : 1 box :: *x* ampules : 2 boxes

as a fraction:

$$\frac{24}{1} = \frac{x}{2} \text{ or } 24 : 1 :: x : 2$$

STEP 2: Solve for *x* by cross-multiplication:

$$1 \times x = 2 \times 24$$

$$x = 48$$

STEP 3: Prove by replacing *x* in equation with your answer:

$$\frac{24}{1} = \frac{48}{2} \text{ (a true proportion)}$$

When working with ratios and proportions that contain unit of measure descriptions such as mg, mL, inches, and teaspoons, both ratios in the proportion must contain the same units:

$$\frac{\text{mg}}{\text{mL}} = \frac{\text{mg}}{\text{mL}} \text{ or mg : mL :: mg : mL}$$

If the units of measure are not the same, conversion must be performed to find like units.

EXAMPLE 55: A dosage of 0.5 g of amoxicillin sodium is prescribed. On hand is amoxicillin sodium 250 mg/5 mL. How many mL would be given for the order using the dosage strength on hand?

STEP 1: Write the proportion:

0.5 g : 1 mL :: 250 mg : *x* mL

STEP 2: Change g to mg using the following information:
1 g = 1000 mg, so 0.5 g = 500 mg.

STEP 3: Rewrite the problem in the same units. Measure and then solve.

500 mg : 1 mL :: 250 mg : x mL

or $\dfrac{500 \text{ mg}}{1 \text{ mL}} = \dfrac{250 \text{ mg}}{x \text{ mL}}$

STEP 4: Multiply the means and the extremes.

$500x = 250$

STEP 5: Isolate the x.

$x = \dfrac{250}{500}$

$x = \dfrac{1}{2}$ or 0.5

STEP 6: Determine what the problem is asking for (milliliters). Be sure to include the proper measurement in your answer. The correct answer is 0.5 mL because mL is a unit of the metric system.

CHECK YOUR UNDERSTANDING—RATIO AND PROPORTION REVIEW   6-22

Solve for x.

1. 1 : x :: 3 : 12   x = _____

2. $x : \dfrac{1}{2} :: 7 : 3\dfrac{1}{2}$ x = _____

3. 4 : 5 :: 16 : x   x = _____

4. 4 : 5 :: x : 15   x = _____

5. 0.2 : 0.8 :: x : 0.16   x = _____

Solve these word problems. Set each one up as a ratio and a proportion.

6. A patient has ibuprofen that is available in 100 mg/5 mL. The physician desires ibuprofen 50 mg be administered. What quantity of ibuprofen should be administered to the patient? _____

7. A prescription reads "take two tablets four times a day." If the patient takes the prescription correctly, how many tablets will he or she have taken by the end of 1 week? (*Hint*: Figure the number of tablets needed in a day first.) _____

8. To reconstitute a medication, the instructions read "add 0.5 mL of sterile water to the vial to obtain a 300-mg dosage strength." If a 200-mg dosage strength is prescribed, how much sterile water would need to be added to the vial? _____

9. If $2\dfrac{1}{2}$ tablets of dextro-amphetamine contain 25 mg of medication, how many tablets equal 15 mg? _____

(continued)

CHECK YOUR UNDERSTANDING (cont'd) 6-22

10. A dosage of Prozac 60 mg is prescribed. On hand is Prozac 20 mg/5 mL. How many milliliters of Prozac would be given for the order using the dosage strength on hand? _____

11. When Humulin R is 100 U/1 mL, how many milliliters would 20U of Humulin R be? _____

12. When Acthar Gel 80 U/1 mL is used for an order, how many milliliters would be needed for Acthar Gel 60 U? _____

13. One kilogram is equivalent to 2.2 pounds. How many kilograms would a person weighing 209 pounds be? _____

14. How many pounds would an 80-kilogram person weigh? _____

15. The patient's total daily dose of sulfamethoxazole is 1 g. The drug is available in 500-mg tablets. How many tablets would the patient take daily? (*Hint*: 1 g = 1000 mg.) _____

16. The cleaning solution is to be diluted one teaspoon to 64 oz of water. How much water would be added to a container containing $\frac{1}{4}$ teaspoon of cleaning solution? _____

17. One hour is 60 minutes. What fractional part of an hour is 45 minutes? _____

CHECK YOUR UNDERSTANDING (cont'd)   6-22

 18. If 1 tablet of chlorothiazide (Diuril) is equivalent to 250 mg, how many milligrams would $2\frac{1}{2}$ tablets be? _____

19. 1000 mg is equivalent to 1 g. What is the milligram equivalent for 0.9 g? _____

 20. Amoxicillin/clavulanate potassium (Augmentin) is supplied in the solution of 200 mg/5 mL. If amoxicillin/clavulanate potassium 300 mg is ordered every 8 hours, how many milliliters would be prepared for one dose? _____

Measurement Systems and Their Equivalents

OBJECTIVES

After studying this chapter, you should be capable of doing the following:
- Identifying the basic units of measure in the metric system and their abbreviations.
- Writing metric measurements in correct notation.
- Converting within metric measurement units.
- Discussing the limited use of the apothecary system.
- Using symbols and Roman numerals in the apothecary system.
- Identifying the basic units of measure in the household system and their abbreviations.
- Explaining milliequivalents and units in determining drug measurements.
- Identifying current trends in the use of symbols and abbreviations.

KEY TERMS

Apothecary	Gram	Metric system
Apothecary system	Household system	Milliequivalent
Dram	Liter	Minim
Grain	Meter	Unit

CHAPTER 7 PRETEST: MEASUREMENT SYSTEMS AND THEIR EQUIVALENTS

Part I. Answer the following questions.

1. Name the three base metric units of measure. _____

2. Identify the metric abbreviation:

kilogram _____   microgram _____

centimeter _____   milliliter _____

3. Write the correct metric notation for three hundred twenty centimeters. _____

4. Determine the answer:

2.8 m = _____ cm   2500 mcg = _____ mg

3250 cc = _____ mL   850 mg = _____ g

0.78 kg = _____ g   2.8 L = _____ cc

CHAPTER 7 PRETEST: MEASUREMENT SYSTEMS AND THEIR EQUIVALENTS—cont'd

Part II. Explain each line of a prescription in language an adult patient would understand.

5. Drug classification

_____
_____
_____
_____
_____
_____
_____
_____

> Lawrence Merry, M.D.
> 4th Street and Jones Ave.
> Holly, GA 00111
> Phone # - 001-555-2176
>
> Patient Name_____ Date _____
> Address_____
>
> Rx   Synthroid 0.1 mg
>   #90
>   SIG: i tab po daily
>
> _____ Refill _____
> DEA#_____

6. Drug classification

_____
_____
_____
_____
_____
_____
_____
_____

> Lawrence Merry, M.D.
> 4th Street and Jones Ave.
> Holly, GA 00111
> Phone # - 001-555-2176
>
> Patient Name_____ Date _____
> Address_____
>
> Rx   Pen Vee K 250 mg
>   # 30
>   SIG: i tab po q6h
>
> _____ Refill _____
> DEA#_____

7. Drug classification

_____
_____
_____
_____
_____
_____
_____
_____

> Lawrence Merry, M.D.
> 4th Street and Jones Ave.
> Holly, GA 00111
> Phone # - 001-555-2176
>
> Patient Name_____ Date _____
> Address_____
>
> Rx   Benadryl elix 12.5 mg/5 mL
>   ℥ iv
>   SIG: 5 mL po qid
>
> _____ Refill _____
> DEA#_____

Hint: 5 mL ≈ 1 teaspoon.

Metric System

The **metric system** originated in France more than 200 years ago. It is sometimes referred to as the SI system, from the French words, *Système International*. The metric system, used in more than 90% of developed countries, is based on the decimal system and is the international standard for scientific and industrial measurements. The United States has been slow to adopt the metric system and still relies heavily the household method of measurement (sometimes referred to as the *English measurement system*). Today in the United States, many items are labeled in the metric, apothecary, and household system. The metric system is much easier to use than either the apothecary or household system because the metric system uses the decimal (or base 10) numbering system (Figure 7-1). By simply moving the decimal point, one can convert units in within the metric system to other metric units (e.g., 12 mm = 1.2 cm).

Three basic units of measure exist in the metric system. The basic unit of weight is the **gram.** The basic unit of volume is the **liter.** The basic unit of length is the **meter.** In medical applications, weight usually references a mass (such as the weight of a pathology specimen) or a solid (such as the amount of medication in a tablet or capsule of medicine).

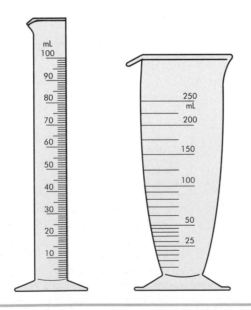

Figure 7-1 Examples of containers commonly found in medical offices that are marked in milliliters for measuring volume. (From Dison N: *Simplified drugs and solutions for health care professionals,* ed 11, St Louis, 1997, Mosby.)

Volume usually references a liquid or a gas, and length references distance.

A prefix may be added to each of the root words (gram, liter, and meter). Figure 7-2 shows the relationships of the common prefixes to their decimal value. As Figure 7-2 shows, deci-, centi-, milli-, and micro units are all less than one whole unit. The following should be memorized:

> *deci* = 0.1 (one tenth of one unit)
> *centi* = 0.01 (one hundredth of one unit)
> *milli* = 0.001 (one thousandth of one unit)
> *micro* = 0.000001 (one millionth of one unit)

To reduce medication errors, a zero is always used *before* the decimal point if the unit is less than one whole unit. For example, .78 would be written as 0.78. Extra zeros to the right of the numbers at the end decimal point should be deleted. For example, 1.0100 should read 1.01.

The base units are abbreviated as follows: gram (g), liter (L), and meter (m). Common units with prefixes used in medicine for weight are kilogram (abbreviated kg; 1 kilogram = 1000 grams, or 1 kg = 1000 g), milligram (abbreviated mg; one thousandth [0.001] of a gram; 1000 mg = 1 g), and microgram (abbreviated mcg; one millionth of a gram [0.000001 g]; 1,000,000 mcg = 1 g). A common prefixed unit used for liquids is the milliliter (abbreviated mL; one thousandth of a liter [0.001 L]; 1000 mL = 1 L). Common prefixed units used for measuring length are the centimeter (abbreviated cm; one hundredth of a meter [0.01 m]; 100 cm = 1 m), and the millimeter (abbreviated mm; one thousandth of a meter [0.001 m]; 1000 mm = 1 m). Clinical applications of these different units of measure include measuring a patient's weight (in kilograms), measuring the concentration of a drug (in g, mg, or mcg), and measuring a surgical wound (in centimeters or millimeters).

In the metric system, decimals are used instead of fractions (e.g., 0.1, not $^1/_{10}$). Because decimals are used, it is simple to convert from one unit to another in the metric system. Moving the decimal point to the right (and adding a zero) raises the value by a power of 10. For example, 1.20 m = 120 cm = 1200 mm. Moving the decimal point to the left lowers the value by a power of 10 for each unit moved. For example, 20 mm = 2 cm = 0.02 m.

When a metric measurement is written, the Arabic number is written first, followed by the metric abbreviation for units. For example, three hundred twenty-five milligrams is written as 325 mg, one hundred sixty-five centimeters is written as 165 cm, and three liters is written as 3 L.

Prefixes

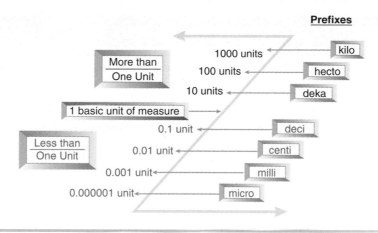

Figure 7-2 The basic units of measure—gram, liter, and meter—with prefixes indicating larger or smaller measures. Thus *deka-* ("ten") refers to ten basic units, and deci- ("tenth") refers to one tenth of the basic unit.

In 1960 the International Bureau of Weights and Measurements adopted the International System of units to reduce possible errors in drug transcriptions. A few common abbreviations may still be written the old way. For example, *gram* is often abbreviated as gm instead of g, as in the SI system. Either is appropriate. This book uses g. *Liter* may be abbreviated as L (in the SI system) or as lowercase l; either may be used. Table 7-1 shows the metric units most often used in clinical medicine, along with their unit value and abbreviation.

The cubic centimeter (cc) is a measurement that may still be seen on measuring devices for over-the-counter (OTC) cough syrups, syringes used for oral medications, and input measuring devices such as patient hospital cups and urine collection containers. One cubic centimeter (cc) is equivalent to one milliliter (mL). The "cc" may possibly be phased out of medical documentation in the future because "cc" may be mistaken for units when poorly written. Milliliter (mL) is the preferred abbreviation.

TABLE 7-1 *Common Metric Units Used in Medicine*

METRIC TERM	UNIT VALUE	ABBREVIATION
WEIGHT OR MASS		
kilogram	1000 units or grams	kg
gram	**base unit**	**g**
milligram	0.001 of a gram	mg
microgram	0.000001 of a gram	mcg
VOLUME OR LIQUID		
liter	**base unit**	**L**
milliliter*	0.001 of a liter	mL
LENGTH		
meter	**base unit**	**m**
centimeter	0.01 of a meter	cm
millimeter	0.001 of a meter	mm

Note: Basic units are in **boldface**.
*One milliliter (mL) = 1 cubic centimeter (cc).

 LEARNING TIP
Memorize the equivalency: 1 cc = 1 mL.

Using a Mnemonic to Make Conversions Within the Metric System

Students may find the mnemonic shown on page 132 useful as a means to identify the metric prefixes and a way to make conversions within the metric system. A mnemonic is designed to assist in memorizing or using difficult material. The purpose of this mnemonic is to assist the student in performing the decimal point movement within the metric system. The metric prefixes are written from largest to smallest. The largest metric unit, the kilo, is used in medicine, but the hecto, deka, and deci prefixes are generally not used. The mnemonic includes hecto, deka, and deci to show the relationship between a basic unit and the units on base 10.

CHECK YOUR UNDERSTANDING—METRIC SYSTEM BASICS   7-1

Identify whether the prefix is greater than or less than one basic unit.

1. centi _____

2. deci _____

3. deka _____

4. hecto _____

5. kilo _____

6. micro _____

7. milli _____

Identify the three basic units of measure in the metric system.

8. Basic unit of length _____

9. Basic unit of weight _____

10. Basic unit of volume _____

Write the decimal correctly.

11. 1.00100 _____

12. .001 _____

13. 0.00110 _____

14. 1.010 _____

15. .101010 _____

CALCULATION REVIEW: Two answers are required for each of the following. On the first line, identify the unit of measure as a weight, volume, or length measurement. Then write the metric notation using abbreviations.

	UNIT	METRIC NOTATION
16. Four tenths of a milliliter	_____	_____
17. One hundred twenty centimeters	_____	_____
18. Six hundred twenty-four milligrams	_____	_____
19. Three thousand and seventy-five-hundredths meters	_____	_____
20. Two and three-tenths liters	_____	_____
21. One thousand micrograms	_____	_____
22. Ten grams	_____	_____
23. Five kilograms	_____	_____
24. One and one-half liters	_____	_____
25. Seven hundred fifty kilometers	_____	_____

Mnemonic

K	H	D	B	D	C	M	—	—	M
Kilo	Hecto	Deka	Base	Deci	Centi	Milli			Micro
0	0	0	•	0	0	0	0	0	0
Kids	Hate	Dogs	Because	Dogs	Chase	Mailmen	(many)	(many)	Mailmen
1000 Thousand	100 Hundred	10 Ten	Base	0.1 Tenths	0.01 Hundredths	0.001 Thousandths			0.000001 Thousand-thousandths or millionths

Rules for Converting Within the Metric System Using the Mnemonic

- Using the mnemonic, construct the horizontal metric line from kilo- to micro- (KHDBDCM_ _M).
- Circle the known metric unit and the desired metric unit that are found in the problem.
- Place the decimal point of the known number in the correct place on the metric line.
- Place the decimal point of the unknown number in the correct place on the metric line.
- Fill in the spaces between the decimal points on the metric line with zeros.
- Avoid using decimal when whole numbers can be used (e.g., 0.5 g would be better expressed as 500 mg).

 LEARNING TIP

Remember that the base units are gram, liter, and meter.

EXAMPLE 1: 500 g = _____ kg

K. H D B. D C M _ _ M
0. 5 0 0.

500 g = 0.5 g

EXAMPLE 2: 5.4 kg = _____ mg

K. H D B D C M. _ _ M
5. 4 0 0 0 0 0.

5.4 kg = 5,400,000 mg

EXAMPLE 3: 0.1 mg = _____ g

K H D B. D C M. _ _ M
0. 0 0 0. 1

0.1 mg = 0.0001 g

EXAMPLE 4: _____ cm = 75 mm

K H D B D C. M. _ _ M
7. 5.

7.5 cm = 75 mm

EXAMPLE 5: _____ mm = 2.5 m

K H D B. D C M. _ _ M
2. 5 0 0.

Length Measurement and Conversion in the Metric System

The basic unit of length in the metric system is the meter. A meter is 39.37 inches, or slightly longer than a yardstick (36 inches). Other than for height, a meter is too long to be useful for most measurements in medicine, so subdivisions of a meter, or smaller units, are used. The centimeter (one-hundredth of a meter; 1 cm = 0.01 m) is most commonly used. Approximately 2.5 cm equals 1 inch. Centimeters may be used to measure a person's height, to measure the circumference of a newborn baby's head, or to measure the length of a wound. The millimeter (one thousandth of a meter; 1 mm = 0.001 m or about the size of the head of a straight pin) is used for small measurements such as sizes of small lesions.

 LEARNING TIP

The conversions to memorize for length include the following:

Meter to millimeter	1 m = 1000 mm
Meter to centimeter	1 m = 100 cm
Centimeter to millimeter	1 cm = 10 mm

Notice that the conversion factor is always in multiples of 10; therefore you can simply move the decimal point in the direction needed to obtain the desired unit. Recall that a basic length unit is a meter, and both the centimeter and the millimeter are subdivisions of *one* basic unit. To convert measurements between centimeters and millimeters, either *divide* if a smaller unit is given and a larger unit needs to be found or *multiply* if a larger unit is given and a smaller unit needs to be found. To divide by 10, move the decimal point to the left one unit place for each difference in conversion of smaller units to larger units. To multiply by 10, move the decimal point to the right for each unit needed for conversion of larger units to smaller units. In some cases, to get the desired value in the new unit, the decimal point is moved more than one place to the right or left.

In moving the decimal point to the right, we are multiplying by 10 for each space the decimal point moves. Because a millimeter is very small, only one thousandth of a meter, we need many of them (1000) to equal a meter (length). Moving the decimal point to the right, or multiplying by 10, gives the larger value wanted for the millimeter measurement quickly. And, of course, the same thing works in reverse. If we start with 50.2 millimeters and want to know the amount in meters, we move the decimal place three places to the left (divide), bypassing centimeters and decimeters:

EXAMPLE **6:** 50.2 mm = _____ m

50.2 mm = 0.0502 m

K H D B. D C M. _ _ M
          0. 0 5 0. 2

Because a meter is large in relation to a millimeter, the value for the meter measurement appears small.

 LEARNING TIP
Moving the decimal left = divide or lower the number
Moving the decimal right = multiply or increase the number.

EXAMPLE **7:** _____ cm = 75 mm

Centimeters are larger than millimeters, and therefore the value for a larger unit needs to be found. Remember: 1 cm = 10 mm. *Divide* by 10 (move the decimal point one place to the left).

$75 \div 10 = 7.5$, so 75 mm = 7.5 cm

K H D B D C. M. _ _ M
                7. 5.

EXAMPLE **8:** _____ mm = 2.5 m

Because millimeters are smaller than meters, the value of a smaller unit needs to be found. Remember: 1 m = 1000 mm. *Multiply* by 1000 (move the decimal point three places to the right).

$2.5 \times 1000 = 2500$, so 2.5 m = 2500 mm

K H D B. D C M. _ _ M
          2. 5 0 0.

Note: Two methods for conversion within the metric system have been presented. Find the method that you find easiest to use and use it consistently.

CHECK YOUR UNDERSTANDING—LENGTH CONVERSIONS   7-2

Convert the following from larger to smaller units by multiplying or by using the mnemonic.

1. 4.5 m = _____ mm

2. 5.75 cm = _____ mm

3. 6.5 m = _____ cm

4. 7 cm = _____ mm

5. 9.2 m = _____ cm

Convert the following from smaller to larger units by dividing or by using the mnemonic.

6. 1000 mm = _____ cm

7. 120 cm = _____ m

8. 1500 mm = _____ m

9. 1450 cm = _____ m

10. 950 mm = _____ cm

CALCULATION REVIEW: Determine whether to multiply, divide, or use the mnemonic to complete the following.

11. 6900 mm = _____ m

12. 4.3 cm = _____ mm

13. 4.3 cm = _____ m

14. 5 m = _____ mm

15. 90 mm = _____ cm

16. 3 m = _____ cm

17. 8.8 cm = _____ mm

18. 1.7 cm = _____ m

19. 1200 mm = _____ cm

20. 12 mm = _____ cm

CHECK YOUR UNDERSTANDING—LENGTH CONVERSIONS (cont'd)   7-2

PRACTICAL APPLICATION: Answer the following questions.

21. A 1-month-old child has a head circumference of 42.5 cm. What is the child's head circumference in millimeters? _____

22. An emergency room patient needs sutures to close a wound that is 8 cm long. How many millimeters long is the wound? _____

23. An infant is measured from head to foot. The measurement is 500 mm. What is the height in centimeters? _____

24. A premature baby has a head circumference of 13 cm. How many millimeters is the circumference? _____

25. A child stands 1 meter tall. Calculate the height in centimeters. _____

Volume Measurement and Conversion in the Metric System

The basic unit of volume in the metric system is the liter. In medicine, liquid volumes are expressed in liters or units of liters. Gas volumes, such as volume of oxygen, are also measured in liters. For comparison, many soft drinks are now sold in 1-, 2-, or 3-liter bottles. The 1-liter bottle is approximately equivalent to (slightly more than) 32 ounces or 1 quart in the household system. A gallon of milk is approximately equivalent to 4 liters (3.78 liters). Many OTC cough medicines now come with a medicine cup calibrated in milliliters (mL), cubic centimeters (cc), and teaspoons (t) or tablespoons (T).

This section explores the volume (liquid or gas) measurements of the milliliter and liter, which in medicine measure a patient's liquid intake and output. IV solutions are usually measured in liters with the drip volume measured in drops per milliliter.

The conversions to be remembered for volume include the following:

Liter to milliliter   1 L = 1000 mL
Milliliter to cubic centimeter 1 mL = 1 cc

The same procedure used for converting meters is used for converting liters. To convert a larger unit to a smaller unit, multiply by 10 (by 10, by 10, and so on), which is effected by moving the decimal place to the right the appropriate num-

ber of spaces and adding the necessary zeros. If you prefer to use the mnemonic, it can be used here also. The same prefixes are used with volume as found with weight.

EXAMPLE 9: _____ mL = 4 L

A milliliter is one thousandth of a liter, so you will be converting from a larger unit to a smaller unit.
Remember: 1 L = 1000 mL. *Multiply* by 1000 (move the decimal point three places to the right).

$1000 \times 4 = 4000$, so *4000 cc = 4 L*

or

K H D B D C M. _ _ M.
                    4. 0 0 0.

EXAMPLE 10: _____ L = 200 mL

A liter is 1000 milliliters, so you will be converting from a smaller unit to a larger unit.
Remember: 1 L = 1000 mL. Divide by 1000 (move the decimal point three places to the left).

$200 \div 1000 = 0.2$, so *0.2 L = 200 mL*

or

K H D B. D C M. _ _ M
         0. 2 0 0.

Always remember to place a 0 to the left of the decimal (.2 is written as 0.2).

CHECK YOUR UNDERSTANDING—VOLUME CONVERSIONS · 7-3

Convert the following from larger to smaller units by multiplying or by using the mnemonic.

1. 1.4 L = _____ mL

2. 1.5 L = _____ mL

3. 5 L = _____ mL

4. 7.5 L = _____ mL

5. 6.6 L = _____ mL

Convert the following from smaller to larger units by dividing or by using the mnemonic.

6. 240 mL = _____ L

7. 200 mL = _____ L

8. 480 mL = _____ L

9. 1000 mL = _____ L

10. 60 mL = _____ L

CALCULATION REVIEW: Determine whether to multiply, divide, or use the mnemonic to complete the following.

11. 1 mL = _____ L

12. 0.5 L = _____ mL

13. 6.4 L = _____ mL

14. 14 mL = _____ L

15. 500 mL = _____ L

16. 2500 mL = _____ L

17. 1450 mL = _____ L

18. 4 L = _____ mL

19. 100 mL = _____ L

20. 3000 mL = _____ L

PRACTICAL APPLICATION: Supply answers to the following questions.

21. A patient is instructed to drink 2 L of water every day to replace body fluids. How many milliliters is this? _____

22. You are instructed to measure the urine output of a patient with a Foley catheter. If the urine collection bag contains 1.5 L of urine, what volume in cubic centimeters will you record upon emptying the bag? _____

23. A standard IV bag contains 1000 mL of liquid. How many liters is that? _____

24. A patient is to receive 250 mL of fluids. How many liters will the patient receive? _____

25. A patient is to receive 3000 mL of IV fluids. How many liters should be ordered from the pharmacy? _____

Weight Measurement and Conversion in the Metric System

The base unit used to measure weight (mass) in the metric system is the gram. Other units of interest are the kilogram (kg; 1000 g), milligram (mg; one thousandth of a gram [0.001 g]), and the microgram (mcg; one millionth of a gram [0.000001 g]). A kilogram is approximately equal to 2.2 pounds. Newborn babies are weighed in kilograms unless they are premature, in which case they may be so small that their weight must be expressed in grams. A gram is about the weight of one large paper clip. Drug weights are usually found in milligrams and micrograms.

The conversions to be remembered for weight include the following:

Kilogram to gram	1 kg = 1000 g
Gram to milligram	1 g = 1000 mg
Milligram to microgram	1 mg = 1000 mcg

These weight units are commonly used in medicine, and they have an interesting relationship: each is one thousandth of the next higher (used) weight. The same ratio of 1:1000 exists between the kilogram and the gram, between the gram and the milligram, and between the milligram and the microgram (thus a microgram is a thousandth of a milligram or a millionth of a gram). Memorizing this feature of weights should help you remember the conversions. (Other units such as the decigram, centigram, dekagram, and so on exist but are used infrequently in the medical field.) As with length and volume, to convert from a larger unit to a smaller unit, multiply. If the smaller unit is given and the value of the larger unit is wanted, divide.

EXAMPLE 11: _____ mg = 8 g

Milligrams are smaller than grams, so the value of the smaller unit is wanted.
Remember: 1 g = 1000 mg. Multiply by 1000 (move the decimal point three places to the right and add zeros).

8 × 1000 = 8000, so 8000 mg = 8 g
or

K H D B. D C M. _ _ M
         8. 0 0 0.

EXAMPLE 12: _____ mg = 635 mcg

Milligrams are larger than micrograms, so you will convert from a smaller unit to a larger unit.
Remember: 1 mg = 1000 mcg. Divide by 1000 (move the decimal point three places to the left).

635 ÷ 1000 = 0.635, so 0.635 mg = 635 mcg
or

K H D B D C M. _ _ M.
               0. 6 3 5.

Remember: Add the zero in front of the decimal.

EXAMPLE 13: _____ g = 4.5 kg

Grams are smaller than kilograms, so you will convert from a larger unit to a smaller unit.
Remember: 1 kg = 1000 g. Multiply by 1000 (move the decimal point three places to the right and add zeros).

4.5 × 1000 = 4500, so 4500 g = 4.5 kg
or

K. H D B. D C M _ _ M
4. 5 0 0.

EXAMPLE 14: _____ g = 3250 mg

Grams are larger than milligrams, so you will convert from a smaller unit to a larger unit.
Remember: 1 g = 1000 mg. Divide by 1000.

3250 ÷ 1000 = 3.25, so 3.25 g = 3250 mg
or

K H D B. D C M. _ _ M
            3. 2 5 0.

Notice that the zero following 3.25 is a trailing zero and has therefore been dropped.

CHECK YOUR UNDERSTANDING—WEIGHT CONVERSIONS   7-4

Convert the following from larger to smaller units by multiplying or by using the mnemonic.

1. 4 kg = _____ g

2. 8 g = _____ mg

3. 9 mg = _____ mcg

4. 0.6 kg = _____ g

5. 0.003 g = _____ mg

Convert the following from smaller to larger units by dividing or by using the mnemonic.

6. 234 mcg = _____ mg

7. 25 mg = _____ g

8. 2750 mcg = _____ mg

9. 330 g = _____ kg

10. 4800 mg = _____ g

CALCULATION REVIEW: Determine whether to multiply or divide or use the mnemonic to determine the following. Drop or add zeros as appropriate.

11. 1500 mcg = _____ mg

12. 400 mg = _____ g

13. 6.5 g = _____ mg

14. 4800 mcg = _____ mg

15. 0.34 kg = _____ g

16. 500 g = _____ kg

17. 0.09 g = _____ mg

18. 2.75 mg = _____ mcg

19. 0.03 kg = _____ g

20. 225 mg = _____ g

(continued)

CHECK YOUR UNDERSTANDING—WEIGHT CONVERSIONS (cont'd)   7-4

PRACTICAL APPLICATION: Answer the following questions.

21. A premature baby weighs 2.2 kg. How many grams does the baby weigh? _____

22. A lab specimen weighs 1850 g. Convert the gram weight into kilograms. _____

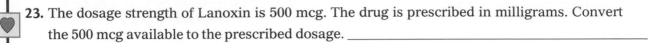

23. The dosage strength of Lanoxin is 500 mcg. The drug is prescribed in milligrams. Convert the 500 mcg available to the prescribed dosage. _____

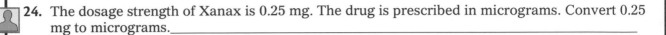

24. The dosage strength of Xanax is 0.25 mg. The drug is prescribed in micrograms. Convert 0.25 mg to micrograms._____

25. A medication comes in a tablet with dosage strength of 88 mcg. The medication bottle reads milligrams. What would you expect the dosage to read in milligrams? _____

Apothecary System

A pharmacist was once known as an apothecary—a person who compounds, prepares, or sells drugs for medicinal purposes. The **apothecary system** is one of the oldest systems for indicating drug mass or volume, but is nearly obsolete today because it has been gradually replaced by the metric system. Apothecary symbols such as gr (grain), ♏ (minim), ʒ (dram) and ℥ (ounce) are still found occasionally so the information is presented here. The basic unit of measure for solid weight is the **grain** (gr).

> 1 grain = approximately the weight
>
> of 1 grain of wheat or rice

When measuring liquids, the volume may be expressed as minim, drams, or ounces. A minim (♏) is still found on some syringes, especially tuberculin syringes, and is approximately the size of a drop. The most commonly used apothecary symbol for a liquid is a dram (ʒ) that is approximately the size of a teaspoon. This symbol is most often found on a prescription for the household measure for the teaspoon. Many physicians still use the ounce symbol (℥) on prescriptions. See Table 7-2 for the commonly used apothecary measures.

Numbers and symbols in the apothecary system are written in reverse order from the metric system. In the metric system, quantity is written first, followed by the unit (e.g., 3 liters, 3 L). In the apothecary system, the symbol or abbreviation comes first, followed by the quantity, which is expressed in lowercase Roman numerals. An exam-

TABLE 7-2 *Units of Measure in the Apothecary System*

LIQUID VOLUME	SOLID WEIGHT
60 minims (♏) = 1 fluid dram (fʒ)	60 grains = 1 dram
8 fluid drams (fʒ viii) = 1 fluid ounce (f℥ i)	

ple is gr iv, which means 4 grains. Usually only the digits 1 through 10, 20, and 30 are expressed in Roman numerals. Most other quantities are expressed in Arabic numbers. However, all numerals are written in Arabic if the entire unit measurement is written in full. For example, 8 grains would not be written viii grains because the word "grain" is written out; it is either "8 grains" or "gr viii."

Another difference between the metric system and the apothecary system is that fractions are used in the apothecary system when necessary. (Remember that metric quantities are expressed in decimals.) For example, the fraction three-quarters is notated as $3/4$ in the apothecary system but as 0.75 in the metric system.

Household Measurement System

The **household system** is also called the U.S. Customary System of Measurement. This system is often used in patient education, especially with diabetic and weight control management. It is used to increase patient compliance when comparing amounts of food and liquids that make up one serving of a food or liquid. The household measurement system is usually based on the number of ounces in a measuring device when measuring quantities of weight or volume. The household system of measuring volume (liquids) uses the measuring devices of the dropper, teaspoon, tablespoon, ounce, and cup. The pint, quart, and gallon are also household measurements, but these measurements are not often associated with medical use because the metric measurements are becoming better known. Although the household system is applicable primarily to liquid medications, the ounce and pound could also be used to measure a patient's solid food intake or a patient's weight. The common household measures of length include the inch, the foot, and the yard. Table 7-3 shows the household measurement units most often used. Note that the table identifies the smallest measure first. When discussing food intake with a patient, the health professional should clearly define the content amount of a "cup," because there are teacups, coffee cups, measuring cups, and many more, all with different capacities.

The household system is not recommended for medical measurements in a medical facility because of the different sizes of the measuring devices. For example, a dropper may have a large or small hole (aperture) for the medicine to pass through, and the medication itself could be either viscous or aqueous, which would change the amount contained in a drop unless a dropper is provided with the medication. Therefore to instruct the patient to use a few drops would not be appropriate without specifying exactly what dropper the person needs to use. Another problem with droppers is that different patients using the same dropper may exert a different amount of force when pinching the plunger of the dropper, thus dispensing different amounts of medication. For OTC drugs that prescribe a teaspoonful of medicine, most pharmaceutical companies are now packaging the medicine with a graduated medication cup, a calibrated hollow-handle spoon, or a calibrated dropper. Consumers who measure drugs

TABLE 7-3 *Household Measurement System*

HOUSEHOLD TERM	UNIT VALUE	ABBREVIATION
WEIGHT OR MASS		
ounce		oz
pound	16 oz	lb; #
VOLUME OR LIQUID		
drop		gtt
teaspoon	60-75 gtt	tsp; t
tablespoon	3 t	Tbs; T
ounce	2 T	oz
cup	8 oz	c
pint	2 c; 16 oz	pt
quart	2 pt; 4 c; 32 oz	qt
gallon	4 qt; 8 pt; 16 c; 128 oz	gal
LENGTH		
inch		in
foot	12 in	ft
yard	3 ft; 36 in	yd

CHECK YOUR UNDERSTANDING—HOUSEHOLD SYSTEM | 7-5

Identify the household abbreviation.

1. T _____

2. gtt _____

3. c _____

4. t _____

5. tbs _____

Write greater than, less than, or equals to make each household measurement a true statement.

6. t _____ tbs

7. tsp _____ gtt

8. T _____ t

9. T _____ c

10. gtt _____ tbs

(continued)

CHECK YOUR UNDERSTANDING—HOUSEHOLD SYSTEM (cont'd)   7-5

PRACTICAL APPLICATION: Instruct the patient on how to use the following OTC remedies.

11. For the relief of occasional constipation, dissolve 2 level tsp of magnesium sulfate, USP, into 1 c of H_2O and take po. _____

12. Add 1-2 c of Epsom salts to warm bath to soothe and refresh your entire body.
_____

13. For temporary relief of cough caused by bronchial irritation, take 1 tsp of elix Benadryl q4h not to exceed 6 doses daily. _____

14. Take 1 cap po daily of 400 units of vitamin E. _____

15. To increase moisture, instill 2 gtts Liquifilm tears in each eye prn. _____
_____

at home most often use the household measurement system because of ease of availability.

Unlike the metric system, which uses the movement of decimals to identify equivalents within the metric system, the unit values must be memorized to find household equivalents. For example, to determine how many ounces are found in a gallon, you must first remember how many ounces are in a cup, how many cups are in a pint, how many pints are in a quart, and how many quarts are in a gallon or memorize all the conversions found in this system.

Units

Some drugs are measured in **units.** Units may be expressed as IU (International Units) or USP (United States Pharmaceutical) units. Drugs measured in units may be derived from plant or animal sources or manufactured in a laboratory (synthetic drugs). This section considers drugs made from animal sources because these drugs are usually measured in units. The strength of the raw material obtained from animal sources used with these medications can vary each time the material is obtained. Factors such as the conditions of growth or the manner in which the drug was obtained, and even the source, can vary greatly. After purification, and by dispensing these drugs in units, they are measured according to their strength and de-

sired effect. Common drugs dispensed in units include heparin (a powerful anticoagulant that prevents blood clots), insulin (for people with inadequate insulin production, such as those with diabetes mellitus), and penicillin G and penicillin V (antibiotics). Some fat-soluble vitamins such as vitamins A, D, and E are also dispensed in units.

CLINICAL TIP
Always read the label carefully to obtain the correct dosage strength desired!

Milliequivalents

The term **milliequivalent** pertains to the amount of a solute contained in a solution. Milliequivalent is abbreviated mEq and is usually expressed as milliequivalent per volume, mEq/L or mEq/mL, mEq/tab, or mEq/cap.

To express drugs in units or milliequivalents, the Arabic numbers are written first, followed by the unit or milliequivalent indicator. For example, if the doctor orders 100 units of insulin, this is written as 100 units; and 2 milliequivalents is written as 2 mEq.

CLINICAL TIP
Weight = strength or mass
Volume = amount or liquid

Current Trends for Symbols and Abbreviations

In 2001 The Joint Commission (TJC) began a movement to reduce medication errors related to the misinterpretation of certain abbreviations, acronyms, and symbols used in handwritten clinical medication documentation. In 2004 it was determined that in order to meet the National Patient Safety Goal (NPSG), an official list of "Do Not Use" abbreviations would be developed (Table 7-4). In May of 2005, TJC mandated that all medical facilities adhere to the changes on the "Do Not Use" list. It was also determined that each year TJC would review and possibly implement further changes in additional abbreviations, acronyms, and symbols. Those changes currently under consideration may be found in Table 7-5. Updated information can be found on the TJC website (www.jointcommission.org) under the tab of Patient Safety. A second website from the Institute for Safe Medication Practices (www.ismp.org) includes not only the abbreviations and symbols, but also dose designations and drug abbreviations that should be avoided.

TABLE 7-4 *Official "Do Not Use" List**

DO NOT USE	POTENTIAL PROBLEM	USE INSTEAD
U (unit)	Mistaken for "0" (zero), the number "4" (four), or "cc"	Write unit
IU (International Unit)	Mistaken for IV (intravenous) or the number 10 (ten)	Write "International Unit"
Q.D., QD, q.d., qd (daily)	Mistaken for each other	Write "daily"
Q.O.D., QOD, q.o.d., qod (every other day)	Period after the Q mistaken for "I" and the "O" mistaken for "I"	Write "every other day"
Trailing zero (X.0 mg)†	Decimal point is missed	Write X mg
Lack of trailing zero (.X mg)	Decimal point is missed	Write 0.X mg
MS	Can mean morphine sulphate or magnesium sulfate	Write "morphine sulfate" Write "magnesium sulfate"
MSO_4 and $MgSO_4$	Confused for one another	

†Exception: A "trailing zero" may be used only where required to demonstrate the level of precision of the value being reported, such as for laboratory results, imaging studies that report the size of lesions, or catheter/tube sizes. It may not be used in medication orders or other medication-related documentation.
From www.jointcommission.org
*Applies to all orders and all medication-related documentation that is handwritten (including free-text computer entry) or on preprinted items.

TABLE 7-5 *Additional Abbreviations, Acronyms, and Symbols (for Possible Future Inclusion in the Official "Do Not Use" List)*

DO NOT USE	POTENTIAL PROBLEM	USE INSTEAD
> (greater than)	Misinterpreted as the number "7" (seven) or the letter "L"	Write "greater than"
< (less than)	Confused for one another	Write "less than"
Abbreviations for drug names	Misinterpreted due to similar abbreviations for multiple drugs	Write drug names in full
Apothecary units	Unfamiliar to many practitioners Confused with metric units	Use metric units
@	Mistaken for the number "2" (two)	Write "at"
cc	Mistaken for U (units) when poorly written	Write "mL" or "milliliters"
μg	Mistaken for mg (milligrams) resulting in one thousand fold overdose	Write "mcg" or "micrograms"

From www.jointcommission.org

Summary

Several systems of measure are encountered in clinical medicine for measuring mass, volume, and length. The metric system is most common and is accepted worldwide. OTC drug instructions frequently refer to household measures such as a drop or cup. Certain medications, such as insulin and penicillin, are measured in units. Finally, the apothecary system, one of the oldest systems of measure devised, is discussed. Because it is important for allied health professionals to know and be able to use all systems, the next chapter introduces conversions between the commonly used metric system and the less frequently used household system and apothecary systems.

Abbreviations are important in most of the measurement systems. Being able to recognize the differences among the various systems will help the student to understand how to read and interpret medication orders, prepare drug inventory records and Material Safety Data Sheets, and assist in patient education when reading and interpreting patient charts.

Critical Thinking Exercises

Supply the missing information in the following table of metric terms and abbreviations. The first row is completed as an example.

METRIC TERM	UNIT VALUE	PREFIX	ROOT WORD	ABBREV.	TYPE OF UNIT
kilogram	1000 units	kilo	gram	kg	weight (solid)
		micro		mcg	weight (solid)
	1 unit	—			length
	0.001 of a unit	milli			volume (liquid)
	1 unit	—		g	
			meter	cm	length
milligram		milli	gram		
	1 unit		liter		volume (liquid)
millimeter		milli		mm	

REVIEW QUESTIONS

Write apothecary, household, or metric to identify the measurement system of each given term.

1. Microgram _____

2. Teaspoon _____

3. Centimeter _____

4. Cup _____

5. Liter _____

6. Gram _____

7. Ounce _____

8. Drop _____

9. Grain _____

10. Meter _____

Fill in the blank.

11. A drug derived from an animal source, such as insulin, is measured in _____.

12. The term _____ refers to the weight of a drug contained in a normal solution.

13. Consumers who measure drugs at home most often use the _____ measurement system.

14. A microgram is abbreviated _____ .

15. _____ (system) quantities are expressed in decimals.

16. One cubic centimeter is equivalent to _____ _____.

17. The three basic units in the metric system are a _____, _____, and _____.

Circle the correct notation.

18. 100 U or 100 units

19. ii milliequivalents or 2 mEq

Match the correct prefix with the unit given.

20. 1000   _____   centi

21. 0.1   _____   deci

22. 0.01   _____   kilo

23. 0.001   _____   micro

24. 0.000001 _____   milli

All of the following statements are *false*. Determine the errors, and then write the correct answers in a complete sentence.

25. A kilogram is a household measure for solid weight. _____
_____
_____

26. A milliliter is equal to a cubic millimeter. _____
_____
_____

27. Consumers who measure drugs at home most often use the apothecary system. _____
_____
_____

28. The household system is considered the international standard of measurement systems. _____
_____
_____

29. Micrograms are larger than milligrams. _____
_____
_____

30. The metric system sometimes has a conversion factor that is a power of 10. _____
_____
_____

31. Medications prescribed in the metric system are measured in teaspoons and tablespoons. _____
_____
_____

32. Drops are usually compared with ounces. _____
_____
_____

33. Milliliters are used to measure solids. _____
_____
_____

34. Drugs measured in units must be manufactured in a laboratory. _____
_____
_____

35. Drops are easy to measure because the size of the aperture of the dropper prevents overdosing.
_____
_____

36. All measurement systems discussed in this chapter are still in use today. _____
_____
_____

37. The meter and the yard are the same length. _____
_____
_____

38. Premature babies are often weighed in metric pounds. _____
_____
_____

39. When referring to insulin, the term milliequivalent identifies the weight of the solution. _____
_____
_____

Converting Between Measurement Systems

OBJECTIVES

After studying this chapter, you should be capable of doing the following:
- Reading the time of day on the international standard 24-hour clock and the 12-hour clock and converting time between the two time standards.
- Reading a thermometer in Fahrenheit scale and in Celsius scale and converting measurements between the two systems.
- Converting from one length unit to another within and between the metric and household systems.
- Converting from one weight or volume unit to another within and between the metric system and the household system or the metric system and the apothecary system.
- Computing approximate equivalents between the metric and household systems.
- Converting approximate equivalents between the metric and apothecary systems.
- Converting approximate equivalents between the household and apothecary systems.

KEY TERMS

Celsius
Convert
Dimensional analysis
Fahrenheit
International Standard ISO 8601
Reconstitution

CHAPTER 8 PRETEST: CONVERTING BETWEEN MEASUREMENT SYSTEMS

Part I: Answer the following questions.

1. Convert the following English standard times into international standard notation.

   10:15 pm = _____   5:47 pm = _____

   9:20 am = _____   1:25 am = _____

2. Convert the following temperatures between Fahrenheit and Celsius.

   18° C = _____°F   80° C = _____°F

   104° F = _____°C   100° F = _____°C

3. Convert the following volume units between systems.

   ℨ ii = _____ tsp   ℥ ii = _____ mL

   $\frac{1}{2}$ qt = _____ mL   3 tbs = _____ mL

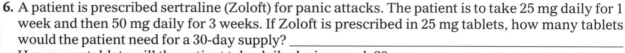

CHAPTER 8 PRETEST: CONVERTING BETWEEN MEASUREMENT SYSTEMS—cont'd

4. Convert the following weight units between systems.

   30 mg = gr _____   5 lb = _____ g

   gr i$\overline{ss}$ = _____ mg

5. Convert the following length units.

   35 cm = _____ ft _____ in   2.5 m = _____ cm

   150 mm = _____ in   40 mm = _____ cm

   17.5 cm = _____ in

   Part II: Determine the answer from the information given.

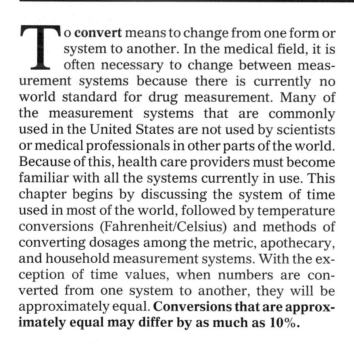

6. A patient is prescribed sertraline (Zoloft) for panic attacks. The patient is to take 25 mg daily for 1 week and then 50 mg daily for 3 weeks. If Zoloft is prescribed in 25 mg tablets, how many tablets would the patient need for a 30-day supply? _____
   How many tablets will the patient take daily during week 2? _____

7. A patient is given a 30-day supply of propranolol (Inderal) for prevention of migraine headaches. If the patient is to take 80 mg a day, and the tablet is supplied in 40-mg dosage strength, how many tablets would the patient be given? _____
   How many tablets will the patient take with each dose? _____

To **convert** means to change from one form or system to another. In the medical field, it is often necessary to change between measurement systems because there is currently no world standard for drug measurement. Many of the measurement systems that are commonly used in the United States are not used by scientists or medical professionals in other parts of the world. Because of this, health care providers must become familiar with all the systems currently in use. This chapter begins by discussing the system of time used in most of the world, followed by temperature conversions (Fahrenheit/Celsius) and methods of converting dosages among the metric, apothecary, and household measurement systems. With the exception of time values, when numbers are converted from one system to another, they will be approximately equal. **Conversions that are approximately equal may differ by as much as 10%.**

Time Conversions

The *International Standard ISO 8601* has been recognized in most countries of the world as the universal standard for telling time and writing the date. The United States has not widely adopted this standard except in the military, in the computer industry, in scientific publications, and in hospitals. The international standard notation for the time of day is hh:mm:ss. (The colons are not written). The *hh* signifies the total complete hours that have passed since midnight; the *mm* states the total minutes that have passed since the start of the hour; and the *ss* identifies the total seconds that have passed since the start of the minute. For example, 25 seconds after 10:20 AM would be written as 102025. (In most cases seconds are not included in the conversion so only the hour and minutes would be documented, such as 1020.) Most countries do not use the abbreviations "AM" and "PM" because they do not recognize the 12-hour notation that is used in the United States. The history of the 12-hour clock dates back to the dark ages when Roman numerals were used and there was no symbol for the digit "zero." A good example of how the 12-hour clock is still used is the analog watch, which displays the numbers 1 through 12. Because digital watches did not become widely available in the United States prior to 1971, health care providers have been trained to take vital signs using the second hand of the analog watch.

The 12-hour clock has only the numbers 1 through 12, so to differentiate between morning and evening, the time between midnight and noon is followed by the letters AM. The hours from noon to midnight are written with the letters PM after

BOX 8-1 THE 12-HOUR CLOCK AND THE 24-HOUR CLOCK

12-HOUR CLOCK	24-HOUR CLOCK
12 midnight	0000 (= 2400)
1 am	0100
2 am	0200
3 am	0300
4 am	0400
5 am	0500
6 am	0600
7 am	0700
8 am	0800
9 am	0900
10 am	1000
11 am	1100
12 noon	1200
1 pm	1300
2 pm	1400
3 pm	1500
4 pm	1600
5 pm	1700
6 pm	1800
7 pm	1900
8 pm	2000
9 pm	2100
10 pm	2200
11 pm	2300
12 midnight	2400 (= 0000)

the numbers 1 through 12. To understand how to convert from the 12-hour (AM/PM) format to the 24-hour format, refer to Box 8-1. (For ease in understanding, the seconds are not shown.) Note that midnight starts the 24-hour clock at 0000. Each hour is shown by the first two digits, which are numbered from 00 to 24. When you get to noon (1200), keep increasing by one digit for each hour. On the 24-hour clock, "AM" and "PM" are not used because one o'clock in the afternoon is written "1300," two o'clock is written "1400," and so on. Minutes are written as the two digits following the hour and are numbered from 00 to 59, just as in the familiar 12-hour system. (Seconds do not vary among the systems either). The clock in Figure 8-1 shows the comparison of hours between the two systems.

EXAMPLE 1: 8:20 AM = _____ international time

The AM symbol tells you that this is in 12-hour format, so change the format to 24-hour notation by dropping the AM, adding a zero before the 8, and deleting the colon.

So, 8:20 AM is 0820 in 24-hour notation.

EXAMPLE 2: 11:55 PM = _____ international time

The PM symbol tells you that this is in the 12-hour format and that it is in the evening, so add one digit for each hour after noon, drop the PM symbol, and delete the colon.

$12 + 11 = 23$. Therefore the time is 2355.

Several valid reasons to use the international standard time in the medical field instead of the old English 12-hour clock exist. With the 24-hour clock there is less chance for human error because there is no duplication in the hours of the day. With the 12-hour clock, if the symbols AM and PM are not used, mistakes can be made, especially on dosages that are meant to be given only once every 24 hours.

Another way to remember how to change from the English 12-hour clock to the 2400 international clock is described as follows (see Figure 8-1).

Draw two circles.
On the first circle, draw a second circle inside the larger circle and label the 12-hour clock.
On the second circle using the number 12, add each number from the 12-hour English clock to obtain the 2400 clock. 2400 is midnight on the international clock, and 0001 is 1 minute after midnight. The first 12 hours after midnight are written the same on both clocks; however, the English clock will identify AM and the international clock is always written using four digits.

Measuring Temperature

In Chapter 7 the metric system was introduced as the international standard for scientific and industrial measurements. In the metric system, temperature is measured as Celsius whereas the Fahrenheit scale is predominant in the United States. The Celsius scale was introduced in the mid-1700s and is often referred to as the *centigrade* scale. Because the metric system is the predominant mathematical system used in much of the rest of the world, it is important to be able to convert from the Fahrenheit scale to the Celsius scale.

The Celsius scale is always the lower number when it is shown with the equivalent degrees on the Fahrenheit scale. Temperatures are always measured in degrees. For example, 0° Celsius is equivalent to 32° on the Fahrenheit scale. (The small ° symbol stands for "degrees). Table 8-1 shows a comparison of some common equivalents between the Celsius and Fahrenheit scales.

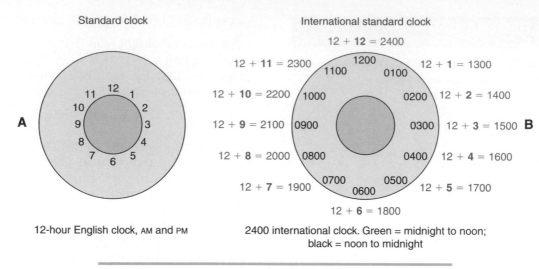

Standard clock

International standard clock

A

12-hour English clock, AM and PM

2400 international clock. Green = midnight to noon;
black = noon to midnight

Figure 8-1 **A**, Standard clock and **B**, international standard clock.

CHECK YOUR UNDERSTANDING—TIME CONVERSION   8-1

Convert the time shown into international standard time.

1. 4:40 AM = _____

2. 6:25 PM = _____

3. 11:02 AM = _____

4. 2:56 AM = _____

5. 10:45 PM = _____

6. 8:10 PM = _____

7. 12:33 AM = _____

8. 10:00 AM = _____

9. 3:33 PM = _____

10. 7:17 AM = _____

Convert the international time to the 12-hour English time.

11. 2121 = _____

12. 1615 = _____

13. 0045 = _____

14. 1234 = _____

15. 2400 = _____

16. 1830 = _____

17. 0210 = _____

18. 1605 = _____

19. 1515 = _____

20. 1357 = _____

TABLE 8-1 *Common Baselines for Fahrenheit and Celsius Temperatures*

	CELSIUS	FAHRENHEIT
Water boils	100°	212°
Normal body temperature	37°	98.6°
Room temperature	20°	68°
Water freezes	0°	32°

Some special considerations should be remembered when placing a decimal in the answer when converting temperatures. The decimal place in Celsius is used in tenths only and may need to be rounded off. For example, if the answer is 35.55°, in the Celsius system the answer is written as 35.6° C. In Fahrenheit, on a thermometer that is not digital, the decimal place is only shown in multiples of two tenths. Look at the thermometer shown in Figure 8-2. Notice that the calibration is by even numbers, so the degrees are recorded as

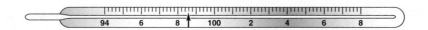

Figure 8-2 Calibration of a thermometer. (Modified from Hunt S: *Student mastery manual to accompany Saunders' fundamentals of medical assisting*, Philadelphia, 2002, Saunders.)

CHECK YOUR UNDERSTANDING—MEASURING TEMPERATURE   8-2

PRACTICE PROBLEMS

Identify the following temperatures in Fahrenheit.

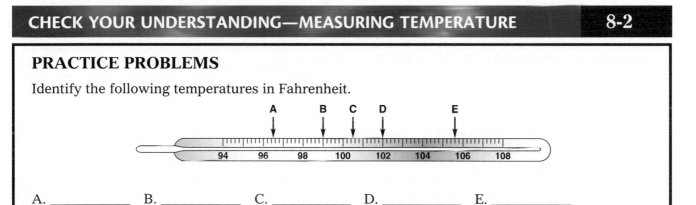

A. _____   B. _____   C. _____   D. _____   E. _____

101.0° F, 101.2° F, 101.4° F, 101.6° F, or 101.8° F. Today medical facilities use digital thermometers which accurately record the temperature in decimal format using all decimals, from one tenth through nine tenths.

Temperature Conversions

There are two ways to convert between Celsius and Fahrenheit. Although both methods obtain the correct results, you should memorize only one of them and consistently use that method to avoid confusion when converting between Celsius and Fahrenheit. Both methods are explained, and you should choose the one that works best for you. Always round your answer to the nearest tenth.

Method 1

To change from Fahrenheit to Celsius, use this formula:

$$C° = \frac{5}{9}(F° - 32)$$

EXAMPLE 3: _____ ° C = 104° F

Using the formula, the first step would be to do the calculation in parentheses by taking 104° F − 32 = 72. The second step is to take the 72 × 5 = 360. The final step would be to divide the 360 by 9 = 40.

Therefore, 40° C = 104° F.

To change from Celsius to Fahrenheit, use this formula:

$$F° = \left(\frac{9}{5}C°\right) + 32$$

EXAMPLE 4: _____ ° F = 38.3° C

Using the formula, the first step would be to do the calculation in parentheses by taking 38.3 × 9 = 344.7. The second step would be to divide: 344.7 ÷ 5 = 68.94.

The final step is to add: 68.94 + 32 = 100.94. Round to 100.9° F, so 100.9° F = 38.3° C.

Review the two formulas:

$$C° = \frac{5}{9}(F° - 32) \qquad F° = \left(\frac{9}{5}C°\right) + 32$$

Method 2

Use the formula C° = (F° − 32) ÷ 1.8 to change from Fahrenheit to Celsius. (In the formula, 1.8 is the decimal equivalent of $^9/_5$.)

EXAMPLE 5: _____ C° = 99.8° F

Using the formula C° = (F° − 32) ÷ 1.8, the first step would be to subtract (99.8° F − 32) = 67.8. The second and final step is to divide 67.8 ÷ 1.8 = 37.67. Remember to round your answer to tenths.

Therefore, 37.7° C = 99.8° F.

Some students find that Method 2 is easier because only two steps instead of three are necessary to find the correct answer. Method 2 can also be used to convert from Fahrenheit to Celsius using the formula $F° = 1.8 (C°) + 32$.

EXAMPLE 6: _____ $F° = 22° C°$

Using the formula $F° = 1.8(C°) + 32$, the first step would be to multiply $(1.8 \times 22° C) = 39.6$. Then just add 32 to your answer $39.6 + 32 = 71.6$.

Therefore, $22° C = 71.6° F$.

When changing *from* Fahrenheit *to* Celsius, you must remember to do what is in parentheses first $(F° - 32)$ before attempting to divide by 1.8. When changing *from* Celsius *to* Fahrenheit, remember to multiply $1.8 \times C°$ before adding the 32.
Review the two formulas again.

From C° to F°	From F° to C°
Multiply C° by 1.8	*Subtract* 32 from F°
Add 32	*Divide* by 1.8

 LEARNING TIP
When performing temperature calculations, remember to complete the steps *in the order given,* by first removing the parentheses.

Converting Between Measurement Systems Using Ratio and Proportion

Sometimes a medication will be ordered in an amount that is not in the measurement system of the medication on hand. When this occurs, you must be able to convert between the systems to obtain the correct amount of medication for administration.

Several methods are used to convert between measurement units. The easiest conversion method is using ratio and proportion. To solve for an unknown variable, a comparison of ratios will provide an answer for solving for *x*. Be sure that the unit values in both ratios are identified. The numerators must be in the same units and the denominators must be in the same units for ratio and proportion to be used. For example: 1 mL is to 15 gtts is the same as 2 mL is to 30 gtts. (Notice that both mL are in the same place in the ratios and the gtts are in the same place.) This can also be written with both numerators in fractional units being in mL and both denominators being in gtts $\left(\dfrac{1 \text{ mL}}{15 \text{ gtts}} = \dfrac{2 \text{ mL}}{30 \text{ gtts}} \right)$. This is can also be written as a linear proportion as follows: 1 mL : 15 gtts :: 2 mL : 30 gtts. When the proportion contains an unknown measurement, this should be identified with *x*. After determining the unknown measurement, a proportion, either fractional or linear,

---

CHECK YOUR UNDERSTANDING—TEMPERATURE CONVERSIONS   8-3

PRACTICE PROBLEMS

Remember to round to the nearest tenth. Using the one method that is most comfortable for you, convert the following:

1. _____ ° C = 99.6° F

2. _____ ° C = 76° F

3. _____ ° C = 103° F

4. _____ ° C = 100.8° F

5. _____ ° C = 80° F

6. _____ ° C = 98.6° F

7. _____ ° C = 212° F

8. _____ ° C = 68° F

9. _____ ° C = 0° F

10. _____ ° C = 97.2° F

11. _____ ° F = 14° C

12. _____ ° F = 30° C

13. _____ ° F = 5° C

14. _____ ° F = 21° C

15. _____ ° F = 96° C

16. _____ ° F = 50° C

17. _____ ° F = 42.3° C

18. _____ ° F = 18.8° C

19. _____ ° F = 11° C

20. _____ ° F = 83° C

may be formed. In the proportion, set the first ratios as the known element that corresponds to the unknown desired and the second ratio with the identified unknown. To solve for x in the second ratio, cross-multiply the fractions or multiply the means and extremes.

LEARNING TIP
When setting up both ratios, be sure to label all of the terms, including the x, with the correct measurement to ensure that the equations are equivalents.

EXAMPLE 7:

$$\frac{1\,g}{2\,mL} \bowtie \frac{x\,g}{4\,mL} \quad \text{OR} \quad 1\,g : 2\,mL :: x\,g : 4\,mL$$

$$2x = 4 \qquad\qquad (2\,mL \times x\,g = 4\,mL \times 1\,g)$$

$$x = 4 \div 2$$

$$x = 2\,g$$

System Conversions

This section will compare approximate equivalents among three different systems—metric, apothecary, and household—commonly used to weigh, find length, and find volume in the medical field. The metric system is the most often used

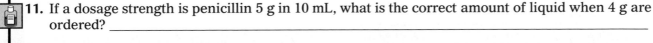
CHECK YOUR UNDERSTANDING—RATIO AND PROPORTION   8-4

CALCULATION REVIEW: Review the following ratios with the fractional equivalent.

1. 1:5 = _____

2. 3:6 = _____

3. 2:5 = _____

4. 4:5 = _____

5. 9:10 = _____

Replace the following fractions with the ratio equivalent.

6. $\dfrac{3}{4}$ = _____

7. $\dfrac{1}{2}$ = _____

8. $\dfrac{1}{10}$ = _____

9. $\dfrac{1}{100}$ = _____

10. $\dfrac{4}{9}$ = _____

PRACTICAL APPLICATION: Determine the following calculations.

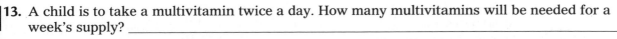

11. If a dosage strength is penicillin 5 g in 10 mL, what is the correct amount of liquid when 4 g are ordered? _____

12. A physician orders ibuprofen 650 mg. The available medication is ibuprofen 325 mg/tablet. How many tablets should the patient take? _____

13. A child is to take a multivitamin twice a day. How many multivitamins will be needed for a week's supply? _____

14. A physician orders KCl (potassium chloride) 80 mEq daily. The available tablets are 40 mEq per tablet. How many tablets should the patient take? _____

15. A physician orders Valium 5 mg at night for rest. The available tablets at the time the prescription is filled are Valium 2.5 mg. How many tablets should the patient take with each dose?

_____

system of measurement for drug labels in the United States. It is important that you be able to convert these units among the systems. The first two measurement systems, volume and weight, are used primarily in the field of medicine for dosage calculations. Volume, measured in mL or L, is usually associated with oral liquid medications, contents in a syringe, intake and output of a patient, and intravenous (IV) medications. Weight, used to measure solid mass, is usually associated with medications measured in milligrams, grams, or micrograms, whereas body weight is usually measured in kilograms or pounds. Except in a few cases, such as with nitroglycerin ointment, length measurements are not usually associated with dosage calculations. Length is primarily used for measuring body surface areas and medical equipment such as needles or suture thicknesses and to measure medical appliances for specific patients. Understanding that there will be as much as a 10% variation for dosage calculations when converting among the systems is *very important*. Also, do not forget to consider the 10% variance is considered equivalent when comparing the approximate equivalents.

Volume

Table 8-2 compares the *approximate* equivalents found among the different units of liquid volume. These equivalents are known as the *conversion factor*. Although it is best to memorize the equivalents, some facilities will have equivalency tables available.

As previously stated, this table shows approximate equivalents. Three generally accepted amounts in the metric system are used and are usually rounded for ease of calculations. For example,

TABLE 8-2 *Volume Measurements*

METRIC SYSTEM	HOUSEHOLD SYSTEM	APOTHECARY SYSTEM
0.06 mL	1 drop (gtt)	♏ i
1 mL = 1cc*	15 or 16† drops	♏ 15-16
4 mL (5 mL)†	1 teaspoon (t)	ʒ i
15 mL	1 tablespoon (tbs)	ʒ ss
30 mL	2 tablespoons, 1 oz	ʒ i
240 mL (250 mL)†*	1 cup (c)	
480 mL (500 mL)†	1 pint (pt)	
960 mL	1 quart (qt)	
(1000 mL)†, 1 L		
3480 mL (3.48 L)	1 gallon, 4 qt	

* cc (cubic centimeters) are being phased out. Use milliliters instead.
† Remember that conversions are approximate measurements.

regarding the equivalents between metric, household, and apothecary systems, 5 mL in the metric system is usually accepted as being equivalent to a teaspoon in the household system and 1 dram in the apothecary system. In the household system, 480 mL is usually rounded up to 500 mL, or is equivalent to a pint; and 960 mL is usually rounded up to 1000 mL, or is equivalent to a quart. Examples in this text use the rounded equivalents (5 mL, 250 mL, 500 mL, and 1000 mL). Remember to use the correct expression (such as decimals or fractions) in your answer when converting between systems. In the metric system, answers are shown in decimal format using only Arabic numerals, whereas the apothecary system uses fractions with Arabic numerals but also uses Roman numerals for the digits 1-10, 20, and 30, and the abbreviation $\overline{ss}$ for ½.

Converting Volume Measurement Units Between Systems

Use the information provided in this section for ratios, proportions, and conversions to determine the volume measurements between metric, household, and apothecary systems.

EXAMPLE 8: fʒ x = _____ mL

Recall that in the apothecary system fʒ x means 10 fluid drams because the apothecary system uses Roman numerals.

Set up the known ratio: 4 mL = fʒ i
Write as either a fraction or a linear ratio:

$$\frac{4\ mL}{f\mathentry{ʒ}\ i} \quad OR \quad 4\ mL : f\mathentry{ʒ}i$$

Next set up the second ratio with the unknown information so the proportion will look as follows:

$$\frac{4\ mL}{f\mathentry{ʒ}\ i} = \frac{x\ mL}{f\mathentry{ʒ}x} \quad OR \quad 4\ mL : f\mathentry{ʒ}i :: x\ mL : f\mathentry{ʒ}\ x$$

Now cross multiply, changing the apothecary Roman numerals to Arabic numbers

$$\frac{4\ mL}{f\mathentry{ʒ}\times1} \bowtie \frac{x\ mL}{f\mathentry{ʒ}\ 10} \quad OR \quad 4\ mL : f\mathentry{ʒ}\ 1 :: x\ mL : f\mathentry{ʒ}\ 10$$

$1 \times x = x$
$4 \times 10 = 40$
$x = 40\ mL$

x is expressed in mL so the answer will be in mL.

Notice that when setting up the proportion with the second ratio, you must use the same unit order that you chose in the first ratio,

EXAMPLE 9: 750 mL = _____ pint(s)

Set up the known ratio first. Known ratio: 500 mL = 1 pint. Next, set up the second ratio with the given and unknown information. Your problem now looks like these linear or fractional proportions:

$$\frac{500 \text{ mL}}{1 \text{ pint}} = \frac{750 \text{ mL}}{x \text{ pint}}$$

OR

500 mL : 1 pint :: 750 mL : x pint

Cross-multiply:

$$\frac{500 \text{ mL}}{1 \text{ pint}} \times \frac{750 \text{ mL}}{x \text{ pint}}$$

OR

500 mL : 1 pint :: 750 mL : x pint

$$500 \times x = 500x$$
$$1 \times 750 = 750$$

The problem now looks like this:

$$500 x = 750$$

Next, solve for x by dividing both sides by 500.

$$\frac{500x}{500} = \frac{750}{500}$$

We now have $x = \dfrac{750}{500}$

Simplifying, we find the answer is $x = 1.5$. x was expressed in pints, so the answer remains in pints.

750 mL = 1.5 pints or 1½ pints.

LEARNING TIP
- Remember the answer may be written as 750 mL = 1½ pints or 750 mL=1.5 pints because pints are household measurements and either fractions or decimals may be used.
- Also, notice that if you try to use the exact equivalent of 480 mL = 1 pint, instead of the approximation that 500 mL = 1 pint, your final answer becomes more difficult to calculate.

Although not used often, a conversion of liquids in the apothecary system includes 60 minims (℥ 60) to a fluid dram (fʒ). Think of a clock with 60 minutes to an hour. A fourth of a dram is 15 minims just as 15 minutes is a fourth of an hour (Figure 8-3). Please notice that HR and DR (abbreviations with "r") are on the outside of the clock with minims and minutes (abbreviations

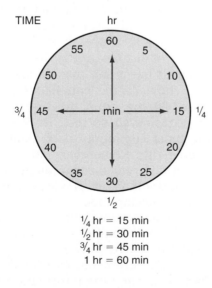

¼ hr = 15 min
½ hr = 30 min
¾ hr = 45 min
1 hr = 60 min

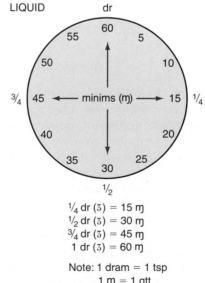

¼ dr (ʒ) = 15 ℥
½ dr (ʒ) = 30 ℥
¾ dr (ʒ) = 45 ℥
1 dr (ʒ) = 60 ℥

Note: 1 dram = 1 tsp
1 ℥ = 1 gtt

Figure 8-3 Conversion clock for liquid medications for metric and apothecary systems. (Fulcher R, Fulcher E: *Math calculations for pharmacy technicians: a worktext,* St Louis, 2007, Saunders.)

CHECK YOUR UNDERSTANDING—VOLUME CONVERSION   8-5

CALCULATION REVIEW: Convert the following volume units to the requested equivalent measurements.

1. 45 mL = _____ tbsp

2. 2 pt = _____ c

3. 1 mL = _____ gtt

4. 30 mL = _____ oz

5. 3 oz = _____ mL

6. 1000 mL = _____ pt

7. 250 mL = _____ c

8. 4 t = _____ mL

9. 1 pt = _____ mL

10. 30 gtt = _____ mL

PRACTICAL APPLICATION: Determine the following conversions.

11. A patient calls stating that he misplaced the medicine cup to his nighttime medicine. The directions say to take 30 mL before bedtime. How many tablespoons would you direct the patient to take? _____

12. A physician tells the patient that he needs to drink two pints of GoLytely. Record this amount in his chart, using the metric system. _____

13. Dr. Haus, a German physician, wants his patient to force fluids. He requests that you convert 2000 mL into a household equivalent for the patient's information. _____

14. A patient is instructed to instill 2 drops of medication into each eye. How many mL would you use if you had a dropper measured in the metric system? _____

15. You are directed to give a patient 30 mL of medication, but the medicine cup is calibrated in ounces. How many ounces are equivalent to 30 mL? _____

with "m") are in the center of the clock. This may assist you in remembering the known elements needed for changing minims and drams.

Weight

Most of the conversions done in the medical field are for converting different weights or solid measurements. The same rules apply for converting weights as for volume. Remember to always *first convert the quantities to be used into the same unit of measure within a system as you convert.* If you are converting among the metric, household, or apothecary systems, you will need to set up a ratio and proportion problem to obtain the equivalent weights first. Then do the math conversion. The most common weight conversion between systems is from pounds to kilograms for both adults and children. However, in the administration of medications, often the amount prescribed and the dosage available may be converted, such as grains to milligrams or grams.

Another important fact to remember is that drug companies sometimes use different equivalents for a measure. In weight, the most common source of discrepancy is the grain, the apothecary system's basic unit of solid measure. Some tables will show 65 mg equal to 1 grain; other tables show 60 mg equal to 1 grain. Both measures are considered correct. In this text, we will use the most commonly used equivalence of 60 mg equals 1 gr. Remember that when converting between different measurement systems, the measurement obtained is only approximate, not an exact measurement. Table 8-3 identifies the most common weight equivalencies. The table may look difficult to remember, but there are basically only two conversions to memorize, and all other measurements can be derived from these formulas, using the information on ratio and proportion provided in chapter 6. The conversion needed for converting from apothecary to metric system is one grain = 60 milligrams or one gram = 15 grains.

TABLE 8-3 *Weight Measurements*

METRIC SYSTEM	APOTHECARY SYSTEM	HOUSEHOLD
0.008 gram (g) = 8 mg	gr $\frac{1}{8}$	NA
0.01 g = 10 milligrams (mg)	gr $\frac{1}{6}$	NA
0.015 g = 15 mg	gr $\frac{1}{4}$	NA
0.06 g = 60 mg	gr 1	NA
0.1 g = 100 mg	gr $\frac{1}{2}$	NA
1 g = 1000 mg	gr 15	NA
30 g	NA	1 ounce (oz)
0.45 kilogram (kg)	NA	1 pound (lb)
1 kg = 1000 g	NA	2.2 lb

 LEARNING TIP

Weight measurement comparisons are easier to remember using the conversion clock shown. Think of 1 hour = 60 minutes (1 hr = 60 min), just as 1 grain = 60 milligrams (1 gr = 60 mg) Use Figure 8-4 to make the conversion easier. Finally you may place all three clocks together to assist with conversion of liquid and solid measurement found with the apothecary system. Remember that the abbreviations containing "r" remain outside the clock while the abbreviations containing "m" remain inside the clock (Figure 8-5).

Converting Weight Measurement Units Between Systems

Converting weight units between systems is similar to converting volume units among systems. The safest way is by setting up a ratio and proportion equation. Then solve the problem using basic math.

 LEARNING TIP

Do not forget to use the correct notation in the apothecary system. The abbreviation "gr" is written first, followed by the quantity, which is written in lowercase Roman numerals, if the number used is $\overline{ss}$ or $\frac{1}{2}$, 1-10, 15, 20, or 30. In the metric and household systems, the quantity is written first, followed by the abbreviation. The following examples illustrate this.

EXAMPLE 10: 300 mg = gr _____

Set up the known ratio first.
Known ratio: 60 mg = gr i.

Write as a fraction or ratio:

$$\frac{60 \text{ mg}}{\text{gr i}} \text{ OR } 60 \text{ mg : gr i}$$

Next, set up the second ratio as a fraction with the given and unknown information. The problem now looks like this proportion:

$$\frac{60 \text{ mg}}{\text{gr i}} = \frac{300 \text{ mg}}{x \text{ gr}} \text{ OR } 60 \text{ mg : gr i :: } 300 \text{ mg : } x \text{ gr}$$

Cross-multiply, cancelling the abbreviations, as appropriate, and change apothecary Roman numerals to numbers.

$$\frac{60 \text{ mg}}{\text{gr 1}} \bowtie \frac{300 \text{ mg}}{x \text{ gr}} \text{ OR}$$

$$60 \text{ mg : gr 1 :: } 300 \text{ mg : } x \text{ gr}$$

$$60 \times x = 60x$$

$$300 \times 1 \text{ gr} = 300 \text{ gr}$$

Rewrite the equation as:

$$60x = 300 \text{ gr}$$

Solve for x by dividing both sides by 60.

$$\frac{60x}{60} = \frac{300 \text{ gr}}{60}$$

Be sure to remember that the abbreviation for x was gr; therefore your answer will be found in grains. When completing the math, $x = 5$. Therefore 300 mg = gr v. The answer is expressed in Roman numerals because the answer is in the apothecary system.

EXAMPLE 11: 206 lb = _____ kg

Set up the known ratio first. Known ratio: 2.2 lb = 1 kg. Write as a fraction or ratio:

$$\frac{2.2 \text{ lb}}{1 \text{ kg}} \text{ OR } 2.2 \text{ lb : 1 kg}$$

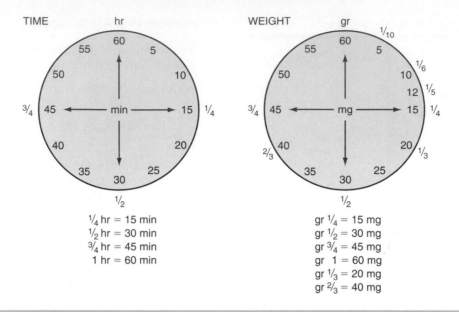

Figure 8-4 Conversion clock for weight or solid measurements. (Fulcher R, Fulcher E: *Math calculations for pharmacy technicians: a worktext*, St Louis, 2007, Saunders.)

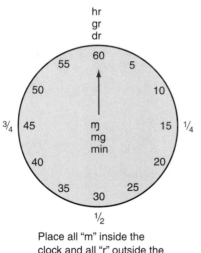

Place all "m" inside the clock and all "r" outside the clock.

Figure 8-5 Conversion clock for liquid and solid measurement. (Fulcher R, Fulcher E: *Math calculations for pharmacy technicians: a worktext*, St Louis, 2007, Saunders.)

Next, set up the second ratio as a fraction with the given and unknown information. Your problem now looks like this proportion:

$$\frac{2.2 \text{ lb}}{1 \text{ kg}} = \frac{206 \text{ lb}}{x \text{ kg}} \quad \text{OR} \quad 2.2 \text{ lb} : 1 \text{ kg} :: 206 \text{ lb} : x \text{ kg}$$

Cross-multiply, leaving off the abbreviations:

$$\frac{2.2 \text{ lb}}{1 \text{ kg}} \diagdown \frac{206 \text{ lb}}{x \text{ kg}}$$

OR

2.2 lb : 1 kg :: 206 lb : x kg

$206 \times 1 = 206$ kg
$2.2 \times x = 2.2$

Rewrite the equation as $2.2x = 206$.
Solve for x by dividing each side by 2.2:

$$\frac{2.2x}{2.2} = \frac{206 \text{ kg}}{2.2}$$

Remember x was in kg; therefore your answer will be found in kg.

$x = 93.6$; therefore 206 lb = 93.6 kg. The kilograms can be rounded to a whole number so that dosage calculations will be easier, so 93.6 kg would be rounded to 94 kg.

Sometimes the conversion cannot be immediately calculated because you may need to determine the correct unit conversions before solving the problem. This occurs if you are given a problem where you must first change the measurement units, such as changing ounces to pounds or milligrams to grams or micrograms to milligrams, so the units you are seeking are the same. After you find the same units, then set up the proportion. Study the following examples. Notice that the requested answer was not in the same unit as the given information, so an extra step was made at the beginning of the problem to convert the numerators and denominators to the same units. After making the units the same, proceed to solve the problem by setting up the proportions as previously shown.

 EXAMPLE 12: A physician orders 600 mcg of nitroglycerin to be given to a patient with angina.

The medicine label reads gr $^1/_{100}$ per tablet. To convert, you must first change micrograms to milligrams; then convert to grains. First change mcg to mg.

600 mcg = 0.6 mg
Known: 60 mg = 1 gr
Set up the problem like this:

$$\frac{60 \text{ mg}}{1 \text{ gr}} = \frac{0.6 \text{ mg}}{x \text{ gr}} \quad \text{OR } 60 \text{ mg} : 1 \text{ gr} :: 0.6 \text{ mg} : x \text{ gr}$$

Cross-multiply, leaving off the abbreviations:

$$\frac{60 \text{ mg}}{1 \text{ gr}} \bowtie \frac{0.6 \text{ mg}}{x \text{ gr}} \quad \text{OR}$$

$$60 \text{ mg} : 1 \text{ gr} :: 0.6 \text{ mg} : x \text{ gr}$$

$$60x = 0.6$$

$$x = \frac{0.6}{60} \text{ or } \frac{6}{600}$$

$$x = \frac{1}{100} \text{ gr}$$

The dose of medication would be one tablet because each tablet is gr $^1/_{100}$.

Another method of completing this example is to calculate the entire problem using dimensional analysis. Dimensional analysis is a mathematical means of canceling unwanted units in conversion of unit equivalency or an extended ratio and proportion. Instead of two calculations of mcg to mg and then the conversion to the apothecary system, the calculation may be performed using several ratios in the fractional equation. Each factor is written as a fraction and the factors must be related to each other for the problem to be solved. If the units are not in the same measurement system the conversion may be made within the one proportional equation. Following are the steps needed to use dimensional analysis. These have been related to the problem given above.

 EXAMPLE 13: A physician orders 600 mcg of nitroglycerin to be given to a patient with angina.

There are six distinct steps in setting up dimensional or fractional analysis here and with all dimensional analysis problems.

1. Find the known quantity: gr $^1/_{100}$

2. What is the desired amount: 600 mcg

3. What is the conversion factor? gr i = 60 mg and 1000 mcg = 1 mg

4. Set up the problem with the available conversion factors placing the desired amount in the first fraction over 1.

$$x = \frac{600 \text{ mcg}}{1} \times \frac{1 \text{ mg}}{1000 \text{ mcg}} \times \frac{1 \text{ gr}}{60 \text{ mg}}$$

5. Cross out unwanted units that are in both the numerator and denominator

$$x = \frac{600 \text{ mcg}}{1} \times \frac{1 \text{ mg}}{1000 \text{ mcg}} \times \frac{1 \text{ gr}}{60 \text{ mg}}$$

6. Multiply the numerators and denominators and solve the calculation.

$$x = \frac{600}{1} \times \frac{1}{1000} \times \frac{1 \text{ gr}}{60}$$

$$x = \frac{600 \text{ gr}}{60000}$$

$$x = \frac{600 \text{ gr}}{60000}$$

$$x = \text{gr } \frac{1}{100}$$

Give one tablet because gr $\frac{1}{100}$ = 600 mcg.

 LEARNING TIP
Dimensional analysis is helpful when more than one conversion is needed to complete a calculation. This will be discussed again in Chapter 9.

The physician desires the weight of a premature baby to be converted to kilograms to be able to calculate the needed dosage for a medication. The physician asks you to convert the pounds and ounces to kilograms.

EXAMPLE 14: A premature baby weighs 4 lb 3 oz. Convert this weight to kilograms.

Household System:
Known: 16 oz: 1 lb

To solve, first change the 4 lb to ounces, then add 3 oz.

$4 \times 16 = 64 + 3 = 67$ oz.

You want to convert ounces to kilograms.

Metric System:
Known: 1 kg: 2.2 lb
And 0.45 kg: 1 lb
Now you can set up the proportion, and solve.

$$\frac{16 \text{ oz}}{0.45 \text{ kg}} = \frac{67 \text{ oz}}{x \text{ kg}} \text{ OR } 16 \text{ oz} : 0.45 \text{ kg} :: 67 \text{ oz} : x \text{ kg}$$

Cross-multiply, leaving off the abbreviations:

$$\frac{16 \text{ oz}}{0.45 \text{ kg}} \diagdown\diagup \frac{67 \text{ oz}}{x \text{ kg}} \text{ OR}$$

16 oz : 0.45 kg :: 67 oz : x kg

$16 \times x = 16x$
$0.45 \times 67 = 30.15$

Write as an equation: $16x = 30.15$

Divide each side by 16 to find x.

$$\frac{16x}{16} = \frac{30.15}{16}$$

$$x = 1.88$$

Finally, round the answer to a whole number for easier dosage calculation: $1.88 \sim 2$. So the final answer is 4 lb 3 oz $= 2$ kg.
Remember that x was expressed in kg, so your answer will be in kg.

To use dimensional analysis:

$$x = \frac{67 \text{ oz}}{1} \times \frac{1 \text{ lb}}{16 \text{ oz}} \times \frac{1 \text{ kg}}{2.2 \text{ lb}}$$

$$x = \frac{67 \text{ o\!z}}{1} \times \frac{1 \text{ l\!b}}{16 \text{ o\!z}} \times \frac{1 \text{ kg}}{2.2 \text{ l\!b}}$$

$$x = \frac{67}{1} \times \frac{1}{16} \times \frac{1 \text{ kg}}{2.2}$$

$$x = \frac{67 \text{ kg}}{35.2}$$

$$x = 1.88 \text{ or } 2 \text{ kg}$$

CHECK YOUR UNDERSTANDING—WEIGHT CONVERSIONS   8-6

PRACTICE PROBLEMS

CALCULATION REVIEW: Convert the following weight units to the requested equivalent measures.

1. gr $\frac{3}{4}$ = _____ mg

2. 12 lb = _____ kg

3. gr xv = _____ mg

4. 0.015 g = _____ mg

5. gr v = _____ g

6. 2.45 kg = _____ g

7. 360 mg = _____ g

8. gr $\frac{1}{60}$ = _____ mg

9. gr vi = _____ mg

10. 15 kg = _____ g

PRACTICAL APPLICATION: Solve the following conversions.

11. A premature infant weighs 1426 g. How many pounds does the baby weigh? (Round to the nearest pound.) _____

12. A patient weighs 45 lb. What is the patient's weight in kilograms? _____

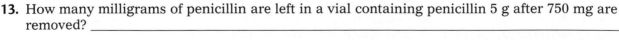

13. How many milligrams of penicillin are left in a vial containing penicillin 5 g after 750 mg are removed? _____

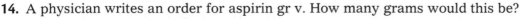

14. A physician writes an order for aspirin gr v. How many grams would this be?

_____

15. A biopsy sample weighs 2½ ounces. Record this in grams. _____

Length

The unit measurement of length is the most versatile of the three conversions we study because length can be measured for many different reasons and in many different ways. For example, patient supplies such as medical garments, elastic stockings, Ace bandages, and even gauze pads are all made to specified sizes that could be measured in terms of a body area circumference, length, or height. Linear measurements are recorded in medical records for lengths of surgical incisions; wounds being sutured; baselines for tests such as the PPD test for TB; and even the diameter of moles and other lesions. The newborn's length, chest, and head circumference are measured. Orthopedic appliances are measured to fit a specific patient usually by girth, length, or both. Table 8-4 shows the length measurement conversions practitioners must know. As with the other conversions, these are approximations.

Converting Length Measurement Units Between Systems

With medical measurements, many of the instruments used are calibrated in metric and household units, but you may occasionally need to convert between measurement systems using Table 8-4. The metric units are used in measuring lesions and lacerations for insurance coding, whereas household measurements are used to measure height and hypodermic needle lengths.

> **EXAMPLE 15:** An abdominal cavity was opened using a 14-inch incision. Convert this measurement into a metric length.

Set this problem up as a proportion. Known ratio: 2.5 cm = 1 in. Set up a proportion with the known and unknown information to look like this:

$$\frac{2.5 \text{ cm}}{1 \text{ in}} = \frac{x \text{ cm}}{14 \text{ in}} \quad \text{OR } 2.5 \text{ cm} : 1 \text{ in} :: x \text{ cm} : 14 \text{ in}$$

Cross-multiply, dropping the abbreviations.

$$\frac{2.5 \text{ cm}}{1 \text{ in}} \diagdown\!\!\!\diagup \frac{x \text{ cm}}{14 \text{ in}} = \quad \text{OR}$$

TABLE 8-4 *Length Measurements*

METRIC	HOUSEHOLD
10 millimeter (mm) = 1 cm	0.4 inch (in)
2.5 centimeters (cm)	1 inch
30 cm	1 foot (ft) = 12 in
90 cm	1 yard
100 cm = 1 meter (m)	39.4 in

$$2.5 \text{ cm} : 1 \text{ in} :: x \text{ cm} : 14 \text{ in}$$

$$2.5 \times 14 = 35$$

$$1 \times x = x$$

$x = 35$. Therefore 14 inches = 35 cm. Remember x was expressed in cm; therefore the answer is in cm.

> **EXAMPLE 16:** A patient is 185 cm tall. Record this using the household measurement of feet and inches.

This problem can also be set up as a proportion. Known ratio: A) 30 cm = 12 in or B) 2.5 cm = 1 in. Either ratio can be used; both are shown below. Set up a proportion with the known and unknown information, using the conversion that you most easily remember. Your problem will look like either of these:

$$\text{A)}\ \frac{30 \text{ cm}}{12 \text{ in}} = \frac{185 \text{ cm}}{x \text{ in}} \quad \text{or } 30 \text{ cm} : 12 \text{ in} :: 185 \text{ cm} : x \text{ in}$$

OR

$$\text{B)}\ \frac{2.5 \text{ cm}}{1 \text{ in}} = \frac{185 \text{ cm}}{x \text{ in}} \quad \text{or } 2.5 \text{ cm} : 1 \text{ in} :: 185 \text{ cm} : x \text{ in}$$

Cross-multiply, dropping the abbreviations.

$$\text{A)}\ \frac{30 \text{ cm}}{12 \text{ in}} \diagdown\!\!\!\diagup \frac{185 \text{ cm}}{x \text{ in}} \quad \text{or}$$

$$30 \text{ cm} : 12 \text{ in} :: 185 \text{ cm} : x \text{ in}$$

OR

$$\text{B)}\ \frac{2.5 \text{ cm}}{1 \text{ in}} \diagdown\!\!\!\diagup \frac{185 \text{ cm}}{x \text{ in}} \quad \text{or}$$

$$2.5 \text{ cm} : 1 \text{ in} :: 185 \text{ cm} : x \text{ in}$$

A) $30 \times x = 30x$ or   B) $2.5 \times x = 2.5x$

A) $12 \times 185 = 2220$ or   B) $1 \times 185 = 185$

Solve for x by dividing both sides.

$$\text{A)}\ \frac{30x}{30} = \frac{2220}{30} \quad \text{or B)}\ \frac{2.5x}{2.5} = \frac{185}{2.5}$$

By either method, $x = 74$ inches, but remember that this measurement is in inches because x was in inches. Because the problem asks you to identify feet and inches, the next step is necessary.

Known equivalent: 12 in = 1 ft.

Set up the problem to determine how many feet are in 74 inches.

$$\frac{1 \text{ ft}}{12 \text{ in}} = \frac{x \text{ ft}}{74 \text{ in}} \quad \text{OR} \quad 1 \text{ ft} : 12 \text{ in} :: x \text{ ft} : 74 \text{ in}$$

Cross-multiply.

$$\frac{1 \text{ ft}}{12 \text{ in}} \diagup\!\!\!\!\diagup\ \frac{x \text{ ft}}{74 \text{ in}} \quad \text{OR}$$

$$1 \text{ ft} : 12 \text{ in} :: x \text{ ft} : 74 \text{ in}$$

$$12 \times x = 12x$$

$$74 \times 1 = 74$$

Solve for x by dividing both sides by 12.

$$\frac{12x}{12} = \frac{74}{12}$$

$x =$ 6 feet with 2 inches left over.

Remember this must be in feet, as x was expressed in feet.

185 cm = 6 ft 2 in.

Using dimensional analysis the equation would be as follows:

$$x = \frac{185 \text{ cm}}{1} \times \frac{1 \text{ in}}{2.5 \text{ cm}} \times \frac{1 \text{ ft}}{12 \text{ in}}$$

$$x = \frac{185 \text{ cm}}{1} \times \frac{1 \text{ in}}{2.5 \text{ cm}} \times \frac{1 \text{ ft}}{12 \text{ in}}$$

$$x = \frac{185}{30}$$

$x = 6.16$ ft or 6 ft 2 in

CHECK YOUR UNDERSTANDING—LENGTH CONVERSIONS   8-7

PRACTICE PROBLEMS

CALCULATION REVIEW: Solve these length conversions. Round answers to tenths if necessary.

1. 8 in = _____ cm

2. 5 ft 6 in = _____ cm

3. 3 m = _____ ft

4. 28 mm = _____ cm

5. 60 cm = _____ ft

6. 80 cm = _____ m

7. 75 in = _____ m

8. 2 in = _____ mm

9. $3\frac{1}{2}$ ft = _____ m

10. 13 mm = _____ cm

PRACTICAL APPLICATION: Determine the following conversions.

11. A patient needs a dressing changed when her wound drainage on the bandage measures 2.5 cm. The current bandage drainage measures 50 mm. What is the difference in millimeters between the measurements? Does the dressing need to be changed? _____

12. A physician needs 75 cm of suture material to close a long laceration. What is the minimum number of feet of suture material you would need to place on the suture tray? (Round to whole number.) _____

13. A small newborn is 18 inches long. Record this in centimeters. _____

14. A pediatric chart to measure height measures up to 120 cm. How many inches is this? _____

15. A physician orders 1.5 cm of nitroglycerin ointment. The measurement paper for the ointment is in inches. How many inches should be applied to the paper for administration? _____
_____

Summary

This chapter begins by introducing the international standard for time, the 24-hour clock. Temperature conversions between Fahrenheit and Celsius are then discussed. The majority of the chapter focuses on conversions between the metric, household, and apothecary measurement systems for units of volume, weight, and length. The conversion methods shown in this chapter are ratio and proportion and dimensional analysis. Symbols discussed in the previous chapter have been incorporated when appropriate to give more exposure to real-life situations. Although most people are most familiar with household measurements, the metric system is the predominant method used by health care providers. A general knowledge of all three measurement systems is necessary in order to work accurately with patients, to complete accurate medical documentation, and to read medical information.

The next chapter introduces calculating dosages of nonparenteral medications. The information learned in this chapter will be used to understand how nonparenteral dosages can be calculated using actual drug dosages and drug names.

Critical Thinking Exercises

Study each case independently. The icon for the body system in which the drug is used is shown. Determine each answer by solving for the missing information. Be sure to show your calculations on a separate sheet of paper.

1. Cyclophosphamide (Cytoxan) is used intravenously in chemotherapy to inhibit the growth of neoplasms. The vial of medication contains Cytoxan 1 g. Could you prepare a dose of 750 mg from this container? _____

2. The physician orders phenobarbital 100 mg. Available are phenobarbital gr ss tablets. Can you administer this medication with the tablets supplied? Show your work.

   _____

3. A patient is prescribed fexofenadine (Allegra) for seasonal allergic rhinitis. If the patient is to take 2 tablets a day, half of the dose in the morning and the other half 12 hours later, give the international standard time for the second dose if the first one was taken at 10:30 AM. _____

4. For juvenile arthritis, the doctor might prescribe ibuprofen (Motrin). If the usual dosage for a child is based on weight in kilograms and the child weighs 66 pounds, how many kilograms does the child weigh? _____

5. The physician's office has scales that weigh in kilograms. The patient asks you how much weight he has lost when the scale shows 22 kg of weight loss. _____

6. Testosterone (Depo-Testosterone) is a hormone used for replacement in the hypogonadal male. This medication is administered by injection with vials that need to be stored at 20° C to 25° C. Convert this temperature to Fahrenheit. Would this medication be stored in a refrigerator? Show your work.

   _____

REVIEW QUESTIONS

PRACTICAL APPLICATION: Solve by using the method of calculation you feel most comfortable using.

1. If a dosage strength is 2 g in 10 mL, what is the correct amount of liquid when 4 g are ordered?
   _____

2. When preparing surgical packs for autoclaving, you need one Allis tissue forceps and three hemostats for each pack you prepare. What are your proportions for 6 packs? _____
   _____

3. A medication contains 1 part pure drug to 25 parts of solute. What is the ratio and what is the fraction?_____

   How many parts of pure drug are in 150 parts of solute? _____

4. The dosage of phenobarbital ordered is gr ¼. The tablets available are phenobarbital gr ½ in a scored tablet, how many tablets would you administer to the patient? _____

5. The doctor orders phenobarbital elixir gr xv. The available medication is phenobarbital gr v per fluid dram. How many teaspoons would you administer? _____

All of the following statements are *false*. Determine the error(s) and rewrite the statement, giving completely correct information in the space provided.

6. A medication that was to be given once a day before bedtime (10:00 PM) is given at 2000.
   _____
   _____

7. The approximate value of 500 mL is 1 quart. _____
   _____

8. In the metric system the primary measurements used for dosage calculations are volume and length. _____
   _____

9. In the apothecary system, 16 oz is equal to 1 lb. _____
   _____

10. A scar that measures 14 cm is approximately 2 inches long. _____
    _____

11. A biopsy specimen weighs 45 g. This would be approximately a half pound in the household system. _____
    _____

12. A ratio is a comparison of two fractions that are considered equivalent. _____
    _____

13. Conversions can be immediately calculated because you do not need to determine unit proportions before solving. _____
    _____

14. A metric-sized orthopedic appliance measures 6 inches in length. _____
    _____

15. A medication weighing gr v would be equivalent to 200 g. _____
    _____

16. The 24-hour clock is often used in the United States. _____
_____

17. When converting between measurement systems, answers will usually vary by ± 1%. _____
_____

18. Volume refers to weight. _____   _____
_____

19. 50° Celsius would be a comfortable room temperature. _____
_____

20. When converting from Celsius to Fahrenheit, remember to multiply first because Fahrenheit is
the smaller number. _____   _____
_____

21. 15 drops in the apothecary system is the equivalent of 1 metric mL. _____
_____

22. 45 kg is equivalent to 1 lb. _____
_____

23. The acceptable metric equivalency of one-half teaspoon is 2 mL. _____   _____   _____
_____

24. A centimeter is smaller than a millimeter, and a centimeter is smaller than an inch. _____
_____

25. A medication is ordered for gr $^3/_4$, and the available amount is 30 mg. The proper amount to administer is one tablet. _____
_____

Calculating Doses of Nonparenteral Medications

OBJECTIVES

After studying this chapter, you should be capable of doing the following:

- Determining the correct dose of medication to be administered, based on a drug order.
- Calculating the dosages of nonparenteral drugs administered in solid form, using ratio and proportion, formula, or dimensional analysis method.
- Calculating the dosages of nonparenteral drugs administered in liquid form, using ratio and proportion, formula, or dimensional analysis method.
- Calculating doses on the basis of body surface area and weight in kilograms.

KEY WORDS

Body surface area (BSA) calculation

Conversion factor

Factors

Formula method

Nomogram

Nonparenteral medications

Reconstitution

Unit

CHAPTER 9 PRETEST: CALCULATING NONPARENTERAL DOSES

Calculate the following dosages.

1. Fill in 1 teaspoon.

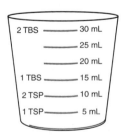

2. Fill in 25 mL.

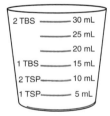

Directions: On the provided lines, explain exactly what quantity of medication in tablets or liquid and the number of doses of medication that should be taken per day.

3. Ordered: hydrochlorothiazide 50 mg daily, to be taken in divided doses with morning and early afternoon meal.
Available: hydrochlorothiazide 25 mg tablets.
Dose to be given: _____
How often? _____

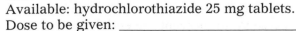

4. Ordered: allopurinol 300 mg daily.
   Available: allopurinol 100 mg tablets.
   Dose to be given: _____
   How often? _____

5. Ordered: Zyrtec 10 mg po daily.
   Available: Zyrtec 1 mg/1 mL syrup. Please give the answer in metric and household measures.
   Dose to be given: _____
   How often? _____

6. Ordered: warfarin sodium 6 mg po daily.
   Available: warfarin sodium 4 mg scored tablets.
   Dose to be given: _____
   How often? _____

7. Ordered: Amoxil 400 mg chewable tablets q12h.
   Available: Amoxil 200 mg chewable tablets.
   Dose to be given: _____
   How often? _____

8. Tina has an infection with moderate pain and was prescribed Lortab Elixir 15 mg/1000 mg tid
   in divided doses. Using the label below, calculate the desired dose to be given:
   Dose to be given: _____
   How often? _____

ucb Pharma

PHARMACIST: Dispense in a tight, light-resistant container with a child-resistant closure.

NDC 50474-909-16   1 Pint (473 mL)

USUAL DOSAGE: See package insert for complete dosage recommendations.

Store at controlled room temperature, 15-30°C (59-86°F) [see USP].

WARNING: May be habit forming.

WARNING: Keep this and all medications out of the reach of children.

LORTAB® ELIXIR

HYDROCODONE BITARTRATE AND ACETAMINOPHEN ORAL SOLUTION
7.5 mg/500 mg per 15 mL

Contains:	Per 5 mL	Per 15 mL
Hydrocodone Bitartrate	2.5 mg	7.5 mg
Acetaminophen	167 mg	500 mg
Alcohol	7%	7%

Lot No.:
Exp. Date:

Manufactured for
UCB Pharma, Inc.
Smyrna, GA 30080
by Mikart, Inc.
Atlanta, GA 30318

℞ only

3 50474-909-16 4

Rev. 2E 10/2001
P/N 1003813   540A16

Introduction to Methods of Dosage Calculation

In this chapter, a comparison of three different methods of calculating dosages for nonparenteral medications is shown. It is not important that you memorize all three methods. It is more important that you choose **one** method and use that method to prevent potential medication errors that could result from switching between the methods. With the first two methods (ratio and proportion and the formula method), the most important concept is *always* to be sure that the units requested and the units on hand are measured in the same system and the same weight or volume measurement. For example, if the drug requested is given in grams but you only have milligrams, the first step must be to convert milligrams to grams or vice versa. In another example, the physician may write the medication in the apothecary system for a drug that is available in the metric system. Then grains (apothecary measure) must be converted to mg, mcg, or a measure of the metric system or vice versa. *As a rule of thumb, when deciding which measurement to find in the final conversion, the final dosage or unit of measure should be that found on the container of available medication. The conversion should be to that measurement.*

In a perfect world, all drugs would come in the same measurement system and would be found in a unit-dose system. Then no calculations would be necessary to find a specific dose. Administration errors would be decreased to a minimum. Sometimes the health care provider will need to determine and prepare the proper doses using conversions between systems when the amount of medication ordered does not match the medication on hand. By reviewing a few of the basic guidelines about the various medications, you can make sure that administration of drugs is still safe. Box 9-1 covers the basic guidelines.

It is important to prevent math errors when calculating the drug dose. A few basic rules can help you remember to calculate with confidence at all times. First, always be sure to use the same units of measure when setting up the problem unless conversion is needed, and then first make the needed conversion when using the ratio and proportion or the formula method. Next, even if the problem seems easy, work the math on paper to find a solution. Although it is always important to take the time to do the calculations, thinking ahead can prevent errors. *If your calculations do not result in the solution you anticipated or do not seem sensible, recheck all calculations.* After calculating the dosage, always be sure to check and recheck decimals or fractions. If the dose is calculated in BSA or for intravenous fluids insert the appropriate factors into the formula and then make the calculations; use a calculator with these measurements to determine the appropriate dose, as many of these may be long and complicated. Finally, read the health care provider's order one more time to ensure you are calculating for the dose requested before administering the medication. Most medications are designed to be adminis-

| BOX 9-1 | NONPARENTERAL DOSAGE GUIDELINES |

- Do not open or divide a capsule.
- Tablets that are not scored are not intended to be divided.
- A tablet that is scored may be divided or broken.
- An enteric-coated tablet or caplet should not be broken or crushed.
- Buccal and sublingual tablets should not be broken, crushed, or swallowed.
- Sustained- or extended-release tablets should not be broken or crushed.
- Before crushing or breaking any tablet or caplet, always check to be sure this action will not affect the drug's purpose.

tered as a whole tablet or capsule, so if you are dividing the medication form, it should be available as a scored tablet or a pourable liquid.

A few additional words of warning about combining different dosages to substitute for the strength on hand: Different strengths must be considered before starting dose calculations. With some oral medications, using combination dosages of medication is appropriate; however be careful with delayed-release and sustained-release dosage strengths because with these types of medications, adding two 5-mg tablets to make a 10-mg dosage is not equivalent because the release time is not the same. Therefore as a rule of thumb, because time-release medications—whether delayed or sustained—are not interchangeable, the dose should be given only in the dosage strength and in the form prescribed.

Remember, when using conversions between measurement systems, the answer will only be *approximate*. In reality, today most doctors prescribe medications in the manufactured dosage strength and form. However, you will have to convert from grains to grams or milligrams on some occasions. With prescriptions from ambulatory care facilities, the pharmacist will usually make the calculation per the physician's order. However, the allied health professional may be expected to make the conversion when administering medications in the ambulatory care setting or when providing samples that are not in a strength that has been ordered. If you have any doubts about the medication calculation, always ask that someone verify your calculations prior to administering the medication. This may mean that you verify the calculation with a fellow employee or that you verify the medication order and the calculation of the dose with the physician.

Each drug calculation problem will have two parts. The first part of the problem tells you what the physician has ordered and is sometimes referred to as "dose desired" or "dose ordered" (DO). The second part of the problem tells you the medication you have on hand and is usually referred to as "dose available" (DA). Regardless of the method you choose to use, remember that this basic method applies to all dose calculations.

The following steps are necessary to calculate dose questions:

1. Note the information provided on the medication bottle on hand, or what the *available* medication is (DA). This is also referred to as what you have.
2. Determine what is asked for on the physician's order, or what dose is *ordered* (DO). This is also referred to as what you want.
3. Identify the available unit of measure or form that will be used to supply the desired dose (DO), or dose to be given, such as tablets, capsules, milliliters, and ounces.
4. Be sure all units are in the same measurement system. The conversion should be to the units found on the available medication bottle.

Conversion between systems must be done prior to the calculation of the dose except with dimensional analysis.

5. Calculate the desired dose.
6. Verify the dose calculation with the medication order using the correct measurement system for your answer.

Dosage Forms for Nonparenteral Medications

Dosage forms are presented in Chapter 3. This section is added as a short review of medication forms and the dosages used for calculating doses given orally. Solid medications are designated as the weight of medication per dosage form, such as milligram/tablet or milligram/milliliter in liquids. Because most people do not have utensils for measuring in the metric system, conversion to the household systems of teaspoons and tablespoons is appropriate. Always be sure that patients understand exactly how to measure a dose for administration.

CHECK YOUR UNDERSTANDING—DOSAGE MEASUREMENTS   **9-1**

CALCULATION REVIEW: Identify the amount of solution in each calibrated medication container.

1. _____ tsp

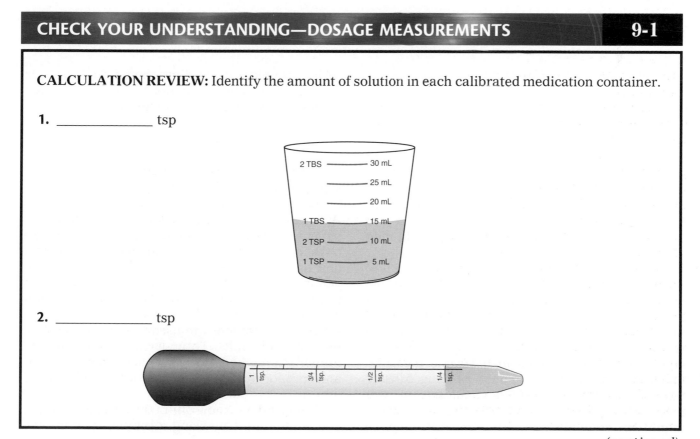

2. _____ tsp

(continued)

CHECK YOUR UNDERSTANDING—DOSAGE MEASUREMENTS (cont'd)   9-1

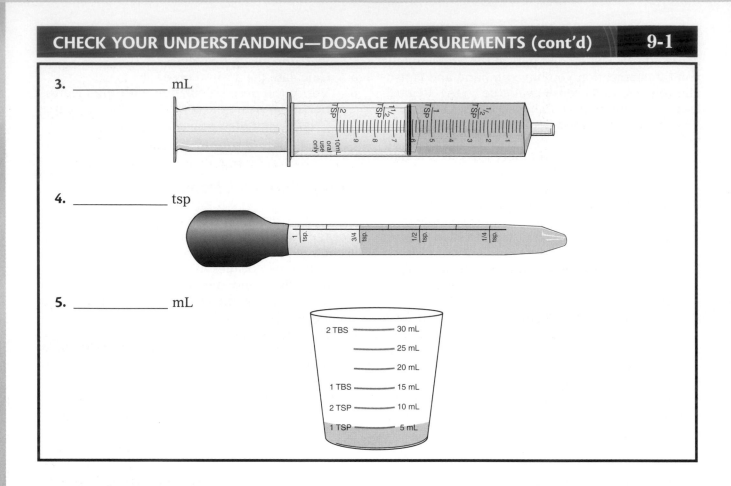

3. _____ mL

4. _____ tsp

5. _____ mL

2 TBS	30 mL
	25 mL
	20 mL
1 TBS	15 mL
2 TSP	10 mL
1 TSP	5 mL

Three Methods of Calculating Nonparenteral Doses

The next three sections will show you how to calculate drug doses by using different methods of calculations. It is important to review each method independently, then choose the method that is easiest for you to use to calculate. To help prevent calculation errors, use *only one* of the three methods. Always keep in mind that if the answer you computed does not seem logical, you should redo the math.

The first method described uses *ratio and proportion* and requires the preparer to convert the problem so that the measurements in the problem are in the same measurement system. The second method is called the *formula method*, which also requires conversion so factors are converted to equivalent measurements in the same measurement system. The third method of drug calculations is called *dimensional analysis*. In this method the problem does NOT convert measurements into equivalent units as a separate step. To

solve a problem using dimensional analysis, one extended fractional equation is necessary and units are cancelled. The following sections explain the three methods further.

Calculating Doses Using Ratio and Proportion

When a doctor requests that a drug be given to a patient, sometimes the dosage available (dosage on hand) will not be in the same measurement unit as the doctor prescribed. When this occurs, you must be able to convert, or change, measurement systems to provide the patient with the correct dose.

Several methods are used to convert between measurement units. To understand the ratio and proportion method, first analyze the terms "ratio" and "proportion." See Box 9-2 for the terminology used with this method.

If you did not know one of the parts of the ratio, you could find it by using a symbol such as *x* to

BOX 9-2	UNDERSTANDING THE TERMINOLOGY OF RATIO AND PROPORTION

Ratio
2 : 1

Means

$$2:1::4:2 \;\leftarrow\; \text{or} \quad \frac{2}{1} = \frac{4}{2} \left(\begin{array}{c} \frac{2}{1} = \frac{4}{2} \\ (2:1::4:2) \end{array} \right)$$

Proportion
2 : 1 :: 4 : 2

Extremes

A ratio is a comparison between 2 numbers (2 : 1).
A proportion is a comparison between 2 ratios (2 : 1 :: 4 : 2).
Means are the two inner numbers in a proportion.
Extremes are the two outer numbers in a proportion.

As you previously learned in conversions, these ratios may be written as fractions such as $^2/_1 = {}^4/_2$ and cross multiplied.

stand for the unknown number. Suppose you only know the first complete ratio to be 3 : 1. In the second ratio you know the first number is 6. You can find the second ratio by replacing the second number with x. It would look like this: 3 : 1 :: 6 : x. Now use cross-multiplication or multiply the means and the extremes to solve for x : 3 is to x as 6 is to 1 or $3x = 6$, so x is equal to 2. Put the number 2 into the second ratio and you have 3 : 1 :: 6 : 2, or $^3/_1 = {}^6/_2$, which shows an equivalency when you multiply means and extremes. Be sure to identify the unit values of both of the ratios. *The numerators and denominators must be of the same measurement units respectively.* For example, 1 mL : 15 gtts is the same as 2 mL : 30 gtts and would be written with both numerators expressed in "mL" and both denominators expressed in "gtts," or

$$\frac{1\;mL}{15\;gtts} = \frac{2\;mL}{30\;gtts} \quad \text{OR} \quad 1\;mL : 15\;gtts :: 2\;mL :: 30\;gtts$$

Use the following formula to find medication doses using ratios or proportions.
Dosage Available (DA) **:** Dosage Form (DF) **::** Dosage Ordered (DO) **:** Dose to be Given (DG)
If using fractions, the formula would be as follows:

$$\frac{DA}{DF} = \frac{DO}{DG}$$

 PROBLEM: Sulfamethoxazole is supplied as 1 g/10 mL. The doctor orders sulfamethoxazole 2 g. How many milliliters would be administered? How many teaspoons would be given?

The easiest way to show proportion between measurement systems is by comparing the known ratio to the unknown ratio. To set up the problem, first identify the known ratio. Next, set up the second ratio using x to signify the unknown unit. Be careful to use the same order for the units in setting up the second ratio as that you used in the first ratio. Then solve for x in the second ratio by using cross-multiplication, reducing when necessary.

EXAMPLE 1:

$$\frac{1\;g}{10\;mL} \bowtie \frac{2\;g}{x\;mL} \quad \text{OR} \quad 1\;g : 10\;mL :: 2\;g : x\;mL$$

$1 \times x = 2 \times 10$

$1x = 20$

Therefore, sulfamethoxazole 20 mL is the dose to be given.

In this problem, x is stated in mL because milliliters were the unknown.

Now solve for the teaspoons

$$\frac{1\;tsp}{5\;mL} = \frac{x\;tsp}{20\;mL} \quad \text{OR} \quad 1\;tsp : 5\;mL :: x\;tsp : 20\;mL$$

$5 \times x = 1\;tsp \times 20$ (Notice that the appropriate abbreviations for measurement systems have been cancelled)

$5x = 20\;tsp$

$x = 4\;tsp$

The dose in household measurements to be given is 4 tsp.

> ✎ **LEARNING TIP**
> When setting up both ratios, be sure to *label all* of the terms including the x with the correct measurement unit to be sure equations are equivalents.

Calculating Doses Using the Formula Method

The first step to calculating drug dosage when using the formula method is to check that the strength of the drug ordered and the strength of the drug available are in the same unit of measure. For example, if the drug is ordered as 0.5 g and the available drug is in milligrams, the first step would be to change the grams to milligrams. Then set up the formula. However, if the drug is ordered in grams and the available drug is in grams, then skip the first step and go directly to the formula.

CHECK YOUR UNDERSTANDING—RATIO AND PROPORTION   9-2

CALCULATION REVIEW: Replace the following ratios with the correct fractional equivalent. Do not simplify.

1. 2:3 = _____

2. 1:50 = _____

3. 1:150 = _____

4. 2:800 = _____

5. 2:7 = _____

Replace the following fractions with the correct ratio equivalent. Do not simplify.

6. $\frac{2}{500}$ = _____

7. $\frac{1}{250}$ = _____

8. $\frac{1}{3}$ = _____

9. $\frac{1}{1000}$ = _____

10. $\frac{2}{7}$ = _____

PRACTICAL APPLICATION: Set up the problem using the ratio and proportion method. Be sure to use a conversion ratio if necessary. Then solve.

 11. Zoloft 75 mg is ordered. The strength available is 50 mg tablet. How many tablets would provide the desired amount? _____

 12. Metformin 750 mg is ordered. The strength available is 0.5 g/tablet. How many tablets would be necessary to administer the desired order? _____

 13. K-Clor 40 mEq is ordered. The strength available is K-Clor 20 mEq tablets. How many tablets would be necessary for the desired order? _____

 14. Amoxicillin 500 mg is ordered. Available is amoxicillin 125 mg/5 mL. How many milliliters would be administered for the desired order? _____
How many teaspoons would be administered? _____

15. Levothyroxine 0.5 mg is ordered. Strength available is 125 mcg/tablet. How many tablets would be necessary for the desired order? _____

The formula is as follows:

$$\frac{\text{Dosage Ordered (DO)}}{\text{Dosage Available (DA)}} \times \text{Quantity (form or unit of measure) (DF)} = \text{Dose to be Given (DG)}$$

The formula can be abbreviated as:

$$\frac{\text{DO}}{\text{DA}} \times \text{DF} = \text{DG}$$

Here is how the formula method can be analyzed:

(DO) To find the desired part of the formula, answer this question: "What did the doctor order?"

(DA) The dosage available part of the formula answers the question "What dosage strength of medication is available?"

(DF) Dosage form identifies the volume or dosage strength the available medication comes in. An example of the quantity in a solid medication would be the number of tablets or capsules for the strength of the dosage form. In a liquid medication, quantity could be shown as a liquid measure such as mL.

(DG) The amount to give represents the unknown amount of the drug that you will want to administer. Like the quantity, the dose given will be stated in the volume or dosage form the available drug comes in.

LEARNING TIP

Always remember to perform dosage calculations in writing and not in your head. Written calculations reduce the chance of error and thus of possible harm to the patient. It is always important to check calculations with a calculator.

PROBLEM: Sulfamethazoxazole 1 g/10 mL is the available medication. The doctor orders 2 g. How many milliliters would be prepared? How many teaspoons should be administered? Determine what the desired, have, quantity, and unknown are:

DO = 2 g; DA = 1 g; DF= 10 mL; DG = x mL

Now set up the formula.

EXAMPLE 2:

$$\frac{2 \text{ g (DO)}}{1 \text{ g (DA)}} \times 10 \text{ mL (Qty or DF)} = x \text{ mL (DG)}$$

$$\frac{2\cancel{g}}{1\cancel{g}} \times 10 \text{ mL} = x \text{ mL}$$

$$\frac{2}{1} \times 10 = x \text{ mL}$$

$$\frac{20}{1} = x \text{ mL}$$

$$x = 20 \text{ mL}$$

Now solve for the teaspoons:

$$\frac{5 \text{ mL}}{1 \text{ tsp}} \diagdown\!\!\!\!\diagup \frac{20 \text{ mL}}{x}$$

$$5x = 20 \text{ tsp}$$

$$x = 4 \text{ tsp}$$

LEARNING TIP

Remember that the medication on hand and the medication ordered must be in the same unit measurement before solving using the formula method.

Here are some additional examples using the guidelines provided.

 EXAMPLE 3: Ordered: Glucophage 850 mg po daily with meal.
Available: Glucophage 850 mg tablets.

Are the units the same measurement? (Yes)

What is the desired unit? 850 mg tablet daily

$$\frac{850 \text{ mg (DO)}}{850 \text{ mg (DA)}} \times 1 \text{ tablet (DF)} = x \text{ tablet (DG)}$$

$$\frac{850\cancel{\text{ mg}} \text{ (DO)}}{850\cancel{\text{ mg}} \text{ (DA)}} \times 1 \text{ tab (DF)} = x \text{ tablet (DG)}$$

$$\frac{1}{1} \times 1 \text{ tab} = x$$

$$x = 1 \text{ tab}$$

Because the amount of medication desired and the amount available are equal to one tablet, the dose to be given is one tablet.

 EXAMPLE 4: Ordered: phenobarbital gr iii po daily hs.

Available: phenobarbital l00 mg scored tablets.

Are the units in the same measurement? (No)

What is the equivalency for conversion? gr i = 60 mg or gr i$\overline{\text{ss}}$ = approximately 100 mg (see Table 8-3).

First convert to the same measurement system using one of the following conversions. Using gr $\overline{ss}$ as the conversion factor:

$$\frac{gr\ 1\frac{1}{2}}{100\ mg} = \frac{gr\ 3}{x\ mg} \quad OR \quad gr\ 1\frac{1}{2}:100\ mg :: gr\ 3:x\ mg$$

$$\frac{gr\ 1\frac{1}{2}}{100\ mg} = \frac{gr\ 3}{x\ mg} \quad OR \quad gr\ 1\frac{1}{2}:100\ mg :: gr\ 3:x\ mg$$

Change 1½ to an improper fraction (³⁄₂) and solve for x (cross-multiply).

$$\frac{3}{2} \times x\ mg = 3 \times 100\ mg \quad OR \quad \frac{3}{2}:100::3::x$$

$$x = \frac{300}{1} \diagup\!\!\!\!\diagdown \frac{2}{3}$$

$$x = \frac{\overset{100}{\cancel{300}}}{1} \times \frac{2}{\underset{1}{\cancel{3}}}$$

$$1\frac{1}{2}\ x = 300\ mg$$

$$x = 200\ mg$$

Therefore, the dose to be given is 200 mg. Using gr i = 60 mg as the conversion factor:

$$\frac{gr\ i}{60\ mg} = \frac{gr\ iii}{x\ mg} \quad OR \quad 1:60\ mg = 3:x$$

$$x = 3 \times 60\ mg$$

$$x = 180\ mg$$

gr iii = 180 mg or rounded to 200 mg

Now solve the problem by the formula method.

$$\frac{200\ mg\ (DO)}{100\ mg\ (DA)} \times 1\ tablet\ (DF) = x\ (DG)$$

$$\frac{200\ mg}{100\ mg} \times 1\ tab = x$$

$$\frac{200\ \cancel{mg}}{100\ \cancel{mg}} \times 1\ tab = x$$

$$\frac{2}{1} \times 1\ tab = x$$

$$2\ tab = x$$

The dose to be given is 2 tablets.

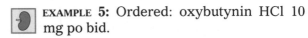 **EXAMPLE 5:** Ordered: oxybutynin HCl 10 mg po bid.

Available: oxybutynin HCI 5 mg scored tablets. Are the units in the same measurement? (Yes)

$$\frac{10\ mg\ (DO)}{5\ mg\ (DA)} \times 1\ tablet\ (DF) = x\ (DG)$$

$$\frac{10\ mg}{5\ mg} \times 1\ tab = x$$

$$\frac{\overset{2}{\cancel{10\ mg}}}{\underset{1}{\cancel{5\ mg}}} \times 1\ tab = x$$

$$2 \times 1\ tab = x\ (DG)$$

$$2\ tab = x$$

The dose to be given is 2 tablets

CHECK YOUR UNDERSTANDING—FORMULA METHOD   9-3

Show your work on a separate sheet of paper. Save your worksheet.

1. Using the following formula equation, $\dfrac{Keflex\ 500\ mg}{Keflex\ 1000\ mg} \times 5\ mL = 2\ mL$, identify:
   a. What the doctor ordered _____
   b. What strength is on the shelf _____
   c. What is the unit of measure _____
   d. How much of the drug will be administered _____

2. Using the following formula equation, $\dfrac{warfarin\ sodium\ 10\ mg}{warfarin\ sodium\ 20\ mg} \times 1\ tab = \frac{1}{2}\ tab$, identify:
   a. What the doctor ordered _____
   b. What strength is on the shelf _____
   c. What is the unit of measure _____
   d. How much of the drug will be administered _____

CHECK YOUR UNDERSTANDING—FORMULA METHOD (cont'd)   9-3

3. Using the following formula equation, $\dfrac{\text{Diorane } 160 \text{ mg}}{\text{Diorane } 320 \text{ mg}} \times 1 \text{ tab} = \frac{1}{2}$ tab, identify:
   a. What the doctor ordered _____
   b. What strength is on the shelf _____
   c. What is the unit of measure _____
   d. How much of the drug will be administered _____

4. Using the following formula equation, $\dfrac{\text{dimenhydrinate } 22.5 \text{ mg}}{\text{dimenhydrinate } 15 \text{ mg}} \times 5 \text{ mL} = 7.5 \text{ mL}$, identify:
   a. What the doctor ordered _____
   b. What strength is on the shelf _____
   c. What is the unit of measure _____
   d. How much of the drug will be administered _____

5. Using the following formula equation, $\dfrac{\text{guaifenesin } 400 \text{ mg}}{\text{guaifenesin } 200 \text{ mg}} \times 5 \text{ mL} = 10 \text{ mL}$, identify:
   a. What the doctor ordered _____
   b. What strength is on the shelf _____
   c. What is the unit of measure _____
   d. How much of the drug will be administered _____

PRACTICAL APPLICATION: Using the same set of problems found in the ratio and proportion method, set up the problem this time using the formula method. Be sure to use a conversion ratio if necessary, then solve.

6. Zoloft 75 mg is ordered. The strength available is 50 mg tablet. How many tablets would provide the desired amount? _____

7. Metformin 750 mg is ordered. The strength available is 0.5g/tablet. How many tablets would be necessary to administer the desired order? _____

8. K-Clor 40 mEq is ordered. The strength available is K-Clor 20 mEq tablets. How many tablets would be necessary for the desired order? _____

9. Amoxicillin 500 mg is ordered. Available is amoxicillin 125 mg/5 mL. How many milliliters would be administered for the desired order? _____
   How many teaspoons would be administered? _____

10. Levothyroxine 0.5 mg is ordered. Strength available is 125 mcg/tablet. How many tablets of the drug would be necessary for the desired order? _____

Calculating Doses Using Dimensional Analysis

The dimensional analysis method of dose calculation is different than the previous two methods discussed because this method does not require the conversion between units in order to solve the problem. Recall in the ratio and proportion method and in the formula method, the first step is to change the strength of the drug ordered and the strength of the drug available to the same unit of measure, and then the problem can be solved. In the dimensional analysis method, only one *linear equation* is used. Linear equations have a right side and a left side separated by an equal sign. A simple example of a linear equation is $x = 2$.

In dimensional analysis, the multiplication of a series of fractions (or ratios) in which the numerator and denominator contain related conversion factors are used. This prevents the need to perform multiple calculations to solve drug dosages. The process involves writing fractional factors that include the conversion factors that are needed to solve the calculation. As previously stated, the starting factor is the known or the quantity given for solving. Next determine what is desired and then find the conversions factors needed to make the calculation. Remember that the numerator abbreviation in the starting factor will be the denominator in the next conversion factor with the same happening throughout the equation.

The most difficult task in computing problems using dimensional analysis is to set up the original linear equation correctly. On the left side of the equation is an *x*. The entries on the right side of the linear equation are written as common fractions. In dimensional analysis, the common fractions are called **factors.** The first factor on the right side is usually "dose ordered" in the problem and is referred to as the *starting factor*.

Place an *x* on the left side of the equation and the starting factor as the first conversion factor on the right side of the equation. To set up the common fraction correctly, the numerator will show the name or abbreviation of the ordered medication. Then continue to add factors, one at a time as needed so that the linear equation can be cancelled out and the answer becomes obvious. Most of the time, the wrong answer for the dose ordered (DO) can be recognized because the answer does not make sense.

EXAMPLE **6:** Ordered: phenobarbital gr iii mg po hs

Available medication: phenobarbital 100 mg scored tablets

Starting factor: gr iii

Conversion factors: 60 mg = gr i or 100 mg = gr iss

$$DA = \frac{100 \text{ mg}}{\text{tab}}$$

Using 60 mg = gr i as conversion:

$$x = \frac{\text{gr iii}}{1} \times \frac{60 \text{ mg}}{\text{gr i}} \times \frac{1 \text{ tab}}{100 \text{ mg}}$$

$$x = \frac{3 \text{ gr}}{1} \times \frac{60 \text{ mg}}{1 \text{ gr}} \times \frac{1 \text{ tab}}{100 \text{ mg}}$$

$$x = \frac{3}{1} \times \frac{60}{1} \times \frac{1 \text{ tab}}{100}$$

$$x = \frac{180 \text{ tab}}{100}$$

$$x = 1.8 \text{ or } 2 \text{ tab}$$

OR using 100 mg = gr iss as conversion:

$$x = \frac{\text{gr iii}}{1} \times \frac{100 \text{ mg}}{\text{gr iss}} \times \frac{1 \text{ tab}}{100 \text{ mg}}$$

$$x = \frac{3 \text{ gr}}{1} \times \frac{100 \text{ mg}}{1\frac{1}{2} \text{ gr}} \times \frac{1 \text{ tab}}{100 \text{ mg}}$$

$$x = \frac{3}{1} \times \frac{1}{1.5} \times \frac{1 \text{ tab}}{1}$$

$$x = \frac{3 \text{ tab}}{1.5}$$

$$x = 2 \text{ tab}$$

LEARNING TIP

For each factor added, the numerator should match the previous factor's denominator so that you can cancel the unnecessary units.

EXAMPLE **7:** Sulfamethoxazole is supplied as 1 g/10 mL. The doctor orders 2 g. How many milliliters would be prepared and how many teaspoons would be administered?

Using dimensional analysis to solve this problem, first set up the linear equation. On the left side of the equation place an *x*. The starting factor is 2 g and the other factors are that 10 mL = 1g and 1 tsp = 5 mL.

$$x = \frac{2 \text{ g}}{1} \times \frac{10 \text{ mL}}{1 \text{ g}} \times \frac{1 \text{ tsp}}{5 \text{ mL}}$$

$$x = \frac{2 \text{ g}}{1} \times \frac{10 \text{ mL}}{1 \text{ g}} \times \frac{1 \text{ tsp}}{5 \text{ mL}}$$

$$x = \frac{2}{1} \times \frac{\overset{2}{10}}{1} \times \frac{1 \text{ tsp}}{\underset{1}{5}}$$

$$x = \frac{4 \text{ tsp}}{1}$$

$$x = 4 \text{ tsp}$$

Notice that when the second factor was added, grams became the denominator so that the starting factor numerator grams could cancel out. You would repeat this method of adding factors and canceling the previous factor until you could solve the problem because all measurement factors except the desired measurement are cancelled out. Remember, in dimensional analysis, do not convert between measurement units but rather make the measurement units as factors in the equation.

Choosing a Calculation Method

Three methods of dosage calculation have been identified in this chapter. The example problem under each method is the same so that you will

CHECK YOUR UNDERSTANDING—DIMENSIONAL ANALYSIS   9-4

Show your work on a separate sheet of paper. Save your worksheet.

The starting factor is given first. Using the guidelines for dimensional analysis, circle the correct second factor.

1. $x \text{ mL} = \dfrac{3 \text{ mL}}{250 \text{ mg}}$ $\dfrac{500 \text{ mg}}{1}$ or $\dfrac{1}{500 \text{ mg}}$

2. $x \text{ caps} = \dfrac{1 \text{ cap}}{500 \text{ mg}}$ $\dfrac{250 \text{ mg}}{1}$ or $\dfrac{1}{250 \text{ mg}}$

3. $x \text{ mg} = \dfrac{1000 \text{ mg}}{2 \text{ tab}}$ $\dfrac{500 \text{ mg}}{1 \text{ tab}}$ or $\dfrac{1 \text{ tab}}{500 \text{ mg}}$

4. $x \text{ kg} = \dfrac{100 \text{ lb}}{1}$ $\dfrac{2.2 \text{ kg}}{1 \text{ lb}}$ or $\dfrac{1 \text{ lb}}{2.2 \text{ kg}}$

5. $x \text{ gtt} = \dfrac{2 \text{ mL}}{1}$ $\dfrac{15 \text{ gtt}}{1 \text{ mL}}$ or $\dfrac{1 \text{ mL}}{15 \text{ gtt}}$

PRACTICAL APPLICATION: Using the same set of problems found in the ratio and proportion method and in the formula method, solve using dimensional analysis. Show your work on a separate sheet of paper. Save your worksheet.

6. Zoloft 75 mg is ordered. The strength available is 50 mg tablet. How many tablets would provide the desired amount?_____

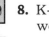

7. Metformin 750 mg is ordered. The strength available is 0.5 g/tablet. How many tablets would be necessary to administer the desired order?_____

8. K-Clor 40 mEq is ordered. The strength available is K-Clor 20 mEq tablets. How many tablets would be necessary for the desired order? _____

9. Amoxicillin 500 mg is ordered. Available is amoxicillin 125 mg/5 mL. How many milliliters would be administered for the desired order? _____
How many teaspoons would be administered? _____

10. Levothyroxine 0.5 mg is ordered. Strength available is 125 mcg/tablet. How many tablets would be necessary for the desired order? _____

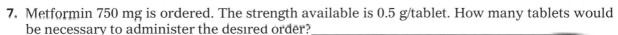

be able to see how each method differs. It is strongly suggested that you choose only *one* of the three methods and always use that method to avoid confusion and math errors.

Reconstituting a Powder

Some medications must be reconstituted from powder to liquid form prior to administration. The label on these medications will give the total strength of the medication in the bottle and the strength/volume of the medication after it has been reconstituted with the required diluents (Figure 9-1). Zithromax suspension will contain azithromycin 200 mg in every 5 mL when the medication has been reconstituted. The label on Zithromax shows the total strength of medication, the volume of sol-

ute to be used, and the strength of medication per volume when the solute is added.

Table 9-1 shows the reconstitution of Zithromax by total strength and volume of medication in the bottle. The weight (amount) of drug is measured in milligrams, so the azithromycin is available with the contents per bottle being either 300 mg, 600 mg, 900 mg, or 1200 mg. The amount of solute (water) added to the available drug makes the solution a dosage strength. If 9 mL of water is added to either the 300-mg or 600-mg bottle, the total volume after reconstitution will be 15 mL of suspension. The difference between the two bottles with 15 mL of oral suspension is that the dosage strength in the azithromycin 300 mg bottle is 100 mg/5 mL, and in the azithromycin 600 mg bottle, the oral suspension is 200 mg/5 mL after reconstitution.

CHECK YOUR UNDERSTANDING—DOSAGE CALCUATIONS   9-5

Show your work on a separate sheet of paper. Identify the method you use. Each answer has three parts. Save your worksheet.

CALCULATION REVIEW: Using only one of the calculating methods, calculate the following solid drug doses. Then write in the number of tablets or capsules for each dose. Interpret the orders to show the number of times the dose is taken each day.

1. Ordered: glucophage 1 g po bid with meals. Available: 500 mg tablets.
   Dose to be given: _____

2. Ordered: theophylline, 300 mg po 1h pc q6h. Available: 100 mg tablets.
   Dose to be given: _____

3. Ordered: dipyridamole 100 mg po qid. Available: 50 mg tablets.
   Dose to be given: _____

4. Ordered: phenytoin sodium 300 mg cap po daily. Available: 100 mg capsules.
   Dose to be given: _____

5. Ordered: griseofulvin 1 g po daily. Available: 250 mg tablets.
   Dose to be given: _____

6. Ordered: furosemide 40 mg po daily. Available: 20 mg tablets.
   Dose to be given: _____

7. Ordered: levothyroxine sodium 0.025 mg po daily. Available: 0.05 mg tablets.
   Dose to be given: _____
   _____

8. Ordered: bupropion hydrochloride 200 mg po q12h. Available: 100 mg tablets.
   Dose to be given: _____

9. Ordered: allopurinol 600 mg po daily in divided doses to be given bid.
   Available: 300 mg tablets.
   Dose to be given: _____

10. Ordered: cimetidine 300 mg po q8h. Available: 100 mg tablets.
    Dose to be given: _____

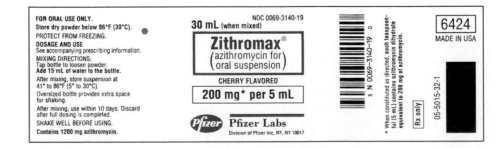

Figure 9-1 Label for Zithromax.

TABLE 9-1 *Constituting Instructions for Zithromax*

TOTAL AMOUNT OF ZITHROMAX	AMOUNT OF WATER TO BE ADDED	TOTAL VOLUME AFTER RECONSTITUTION (AZITHROMYCIN CONTENT)	AZITHROMYCIN CONCENTRATION AFTER RECONSTITUTION
300 mg of drug	9 mL	15 mL	100 mg/5 mL
600 mg of drug	9 mL	15 mL	200 mg/5 mL
900 mg of drug	12 mL	22.5 mL	200 mg/5 mL
1200 mg of drug	15 mL	30 mL	200 mg/5 mL

CHECK YOUR UNDERSTANDING—RECONSTITUTING A POWDER 9-6

PRACTICAL APPLICATION: Using the label in Figure 9-1 and Table 9-1, answer the following questions.

1. According to the label, how much azithromycin is available in the bottle if it is properly reconstituted? _____

2. According to the label, what dosage strength is available if properly reconstituted?_____
_____

3. According to the label, what is the total volume of the bottle after reconstitution? _____
_____

4. Does this medication expire as soon as the suggested dosage of "once daily for 5 days" is over? _____

5. Would you instruct a patient to use a teaspoon for the 5 mL dose? Explain your answer._____
_____

6. What specific instructions would you give to the patient? (two answers)_____
_____
_____

Using the label in Figure 9-1 *and* assuming the medication is properly reconstituted, answer the following questions.

7. If the doctor instructs the patient to take a teaspoon a day, how many mg would the patient be taking per day? _____

8. How many mL of water were added to the drug powder? _____

9. How many days would this medication last if the patient takes 5 mL a day? _____

10. Could you add less fluid to make a stronger dose? Why or why not? _____
_____

Use the following reconstituting instructions for Augmentin 400 mg/5 mL suspension. Answer questions 11-12.

BOTTLE SIZE	AMOUNT OF WATER REQUIRED FOR SUSPENSION TO OBTAIN **400 mg/5 mL**
50 mL	44 mL
75 mL	66 mL
100 mL	87 mL

(continued)

CHECK YOUR UNDERSTANDING—RECONSTITUTING A POWDER (cont'd)   9-6

11. How much water would you need to add to a 100 mL bottle in order to have the suspension of 400 mg/5 mL of Augmentin? _____

12. What size bottle would you need to use if you were only adding 66 mL of water to obtain a suspension of 400 mg/5 mL of Augmentin? _____

Use the following constituting instructions for cefdinir oral suspension. Answer questions 13-15.

FINAL CONCENTRATION	FINAL VOLUME	AMOUNT OF WATER	DIRECTIONS
125 mg/5 mL	60 mL	38 mL	Tap bottle to loosen
125 mg/5 mL	100 mL	63 mL	powder; then add water in two portions. Shake well after each addition.

13. Exactly how do you reconstitute cefdinir? _____
_____

14. What is the maximum dosage strength if this medication is reconstituted correctly?
_____

15. Because the dosage strength is the same on both final concentrations, would you predict that the bottle is the same size also? Explain. _____
_____

Special Calculations

Infants and children, because of their small size and their body function, cannot tolerate adult medications that are simply reduced in volume or amount of drug. In pediatric patients, this is referred to as "immature body systems," meaning that the body systems may not tolerate adult medications. Infants' body systems are not fully developed, and they lack the enzymes necessary to metabolize drugs. Also, the child's volume of total body water, when compared with that of an adult, is much greater, so the medication will be distributed differently, thus altering the effects of the drugs. The geriatric patient may require more specific calculation of medication dosage because of the potential toxicity due to the decrease in body functions. Finally, because of the toxicity of chemotherapeutic agents, the patient's height and weight become factors in the safe administration of these drugs.

Calculations Using the Body Surface Area Method

Infants and children can receive medications via the same routes as adults—parenteral and nonparenteral—but the method of using **body surface area (BSA) calculation** to determine correct dosage is used for calculating special dosages for children and geriatric patients, and with toxic drugs such as antineoplastics.

Calculating BSA

BSA is found by placing the patient's height and weight on a nomogram that calculates the body surface area rather than prescribing medications based on "normal adult" size. If a child is of normal height for weight, the BSA can be determined by weight alone, as is calculated on the box found in the center of the nomogram (Figure 9-2). However if the height and weight are not proportional, the nomogram may be used. The purpose of the **nomogram** is to measure the total surface area in square meters (m^2). Notice that height is measured in both cm (centimeters) and in (inches) and weight is in lb (pounds) and kg (kilograms). When using the nomogram, be careful that you read the appropriate calibration for both height and weight. To read a nomogram, use a ruler to line up the height (extreme left) and weight (extreme right) to obtain the BSA in m^2 that is found between these two columns. (All patients that require the use of a nomogram should be weighed and measured for

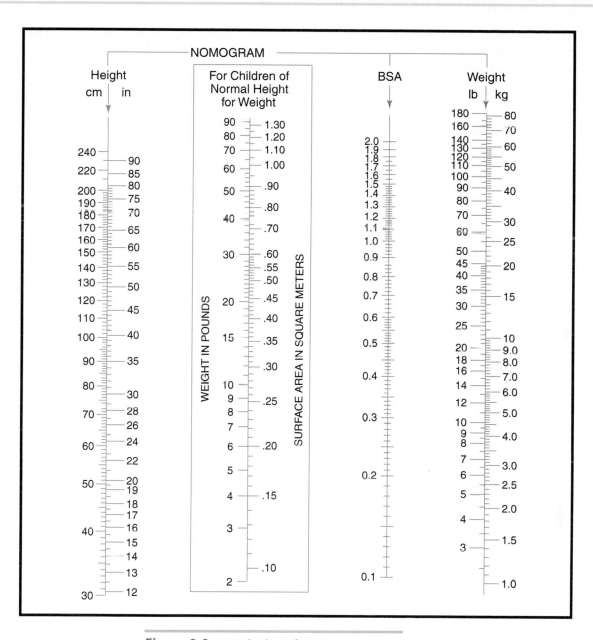

NOMOGRAM

Figure 9-2 West body surface area nomogram.

height prior to calculating with the nomogram.) Read the BSA at the point where the ruler intersects the graph. The number found in the BSA column is the BSA you will record. Note that the calibrations between designated numbers on BSA are not consistent from the top to the bottom of the graph. Some of the calibrations are in 0.01, others are in 0.1 markings, and some are even in 0.2 increments. Now try a few examples of calculating the BSA.

EXAMPLE 8: A child weighs 55 lb and is 85 cm tall. Determine this child's BSA using the nomogram.

Using the nomogram in Figure 9-2, do the following:

STEP 1. Find and mark the child's height in the first column. Be sure to find the height in centimeters, not inches.

STEP 2. Find and mark the child's weight in pounds (not kilograms) in the last column.

STEP 3. Use a ruler to align the marks. Then look on the column marked BSA at the top, and read the BSA from that column.

The answer is 0.82 m^2.

EXAMPLE 9: A child is of normal height for weight and weighs 32 lb. Determine this child's BSA using the nomogram.

Using the nomogram in Figure 9-2, do the following:

STEP 1. Find the middle column that is headed "For Children of Normal Height and Weight," which is enclosed within a box.

STEP 2. Find and mark the child's weight on the left side of the centerline.

STEP 3. Use a ruler to read the corresponding number on the right side of the centerline. This is the BSA.

The answer is 0.62 m^2.

Using BSA

After determining the BSA of the patient, the dosage calculation is completed by entering this information into a given formula. In the metric system, m^2 is the size of the body in height and weight. The assumption is that the BSA of an average adult weighing 140 lb is 1.7 m^2. Because most medications are based on average adult dosage, this dose must be adjusted for the person who needs a special amount of medication, such as an infant or child, an older person who no longer has the average weight for height, or a person taking very toxic medications such as antineoplastics.

The formula for calculating the dose is

$$\frac{\text{BSA m}^2}{1.7} \times \text{adult dose} = \text{desired dose}$$

 EXAMPLE 10: A child weighs 55 lb and is 85 cm tall. The physician orders amoxicillin to BSA for the child. BSA for this child on the nomogram is 0.82 m^2. The adult dose of amoxicillin is 500 mg. What is the dose for the child?

$$0.82 \text{ m}^2 (\text{BSA})/1.7 \times 500 \text{ mg} = 241 \text{ mg}$$

Now calculate the dose of amoxicillin that is to be given using the formula or the ratio and proportion method. The example below uses the formula method.

The child's dose would be 241 mg. Amoxicillin is available in 250 mg/5 mL.

$$\frac{241 \text{ mg (DO)}}{250 \text{ mg (DA)}} \times 5 \text{ mL (DF)} = 4.8 \text{ mL},$$
$$\text{or 5 mL (DG)}$$

This child would receive 1 teaspoon of amoxicillin.

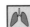 EXAMPLE 11: A child weighs 70 lb and is 45 inches tall. The physician orders albuterol for the child based on the BSA. The BSA is 1.2 m^2. The normal adult dose is albuterol 4 mg. What is the dose for the child?

$$\frac{1.2 \text{ m}^2 \text{ (BSA)}}{1.7 \text{ m}^2} \times 4 \text{ mg (adult dose)} = 2.8 \text{ mg},$$
$$\text{or 3 mg}$$

The child's dose would be albuterol 3 mg. Albuterol syrup available is 2 mg/5 mL.

$$\frac{3 \text{ mg (DO)}}{2 \text{ mg (DA)}} \times 5 \text{ mL (DF)} = 7.5 \text{ mL (DG)}$$

The child would be administered 7.5 mL or 1½ tsp of albuterol.

CHECK YOUR UNDERSTANDING—USING A NOMOGRAM   9-7

CALCULATION REVIEW: Use the nomogram in Figure 9-2 to calculate the BSA in m^2.

1. A child is 60 cm and weighs 7 kg. _____

2. A child is 35 lb and 72 cm. _____

3. A child is 45 inches and weighs 70 lb. _____

4. A child is 20 kg and 90 cm. _____

5. A child is of normal weight and height and weighs 75 lb. _____

CHECK YOUR UNDERSTANDING—BODY SURFACE AREA   9-8

Show your work on a separate sheet of paper. Save your worksheet.

CALCULATION REVIEW: Calculate the following dosages using BSA.

1. A child weighs 65 lb and is 42 inches tall. The physician orders Ilosone for the child. The normal adult dose is Ilosone 250 mg. Available Ilosone oral suspension 250 mg/5 mL. What is the BSA? _____
   What dose and volume of medication should be administered? _____

2. A child is 30 inches tall and weighs 27 lb. The physician orders Claritin syrup for the child. The normal adult dose is Claritin 10 mg. Available is Claritin syrup 10 mg/10 mL.
   What is the BSA? _____
   What dose and volume of medication should be administered? _____

3. A child is 65 inches tall and weighs 95 lb. A physician orders prednisone for the child. The normal adult dose is prednisone 5 mg. Available is prednisone 5 mg/5 mL.
   What is the BSA? _____
   What dose and volume of medication should be administered? _____

4. A child who weighs 30 lb and is the normal height for this weight has an order for Zantac syrup. The normal adult dose is Zantac 150 mg. Available is Zantac syrup 15 mg/mL.
   What is the BSA? _____
   What dose and volume of medication should be administered? _____

5. A child is 53 inches tall and weighs 70 lb. A physician orders cephalexin. The normal adult dose is cephalexin 500 mg. Available is cephalexin suspension 250 mg/5 mL.
   What is the BSA? _____
   What dose and volume of medication should be administered? _____

6. A baby who weighs 55 lb and is the normal height for this weight needs Demerol for pain following surgery. The usual adult dose is Demerol 100 mg. Available is meperidine syrup 50 mg/5 mL.
   What is the BSA? _____
   What dose and volume of medication should be administered? _____

7. A baby who weighs 10 lb and is 20 inches tall has an order for Keflex. The usual adult dose is Keflex 500 mg. Available is Keflex suspension 125 mg/5 mL.
   What is the BSA? _____
   What dose and volume of medication should be administered? _____

8. A child who weighs 30 lb and is the normal height for this weight has seizures. The physician orders Dilantin. The usual adult dose is Dilantin 100 mg. Available is Dilantin suspension 30 mg/5 mL.
   What is the BSA? _____
   What dose and volume of medication should be administered? _____

Calculating Dose Using Mg/Kg

In many pediatric settings the use of mg/kg/day is used to determine a standard dose. For example, in the Health Maintenance Organization's (HMO) formulary the dose information for amoxicillin is given as 30 to 50 mg/kg/day for a standard dose and 80 to 100 mg/kg/day for a high dose.

The first step is to change pounds to kilograms if the weight has been obtained in pounds. Remember that 2.2 lb = 1 kg. The easiest method for converting these measurements is by using ratio and proportion.

> **LEARNING TIP**
>
> The "/" in mg/kg means to multiply the numbers. Therefore the equation actually reads mg × kg × frequency of administration or dose.

EXAMPLE 12: 2.2 lb : 1 kg :: 22 lb : x

$$2.2\,x = 22 \text{ kg}$$
$$x = 10 \text{ kg}$$

Medication ordered: amoxicillin 50 mg/kg/day in three divided doses.

The child weighs 10 kg.

Calculation: $10 \times 50 \text{ mg} \times 1 \text{ day} = 500 \text{ mg per day}$

Now divide the total amount by three doses so that each dose will be 167 mg. (500 mg : 3 doses [3 times a day] :: x : 1 dose)

CHECK YOUR UNDERSTANDING—Mg/Kg   9-9

Show your work on a separate sheet of paper. Save your worksheet.

1. Ordered: Veetids 10 mg/kg/q8h for a child who weighs 55 lb.
   Available medication: Veetids 250 mg/5 mL.
   What is the strength of medication for one dose? _____
   What is the volume of medication to be given with that dose? _____

2. Ordered: Dilantin 2.5 mg/kg/per dose for a child who weighs 53 lb.
   Available medication: Dilantin Kapseals 30 mg
   What is the strength of medication for one dose? _____
   How many kapseals should be given with each dose? _____

3. Ordered: amoxicillin 20 mg/kg/day in three divided doses for a child who weighs 42 lb.
   Available: amoxicillin 125 mg/mL
   What is the strength of the medication for a day? _____
   What is the strength of the medication for a dose? _____
   What is the volume of medication for a dose? _____
   What is the volume of the dose in household measurement? _____

4. Ordered: Zyrtec syrup 0.1 mg/kg/daily for a child weighing 55 lb.
   Available medication: Zyrtec syrup 5 mg/5 mL
   What is the strength of medication to be administered for a day? _____
   What is the volume of medication to be administered daily? _____

5. Ordered: Zarontin syrup 20 mg/kg bid for a child who weighs 54 lb.
   Available medication: Zarontin syrup 250 mg/5 mL
   What is the strength of the medication to be given with each dose? _____
   What is the volume of medication to be given with each dose? _____
   What is the volume of medication to be given in household measurements? _____

Other Nonparenteral Medications

Medications used for nonparenteral routes come in several dosage forms other than the oral liquid and solid forms. Examples include ophthalmic and otic drops, which are almost always prescribed with a dropper because they are instilled into a body cavity; nasal sprays, inhalation solutions, and aerosols, which are prescribed in metered doses; aerosol powders, lotions, creams, ointments, and transdermal patches, which are applied topically; and chewable tablets for children, which are prescribed like other tablets, except that the patient is instructed to chew the medication. The importance of patient education cannot be stressed enough, especially with a drug form that the patient may be unfamiliar with leading to the chance that the patient may use it incorrectly. For example, the patient instruction sheet for the nasal spray triamcinolone acetonide tells the patient to "prime" the medication and then goes into detail about how the patient should do this. However, most patients do not take the time to read the accompanying literature. The allied health care professional should explain and demonstrate the correct procedure and allow the patient to ask questions to confirm understanding of the correct administration of the medication.

Summary

Medication is most frequently administered orally because of the ease of administration and dosage calculation. Nonparenteral medications usually come in solid or liquid form. Some medications, such as lotions and sprays, are prescribed for use on the skin that will be prescribed by the number of doses to the area per day.

This chapter shows three methods to calculate doses. The first two methods, called the ratio and proportion method and the formula method, require you to first convert to like measurement systems when necessary in order to solve the drug calculation. The third method, called dimensional analysis, uses common fractions that include the conversion for measurement systems as factors to allow cancellation of unnecessary units to solve the calculation using only one linear fraction. It is recommended that you choose only one method and that the method be the one with which you are most comfortable to lessen math errors.

Solid medications, such as tablets, may be prescribed in either of ½ to whole tablets per dose but are usually not divided into other measurements. Capsules cannot be divided, and time-release medications should be given in the prescribed dosage only. Liquid medications can easily be administered in the incorrect dosage if proper measuring devices are not used. Some patients are not what is considered "normal adults" and may not tolerate adult medications that have not been clinically approved for their body systems. Sometimes the BSA is measured to determine the amount of medication to administer to children, older adults, and persons taking highly toxic chemotherapy. The BSA method for calculating doses is based on the weight/height of the patient. This calculation is then compared to the normal adult BSA of 1.7 m^2 and the normal adult dose.

Critical Thinking Exercises

Using the medication label provided, calculate the oral dosage of each medication. Show your work. On the dosage line, explain exactly how much medication is taken and how often the medication is taken.

1. Mr. Walters is taking an antiulcer medication in an effort to manage an acute duodenal ulcer. He is currently taking ranitidine 150 mg po bid.
Dose to be given: _____

NDC 0093-8544-06
RANITIDINE
Tablets, USP
150 mg*
* Each tablet contains: Ranitidine Hydrochloride equivalent to 150 mg of Ranitidine
℞ only
60 TABLETS
TEVA

2. Ms. Lechuga has type 2 diabetes mellitus and has been prescribed Prandin 2 mg by mouth bid, with a meal, to regulate her blood glucose.
Dose to be given: _____

Prandin™ (repaglinide) Tablets 2 mg 100 tablets Do not store above 77°F (25°C) NDC 0169-0084-81 List 008481 Marketed by: *Novo Nordisk Pharmaceuticals, Inc.* Princeton, NJ 08540 Exp. Date: 10/2003 Control: 9K21020

3. Mr. Bates has been prescribed the antidepressant drug fluoxetine and is instructed to take fluoxetine 20 mg every morning.

Dose to be given: _____

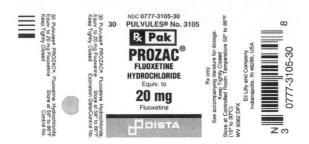

4. Ms. Allison is on a trip, and her purse with her heart medication in it has been stolen. She is taking the anticoagulant Coumadin 5 mg daily.

Dose to be given: _____

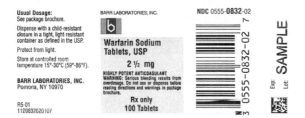

5. Mr. Davis is being treated for Paget's disease with risedronate 30 mg daily at least 30 minutes before the first food or drink of the day, for the next 2 months.

Dose to be given: _____

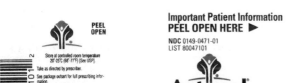

6. After her thyroidectomy, Bernadette was instructed to take levothyroxine tablets once a day for the rest of her life. She currently takes levothyroxine 100 mcg daily.

Dose to be given: _____

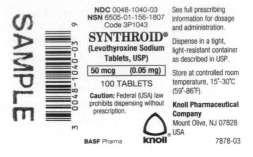

7. Mr. Rockwell has been diagnosed with congestive heart failure and will be prescribed lisinopril 10 mg daily to control his hypertension.

Dose to be given: _____

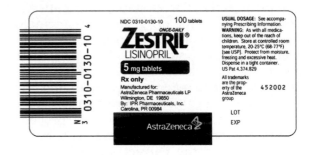

8. Mark White experienced constant muscle hyperactivity after his car accident, and Dr. Merry prescribed metaxalone 800 mg tid.

Dose to be given: _____

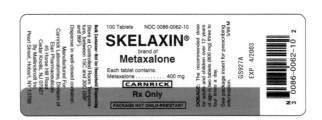

9. Ms. Marta had moderate pneumonia and was prescribed azithromycin 400 mg the first day and 200 mg for days 2 through 5.

Dose to be given on first day:_____

Dose to be given on days 2 through 5: _____

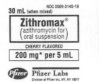

CALCULATION REVIEW: Calculate the following problems using *only* one method. Be sure that the dose is in the correct dosage form. Show your work on a separate sheet of paper. Save your worksheet.

Dose to be given

1. Ordered: Benadryl 50 mg
   Available: Benadryl 25 mg caps

   _____

2. Ordered: chlorpromazine HCl 20 mg
   Available: Thorazine 10 mg tabs

   _____

3. Ordered: warfarin sodium 10 mg
   Available: warfarin sodium 5 mg tabs

   _____

4. Ordered: Proventil syrup 4 mg
   Available: Proventil syrup 2 mg/5 mL
   How would you give this in household measure?

   _____

   _____

5. Ordered: Captopril 25 mg
   Available: Captopril 12.5 mg tabs

   _____

6. Ordered: amoxicillin 500 mg
   Available: Amoxil 250 mg caps

   _____

7. Ordered: Biaxin 150 mg
   Available: Biaxin 250 mg/tsp
   What is the dose in mL?

   _____

   _____

8. Ordered: K-Dur 10 mEq
   Available: K-Dur 20 mEq scored tabs

   _____

9. Ordered: dimenhydrinate HCl 25 mg
   Available: Dramamine 12.5 mg tabs

   _____

10. Ordered: Ativan 1.5 mg
    Available: Ativan 1 mg tabs

    _____

REVIEW QUESTIONS

All of the following statements are *false*. Determine the error(s) and rewrite the answer, giving complete and correct information in the space provided.

1. BSA is calculated by measuring weight alone. _____
   _____

2. A comparison of the relationship between two ratios is called the *formula method* of dosage calculation. _____
   _____

3. One household teaspoon is approximately equal to 15 milliliters. _____
   _____
   _____

4. A value in a measurement system is called a *nomogram*. _____
   _____

5. When a medication needs to be reconstituted, adding more fluid than required will give you a better dosage unit. _____
   _____

6.   10 mL given as one tablespoon is the correct dosage when the drug order states give 80 mg and the label reads 40 mg/5 mL. _____

7.   When using the proportional method, the dosage form is compared with the dose to be given. _____

8.   Capsules can be divided in half. _____

9.   When reconstituting a drug, the only facts you need to remember are the desired strength and the total volume after reconstitution. _____

10. The apothecary system uses teaspoons and tablespoons. _____

11. The dosage ordered of a drug is also called the *dosage* to be given. _____

12. When using the proportional method, in order to read the proportion, you should compare the means with the extremes. _____

13. The most important concept when calculating dosages is to be sure that the units requested and the units you have on hand are metric measurements. _____

14. If the dosage ordered stated 40 mg tablet, and the available was a 20 mg tablet, you would give ½ of one tablet. _____

15. The nomogram is used to calculate a child's dosage on the basis of body fat. _____

16. To reduce possible calculation errors, it is best to use several methods of calculating dosages. _____

17. A conversion factor refers to the unknown equivalency of two values. _____

18. A reconstituted drug is one that has had a liquid added to make an approximate dosage strength. _____

19. It is most cost effective to use the unit-dose system. _____

20. All dosage problems have two parts: knowing what the physician has ordered and knowing what dosage is to be given. _____

CALCULATION REVIEW: A prescription medication comes in tablet form with dosage strengths of 5 mg, 10 mg, 20 mg, 40 mg, and 80 mg. Determine the best combination for each total dose. (This is not time-release medication.)

21. 60 mg daily dosage, to be given in divided doses tid. _____

22. 15 mg daily dosage, to be given as a single dose daily. _____

23. 100 mg daily dosage, to be given in divided doses qid. _____

24. 90 mg daily dosage, to be given in divided doses bid. _____

25. 90 mg daily dosage, to be given in divided doses tid. _____

Estimate the correct dosage (number of tablets or capsules) without working out the math.

26. On hand is a capsule containing 100 mg; 300 mg is ordered. _____

27. On hand is a scored tablet containing 500 mcg; 250 mcg is ordered. _____

28. On hand is a scored tablet containing gr ¼; gr ½ is ordered. _____

29. On hand is a scored tablet containing 8 mg; 12 mg is ordered. _____

30. On hand is a capsule containing 325 mg; 650 mg is ordered. _____

Calculate the following problems using only one method. Be sure that the dose is in the correct form. Show your work on a separate sheet of paper. Save your worksheet.

31. Ordered: Dilantin 60 mg
     Available: Dilantin 30 mg caps
     Dose to be given: _____

32. Ordered: Maalox 15 mL
     Available: Maalox liquid
     How much would you give in a household dose? _____

33. Ordered: Lanoxin 0.25 mg
     Available: Lanoxin 0.125 mg tabs
     Dose to be given: _____

34. Ordered: Inderal 80 mg
     Available: Inderal 20 mg tabs
     Dose to be given: _____

35. Ordered: amoxicillin 0.25 g
     Available: Amoxil 125 mg caps
     Dose to be given: _____

36. Ordered: Zyloprim 0.1 g
     Available: Zyloprim 25 mg tabs
     Dose to be given: _____

37. Ordered: thyroid gr 1/300
     Available: thyroid 0.2 mg tabs
     Dose to be given: _____

38. Ordered: aspirin 0.6 g
     Available: acetylsalicylic acid gr v tabs
     Dose to be given: _____

39. Ordered: ampicillin 500 mg
     Available: ampicillin 125 mg/5 mL
     Dose to be given: _____
     How much would you give in a household dose? _____

40. Ordered: furosemide 80 mg
     Available: furosemide 40 mg/5 mL
     Dose to be given: _____
     How much would you give in a household dose? _____

41.   Ordered: ascorbic acid 0.5 g
Available: ascorbic acid 250 mg tabs
Dose to be given: _____

42.   Ordered: Inderal 60 mg
Available: Inderal 20 mg tabs
Dose to be given: _____

43.   Ordered: mineral oil 10 mL
Available: mineral oil 180 mL bottle
Dose to be given: _____
How much would you give in a household dose?_____

44.   Ordered: levothyroxine 0.3 mg
Available: levothyroxine 100 mcg tabs
Dose to be given: _____

45.   Ordered: Zantac 300 mg
Available: Zantac 15 mg/mL
Dose to be given: _____

46.   Ordered: Norvasc 7.5 mg
Available: Norvasc 2.5 mg tabs
Dose to be given: _____

47.   Ordered: colchicine 1.2 mg
Available: colchicine 0.6 mg tabs
Dose to be given: _____

48.   Ordered: Elix. phenobarbital gr i
Available: Elix. phenobarbital 20 mg/5 mL
Dose to be given: _____
How much would you give in a household dose? _____

49.   Ordered: Atarax 25 mg
Available: Atarax 10 mg/tsp
Dose to be given: _____
How much would you give in a metric dose? _____

50.   Ordered: Elix. Lanoxin 0.025 mg
Available: Elix. Lanoxin 0.05 mg/5 mL
Dose to be given: _____
How much would you give in a household dose? _____

Calculating Doses of Parenteral Medications

OBJECTIVES

After studying this chapter, you should be capable of:
- Determining the correct syringe for administration of parenteral dosages.
- Calculating doses of parenteral medications in the metric system.
- Calculating doses of parenteral medications in units.

KEY TERMS

Agitate
Parenteral
Unit

CHAPTER 10 PRE-TEST CALCULATING DOSES PARENTERAL MEDICATIONS

Identify the most appropriate syringe size to use to administer the medication given in Column A. Use the choices in Column B as many times as necessary but use only one answer per question.

COLUMN A	COLUMN B
1. _____ 1.1 mL	A. insulin syringe
2. _____ 86 units of U-100	B. tuberculin syringe
3. _____ 2.4 mL	C. 3 mL syringe
4. _____ 0.22 mL	
5. _____ 0.86 mL	
6. _____ 0.25 units	
7. _____ 0.25 units of U-100	

Calculate the answers to the following problems, then shade in the syringe with the exact dose you would administer.

8. A patient comes to Dr. Merry complaining of shortness of breath after ingesting mushrooms found near his home. The doctor diagnoses mushroom poisoning and prescribes atropine 0.5 mg SC, as an antidote. The available atropine vial is labeled 0.4 mg/mL

Volume of dose to be administered: _____

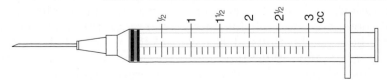

CHAPTER 10 PRE-TEST CALCULATING DOSES PARENTERAL MEDICATIONS—cont'd

9. After confirming that the patient has no known allergies, Dr. Merry prescribes V-Cillin K 400,000 units IM to combat the patient's pneumococcal infection. Available: a vial of V-Cillin K powder 1 million units. Directions for reconstitution state to: add 4.5 mL normal saline solution to the powder to provide a dosage of 1 million units/5 mL.

Volume of medication to be administered: _____

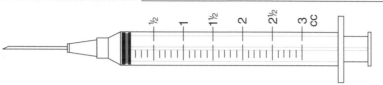

Parenteral Medications

Parenteral medications are administered to provide quick absorption of the drug into the blood stream or when a patient cannot take oral medications, such as when the patient is uncooperative or unconscious. Also, some medications cannot be administered orally because the gastrointestinal tract enzymes and acids do not allow for proper absorption of the medication. This chapter concentrates on calculating doses for parenteral medications in the metric system or in units. Intravenous (IV) medications and their calculations are covered in Chapter 11. Also included is knowledge of the proper needle size and syringe use when calculating parenteral medications and the use of reconstituted powders (see Chapter 9 for the initial discussion of reconstitution of powders). Finally calculations of medications found in units per volume and reading percentages of solutions that are also indicated in the metric system are presented. Drugs may be labeled in both percentage strengths and in the metric system. For example, lidocaine HCl inj. 1% USP will also have the amount of medication as 10 mg/mL, included on the label.

Many drugs, such as some antibiotics, come in a solid powdered form and must be reconstituted to a liquid for parenteral administration. These drugs are packaged in dry form because they are unstable for prolonged periods of time in liquid form. After reconstitution, the shelf-life is short with rapid loss of potency and effectiveness. When reconstituting these medications, it is extremely important to read and understand the vial label or package insert because different dosage strengths are determined by the amount of diluent added. A medication can have only one dosage strength per vial once it has been reconstituted. In other words, more fluid cannot be added to the vial to make the dose weaker after the powder has been reconstituted if any amount of the medication has been withdrawn from the vial for administration. During reconstitution, the directions will specifically instruct the allied health professional either to roll the medication to dissolve the powder or to shake (agitate) the vial to place the dry ingredients into the needed liquid state for injection. Some of these medications, when found as a suspension, will have to have the precipitate placed back into the liquid before preparing the medication for injection; in other cases, the medication becomes a solution that does not need agitation with each administration.

Drugs are usually reconstituted with sterile water or 0.9 percent sodium chloride (normal saline [NS] solution). If a drug comes packaged with a specific solution to be used in reconstituting the medication, never substitute another liquid. Some medications for reconstitution will come in single-dose vials that are reconstituted for immediate use. Single dose vials should never be reconstituted prior to the time for use. When multiple-dose vials are prepared, the reconstituted medication should be labeled with the reconstituted dosage strength, reconstitution date and time, and the expiration date. The person doing the reconstitution should initial the vial for safety of the patient. Labeling of medication should be done consistently by all personnel. (Note: Chapter 15 presents the technique for administering parenteral medications.)

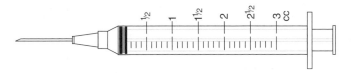

Figure 10-1 Typical 3-mL syringe.

Reading Syringes for Parenteral Drug Administration

Intramuscular (IM) medications are administered directly into a muscle for rapid absorption. Antibiotics, antihistamines, steroidal antiinflammatory drugs, pain medications, and immunizations are all examples of types of medications that are administered by this route. Intramuscular injections are typically administered in volumes up to 3 mL depending on the site of the injection. In most cases, syringes used for IM injections are calibrated in tenths of a milliliter (mL) with the 3 mL syringe being the typical choice (Figure 10-1).

Calculations to find doses of parenteral medications are performed in a manner similar to that introduced in Chapter 9 for nonparenteral medications. However, instead of calculating how many tablets, capsules, teaspoons, or even milliliters to administer orally, you will be calculating the number of mL, or how much volume of medication (liquid) will be drawn into a syringe. To calculate the dosage using the 3 mL syringe, first observe that the numbers on the syringe start with ½ and are in increments of ½, so they include the numbers, ½, 1, 1½, 2, 2½, and 3. Between each number are markings that signify one tenth of 1 mL. Therefore, the syringe has four short markings for tenths between the longer markings that show ½-mL increments. Medication dose would not typically be written as ½; it would be written as 0.5 mL because the designation is in the metric system and 0.5 is the decimal equivalent of ½. Recall that when no number appears before the decimal a zero should be placed in front of the decimal place to aid in reducing calculation errors.

EXAMPLE 1: 2.2 mL is shown below:

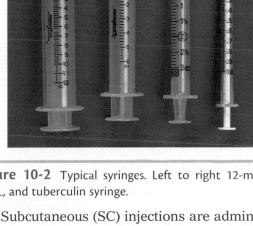

Figure 10-2 Typical syringes. Left to right 12-mL, 6-mL, 3-mL, and tuberculin syringe.

Subcutaneous (SC) injections are administered into the subcutaneous layer of tissue, which is between the muscle and epidermal layer of skin. The volume of a subcutaneous injection is usually between 0.5 and 1 mL; the maximum amount of fluid that can be injected by this route is 2 mL, depending on the size of the person. The 3-mL syringe may be used for subcutaneous (SC) injections but in specific instances tuberculin syringes may be used when small amounts of medication are ordered. Insulin syringes are used only for the administration of insulin (Figures 10-2 and 10-3).

Intradermal (ID) injections are used to administer medications into the epidermal layer of the skin. This area is located just under the epidermis, above the subcutaneous layer. The volume of drug administered is usually 0.1 mL or less, but is always less than 0.2 mL. The syringe used is the 1-mL tuberculin syringe that is calibrated in 0.01 increments from 0.01 mL to 1 mL. The calculations of the medications for intradermal use are performed in the same manner as other parenteral medications.

Some medications such as penicillin are given in units per mL. When you see units per mL, always check to see how many units of medication are equivalent to 1 mL. Then work the problem by calculating units per volume or milliliters to provide the needed dose.

If a medication has to be reconstituted, the calculation is performed in the same manner as for other medications in strength per volume or mg per mL after reconstitution.

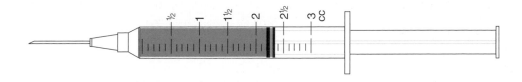

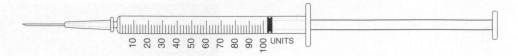

Figure 10-3 Typical U-100 insulin syringe.

CHECK YOUR UNDERSTANDING—READING SYRINGES

10-1

CALCULATION REVIEW: Read the syringe and write the amount of medication that is indicated.

1. _____

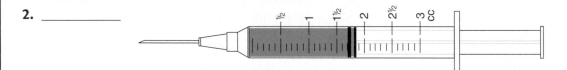

2. _____

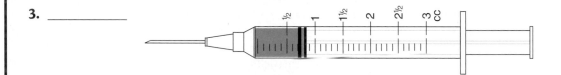

3. _____

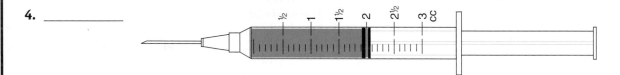

4. _____

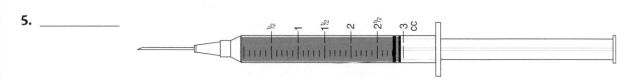

5. _____

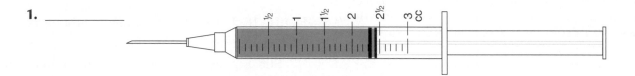

You are given the dose. Draw a line and shade in the exact number of mL that would show in the syringe.

6. 1.4 mL

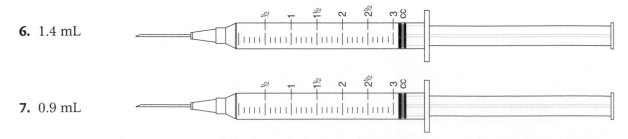

7. 0.9 mL

CHECK YOUR UNDERSTANDING—READING SYRINGES (cont'd)   10-1

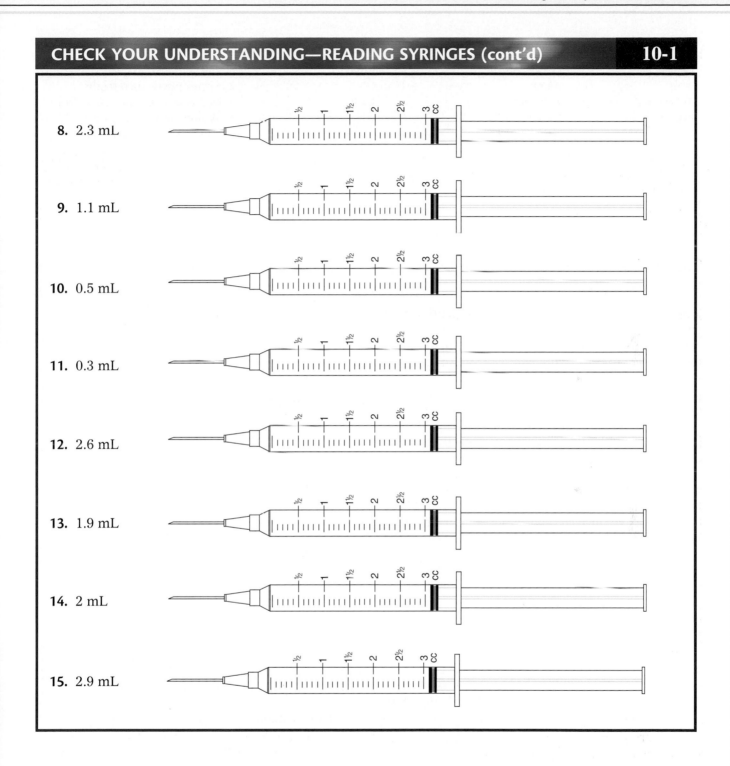

8. 2.3 mL

9. 1.1 mL

10. 0.5 mL

11. 0.3 mL

12. 2.6 mL

13. 1.9 mL

14. 2 mL

15. 2.9 mL

Insulin is manufactured in units per mL; therefore, insulin should always be administered using an insulin syringe that is calibrated in units, not milliliters.

When finding the answer to dosage calculations, a few points should be remembered. First, all calculations in milliliters requiring the use of a 3-mL syringe are carried out two decimal places and then rounded to the nearest tenth if necessary. For example, 1.25 mL would be rounded to 1.3 mL, and 1.24 mL would be rounded to 1.2 mL. For tuberculin syringes, when calculating milliliters, carry calculation out to three decimal places and round to the nearest one-hundredth, because the tuberculin syringe is marked in hundredths (0.01) of a mL. For example, 0.836 mL would be rounded to 0.84. Table 10-1 shows the comparison between syringes and dosage volumes.

TABLE 10-1 *Syringe and Dosage Volume Comparison*

SYRINGE SIZE	TYPICAL VOLUME	CALIBRATION	ROUND CALCULATIONS TO:
3 mL	1-3 mL	Tenths	2 decimal places, then tenths
Tuberculin	0.01-1.0 mL	Hundredths	3 decimal places, then hundredths
Insulin	1-100 units (0.01 cc = 1 unit)	May be in 1- or 2-unit calibration	Medication ordered in even units; either syringe may be used. If ordered in odd-unit amounts, the syringe used must be calibrated in one-unit increments.

Calculating Parenteral Medications Using the Metric System

Unlike calculating a dose of oral medication that can be in several solid and liquid forms, parenteral medications will always be in a liquid form—in most cases in mL. The basic strength unit for parenteral medications is usually the milligram although units, grams, or milliequivalents may be used. When using any of the weight designations, the cancellation of the designation during calculation will allow the final dose to be in a liquid form.

Once you have practiced reading the volume in syringes, the next step is to calculate the dose using one of the methods learned in Chapter 9. If the medication requires conversions between measurement systems, use the conversion information found in Chapter 8. Because the actual steps for calculating medications using ratio and proportion, the formula method, and dimensional analysis were presented in Chapter 8, the exact calculations will not be placed below. If you need to review the exact steps for solving dose calculations, please review Chapter 8.

 EXAMPLE 2: Ordered: meperidine (Demerol) 100 mg every 3-4 hours IM for pain management.

Available: meperidine 50 mg/1 mL.

Calculating Dose Using the Ratio and Proportion Method

Compare the known ratio to the unknown ratio.
Known: 50 mg : 1 mL
Unknown: 100 mg : x mL

Set up the proportional equation:

50 (DA) : 1 (DF) :: 100 (DO) : x (DG)

Administer Demerol 2 mL every 3 to 4 hours.

Calculating Dose Using the Formula Method

Set up the formula:

$$\frac{DO}{DA} \times DF = DG$$

$$\frac{100 \text{ mg (DO)}}{50 \text{ mg (DA)}} \times 1 \text{ mL (DF)} = x \text{ (DG)}$$

$$DG = \text{Demerol 2 mL q 3-4h}$$

The volume of the drug to draw into the syringe is 2 mL.

Calculating Dose Using the Dimensional Analysis Method

The first step is to set up the equation with x on the left and the starting factor in the linear equation being the dose to be found. This should be followed by the available medication.

The problem looks like this:

$$x = \frac{100 \text{ mg}}{1} \times \frac{1 \text{ mL}}{50 \text{ mg}}$$

The dose to be given is Demerol 2 mL q 3-4 h

 LEARNING TIP

Regardless of the method of calculation, the dose to be drawn into the syringe must be a liquid volume, so the answer must be expressed as a liquid (in milliliters).

CHECK YOUR UNDERSTANDING—CALCULATING DOSES IN THE METRIC SYSTEM   10-2

CALCULATION REVIEW: Calculate the following parenteral doses. Then draw the correct amount of fluid in the syringe. Show your work on a separate sheet of paper. Save your worksheet. (Label your answer on the syringe with the correct number of mL.)

1. Ordered: hydrocortisone sodium phosphate 125 mg IM.
   Available: hydrocortisone sodium phosphate 50 mg/mL.
   Desired dose: _____
   Show this amount on the syringe.

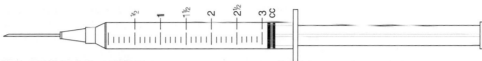

2. Ordered: furosemide 25 mg IM.
   Available: furosemide 10 mg/mL.
   Desired dose: _____
   Show this amount on the syringe.

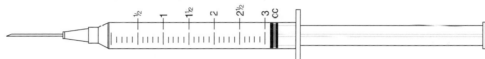

3. Ordered: atropine sulfate 0.5 mg IM.
   Available: atropine sulfate 1 mg/mL.
   Desired dose: _____
   Show this amount on the syringe.

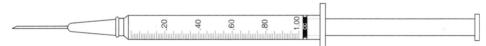

4. Ordered: diazepam 2 mg IM every 3-4 hours.
   Available: diazepam 5 mg/mL.
   Desired dose: _____
   Show this amount on the syringe.

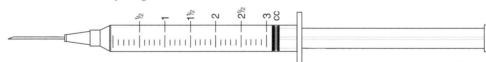

5. Ordered: digoxin 375 mcg IM stat.
   Available: digoxin 0.125 mg/1 mL.
   Desired dose: _____
   Show the amount on the syringe.

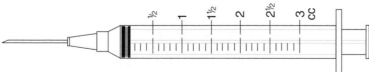

6. Ordered: methylprednisolone (Solu-Medrol) 125 mg.
   Available: methylprednisolone reconstituted to 62.5 mg/mL.
   Desired dose: _____
   Show the amount on the syringe.

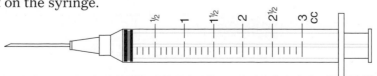

Calculating Doses of Parenteral Drugs in Units

Aqueous based medications, such as analgesics (opioids), vitamin B_{12}, epinephrine, certain vaccines, insulin, heparin, and anticoagulants, of less than 2 mL may be given subcutaneously. Medications that are injected intradermally or are less than 1 mL, including those in units (except for insulin) are prepared in a tuberculin syringe. Insulin, however, should always be prepared in an insulin syringe that is marked in units. Heparin is designated in units but the doses are indicated in mL,

so the medication is prepared in a tuberculin syringe for doses less than 1 mL.

The tuberculin syringe has a capacity of 1 mL and is calculated in hundredths of a mL (0.01). The U-100 insulin syringe holds either 50 U (0.5 mL) or 100 U (1 mL) of medication and is calibrated in units. The number of units of insulin indicates the amount of insulin being given. The standard insulin syringe used today is the U-100 1 mL (100 units), but insulin syringes also come in a 0.5-mL (50-unit) size and a 0.3-mL (30-unit) size. The U-50 insulin syringes are marked off in "ones" and are therefore more precise when

---

CHECK YOUR UNDERSTANDING—DOSES IN UNITS   10-3

CALCULATION REVIEW: Read the syringe and write the amount of medication that is indicated.

1. _____

2. _____

3. _____

4. _____

5. _____

CHECK YOUR UNDERSTANDING—DOSES IN UNITS (cont'd)   10-3

You are given the dose. Draw a line and shade in the exact amount (volume) that would show in the syringe.

6. 80 units insulin

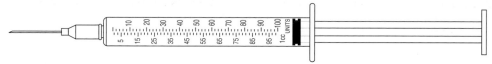

7. 46 units insulin

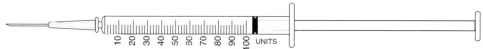

8. 36 units insulin

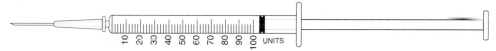

9. 5000 units heparin (10,000 units/mL)

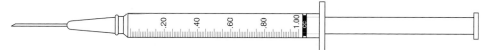

10. 2500 units heparin (5000 units/mL)

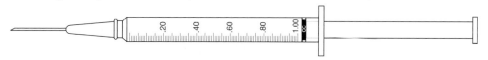

insulin is ordered in an odd number of less than 50 units. The syringes holding the smaller volume are for use by people with visual impairment and are using only small dosages.

Calculating a Parenteral Medication Available In Units

To calculate units, set up the problem as shown previously using one of the three methods of calculation.

 LEARNING TIP
When calculating with numbers with multiple zeros at the end, such as 200,000, cancel as many zeros as possible to make the calculations easier.

 EXAMPLE 3: Ordered: penicillin G 200,000 units IM.

Available: penicillin G 250,000 units/mL.

Calculating Units Using the Ratio and Proportion Method

Known: 250,000 units : 1 mL
Unknown: 200,000 units: x mL

$250\cancel{000}$ U (DA) : 1 mL(DF) :: $200\cancel{000}$ U (DO): x (DG)

$x = 0.8$ mL

Administer penicillin G 0.8 mL

Calculating Units Using the Formula Method

$$\frac{DO}{DA} \times DF = DG$$

$$\frac{200\cancel{000} \text{ units (DO)}}{250\cancel{000} \text{ units (DA)}} \times 1 \text{ mL (DF)} = x \text{ (DG)}$$

Administer penicillin G 0.8 mL IM

Calculating Units Using the Dimensional Analysis Method

$$x = \frac{20\cancel{0}\cancel{0}\cancel{0}0 \text{ U}}{1} \times \frac{1 \text{ mL}}{25\cancel{0}\cancel{0}\cancel{0}0 \text{ U}}$$

Administer penicillin G 0.8 mL IM

Remember to complete the additional steps for parenteral doses:

What size syringe would you choose? (1 mL tuberculin or 3 mL syringe)

How much penicillin G would you draw into this syringe? (0.8 mL)

What parenteral route is used? (Intramuscular [IM])

Calculating Heparin Doses in Units

Heparin is available in units/mL. Orders for heparin are written in units but the dose to be given will be in mL. If the dose is less than 1 mL, the medication should be prepared in a tuberculin syringe for accuracy. If the dose is larger than 1 mL, the medication will be prepared in a 3-mL syringe.

> **Example 4:** Dose ordered: heparin 2500 U.
> Available medication: heparin 10000 U/mL.

Calculating Heparin Units Using Ratio and Proportion

Known: 10000 U/1 mL

Unknown: 2500 U

10$\cancel{0}\cancel{0}\cancel{0}$0 U (DA) : 1 mL (DF) :: 25$\cancel{0}\cancel{0}$00 U (DO) : x (DG)

Dose to be given is heparin 0.25 mL.

Calculating Heparin Units Using the Formula Method

$$\frac{DO}{DA} \times DF = DG$$

25$\cancel{0}$0 U/10$\cancel{0}\cancel{0}$00 U × 1 mL = x

Dose to be given: heparin 0.25 mL.

Calculating Heparin Units Using Dimensional Analysis

$$x = \frac{25\cancel{0}\cancel{0}0 \text{ U}}{1} \times \frac{1 \text{ mL}}{10\cancel{0}\cancel{0}\cancel{0}0 \text{ U}}$$

Dose to be given: heparin 0.25 mL.
Because this is a small dose volume, a tuberculin syringe should be used.

Measuring Insulin in Units

Insulin is measured in units and some forms of insulin may be mixed for administration. When calculating the total amount of insulin to be drawn into the syringe, individual dose units of each insulin type must be added together to find the total dose unit volume to be administered.

> **EN DO** **EXAMPLE 5:** Ordered: Humulin R 22 units and Humulin N 26 units.
> Available: 10-mL vials of Humulin R U-100 and Humulin N U-100.
> How much insulin would you draw into a U-100 syringe? Humulin R 22 U and Humulin N 26 U for a total of 48 units.

CHECK YOUR UNDERSTANDING—CALCULATING DOSES IN UNITS   10-4

CALCULATION REVIEW: Compute the following doses in units. Then draw in the correct amount of fluid on the syringe. Show your work on a separate sheet of paper. Save your worksheet.

EN DO **1.** Ordered: Humulin R 35 units SC.
Available: Humulin R U-100 insulin 10-mL vial.
Desired dose: _____

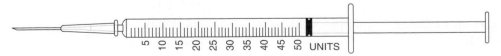

CHECK YOUR UNDERSTANDING—CALCULATING DOSES IN UNITS (cont'd)   10-4

2. Ordered: Lente insulin 66 units SC ac 8:00 AM.
Available: Lente insulin U-100 10-mL vial.
Desired dose: _____

3. Ordered: Humulin-L 34 units and Humulin R 50 U SC ac 7:30 AM.
Available: Humulin-L insulin U-100 and Humulin R U 100 in 10-mL vials.
Desired total dose: _____

4. Ordered: Novolin-N 25 U and Novolin R 20 U SC.
Available: Novolin-N U 100 and Novolin R U-100 10-mL vials.
Desired dose: _____

5. Ordered: Humulin 70/30 15 U q AM and q PM.
Available: Humulin 70/30 insulin U-100 10-mL vial.
Desired dose: _____

6. Ordered: tetanus immune globulin 150 units IM.
Available: tetanus immune globulin 250 units/mL.
Desired dose: _____
Show this amount on the syringe.

(continued)

CHECK YOUR UNDERSTANDING—CALCULATING DOSES IN UNITS (cont'd)   10-4

Using the information provided, determine the answers to questions 7 to 10.

Penicillin G potassium powder, 1,000,000 Units

DESIRED CONCENTRATION	VOLUME (ML) OF DILUENT TO BE ADDED
50,000 units/mL	20 mL
100,000 units/mL	10 mL
250,000 units/mL	4 mL
500,000 units/mL	1.8 mL

7. Calculate the number of mL to be given per dose for a patient who was prescribed penicillin G potassium 400,000 units daily IM in four divided doses when the volume of diluent added was 10 mL.
   Desired dose: _____
   Show this amount on the syringe.

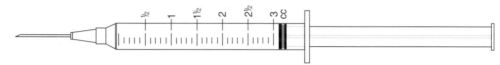

8. The physician prescribed penicillin G potassium 400,000 units to be administered IM bid. Diluent added: 4 mL to obtain the desired dosage strength. Identify the dosage strength per mL and calculate the volume per dose to be administered.
   Dosage strength: _____
   Volume per dose: _____

9. How much diluent should be added to the penicillin G to make a concentration of 500,000 units/mL dosage strength? _____

10. Explain how so many dosage strengths are possible with just one vial of medication. _____
    _____

Summary

This chapter concludes the calculation of medications (except IV medications) section of this textbook. At this point, the successful student should feel comfortable with calculating doses for parenteral and nonparenteral medication delivery. This chapter emphasizes the importance of first reading the label, taking the time to understand the medication asked for and observing the medication available, then following directions, calculating dosages, and reconstituting as necessary. Throughout this section, all math calculation examples are shown using either ratio and proportion, the formula method, or dimensional analysis. If a review of the exact steps necessary in these calculations is needed, the student should go back to Chapters 8 and 9 for the information. Students should find a method that they are most comfortable with and that produces the correct results, and then they should use that method with consistency. Dose calculation errors are less likely to occur if the student consistently computes dose calculations using only one method.

Three basic syringes are used to administer most parenteral medications. Choosing the correct syringe is extremely important, especially with the use of tuberculin or insulin syringes. Insulin and heparin are both calibrated in units and must be administered in exact doses. Insulin units should be administered with an insulin syringe that is standard at U-100/mL, whereas heparin units should be administered with a tuberculin syringe. Most other medications are administered in calibrated syringes using milliliters. The syringe size that is most frequently used is a 3-mL (3-cc) syringe.

CHECK YOUR UNDERSTANDING—REVIEW   10-5

CALCULATION REVIEW: Calculate the following problems. Show your work on a separate sheet of paper. Save your worksheet.

1. Ordered: conjugated estrogens 2.5 mg SC
   Available: conjugated estrogens 5 mg/mL
   Desired dose: _____

2. Ordered: Demerol 75 mg IM
   Available: Demerol 50 mg/mL
   Desired dose: _____

3. Ordered: procaine penicillin G 1,200,000 units IM
   Available: procaine penicillin G 600,000 units/mL
   Desired dose: _____

4. Ordered: ampicillin 1 g IM
   Available: ampicillin reconstituted to 2 g/6.8 mL
   Desired dose: _____

5. Ordered: furosemide 2 mg IM
   Available: furosemide 10 mg/mL
   Desired dose: _____
   What syringe would you use?_____

Critical Thinking Exercises

Name each of the syringes shown below and then identify the characteristics of each. Then circle the appropriate injection route(s) for each.

1. Type of syringe: _____
   Volume capacity: _____
   Calibration: _____
   Typically used for: Intradermal Subcutaneous
       Intramuscular

2. Type of syringe: _____
   Volume capacity: _____
   Calibration: _____
   Typically used for: Intradermal Subcutaneous
       Intramuscular

3. Type of syringe: _____
   Volume capacity: _____
   Calibration: _____
   Typically used for: Intradermal Subcutaneous
       Intramuscular

REVIEW QUESTIONS

All of the following statements are *false*. Determine the error(s) and rewrite the answer giving completely correct information in the space provided.

1. To calculate a syringe dose, read the fluid level from the tip of the plunger just above the calibration mark. _____
    _____
    _____

2. A tuberculin syringe is calibrated in units only. _____
    _____
    _____

3. Only viscous solutions are given subcutaneously. _____
    _____
    _____

4. The most common insulin syringe is called the U-50. _____
    _____
    _____

5. Heparin is normally given using an insulin syringe._____
    _____
    _____

6. The typical intramuscular syringe holds 100 units of medication. _____
    _____
    _____

7. A viscous injectable fluid is usually considered thin or watery. _____
    _____
    _____

8. Typically, a tuberculin syringe is used to administer an antibiotic. _____
    _____
    _____

9. Many medications given IM are aqueous and irritating to the tissues. _____
    _____
    _____

10. Insulin may be administered in a 3-cc syringe if it is calibrated in units. _____
    _____
    _____

11. When using a 2- or 3-mL syringe, always round calculations to the nearest whole number.
    _____
    _____

Calculate the following problems. Show your work on a separate sheet of paper. Save your worksheet.

12. Ordered: furosemide 10 mg IM
    Available: Lasix 40 mg/5mL
    Desired dose: _____

13. Ordered: procaine penicillin G 500,000 units IM
    Available: procaine penicillin G 250,000 units/mL
    Desired dose: _____

14. Ordered: Benadryl 25 mg IM
Available: Benadryl 50 mg/mL
Desired dose: _____

15. Ordered: Phenergan 75 mg IM
Available: Phenergan 50 mg/mL
Desired dose: _____

16. Ordered: heparin 4000 U SC
Available: heparin 10,000 units/mL
Desired dose: _____

17. Ordered: Humulin-R 35 units
Available: Humulin-R U-100
Desired dose: _____

18. Ordered: Rocephin 500 mg IM
Available: Rocephin 1000 mg/4 mL
Desired dose: _____

19. Ordered: morphine sulfate gr ¼ IM
Available: morphine sulfate 15 mg/mL
Desired dose: _____

20. Ordered: morphine sulfate gr ¼ IM
Available: morphine sulfate gr ½ /mL
Desired dose: _____

21. Ordered: Reglan 7.5 mg IM
Available: Reglan 10 mg/mL
Desired dose: _____

22. Ordered: Vistaril 75 mg IM
Available: Vistaril 50 mg/mL
Desired dose: _____

23. Ordered: Depo-Estradiol 10 mg IM
Available: Depo-Estradiol 5 mg/mL
Desired dose: _____

24. Ordered: epinephrine 1:200 SC
Available: epinephrine 1:200/0.3 mL amp
Desired dose: _____

25. Ordered: morphine sulfate 8 mg IM
Available: morphine sulfate gr ⅙ per mL
Desired dose: _____

26. Ordered: Phenergan 12.5 mg IM
Available: Phenergan 50 mg/2 mL amp
Desired dose: _____

27. Ordered: neomycin 400 mg IM
Available: neomycin 500 mg/2.5 mL
Desired dose: _____

28. Ordered: meperidine 15 mg IM
Available: meperidine 50 mg/mL
Desired dose: _____

29. Ordered: vitamin B_{12} 1 mg IM
Available: vitamin B_{12} 1000 mcg/mL
Desired dose: _____

30. Ordered: Toradol 60 mg IM
Available: Toradol 30 mg/mL and 15 mg/mL
Calculate the amount for each and tell which you would administer.
Desired dose: _____

31. Ordered: Depo-Provera 150 mg IM
Available: medroxyprogesterone acetate 100 mg/mL
Desired dose: _____

32. Ordered: Thorazine 37.5 mg IM
Available: Thorazine 25 mg/mL in 10 mL vial
Desired dose: _____

33. Ordered: cefoxitin sodium 1000 mg IM
Available: Mefoxin 1000 mg/2 mL
Desired dose: _____

34. Ordered: Nembutal 100 mg IM
Available: Nembutal 50 mg/mL
Desired dose: _____

35. Ordered: codeine gr ½ IM
Available: codeine 60 mg/mL
Desired dose: _____

36. Ordered: Talwin 30 mg IM
Available: Talwin 60 mg/mL
Desired dose: _____

37. Ordered: Cleocin 225 mg IM
Available: Cleocin 150 mg/mL
Desired dose: _____

38. Ordered: Fragmin 2500 U SC daily
Available: Fragmin 7500 U/mL
Desired dose: _____

39. Ordered: Zofran 2 mg IM 30 minutes prior to chemotherapy
Available: Zofran 4 mg/5 mL
Desired dose: _____

40. Ordered: Lanoxin 0.25 mg IM stat
Available: Lanoxin 500 mcg/2 mL
Desired dose: _____

CHAPTER 11

Principles and Calculations in Intravenous Therapy

OBJECTIVES

At the completion of this chapter, you should be capable of doing the following:

- Defining the key terms associated with basic intravenous (IV) therapy.
- Providing information about the evolution of IV therapy.
- Explaining the physiology of fluids in maintaining homeostasis and electrolyte balance.
- Describing the indications for and advantages of IV therapy.
- Identifying the dangers of IV therapy.
- Identifying the types of fluids used for IV replacement therapy.
- Listing the factors used in determining the types of IV fluids used in therapy.
- Identifying the equipment and delivery systems needed for IV therapy.
- Knowing the basic formulas for calculating intravenous flow rates, drip rates, and amount of medication for administration and calculating IV medication using these factors.
- Explaining why the allied health professional must assess the patient and the related medical conditions before initiating IV therapy.
- Discussing the legal and ethical issues of beginning IV therapy.

KEY TERMS

Bolus
Cannula
Catheter
Chemotherapy
Diuresis
Drip chamber
Drop factor
Drop orifice
Electrolytes
Embolus, emboli
Extracellular fluids
Flow rate
Hematoma
Hypertonic solution
Hypotonic solution

Infiltration
Infusate
Infusion pump
Infusion therapy
Injection port
Intracellular fluids
Isotonic solution
IV flush
IV piggyback (IVPB)
IV therapy
Lethargy
Macrodrip
Maintenance therapy
Metabolic acidosis
Microdrip

Needleless systems
Overload
Over-the-needle catheter
Phlebitis
Replacement therapy
Respiratory acidosis
Restoration therapy
Solute
Solvent
Spike
Stylet
Thrombus, thrombi
Venous spasm
Winged-infusion scalp or butterfly
   needle

Although many allied health professionals may not be expected to provide IV therapy on a regular basis, the principles of **IV therapy** are necessary for patient education and for understanding patient care. The scope of practice in the locale of employment will be the guide for the actual practice of this technique.

Brief History of Intravenous Therapy

Intravenous therapy includes the administration of fluids, nutritional support, and transfusion therapy. When IV therapy is discussed, the concept is considered a relatively new practice in the medical field. In actuality, the use of IV therapy began in the seventeenth century with experiments using blood transfusions to treat illnesses. With the discovery of the circulation of blood by Sir William Harvey in 1616 and the production of the first hypodermic needle by Sir Christopher Wren in 1660, the first use of injecting substances such as wine and opium into the bloodstream through a vein using a quill and bladder was tried. Later, these experiments were banned and the next use of IV therapy was in the nineteenth century when blood transfusions were administered to women who were hemorrhaging during childbirth. Because newly found infection-control procedures such as handwashing and the germ theory had been introduced, the ban was lifted and IV therapy was again an interest in the medical field.

The earliest fluids used included infusions of 0.9% sodium chloride solutions because of their isotonic nature with blood. When pyogens were found in distilled water, the researchers worked to remove the bacteria, making fluids much safer and more widely accepted. In 1925, dextrose was added to fluids as a source of calories, but only the most critically ill persons in hospital settings received the treatment.

In the mid-1950s, the two indications for IV therapy were surgery and dehydration, with less than 20% of hospital patients receiving intravenous therapy. The most common site for infusion of dextrose 5% in water (D-5-W) or in 0.9% normal saline (D-5-NS) was the antecubital space of the elbow with the arm restrained on a flat padded board. The solutions ran for 3 to 4 hours but were discontinued at night. Because of the frequent infiltrations using nondisposable needles, a flexible plastic **cannula** that could be inserted into the vein through the needle was introduced. This cannula led to less tissue injury and more comfort and mobility for the patient.

During the 1960s, fluids were refined, so the choices now consisted of about 200 different types available for use; thus the field of IV therapy accelerated. Added to the field were piggyback medications, filters, and electronic infusion devices that made IV infusions safer and more commonly used. Medications were made available for IV use for patients at all levels of care with the increase in use of IV therapy in the last half of the twentieth century as a result. Today the medications for such areas as **chemotherapy** are available only with IV use.

Today, IV therapy can be very technical and specialized with approximately 90% of all hospitalized patients receiving IV fluids during a hospital stay. More importantly, this therapy is no longer confined to hospital use but is becoming more common in the ambulatory care setting such as home health care and in physicians' offices.

Physiology and Intravenous Therapy

Water, accounting for approximately 60% to 75% of total body weight, is the single largest constituent of the body's mass and is essential to life. Fat cells contain less water, making the percentage of body water dependent on the fat distribution of the person. Age, gender, ethnic origin, and weight also are factors that influence the amount and distribution of body fluids.

Continually moving in the body, water is given different names in various locations such as **intracellular fluid,** extracellular fluid, plasma, lymph, and interstitial fluid. Homeostasis depends on fluid and electrolyte intake and physiologic factors, disease processes, external factors, and pharmacologic interventions. **Electrolytes** for homeostasis are dissolved in the blood plasma, a body **solvent,** for transport throughout the body. Body fluids are continuously exchanged in the intracellular and interstitial spaces and plasma. For a person to remain in fluid homeostasis, that person must maintain an approximately equal intake to output of fluids.

Functions of Body Fluids

Fluids function to maintain blood volume, regulate body temperature, and transport needed nutrients to and from cells for cell metabolism. Body fluids also aid in digestion through hydrolysis, act as a medium for excretion, and act as solvents in which **solutes** are transported for cell function.

- Body fluids contain 0.9% sodium chloride, and IV fluids are described as isotonic when they contain the same salt concentration as found in normal body fluids. For the person who needs only replacement of normally lost body fluids, isotonic fluids are used.
- Fluids that contain less salt (sodium chloride) than fluids found in the body are referred to as *hypotonic*. When **hypotonic solutions** are administered, the normal fluids in blood vessels shift from the circulating blood into the interstitial spaces and the interstitial tissue and cells. This action hydrates cells but can deplete the circulatory system fluids.
- **Hypertonic solutions** contain greater concentrations of salt (sodium chloride) than those found in body fluids. Thus these solutions cause **extracellular fluids** to shift from the cells into the blood. This action reduces body edema but increases the pressure in blood vessels, causing elevated blood pressure, hypertension, and increased work for the heart and lungs.
- Therefore the physician will carefully choose IV fluids to meet the specific needs of each person so that the body will remain in or quickly return to homeostasis. IV therapy has specific indications and must be carefully chosen to meet the needs of the patient. The health professional who participates in IV therapy in any manner must be just as careful that the order is properly prepared for administration.

Reasons for Intravenous Therapy

For any medication to be effective, it must reach the blood for distribution throughout the body. Oral medications are absorbed through the digestive tract, and parenteral medications other than those given intravenously cross tissue barriers before absorption. With IV therapy, these barriers do not exist and the loss of potency of medication is avoided, allowing the entire dose of medication to be distributed through the bloodstream to the body immediately following administration. Thus one of the major indications for and possible advantages of IV therapy is the rapid absorption of medication.

For patients who are unable to take medication by mouth or for whom the ordered parenteral injection would cause irritation of tissues, such as with chemotherapy medications, the IV route is often indicated. When drugs are altered by the gastrointestinal tract to make the medication less effective, the preferred route also is parenteral. The preferred route is parenteral—perhaps specifically intravenously—in patients who are unconscious, vomiting, or uncooperative in oral intake.

Another goal of IV therapy is to maintain or restore normal fluid volume and electrolyte balance for homeostasis and for nutritional therapy. The infusing of supplements that contain amino acids and other needed nutrients allow the body to build tissue, whereas solutions containing dextrose only contain sufficient carbohydrates to minimize tissue breakdown and prevent starvation. The type of fluid prescribed depends on the patient's state of homeostasis, the need for nutrition, or both.

Most indications for providing IV therapy are divided into three categories: **maintenance therapy, replacement therapy,** and **restoration therapy.** Each type of therapy has a direct influence and a specific rationale for the type of IV fluids ordered by the physician.

- Maintenance therapy provides the necessary nutrients to meet the daily needs for water, electrolytes, and nutritional replacement. The amount of fluid is determined by the patient's age, height, weight, and amount of body fat. Maintenance therapy is used for patients who have either no intake of fluids by mouth or a limited oral intake and require supplements of fluids and nutritional elements.
- When a patient has had a deficit of fluids and electrolytes over time, usually 48 hours or more, replacement therapy may be necessary. Patient indications include vomiting and diarrhea, starvation, and hemorrhage. Before replacement fluids are instituted, kidney function should be evaluated. Because of the increased volume of fluids added to the body and the inherent loss of potassium, potassium replacement also may be necessary to maintain homeostasis if the level is found to be deficient.
- Finally, restoration therapy is daily restoration of vital fluids and electrolytes. With this therapy, the fluids used are physiologically the same as the fluids being lost as determined by laboratory testing. Often several types of fluids are ordered for administration on the same day. This is more often seen in inpatient settings because of the dangers associated with fluid **overload.**

In an ambulatory care center, the most common type of IV therapy is replacement therapy.

The allied health care professional responsible for the fluid IV administration should carefully monitor the person for any signs of overload or toxicity such as increased blood pressure, breathing difficulties, chest discomfort, and other common symptoms of adverse reactions (e.g., itching, rashes, edema).

Dangers of Intravenous Therapy

Contamination

One obvious danger of IV therapy is the possible introduction of microorganisms directly into the bloodstream when sterile aseptic technique is not precisely followed. Because fluids are directly transported throughout the body, the strictest of aseptic technique is necessary. Remember, sterility is not measured in degrees.

Infection or Inflammation at Injection Site

Another major danger is infection or inflammation at the injection site including local infection and **phlebitis.** The care of the injection site and bandaging around the site must be performed using medical and surgical asepsis to prevent the spread of bacteria from the dressings to the vein at the injection site. Phlebitis at the site may result from IV fluid irritation, needle movement because of patient activity, and improper handling of fluids and equipment. The signs of phlebitis are discomfort, swelling, and inflammation radiating from the administration site along the route of venous circulation.

Wrong Solutions

The use of hypertonic or hypotonic solutions may cause destruction of blood cells, resulting in an **embolus** formation from the debris of these cells. Particles of undiluted medications that have not dissolved in the fluid also may result in an embolus.

Overload

If the physician's order is not carefully followed or if the fluids are given too rapidly and in large volumes over a short time, fluid overload in the body may occur. This condition is especially dangerous for patients with kidney disease, hypertension, and heart disease such as congestive heart failure.

Medication Error

Finally, the introduction of medications using IV fluids is not reversible. Once the medication or fluids have been injected into the veins, the medication will travel immediately throughout the body. Blood needs only 1 minute to circulate through the body. Even the immediate discontinuation of an injected fluid does not prevent transportation throughout the body for absorption.

The allied health professional must use strict aseptic technique, meet all infection-control standards, continually observe the injection site, and follow the physician's orders exactly. Only with a competent level of education and technical competence should any health care professional begin IV therapy or monitor an infusion. The danger to the patient is great, and the ability to evaluate a situation for possible adverse reactions is a necessity before the responsibility of administering IV therapy should be accepted.

Introduction to Basic Intravenous Equipment

Types of fluids and equipment for IV therapy are based on the needs of the patient, the proper selection of equipment to meet the physician's order, and the safety of the patient. The selection of fluids is based on the physician's order. The person performing the infusion must be sure that patient safety is promoted and that the infusion is effectively delivered.

Types of Fluids and Reasons for Intravenous Therapy

In ambulatory care, IV fluids are administered as intermittent infusions to care for an acute condition that does not require hospitalization. IV fluids are also given to maintain fluid intake during illness, reestablish plasma volume, replace electrolyte losses resulting from gastrointestinal diseases, and provide nutrition in patients who cannot consume adequate calories daily. Parenteral fluids can contain dextrose, sodium chloride, and other electrolytes with added nutritional supplements.

- One simple IV solution is 0.9% sodium chloride, or normal saline. This isotonic solution maintains body fluid levels and does not result in a shift in the fluid in the intracellular, intravascular, and extracellular spaces.

- IV fluids are usually combined with glucose (e.g., dextrose 5% in water [D-5-W] or saline [D-5-NS]) to supply nutritional needs and provide part of the daily caloric requirement. The higher the concentration of dextrose, the more likely the solution will cause a shift in body fluids. Higher concentrations of dextrose (≥5%) tend to be more characteristic of hypotonic solutions that decrease intravascular fluid loss and increase cellular edema.
- A third common type of IV fluid is a multiple electrolyte solution such as Ringer's or lactated Ringer's, which contains sodium, potassium, calcium, and chloride ions. Unless dextrose is added to Ringer's solutions, no calories are supplied. Because of the increase in electrolytes, Ringer's solutions are contraindicated in patients with congestive heart failure, renal impairment, and liver disease (Tables 11-1 and 11-2).

Figures 11-1 to 11-7 illustrate only the infusion fluids most commonly seen in ambulatory care facilities. These include parenteral fluid containers

TABLE 11-1 *Fluids for Maintaining Homeostasis*

COMMON IV FLUID	COMMON USE	CONTRAINDICATIONS
Isotonic saline (0.9%)	Replace sodium losses in such conditions as gastrointestinal fluid loss and burns	Congestive heart failure, pulmonary edema, renal impairment
Isotonic 5% dextrose in water (D-5-W)	Maintain fluid intake and provide daily need of calories; peripheral nutrition; does not replace electrolyte deficiencies	Head injuries; may need insulin added for persons with diabetes mellitus
Isotonic 5% dextrose in 0.3% NaCl		
Hypotonic 10% dextrose in water (D-10-W)	Supply calories for nutritional needs	No typical contraindications; may need insulin added for persons with diabetes mellitus
Hypotonic 5% dextrose in 0.9% NaCl	Maintain fluid intake; maintenance fluid of choice if no electrolytes necessary	No typical contraindications; may need insulin added for persons with diabetes mellitus
Isotonic Ringer's solution	Replace electrolytes in concentrations similar to normal plasma levels; no calories	When electrolytes are not necessary
Isotonic lactated Ringer's solution	Similar electrolytes as plasma; lactated to correct metabolic acidosis; replaces fluid losses of diarrhea, burns, etc.	Congestive heart failure, renal impairment, liver disease, respiratory alkalosis

TABLE 11-2 *Advantages and Disadvantages of Common Fluids*

COMMON SOLUTION	ADVANTAGES	DISADVANTAGES
Dextrose in water	Provides carbohydrates and nutrition; can be used to treat dehydration	Must be used carefully with patients with diabetes
Saline solutions	Provides replacement of extracellular fluids; is used to treat patients with sodium depletion	May provide more sodium and potassium than needed by the patient; can lead to circulatory overload
Dextrose in normal saline	Can be used to treat circulatory insufficiency; replaces nutrients and electrolytes; is a hydrating solution	May provide more sodium and potassium than needed by the patient; can lead to circulatory overload
Ringer's solution	Acts as a fluid and electrolyte replacement; is a replenisher after dehydration; is similar to normal saline	Can be incompatible with medications, has no calories, causes sodium retention with subsequent congestive heart failure and renal insufficiency
Lactated Ringer's solution	Acts much like extracellular electrolytes	Has no calories, can be incompatible with medications, can increase sodium levels in person with normal sodium levels

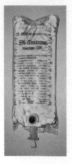
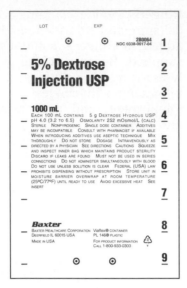

Figure 11-1 Five percent dextrose in water. (From Brown M, Mulholland JM: *Drug calculations: process and problems for clinical practice*, ed 7, St Louis, 2004, Mosby.)

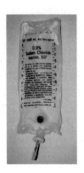
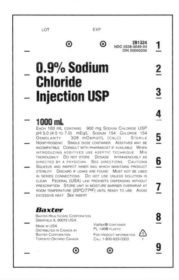

Figure 11-2 Normal saline 0.9%. (From Brown M, Mulholland JM: *Drug calculations: process and problems for clinical practice*, ed 7, St Louis, 2004, Mosby.)

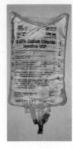
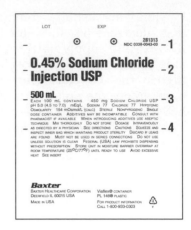

Figure 11-3 Normal saline 0.45%. (From Brown M, Mulholland JM: *Drug calculations: process and problems for clinical practice*, ed 7, St Louis, 2004, Mosby.)

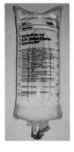
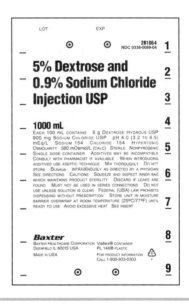

Figure 11-4 Five percent dextrose in normal saline. (From Brown M, Mulholland JM: *Drug calculations: process and problems for clinical practice*, ed 7, St Louis, 2004, Mosby.)

in 500 mL and 1000 mL. Infusion fluids are also available in 50-, 100-, and 250-mL containers that are most often used for administering medications as **intravenous piggyback (IVPB).** Many different types of parenteral solutions are available. Most physicians in the ambulatory setting use the fluids that have the least chance of causing adverse reactions. For a more acutely, chronically, or critically ill person, the physician may order that drugs, supplements, or fluids be added to the parenteral fluids in inpatient facilities.

Tonicity of Fluids

The tonicity of fluids is based on the concentration of solutes in the solvent or the ability of the solvent to pass through the semipermeable membranes that separate solutions of different concentrations. The solvent passes from areas of higher solute concentration to those of lower solute concentration to attempt to equalize the concentrations of solutes on both sides of the membrane.

Hypotonic fluids hydrate cells and deplete the amount of fluid in the circulatory system. Because

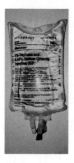
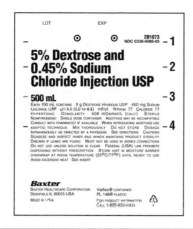

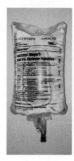
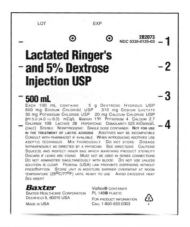

Figure 11-5 Five percent dextrose in ½ normal saline. (From Brown M, Mulholland JM: *Drug calculations: process and problems for clinical practice,* ed 7, St Louis, 2004, Mosby.)

Figure 11-7 Lactated Ringer's and 5% dextrose. (From Brown M, Mulholland JM: *Drug calculations: process and problems for clinical practice,* ed 7, St Louis, 2004, Mosby.)

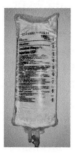
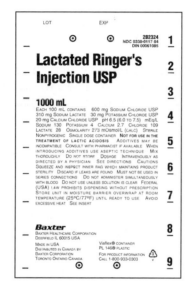

Figure 11-6 Lactated Ringer's solution. (From Brown M, Mulholland JM: *Drug calculations: process and problems for clinical practice,* ed 7, St Louis, 2004, Mosby.)

hypotonic fluids have lower solvent concentrations than the surrounding tissues, fluid moves from the vascular system into the intracellular spaces. The person administering these fluids must remember that a fall in circulating plasma results in lowered blood pressure.

Hypertonic fluids are used to replace electrolytes because the fluids contain stronger concentrations of electrolytes, causing a shift of electrolytes to the tissues and a shift of fluids to the vascular system. Administration causes a shift of extracellular fluids from the interstitial spaces into the plasma for increased blood volumes. These fluids can be used when the extracellular

fluids need to be shifted into the plasma, such as with severe edema. These fluids must be given slowly, and the patient must be monitored closely for circulatory overload with symptoms such as shortness of breath, cough, and pitting edema in dependent areas.

Isotonic solutions are similar to body fluids and are used to expand the extracellular fluid space. These fluids do not cause the shift of body fluids into other compartments, but circulatory overload is a danger.

Equipment for Infusion Therapy

Containers for IV infusions are open systems in which the air entering the container displaces the fluids for the infusion or closed containers in which atmospheric pressure is the factor for fluid displacement. In either case, the appropriate infusion set must be used for the containers to function correctly. When infusion administration equipment does not match the type of fluid container, the infusion will not be as safe and effective and may even be dangerous for the patient.

The equipment used for IV therapy must be sterile and specific for the physician's order. The allied health professional should always check the equipment closely prior to initiating the infusion therapy.

Containers

Open containers are rigid and are usually made of glass. These are seldom used today except when the incompatibility of medications with plastic does not allow the use of closed bag plastic containers. Glass containers must be air vented, and the specific infusion set for these containers must be used. Plastic or closed containers are made of flexible plastic and do not require venting. With this system, the plastic bag collapses as the fluid is infused and the chance of contamination is reduced because air does not enter the fluid. Before use, fluids for IV infusion therapy should be carefully inspected for clarity to ensure that no precipitates are present. Any discoloration or precipitate indicates contamination. Only fluids that have not passed the expiration date should be used. The date and time of administration are noted and placed on the bag, but do not write directly on the bag to prevent puncturing it. If the plastic bag has been refrigerated, bubbles may be present and the fluid should be agitated to remove the bubbles prior to administration.

Interpreting Intravenous Fluid Labels

When interpreting the fluids that the patient is to receive, the commonly used infusates are available in percentage strengths in specific fluid amount. The first letter indicates the chemical that will be found in the fluid, the second number is the percentage strength of that chemical, and the third designation is the fluid in which the chemical is found. When a label reads 1000 mL NS, it indicates that 0.9% sodium chloride (NaCl) (or normal saline) is in a 1000-mL container. This actually means the parts per hundred of the solvent (NaCl) in the solute (water). The use of percentage states that 0.9 g of NaCl is found in each 100 mL of solute (usually water) or 9 g of NaCl are found in 1000 mL of solute or water. Another example of the use of percentage is 5% dextrose in ½ NS (D-5-½ NS). In this case, 50 g of dextrose and 4.5 g of NaCl (½ NS indicates that the NaCl is 0.45% rather than the 0.9% found in NS) would be found in each 1000 mL of water. Understanding the percentage of solute in a solvent is important for patient safety when administering fluids. When choosing the correct fluids for the patient, be sure that the percentages agree with the physician's order.

This information is just a reminder of the necessary background for administering medications and fluids. In most cases in which drugs are added to IV fluids, this is accomplished by a pharmacist, so the actual calculation of the medication dose has been done. However, the person infusing the medication has the responsibility of being sure that an accurate dosage has been calculated and prepared. Therefore all fluids administered with medications added should be rechecked for the accuracy of preparation

and should be checked to the physician's order prior to hanging the infusate. Again, the triangulation of health care professionals provides quality assurance for patient safety.

Administration Equipment

Administration equipment for infusion therapy is usually in packages that contain the cannula and needle needed for the injection and IV tubing with the associated equipment for attachment to the container of fluids. Each set is individually labeled with the name, description of the equipment, lot number, drops-per-milliliter rate for the **drip chamber** and **drop orifice,** usage description, and manufacturer's name. Each administration set should be carefully chosen by the person starting the infusion to ensure that the kit provides the ordered IV infusion rate. It should also be inspected for maintenance of sterility.

Fluid administration sets come in several types such as primary administration sets used to provide medications directly into the bloodstream, secondary infusion sets used to add intermittent medications through secondary tubing, and blood administration sets. In most ambulatory care settings, primary administration sets will be used for infusion (Figure 11-8). These sets are labeled individually with the information showing the name;

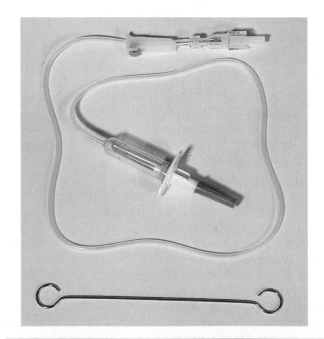

Figure 11-8 Intravenous equipment including tubing, drip chamber, spike, flow-control clamp, and Luer-Lok connector. (From Leahy JM, Kizilay PE: *Foundations of nursing practice: a nursing process approach*, Philadelphia, 1998, Saunders.)

drops per milliliter; use (primary, secondary, or specialty set); and gauge and length of the needle/cannula. The most frequently used are single line sets that include the primary line and ability to add secondary lines such as IV piggyback (IVPB).

The administration set has a **spike** or piercing pin that is sharply tipped to allow for insertion into the solution container. It is an extension of the drop orifice and drip chamber. The spike must remain sterile, so it is manufactured with a cover to maintain sterility. When the tubing is inserted into the bag, this spike can perforate the side of the bag, so care must be taken to prevent fluid contamination and prevent damage to the fluid container. Directly under the spike is a vent, which permits the movement of air to displace the infusing fluids. The drip chamber, which is a pliable enlarged plastic tube, holds the fluids before infusion. The opening of the drip chamber from the spike contains the drop orifice, which determines the size and shape of the drop of fluids.

Primary (standard) sets are available with a drip chamber that may be in either **macrodrip** form to administer 8 to 20 drops/mL or **microdrip** form to administer 50 to 60 drops/mL (Figure 11-9). (The microdrip administration set has a smaller drop orifice diameter, so it supplies more drops per milliliter and has a slower rate of infusion.) The macrodrip set, with its large drop size, is more commonly used in adults, and the microdrip or minidrip set is more frequently used when small amounts of fluids are required such as in pediatric patients or with medications that require slow administration.

Infusion tubing that connects to the drip chamber varies in length from 60 to 110 inches and varies in flexibility relative to the internal diameter or lumen. Most tubing is relatively flexible, except macrotubing that is used for rapid **flow rates.** The amount of tubing needed for the patient to have some mobility and the placement of the fluids in relation to the patient's position are the determining factors for the length of tubing used.

Clamps, **injection ports,** and back-check valves may be found on tubing, depending on the manufacturer. A flow control clamp may be used to compress the tubing to regulate the rate of infusion and is located on the tubing that descends from the drip chamber (Figure 11-10). Most clamps are either roller or screw clamps, although the less reliable sliding clamp may also be found, depending on the administration set used in the medical setting. Most tubing has a Luer-Lok connector at the needle to prevent the accidental disconnection of the needle from the tubing and to serve as the

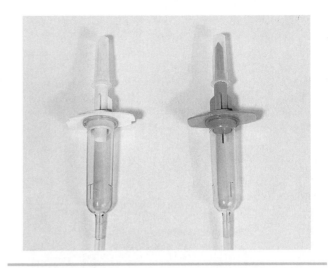

Figure 11-9   *Left,* Intravenous macrodrip set. *Right,* Microdrip set. (From Leahy JM, Kizilay PE: *Foundations of nursing practice: a nursing process approach,* Philadelphia, 1998, Saunders.)

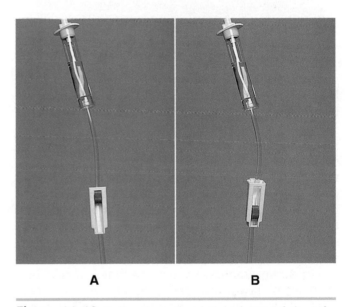

A   **B**

Figure 11-10   Roller clamp for the regulation of the infusion rate. **A,** Open position. **B,** Closed position. (From Perry AG, Potter PA: *Clinical nursing skills and techniques,* ed 6, St Louis, 2006, Mosby.)

attachment of the needle to the tubing. Some tubing has injection ports that act as access points for the addition of other fluids using secondary infusion sets (IVPB) if needed. These ports, located at various sites along the tubing, should ideally be punctured with a needleless system or needle-protective devices to prevent needle stick injuries and ensure resealing of the ports after use. Needleless systems consist of a blunt-tipped plastic insertion tool and a port for injection that opens on activation and immediately reseals (Figure 11-11). As with

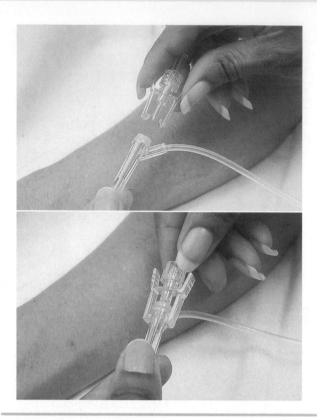

Figure 11-11 Example of a needleless protective system. (From Perry AG, Potter PA: *Clinical nursing skills and techniques*, ed 6, St Louis, 2006, Mosby.)

other injectable devices, the shielded needle prevents accidental needle stick injuries to the health care worker by covering the needle after use. Back-check valves are used to allow the primary infusion to continue when the secondary or IVPB infusion has completed. They also prevent the secondary infusion from entering the primary solution.

In some ambulatory care settings, a **winged-infusion** or **scalp (butterfly)** needle may be used for short-term infusion therapy, especially if therapy is after phlebotomy for laboratory testing. Winged-infusion needles are available from size 25 to size 17 and in lengths from 0.5 to 1 inch. A danger is that the tip of the stainless steel needle can puncture the blood vessel wall after placement, causing the risk of infiltration of fluids if the patient does not remain relatively inactive during the infusion (Figure 11-12, *A*).

Over-the-needle catheters consist of a needle with a plastic or plasticlike sheath covering the distal point of the needle. The needle, or **stylet,** is used to inject the vein and guide the **catheter** (Figure 11-12, *B*). When the catheter is in the vein, a flashback of blood occurs into a chamber behind the catheter hub. The catheter is then threaded off the needle, leaving the softer catheter in place.

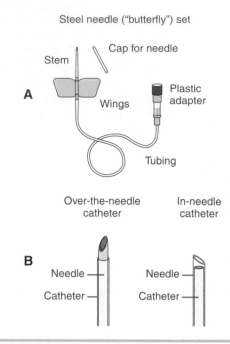

Figure 11-12 Equipment for starting short-term peripheral IV infusions. **A,** Winged-infusion needle. **B,** Over-the-needle catheter. (From Leahy JM, Kizilay PE: *Foundations of nursing practice: a nursing process approach*, Philadelphia, 1998, Saunders.)

The catheter needle comes in lengths from 0.5 to 2 inches and gauges of even numbers from 24 to 12. The shortest catheter with the smallest appropriate gauge should be used to deliver the ordered fluids; 22 or 24 gauges are usually used in ambulatory care. The vein must be large enough or the catheter small enough to allow sufficient flow of blood past the injection site to decrease the irritation to the vein wall.

Methodology

After the venipuncture, the hub of the needle is secured by a dressing to prevent movement in the vein. The choice of the dressing material depends on the needle support needed for the IV equipment and any patient allergies. Gauze is inexpensive, but the dressing must be removed to view the injection site, and then another sterile dressing must be applied. Semipermeable transparent dressings allow moisture to pass from the skin through the dressing, but they may be loosened by perspiration or drainage at the site. These especially designed dressings adhere to the skin and minimize the amount of tape needed to secure the IV equipment.

In some circumstances, an electronic **infusion pump** is used to deliver the fluids to the highest rate of accuracy. These devices may be stationary, such as a pump attached to an IV pole, or ambulatory, such as a battery-operated pump attached to the patient's clothing. In most cases, controllers on the IV infusion tubing are used as infusion-assist devices that rely on gravity for the proper rate of fluid administration. A drop-sensor placed on the drip chamber is also used with controllers to indicate the flow of fluids. The controller monitors the infusion and beeps to alert the patient and health care professional when flow is interrupted. Controllers do not push fluids into the patient but rather allow monitoring of fluid infusion.

The specific equipment needed for infusion therapy varies among offices and patients. The health care professional must know which equipment best suits the patient's condition and must follow the physician's order to provide the ordered fluids with the least discomfort and chance of adverse reactions for the patient.

Information Needed for Calculations of Intravenous Fluids

The physician orders the desired flow rate of fluids. To calculate the rate of infiltration, the allied health professional must know the volume of fluid to be infused, the length of time for the infusion as ordered by the physician, and the manufacturer's drop rate (number of drops per milliliter) on the tubing. The tubing may be microdrip or macrodrip, as previously described, and the manufacturer provides the information in drops per milliliter on the packaging for the drop rate needed for use in each calculation to meet the physician's order.

Calculation of Intravenous Flow Rates

Fluids may be infused without added medications, but in many instances the medication is added for therapeutic reasons. The rate of administration of the fluids will vary depending on the condition of the patient and the medications or fluids that are to be infused. The physician's order may state the number of milliliters per minute the patient should receive, whereas in other cases the physician may designate the time that is necessary for the infusion.

The calculation of drops per milliliter is called flow rate, a mathematical problem that is dependent on the equipment chosen for use. Remember from the section on equipment that the administration set may be designated as either a macrodrip set that provides fluids in 10 to 20 drops per milliliter or a microdrip set that provides 50 to 60 drops per milliliter. Remember that the size of the drop is basically determined by the drop size into the drip chamber. The macrodrip is used for adults in most instances, whereas the microdrip set (sometimes abbreviated as µgtt) is also called the pediatric chamber.

The rate of flow or the infusion rate in drops is also dependent on the amount of pressure on the tubing, whether this is from a clamp device or an infusion pump. Before any calculations of the flow rate can be performed, the size of the drop from the label provided by the manufacturer must be known. This information is found on the box of the administration set, so the correct administration set must be chosen. This **drop factor** will be used for calculating the infusion flow rate. If there is a doubt after the administration set is in place, the tubing also contains the information concerning the drop factor. The attached tubing is not interchangeable with other drip chambers because the lumen of the tubing has been considered with the drop factor.

IMPORTANT FACTS

The four factors to be considered with the administration of fluids follow:
- The total amount of fluids to be administered in milliliters
- The calibration of the administration set in drops/milliliter (gtt/mL)
- The flow rate of the fluids in drops/minute (gtts/min)
- The time for the fluids to infuse in minutes (min)

When the amount of fluid, the calibration of the administration, and the time for fluid infusion are known, the rate of flow or the time for infusion can be calculated using the following formula.

$$\text{Flow rate} = \frac{\text{Amount of fluid} \times \text{Calibration on administration set}}{\text{Time for infusion (minutes)}}$$

OR

$$\text{Flow rate} = \frac{\text{milliliters ordered} \times \text{gtt/mL}}{\text{min for infusion}}$$

 EXAMPLE: A physician orders 1.5 L of lactated Ringer's to be infused over 8 hours. The infusion administration set reads 20 gtt/mL.

$$\text{Flow rate} = \frac{1500 \text{ mL} \times 20 \text{ gtt/mL}}{8 \text{ hr} \times 60 \text{ min/hr}}$$

(The hours must be changed to minutes because the formula indicates minutes for infusion.)

$$\text{Flow rate} = \frac{\dfrac{1500 \text{ mL} \times 20 \text{ gtt}}{1 \text{ mL}}}{\dfrac{8 \text{ hr} \times 60 \text{ min}}{1 \text{ hr}}}$$

$$\text{Flow rate} = \frac{\dfrac{1500 \cancel{\text{ mL}} \times 20 \text{ gtt}}{1 \cancel{\text{ mL}}}}{\dfrac{8 \cancel{\text{ hr}} \times 60 \text{ min}}{1 \cancel{\text{ hr}}}}$$

$$\text{Flow rate} = \frac{1500 \times 20 \text{ gtt}}{8 \times 60 \text{ min}}$$

$$\text{Flow rate} = \frac{30000 \text{ gtt}}{480 \text{ min}} \quad \text{or} \quad \frac{3000\cancel{0} \text{ gtt}}{48\cancel{0} \text{ min}}$$

$$\text{Flow rate} = 62.5 \text{ gtt/min or } 63 \text{ gtt/min}$$

If it is easier for you to complete the infusion rate in two steps, the following two steps may be used:

 EXAMPLE: A physician orders 1.5 L of lactated Ringer's to be infused over 8 hours. The infusion administration set reads 20 gtt/mL.

STEP 1:

$$\text{mL/hr} = \frac{\text{Total volume of fluids (TV)}}{\text{Total time in hours (TTH)}}$$

$$\text{mL/hr} = \frac{1500 \text{ mL (TV)}}{8 \text{ hr (TTH)}}$$

mL/hr = 187.5 or 188 mL/hour should be administered

Notice that the problem at this point is milliliters per hour. Now the time should be converted to minutes.

STEP 2:

$$\text{gtt/min} = \frac{\dfrac{\text{drop factor}}{\text{(gtt/mL)}}}{\dfrac{\text{Time in min}}{\text{(TM)}}} \times \begin{array}{c}\text{total volume}\\\text{per hour}\end{array}$$

$$\text{gtt/min} = \frac{20 \text{ gtt/mL}}{60 \text{ min}} \times 188 \text{ mL/hr}$$

$$\text{gtt/min} = \frac{20 \times 188}{60} \quad \text{or} \quad \frac{\cancel{20}^{1} \times 188}{\cancel{60}_{3}}$$

$$\text{gtt/min} = \frac{188}{3}$$

gtt/min = 62.7 or 63 gtt/min

If dimensional analysis is the preferred means of calculating dosage, the following is the formula for the equations:

 EXAMPLE: A physician orders 1.5 L of lactated Ringer's to be infused over 8 hours. The infusion administration set reads 20 gtt/mL.

The formula needed to use dimensional analysis is as follows:

$$\text{DF} \times \text{CFV} \times \text{DV} \times \text{DT} \times \text{CFT} = \text{FR}$$

DF = Drop factor
CFV = Conversion factor volume
DV = Dose volume
DT = Dose time
CFT = Conversion factor time
FR = Flow rate in gtt/min

The necessary information for using dimensional analysis with this example follows:

Drop factor (DF) = 20 gtt/mL
Dose volume (DV) = 1.5 L
Dose time (DT) = 8 hr
FR (flow rate in gtt/min)= x
Conversion Factors 1 L = 1000 mL (CFV);
    1 hr = 60 min (CFT)

$$\frac{20 \text{ gtt (DF)}}{1 \text{ mL}} \times \frac{1000 \text{ mL (CFV)}}{1 \text{L}} \times \frac{1.5 \text{ L (DV)}}{8 \text{ hr (DT)}}$$
$$\times \frac{1 \text{ hr (CFT)}}{60 \text{ min}} = x \text{ (FR) gtt/min}$$

$$\frac{20 \text{ gtt (DF)}}{1 \cancel{\text{mL}}} \times \frac{1000 \cancel{\text{mL}} \text{ (CFV)}}{1 \cancel{\text{L}}} \times \frac{1.5 \cancel{\text{L}} \text{ (DV)}}{8 \cancel{\text{hr}} \text{ (DT)}}$$
$$\times \frac{1 \cancel{\text{hr}} \text{ (CFT)}}{60 \text{ min}} = x \text{ (FR) gtt/min}$$

$$\frac{20 \text{ gtt} \times 1000 \times 1.5 \times 1}{1 \times 1 \times 8 \times 60 \text{ min}} = x \text{ in gtt/min}$$

$$\frac{30000 \text{ gtt}}{480 \text{ min}} = x \text{ in gtt/min}$$

$$\frac{3000\cancel{0} \text{ gtt}}{48\cancel{0}} \quad \text{or} \quad \frac{3000 \text{ gtt}}{48 \text{ min}}$$

x = 62.5 gtt/min or 63 gtt/min should be administered

CHECK YOUR UNDERSTANDING   11-1

PRACTICE PROBLEMS

1. A physician orders 2 L of RINGER'S LACTATE over 12 hours. The drop factor is 20 drops/mL. How many gtt/min will be infused? _____

2. A physician orders 250 mL D-5-S to be administered over 16 hours to keep a vein open. The drop factor is 60 microdrips/mL. How many gtt/min will be infused? _____

3. A physician orders 150 mL of D-5-S to be infused in 40 minutes. The drip factor is 15 drops/mL. How many drops per minute will be infused? _____

4. A physician orders 500 mL of NS to be infused over 30 minutes. The drop factor is 20 gtt/mL. How many gtt/min will be infused? _____

5. A physician orders 150 mL of NS to infuse over 2 hours. The drop factor is 20 gtt/mL. How many drops per minute will be infused? _____

If the physician orders a variety of fluids for a given period of time, such as over 24 hours, the professional should add all of the fluids for the day and then determine the flow rate unless the time for infusion varies with each fluid ordered.

Calculating Intravenous Infusion Times

In some instances the physician will provide an order for the amount of fluids to be infused and the milliliters per hour without providing the specific running time for the infusion. The problem then becomes to decide how long it will take for the total infusion using the drop factor ordered by the physician. As the person responsible for the infusion, you have a responsibility to have the container of fluids, if ordered, to follow the current infusion ready when needed. These calculations may be used in other circumstances, such as the time needed for ambulatory care or for patient discharge or testing following the completion of infusion.

Basically the formula for determining the time of infusion is the same formula with the unknown being changed.

 EXAMPLE USING FORMULA METHOD:

A physician orders 1000 mL D-5-S to be administered at 20 gtt/min. The drop factor is 15 gtt/mL. What is the running time (or minutes for infusion) for these fluids?

Using the formula shown in the previous section and substituting information into the formula, the calculation can be made:

$$\text{Flow rate} = \frac{\text{mL ordered} \times \text{gtt/mL (drop factor)}}{\text{min for infusion (time for infusion)}}$$

Flow rate = 20 gtt/min

mL ordered = 1000 mL

gtt/mL = 15 gtt/mL

With these numbers, the equation will appear as follows:

$$20 \text{ gtt/min} = \frac{1000 \text{ mL} \times 15 \text{ gtt/mL}}{x}$$

$$20 \text{ gtt/min } x = 1000 \text{ mL} \times 15 \text{ gtt/mL}$$

$$20 \text{ gtt/min } x = 1000 \text{ mL} \times 15 \text{ gtt/mL}$$

$$20 \text{ min } x = 15000$$

$$x = \frac{15000}{20 \text{ min}}$$

$$x = \frac{1500\cancel{0}}{2\cancel{0} \text{ min}}$$

$x = 750$ min or 12.5 hours

EXAMPLE USING DIMENSIONAL ANALYSIS:

A physician orders 1000 mL D-5-S to be administered at 20 gtt/min. The drop factor is 15 gtt/mL. What is the running time for these fluids?

DF = Drop factor
CFV = Conversion factor volume
DV = Dose volume
DT = Dose time
CFT = Conversion factor time
FR = Flow rate in gtt/min

$$DF \times CFV \times DV \times FR = DT$$

Again we will use substitution and complete the equation.

DF = 15 gtt/mL
DV = 1000 mL
DT = x

FR = 20 gtt/min

$$\frac{15 \text{ gtt (DF)}}{1 \text{ mL}} \times \frac{1000 \text{ mL (CFV)}}{1000 \text{ mL}} \times \frac{1000 \text{ mL (DV)}}{\text{Dose}}$$
$$\times \frac{\text{Dose}}{20 \text{ gtt/min (FR)}} = DT$$

$$\frac{15 \cancel{\text{gtt}} \text{ (DF)}}{1 \cancel{\text{mL}}} \times \frac{1000 \cancel{\text{mL}} \text{ (CFV)}}{1000 \cancel{\text{mL}}} \times \frac{1000 \cancel{\text{mL}} \text{ (DV)}}{\cancel{\text{Dose}}}$$
$$\times \frac{\cancel{\text{Dose}}}{20 \cancel{\text{gtt}}/\text{min (FR)}} = DT$$

$$\frac{15 \times 1000 \times 1000}{1 \times 1000 \times 20 \text{ min}} = DT$$

$$DT = \frac{15000000}{20000 \text{ min}}$$

$$DT = \frac{1500\cancel{0000}}{2\cancel{0000} \text{ min}}$$

$$DT = \frac{1500 \text{ min}}{2}$$

DT = 750 min or convert minutes to hours
= 12.5 hrs.

CHECK YOUR UNDERSTANDING   11-2

PRACTICE PROBLEMS

1. A physician orders 500 mL D-5-S to be infused at 15 gtt/min. The drop factor is 10 gtt/mL. What would be the necessary time for the fluids to infuse? ___ min ___ hr

2. A physician orders 100 mL D-5-W to infuse at 25 gtt/min using a 60 gtt/mL infusion set. What is the running time for the infusion? _____

3. A physician orders LR 50 mL to be infused at 50 gtt/min. The infusion set read 10 gtt/mL. What is the infusion time? _____

4. A physician orders 150 mL of NS to be infused at 25 gtt/min. The drop factor is 20 gtt/mL. What is the infusion time in minutes? _____

5. A physician orders 500 mL of D-5-1/2 NS to be administered at 30 gtt/min using a drop factor of 50 gtt/mL. How long will it take for this infusion to occur? _____

Calculating Amount of Medication Infused in Amount of Fluids

In some cases the professional who is monitoring an infusion will be required to determine the amount of medication a patient has already received during a certain period of time. To make this determination using ratio-proportion, the amount of medication in the total solution and the total amount of solution should be placed in one ratio of the proportion and the amount of infused fluids should be placed in the other ratio with "x" being the amount of medication infused.

OR

Total amount of medication : Total of fluid ::
   x (Amount of medication infused) : Amount of fluid infused

 EXAMPLE: A patient receives 750 mL of 1000 mL N/S with 4 mEq KCl added. How many mEq of KCl did the patient receive?

Total amount of medication : Total of fluid ::
   x (Amount of medication infused) : Amount of fluid infused

$$4 \text{ mEq} : 1000 \text{ mL} :: x : 750 \text{ mL}$$

$$4 \text{ mEq} : 1000 \text{ mL} :: x : 750 \text{ mL}$$

$$1000 \, x = 3000 \text{ mEq}$$

$$x = \frac{3000 \text{ mEq}}{1000}$$

$$x = 3 \text{ mEq}$$

With all calculations, the professional should be in a quiet place with as few distractions as possible when doing the mathematics for intravenous infusions. If the calculation appears to be incorrect or if there is a question about the answer, always ask for assistance. To verify medication amounts that are to be infused, check the orders first and then verify with the health care professional or pharmacist if appropriate. If the calculation is questionable, recalculate; if there is still a question, ask another professional to check your calculations. Never infuse fluids if there seems to be an error of any kind. Remember that once the fluids have been infused, removal is impossible.

CHECK YOUR UNDERSTANDING   11-3

PRACTICE PROBLEMS

1. A physician orders FENTANYL CITRATE 50 mcg to be added to D-5-W 500 mL. The medication is available as 10 mcg/mL.
   How many milliliters of FENTANYL should be added to the fluids? _____
   If the patient receives 400 mL of the fluids, how many milliliters of FENTANYL did the patient receive? _____

2. A physician desires that a patient receive LIDOCAINE 1.5 g in D-5-W 200 mL IVPB.
   How many milligrams of LIDOCAINE are in each milliliter of fluids? _____
   If the patient receives 65 mL of IV fluids, how many milligrams of LIDOCAINE would the patient receive? _____

3. A physician orders SOLU-MEDROL 125 mg IV in D-5-S 100 mL for infusion in an hour for a patient with asthma. The medication is available in a vial containing 250 mg/5 mL.
   How many milliliters of SOLU-MEDROL will be added to the fluid to complete the order?
   _____
   If the patient receives the medication for 50 minutes, how many milligrams of the medication will the patient receive? _____

(continued)

CHECK YOUR UNDERSTANDING—cont'd   11-3

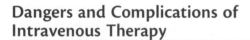

4. A physician orders MAGNESIUM SULFATE 10 g to be added to RINGER'S LACTATE 1 L.
   What is the concentration of MAGNESIUM SULFATE per milliliter? _____
   If this is to infuse over 5 hours, how many milligrams of MAGNESIUM SULFATE will the patient receive each hour? _____

5. A physician orders ERYTHROMYCIN 500 mg in 100 mL NS for IVPB stat. The vial of medication contains 1 g of ERYTHROMYCIN to be diluted with 10 mL of sterile water.
   How many milliliters of ERYTHROMYCIN should be added to the NS? _____
   If the fluids are ordered to infuse in 2 hours, how many milligrams of ERYTHROMYCIN will the patient receive in 1 hour? _____
   How many milligrams of ERYTHROMYCIN will the patient receive in 1 hour and 15 minutes? _____

Dangers and Complications of Intravenous Therapy

Most of the dangers of IV therapy are associated with human error, whereas the complications are from the IV fluids. An obvious danger of IV therapy is the possible introduction of microorganisms directly into the bloodstream when aseptic technique is not followed precisely. Because fluids are introduced directly into the bloodstream for transport throughout the body, strict asepsis must be followed and any possible loss of asepsis should be confronted. Remember that sterility is not measured in degrees—an article is either sterile or it is not.

Dangers include safety measures related to such errors as medication calculations, basic concepts of infection control, or the lack of using the "seven rights" and "three befores" when preparing medications. The allied health professional has the responsibility of continually using good techniques and then continually observing the infusion site and patient's general status to detect any complications that may arise. Patient safety is of utmost importance, and caring for any possible complications in a timely manner prevents any further insult to the patient.

Complications may be local in nature, such as mechanical problems (e.g., infiltration into the surrounding tissue, leak of fluid at the infusion site, or a displaced catheter). Localized infection may occur as phlebitis or local tissue infection. Systemic complications include circulatory overload, phlebitis, **thrombus** formation, pulmonary embolism, air embolism, or generalized infection. The possibility of drug overdose and toxicity also exists with the introduction of medication into the bloodstream. Because of the many chances of complications and possible dangers of IV therapy, careful monitoring of patients receiving IV therapy is crucial. Even after the infusion has been completed, possible complications such as bleeding at the site, and even hemorrhaging, may occur. Mechanical problems during infusion may also lead to delayed local adverse reactions. The allied health professional has the legal responsibility and ethical role of understanding all of the possible complications of IV therapy prior to initiating and for screening patients during the infusion.

Intravenous Screening

Before Administration

Before ordering an IV infusion, the physician performs a baseline screening of the patient. An allied health professional usually assists with tasks as appropriate. An accurate medical history taken before infusion allows health care workers to determine whether changes have occurred in the patient's condition during **infusion therapy.** The history should include both medical conditions and family history.

A clinical screening is equally important. The patient's body weight during or following therapy is compared with the baseline weight; rapid changes usually indicate fluid loss or gain. A total of 1 lb of body weight is approximately 500 mL of fluids. The concentration of urine is determined during the initial screening; a urinalysis allows the medical team to assess the patient's hydration level. In **diuresis,** low specific gravity and dilution of urine occur; in dehydration, a higher specific gravity or urine concentration occurs, necessitating hydration therapy.

Vital signs should also be taken and recorded before, during, and after therapy. Electrolyte changes and fluid loss may cause hypotension, especially during postural changes, and fluid gain may increase blood pressure and cause breathing difficulties.

Behavioral changes such as restlessness and apprehension may indicate fluid deficit. Increased irritability, disorientation, and mental confusion may result from fluid loss or electrolyte imbalance. Although screening for these signs is not legally indicated, such signs should be documented before fluid administration; belligerence, disorientation, and **lethargy** should also be documented.

During Infusion

The health care worker should screen the patient frequently for complications so that early interventions can occur. Complications may be either local or systemic and include infiltration, phlebitis, hematoma, circulatory system overload, and local infection. Problems with equipment can also occur.

Infiltration of fluids is a common local complication. The signs of infiltration include a slowing or stopping of fluid infusion, tissue induration, and swelling around the injection site with tissue remaining cool to the touch. If it does occur, the infusion site is changed and the affected arm is elevated and covered with warm compresses. Infiltration is prevented by observing the IV site at least every hour and anchoring the tubing to prevent movement of the infusion equipment.

Although not common in ambulatory care, phlebitis, an inflammation of the veins, can occur, especially if fluids are given on successive days. Phlebitis is indicated by at least two of the following: redness, pain, swelling, and warmth at the site. Inflammation may cause the vein to feel like a cord. The infusion site should be moved and warm compresses should be applied to the area of induration and redness.

Nicking of the vein during venipuncture, application of a tourniquet above the area of a previously attempted venipuncture site, or a leaky vein from frequent injections may cause a **hematoma,** especially in those who bruise easily. Discoloration of the skin, swelling, and discomfort are typical signs. Careful venipuncture technique and the correct placement of the tourniquet prevent this complication.

If a local infection occurs at the venipuncture site, the site and the catheter, if present, should be cultured.

Redness and a purulent exudate are common signs of infection. The patient may also have a fever and an elevated white blood cell count. The infusion should be stopped and restarted, if appropriate, and the infected site covered with sterile dressings. The best prevention is good aseptic technique at the time of venipuncture and throughout infusion.

Too-rapid infusion of IV fluids causes circulatory system overload. If overload occurs, the physician should be notified immediately and vital signs should be taken. The patient is checked for shortness of breath, pitting edema, a rise in blood pressure, and other signs of cardiac problems. Checking of flow rate calculations at least twice by the person administering the fluids before starting the infusion can help prevent this complication. Controllers or infusion devices should be used in patients at greatest risk. Time-tapes applied to the fluid container indicate the amount of fluid that should be administered each hour. These tapes, which easily indicate whether the fluids are infusing too slowly or rapidly, are attached to the fluid container for quick evaluation and adjustment, as needed, of the infusion rate.

If the infusion becomes sluggish, the tubing should be observed for kinking or another obstruction; the patient also could be lying on the tubing. If correcting these problems does not correct the flow rate, the injection site may need to be repositioned or relocated.

If the tubing is not tightly attached to the needle, leaking may occur at the needle-tubing junction. If the tubing is contaminated because of the leak, it must be changed. The use of Luer-Lok devices and proper connection of the tubing to the needle should prevent this potential problem because the needle is locked into place.

An obstructed IV line may need to be flushed. This should be done only by a professional knowledgeable in the technique. The **IV flush** should not be forced; the infusion site should be changed if minimal pressure fails to reopen the IV line.

The administration of cold IV fluids causes **venous spasm.** Sharp pain may exist along the length of the vein, and the infusion may slow. Thus fluids should be at room temperature when they are administered.

Cultural Beliefs Regarding Intravenous Therapy

As with most areas of the medical field, the cultural beliefs including religious customs of the patient will affect the way the need for IV therapy is accepted. How a patient reacts to IV therapy will depend on his or her cultural perspective, the tenets of his or her lifestyle, and in some cases, his or her religious beliefs. These beliefs are dynamic and cannot be ignored when providing medical care because these are the basis for how patients feel about health and disease and necessary treatment.

The person administering IV therapy must not stereotype patients by cultures or religions because each person is an individual with individual understanding of traditional and nontraditional medical care.

The health care worker's cultural background also has a distinct influence on the acceptance or rejection of IV therapy. The health care worker must take all measures possible to separate his or her beliefs and not influence the patient's health care needs on the basis of cultural beliefs.

The assessment of the patient, including beliefs and cultural practices, is an important factor in obtaining trust and providing competent care. Through the assessment, risky behaviors of the patient may be uncovered and handled without causing further harm to the patient receiving the therapy. Observation of the patient and the use of verbal and nonverbal communication skills are important factors for the health care professional. The patient assessment also allows time for the patient to ask questions and obtain answers to these concerns.

The allied health professional must look at each patient as a whole person and must provide holistic health care for patient safety and professional trust when providing medical treatment. Cultural and spirituality differences need to be considered when providing IV therapy, and the necessary adaptations must be taken as appropriate.

Legal and Ethical Issues

The physician is legally responsible for the actions of the unlicensed professional following his or her orders, but the allied health professional does have the legal responsibility for ensuring that no procedure is attempted for which he or she has no educational or technical background. State medical practice acts or other statutes define which procedures the allied health professional can perform. The allied health professional must always be aware of the changes legislated in each state and must ensure that his or her actions are in compliance with the laws. Ignorance of the law is not an acceptable defense when prohibited procedures are performed or when life-threatening critical errors occur.

Because there is an increasing need for allied health professionals to perform more advanced procedures in ambulatory care settings, these professionals are also being placed in situations that require ethical decision making. Because ethical decisions are essentially moral decisions, they are individual and can change with each professional situation. The health care worker must decide on the "right" course by relying on his or her own educational and technical background.

IV infusion is a highly technical skill that also requires a high-level knowledge base. The exact procedure for performing the initiation of IV fluids is similar to that for performing a venipuncture, but the introduction of fluids or medications into the veins has greater potential for harm. The ethical decisions are therefore much harder to make and must be made with patient safety in the forefront.

The fact that a procedure is legally within the scope of practice in a specific geographic area does not necessarily mean that it should be performed by all personnel who can legally perform it. Critical thinking skills, as well as knowledge of technique and screening, are essential for patient safety, and the allied health professional must be proficient and knowledgeable in these areas before performing IV initiation and infusion therapy. The ethical responsibility of acknowledging limitations in technical skills and knowledge belongs solely to the person asked to perform the task; the allied health professional must make the ethical decision about whether the task is within his or her scope of practice. The health care professional should always ask, "Is this a task that I would do to myself if I could? Would I feel comfortable if I were the patient during this procedure? Are my knowledge and technical bases adequate for patient safety?"

Critical Thinking Exercises

1. A physician orders KEFUROX 1.5 g in D-5-S 100 mL to be infiltrated over 1 hr as IVPB. The drop factor is 20 gtt/mL.

   What is the necessary drip rate (gtt/min) to fulfill this order? _____

   If the patient receives 80 mL of the IVPB, how many milligrams of KEFUROX will the patient receive? _____

   If the patient receives the IVPB for 35 minutes, how many milliliters of solution will the patient receive? _____

2. **EN DO** A physician orders HUMULIN R 60 U added to D-2½-½ NS 100 mL as an IVPB. The drop factor is 60 gtt/mL. The physician desires that the INSULIN infuse at 2.5 U/hour. The label for insulin is Humulin R-100.

   How many milliliters per hour will be infused to complete the order? _____

   How long will the fluids need to infuse as ordered?_____

   How many milliliters of INSULIN will be added to the fluids? _____

3. ♥ A physician orders NITRO-BID IV 50 mg in D-5-W 250 mL to be infused at the rate of 50 mcg/min. The drop factor is 60 gtt/mL.

   What is the amount of medication in micrograms per 1 mL of solution? _____

   How many milliliters of solution will be necessary to fulfill the order for 50 mcg/mL? ___

   _____

   How long will these fluids take to infuse?

   _____

How many milliliters will provide NITRO-BID 5 mg? _____

4. 🍶 A physician orders AMIKIN 5 mg/kg/q8h in 100 mL of fluids IVPB. The patient weighs 176 lb. The drop factor is 20 gtt/mL. The time for infusion is 2 hours.

   How many milligrams of medications should be added to the fluids? _____

   If the medication is available as AMIKIN 50 mg/mL, how many milliliters of medication should be added to the fluids?

   _____

   What is the flow rate in gtt/min to ensure that the medication is given to physician's order? _____

5. ⬭ A physician orders 500 mL D-5-LR to be infused over 12 hours. The drop factor for the infusion set is 60 gtt/mL.

   What is the flow rate in mL/min? _____

   How many milliliters of IV fluid should be infused in an hour? _____

REVIEW QUESTIONS

1. What is the difference among hypotonic, isotonic, and hypertonic solutions? How do these affect the movement of fluids in the body?_____

   _____

   _____

2. What are the three basic types of IV therapy? _____

   _____

   _____

3. What are the two types of drip chambers found on IV tubing? Why are they important?_____

   _____

   _____

4. Why is it important to carefully calculate the infusion rate for IV therapy?_____

   _____

   _____

Medication Administration

CHAPTER 12
Safety and Quality Assurance, 226

CHAPTER 13
Enteral Routes, 237

CHAPTER 14
Percutaneous Routes, 247

CHAPTER 15
Parenteral Routes, 261

Safety and Quality Assurance

OBJECTIVES

After studying this chapter, you should be capable of doing the following:

- Explaining the importance of safety when using over-the-counter (OTC) medications.
- Describing legal, ethical, and other measures to protect health care personnel during medication administration.
- Describing quality assurance in medication administration.
- Explaining the relationship of the medical office and Occupational Safety and Health Administration (OSHA) regulations related to pharmacology.
- Discussing the three "befores" and seven "rights" of administering medications safely.
- Explaining the procedures necessary to prevent medication errors and the documentation required in the event an error occurs when administering medications.
- Describing the routes by which medications are delivered into the body.

Betty, an allied health professional in a physician's office, is asked by a co-worker to administer a physician-ordered dose of Decadron to Joseph, in Room 5, who has arthritis. Betty picks up a bottle that appears to be Decadron from the shelf. She draws the dose and administers it to the patient in Room 2 without asking the patient his name because she thinks she knows the patient. Actually, Betty has drawn an estrogen preparation and given it to Mac. The other allied health professional working in the area realizes that Betty has given the wrong medication to the wrong patient.

    What rules of medication administration has Betty failed to follow?

    What information does Betty need to document?

    Does she need to notify the physician? Why or why not?

KEY TERMS

Enteral route	Parenteral route
Medication administration	Percutaneous route
Medication error	Quality assurance

When teaching patients about OTC drugs, the allied health professional should be sure that the patient realizes these preparations are actually drugs and need to be taken with the same precaution as prescription medicines. This means taking OTC drugs as they are meant to be taken, with the patient reading all instructions and following the manufacturer-recommended dosages for age and weight. All ingredients in an OTC medication should be evaluated by the patient or the person administering the medication before these preparations are used to be sure that harmful ingredients that have caused drug intolerances, allergies, and adverse reactions are not being taken. An important fact is that OTC medications may have changes in inert ingredients so the label should be read with each purchase to ensure allergies and intolerances will not occur because of the changes.

Safety with medications, whether the medication is taken from OTC agents or by prescription, is an important factor for therapeutic patient care. The allied health professional has the responsibility to obtain a list of all medications—prescription, herbal, and OTC—that a patient is taking so that safety in drug usage occurs. A complete list of medications includes both drugs taken regularly and those taken as needed (or prn).

Safety with Medications Taken by Patients

Self-medication may delay needed medical care because OTC drugs can mask important symptoms. When taking OTC medications, the patient does not receive the printouts that supply drug interactions and the patient is therefore not aware of the possible dangers. Furthermore, with self-medication, the chemical ingredients of all OTC substances including drugs and herbals must be evaluated for their potential for detrimental effects caused by the physical condition of the patient and the potential for life-threatening effects. The following are important factors when the patient is providing self-treatment with OTC preparations:

- For safety, document the excessive use of drugs such as alcohol or caffeine (found in coffee, soft drinks, and tea).
- Document nicotine from tobacco products.
- Patients may obtain OTC and herbal drugs without a prescription, and these need to have complete documentation in the medical record.
- Spend extra time with the patient who takes OTC medications to be sure the patient is aware of the possible dangers of self-treatment in conjunction with the use of prescription drugs, and remind the patient that OTC drugs should be used only as directed on the labels and that the label should be read carefully before using the drug.
- Inform the patient that the dosages of many OTC drugs are low, so they may not supply the patient with adequate medication to have an adequate therapeutic effect, depending on the patient's physical condition, such as Aleve one to two tablets twice daily (200 mg) for severe arthritis compared with the prescription strength of naproxen of 375 to 500 mg twice to three times a day. The amount of the OTC medication used may even mask the true severity of the disease.
- OTC medications often contain more than one active ingredient, allowing drug interactions to occur. Remember that only one of the active ingredients may cause an interaction.
- Any adverse or allergic reactions that the patient has experienced should be documented.
- Finally, patients may not be aware of the ingestion of the same medication under different names such as Advil, Motrin, and ibuprofen.

Patient safety is also important with all medications, OTC and prescription. The allied health professional has a responsibility to ensure that patient medication safety is maintained. Box 12-1 lists safety tips for patient administration of medications.

Medication Administration

Many lay people think that administering medications is the main thrust of pharmacology. In reality, pharmacology is the knowledge necessary to give medicines safely. **Medication administration** means giving a dose of a medication to a person. The roles of health care personnel in drug treatment are considered to form a triangle for the protection and efficient medical care of the patient: the physician prescribes a medication, the pharmacist dispenses the medication, and the allied health professional administers the medication. (If the medication has been dispensed, the patient self-administers the drug in most conditions.) All three points of the triangle are necessary for safe drug therapy.

To safely administer medications, proper knowledge of medications is essential. Proper techniques in giving medications using the seven "rights" (right patient, medication, dose, route, time, technique, and documentation) and three "befores" (before removing from storage, before preparing medication, and before returning to storage) and proper safety precautions as determined by regulatory agencies cannot be overemphasized to ensure high-quality patient care.

Quality assurance—establishing standards of excellence in patient care and tailoring practice to those standards—is at the core of applied medicine. Quality assurance is prescribed by a set of policies and procedures found in each office and by various federal regulations that affect medical offices. When followed, these rules provide a safety net for patients and practitioners alike. If they are not followed, a multitude of problems can result: medication errors, personnel exposure to dangerous pathogens, and costly litigation. Allied health professionals who adhere to quality assurance measures as a matter of course can be confident they are helping themselves and their patients in safe medication administration.

BOX 12-1   TIPS TO ENSURE SAFETY IN MEDICATION ADMINISTRATION

1. For safe and effective therapy, explain to the patient how and why the drug is to be taken.
2. Specify a time for the medication to be taken. Some medications need to be taken with meals, whereas others need to be taken on an empty stomach. Some drugs need to be taken at a specific time each day; others may need to be taken several times a day with no relationship to a specific time.
3. If the patient is elderly or has difficulty remembering the schedule, suggest making a chart or calendar to remember when to take medications. A large calendar may be used to check off medications throughout the day. Medications that are dispensed for more than one dose per day may be dispensed in containers with reminder mechanisms such as individual slots for daily medications or different-colored containers for different times of the day.
4. Be sure the patient knows how long the medication is to be taken. Some drugs are prescribed for short-term therapy and others for long-term, even lifetime, use. If short-time medications such as antibiotics are prescribed, the patient should be instructed to complete the entire course of treatment. For chronic conditions, the patient should be instructed to continue taking the medication as directed until the physician stops the medication, if that is the protocol of the physician.
5. Be sure the patient knows that some medications such as antihypertensives may make him or her feel worse while the body is adjusting closer toward homeostasis. Also, the patient should be taught the symptoms of dangerous side effects. The medication should be discontinued only on the advice of the physician.
6. The patient should be instructed that some medications (e.g., prednisone, tranquilizers) cannot be stopped abruptly but must be tapered off.
7. The patient should be taught the side effects of the medication (e.g., drowsiness from antihistamines) and safety measures to follow while taking the medicine (e.g., avoid driving or operating machinery).
8. Inform the patient that all adverse reactions should be reported so that they can be noted in the medical record and adjustments to medications can be made as needed.
9. The patient should be told that misuse of any medication might lead to dangerous side effects, such as bleeding ulcers with aspirin or drug dependence with pain relievers.
10. Proper storage of medications should be discussed with the pharmacist. The warmth and dampness of bathrooms and sunny windowsills make these places inappropriate for storing medicines.
11. Old medicines should be discarded by flushing them down the toilet. Expired medications lose efficacy, and their effects are unpredictable; some may even become toxic with time.
12. Medications are prescribed for a given person with a specific condition and should not be shared with others. A person who takes drugs prescribed for someone else might experience severe adverse reactions.
13. The patient should always check with the pharmacist or physician before mixing medications with alcohol, tobacco, or other medications including OTC drugs and herbals.
14. Medications should be taken in well-lighted areas so that the label can be safely read. Never assume that a bottle of medicine is the correct bottle; always read the label. For a person with poor eyesight, the print on the bottle label should be large, or the patient should have someone else prepare the medications. Ask the pharmacist to assist in providing aids for safe administration with low-vision individuals.

OSHA Standards in Medication Administration

In July 1992 OSHA started to enforce workplace controls concerning bloodborne pathogens. Body fluids may contain pathogenic microorganisms capable of causing disease. Each medical facility must have its own exposure control plan that dictates how the facility will comply with OSHA standards.

Standards that are specific to giving medications include the following:

• Barrier equipment should be worn if a chance of splashing or spraying of body fluids during medication administration is possible.

• When performing injections, health care personnel should wear gloves to protect against possible cross contamination.

• Used needles and other single-use equipment such as vaginal applicators or inhalation devices that have come in contact with potentially infectious body secretions must be disposed of properly in puncture-resistant containers.

• All disposable syringes and needles should have retractable safety caps and should be placed in a puncture-resistant container that is located close to the area of use (Figures 12-1 and 12-2).

• If the needle must be recapped, this should be accomplished by placing one hand behind the

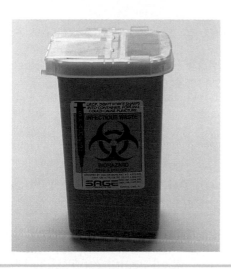

Figure 12-1 Disposable syringes and sharps should be disposed of in a puncture-proof container. (From Young AP, Proctor DB: *Kinn's the medical assistant*, ed 10, St Louis, 2007, Saunders.)

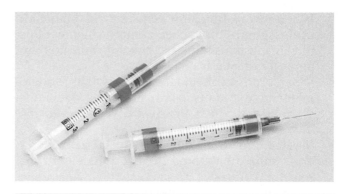

Figure 12-2 The Occupational Safety and Health Administration suggests using syringes with retractable needle covers. (From Young AP, Proctor DB: *Kinn's the medical assistant*, ed 10, St Louis, 2007, Saunders.)

back and "scooping" the cover over the needle (Figure 12-3).

- Sterile needles may be recapped after they have been used to withdraw medications from vials.
- A needle should never be directed toward any part of the body of the allied health professional.
- Contaminated waste must be disposed of in accordance with federal, state, and local regulations.
- Any exposure must be evaluated, and a postexposure follow-up plan for the facility completed including an incident report and a confidential medical evaluation.

In subsequent chapters the icons shown previously are used in procedures illustrating their need with the different routes of medication administration.

IMPORTANT FACTS ABOUT MEDICATION AND OSHA STANDARDS

Medication administration should be done in accordance with the latest appropriate OSHA standards relating to splashes of body fluids and possible contact with body fluids.

Quality Assurance in Medication Delivery

Quality assurance ensures that practices result in the highest possible level of patient care and that the services are consistent with high principles of

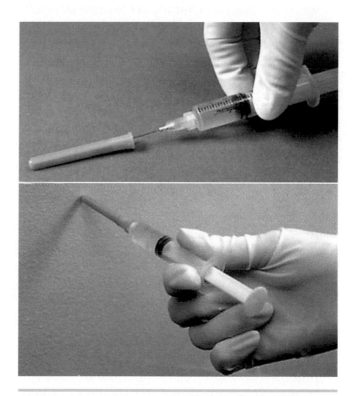

Figure 12-3 To recap needles, use one hand and a scooping technique. (From Young AP, Proctor DB: *Kinn's the medical assistant*, ed 10, St Louis, 2007, Saunders.)

professional conduct. The allied health professional should monitor all aspects of medication administration for quality assurance. This includes developing a written systematic monitoring system to ensure that the medications administered are safe and are of the highest possible quality. To provide quality assurance, the following steps may be necessary:

- When medication shipments arrive, the health professional should check that the medications have been maintained at the appropriate temperature during transport.
- When ordering medications, the facility should avoid having items in transit during weekends or holidays, when timely delivery cannot be made.
- Medications that require special considerations should be stored in accordance with the relevant controls.
- As medications are stocked, the strength, size of the container, and drug itself should be checked against the inventory and packing slip and stored in the appropriate location.
- The medications should be placed in exact locations, with the label facing toward the front, with the same medications of the same strength being stocked as previously found.
- Drugs should be separated by route of administration, especially ophthalmic and otic preparations.
- Drugs with specific uses (e.g., estrogen preparations) should be stocked together.
- Check expiration dates. The possible loss of stock due to expiration or the use of more than one container of stock at a time may occur if stocking is done in an inconsistent manner.
- As new medications arrive at the office, the expiration date, or shelf-life, should be carefully observed. Those with a short shelf-life may need to be returned to the purchase source.
- Supplies should be placed where they are most accessible yet protected from damage and exposure to such elements as heat, light, moisture, and air.
- Check storage requirements with each order. Most drugs should be stored in a cool, dark area away from direct light to avoid deterioration.
- Medications for external use should be stored separately from those for internal use.
- Poisons and chemicals, including disinfectants and other cleaning agents, that may cause harm to a patient if used in error should not be stored with drugs and chemicals used as drugs, either internally or topically.
- Labels should be carefully preserved, and all medications must be stored in their original containers.
- A container without a label or with a label so damaged that it is difficult to know what is in the container should be destroyed.

IMPORTANT FACTS ABOUT QUALITY ASSURANCE
- Quality assurance in medication administration ensures that the patient receives quality drugs given safely in the correct manner.
- Quality assurance provides a medication that has been properly transported and stored and has not expired.

Medication Administration for Patient Safety

Medications may be given only under the direct order and supervision of a health care provider. However, the allied health professional has a responsibility to assess a situation and to address problems related to administering the drugs. The physician performs the physical assessment of the patient, but the allied health professional should again assess the patient and the environment before giving a drug. If changes have occurred that would make administration of the drug undesirable or improper, the allied health professional should notify the health care provider before giving the medication.

Some factors that might cause variance in drug use include the following:

- Size and age of the patient.
- Changes in vital signs.
- Changes in organ system function.
- Possible contraindications to the drug (e.g., previous illness, concurrent use of medications such as heparin or OTC medications) or drug interactions.
- Food or animal allergies that may prohibit the use of a medication (e.g., allergies to eggs, animal dander).
- Possible drug dependency.
- The route of administration and the patient's medical status might make the use of the usual route undesirable (e.g., oral administration for a person who has difficulty swallowing, injuries at the site of parenteral administration).
- The proper dosage of the medication. If in doubt, the allied health professional should not give the medication but should ask the health care provider to confirm the order. Never hesitate to question the possibility of a mistake in interpreting a medication order.
- The presence of an appropriate person in the event that an allergic reaction occurs. Do not give medications without a physician present

(even if the drug has been ordered or given on multiple occasions) in case a situation requiring emergency care should occur.

- The patient should not be at risk of injury from a fall or from inappropriate behavior. Safe surroundings for the patient are especially important after pain medications have been-administered.
- Medications should always be stored in the same place when cleaning or when replacing the drugs. The potential for errors to occur happen when medications are moved from the usual placement.

When administering a drug, certain rules must be followed to ensure safety. Box 12-2 lists these important rules.

IMPORTANT FACTS ABOUT PATIENT SAFETY WITH MEDICATION ADMINISTRATION

- Labels should be present on all drugs and chemicals.
- The health care professional should be sure that he or she understands the drug order. If there is doubt concerning the order, the allied health professional should ask for clarification.

Reducing Medication Errors Using 3 + 7

The administration of drugs should never become routine; it should be an organized, concise pro-cedure to ensure safety for the patient and the provision of quality care by the allied health professional. Medication administration requires 10 steps to ensure a quality process. Throughout this text, these steps are not repeated when each route of administration is discussed. Therefore these rules will be indicated by the icon 3+7. When this icon appears, these rules should be followed.

Before administering a drug, the professional—whether the allied health professional or the health care provider—should use the three "befores" of checking the labels. By being sure that medications are consistently stored by medicinal use and by preference, the "befores" are more easily processed.

Three "Befores"

The three "befores" in preparing a drug for medication administration follow:

1. Read the label on the medication *before* removing the drug from the shelf. Be sure that the correct medication and dosage is obtained from storage for administration.
2. Read the label on the medication *before* preparing the medication for administration. Double-check to be sure the correct drug is being used.
3. Read the label on the medication before returning the drug to storage after preparation of the

BOX 12-2   RULES TO FOLLOW WHEN ADMINISTERING MEDICATIONS

- Give only medications that have been ordered by the health care provider, either in writing or verbally. If there is no order, do not give the medication.
- Know the drug you are giving. If you are not familiar with a certain medication, consult a drug reference before administration. Calculate the needed dose of medication in a quiet area where you will not be interrupted. If you are unsure of the dose, ask someone else to check the medication order.
- Always wash your hands before administering medications. Do not handle the drugs directly.
- All prepared medications should be given immediately or stored safely until administered. Do not give any medications that you did not personally prepare unless prepared in a pharmacy for the patient, then check for proper patient identification.
- Identify the patient and ask about possible allergies even if you think you know the person and his or her medical history.
- Never return medications that have been prepared to their original containers. Any medication not given should be disposed of properly with proper documentation of DEA scheduled medications.
- Never document the administration of any medication before giving it. All documentation should be done immediately following administration.
- Observe the patient for adverse reactions following the administration of the drug.
- Give the person specific information concerning the signs of adverse reactions that need to be reported to the health care provider.
- Patients taking medications such as penicillin or immunotherapeutic drugs that might cause allergic reactions should be carefully monitored to be sure that the allergic reaction does not occur.
- Allergic reactions, no matter how small, should be documented so that future doses of the medication can be carefully evaluated prior to administration.
- If you make an error when administering medications, immediately report the error to the health care provider and document the error in the patient's record.

drug for administration. Never give medications that you have not personally prepared.

Seven "Rights"

The seven "rights" of medication administration should be adhered to without deviation. Before administering medication to a patient, ask yourself whether you have followed the seven "rights" (Figure 12-4).

1. *Right patient*—Even if you believe you know the patient, address the patient by name to identify any discrepancy in identification. Verify the name on the patient record. If the person is not known, ask the patient to provide his or her name by asking, "What is your name?"
2. *Right drug*—Using the three "befores," be sure the medication is the one ordered. Compare the health care provider's order with the medicine on the shelf. When checking the label on the medicine, always check the expiration date. *Never use an expired drug.* Always "palm the

label" to protect it; this is especially important with liquid medications. If the label is damaged but readable, repair the label; if the label is not readable, the medication should be destroyed. Never relabel a medication.

3. *Right dose*—Compare the medication order with the dose prepared for administration. This requires reading the label carefully and ensuring that the dose and the order are the same and in the same measurement system. Be sure that the dose is within the acceptable dose range for the patient. Do the calculations required, and double-check your calculations. Use the proper device to give the most accurate measurement of the dose.
4. *Right time*—Be sure that the medication is being given at the proper time, especially with medications that are given in a series such as allergy injections and immunizations. The time factor is important in maintaining consistent blood levels of drugs, in maximizing the effectiveness of the drug, and in ensuring proper absorption of the medication.

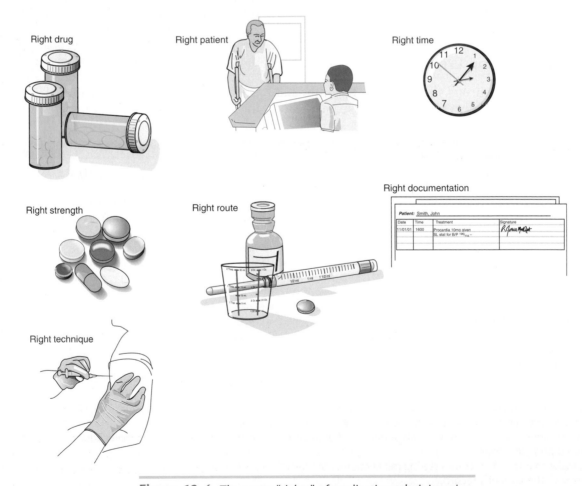

Figure 12-4 The seven "rights" of medication administration.

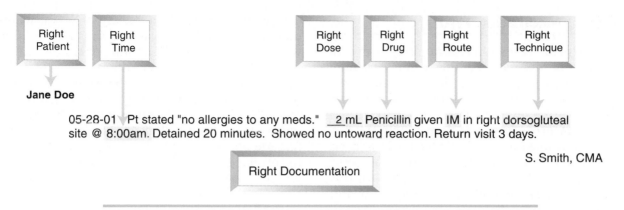

Figure 12-5 Documentation of the seven "rights" of medication administration.

5. *Right route*—Be sure that the medication being prepared matches the route of administration ordered. Check to be sure that the medication is in the form to be administered as ordered and that the route is appropriate for the person receiving the medication.

6. *Right technique*—After a final review of the medical record and an assessment of the patient, select an appropriate site and route and use appropriate delivery techniques. Be sure to use aseptic technique.

7. *Right documentation*—For medicolegal reasons, precisely and accurately enter the documentation in the patient's record *immediately after* giving medication to avoid **medication errors** (Figure 12-5). If adverse reactions occur, record any adverse symptoms and the actions taken as a result. If you document prior to administration, the patient may refuse the medication and an error in charting has then occurred. If you wait to document later, you may forget what was given, or even worse, someone else may repeat the medication (Box 12-3).

If these seven "rights" are followed, the allied health professional will be using the "right knowledge" base for giving drugs safely. To ensure safety in medication administration, the health care professional must comply with the 3 + 7 steps in medication administration.

IMPORTANT FACTS FOR REDUCING MEDICATION ERRORS

- Use the three "befores" and the seven "rights" when preparing medications.
- To reduce the possibility of error, prepare medications in a quiet, well-lit environment.
- Always administer the medications that you prepare.

BOX 12-3   CHECKLIST FOR DOCUMENTING MEDICATION ADMINISTRATION

- Record in the chart any patient assessments that were done before the medication was administered.
- Record the date and time the medicine was given.
- Record the name of the medicine and dose administered.
- If the treatment was an immunization, record the name of the manufacturer, expiration date, and lot number of the vaccine.
- If a parenteral or percutaneous route of administration was used, record the route and site of administration.
- Record any patient reactions that may have occurred. If the medication is associated with possible reactions (such as penicillins), record the waiting time of the patient.
- If patient education was provided, record the education given and the time required to give it.
- If the patient refuses the medication, record the reason for refusal (see Figure 12-5).

IMPORTANT FACTS FOR REDUCING MEDICATION ERRORS—*Cont'd*

- Know the drug that you are administering and the condition for which it is being prescribed.
- After administering a medication, observe the patient for possible unexpected reactions.
- Never return medications that have been prepared to their original containers. If not used, discard these medications properly.
- Always check for possible medication allergies prior to giving a drug. Check the medical record and ask the patient about allergies.
- Identify the patient before giving a medicine.
- Medication errors occur even with the utmost of care. If an error is made when administering a medication, assess the patient, notify the health care provider, proceed with the needed therapy as directed, and document what has happened. Assess the cause of the situation and make the needed adjustments so that the same error does not occur in the future.

Sources of Medication Errors

The goal of medication administration is to give the correct dose of medication to the correct patient by the correct route at the correct time with the correct technique and documentation, on each and every occasion. (Use the seven rights.) If this is done, there should be no error in medication administration. However, mistakes are sometimes made and adverse drug events and medication errors do occur. For example, Celebrex is a medication for arthritis, Celexa is an antidepressant, and Cerebyx is an anti-epilepsy drug. These drug names sound alike and are spelled similarly. A medication error is at best an inconvenience and at worst a tragedy. Each error is potentially tragic and costly for patients and professionals alike.

Medication errors are not trivial. Preventable medication errors cause approximately 2% of all hospitalizations, at a cost of $17 billion to $29 billion per year. The need for extreme care in medication administration to prevent errors is obvious. An inquiring attitude by the patient and the professional may make the difference between a medication error and safety for the patient. When an error occurs, the person committing the error should immediately acknowledge the error. Reporting the mistake to the proper supervisor will initiate the needed measures to counteract the effect of the drug as warranted. Appropriate documentation following an error is essential for patient safety and for medicolegal reasons (Box 12-4).

Delivery of Medications

Drugs may be delivered to the body by several methods. The method of administration depends partly on the purpose of the medication. Some drugs can be given in a variety of ways, whereas others must be administered in specific, limited ways to be effective. Generally, drugs are given either through **enteral** or **parenteral** routes to produce systemic or general effects. **Percutaneous** administration occurs when the drug is placed in direct contact with and is absorbed through the skin, tissue, or mucous membranes. Drugs given for systemic effect are absorbed and circulate in the bloodstream to produce effects on body cells and tissues, whereas those for local effect are given locally to remain at the site of administration and to prevent systemic dosing. The most reliable method for delivery and the precision needed to ensure expected results should be considered when choosing the route and technique of medication administration.

Medication administration denotes the introduction of a drug into the body or its application to the body. The goal is to deliver a precise, reliable dose with the desired effects to the desired site. When choosing the route of medication administration, five factors are considered:

- The chemical properties of the drug
- The physical properties of the drug
- The desired site of action
- How rapidly the drug response is wanted
- The physical and mental health of the person receiving the drug

The routes of administration discussed in this text are gastrointestinal system, or enteral, routes (medications swallowed by mouth or taken through rectal suppository or enema); parenteral routes of administration (subcutaneous, intramuscular, Z-Track, intradermal, and intravenous routes of administration); and percutaneous routes (through the skin; by vaginal applications; through mucous membranes such as the eye, ear, mouth, or nose instillations; and by inhalation). The most commonly used route for ambulatory care medications is the enteral route. Medicines given by the enteral route have the advantages of being safe, convenient for most patients, relatively economical, and, in most cases, readily available. The disadvantages include slowness of action and low dependability of absorption. In addition, some medicines such as insulin are destroyed by digestive fluids and cannot be administered through the gastrointestinal tract.

Generally, the parenteral route is considered to be administration of medications by injection, or under the skin. With parenteral route administration, the drug action is more rapid than with the enteral route but has a shorter duration of action. The

BOX 12-4	WHAT TO DO IF A MEDICATION ERROR OCCURS

- Notify the health care provider of the error and the patient's apparent reaction.
- Observe the patient and evaluate his or her reaction.
- Perform any corrective steps as directed by the health care provider.
- Document the error including filing an incident report if that is the policy of the facility. If a report form is not available, document the incident completely. Use the guidelines of the liability insurance carrier for the placement of documentation.
- Evaluate the circumstances and make any necessary changes in policy or procedure that will prevent the same error from occurring in the future.

dosage with this route tends to be smaller because the absorption is more rapidly accomplished. The disadvantages of the parenteral route include greater cost of supplies, an increase in the chance of adverse patient reaction, and an increase in the chance of such complications as infections and abscesses, which may occur because the skin has been broken.

The percutaneous routes are those in which absorption occurs through the skin or through mucous membranes. In most cases the action of the drug is confined to the site of application; in some cases, however, the medication may be applied transdermally for systemic use. The chance of a systemic reaction is reduced because the action of the medicine is most often confined to the place of application. The disadvantages include a slow rate of absorption (although this may also be a reason to use this route), irritation at the site of application, difficulty in applying the drug, or messy residue that occurs from the drug base. Because the duration of action is less in most instances, these medications may require more frequent applications. However, some of these medications remain in place for several days.

IMPORTANT FACTS ABOUT MEDICATION ADMINISTRATION

- Enteral routes of administration are those in which the drug is absorbed in the gastrointestinal tract.
- Parenteral routes of administration generally refer to injections or medications under the skin.
- Percutaneous (through the skin) routes of administration are those in which the drug is applied to the skin or mucous membranes for absorption.

Summary

Administering a safe dose of a medication is one of the duties of allied health professionals. Administration requires knowledge of the drug being given and the proper route of administration following the seven "rights" and the three "befores," and all health care workers must follow OSHA guidelines for personal safety.

To give medications safely, the professional should demonstrate the ability to follow the health care provider's orders, calculate doses correctly, and assess the patient, drug, and environment prior to administering the medicine. Following administration of medicine, observation of the patient for possible adverse reactions is necessary for safety issues.

When medication errors occur, the person administering the medication must report the error, document the error, document the treatment used to reverse the error (if any), and document the subsequent adverse effects. The goal is error-free medication administration, but in reality errors do occur.

In choosing the route of drug administration by either enteral, parenteral, or percutaneous routes, the health care provider considers the physical and mental condition of the patient. The goal is to deliver a precise, reliable dose of the drug to the target tissues with the fewest side effects. Full documentation is necessary for the task to be complete.

Critical Thinking Exercises

SCENARIO

Judy, a health care professional, is to administer a dose of penicillin to Jim for an upper respiratory tract infection. The physician has ordered a dose that Judy thinks is excessive for Jim, but this is her opinion based on her background, not on actual dosage charts.

1. What should Judy do next?
2. Judy finds that the dose is actually at the high end of the acceptable dosage range. What should Judy do next?
3. After Judy talks with the health care provider and is assured that the dose is acceptable, Jim tells her that in the past, he might have had a rash after taking penicillin, but he guesses it does not matter. Should Judy give the penicillin?
4. If not, what should she do? If so, what reaction should she look for?

REVIEW EXERCISES

Documentation of Medications

Document the following as it should appear in the medical record. All entries will be the date and time the exercise is done. Sign the documentation as a student in the field of study.

1. Sara Medici, age 2, has come to Dr. Merry for a measles-mumps-rubella (MMR) vaccine. Dr. Merry orders that the vaccine be given to Sara in the vastus lateralis muscle. The lot number is no. 12356, manufactured by Sohol Drugs. The expiration date is 10/04/09. The dose for MMR is one vial (or 1 mL) after reconstitution. You informed the patient of the side effects to expect and possible reactions including the possibility of a rash and low-grade fever in 2 to 3 days. _____

2. Mary Alleri has come to the office to receive her injections for allergies. She has a standing order from Dr. Merry to receive the next dose unless she had a reaction to the previous dose. Ms. Alleri tells you that she had no problems with the last dose. Today's dose comes from Allergy Extract Bottle no. 4, 0.2 mL of extract. You give the injection in the right deltoid area subcutaneously as ordered. Ms. Alleri always waits 20 minutes after receiving the injection to be sure no reactions occur. When you check on her, there is no redness or swelling at the sight of injection, and she has no signs of an allergic reaction. _____

REVIEW QUESTIONS

1. What is quality assurance? _____
_____
_____

2. What does "properly storing medications" mean? Where does an allied health professional obtain the needed instructions for this task? _____
_____
_____

3. The physician must order and supervise any medication administration in a medical office setting. Why is this important? _____
_____
_____

4. When should an allied health professional question an order from a health care provider? Why?
_____
_____
_____

5. What are the three "befores" of medication administration? _____
_____
_____

6. What are the seven "rights" of medication administration? _____
_____
_____

CHAPTER 13

Enteral Routes

OBJECTIVES

After studying this chapter, you should be capable of doing the following:

- Explaining what is meant by the enteral route of medication administration.
- Describing the forms of medications that are administered orally.
- Describing the role of the allied health professional in the administration of oral medications.
- Demonstrating procedures for administering oral medications.
- Preparing a solid form of medication.
- Preparing liquid medications using a medicine cup, a dose spoon, and a graduated-dose syringe.
- Discussing the indications for use of a rectal suppository.
- Administering medications using a rectal suppository for absorption in the rectal mucosa.
- Discussing the indications for and contraindications to a rectal enema.
- Demonstrating how to administer a rectal enema.
- Explaining to a patient how to administer medications rectally.

Billy, a 2-year-old with a cough and runny nose, comes to Dr. Merry's office accompanied by his mother. Dr. Merry examines Billy and prescribes liquid medication for his symptoms. Billy's mother tells you that Billy always wants to drink water after taking cough syrup.

Is this a matter that requires patient education? Why or why not?

Should Billy take cough syrup with meals? Why or why not?

What kind of measuring equipment would you tell Billy's mother to buy for accurate administration of the medicine?

Billy's mother also tells you that she has to call medicine "candy" to get Billy to take it. Is this a safe practice? Why or why not?

KEY TERMS

Dose spoon
Dose syringe
Enema
Meniscus

The general rules for drug administration were discussed in Chapter 12 and should be followed when administering medications by any route, but the techniques may differ for different routes of administration. Although the 3+7 icon is present, such common practices as the three "befores" and seven "rights" and basic procedures in medication administration are not included in each procedure because it is expected that you, the allied health professional, are now aware of the necessity of these steps for the safety of both you and the patient.

As with all procedures, current OSHA standards must be followed. With the oral route of administration, OSHA standards may not include any personal protective equipment or special disposal of the products used for administration because body fluids are not expected to be present for cross-contamination. However, with rectal administration of enemas or medications, depending on the condition of the patient, a gown may be necessary and gloves will always be necessary. The allied health professional should always be aware of the latest OSHA regulations and also be aware of any condition of the patient that may require a higher level of protection than expected. The icons for the OSHA standards are also included with the procedures. One of the OSHA standards necessary for administration of any medication is hand sanitization, and the icon 🖐 for this shows on the procedure guidelines.

This chapter considers medications that are absorbed by way of the gastrointestinal (GI) tract (or enterally) through the mouth or rectum through the mucous membranes. *Oral medications* are administered by the patient's swallowing a drug. The drug is absorbed in the GI tract, usually in the intestines—thus the name of enteral medications. *Rectal medications* are administered into the rectum, either by a suppository or by means of an enema, and are included in this chapter because of the absorption in the GI tract.

Medications may also be administered into the GI tract through nasogastric or gastric tubes. These are not as common as oral and rectal administration and are more commonly found in inpatient settings.

Oral Administration Of Medications

The easiest, safest, and most frequently used route of drug administration is by mouth (Procedures 13-1 to 13-3). Most people can self-administer their own medications with few problems when drugs are prescribed for oral use. Occasionally the oral route is not desirable, as indicated in the following cases:

- Drugs may be irritating to the stomach when taken by mouth.
- The effect of drugs may be altered by gastrointestinal juices.
- Vomiting, poor GI absorption, and inability to swallow food or fluids (or drugs).

Even with the possible side effects from oral administration and the length of time for absorption, it is the route of choice for most drug therapy.

The important precaution with oral administration is to avoid aspiration of medications. Aspiration occurs when medications intended for the GI tract are drawn into the respiratory tract. The risk of aspiration can be reduced by first assessing the patient's ability to swallow medications at the time of administration.

When the forms of medicine for oral consumption—tablets, capsules, powders, elixirs, syrups, solutions and suspensions—enter the mouth, the medication must be swallowed to reach the stomach and then the small intestine for absorption. (Forms of medication for oral administration are found in Chapter 3.) Food and digestive disorders will change the rate of absorption and the flow of the medicine through the GI tract. Some medications cannot be given orally because digestive secretions in the GI tract make the drug ineffective or slow the absorption of the drug into the bloodstream. Solid forms (tablets, capsules, and so on) should be taken with water or another fluid, but many liquid preparations such as cough syrups should not be taken with another fluid to avoid diluting the medicine. Be sure that the patient follows directions and reads patient education materials when administering any medication (Box 13-1). Finally, in some instances food may be required for absorption, whereas in others it is contraindicated (see Chapter 4). Always follow the rules for safety with medications found in Chapter 12.

IMPORTANT FACTS ABOUT ADMINISTERING ORAL MEDICATIONS

- All medications should be given according to the general rules of medication administration discussed in Chapter 12.
- The easiest, most desirable, safest, and most frequently used route of drug administration is the oral route because most people can self-administer medications effectively.
- Persons who cannot swallow should not be given oral medications.
- Aspiration of medications into the respiratory tract is the main danger of the oral route.
- Oral medications may be administered in solid or liquid form.
- The presence or absence of food in the GI tract and digestive disorders affect the rate of absorption of oral medications.
- Adequate fluids must be administered with the medication so that the patient can swallow solid preparations, whereas liquids are rarely given after liquid preparations.
- Some medications may be crushed or chewed for ease of administration, whereas enteric-coated or timed-release forms should not be altered before they are swallowed. Scored tablets may be divided to give a partial dose of the medication.

PROCEDURE 13-1   Administering Solid Medications Orally

Objective: To safely administer solid medications by mouth.

Guidelines

Equipment Needed

- Medication order
- Container of the chosen medication
- Cup for measuring or holding medication
- Liquid for swallowing medication
- Tablet splitter if applicable

Methodology `3+7`

1. If giving tablets or capsules, open the container and tap the correct number into the cap of the bottle.

2. If the tablet is scored and needs dividing, break on the score line to provide equal parts for the dose needed.

3. Do not touch the medicine or the inside of the cap or bottle because these areas are considered clean, whereas the countertop is considered contaminated. To prevent further contamination, the inside of the cap of the medication bottle should not be placed on the countertop; the cap should be turned with the inside up if necessary to place on the counter.

4. After dispensing the drug into the bottle cap, transfer the drug to a medicine cup.

5. Give the medicine to the patient with sufficient liquid for swallowing after identifying the patient.

6. Watch the patient take the medicine.

7. Document your assessment and observation of the patient following administration. Answer patient questions and supply patient education as appropriate.

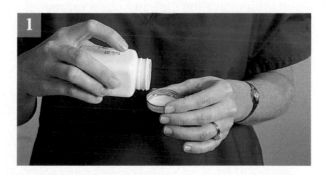

TYPICAL DOCUMENTATION
3/15/0X 9:10 AM acetaminophen, 650 mg po given with no apparent adverse reactions._____
_____G. OLSEN, CMA

PROCEDURE 13-2   Administering Liquid Medications Orally Using a Medicine Cup

Objective: To safely administer liquid medications by mouth using a medicine cup.

Guidelines

Equipment Needed

- Medication order
- Container of the chosen medication
- Calibrated medicine cup for holding medication

Methodology [3+7]

1. When giving a liquid medication, obtain a calibrated medicine cup and the ordered medication. If necessary, shake the medication for even distribution of the drug (mix the medication if necessary. If the medication is a suspension, shake the medication well before pouring it to place the medication back into suspension).

2. Locate the ordered dosage on the medicine cup and place a thumbnail at that line.

3 Hold the cup at eye level and pour the correct amount of the liquid into the container, reading to the meniscus. To keep the medicine from dripping on the label, always pour away from the label or "palm" the label.

4. After pouring the medicine, place the cup on a level surface and check the level of the medication for accuracy. If you have poured too much medicine, discard the extra amount. Do not return poured medicine to a stock container.

5. Identify the patient and give the medicine, watching the patient to be sure all the medication has been swallowed. Additional liquids are usually not given following the administration of a liquid medication.

6. Discard the medicine cup and observe the patient for indications of adverse effects.

7. Document the medication administration and any observations of the patient. Answer patient questions and supply any patient education needed.

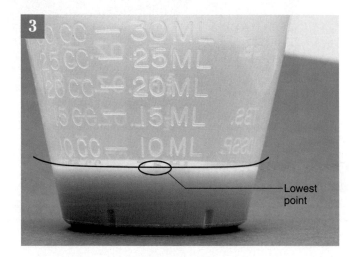

TYPICAL DOCUMENTATION

3/15/0X 10:00 AM ibuprofen liquid, 100 mg (1 tsp) po given with no apparent adverse reactions._____
_____G. OLSEN, CMA

PROCEDURE 13-3   Administering Liquid Medication Orally Using an Oral Syringe or Dose Spoon

Objective: To safely administer liquid medications by mouth using an oral syringe or dose spoon.

Guidelines

Equipment Needed
- Medication order
- Container of the chosen medication
- Oral syringe or dose spoon

Methodology 3+7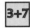

1. Placing the syringe into the liquid medicine, draw the desired amount of medication into the syringe or pour the correct amount of medication to the meniscus into the dose spoon holding the spoon upright.

2. After identifying the patient slowly squirt the medicine into the side of the patient's mouth to prevent choking. If using the dose spoon, allow the person to slowly swallow the medicine.

3. Care should be taken that the person taking the medicine does not aspirate the drug.

4. Immediately wash the utensil to keep medicine from drying in the syringe or dose spoon.

5. Document the medication administration and any observations of the patient. Answer patient questions and supply any patient education needed.

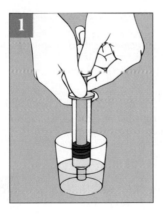

TYPICAL DOCUMENTATION
3/15/0X 9:15 AM amoxicillin 500 mg (10 mL) given po with no apparent adverse reactions._____

_____G. OLSEN, CMA

Rectal Administration Of Medications

Rectal medications are usually given as suppositories, by enema, or as ointments. The rectal mucosa allows rapid absorption of drug by the bloodstream because the blood supply to a relatively small area is great. Medications inserted into the rectum are not changed by the digestive juices and do not irritate the lining of the GI tract except possibly at the site of insertion. Many rectal medications relieve discomfort locally (e.g., anesthetic ointments and creams used to treat rectal discomforts) or may be used to stimulate evacuation of the bowel or as a stool softener. Other suppositories have systemic action and are used in patients with nausea and vomiting or fever. The rectal route is not as reliable as the oral or parenteral route, but it is safe because except for local irritation, side effects are rare.

Rectal ointments and creams are usually administered by means of an applicator attached to

BOX 13-1   SAFETY IN ADMINISTRATION OF ORAL MEDICATIONS

- Tell the patient to place oral medications in solid form (tablets, caplets) on the back of the tongue for ease of swallowing. Then the patient should tilt the head forward to stimulate the tongue and the swallowing reflex followed by tilting the head back for actual swallowing.
- The mouth should be moist to prevent the solid medication from adhering to the inside of the dry mouth. A dry mouth tends to make swallowing more difficult, increasing the chance of the medication's dissolving in the mouth.
- Oral medications should not be stored in strong light, high humidity, or open air. Discard medications that have changed color, are out of date, or have an unexpected odor such as the vinegar odor that occurs with out-of-date aspirin.
- If the medication has the potential to stain teeth (iron preparations, iodides), the liquid medication should be ingested through a straw. If the person has dentures, the dentures should be removed before the person ingests staining medications. Patients should always rinse the mouth with water after taking these medications.
- If a medication in a solid form cannot be swallowed whole by the patient, some tablets may be crushed or split for ease of administration. *Medications with enteric coating, sustained release, or other special release capabilities should never be crushed, chewed, or split.* Consult a drug reference to determine if the medicine may be crushed, split, or chewed.
- Effervescent tablets or powders should be given immediately after the solid form has dissolved in water so that the desired effervescence is maintained.
- Some medications come in solid sprinkles that are dispersed on food for administration, such as Depakene for seizures and theophylline for asthma. All food on which the sprinkles are applied must be eaten for the desired dosage to be administered.
- Sprinkles should not be applied to hot food because this activates the medication; the drug should only be applied to food at room temperature or colder to allow for absorption in the GI tract.
- Unless contraindicated, medications that are difficult to swallow may be placed in thick liquids such as applesauce or pudding to make swallowing easier. A product, Thick-It, is available over the counter to thicken liquids and make them easier to swallow.
- A scored tablet is usually a sign that the tablet may be split or divided.

Oral Medication Safety with Children and the Elderly
- Young children and older adults may have difficulty swallowing. If this is the case, check to see if the solid preparation is available in a liquid form.
- To give oral medications to children, approach them as if you expect cooperation and praise the child for cooperating and taking the medication.
- Never tell a child that medicine is "candy."
- Never trick a child about taking medicines.
- Never try to force a child to swallow medicine or hold the child's nose or mouth shut because this may cause choking.
- Never give medicine to a crying child because this may cause aspiration.

the medication tube. The medication order reads to apply the ointment or cream to the area, with no specific dosage given.

Rectal suppositories are manufactured in a glycerin or cocoa butter base that melts on contact with the body. Most suppositories are bullet shaped (Figure 13-1) with rounded ends to prevent trauma to the rectal mucosa on insertion. Most suppositories administered in the ambulatory care facility are for the treatment of nausea and vomiting and to reduce fever in young children (Procedure 13-4).

Enemas are liquids instilled into the rectum that may be used to soften hard feces, relieve fecal impactions, or evacuate the bowel or as a means of administering medication (Procedure 13-5). Single-use enemas such as Fleet enemas may be prescribed for use prior to diagnostic tests (Figure 13-2). Although enemas are rarely performed in

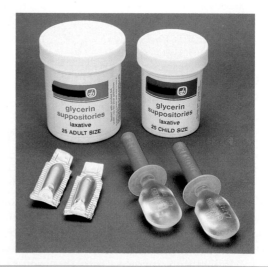

Figure 13-1 The shape and packaging of a rectal suppository and small enemas for infants. (From Perry AG, Potter PA: *Clinical nursing skills and techniques,* St Louis, Mosby.)

PROCEDURE 13-4   Administering Medications Rectally by Suppository

Objective: To safely administer a rectal suppository.

Guidelines

Equipment Needed
- Medication order
- Appropriate rectal suppository for the medical order
- Gloves
- Drape to cover the body for privacy
- Water-soluble lubricant
- Tissues

Methodology

1. Identify the person and place the patient in the Sim's position, being sure the patient is draped for privacy. (Children may be placed in the dorsal recumbent position. Infants and small children may be placed supine so that both legs can be elevated to observe the rectum.)

2. Remove the wrapper from the suppository if necessary. Do not handle the suppository more than necessary because body warmth may lead to softening of the suppository and insertion of the medication into the rectum may be hindered.

3 Lubricate the rounded end of the suppository with water-soluble jelly or water.

4. Lubricate the tip of the gloved finger to be used for insertion.

5. Elevate the upper buttocks to show the anal opening. Ask the patient to take deep breaths through the mouth to relax the rectal sphincter.

6 With a gloved hand, gently push the suppository past the anal sphincter into the rectum (about 4 inches). Do not insert the suppository into fecal matter because the medication will not be absorbed.

7. Wipe excess lubricant from the anal area with tissues.

8. Ask the patient to remain quiet for about 5 to 10 minutes to allow the medication to be absorbed without a bowel movement occurring.

9. Remove the gloves.

10. Observe the patient for reactions, both expected and possibly adverse.

11. Document the medication administration. If the medication is for bowel evacuation, document the results obtained.

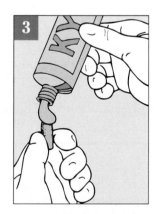

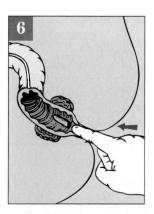

(continued)

PROCEDURE 13-4 — Administering Medications Rectally by Suppository—cont'd

TYPICAL DOCUMENTATION

3/15/0X 3:15 PM Phenergan 25-mg suppository inserted into rectum with no apparent side effects. Suppository retained and symptoms of nausea decreased in 30 min. _____ G. OLSEN, CMA

PROCEDURE 13-5 — Administering Medications Rectally Using an Enema

Objective: To safely administer a rectal enema.

Guidelines

Equipment Needed
- Medication order
- Appropriate ordered enema
- Gloves
- Water-soluble lubricant
- Tissues

Methodology 3+7

1. Identify the patient and place in the Sim's position, or other appropriate position, and drape for privacy.

2. Remove the plastic cap and lubricate the tip of the enema, if necessary. (Some enemas come prelubricated.)

3. Locate the rectum and ask the patient to breathe deeply and slowly to relax the rectal sphincter.

4. Gently insert the tip of the enema into the rectum. If using a prepackaged enema, roll the bottle from the bottom to the tip until the liquid has been delivered into the rectum. If using a non-disposable enema, hold the enema bag six to eight inches above the rectum and slowly administer the liquid into the rectum.

5. Instruct the patient to retain the enema for at least 5 to 10 minutes before expelling the fluid and any waste materials from the rectum.

6. Remove the gloves.

7. Assist the patient to the bathroom at the proper time.

8. Observe the return from the enema.

9. Observe the patient for any adverse effects.

10. Document the procedure including the return from the enema, as well as any adverse effects.

TYPICAL DOCUMENTATION

3/16/0X 1:15 PM Fleet enema administered with no adverse effects. Return of enema contained large amounts of hard, constipated feces. _____G. OLSEN, CMA

an ambulatory care setting, it may be necessary to teach the patient the technique for home use. The patient should be told to remove the wrapper and insert the enema tip followed by the administration of the liquid into the rectum. The patient should then hold the medication in the rectum for as long as possible to obtain the best possible results. The fluid of the enema breaks up the fecal mass, stretches the rectal wall, and induces the defecation reflex.

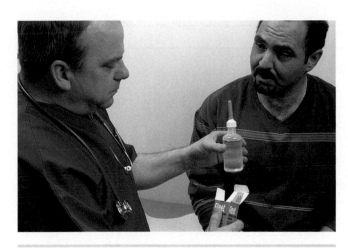

Figure 13-2 Prepackaged enemas. (From Perry AG, Potter PA: *Clinical nursing skills and techniques*, St Louis, Mosby.)

IMPORTANT FACTS ABOUT RECTAL MEDICATIONS

- Be sure that the wrapper covering the suppository is removed prior to insertion of the suppository. Lubricate the end of the suppository with either water-soluble jelly or water.
- Keep a suppository cool before inserting it because a soft suppository is difficult to insert. To keep the medication from melting, do not hold the suppository in the hand. If the suppository is soft, place it in the freezer for a few minutes to harden, but do not let the medication freeze.
- Gently insert the rounded end of the suppository past the anal sphincter for retention. Wear a glove on the hand used for insertion.
- Remain lying down for approximately 5 to 10 minutes to allow the suppository to melt. Resist the urge to have a bowel movement immediately so that the medication can melt and be absorbed.
- Medications inserted into the rectum are not changed by digestive juices and do not irritate the GI tract, except possibly at the site of insertion.

Summary

Oral administration of medicines is the easiest and most frequently used route because it is the safest. The drug is placed in the mouth and swallowed into the stomach for absorption in the GI tract, usually the intestines. Some solid forms of oral medications may be crushed or divided for administration; others have specific coatings or forms that should not be altered. Medications may irritate the GI tract or may be altered by the juices found in the stomach and intestines. In these cases the drug may not be given through oral administration. The danger of aspiration should be evaluated before oral medications are given. Patients who cannot swallow should not be given drugs by mouth.

Rectal medications may be administered by either suppository or enema, with neither route being irritating to the GI tract except at the site of administration. The base for suppositories is usually either glycerin or cocoa butter for ease of melting in the rectum. Therefore suppositories should not be handled any more than necessary, to prevent changes in shape or melting prior to insertion. Enemas may be used for cleansing purposes or to soften hardened feces. Medications are infrequently administered rectally in the ambulatory care setting, so the allied health professional's responsibility may be focused on teaching the patient how to administer an enema at home. For a person who cannot swallow medications, rectal administration, especially in a patient with vomiting, may be the route of choice.

Critical Thinking Exercises

SCENARIO

Sally is providing patient education to an older patient, Mrs. Campo, who is having difficulty swallowing the large tablets needed for her medical condition. She tells you that two of the tablets have "deep lines" through the tablet and one has a very hard coat. Mrs. Campo wants to know if there is any way she can make swallowing the medicine easier.

1. What information can Sally give her about the scored tablets?
2. Can these tablets be crushed or divided for easier administration?
3. What about the tablet that seems to have an enteric coating?
4. Mrs. Campo states that the tablets seem to stick to her mouth because her mouth is so dry. What instructions should Sally give Mrs. Campo that will make swallowing easier?

REVIEW QUESTIONS

1. Why is oral administration of a medication the most desirable route? _____
   _____
   _____

2. Why can some medications not be given orally? _____
   _____
   _____

3. What medications can be divided for doses? What medications should not be crushed for administration? _____
   _____
   _____

4. What does it mean to "pour a medication to the meniscus"? _____
   _____
   _____

5. Why are medications given by rectal suppository? _____
   _____
   _____

6. "All medications given by rectum are for local effect." Why is this statement false? _____
   _____
   _____

CHAPTER 14

Percutaneous Routes

OBJECTIVES

After studying this chapter, you should be capable of doing the following:

- Describing the percutaneous routes of medication administration.
- Administering topical forms of medications.
- Administering nitroglycerin ointment.
- Describing patch testing for allergens.
- Explaining how to apply transdermal drugs.
- Discussing the use of sublingual and buccal forms of medicine.
- Administering ophthalmic drops and ointments.
- Administering otic medications.
- Describing how to use nasal medications.
- Administering inhalation medicines using a metered dose inhaler.
- Describing the use of vaginal suppositories and douches.

Allie, age 2, has an earache and no other symptoms. Dr. Merry looks in Allie's ear and sees that ear tubes are in place but the ear canal is red. He orders otic drops for use in the ear four times a day.

At what temperature should Allie's mother keep the drops to stop further pain on instillation?

How should you tell Allie's mother to hold Allie's ear to get maximum effect of the drops?

With tubes in Allie's ears, can Allie's mother use any ear drops, or do the drops need to be sterile? Why or why not?

Why should Allie's mother massage Allie's ear after inserting the drops?

KEY TERMS

Aerochamber	Percutaneous	Transdermal
Excoriation	Spacer	
Nebulizer	Topical	

Medications for **percutaneous** use are absorbed through the skin or mucous membranes. Rectal medications are included and discussed in Chapter 13 because of the gastrointestinal (GI) tract site. However, rectal medications are absorbed through the mucous membranes of the rectum. Both over-the-counter (OTC) and prescription drugs may be given percutaneously, and percutaneous medications may have local or systemic effects and sometimes both. The route of administration includes sublingual and buccal medications, which are absorbed through the mucous membranes of the mouth; **topical** or surface preparations in the form of ointments and liniments; and **transdermal** or through-the-skin delivery patches. Percutaneous routes of administration are chosen when direct contact of the medication with the skin is necessary and because of ease of administration and the low risk of systemic adverse reactions. Because the absorption of some topical agents has unreliable systemic action due to differences in drug absorption, percutaneous routes are seldom used for treating systemic diseases. Drugs absorbed percutaneously, except those absorbed through the mucous membranes of the mouth and lungs, are slow acting and are used when slow, steady, extended medication administration is desired.

Topical Medications

Medications may be applied topically for local effect, such as to relieve itching or provide warmth, or for systemic action, such as to relieve unstable angina with nitroglycerin ointment or patches. Topical medications can cause systemic adverse reactions and for safety should be applied as prescribed. Types of skin preparations range from such common forms as creams, ointments, and powders to wet dressings and soaks for wound care and patches for hormone replacement therapy. (For discussion of forms of medication, see Chapter 3.)

Except in the specific treatment of rashes and wounds, the skin should be clean, dry, and free of infection, rashes, encrustations, open areas, and dead tissue. Before topical medications are applied, the skin should be inspected for integrity and cleansed with water. Soap can alter the absorption of medications, so the skin should be free of all soap residues before topical preparations are applied, especially patches. If the medication is indicated to reduce itching, it should be applied with gentle strokes. If the drug is rubbed vigorously, the friction will heat the skin, increasing the itching.

For optimal absorption to be maintained without a protective covering, such as a bandage or a patch, adequate skin hydration is necessary. Transdermal medications should be applied behind the ear for fastest absorption. The back, chest, and abdomen are the next most rapid sites of absorption. The slowest sites of absorption are the thigh and forearm.

Powders, Soaks, Compresses, and Dressings

To use powders such as Tinactin powder for fungal infections, follow these steps:

- The skin surface should be thoroughly dry, to minimize crusting and caking of the powder.
- The skin surface to which the powder is to be applied should be fully exposed with the folds of skin spread open.
- The powder is lightly dusted onto the surface, leaving a fine, thin layer of powder. A thin layer of powder is more absorbent than a thick layer and reduces friction by increasing the evaporation of moisture.

For soaks, compresses, and wet dressings such as Betadine, the following points apply:

- An active ingredient dissolves in water-based solutions to leave a film on the skin after application.
- These substances contain a mild astringent that provides a soothing, cooling, and antipyretic effect when used on blistered or oozing skin areas.
- Bandages may be soaked in the solution and then applied to the skin. An extremity may be soaked in the solution. For a wet dressing, a plastic wrap may be placed over the dressing to keep the dressing damp.

Creams, Ointments, Gels, and Lotions

Creams and ointments are semisolid preparations used for topical applications such as Neosporin and Triple Antibiotic Cream or Ointment.

- Creams are active ingredients in a water base.
- Creams are used to deliver drugs directly to or into the skin.
- Creams are absorbed into the skin and vanish, and usually have a cooling effect.
- Ointments are soft, fatty substances with the active ingredient carried in an oil, lanolin, or petroleum base.
- Ointments deliver drugs to the surface of the skin, and the drug stays in contact with the skin longer than a drug carried in a cream.
- Creams may be used to deliver antipyretics, antimicrobials, and softening compounds. The application of an antimicrobial ointment or cream is described in Procedure 14-1.

Nitroglycerin ointment, used in the treatment of angina pectoris or cardiac ischemia, is applied directly to the skin on the chest, back, upper arms, or thighs. The site should be dry and relatively free of hair and scar tissue. The allied health professional should avoid contact with nitroglycerin because it can cause a headache if it is absorbed during administration. To prevent overdose, any ointment remaining from previous applications should be removed before a new dose is applied. The procedure for applying nitroglycerin ointment is described in Procedure 14-2.

PROCEDURE 14-1   Administering Topical Medications

Objective: To apply topical medications appropriately.

Guidelines

Equipment Needed

- Medication order
- Medication ordered
- Gloves
- Supplies to cleanse skin
- Dressing and bandages as needed

Methodology 3+7

1. After identifying the patient, cleanse the skin and pat dry, using good aseptic technique.

2. Change your gloves if they are wet or contaminated after cleansing the skin.

3. If a cream or ointment is to be applied to the skin, place the medication in a cleanly gloved hand. The applicator tip should not touch the glove or the skin site. If the medication is sterile, sterile technique using a sterile tongue blade to apply the medication to sterile gauze should be used.

4. Hold the medication in your hand to allow the preparation to soften to body temperature. Softening the ointment helps the medication spread easily and evenly.

5. Apply the medication using long, even strokes. This technique avoids irritating hair follicles.

6. A dressing and bandage may be applied to keep the medication in contact with the skin.

7. In some instances the ointment may be applied to the dressing and then applied to the skin.

8. Document the procedure.

TYPICAL DOCUMENTATION

6/30/0X 11:25 AM Abrasion on left knee cleansed with soap and water and dried. Polymyxin B sulfate/neomycin sulfate/bacitracin ointment applied to lesion. Dry dressing applied. No apparent sign of adverse reaction. _____ G. OLSEN, CMA

Gels such as K-Y Jelly are thick water-based substances for lubrication or for ease of applying the active drug to the skin. Some gels have an oil ingredient added for better coverage of an area to help the medication application last for longer periods of time.

Pastes are either thick oil- or water-based compounds such as zinc oxide that are often used as sun blocks and to deliver medications.

Lotions such as calamine lotion are water-based compounds.

- Lotions are used to control itching (e.g., calamine lotion) or to relieve muscle and joint pain.
- Lotions are applied lightly to the skin surface using a gauze pad and stroking in the direction of hair growth. Rubbing rather than stroking

lightly may increase itching rather than relieve discomfort.

- Evaporation of water from the lotion leaves the area feeling cool.
- Some lotions contain powder and leave a thin film of powder at the site of application.
- If the lotion is in the form of a suspension, the container should be shaken vigorously for mixing the solute in the solvent.

Patches, Disks, and Transdermal Dots

Some topical medications come prepackaged in transdermal disks, patches, or dots that provide extended effect—up to several days. An example is scopolamine patches for motion sickness.

PROCEDURE 14-2   Application of Nitroglycerin Ointment

Objective: To properly apply nitroglycerin ointment.

Guidelines

Equipment Needed
- Medication order
- Nitroglycerin ointment with measured application papers
- Gloves
- Supplies to cleanse skin (if needed)
- Tape as appropriate

Methodology **3+7**

1. After identifying the patient, cleanse the skin of residual nitroglycerin ointment. The site should be dry, relatively free of hair, and without scar tissue. The site of application must be rotated on a daily basis.

2. The prescribed dose of nitroglycerin in inches should be squeezed and measured directly to the manufacturer's applicator paper.

3. Check the patient's pulse and ensure that the rate is greater than 60 beats/min. If below 60 beats/min, consult with a physician before applying ointment.

4. Apply the ointment to the skin and hold in place for 10 seconds. A strip of adhesive tape may be applied to prevent slippage of the paper.

5. A plastic or wax occlusive dressing that comes with the ointment may be added if the desired effect is not achieved.

6. Document the procedure.

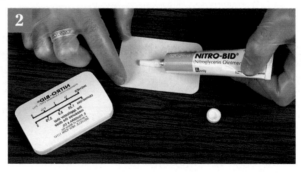

TYPICAL DOCUMENTATION

7/13/0X 9:15 AM Pulse 72. Nitroglycerin ointment, 2 inches applied to left upper chest after skin cleaned of residue. Tape applied to application paper. No apparent adverse reactions._____ G. OLSEN, CMA

- These forms are a painless, convenient method of administering medications for many medical conditions.
- The medication released from transdermal patches passes through the skin and into the circulatory system for continuous treatment without repeated dosing during the day.
- The transdermal medication form must be reapplied as indicated to maintain the dosage desired.

- When a patch, dot, or disk is applied, the date and time of application should be written on the application material or noted on a calendar when self-administered.
- Transdermal forms of medication should be applied by the patient and should be handled carefully to avoid getting the medication on the fingers, where the drug may be absorbed (Figure 14-1). Each person touching these

patches or dots should wash his or her hands immediately to avoid undesirable absorption of medicine and undesired side effects.

- Soap should not be used at the application site because soap enhances and prolongs absorption.

See Box 14-1 for medications that typically come in transdermal patch applications.

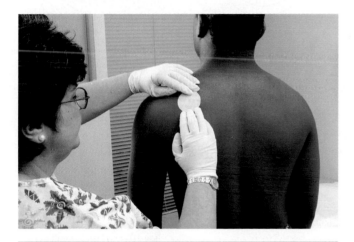

Figure 14-1 Application of a transdermal medication patch. (From Chester GA: *Modern medical assisting*, Philadelphia, 1998, WB Saunders.)

Sprays and Aerosols

Some medications come in aerosol or spray applications such as ethyl chloride. Prior to application the skin must be clean and dry. The container must be vigorously shaken to ensure the medication and the propellant are evenly distributed prior to application. The container label will specify the distance to hold the medication from the skin with the usual distance being 6 to 12 inches. The spray should be fine and even, applying a thin coating of the medication to the skin. Holding the container too close to the skin may result in a thin, watery distribution.

Special Considerations for Topical Medications in Geriatric Patients

The skin of older people is fragile, and the blood supply is close to the thin skin, increasing the risk of bruising. Application of medication directly to the skin should be done with minimal friction. The elderly also have diminished sensations including those of pain, temperature, and itching. The skin should be observed on a regular basis to ensure that the medication is not causing irritation and breakdown of the skin itself. Dry flaky skin is easily **excoriated,** and any changes in the skin condition should be observed when applying topical medications.

BOX 14-1 COMMON MEDICATIONS IN TRANSDERMAL PATCHES, DOTS, OR DISKS

- Nitroglycerin, supplied as Transderm-Nitro for angina pectoris, is applied to the upper chest, with the site rotated on a daily basis.
- Female hormones in the form of estradiol dots to relieve menopausal symptoms such as hot flashes, night sweats, and vaginal dryness should be applied to the thighs and buttocks for slow absorption and are rotated on a schedule provided by the manufacturer.
- Scopolamine, supplied as Transderm-Scop, is used to prevent the nausea and vomiting of motion sickness and is applied behind the ear. For maximum effectiveness, this medication should be applied 4 hours prior to travel.
- Duragesic (fentanyl citrate) patches are used for the continuous analgesia of chronic pain. These patches remain in place for 3 days, and the site of application is changed with each application to prevent skin irritation and possible lack of absorption in the tissues.
- Nicotine patches are used to assist with smoking cessation. Prescribed as a 3-month supply, the patch is changed every 24 hours. The nicotine patches are expensive but are a sound investment in better health. The patient should be warned against smoking while wearing the patch because the increased nicotine may cause coronary symptoms.
- Allergy testing patches are for diagnosing contact dermatitis. Small amounts of the suspected 20 to 30 allergens are individually placed on the forearm or back, covered with cellophane, and read 24 to 48 hours later. As with all patches, the allergen and the date and time of application should be on the patch.
- Contraceptives, such as Ortho-Ever Patch, are applied to the hips for 7 days for 3 weeks. During the fourth week, no patch is applied.
- Methylphenidate (Ritalin) is applied as a patch in the morning and removed midafternoon.
- Testosterone, a male hormone, is found in two different application-site patches for daily application. This medication is also available in creams and gels for topical application.

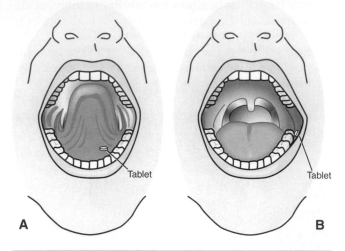

IMPORTANT FACTS ABOUT TRANSDERMAL MEDICATIONS

- Percutaneous routes of medication administration are those through the skin and through mucous membranes.
- The percutaneous route is used because of ease of administration, the low risk of systemic adverse reactions, and for slow, steady, extended-duration effect.
- Because the amount of medication is not delivered with the same absorption, percutaneous administration cannot be used when reliable amounts of medication must be absorbed systemically.
- When a topical medication is applied in powder form, the skin should be dry to prevent caking and crusting of the powder and only a thin layer should be applied.
- Creams are absorbed into the skin because of the water base, whereas ointments have an oily base and tend to remain on the surface of the skin, where absorption is prolonged.
- Nitroglycerin ointment is applied directly to the skin of the chest to maintain a slow, continuous supply of medication for angina pectoris. When nitroglycerin ointment is used, any residual ointment should be removed before the new dose is applied. The person applying nitroglycerin ointment should not allow the medication to touch his or her own skin because headaches and other side effects of the medication may occur if the nitroglycerin is absorbed through the fingers.
- Lotions, used to control itching and relieve joint pain, should be applied lightly to prevent increased irritation.
- Prepackaged disks and patches are used for multiple medical conditions including allergy testing. Application sites are determined by the indication for the medication.
- Topical medications should be applied gently to older persons. Their skin is fragile, and the blood supply is near the surface, which causes easy bruising.

Figure 14-2 **A,** Sublingual administration of medication. **B,** Buccal administration of medication. (From Leahy JM, Kizilay PE: *Foundations of nursing practice: a nursing process approach*, Philadelphia, 1998, WB Saunders.)

Buccal And Sublingual Medications

The sublingual administration of medications involves placing the medication form, such as tiny porous tablets, a liquid squeezed from a capsule, or an aerosol spray, under the tongue for rapid absorption into the bloodstream through the mucous membranes (Figure 14-2, *A*). Nitroglycerin is a typical drug given in this manner. The buccal administration of medications involves placing the drug between the cheek and gums for local absorption by the mucous membranes. Buccal medications such as Mycelex may also be absorbed systemically when the drug is absorbed in saliva and swallowed (Figure 14-2, *B*). The patient's mouth should be damp prior to administration, and the patient should avoid eating, drinking, or chewing while the medication is in place. Sublingual and buccal medications should not be swallowed but should be retained in the desired location until they have dissolved. If these medications are swallowed, the time for absorption will be prolonged or the medication may be changed by the gastric juices and be ineffective.

Ophthalmic Medications

Common ophthalmic preparations come in the form of ointments and drops and intraocular disks for a longer-lasting medication effect. The disk resembles a contact lens and is placed in the conjunctival sac, where it remains in place for a desired period of time. The lower lid is pulled away from the eye, and the disk is inserted so that it floats on the sclera. The patient should be instructed not to rub the eyes when the medication disk is in place to prevent too rapid absorption or eye irritation.

Drugs applied to the eye must be sterile, and only medications marked "ophthalmic" should be used in eyes. These drugs should not be applied directly to the cornea because of the rich supply of nerve fibers in the cornea. The conjunctival sac is much less sensitive and is a more appropriate site for administering a drug. Eye drops should be warmed before they are instilled to make the drops less irritating. Procedure 14-3 outlines how to instill ophthalmic medications.

Otic Medications

The internal ear structures are sensitive to temperature extremes, so all ear medications should be administered at room temperature. If cold drops are placed in the ear, the patient may experience vertigo and nausea. Drops can be warmed by

PROCEDURE 14-3   Instillation of Ophthalmic Medications

Objective: To instill sterile ophthalmic eye medications.

Guidelines

Equipment Needed
- Medication order
- Gloves
- Ophthalmic medication as ordered
- Supplies to cleanse eye as needed

Methodology `3+7`

Instilling Eye Drops

1. After identifying the patient, cleanse any drainage from the eye moving from the inner to outer canthus.

2. Warm eye drops by holding in the hands prior to instillation to prevent eye irritation. Be sure that the medication has an "ophthalmic" label.

3. Hold the medication dropper approximately $\frac{1}{2}$ to $\frac{3}{4}$ inch above the conjunctival sac, taking extreme care not to contaminate the dropper by allowing the tip to touch the eye.

4. Drop the prescribed amount of medication into the conjunctival sac to prevent irritation to the cornea. If the person blinks or closes the eye prior to administration, repeat the procedure.

5. When administering a medication that may have a systemic effect, apply gentle pressure to the nasolacrimal duct for 30 to 60 seconds following administration to prevent overflow of the medication into the nasal and pharyngeal passages.

6. Instruct the patient to close the eye to help distribute the medication from the conjunctival sac.

7. Document the procedure.

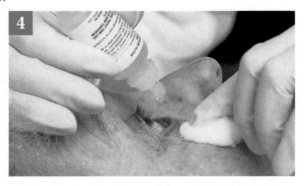

Instilling Eye Ointment

1. After identifying the patient, cleanse any drainage from the eye, moving from the inner to outer canthus.

2. Be sure that medication has an "ophthalmic" label.

(continued)

PROCEDURE 14-3   Instillation of Ophthalmic Medications—cont'd

3 Ask the patient to look at the ceiling. Hold the ointment applicator $\frac{1}{2}$ inch above the lower lid and apply a thin stream of ointment along the inner edge of the lower lid from the inner to outer canthus.

4. Ask the patient to close the eye slowly, then open and close the eye several times to further melt the ointment and distribute the medication across the eye.

5. If there is excess medication on the eyelid, remove with a tissue from the inner to outer canthus.

6. If an eye patch is necessary, apply a clean one over the eye and tape it securely without applying pressure to the eye. Most ointments may blur vision for up to 30 minutes.

7. Document the procedure.

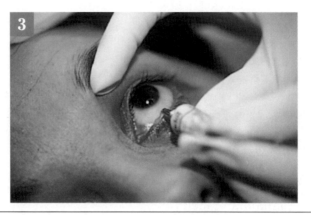

TYPICAL DOCUMENTATION
7/22/0X 3:15 PM Pilocarpine hydrochloride ophthalmic drops, gtt i OU, with no apparent adverse reactions. _____ G. OLSEN, CMA

holding the medication bottle between the hands for approximately 2 minutes. Although the outer ear is not sterile, sterile drops and solutions should be used if the eardrum is ruptured or if tympanic tubes are present. Nonsterile solutions that reach the middle ear may cause serious infections. Never force any solutions into the ear. *Sterile ophthalmologic drops may be used as otic medications, but otic medications cannot be used for ophthalmic use.* Never fill the ear canal with a medicine dropper because this can cause pressure in the canal during instillation of medications and can cause further injury to the eardrum. The procedure for instilling otic medications is outlined in Procedure 14-4.

Nasal Medications

Nasal medications, administered by atomizer, dropper, or aerosol spray for local effect, may be absorbed into the bloodstream for systemic effects, but are usually considered topical or local medi-cations. Nasal drugs are commonly used as decongestants for blocked nasal passages due to sinusitis or upper respiratory symptoms or to stop nosebleeds. Nasal drugs are relatively safe when administered in small doses as needed; however, these drugs may change vital signs either intentionally or accidentally. Repeated use of decongestant sprays can worsen nasal congestion because of the rebound effect. To instill nasal drops:

- Tilt the patient's head back or place the patient in a supine position with the head tilted backward.
- After instillation, tilt the head forward to distribute the medication properly. Taking short, quick breaths will help spread the medication evenly.
- Any nose drops that spill down the throat should be expectorated to prevent systemic side effects.

Nasal sprays are increasingly used to administer various medications because of the rapid

PROCEDURE 14-4   Instilling Otic Medications

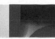

Objective: To instill ear medications.

Guidelines

Equipment Needed
- Medication order
- Otic medication
- Gloves
- Cotton to fill external auditory canal

Methodology 3+7

1. After identifying the person, ask the patient to lie still to prevent injury from the ear dropper. The head should be turned to the side and the affected ear should face up.

2. Hold the medication to warm the solution.

3. For the older child or adult ear, straighten the ear canal by pulling the external ear up and out or back. If the patient is 3 years of age or younger, gently pull the external ear down and back.

4. Slowly administer the prescribed amount of medication, holding the dropper about $\frac{1}{2}$ inch above the ear and aiming the drops toward the wall of the canal rather than toward the eardrum.

5. Gently massage the outer ear to move the medication inward.

6. Ask the patient to remain in the same position for 5 minutes so that the medication can be absorbed.

7. Document the procedure.

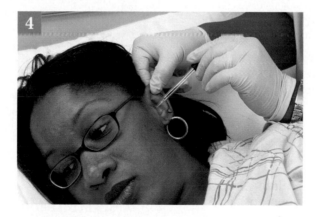

TYPICAL DOCUMENTATION
7/13/0X 2:45 PM Cortisporin Otic Solution, gtts iii AS, with no apparent adverse reaction. Patient instructed in proper method of instilling ear drops at home. _____G.OLSEN, CMA

absorption into the vast capillary supply in the nasal passages. Drugs for migraine headaches, insulin preparations, smoking cessation agents, and cortisone and decongestants for sinus conditions are just a few of the medications being used for administration by means of the nasal spray. Use of nasal sprays and atomizers involves the following:

- The patient should be sitting upright with the head tilted backward.
- Prior to application, the nasal passages should be cleared as much as possible.
- To administer the medication, occlude one nostril and have the patient inhale through the other.

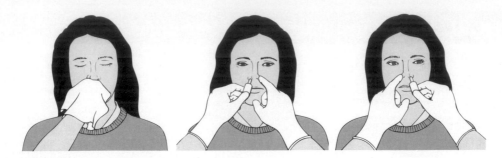

Figure 14-3 Administration of nasal medication. (From Chester GA: *Modern medical assisting*, Philadelphia, 1998, WB Saunders.)

- Be certain that the spray tip is centered in the nostril and not against the nasal cavity wall.
- To deliver the medication, squeeze the container while the applicator is inside the nostril.
- The head should remain tilted back for about 5 minutes, and the patient should not blow the nose.
- If the aerosol delivers a metered dose, shake the container well and insert the tip into the nostril. Instruct the patient to hold his or her breath during administration of the medicine (Figure 14-3).

Vaginal Medications

Vaginal medications occur in the form of suppositories, tablets, creams, and solutions and are absorbed through the mucous membranes for treating local infections.

- Solutions used for irrigating, or douches, may be antiinfectants. Douches may be either prescription or OTC preparations.
- Creams and foams are available for contraception and to treat fungal infections. These medications are inserted with applicators.
- Suppositories may require an applicator or may be inserted by hand after being lubricated or moistened with water for ease of insertion.
- Most vaginal medications are prescribed for use at bedtime and are best used when the woman is lying down. The woman should remain flat for at least 10 minutes following the insertion of a cream or suppository.
- The medication course as prescribed by the physician must be completed because the causative condition may return if medication is stopped early even though it seems to have improved.

- Vaginal medications tend to result in drainage, and use of panty liners or a tampon, if acceptable to the physician, will help hold the medication in the vagina.
- Vaginal suppositories should not be handled more than necessary prior to insertion, to prevent premature melting of the medication. The covering on the suppository should be removed before insertion.

DID YOU KNOW?
The vagina produces its own secretions for an antiseptic effect, and frequent douching may change the acidity of the vaginal canal, making the woman more prone to vaginal infections from either resident body flora or invading bacteria. Advertising campaigns have caused women to believe that douching is necessary; in reality, daily bathing should be sufficient for cleanliness. Excessive odor and vaginal discharge are symptoms of infection that may require medical attention.

IMPORTANT FACTS ABOUT MEDICATIONS ABSORBED THROUGH MUCOUS MEMBRANES
- Buccal and sublingual medications are absorbed through the mucous membranes of the mouth.
- Sublingual medications are absorbed rapidly because of the rich blood supply under the tongue.
- Ophthalmic medications, usually drops or ointments, are for topical administration, although some have systemic absorption. Medication discs resembling contact lenses are also used to provide prolonged medication application to the eye.
- When administering medications for the eye, be sure that the medication label reads "ophthalmic."
- Otic medications should be at room temperature prior to administration into the ear. If the drops are cold, nausea and dizziness may result.

IMPORTANT FACTS ABOUT MEDICATIONS ABSORBED THROUGH MUCOUS MEMBRANES—
Cont'd

- After instilling ear medications, the patient should remain in a lying position with the affected ear facing up for at least 5 minutes.
- Before instilling nasal medications, be sure the nasal passages are cleared of mucus. Nasal medications may enter the systemic blood supply and change vital signs, although nasal preparations are considered topical medications. This is especially true if the medication is swallowed.
- Rebound congestion may occur if nasal preparations are used too often or inappropriately.
- Nasal preparations are now available for many types of medications including insulin, smoking cessation agents, corticosteroids, and hormone therapy.
- Vaginal medications include suppositories, creams, tablets, and solutions. Many of these preparations can be purchased OTC.
- Women should be taught that excessive douching is not necessary because the vagina is self-cleansing. Excessive douching can change the pH of the vagina and lead to infections.

Inhaled Medications

Inhalation medications are supplied in the form of gases, sprays, powders, and liquids to be inhaled into the respiratory tract. Because of the rich blood supply to the respiratory tract through the alveolar-capillary network, medications are absorbed more rapidly than with any other mucous membrane. Drugs for inhalation may be used to liquefy bronchial secretions for expectoration or to dilate bronchi to ease breathing. Inhalation is also used for oxygen therapy and general anesthesia.

Metered dose inhalers (MDIs) are hand-held devices that disperse the medications into the airways and lungs. Each measured dose requires about 5 to 10 lb of pressure to activate the aerosol. Older people may have insufficient hand strength to activate the application, so adapters or aerochambers are available to assist with coordination for accurate administration (Figure 14-4).

Use of an MDI also requires coordinating breathing with the administration of the medication; if this coordination is not present, the medication may be sprayed only into the back of the throat, and only a small amount of medication will reach the desired site. For the full amount of medicine to reach the lungs, the inhaler must be depressed just as the person breathes. The procedure for using an MDI is outlined in Procedure 14-5.

The first inhalation of medication opens the airways and reduces inflammation, whereas the second dose penetrates the deeper airways. MDI medications should be administered at regular

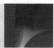

Figure 14-4 A metered dose inhaler. (From Perry A, Potter P: *Clinical nursing skills and techniques*, ed 4, St Louis, 1998, Mosby.)

PROCEDURE 14-5 Administration of Medication Using a Metered Dose Inhaler

Objective: To effectively administer medications using an MDI.

Guidelines

Equipment Needed
- Medication order
- Medication ordered
- Gloves
- MDI
- Spacer if indicated by age or physical condition

(continued)

PROCEDURE 14-5   Administration of Medication Using a Metered Dose Inhaler—cont'd

Methodology  **3+7**

1 Identify the patient and remove the cover from the MDI, gently shaking it to ensure the particles in the medication are aerosolized.

2. Instruct the patient to take a deep breath and exhale in order to prepare the airways for the medication.

3 Position the inhaler either in the mouth with the opening toward the back of the throat or, preferably, with the mouthpiece 1 to 2 inches from the mouth, holding the inhaler with the thumb and the index finger with the middle finger at the top for compression of inhaler. A spacer may be needed.

4. Instruct the patient to tilt the head back slightly to distribute the medication into the airways and then to inhale slowly and deeply through the mouth.

5 Depress the medication canister fully and instruct the person to hold his or her breath for approximately 10 seconds to allow the released medication to reach the deeper airway branches.

6. The patient should exhale through pursed lips to keep the small airways open during exhalation. If a second dose of the medication should follow, the person should wait 2 to 5 minutes to allow the full distribution of the medication.

7. Cleanse the MDI immediately after use because an accumulation of medication around the mouthpiece may interfere with the medication reaching the desired locations. Some brands of MDIs have different directions, so the manufacturer's package insert should be read carefully to ensure proper use of the inhaler.

8. If the patient is to administer this medication at home, have the patient repeat the instructions to you and provide the patient with printed instructions for his or her use.

9. Document the procedure.

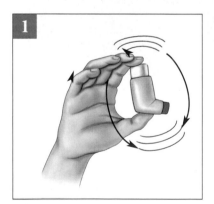
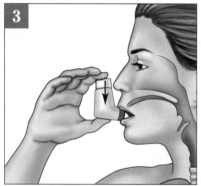
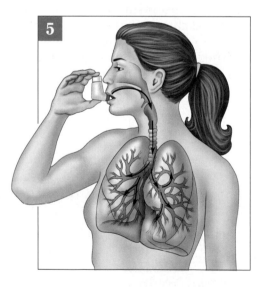

TYPICAL DOCUMENTATION
7/12/0X 9:15 AM Albuterol inhaler, 2 puffs as directed, with no apparent adverse reactions. Instructions given for use at home with return demonstration by patient. _____G. OLSEN, CMA

intervals throughout the day to provide constant drug levels. "Extra" doses of MDI aerosols should not be administered because these may cause harmful side effects. If the aerosol has not been administered correctly, the person may have a gagging sensation caused by the droplets of medication on the tongue or pharynx.

Nebulizers provide a spray or mist of medication. These type medications may also be called aerosols or atomizers. With a nebulizer, the patient inserts the mouthpiece into the oral cavity and sprays the medication while inhaling.

Rotadisk contains a powder of medication. The patient should exhale as deeply as possible, insert the mouthpiece into his or her oral cavity, puncture the medication pouch, and inhale the powder. Each Rotadisk contains one dose of medication.

DID YOU KNOW?

Current trends in medications include the introduction of antibiotics that are inhaled for the treatment of lung infections. These inhaled antibiotics would provide local action rather than systemic response as found today with oral or parenteral administration of these drugs.

IMPORTANT FACTS ABOUT INHALED MEDICATIONS

- Drugs for inhalation come in the form of powders, gases, sprays, and liquids.
- Medications given by inhalation are rapidly absorbed because of the blood supply to the lungs.
- MDIs are hand-held inhalers that disperse inhalation medications to the lungs. Use of an MDI requires coordination and strength to push the canister and breathe at the same time. Thus elderly patients may have difficulty using an MDI.

Summary

Percutaneous medication administration is easily accomplished and results in absorption of the drug through the skin, mucous membranes, or alveoli in lungs. The chance of systemic reactions is reduced because the medication is administered at the desired site, rather than having to reach the site through systemic absorption. The site of administration should be intact and adequately hydrated to absorb the medication. Use of percutaneous drugs to treat systemic illnesses is infrequent because topical agents are absorbed slowly and the dose absorbed is unreliable. The percutaneous route may be the route of choice when a slow, steady, extended-duration effect is desired.

Critical Thinking Exercises

SCENARIO

George has a large abrasion on his lower leg from falling while playing baseball. After the wound is cleaned, the area is covered with an antibiotic-impregnated dressing. The allied health professional should teach George how to change this dressing twice a day. George first asks why a systemic antibiotic has not been ordered. During the teaching, George informs you that he has the same antibiotic cream at home and wants to use that rather than buy the medication in an ointment form.

1. What do you tell him?
2. What do you tell George about the residue from previous dressings?
3. What can George do to make the medication go on smoothly and with little jerking motion to the skin?

REVIEW QUESTIONS

1. What is percutaneous medication administration? Why are these routes used? _____
    _____
    _____

2. What are the disadvantages to percutaneous medication administration? _____
    _____
    _____

3. Why are medications applied topically? What precautions should be taken? _____
    _____
    _____

4. What precautions should be taken with percutaneous applications of medications in the older person? _____
_____
_____

5. What label must be on medications that are used in the eye? _____
_____
_____

6. What is the proper position of the ear when instilling drops in a young child? In an adult? _____
_____
_____

7. What are the common indications for nasal medications? What are some of the newer indications for nasal sprays? _____
_____
_____

8. What are the forms of medications for vaginal administration? What documentation is necessary to show the patient was taught how to use the medication correctly? _____
_____
_____

CHAPTER 15

Parenteral Routes

OBJECTIVES

After studying this chapter, you should be capable of doing the following:

- Explaining the parenteral routes of medication administration.
- Describing how to select the appropriate syringe and needle for administering a parenteral medication.
- Preparing medications for parenteral administration from a vial or ampule.
- Mixing medications properly for injection.
- Reconstituting powders to liquid form for parenteral administration.
- Administering medications by intradermal (ID), subcutaneous (SC or SQ), and intramuscular (IM) routes.

Dr. Merry has ordered cyanocobalamin 1 mL subcutaneously once weekly, for Lynda, who has pernicious anemia. Dr. Merry has asked you to show Lynda how to give herself the injections.

What are the appropriate sites for these injections?
How often should the sites be rotated?
Which syringe should Lynda use?
What length needle should be used?
What gauge needle should be used with this aqueous solution?
What do you need to teach Lynda about aseptic technique?

KEY TERMS

Ampule	Filter needle	Lumen
Aqueous	Gauge	Subcutaneous
Aspirate	Intra-articular	Vial
Bevel	Intradermal	Viscous
Compatible	Intramuscular	Wheal
Diluent	Intravenous	

The word *parenteral* means outside the alimentary canal (Greek: *para* plus *enteron,* intestine). Parenteral administration of a substance such as a drug entails giving that substance by a route other than through the gastrointestinal (GI) tract and by injection, which is an invasive procedure with greater risks of administration than the oral or percutaneous routes. For this reason, injectable medications should only be given if a physician or other designated health professional is available to intervene in case of adverse reactions. The allied health professional in an ambulatory care setting may prepare medications and administer the medication, depending on the medical practice act of the state of employment. Parenteral injections are commonly given into the dermis of the skin, or **intradermally;** into the SC tissue, or **subcutaneously;** into the muscle, or **intramuscularly;** into joints, or **intra-articularly** (IA); or into veins, or **intravenously.** (See Chapter 11 for principles of intravenous [IV] therapy). Physicians may ask the assistance of allied health professionals when giving intra-articular injections because giving injections into joints is beyond the scope of practice for allied health professionals (Figure 15-1).

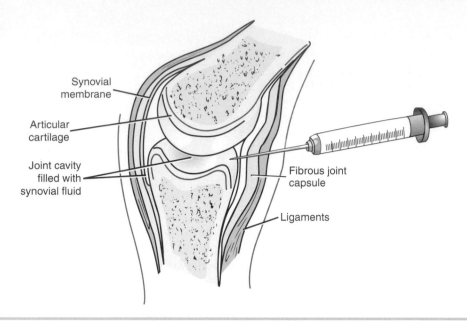

Figure 15-1 Intra-articular joint injections are performed by the physician with assistance from an allied health professional.

Advantages of Parenteral Administration

Drugs injected under the skin are not absorbed in the GI tract and are not initially metabolized in the liver. Therefore lower doses than those needed with oral administration are often given. The following are reasons for using parenteral medications:

- When medicines are inactivated by digestive juices, the parenteral route is the desired means of administration.
- The availability of the drug is increased because the medication enters circulation faster and with less inactivation due to metabolism prior to absorption.
- Duration of action of injected medications may be shorter than that of enteral medications.
- Injectable medications may be used in a patient unable to swallow because of unconsciousness or physical incapacity.
- Injections eliminate the loss of medicine when patients are vomiting or have gastric disorders that affect the absorption of medicines.
- Agents may be added to injectable medicines to prolong the desired effects.

Disadvantages of Parenteral Administration

The drawbacks to parenteral administration include the following:

- Pain occurs on administration.
- Infection is possible because the protective barrier provided by the skin has been broken.
- Once delivered under the skin, the drugs cannot be retrieved.
- Strict adherence to aseptic technique is necessary when administering medications parenterally.

Once the drug is under the skin, absorption occurs. Because of the dangers associated with injectable medications, the allied health professional should prepare these medications with extreme caution using 3 + 7 (Chapter 12), full knowledge of the drug and its route of administration, and aseptic technique. Failure to inject the medication properly may result in damage to nerves, an overly rapid response to the drug, pain, localized bleeding into the skin, sterile abscesses, and death of the tissue.

Special Precautions with Parenteral Medications

The following precautions are essential with parenteral medications:

- Parenteral medications must be sterile and in liquid form, except for some implants that are surgically inserted.

- A parenteral drug is usually administered in a solution that is minimally irritating to tissue such as physiologic saline or sterile water. The liquid may contain a preservative or a small amount of an antibiotic agent to prevent bacterial growth.
- *Always be sure that the patient receiving the injectable medication is not allergic to the additives or the base for the medicine being administered.*

IMPORTANT FACTS ABOUT PARENTERAL MEDICATIONS

- Medications given parenterally are delivered through the skin.
- The parenteral administration of medications requires strict sterile technique and care in selecting the correct gauge of needle, syringe, and site for administering the medication.
- Parenteral routes of medication administration that are most frequently seen in ambulatory care settings are intradermal, SC, and IM. A Z-track IM injection may be used for irritating medications or for drugs that stain the skin.
- Parenteral medications are used when enteral forms of drugs cannot be used, such as in patients who are vomiting, when a more rapid rate of action is desired, or when the drug would be inactivated by digestive juices.
- Drawbacks to the parenteral administration of drugs (i.e., injections) include pain on administration, inability to retrieve medications given in error, and the possibility of infection if aseptic technique is not followed.
- Parenteral medications must be sterile and in a liquid form. Additives are found in some parenteral medications, and the patient's sensitivity to such additives should be checked.

Equipment Selection for Injectable Medications

Medication Containers

Injectable medicines are supplied in dated, single-dose **ampules,** in single-dose or multidose **vials,** or in prefilled syringes. The person administering the drug should be sure that the expiration date has not passed and that the liquid has not deteriorated from improper storage. Safety of the patient and self should always be on the mind of the person administering medications, especially when the medicine is administered parenterally. Occupational Safety and Health Administration (OSHA) standards for needle handling should be followed at all times to prevent injury to the person giving the medicine.

Syringes

Syringes, both nondisposable glass types and disposable one-use types, come in a variety of sizes, from 60 mL to insulin syringes to some that hold only 0.5 mL (Figure 15-2). Some syringes are packaged with the needle attached (Figure 15-3). The most commonly used syringes in an ambulatory setting are 3-mL syringes and tuberculin syringes. A 5-mL syringe may be used when larger doses of medication are required, although the largest usual acceptable amount of medication to be given to an adult intramuscularly is 4 mL. An insulin syringe is commonly used for administration of insulin. Knowledge of how to choose the proper syringe for the amount of medication to be administered and its proper use is essential when administering an injectable drug. The improper choice of syringe may prohibit the correct dosage, especially when the amount to be given is small.

Syringe Selection

The appropriate syringe for injections is the smallest syringe that will hold the prescribed amount of medication. This determination ensures the most accurate measurement because the calibrations on the syringe will accurately show the amount to be given.

Safety with syringes includes the following:

- Retractable needle covers to prevent needle sticks from contaminated syringes (Figure 15-4).
- Injector pen, used most frequently for insulin administration (Figure 15-5). The type of injector pen depends on the medicine to be given and amount dispensed with each dose.
- Use disposable syringes to prevent cross-infection.
- Disposable syringes do not sustain damage from continuous use and do not require cleaning and sterilization following use. Specialty syringes may be found in nondisposable forms, but most syringes used in the ambulatory care setting are disposable.

Syringes consist of a cylindrical barrel with a tip designed to hold the needle and a plunger for delivery of the medicine (Figure 15-6). Syringe variations include the following:

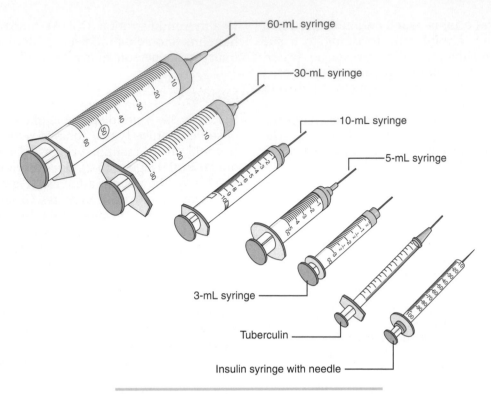

60-mL syringe

30-mL syringe

10-mL syringe

5-mL syringe

3-mL syringe

Tuberculin

Insulin syringe with needle

Figure 15-2 Disposable syringes in various sizes.

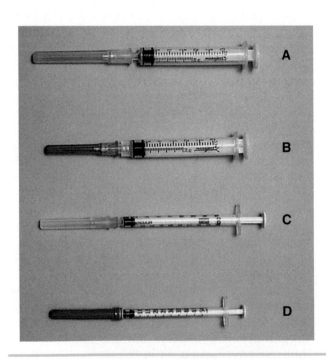

A

B

C

D

Figure 15-3 Various types of syringes with attached needles. **A,** Plain tip marked in 0.1 (tenths). **B,** Luer-Lok syringe marked in 0.1 (tenths). **C,** Tuberculin syringe marked in 0.01 (hundredths). **D,** Insulin syringe marked in units (50). (From Lilley L, Harrington S, Snyder J: *Pharmacology and the nursing process,* ed 4, St Louis, 2005, Mosby.)

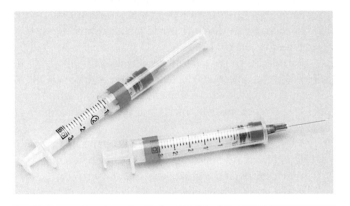

Figure 15-4 Disposable syringe with a retractable needle cover, as required by Occupational Safety and Health Administration standards.

- A tip that may be a plain tip where the needle slips onto the tip or a Luer-Lok tip used to prevent unwanted removal of the needle from the syringe, requiring the needle to be twisted onto the tip and locked in place.
- A barrel that indicates the amount of medication to be delivered by the specific syringe. The barrel, which holds the medication, is calibrated for measuring the dose. The inside of the barrel must remain sterile; the outside of the barrel may be touched (Figure 15-7).

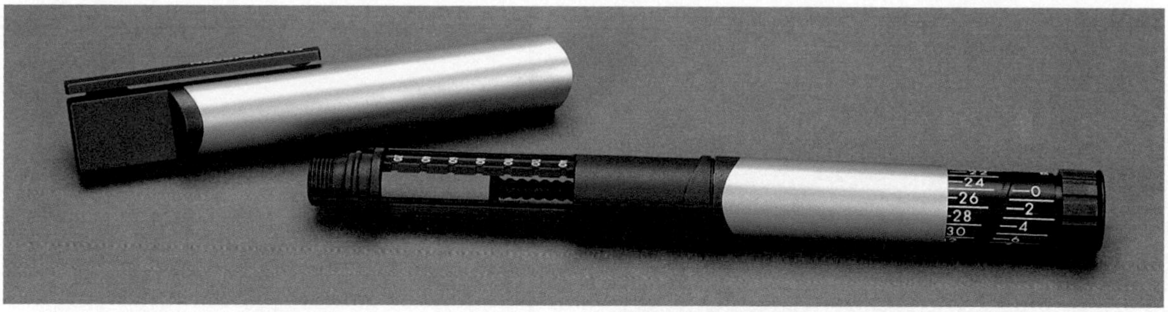

Figure 15-5 Injector pen for needleless administration of medication.

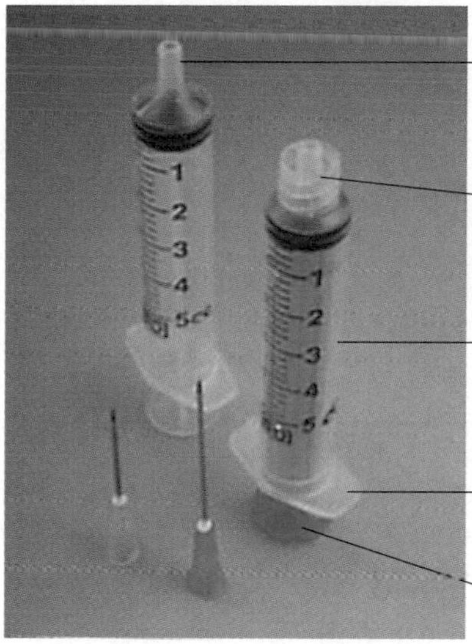
Plain tip
Luer-Lok tip
Barrel with measurements marked
Flange
Plunger

Figure 15-6 Parts of a syringe.

- A flange that keeps the cylindrical syringe from rolling when placed on a flat surface. The flange is also used to steady the hands when administering the injection.
- A plunger that is used to deliver the medication. The plunger must remain sterile within the barrel and should not be touched when outside the barrel (see Figure 15-7). The plunger fits inside the barrel and moves back and forth, forming a tight seal against the interior walls to draw and expel the medication.

Some syringes such as the 3-mL syringe are scaled in tenths of a milliliter (mL), cubic centimeters (cc), or minims (♏). Those with specific applications are scaled in hundredths of a milliliter, such as tuberculin syringes that hold 1 mL of liquid. Likewise, the U-100 insulin syringe holds 100 units of insulin to 1 mL. Insulin syringes that are designated as Lo-Dose syringes contain 50 units of insulin in 0.5 mL for persons with visual

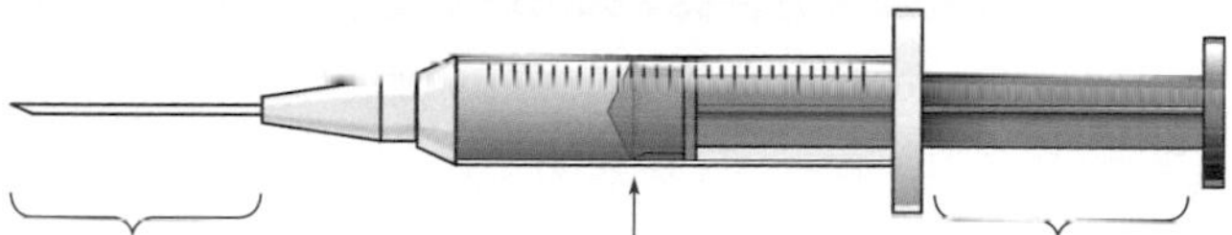
Keep sterile
Measure dose here
Avoid touching

Figure 15-7 Parts of a syringe that must not be touched. (From Perry A, Potter P: *Basic nursing skills*, ed 5, St Louis, 2003, Mosby.)

difficulties. If the latter type of syringe is used, the medical record should include specific documentation of the patient's preference and uses in case a prescription is necessary.

IMPORTANT FACTS ABOUT SYRINGES

- Syringes may be disposable or nondisposable and may hold from 0.5 mL to 60 mL. The syringes most commonly used in the ambulatory care setting are 3-mL syringes and tuberculin syringes.
- The smallest syringe that will hold the amount of medication to be given should be used.
- Injector pens are available for use with insulin or for allergic reactions such as the EpiPen.

Needles

Needles for injection are made in many lengths and widths/diameters, or **gauges** (Figure 15-8). The proper choice of needle depends on the depth needed for placement of the injection and the **viscosity** or thickness of the medication to be administered. The needle is actually a hollow metal tube with a sharp point that pierces the skin to deliver the medication. Needles may be purchased separately, or the needle may come attached to the syringe. In other cases the syringe and needle are separate but are prepackaged together as a needle-syringe unit for specific uses.

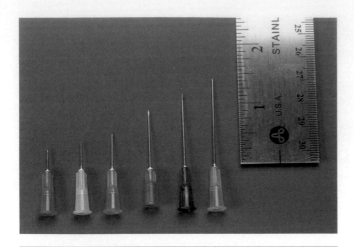

Figure 15-8 Needle lengths used in ambulatory care settings.

Four factors are important in needle selection: safety, rate of flow of the medication, comfort for the patient, and the depth to which the needle must penetrate to deliver the drug to the appropriate site.

Needles are constructed with three specific points—regular point for general injection use, short **bevel** for use with subcutaneous injections, and intradermal bevel for intradermal injection use (Figure 15-9).

Needle Selection

Needle gauges range from size 14, which has the largest lumen or opening, to size 31, which has the smallest lumen. The smallest possible needle that will administer the desired medication with the least pain is the needle of choice. Thirty-one-gauge needles are short and most frequently used on injection pens for insulin and in dermatology and plastic surgery. The gauge with the highest number (29 or 27) has a small lumen and is short ($3/8$ to $5/8$ inch) to prevent the needle bending with injections.

The needles with small lumens (large gauges) are used for **aqueous** medications that are delivered just under the surface because the length of the needle is usually short. Needles with gauges 27 to 25 and $5/8$ to $7/8$ inch long are commonly used for aqueous SC injections. These needles cause minimal pain and less tissue damage. A person with thick skin may find a 25-gauge needle more comfortable than a 29-gauge needle because the needle will not bend on insertion. Larger needles, gauges 23 to 20, are used for IM injections of thicker, or **viscous,** medications into muscular tissue. The needle must be at least 1 inch long and of thicker gauge for the support needed to reach the muscle. The patient

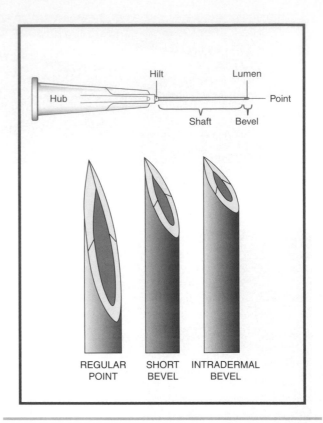

Figure 15-9 Types of needle points. (From Young AP, Proctor DB: *Kinn's the medical assistant: an applied learning approach,* ed 10, St Louis, 2007, Saunders.)

cannot feel the difference between a 20-gauge and a 22-gauge needle, and the 20-gauge needle will supply medications with less resistance from the skin when administering medications that are fairly viscous (see Figure 15-8). The general rules for selecting needles and syringes are reviewed in Box 15-1.

IMPORTANT FACTS ABOUT NEEDLES

- Needles for injection come in many lengths and gauges. The choice of needle depends on the site and route of injection, as well as the viscosity of the medication to be given.
- Needles have retractable covers to meet OSHA standards.
- The four factors in needle selection are safety, comfort for the patient, rate of flow of the medication, and the depth of injection needed to deliver the drug to the proper site.
- Needles come with three specific points—regular point (for general injection use), short bevel (for use with SC route injection), and intradermal bevel (for ID use).

BOX 15-1   GENERAL RULES FOR INJECTIONS

- Use disposable syringes when possible to prevent cross contamination.
- Use aseptic technique when preparing medications for injection. If contamination occurs, discard the medication being prepared and start over.
- Remember that disposable needles are sharp and coated with silicon for smooth injection.
- Observe that disposable needle-syringe units are color coded for needle gauge/length and packaged in paper wraps or rigid plastic containers with shields over the needle.
- Never swab the shaft of the needle.
- Always use a filter needle to withdraw medication from a glass ampule to prevent glass particles from being aspirated into the fluid for injection.
- Know the volume and characteristics of the medication to be administered. Giving volumes too large for the site will cause pain and destruction of the tissue involved.
- Recap needles on medications for injection for delivery to the room where the administration will take place. Do not wrap the needle in a cotton ball or wipe.
- Never combine two medications in a syringe unless specifically ordered to do so.
- When preparing medications for the physician to give, place the container from which medication was obtained beside the filled syringe.
- Choose sites of injection that are free of restrictive clothing and are not in areas where lymph nodes have been surgically removed. With a postmastectomy patient, the arm on the side of the mastectomy should be avoided, as should an area of trauma or burn.
- Use correct technique and identify the correct landmarks when administering medications by injection.
- Tell the patient that a little discomfort is to be expected but will last only a short time.

IMPORTANT FACTS ABOUT NEEDLES—*Cont'd*

- Needle gauges found in ambulatory care are from 18 (a large lumen) to 31 (smallest lumen). Lengths found in the ambulatory care setting are $3/8$ inch to 2 inches and are selected according to the size of the patient, the site of injection, and the viscosity of the medication.
- Aqueous medications require a smaller lumen, while drugs in oil or viscous bases are administered through a needle with a larger lumen.
- All contaminated needles should be discarded in puncture-proof biohazard waste containers.

Containers for Injectable Medications

Parenteral medications must be sterile and come in three types of containers—vials, ampules, and prefilled syringes (Figure 15-10). Before using any injectable medications, be sure to check the expiration date.

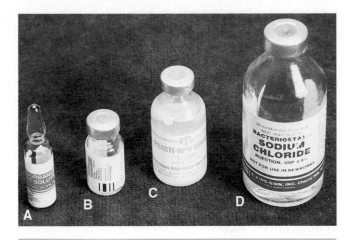

Figure 15-10 A, Ampule. **B,** Single-dose vial. **C** and **D,** Multidose vials. (From Young AP, Proctor DB: *Kinn's the medical assistant: an applied learning approach*, ed 10, St Louis, 2007, Saunders.)

Ampules

Ampules are small, hermetically sealed glass containers that hold a single dose of sterile medication. The neck of an ampule is thin and is broken just before use. Medications in ampules that are not used in entirety should never be kept for later use because sterility cannot be assured once the ampule is broken (Procedure 15-1).

Vials

Vials come in both single-dose and multidose sizes. A single-dose vial, a small glass container with a rubber stopper on top, holds only one dose of an injectable medication or diluent for reconstitution. A sterile needle is inserted through the rubber stopper to withdraw the fluid. Some single-dose vials may contain a powder that must be reconstituted to liquid form. If reconstitution is required, follow the directions with the medication *exactly*. Each vial is labeled with the name of the medication and the weight of medication per liquid volume (in milliliters), after reconstitution if applicable.

Multidose vials contain enough medicine for multiple injections from the same container. Multidose vials may contain from 1 mL to 100 mL or more. When multidose vials are used, great care must be exercised each time the vial is entered to prevent contamination of the solution. If you suspect that contamination of a multidose vial has occurred or if an error in preparing the medication occurs, discard the vial and start over. When withdrawing medications from a multidose vial, the drug should be withdrawn to the exact amount and excess waste

PROCEDURE 15-1   Preparing a Medication from an Ampule

Objective: To accurately prepare a medication from an ampule.

Guidelines

Equipment Needed
- Medication order
- Ampule of medication to meet medication order
- Syringe and filter needle
- Alcohol swab
- Sterile gauze
- Needle of proper length

Methodology 3+7

1. To open an ampule, gently tap above the neck to release the medication into the larger bottom section of the glass container.

2. Wipe the neck of the ampule with an alcohol wipe to disinfect the outside of the container.

3. With sterile gauze around the ampule, forcefully snap your wrists away from you so that the neck of the ampule snaps to break in two. If the glass does not break easily, rotate the ampule a quarter turn and try again. If that does not allow opening, or if the ampule does not have a scored line, score the neck with a file and disinfect again. The glass of the ampule is designed not to shatter so that the medication will not spill.

4. When the ampule opens, you will hear a pop as the vacuum on the container is released. Discard the top of the ampule in the sharps container.

5. Uncap the filter needle and insert it into the ampule opening without touching the sides of the ampule. Gently pull back on the syringe plunger, keeping the tip of the needle in the liquid medication. If necessary, turn the ampule to the side to obtain all available drug or amount of drug needed for the desired dose. The container is designed to prevent spillage on tipping.

6. Recap the filter needle and dispose of it in the sharps container.

7. Place the proper gauge and length needle for administration on the syringe.

8. Discard the used supplies in the biohazard container.

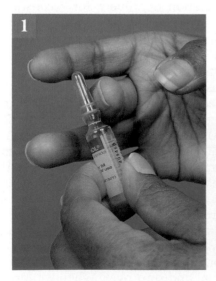
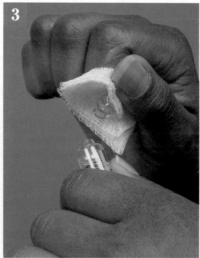
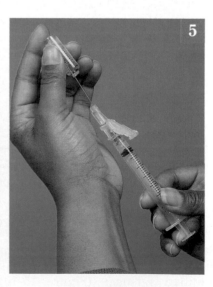

should be avoided. Of importance for ease of with-drawing medications, the pressure within the vial must be kept equal by adding air to replace the medication being withdrawn (Procedure 15-2).

Prefilled Syringe

A prefilled syringe is a sterile, disposable syringe-and-needle unit that is packaged to supply a single dose of a given medication. A prefilled syringe should never be used to administer a second dose, except with the new methods of insulin administration, where the prefilled unit is designed to be used repeatedly by the same patient.

Disposable Injection Units

Some medications come in single-dose prefilled syringes that require the use of a medication cartridge for administration. With these units, the health professional does not need to prepare the dose except perhaps to expel a volume of medication that is in excess of the dose ordered by the physician. The prefilled medication injection systems are purchased by the box, and the cartridge loader is reused. Tubex and Carpujet injection systems provide a cartridge that slips onto the cartridge loader for injection (Figure 15-11, Procedure 15-3).

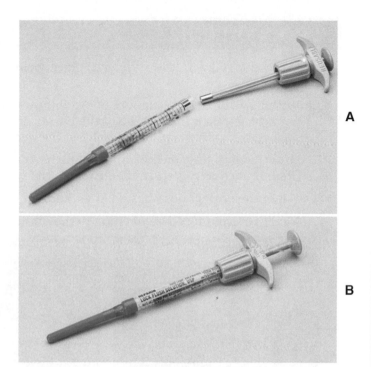

Figure 15-11 Components of a closed prefilled medication injection syringe. **A,** Unassembled. **B,** Assembled. (From Young AP, Proctor DB: *Kinn's the medical assistant: an applied learning approach*, ed 10, St Louis, 2007, Saunders.)

PROCEDURE 15-2   Preparing a Medication from a Vial

Objective: To accurately prepare a dose of medication from a vial.

Guidelines

Equipment Needed
- Medication order
- Vial of desired medication to meet medication order
- Syringe and needle
- Alcohol swab

Methodology 3+7

1. If the vial is being used for the first time, the metal or plastic cap covering the rubber stopper must be removed.

2. Cleanse the stopper, from center outward, with an alcohol wipe to prevent contamination of the fluid in the vial.

3. To withdraw medication from a vial, the pressure in the vial must be kept equal. After removing the cover on the needle, draw air into the syringe in a volume that will equal the volume of liquid to be withdrawn from the vial. The withdrawn medication must be replaced with an equal amount of air to maintain equal pressure within the vial to prevent a vacuum from forming, and for ease of aspiration. If too little air is injected, the medication will be difficult to remove because of the vacuum. If too much air is injected, the air will force the medication into the syringe without pulling on the plunger to withdraw it.

4. Insert the needle into the rubber cap and inject the air into the vial.

(continued)

PROCEDURE 15-2   Preparing a Medication from a Vial—cont'd

5   Invert the vial with the syringe in place, being sure that the needle remains below the surface of the liquid.

6   Withdraw the desired amount of medicine and withdraw the needle from the vial. If air remains in the syringe, flick the outside of the barrel. The bubbles should float into the needle hub to be pushed out with the plunger, holding the needle pointing straight up.

7.   Draw back slightly on the plunger and then push the plunger to expel air, being careful not to expel fluid. If necessary, return the needle to the vial to obtain the correct dosage.

8.   When the correct dose has been withdrawn into the syringe, remove the needle from the vial.

9.   Never return unused medication to the multidose vial.

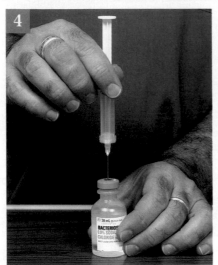
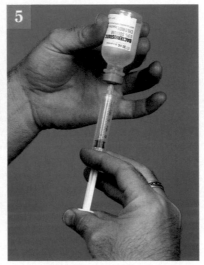
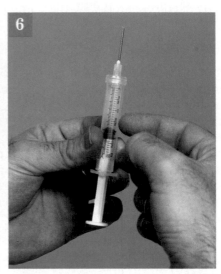

PROCEDURE 15-3   Preparing a Medication Using a Disposable Injection Unit

Objective: To accurately prepare a dose of medication using a disposable injection unit.

Guidelines

Equipment Needed
- Medication order
- Prefilled disposable injection unit to meet medication order
- Tubex or Carpujet injector

Methodology 3+7

1   To load the injector, hold the injector in a vertical position with the plunger rod in one hand. With the other hand, turn the injector clockwise until it stops. This places the assembly in the open position for loading.

2.   Insert the cartridge with the covered needle attached to the open end.

3   Turn counterclockwise until the prefilled syringe is tight and the cartridge is in the closed position.

4.   Engage the plunger rod onto the threads of the cartridge plunger of the sterile medication cartridge.

5   Rotate the plunger clockwise until resistance is felt. This indicates that the system is ready for use and is secure.

PROCEDURE 15-3 | Preparing a Medication Using a Disposable Injection Unit—cont'd

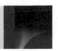

6 Following administration of the drug to the patient, remove the plunger rod from the cartridge.

7 The entire prefilled cartridge is deposited of in a sharps container, holding the injector with the needle down. The loader is reusable and should be sanitized and saved. This system is designed to reduce the risk of needle-stick injuries.

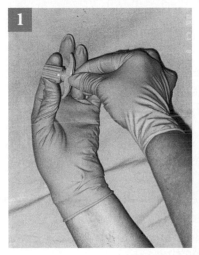
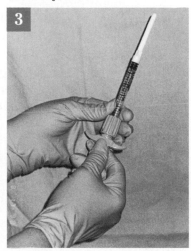
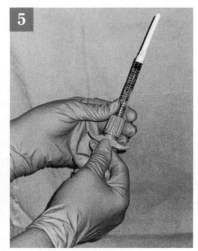

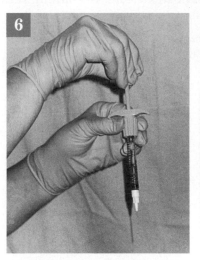
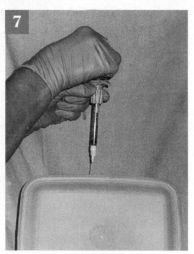

Preparation of Medications for Injections

Reconstitution of Powder Forms of Medication

Some medications that are unstable in liquid form are packaged as a powder for reconstitution at the time of administration. The vial label specifies the amount of diluent to be used to dissolve the powdered drug to prepare the correct concentration of the medication. Both the powder and the diluent must be sterile because these will be injected under the skin. After reconstitution, the weight/volume of medication should be designated on the vial. The expiration and reconstitution dates should also be shown (Procedure 15-4).

Mixing Two Medications for Administration

Occasionally two medications from vials or ampules are mixed for ease of administration and to prevent more than one injection. Before mixing medications,

PROCEDURE 15-4   Reconstituting Medications from Powders

Objective: To accurately reconstitute powdered medications to the appropriate strength.

Guidelines

Equipment Needed

- Powder to be reconstituted to meet medication order
- Vial of specified diluent as designated by manufacturer
- Alcohol wipes
- Proper syringe and needle

Methodology   3+7

1. Using the indicated diluent (as specified on the medication package), withdraw the correct amount (as specified on the medication package to provide the proper strength) from the vial. (Note: Some medications require bacteriostatic water as a diluent, some call for sterile normal saline, and yet others have the needed diluent provided with the medication.)

2. Use the same precautions to maintain sterility as when opening an ampule or vial—cleanse the ampule top with alcohol and ensure sterile aseptic technique. Remember to add air to allow for withdrawal of the diluent.

3. Invert the vial for ease of withdrawal. After cleaning the top of the powder vial, insert the needle into the powdered medication vial and inject the diluent.

4. Mix the powder and diluent by gently rolling the vial between your hands until the powder and diluent are completely mixed. (Note: Some medications require shaking rather than rolling; be sure to read the medication label for directions.)

5. If the reconstituted medication is in a multidose vial, write the reconstituted strength, the date of reconstitution, and your initials on the vial. Store according to label directions. (Note that some medications must be refrigerated after reconstitution.)

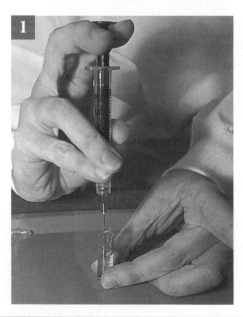

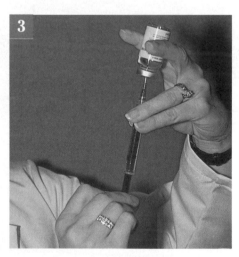

the health care professional should be sure that the medications to be mixed are **compatible.** Each vial of medication must have the correct amount of air added and then aspirated correctly to prevent a vacuum. Care must be taken to prevent cross contamination of the medications when using multidose vials.

When mixing medications in an ampule and a vial or in two single-dose vials, the mixing is relatively easy because it is not necessary to add air to the ampule. In the case of an ampule and a vial, prepare the medication from the vial first and then from the ampule. When mixing from two single-dose vials, add air to each and withdraw medications as if preparing an injection using one vial. When mixing medications from two multidose vials, follow the steps outlined in Procedure 15-5.

If insulin is to be prepared, special guidelines apply when mixing two types of insulin. This order is necessary to prevent precipitation of insulin in the barrel (Figure 15-12).

1. Regular insulin may be mixed with any other type of insulin but should be drawn into the syringe first.
2. NPH insulin may be mixed only with regular insulin.
3. Lente insulins may be mixed together or with regular insulin but should not be mixed with other types of insulin.
4. Humulin insulin preparations may be mixed only with other Humulin insulin preparations.

IMPORTANT FACTS ABOUT MIXING MEDICATIONS
- Occasionally two medications may be mixed for a single injection. Be sure that the medications are compatible prior to mixing.
- When mixing medications from an ampule and a vial, draw the medicine from the vial first and then the ampule. If drawing from two vials, inject the air into vial A prior to injecting air into vial B, followed by preparing the drug from vial B. Finally, return to vial A to withdraw the needed medicine.

PROCEDURE 15-5   Mixing Medications Using Two Multidose Vials

Objective: To accurately prepare two medications from two multidose vials for administration as one injection.

Guidelines

Equipment Needed
- Medication order
- Two medication vials to meet medication order
- Syringe with needle
- Extra needles
- Alcohol wipes

Methodology 3+7

1. Using a sterile syringe, aspirate the volume of air needed to replace the medication to be removed from vial A.

2. Inject air into vial A. Be sure the needle does not touch the solution in vial A.

3. Hold the plunger and remove the syringe from vial A. Aspirate the air needed to replace the volume of fluid to be removed from vial B.

4. Insert the syringe into vial B, injecting the air and removing the proper amount of medication for the ordered dose.

5. Withdraw the syringe and needle from vial B and check the dosage to ensure the proper volume has been obtained. Change the needle.

6. Find the point on the syringe where the total of both medications should measure. Insert the needle into vial A, taking extreme care not to allow the medication from vial B to enter vial A. Hold the plunger and carefully withdraw the amount of medication for the ordered dose.

PROCEDURE 15-5   Mixing Medications Using Two Multidose Vials—cont'd

7. Withdraw the needle and expel any excess air or fluid. Change the needle as appropriate.

8. Prepare the medication for administration by the proper route.

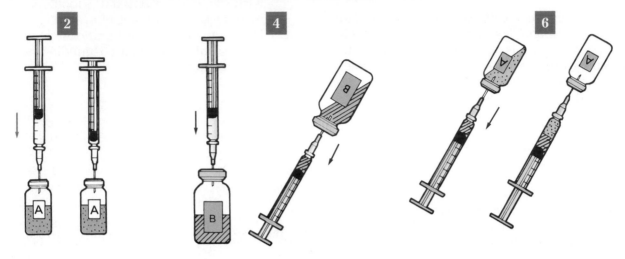

Administering Injectable Medications

When administering injectable medications, technique is important for the following reasons:

1. To prevent injury to nerves, blood vessels, and tissues
2. To prevent the possibility of infection locally or systemically
3. To avoid undue pain for the patient

Always explain the procedure to the patient for the following reasons:

- To relieve anxiety
- To be honest with the patient. Tell the person that the injection may hurt for a short time, not that it will not hurt at all.

Having assistance in holding a child is advisable.

As a health care professional, you may need to explain to parents how to explain the need for injections to the child. Injections should never be used as a threat for disciplinary actions. Box 15-2 lists tips for administering medications by injection. When injectable medications are given using incorrect methodology, legal repercussions may occur.

Routes of Administration and the Common Indications

Certain indications for medications designate the route of administration (Table 15-1).

Administering Intradermal Injections

Intradermal injections are most frequently used for tuberculin skin testing and allergy testing. The drug is injected into the top layer of skin, where many nerves are present, thus causing momentary burning or stinging (Procedure 15-6).

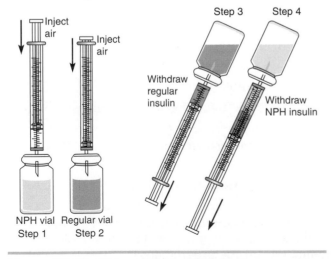

Figure 15-12 Mixing regular and NPH insulin in one syringe.

- The needle is inserted at a 10- to 15-degree angle into the dermis of the skin.
- The injection is administered using a tuberculin syringe or a small syringe with a short (generally $3/8$ inch), fine-gauge needle (26 to 28 gauge or possibly smaller) with an intradermal bevel.
- Use only small amounts of the medication (usually ≤ 0.1 mL) to form a **wheal** (Figure 15-14).
- The sites for intradermal injection are the forearm, upper back, upper dorsal aspect of the arm, and upper chest (Figure 15-15).
- Avoid scarred, blemished, or hairy areas.

Administering Medications Subcutaneously

Subcutaneous medications are injected into the adipose tissue (see Figure 15-13) (Procedure 15-7). SC tissue is not as richly supplied with blood vessels as muscle is, so drugs administered subcutaneously are not as rapidly absorbed. The following are guidelines for administering SC injections:

- Smaller doses (≤ 2 mL) of nonirritating, nonviscous medications, usually in an aqueous base, are appropriate for SC administration.
- The connective tissue under the skin is sensitive to irritating solutions and may form abscesses as the medication collects under the skin if absorption does not occur.
- The best sites for SC injection include the posterior upper arm (in the fatty tissue over the triceps), the abdomen, and the anterior aspects of the thigh.
- The upper back and upper ventral/dorsal gluteal areas may also be used (Figure 15-16). These areas, except for the upper back, are convenient for the person who self-injects insulin.
- Injection sites should be free of infection, lesions, and scars and be away from bony prominences and large underlying muscle or nerves.
- The injection site should be rotated on a regular basis.
- The amount of adipose tissue determines the choice of needle length and the insertion angle; generally the needle is 25 gauge, $5/8$ inch long, with a regular or short bevel, and the angle of insertion is 30 to 45 degrees.
- If the patient is obese, a longer needle may be necessary to reach the subcutaneous tissue.
- Insulin, heparin, allergy injections, and some therapeutic medications are given by SC administration.

BOX 15-2 GUIDELINES FOR INJECTING MEDICATIONS

- Use the smallest gauge and shortest length needle that is appropriate.
- If the liquid has coated the needle while preparing the injection, change the needle so that the medication will not be uncomfortable going through the subcutaneous tissue.
- Position the injection site to reduce the muscle tension.
- Medications should not be given near bones or blood vessels, nor should they be injected into areas where lymph nodes have been removed, such as in the arms of postmastectomy patients.
- When giving the injection, try to divert the attention of the patient. If the patient is scared, have the patient look in some place other than the injection site.
- Insert the needle into the tissue smoothly, quickly, and without hesitation. A jerking motion increases the pain.
- When injecting the medication, do so slowly but smoothly.
- When the syringe is in the tissue, hold it steady to prevent damage to the tissue.
- Withdraw the needle at the same angle of insertion into the skin. Be sure to use the proper angle for the type of injection being given (Figure 15-13). Wipe the injection site with an alcohol pad after removing the needle to prevent the chance of infection. The same aseptic techniques as are used in minor surgery should be used to administer parenteral medications.
- Apply gentle pressure at the injection site after administration if appropriate for the medication. Massaging the area will increase the rate of absorption if needed.
- Rotate injection sites to prevent the formation of areas of induration or abscesses and to prevent thickening of the skin from continuous injections.
- Be sure the injection site is free of constrictive clothing. Remove any clothing that may restrict absorption.
- Follow the steps necessary for the preparation of medications (3 + 7). Injections require the use of gloves and the proper disposal of biohazardous waste. OSHA guidelines on recapping needles must be followed.

TABLE 15-1 *Indications for the Routes of Administration*

TECHNIQUE	USE
Intradermal (ID)	Allergy, tuberculin skin testing
Subcutaneous (SC)	Immunizations, insulin
Intramuscular (IM)	Immunizations, analgesics, antibiotics, hormones, corticosteroids
Intramuscular Z-Track	To prevent leakage of medications into subcutaneous tissue, especially when medications will discolor skin

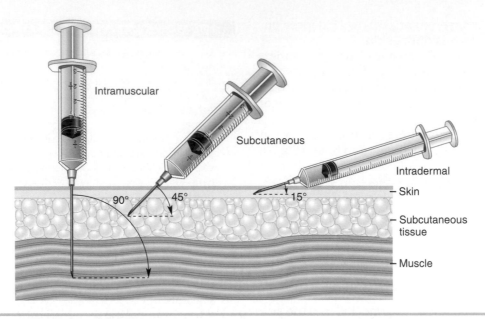

Figure 15-13 Needle angles for injecting medications. (From Hunt SA: *Saunders fundamentals of medical assisting,* St Louis, 2007, Saunders.)

PROCEDURE 15-6   Giving an Intradermal Injection

Objective: To give an intradermal injection that produces a wheal.

Guidelines

Equipment Needed
- Medication order
- Medication appropriate to meet medication order
- Tuberculin syringe
- Short, small-gauge, intradermal beveled needle
- Alcohol wipe

Methodology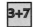

1. Prepare medication dose to the physician's order.

2. Identify the patient, locate the proper site for the injection, and wipe it in a circular motion with alcohol pad, from the center outward. If injecting in the forearm, choose a nonhairy area.

3. Stretch the skin tight with your nondominant thumb and index finger to facilitate injecting just under the skin.

4. Insert the needle, with the bevel up, into the outermost layer of the skin at a 10- to 15-degree angle.

5. Slowly inject the medication just under the skin so that a wheal is formed on the skin.

6. Withdraw the needle and wipe the skin with an alcohol swab. Do not massage the area because this will affect the final reading of the test. Do not apply pressure because this may force medication to leak from under the skin.

7. Discard the syringe and needle in the sharps container. Discard the gloves in the biohazard waste container. Sanitize hands.

PROCEDURE 15-6   Giving an Intradermal Injection—cont'd

8. Document the procedure. Tell the patient to return in the designated time to have the test read.

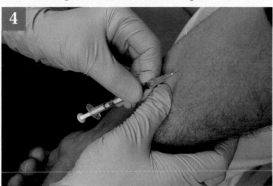
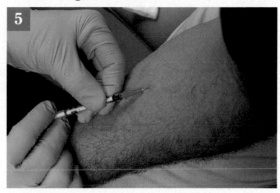

TYPICAL DOCUMENTATION

3/18/0X 10:15 AM PPD 0.1 mL administered ID, RT forearm with no apparent side effects. Told to keep area clean and not to massage the area. Instructed to return in 72 hours for reading of test. Appointment card given for test reading. _____ G. OLSEN, CMA

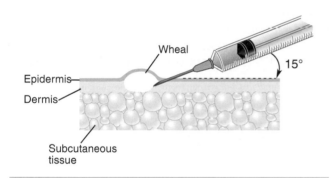

Figure 15-14 A wheal is formed by an intradermal injection. (From Hunt SA: *Saunders fundamentals of medical assisting,* St Louis, 2007, Saunders.)

Administering Medications Intramuscularly

Intramuscular injections are used when a person needs a medication requiring more rapid absorption than through subcutaneous tissue or the medication would be irritating to the subcutaneous tissue. The abundance of blood vessels in the muscle tissue results in faster drug absorption.

- An aqueous solution is absorbed in 10 to 30 minutes.
- The increased danger of injecting the medication into a blood vessel does exist because of increased vascularity.
- IM injections are used when the volume is too large for subcutaneous tissues.

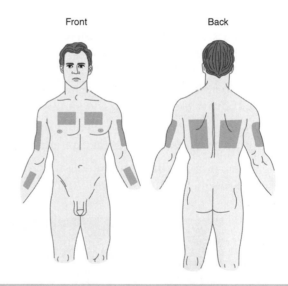

Figure 15-15 Sites for intradermal injections. (From Hunt SA: *Saunders fundamentals of medical assisting,* St Louis, 2007, Saunders.)

- Viscous medications should be injected into muscle.
- The maximum safe dosage for a well-developed adult is routinely 3 mL, although tolerance up to 4 mL of medication is possible in the larger muscles such as the gluteus medius. The thin adult should receive a maximum of 2 mL. Small children, especially those younger than 2 years of age, should receive no more than 1 mL by IM injection.

PROCEDURE 15-7   Giving a Subcutaneous Injection

Objective: To give an SC injection safely.

Guidelines

Equipment Needed
- Medication order
- Appropriate syringe (3-mL, tuberculin, or insulin syringe)
- Appropriate needle gauge and length (usually 25 to 27 gauge, $5/8$ inch length)
- Medication appropriate for the medication order
- Alcohol wipe
- Band-Aid

Methodology 3+7

1. Prepare medication dose according to the medication order.

2. Identify the patient and locate the proper site for the injection (see Figure 15-16). Wipe the area in a circular motion, from injection site outward, using an alcohol wipe.

3. Grasp the skin firmly with your nondominant hand, gently pinching the subcutaneous tissue between the thumb and index finger to minimize the discomfort.

4. Insert the needle at a 45-degree angle. The angle may increase to 90 degrees in an obese person and may decrease to 15 to 45 degrees for the thin or pediatric person.

5. Release the skin and aspirate on the plunger to be sure no blood enters the hub. If no blood appears, slowly and steadily inject the medication. If blood enters the hub, immediately withdraw the syringe and compress the site. If blood has mixed with the medication, prepare the medication again. If the needle is removed from the site and the medication is not contaminated with blood, change the needle prior to injecting in another site.

7. Withdraw the needle at the same angle of insertion.

8. Apply pressure with the alcohol wipe to keep the site from bleeding. Gently massage the site if appropriate for the medication administered. Apply Band-Aid as indicated.

9. Discard the syringe and needle in the sharps container. Discard the gloves in the biohazard waste container. Sanitize hands.

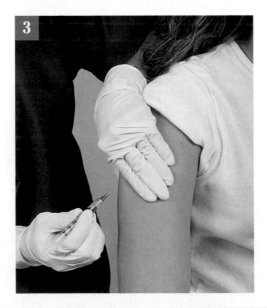

PROCEDURE 15–7   Giving a Subcutaneous Injection—cont'd

10. Document the procedure. If the injection given was desensitization for allergies or other medication with increased possibility for allergic reactions, the patient must stay for 20 minutes following the injection, depending on office policy.

TYPICAL DOCUMENTATION

3/18/0X 11:00 AM cyanocobalamin 0.5 mL SC in the RT upper arm with no apparent adverse reactions.
_____G. OLSEN, CMA

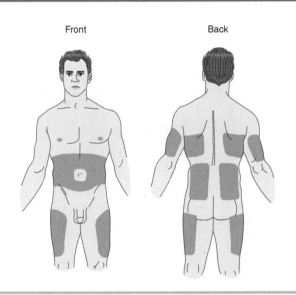

Front   Back

Figure 15-16 Sites for subcutaneous injections. (From Hunt SA: *Saunders fundamentals of medical assisting,* St Louis, 2007, Saunders.)

- When choosing the injection site, the appropriate needle selection must penetrate beyond the fat layer.
- A longer and heavier-gauge needle is necessary to pass into the muscle tissue. Generally for the adult, a 20- to 23-gauge, 1- to 1½-inch needle is used to enter the deeper tissue at a 90-degree angle (see Figure 15-13).
- Pediatric, geriatric, or thin, emaciated persons may require a smaller-gauge, shorter needle because of less muscle mass.
- Muscle tissue that has lost muscle mass should be avoided if at all possible.
- Always aspirate before injecting medication to be sure the needle is not in a blood vessel.

A special type of IM injection is the Z-track technique, which is recommended for irritating or staining medications such as iron dextran. A zigzag path of insertion seals the needle track to prevent leakage back into the subcutaneous tissue and to minimize pain.

- The tissue is displaced downward or laterally for about 1 to 1½ inches by holding it to the side of the injection site (Figure 15-17).
- After medicine to be given by the Z-track technique has been prepared, the needle on the syringe should be changed to prevent irritation to the tissue as the needle passes into the muscle.
- Inject the drug slowly and release the skin after removing the needle.

Sites for Intramuscular Injections

The common sites for IM injections are the deltoid area of the upper arm, the dorsogluteal or upper outer portion of the hip, the ventrogluteal or lateral outside portion of the hip, and the vastus lateralis or midportion of the thigh. When administering IM injections, positioning of the patient for observation of the entire site is of utmost importance.

Deltoid Site

The deltoid area of the arm is often used only in the adult for IM injections because it is easily accessible for injections of less than 2 mL. The ideal amount of a medication given in the deltoid area is 0.5 to 1 mL.

- Preferably, the person is seated, although the injection can also be given with the patient standing or lying down.
- The patient's arm should be flexed and relaxed.

To locate the deltoid muscle (the radial and ulnar nerves and the brachial artery lie within this area), expose the upper arm and shoulder, removing a tight-fitting garment. Relax the arm at the side and then flex the elbow to find the

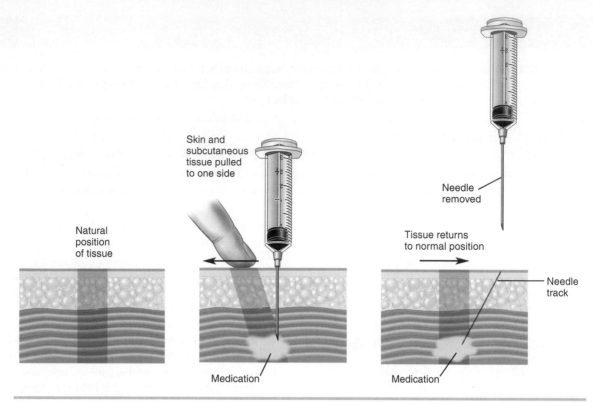

Figure 15-17 Administering medication using the Z-track method. (From Hunt SA: *Saunders fundamentals of medical assisting,* St Louis, 2007, Saunders.)

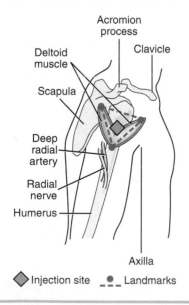

Figure 15-18 Site for an intramuscular injection in the deltoid area. (From Leahy JM, Kizilay PE: *Foundations of nursing practice: a nursing process approach,* Philadelphia, 1998, Saunders.)

triangle-shaped area formed by the deltoid muscle. The injection site is in the center of the triangle, or about 1 to 2 inches below the acromion process. Figure 15-18 shows the site of needle insertion for injections into the deltoid muscle.

Dorsogluteal Site

Traditionally, IM injections have been given in the dorsogluteal muscle. Extreme caution is necessary when using this area because of the underlying sciatic nerve and the major blood vessels of the gluteal trunk. Penetrating the sciatic nerve with a needle may cause permanent or partial paralysis of the involved leg. Therefore, the current recommendation is that this site should not be used routinely.

- This site should not be used in infants or in small children younger than 12 years old who have small muscle mass.
- Always protect the patient's privacy when using the dorsogluteal site for injection.
- Be sure the person receiving the injection can move his or her leg after administering the injection.

To locate the exact site, the patient should be prone with the toes pointed inward to relax the muscles. Draw an imaginary diagonal line starting at the greater trochanter of the femur, across the buttocks, to the posterior spine of the ilium. Locate the bony prominences to be sure you have the correct site. The injection is made into the gluteus medius muscle several inches below the iliac crest (Figure 15-19).

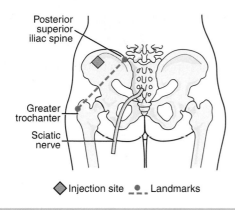

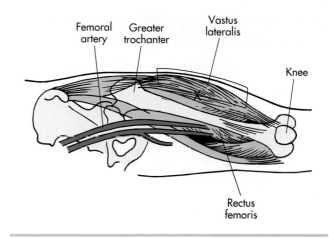

Figure 15-19 Site for an intramuscular injection in the dorsogluteal area. (From Leahy JM, Kizilay PE: *Foundations of nursing practice: a nursing process approach*, Philadelphia, 1998, Saunders.)

Figure 15-21 Site for intramuscular injection in the vastus lateralis. (From Perry AG, Potter PA: *Clinical nursing skills and techniques*, ed 6, St Louis, 2006, Mosby.)

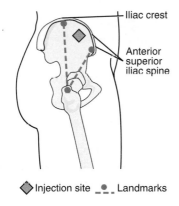

Figure 15-20 Site for an intramuscular injection in the ventrogluteal area. (From Leahy JM, Kizilay PE: *Foundations of nursing practice: a nursing process approach*, Philadelphia, 1998, Saunders.)

To locate this area, place the heel of the hand over the greater trochanter of the hip with the wrist almost perpendicular to the femur, using the right hand for the left hip and the left hand for the right hip. The index finger should be on the anterior iliac spine. Spread the middle finger back as far as possible from the index finger, attempting to touch the crest of the ilium (Figure 15-20). The center of the triangle formed by the index finger and middle finger is the site for the injection.

Vastus Lateralis and Rectus Femoris Sites

The vastus lateralis and rectus femoris are parts of the quadriceps muscle group, one of the largest muscle groups, and are found in the thigh.

Ventrogluteal Site

This site including the gluteus medius and minimus muscles is considered safe, although it is not used as often as other muscle tissue.

- It is free of major nerves and blood vessels and has a relatively large muscle mass.
- The site is considered safe for infants, children, and adults.
- All IM medications may be injected here including thick, viscous medications.
- The ventrogluteal site is not associated with some of the injuries, such as fibrosis, tissue necrosis, and nerve damage, that are associated with other IM injection sites.
- For a child, a 1-inch needle may be used, whereas for an obese adult, the needle may need to be 2 to 2½ inches long.

- These muscles are considered safe for use in infants less than 7 months old because the muscles are well developed at birth.
- This is considered a safe site in adults because it contains few major nerves and blood vessels.
- The adult may stand or sit, but the site is easier to find with the person in supine position.

The vastus lateralis fills the midportion of the upper outer thigh from one handbreadth above the knee to one handbreadth below the greater trochanter (Figure 15-21). The rectus femoris is on the anterior thigh. The middle third of the muscle group is the preferred site for the injection. In infants and children, the acceptable site lies below the greater trochanter of the femur and within the upper lateral quadrant of the thigh (Procedure 15-8).

PROCEDURE 15-8   Giving an Intramuscular Injection

Objective: To give an intramuscular injection safely in one of four acceptable sites for this type injection.

Guidelines

Equipment Needed
- Physician's order
- Medication to meet medication order
- Syringe of appropriate size
- Needle of appropriate length and gauge for medication
- Alcohol wipe
- Bandage

Methodology 3+7

(Refer to Figures 15-18 through 15-21 for the sites for administering IM medications.)

1. Prepare the medication dose to the medication order.

2. After patient identification locate the deltoid, dorsogluteal, ventrogluteal, vastus lateralis, or rectus femoris site indicated by age, size, and general physical condition of the person and the viscosity of the medication.

3. Choose needle of the appropriate length to reach the muscle tissue at the chosen site.

4. Position the person correctly to access the site of injection.

5. Wipe the site with an alcohol wipe in a circular motion from the injection site outward.

6. Hold the skin at the injection site for dorsogluteal or ventrogluteal injection taut with nondominant hand to prevent pulling of the skin during the insertion of the needle. When using the vastus lateralis, rectus femoris, or deltoid sites, pinching of the tissue with the nondominant hand is acceptable.

7. Hold the barrel of the syringe like a dart in your dominant hand and insert the entire needle into the skin at a 90-degree angle. This depth ensures that the medication is inserted into the muscle and not subcutaneous tissue.

8. Aspirate the plunger to ensure that blood does not appear in the hub. If blood appears, you have entered a blood vessel, and the entire process should be started again with another needle and syringe. If there is no blood, inject the medication slowly and smoothly to minimize discomfort and distribute the medication into the muscle evenly.

9. Quickly withdraw the needle at the same angle as insertion to prevent further trauma to tissue.

10. Apply pressure to the site using the alcohol swab to prevent seepage into the subcutaneous tissue. If rapid absorption is desired, massage the site for 1 to 2 minutes. Cover with bandage as needed.

11. Discard used equipment in proper biohazard containers. Sanitize hands.

12. Document the procedure.

13. Watch the patient for any signs of adverse reactions when giving IM injections because of rapid absorption of the medication into the bloodstream. If giving the medication in the dorsogluteal site, be sure the patient is able to move the leg on the side of the body used for the injection as a means of evaluating any damage to the sciatic nerve. Be sure a health care provider is readily available in case of a serious adverse reaction.

PROCEDURE 15–8   Giving an Intramuscular Injection—cont'd

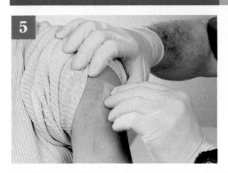
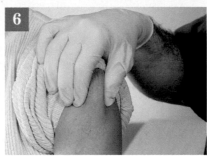
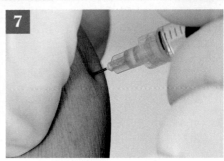

TYPICAL DOCUMENTATION

2/18/0X 11:20 AM Penicillin 300,000 U IM given in LT upper thigh. Able to move left leg. No apparent adverse reaction after waiting 20 minutes. _____ G. OLSEN, CMA

Summary

Parenteral administration of medications—intradermally, subcutaneously, or intramuscularly—requires special processes that must be carried out while maintaining sterile technique because the skin is penetrated. Injections are invasive procedures and should be performed only if allowed by the medical practice act of the state of employment and if a physician or other health care provider is readily available in case adverse reactions occur.

Drugs given by injection are absorbed and activated at a faster rate and may not have the duration of action of enteral administration. Injections are used for persons who cannot swallow or who may be unable to take drugs because of gastric disorders or with medications that cannot be administered by enteral means.

Each route of administration requires special skills to be sure that the medication reaches the desired location. Any medication given parenterally must be in a sterile liquid form. The liquid is usually one that is minimally irritating to tissue and may contain preservatives or a small amount of antibiotic. Always be sure that the patient is not allergic to the additives or the base fluid for the medication being administered. Safety should be of utmost importance with parenteral administration of medications.

Syringes, chosen according to the type and volume of medication to be given, come in nondisposable and disposable types in sizes from 60 mL to those that hold only 0.5 mL in unit increments for insulin. Needles come in different lengths and gauges and are matched to the site of injection, depth needed to give the drug properly, and vis-

cosity of the medication. The smallest possible needle that will produce the least pain is the needle of choice. Needles are gauged from 14 (largest lumen) to 31 (smallest lumen), with gauges between 20 and 27 the most frequently used in ambulatory care.

Sterile parenteral medications come in vials, ampules, and prefilled syringes. Ampules are small sealed glass containers that hold a single dose of medication. Any medication left in an ampule after administration of a dose should be discarded because, on standing open, the medication is no longer sterile. When preparing a dose of medication from an ampule, the needle point must be kept below the meniscus of the liquid in the ampule. Vials are manufactured in single-dose and multidose sizes. To withdraw the drug from a vial, the positive pressure in the vial must remain constant. To prepare the medication, invert the vial, keeping the needle under the liquid line to prevent aspirating air. Never return unused medication to a vial. Prefilled syringes and disposable injection units come with the medication ready for injection. Dosages will be calculated to the prefilled syringe and the medication order. In some cases, some of the medication may have to be discarded prior to administration.

Drugs that are unstable as a liquid come in a powder form for reconstitution to a liquid prior to administration. To reconstitute, be sure that you have the correct diluent in the correct amount to form the correct concentration of medication. After reconstituting powders, always write the date and time on the vial, the reconstituted strength, and your initials to prevent medication errors if the medication is in a multidose vial.

TABLE 15-2 *Parenteral Administration of Medications*

INJECTION METHOD	NEEDLE GAUGE	NEEDLE LENGTH (INCHES)	MEDICATION AMOUNT	INJECTION ANGLE (DEGREES)	SYRINGE SIZE	ADMINISTRATION SITES
Intradermal (ID)	26-29	$\frac{3}{8}$ - $\frac{5}{8}$	Adult/child: 0.05-0.2 mL	10-15	Tuberculin	Forearm, back, upper chest
Subcutaneous (SC)	25-26	$\frac{3}{8}$ - $\frac{7}{8}$	Adult: ↓ 2 mL	45	Tuberculin, insulin, 3 mL	Deltoid, thigh, abdomen
		Same as for adult	Child: 0.5 mL-1 mL	45	Same as for adult	
Intramuscular (IM)	23-19	1-3	Small adult: 1-2 mL Large adult: 2-4 mL	90	3 mL-5 mL	Deltoid, dorsogluteal, Ventrogluteal, vastus lateralis
	Same as for adult	Same as for adult	Child: 1-2 mL	Same as for adult	Same as for adult	Ventrogluteal, vastus lateralis
Intramuscular, Z-track	Same as IM	Same as IM	Same as IM for adult and child	Same as IM	Same as IM	Dorsogluteal, ventrogluteal

Occasionally, two medications may be mixed in one syringe to avoid giving more than one injection. Always be sure that the medicines are compatible. When preparing medicines from a vial and an ampule, always pull from the vial first and then from the ampule. If the medications are in two single-dose vials, add air to one vial (A), then add air to the other vial (B) and draw the medication from this vial (B); finally, draw the medication from the first vial (A). If mixing from two multidose vials, add air to vial A, then add air to vial B and prepare the medication from this vial. After changing the needle, return the syringe and needle to vial A and draw this medicine. If preparing two types of insulin, always draw regular insulin into the syringe first.

When giving injectable medications, correct technique is important to prevent injury to nerves, blood vessels, and tissue. Sterile technique must be used to prevent infection. When given correctly, injectable medications should cause little pain. If given incorrectly, the legal repercussions may be significant and the possibility of injury to tissue increases.

Table 15-2 summarizes the parenteral administration of medications. These guidelines must be followed for the safety of the patient and to prevent tissue damage.

Critical Thinking Exercises

SCENARIO
Sally is 6 months old and needs several IM immunizations as prescribed by the Centers for Disease Control.
1. In what position should Sally be placed?
2. What muscle group should the allied health professional choose for giving this medication?
3. What length needle should be chosen?
4. Should the medications be mixed if the health care provider does not order the mixing? Why or why not?
5. How would the allied health professional choose the size of the syringe?
6. These medications are to be given intramuscularly. What angle should be used for insertion of the needle?

REVIEW QUESTIONS

1. What does parenteral administration of medications mean?_____

   _____

   _____

2. What are the routes used for giving medications parenterally?_____

   _____

   _____

3. What are three reasons for administering medications parenterally rather than orally?_____

_____

4. What are the drawbacks to using parenteral routes of administration?_____

_____

5. What body structures may be damaged by giving injections incorrectly?_____

_____

6. What is the calibration on a 3-mL syringe? On an insulin syringe? On a tuberculin syringe? Give a specific use for each._____

_____

7. What are the factors in choosing a needle for injections? What are the criteria for the needle of choice?_____

_____

8. What containers are used to hold parenteral medications prior to preparation of injections?

_____

_____

9. How much diluent is used to reconstitute powdered medications for injection?_____

_____

10. Why is good technique so important when administering medications parenterally?_____

_____

Pharmacology for Multisystem Application

CHAPTER 16
Analgesics and Antipyretics, 288

CHAPTER 17
Immunizations and the Immune System, 305

CHAPTER 18
Antimicrobials, Antifungals, and Antivirals, 331

CHAPTER 19
Antineoplastic Agents, 365

CHAPTER 20
Nutritional Supplements and Alternative Medicines, 382

Analgesics and Antipyretics

OBJECTIVES

After studying this chapter, you should be capable of doing the following:

- Defining analgesics, antiinflammatory medications, and antipyretics.
- Identifying analgesics that are regulated by the Controlled Substances Act of 1970.
- Describing the therapeutic effects of narcotic and nonnarcotic pain relievers, nonsteroidal antiinflammatory drugs (NSAIDs), and antipyretics commonly used in ambulatory medical care.
- Classifying nonopioid analgesics and antipyretics commonly used into categories by their drug use.
- Providing patient education for safe administration of nonprescription analgesics and antipyretics and the possibilities of overdosage with over-the-counter (OTC) medications.
- Educating patients about drug safety by making them aware of the dangers of mixing OTC and legend (prescription) analgesics.

Jeanne has a history of headaches, for which she takes nonopioid analgesics for relief. Jeanne calls Dr. Merry to ask that the local pharmacy be called to refill her prescription. The pharmacist had informed Jeanne when she last refilled her prescription that the number of approved refills had been used.

What questions do you ask to get her to describe the pain?

Why do you need to ask Jeanne when she last refilled the prescription?

Why do you need to have the medical record available for Dr. Merry to evaluate when you know that Jeanne gets this prescription on a regular basis?

KEY TERMS

Addiction

Adjuvant medication

Aggregation

Analgesic

Antiinflammatory

Antipyretic

Ceiling effect

Coanalgesia

Drug dependence

Endorphin

Narcotic

Nonopioid analgesic

Nonsteroidal antiinflammatory drug (NSAID)

Opiate

Opioid

Pain perception

Pain threshold

Pain tolerance

EASY WORKING KNOWLEDGE OF INDICATIONS AND SIDE EFFECTS

Common Signs and Symptoms of Pain
Contorted facial expressions
Fist clenching
Changes in posture
Holding breath
Increased vital signs
Irritability
Restlessness; lethargy
Guarding of body part
Self-focus
Fatigue

Common Side Effects of Analgesics
Lightheadedness, dizziness
Orthostatic hypotension
Drowsiness
Constipation
Diarrhea
Headaches
Nausea and possibly vomiting

Easy Working Knowledge of Medications Used as Analgesics

DRUG CLASS	PRESCRIPTION	OTC	PREGNANCY CATEGORY	MAJOR INDICATIONS
Opioid (narcotic) analgesics Opiates	Yes; prescriptions for controlled substances in Schedule II must be written; prescriptions for drugs on Schedules III-V may be verbal	Yes, depending on state regulations	B, C	Control of moderate to severe pain
Combination opioid/nonopioid analgesics	Yes; prescriptions for Schedule II drugs must be written; prescriptions for Schedule III-V drugs may be verbal	Yes, depending on state regulations	B, C	Control of moderate pain; cough control; control of diarrhea
Nonopioid analgesics, antipyretics, antiinflammatories	Yes; prescriptions for Schedule III-V drugs may be verbal	Yes	B, C, D—aspirin	Control of mild to moderate pain; reduce fever and inflammation

P ain is one of the most frequent reasons why patients see physicians. Pain management involves relieving symptoms that cause distress and disability. Analgesics are currently available for all levels of pain, and many also have antipyretic action and antiinflammatory action.

What Is Pain?

Pain is whatever a person says it is and exists wherever and whenever the person says it exists. Pain is personal and subjective, with few objective findings. A person's reaction to pain depends on that individual's **pain perception, pain threshold, and pain tolerance,** as well as physiologic changes that may be the cause of pain.

Pain may vary at different times and in different or even similar situations such as time of day. Mental condition, physical stamina, and even ethnic background may affect pain because pain has both psychologic and physiologic elements but under most circumstances the pain threshold remains constant (Box 16-1).

The severity of the pain, the source or cause of pain, and the physiologic and disease characteristics of the patient, as well as an individual's ability to adapt to pain, are factors in deciding what medication is necessary to relieve the discomfort. The fears and myths about addiction or tolerance to pain medications often result in the patient not receiving an adequate dosage to relieve symptoms. The response to medications is individualized, and each person needs to know that the prescribed or OTC pain medicines are safe if taken as prescribed for a particular situation.

When evaluating pain, the patient should be asked where the pain is found, the duration of the pain, and the intensity of the pain on a scale of 1 to 10 with 1 being the least intense pain and 10 being the most intense. Any precipitating factors for pain or for intensification of pain should also be noted.

Pain and Emotional Responses

Pain comes as stimuli to the nervous system and is affected by emotions and cognition, as well as stimuli from somatic and visceral organs. The afferent pathways of the nervous system recognize the stimuli and carry the stimuli from the pain receptors throughout the body to the central nervous system and the brain where the stimuli are interpreted as painful. The brain continues to react until the stimulus causing the pain is removed. Then the efferent nerves carry the messages to the rest of the body via the spinal cord. The response of the nervous system causes a stress response that releases **endorphins.** Prolonged stress of pain, as well as prolonged use of pain relievers, will decrease endorphin levels and increase the individual's perception of pain (Box 16-2).

Some pain is not apparent at the site of the problem but is felt in a different area of the body. This pain is called *referred pain*. Figure 16-1 shows the sites of referred pain.

Pain and Medications

Pain may be acute or chronic.

- Acute pain warns of tissue damage in some part of the body and is usually of short duration, responding to analgesics.
- Chronic pain has a longer duration and does not have the sole purpose of indicating body tissue damage.
- In most cases the body adjusts to chronic pain over a period of time because the nerve endings have decreased sensitivity when stimulated over a prolonged period.

BOX 16-1	FACTORS AFFECTING THE RESPONSE TO PAIN

Factors That Increase Sensitivity
Sleeplessness
Anger
Tiredness
Fear
Anxiety
Isolation
Depression
Hunger

Factors That Decrease Sensitivity
Sleep
Empathy
Diversion
Tolerance
Medications
Addiction

BOX 16-2	WAYS PATIENTS COMMUNICATE PAIN LEVELS

Pain is usually evaluated on the basis of the patient's subjective report of the type, duration, site, and intensity of the pain. When pain is prolonged, the person may turn to folk or unscientific remedies for relief. Pain medications are often prescribed on the basis of these subjective symptoms. However, the allied health professional can evaluate pain and pain management by observing the following:
- Facial expressions
- Posture
- The patient's grasping or holding a body part
- The presence or absence of restlessness or irritability
- Vital signs and their evaluation

The allied health professional may find nonverbal expressions missing in the drug abuser. The lack of the signs listed previously should be reported to the health care provider for further evaluation during the physical examination.

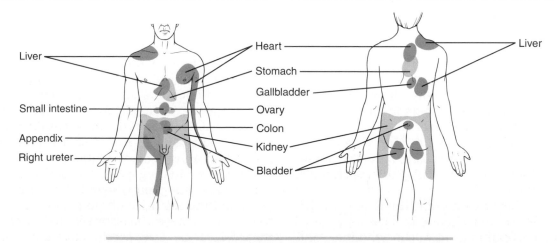

Figure 16-1 Sites of referred pain, anterior and posterior views.

- The patient may not even report chronic pain because it has become a way of life. An example is the patient with arthritis, who may get little relief from routine medications.
- The body may also become less responsive to analgesics, requiring a higher dosage of medication to relieve chronic discomfort as drug tolerance occurs.
- Additional drugs may be added to the primary analgesic to supply greater pain relief.
- The person with chronic pain easily builds up a tolerance to analgesics—a cause-and-effect situation—so analgesics may provide little relief in long-term chronic pain.

Analgesics are, by definition, medications that are used for pain relief. Analgesics include both **opioid/opiate** substances, which are controlled by the Drug Enforcement Administration, and **nonopioid** medications, which may be prescription or OTC medications. Many of the nonopioid and nonopioid/opioid preparations also work for antipyretics and antiinflammatory agents as a desirable therapeutic effect.

Patient Education for Compliance

1. The level of pain is what the patient perceives it to be. Pain is evaluated by the patient on levels from 1-10, with 1 being no pain and 10 being the most intense pain.
2. The patient, family, and significant others (with the permission of the patient) should be oriented to the benefits of adequate pain management. The patient's perception of pain and the use of pain medication in the past are factors that become important in pain control.
3. Addiction and drug dependence (see Chapter 32) are not a problem when pain medication is used over a short period of time and should not be considerations in treating terminal pain. Pain relief is of utmost importance in terminal illness. Addiction and drug dependence become a problem with long-term chronic pain.
4. The goal of using analgesics is to achieve sufficient pain control to ensure the patient's comfort.
5. Patients should be taught that various pain medications are available to manage different levels of pain—from OTC to opioids and opiates. Reporting the severity of the pain correctly and honestly is necessary for choosing the appropriate medication.
6. Pain relief management is individual and must be evaluated by the patient and physician together to ensure that the regimen is appropriate.

Patient Education for Compliance—cont'd

7. The patient should be taught how to self-administer medications—which route, the time between doses, and so on.
8. The patient should be taught that for the best pain management, medications should be taken before the pain becomes severe. Waiting until mild to moderate pain becomes excessive will keep the patient from receiving the full effect of the analgesic. Also, apprehension of further pain can heighten the perception of the pain's intensity.

IMPORTANT FACTS ABOUT PAIN

- Pain is based on the patient's psychologic, physiologic, and cultural background and is one of the most common symptoms that cause patients to seek medical attention.
- The reaction to chronic or acute pain depends on the person's pain perception, pain threshold, and pain tolerance.
- Pain is subjective and is affected by anxiety levels, age, and past experiences, but signs of pain may be objective such as found with the patient's posture and facial expressions.
- Analgesics may also work as antipyretics or antiinflammatory agents, or both.
- The objective of analgesic use is to produce pain relief and is more effective if used prior to the onset of severe pain. Pain is more easily controlled while it is mild to moderate.
- Pain relief must be individualized for each patient.
- Analgesics may be given by mouth, by injection, by suppository, or transdermally, depending on how fast relief from pain is necessary, the intensity of the pain, the ability of the patient to self-administer the medication, and the availability of the medication form.

Types of Analgesics

Analgesics are classified as opioid, nonopioid, and medications used for adjuvant action. **Opioid** (including opiate) medications are strong analgesics capable of reducing pain of any origin. **Nonopioids** may require a prescription or may be bought OTC. Because of the ease and popularity of self-medication, these OTC medications are often used today to relieve mild to moderate pain, fever, and chronic painful conditions such as arthritis.

Nonopioids may also be used in **coanalgesia** or as **adjuvant** medications. The coanalgesics such as codeine and acetaminophen are most often used for chronic pain but may be used for acute pain that requires opioid use. The adjuvant medications are medications such as diazepam given with the administration of opioids that are not true analgesics but are used with analgesics to potentiate pain relief. The use of both of these types of medications is to enhance the effectiveness of the opioids, treat concurrent symptoms, or provide analgesia for some types of concurrent pain.

Opioid and Opiate Analgesics

Narcotic analgesics are derivatives of opium or synthetic chemicals that produce pharmaceutic effects similar to those of opium. If purified opium is naturally found in the medication, the drug is called an **opiate.** Some examples are codeine and morphine. Opioids are synthetic manufactured narcotics; examples are meperidine (Demerol) and fentanyl (Duragesic) (Table 16-1).

> **DID YOU KNOW?**
> Morphine, used for severe pain, is considered the standard for narcotic analgesia. This means that the amount of analgesia achieved with a particular drug is compared with the amount of analgesia achieved with an equivalent of morphine.

Narcotic analgesics alter the patient's perception of pain, thus increasing the pain threshold. These medications vary in their potency, onset of action, and incidence of side effects. Because sedation is one of the side effects of narcotic analgesia, the anxiety that accompanies pain is also reduced as the analgesic activity is increased. Most people stop taking the medication when the pain stops, preferring not to have the sedation and confusion. Tolerance to these medications and the potential for dependence keep the opiate and opioid medications from being routinely used for chronic pain, except in terminally ill patients or those with pain unresponsive to other relief methods. Especially for the terminally ill patient, pain relief, not dependence, is the issue, and combinations of medications may be used to relieve the pain.

Most narcotics are Schedule II drugs because of their danger of addiction and dependence (see Chapter 1 for a list of schedules and the applicable drugs for each schedule). Drugs that contain small amounts of a narcotic in combination with another medication may be placed on Schedules III and IV, meaning that there is less potential for dependence or abuse. Some of the antitussives such as terpin hydrate with codeine contain a narcotic, usually codeine or hydrocodone, to control the cough reflex. Because of their limited abuse potential, these medications are usually found on Schedule V.

> **DID YOU KNOW?**
> Morphine was first isolated from the dried seeds of the opium poppy in 1815. It was named for the Greek god of dreams, Morpheus, who was the son of the Greek god of sleep, Hypnos. Used in the Civil War, many veterans were addicted to the drug following the war. Heroin was introduced in 1898 as a nonaddicting substitute for morphine. In 1939 meperidine was introduced with the same assumption. Both meperidine and heroin were also later found to be addicting.

Uses of Opioids and Opiates

Opiates and opioids are used to treat acute pain of moderate to severe intensity. Opioid and opiate analgesics alter the perception of the pain by mimicking endorphins to block the neurotransmission of the painful impulse.

The World Health Organization (WHO) has described a three-step analgesic ladder in the pharmacologic treatment of pain. Use of adjuvant analgesics in conjunction with opioids and opiates has been linked to use with each type of pain.

- *Mild pain*—Use acetaminophen, aspirin, or another antiinflammatory **NSAID** around the clock.
- *Moderate pain*—If pain persists or increases, adding a mild opioid such as codeine or hydrocodone may be sufficient.
- *Severe pain*—If pain persists or if it is moderate to severe at the outset, discontinue the mild opioid and give a strong opioid or opiate such as morphine, fentanyl, or meperidine. The nonopioid medication may be continued.

The health care provider must remember that pain is a personal response and is best controlled before the severity is too great. The objective of pain medication is to achieve pain relief with an acceptable level of side effects. The allied health professional's assessment of the patient's pain with documentation of the objective signs the patient displays is important in the evaluation of medicinal therapy to relieve the discomfort.

TABLE 16-1 *Select Opiates, Opioids, and Other Controlled Substances Commonly Used in Ambulatory Care*

GENERIC NAME	TRADE NAME	USUAL ADULT DOSE, RATE AND FREQUENCY OF ADMINISTRATION	INDICATIONS FOR USE	MAJOR SIDE EFFECTS	DRUG INTERACTIONS
				Respiratory depression, constipation, urinary retention, confusion, euphoria, sedation, dizziness, lightheadedness, orthostatic hypotension	Respiratory arrest*
morphine sulfate (Schedule II)[†,‡]	MSIR	5-15 mg SC, IM q4h 30-60 mg po SC, IM q4h	Moderate to severe pain		
codeine (Schedule II)[†,‡]	Same	15-60 mg po SC, IM q4h	Moderate to severe pain		
meperidine HCl (Schedule II)[†,‡]	Demerol	50-150 mg po SC, IM q3-4h	Moderate to severe pain		Circulatory collapse* MAO inhibitors
fentanyl (Schedule II)[†]	Duragesic, Sublimaze,	12.5-100 mcg 1 patch q72h 50-100 mcg q1-2h IM, IV	Severe chronic pain		Many IV incompatibilities
	Actiq buccal lozenge	200-800 mcg for breakthrough pain of cancer			
oxycodone HCl (Schedule II)[†]	OxyContin	10-40 mg po q8-12h	Moderate to severe pain		
propoxyphene HCl (Schedule III)[†]	Darvon, Doraphen	65 mg po q4h	Moderate pain		
camphorated opium tincture (Schedule III)[†]	Paregoric	3 i-ii po q4h	Localized pain and diarrhea		
pentazocine (Schedule IV)[§]	Talwin NX	50 mg po q3-4h 30 mg SC, IM q3-4h	Moderate pain	Hypertension	

*Life-threatening adverse reaction.
†Opioid medications interact with central nervous system medications and depressants, such as psychotropics, alcohol, sedatives, hypnotics, muscle relaxants, antihistamines, antiemetics, antiarrhythmics, and antihypertensives.
‡Idiosyncratic reactions include agitation, restlessness, itching, and nausea.
§Not scheduled at present but is being evaluated by the Food and Drug Administration.

The health care provider prescribes analgesic doses on the basis of age, severity of pain, cultural norms, and the patient's pain tolerance and pain threshold. The health care professional must realize that the patient is the only person who can describe the existence of pain and its nature or severity. Some patients need more than a standard dose, and others need less, and the analgesic dosage should be adjusted to these idiosyncrasies. The metabolism of the narcotic—faster in older children and adolescents and slower in the elderly—will determine how often the medication is given. The analgesic must provide relief without unacceptable side effects to be the drug of choice. The **ceiling effect** is seen with opiates but does not affect the pure opioids. The issue of ceiling effect is that side effects often increase in occurrence and intensity if the dose continues to be increased once the ceiling has been reached.

 CLINICAL TIP

The patient must be taught to take medications consistently as ordered to maintain serum levels sufficiently high to produce relief without having breaks in the pain control. This may mean having the patient take the medication on a regular basis for a few days or until the acute pain subsides.

IMPORTANT FACTS ABOUT OPIOIDS AND OPIATES

- Opioids and opiates are derivatives of opium or synthetic opium-like chemicals that produce results resembling opium's effects to elevate pain thresholds and alter the perception of pain.
- Opiates and opioids have antitussive effects and may also cause respiratory depression, especially in the elderly.
- Opioids and opiates are used for acute pain and terminal illnesses with pain of moderate to severe intensity.
- Addiction and psychologic dependence may be a problem with the use of strong analgesics for chronic pain, but these analgesics are effective and safe for short-term usage.
- Round-the-clock dosing of opioids/opiates is beneficial for severe, acute pain and the severe, chronic pain found with terminal illnesses.

Precautions with Opioid and Opiate Analgesics and Drug Interactions

In the geriatric patient, opioid use may have undesirable effects that may be enhanced by age, coexisting medical problems, and polypharmacy.

- The use of opioid/opiate medications may lead to confusion and respiratory depression.
- Liver and kidney impairment may lead to reduced metabolism and excretion; therefore meperidine, propoxyphene (Darvon), and pentazocine (Talwin) should be used with caution because of their slowed excretion time.
- Constipation is often a dangerous side effect, especially in the elderly.
- The cough reflex is suppressed, and the respiratory centers are especially sensitive to narcotics.
- Meperidine and morphine should not be used together because they potentiate each other and are physically incompatible when administered in the same syringe.

BOX 16-3   USE OF TRANSDERMAL FENTANYL

- Skin should be cleansed with water prior to application of the pad. Do *not* use soap, oil, lotion, alcohol, or other products because these alter the absorption of the medication.
- The patch should be applied as supplied, not altered by cutting, trimming, etc., to a nonhairy body surface, preferably on the upper body.
- Do not use heat sources (heating pads, electric blankets, hot tub bath) because they increase the absorption rate and toxic effects.
- Short-term analgesics may be added for pain until the transdermal patch takes effect. The patch has a slow onset of action.
- Fever increases the rate of absorption of the medication by about one third.
- Patches should be kept away from children and pets. To discard the patch, fold it together on the adhesive side and flush it down the toilet. If it is placed in the trash, be careful that children and pets do not come in contact with the patch.

- Because urinary retention occurs with opioid/opiate administration, men with prostatic hypertrophy must be followed closely.

Narcotic antagonists such as naloxone (Narcan) block the action of administered opioid/opiates to treat overdosing and to treat such side effects as itching.

Fentanyl (Duragesic), a transdermal patch, is used for chronic persistent pain in an adult who requires constant analgesia, such as the pain of cancer. These patches provide continuous opioid administration percutaneously over a 72-hour period (Box 16-3).

Patient Education for Compliance

OPIOIDS AND OPIATES

1. Cultural, psychologic, and physiologic aspects of pain are interwoven in the person's pain perception and response to analgesics.
2. Analgesics should be taken before the pain becomes severe to assure the medication will provide the needed relief. The medications should be administered while previous doses are still effective for the maintenance of pain relief.
3. Opioid and opiate analgesics are for the short-term treatment of moderate to severe pain. Prescription items and OTC medications for coanalgesia may be used for mild to moderate pain, and adjuvant medications may be prescribed along with the stronger analgesics to provide a higher degree of pain relief.

Patient Education for Compliance— cont'd

4. Orthostatic hypotension occurs with the use of strong analgesics, and the patient should be warned about sudden changes in position. Changing positions for ambulation may cause dizziness.
5. Diets should be increased in fiber and fluids to relieve the constipation that occurs as a side effect of analgesics.
6. Pain medications should be taken with food to minimize the gastrointestinal (GI) reactions.
7. Sedation is a real side effect. Patients should avoid driving, operating machinery, or other hazardous activities after taking pain medications because the sedation caused by these drugs makes these activities dangerous.
8. Alcohol and other CNS depressants should not be taken with opioids because they tend to enhance the analgesic effect and further suppress the CNS and respiration.

Nonopioid Analgesics

Nonopioid analgesics for mild to moderate pain differ from narcotic analgesics in several ways.

- They are not chemically or structurally related to morphine, although some do produce CNS analgesia.
- Most nonopioid analgesics act on the peripheral nervous system rather than the CNS, as opioids and opiates do. However, acetaminophen is a centrally active medication with little to no peripheral action.
- Nonopioid analgesics are not effective alone for acute, severe, sharp, or visceral pain.
- These medicines do not usually produce physical dependency or tolerance but do have the adverse reaction of GI bleeding.
- A ceiling effect does occur; in these cases the adverse reactions increase in proportion to the increased amount of drug being taken.
- Some of these medications are potent and are scheduled medications under the Controlled Substances Act of 1970.

These nonnarcotic analgesics are usually the first step in pain control and are not as expensive as narcotics or as addictive (Box 16-4). Most of the nonopioid analgesics such as aspirin, ibuprofen, and acetaminophen are available as OTC drugs, although prescription medications for pain that are not considered addictive have recently been approved by the FDA (Table 16-2). These non-addictive medications require a prescription, as do

those OTC preparations that are combined with other pain medications such as opioids/opiates.

BOX 16-4   CHARACTERISTICS OF NONOPIOID ANALGESICS

- Nonopioid analgesics do not alter consciousness or mental function to the degree of opioids/opiates and are used to treat the mild to moderate pain associated with many disease conditions.
- They relieve the inflammation and associated low-intensity pain, dull aches, and vague pains that occur at times throughout the body.
- Most reduce fever.
- Three pharmacologic uses—antiinflammatory, analgesic, and antipyretic—are found with these medications.
  - Aspirin has all three of these qualities, which is why it is so widely used.
  - Acetaminophen has analgesic and antipyretic actions but little antiinflammatory effect.
  - Ibuprofen has antipyretic and antiinflammatory effects with less analgesia.

DID YOU KNOW?

Extra-strength OTC drugs such as Extra-Strength Tylenol and Anacin usually contain 500 mg of analgesic per tablet, whereas regular-strength medication contains 325 mg per tablet.

Salicylate Analgesics

The *salicylates* including aspirin or acetylsalicylic acid are the oldest of the nonopioid analgesics and are still frequently used. Aspirin has fewer side effects than most of the nonopioid analgesics when taken for chronic pain over a long period of time. The salicylates may be combined with caffeine to potentiate their action (e.g., Anacin, Excedrin). Others are combined with antacids or are enteric coated to reduce possible GI problems (e.g., Bufferin, Ecotrin).

Aspirin has four distinct therapeutic actions:

1. It is analgesic, relieving pain by inhibiting the synthesis of prostaglandin from damaged tissue.
2. It is an antiinflammatory, decreasing inflammation by reducing the synthesis of prostaglandin.
3. It is an antipyretic, reducing fever by causing vasodilation and sweating, which, in turn, cause heat loss from the skin. It also resets the temperature control in the hypothalamus to normal.
4. It is an anticoagulant, prolonging clotting time by preventing platelets from **aggregating** or clumping. The public thinks of this as

TABLE 16-2 *Analgesics—Nonscheduled Medications*

GENERIC NAME	TRADE NAME	USUAL ADULT DOSE, RATE AND FREQUENCY OF ADMINISTRATION	INDICATIONS FOR USE	MAJOR SIDE EFFECTS	DRUG INTERACTIONS
tramadol	Ultram	1 or 2 tabs po q4-8h	Moderate chronic pain	Dizziness, hallucinations, GI bleeding	MAOIs, neuroleptics, carbamazepine
pregabalin	Lyrica	150 mg qd in divided doses	Peripheral neuropathy, postherpatic neuralgia	Dizziness, somnolence	oxycodone, lorazepam

GI, Gastrointestinal; *MAOIs*, monoamine oxidase inhibitors.

"thinning the blood." Actually, the platelets cannot clump; therefore blood clots cannot form. Often aspirin is prescribed to decrease the chance of heart attacks.

Aspirin should not be used for fever reduction in children with viral diseases because of the danger of causing Reye's syndrome.

Acetaminophen for Pain

Another common OTC nonopioid analgesic is acetaminophen, which has analgesic and antipyretic action by acting within the CNS to increase the pain threshold. The action of acetaminophen inhibits prostaglandin synthesis in the CNS. Unlike aspirin, it does not have antiinflammatory actions. Acetaminophen is used to treat mild pain and has been found to be effective with osteoarthritis. The advantages of acetaminophen over aspirin include the following:

1. All age groups, from infants to the elderly, may use acetaminophen with relative safety.
2. Acetaminophen can be used by people who are allergic to aspirin and aspirin-like drugs.
3. Acetaminophen rarely causes the GI upset and bleeding problems that can occur with aspirin.
4. Acetaminophen may be used in children because it has not been associated with Reye's syndrome.
5. Acetaminophen can be taken with anticoagulant medications.

The main disadvantage of acetaminophen is liver damage if used for a prolonged period of time for chronic pain or with intake of alcohol. If the medication is dosed at less than 4 g per day with most patients and 2 g or less with the elderly and alcoholics, the medication is relatively safe.

Nonsteroidal Antiinflammatory Drugs

NSAIDs are used for mild to moderate pain when opioids are not indicated. Most NSAIDs are used for inflammatory conditions such as arthritis (see Chapter 24 for medications for orthopedic conditions) and for dysmenorrhea and dental pain. NSAIDs are available OTC in lower dosage and by prescription in stronger doses, such as ibuprofen 200 mg as OTC medications and ibuprofen 600 mg or 800 mg as prescription medications. The difference between OTC drugs and legend drugs is the strength of the drug. NSAIDs should not be taken with any other OTC analgesics (aspirin, acetaminophen, or other NSAIDs). The acceptable time limit for taking NSAIDs is 10 days for pain, 3 days for fever, or as prescribed by a health care provider. These medications should not be used in the last 3 months of pregnancy because they could have an adverse effect on the fetus and may cause complications during delivery. Alcohol with many of these medications may result in drug interactions (Table 16-3).

Combination Nonopioid Medications

Medications may be combinations of several drugs used to enhance the medicinal qualities of each. The more common OTC combinations include acetaminophen with salicylates, buffers, or caffeine such as Goody's Powders or Excedrin.

- Antacids decrease gastric irritation such as found with Bufferin and Alka-Seltzer, although some researchers believe the amount of antacid in these medications is too little to be effective.
- The effervescent antacids found in such medications as Alka-Seltzer speed the dissolution of the medication, resulting in a more rapid absorption of the analgesic.
- Caffeine is thought to produce better pain relief than an analgesic given alone because it slows aspirin excretion and keeps blood levels elevated for longer periods of time.

 CLINICAL TIP

Effervescent drugs often contain large amounts of sodium and should be avoided by patients with cardiac or renal problems.

TABLE 16-3 *Over-the-Counter Nonopioid Analgesics**

GENERIC NAME	TRADE NAME (EXAMPLES)	USUAL ADULT DOSE AND FREQUENCY OF ADMINISTRATION	INDICATIONS FOR USE	MAJOR SIDE EFFECTS	DRUG INTERACTIONS
SALICYLATES				Bleeding, including GI bleeding	
aspirin [†,‡,§]	Bayer,* Bufferin,*‡,¶ Alka-Seltzer*	gr x q4-6h po 1¼ gr-5 qd supp/dose age dependent	Mild to moderate pain; analgesic, antipyretic, antiinflammatory; therapeutic effects— prevent clumping of palates		NSAIDs, anticoagulants, some anticonvulsants, antidiabetic agents, therapeutic effects
	Aspergum	Chew 1 to 2 pieces depending on age			
NONSALICYLATES				Nausea	
acetaminophen	Tylenol, Datril, Tempra	325-650 mg po, suppository q4-6h	Mild to moderate pain Analgesic, antipyretic		Alcohol (causes liver damage)
NSAIDs				GI distress, gastric ulcer, GI bleeding	
ibuprofen	OTC Motrin, Advil, Nuprin R Motrin	200-400 mg po q4-6h 600-800 mg po tid-qid	Mild analgesic, antipyretic		aspirin, Coumadin
naproxen	OTC Aleve R Naprosyn R Anaprox	250 mg po q4-6h 250-500 mg q4-6h 275-550 mg q4-6h	Mild to moderate pain; analgesic, antiinflammatory		Coumadin

GI, Gastrointestinal; *NSAIDs*, nonsteroidal antiinflammatory drugs.

* Major side effects are relatively rare.

[†] Aspirin should not be administered to children with viral diseases, especially chickenpox.

[‡] Bulk-forming laxatives will reduce the absorption of aspirin and reduce the analgesic effect.

[§] Aspirin and Pepto-Bismol (bismuth subsalicylate) both contain salicylates and should not be used together.

[¶] Contains buffering agents, which reduce gastric upset.

Patient Education for Compliance

NONOPIOIDS

1. If the patient is allergic to one nonopioid analgesic, care should be taken prior to taking another OTC analgesic.
2. Patients with liver and kidney disease, as well as pregnant or breast-feeding mothers, should avoid analgesics and should take only the dosage suggested by the health care provider.
3. If symptoms worsen, if new symptoms occur, or if the pain increases, the patient should contact a health care provider.
4. If stomach distress occurs, the medication should be taken with meals.

Patient Education for Compliance— cont'd

5. Aspirin should be avoided in children with viral diseases, especially those with chickenpox or influenza, because of the danger of Reye's syndrome.
6. Aspirin and aspirin-like medications should be stopped at least 5 days before elective surgery. These drugs slow blood clotting by preventing aggregation of platelets, and their use could lead to complications such as hemorrhage.
7. Aspirin should not be placed on the gum or mucous membranes or on teeth because it may irritate (burn) tissues.

Patient Education for Compliance— cont'd

8. If aspirin has a strong vinegar odor, it should not be used. The vinegar odor is a sign of medication deterioration.

9. The health care provider should be notified if pain lasts more than 5 days, if fever lasts more than 3 days, or if redness or swelling develops.

10. These drugs may cause drowsiness and will reduce the coordination needed to drive, operate machinery, or perform manual tasks.

11. Patients should not exceed the recommended daily dosage of an OTC medication, especially those of geriatric or pediatric ages.

12. Acetaminophen may cause a false-positive decrease in blood glucose levels on home testing strips.

13. The use of acetaminophen with the intake of alcohol increases the risk of liver damage.

14. Aspirin and ibuprofen should not be taken during the same period of time because the two medications slow the action of each other and increase side effects such as GI bleeding and decreased antiplatelet effect of aspirin. However, if low doses of aspirin are prescribed to decrease platelet aggregation, the aspirin/ibuprofen combination may be used.

IMPORTANT FACTS ABOUT NONOPIOID ANALGESICS

- Nonopioid analgesics may be prescription or OTC items. Opioid and nonopioid analgesics are given together (coanalgesia) for more effective pain relief and to decrease inflammation in the pain receptors.
- The use of OTC analgesics may lead to polypharmacy, especially in the elderly, because these medications are readily available and widely used for mild to moderate pain.
- OTC analgesics include salicylates, acetaminophen, and NSAIDs. All are antipyretics, but acetaminophen does not have an antiinflammatory effect.
- Salicylates are also used to prolong the clotting time by preventing platelets from binding together.
- NSAIDs are also used for the treatment of musculoskeletal diseases.
- Nonopioids, especially OTC medications, have a therapeutic ceiling effect: when maximum effect is achieved, increasing the dose does not increase the effect.

Combining Analgesics for Greater Effectiveness

Narcotic and nonnarcotic medications are often given in combination because (1) the nonnarcotic agent provides a foundation for analgesic relief, so the narcotics can be more effective; and (2) the combination medication will reduce the pain from the stimulation of nerve endings or that pain intensified by the patient's anxiety. When used together, combination medications are used to provide greater relief of moderate to severe pain than if used separately. Combinations with acetaminophen should not be given with additional acetaminophen; the same is true of aspirin with other salicylate drugs (Table 16-4).

DID YOU KNOW?

Medications with the word *compound* in their name contain aspirin. Drugs that end in *-cet* such as Percocet contain acetaminophen; drugs that end in *-dan* such as Percodan contain aspirin.

Adjuvant Analgesics

Adjuvant analgesics are drugs that enhance the analgesic efficiency of opioid or opiate medications, treat symptoms that might exacerbate pain, and provide analgesia for specific pain. A decrease in the amount of pain medication with an increase in pain control is the object of adjuvant pain therapy. Adjuvant analgesics may also be used to reduce the side effects common to analgesics such as nausea while also acting as synergists to the analgesics (Table 16-5).

The route of administration of analgesics must be considered when administering these medications because of the related side effects. The allied health professional has an ethical duty to be aware of side effects that can occur when administering the medications. Side effects may be rapid if the analgesic is given by injection or slow when it is given by mouth (Table 16-6).

IMPORTANT FACTS ABOUT ADJUVANT ANALGESICS

- Analgesics may be given with drugs that prevent nausea, vomiting, constipation, and other side effects.
- OTC medications may be used as adjuvant drugs to prolong the effect of prescription medications.
- When two analgesics are given together, the action is coanalgesia. When analgesics and medications to enhance the analgesic are given together, adjuvant medication administration occurs.

TABLE 16-4 *Selected Combination Medications for Analgesia*

GENERIC NAME (SCHEDULE)	TRADE NAME (EXAMPLES)	USUAL ADULT DOSE AND FREQUENCY OF ADMINISTRATION	INDICATIONS FOR USE	DRUG INTERACTIONS
COMBINATIONS OF NARCOTICS AND NONNARCOTICS				
acetaminophen/ propoxyphene (IV)	Darvocet N	i or ii tabs po q4-6h	Moderate to severe pain	Alcohol, anticoagulants
aspirin/propoxyphene/ caffeine (IV)	Darvon compound	i or ii caps po q4-6h	Moderate to severe pain	Alcohol, anticoagulants
aspirin with codeine	Empirin with codeine	i or ii tabs po q4-6h	Moderate to severe pain	Alcohol, CNS depressants, anticoagulants
15 mg (IV)	#2			
30 mg (IV)	#3			
60 mg (III)	#4			
Aspirin/hydrocodone (III)	Lortab with ASA	i or ii tabs po q4-6h	Moderate to severe pain	Alcohol, CNS depressants, anticoagulants
acetaminophen/codeine 30 mg/ butalbital (III)	Fioricet with codeine	i or ii tabs po q4-6h	Moderate to severe pain	Alcohol, CNS depressants
aspirin/butalbital/codeine 30 mg (III)	Fiorinal with codeine	i or ii tabs po q4-6h	Moderate to severe pain	Alcohol, CNS depressants, anticoagulants
acetaminophen/hydrocodone (III)	Lortab, Vicodin, Lorcet	i tab po q4-6h	Moderate to severe pain	Alcohol, CNS depressants
meperidine/promethazine (II)	Meprozine	i or ii caps po q4-6h	Severe pain	Alcohol, CNS depressants, anticoagulants
acetaminophen/oxycodone (II)	Percocet, Tylox	i or ii tabs po q4-6h	Moderate to severe pain	Alcohol, CNS depressants
aspirin/oxycodone (II)	Percodan	i or ii tabs po q4-6h	Moderate to severe pain	Alcohol, anticoagulants
ibuprofen/hydrocodone (III)	Vicoprofen	i or ii tabs po q4-6h		
NONNARCOTIC COMBINATIONS				
aspirin/caffeine	OTC Anacin	i or ii tabs po q4-6h	Mild pain	Coumadin
aspirin/sodium bicarbonate	OTC Alka Seltzer	i or ii effervescent tabs in water po q4-6h	Mild pain	Coumadin
acetaminophen/aspirin	Excedrin	i or ii tabs po 1r-6h		
	Goody's powders	i pkg in water po q3-4h		
acetaminophen/butalbital/caffeine *,† (III)	Fioricet	i or ii tabs po q4-6h	Moderate to severe pain	CNS depressants, alcohol
aspirin/butalbital/ caffeine† (III)	Fiorinal	i or ii tabs po q4-6h	Moderate to severe pain	Coumadin, CNS depressants, alcohol
acetaminophen and tramadol	Ultracet	i or ii tabs po q4-6h	Moderate to severe pain	

MAJOR SIDE EFFECTS OF COMBINATION MEDICATIONS: Sedation, dizziness, constipation, lightheadedness, orthostatic hypotension

Note: Medications containing aspirin should not be used in persons taking anticoagulants such as Coumadin.

CNS, central nervous system; *OTC,* over the counter.

*Not scheduled in some states but scheduled in others.

†Drugs such as Fioricet, Ultracet, and Percocet contain acetaminophen; Fiorinal and Percodan contain aspirin.

TABLE 16-5 *Selected Adjuvant Medications*

DRUG CATEGORY/DRUG	TYPICAL DOSE	DESIRED EFFECT	MAJOR SIDE EFFECTS	TYPE OF PAIN
TRICYCLIC ANTIDEPRESSANT				
amitriptyline (Elavil)	10-25 mg po q6-8h	To elevate mood, enhance opioids, direct analgesic effect	Sedation, dizziness, confusion, nausea and vomiting, constipation	Neuropathic pain described as dull, aching, or throbbing, as found in headaches, herpes, arthritis, back pain
doxepin (Sinequan)	25-50 mg po hs			
imipramine (Tofranil)	25-50 mg po bid or hs			
nortriptyline (Pamelor)	50-100 mg po hs			
ANTICONVULSANTS				
carbamazepine (Tegretol)	200 mg po bid-qid	To suppress spontaneous nerve stimuli	Same as above	Neuropathic pain described as sharp, shooting, or burning, as found in neuralgia, cancer, and herpes
phenytoin Na (Dilantin)	100-200 mg po tid (take 1000 mg in first 24 hr)			
lorazepam (Ativan)	0.5-1 mg po qd-bid			
topiramate (Topamax)	25-50 mg po qd			
gabapentin (Neurontin)	900-1800 mg po qd in divided doses			
CORTICOSTEROIDS				
dexamethasone (Decadron)	0.75-2 mg po tid	To elevate mood, strong antiinflammatory action, to stimulate appetite	Nausea and vomiting	Pain of cerebral or spinal cord edema or peripheral nerve pain
prednisone (Deltasone)	10 mg po tid			
ANTIHISTAMINES				
hydroxyzine (Atarax, Vistaril)	10-25 mg po tid-qid	To relieve anxiety, insomnia, nausea, and itching	Constipation	Pain with nausea, and anxiety

Analgesics in Children

Children and adults experience pain, but young children cannot express themselves to describe the degree of pain or the site of the pain. Comfort measures to control pain and fever should be used with children so that they do not suffer unnecessarily. In pediatrics a low level of analgesia appropriate for the age of the child should be administered, and parenteral administration should be avoided if possible.

Poisoning may result from the inappropriate use of analgesics by children, especially because some of these medications are easily obtained without a prescription. Aspirin use in children, in-cluding teenagers with acute viral infections, has been associated with the possible development of Reye's syndrome, so aspirin therapy should be avoided with viral diseases. Table 16-7 lists pediatric uses of OTC analgesics.

DID YOU KNOW?

Pharmaceutical companies are aware of the danger of children taking baby aspirin as candy, so OTC bottles of baby aspirin contain only 36 tablets—less than a lethal overdose if the entire bottle is taken. Federal law requires all aspirin to be in a lock-top bottle for children's safety.

TABLE 16-6 *Advantages and Disadvantages of Selected Medication Routes for Analgesics*

MEDICATION TYPE	ADVANTAGES	DISADVANTAGES
NONPRESCRIPTION		
Oral analgesics (acetaminophen, aspirin, NSAIDs)	Used for many types of mild to moderate pain	Ceiling effect for analgesia
	Easily obtained, some OTC	Gastric and renal side effects
	Used as adjuvant/additive medications with opioids	May affect bleeding time
	Easily administered by patient or family	Increased effects in elderly and children
	Nonaddictive, nonlegend medications	Children: no aspirin for viral diseases
	Relatively inexpensive	
Rectal analgesics (acetaminophen)	Same as above	Same as above
	Can be used with nausea and vomiting	May cause rectal irritation
PRESCRIPTION		
Oral (NSAIDs, legend drugs, [Schedule III, IV] opioids)	For generalized and localized pain	Side effects limit analgesic effects
	Ceiling effect only from possible side effects or long-term use	Regulated by strict prescription codes
	Sedation and anxiety relief useful for moderate to severe effect	Less effective in patients with alcohol or drug dependence
	Multiple drug choices	Stigma or fear of use
	Easily administered by patient or family	Gastric bleeding
	Inexpensive to expensive	
Transdermal opioids (fentanyl)	Long duration of action (24-72 hr)	Side effects not easily reversed because of time of action
	Used in outpatient settings for patients who cannot tolerate morphine or related medications	Slow onset of relief
	Used for chronic severe pain	May require additional medications for breakthrough pain
	Easy use	Skin irritation
	Continuous release without invasive techniques	Expensive
	Easily administered by patient or family	
Rectal opioids	Relatively easy to use as an alternative to oral administration	Rectal suppositories not easily accepted by patients
	Can be administered by family	Rectal irritation
	Moderately expensive	Slower than injectable medications
	Faster onset of action than oral	May be expelled prior to complete absorption due to stimulation of the rectal muscles
	Can be used with nausea and vomiting	

NSAIDs, Nonsteroidal antiinflammatory drugs; *OTC*, over the counter.

TABLE 16-7 *Typical Safe Administration of OTC Analgesics in Children**

OTC DRUG	INFANT	2-3 YR	4-5 YR	6-12 YR	12 YR AND OLDER
aspirin (chewable tablets, 81 mg)	By physician's order	162 mg or 2 tablets	243 mg or 3 tablets	325 mg or 4 tablets (equal to 1 adult aspirin)	650 mg or 2 adult aspirin tablets
acetaminophen 80 mg/2.5 mL liquid (infant's strength) 160 mg/5 mL elixir 160 mg/5 mL liquid 120-mg suppositories 80-mg chewable tablets (children's strength) 160-mg chewable tablets (junior strength) 80- or 160-mg sprinkle	0-3 mo: 40 mg 4-11 mo: 80 mg 1-2 yr: 120 mg	160 mg	240 mg	6-8 yr: 320 mg 9-10 yr: 400 mg 12 yr: 480 mg	660 mg
Ibuprofen 40 mg/mL oral drops 100 mg/5 mL suspension 50-mg chewable tablets 100-mg chewable tablets 200-mg tablets	←	Based on body weight of 5-10 mg/kg, depending on amount of fever or pain, or physician's suggestion; not to exceed 40 mg/kg/24 hr			→

OTC, Over the counter.

* These dosages were determined in children of normal weight for age.

Patient Education for Compliance

Chewable analgesics should not be called candy because children are attracted to the colored tablets and their sweet flavor. The result might be toxic to the child who chews more of the tablets than the recommended dose in the belief that the tablets are candy.

Analgesics in the Elderly

Altered pharmacokinetics and pharmacodynamics in the elderly can result in a greater risk of adverse effects and in drug interactions. Also, the elderly frequently take multiple medications to relieve multiple symptoms of pain, which also leads to interactions and adverse reactions. Non-opioid analgesics, including NSAIDs and acetaminophen, are appropriate for pain management in the elderly. However, a heightened awareness of possible OTC analgesic abuse by the elderly should be evaluated by the health care professional and a thorough assessment of the pain is necessary.

The elderly are more prone to gastric irritation, renal toxicity, and constipation and are at greater risk for GI bleeding. Taking analgesics with food will decrease the possibility. In addition, elderly patients experience higher peak levels and a longer duration of action with opioid medications. Sedation, depression of the respiratory system, and urinary retention may occur in elderly individuals who are given opioids. Confusion, ototoxicity nausea, tinnitus, and orthostatic hypotension are common side effects and need careful evaluation because of the prolonged half-life of pain medications in older adults whose body functions have slowed. Propoxyphene (Darvon) and pentazocine (Talwin) are considered inappropriate for the elderly because of the prolonged excretion time.

Patient Education for Compliance

Polypharmacy in the elderly increases the likelihood of side effects and adverse reactions. Care should be taken to ensure safety with polypharmacy because OTC medications are so readily available for the pain often experienced in the elderly.

Summary

Pain is a major worldwide health consideration that is often disabling. For pain to be properly treated, the intensity and the type of pain must be evaluated so that the proper medication can be prescribed.

Cultural, psychologic, and physiologic considerations play important roles in how a patient perceives pain and responds to pain medication. Analgesics vary from OTC drugs such as aspirin and acetaminophen, which are also antipyretics, and aspirin and nonsteroidal antiinflammatory agents with antiinflammatory effects, to opioids and opiates, which are tightly regulated because of their addictive potential or dependency state. In cases of moderate to severe pain, coanalgesia and adjuvant medications may be used for therapeutic effects.

Some analgesics such as aspirin and propoxyphene are administered by mouth, whereas other medications such as morphine and meperidine are given by injection for faster absorption. The severity of the pain and ease of administration for the patient are important factors to consider in selecting drugs and the route of administration. Polypharmacy in the elderly requires careful analysis of the pain and its relief including any adjuvant or alternative therapies that are available and being used.

Societal attitudes often contribute to the unnecessary undertreatment of pain. The fear of addiction or dependency with opiates and opioids is a consideration in the use of scheduled drugs. An opioid typically is used for moderate to severe pain over a short period of time. For the chronically ill, these medications may lead to dependency. For the terminally ill, the risk of dependence is no reason to withhold medications.

OTC medications are easily obtained and may be abused if taken over long periods of time for those with mild to moderate pain. A common belief is that OTC medications are completely safe, with no chance of overdosage or reaction. Analgesics are perhaps the most frequently administered medications and perhaps the most abused medications because of the ease in obtaining them. Pain should be relieved and evaluated on a personal basis to be sure analgesics are being used properly.

Critical Thinking Exercises

SCENARIO

Mrs. Jones, age 76, takes an aspirin as anticoagulant therapy. When the rheumatologist sees her, she is given a prescription for ibuprofen 800 mg tid for arthritis.

1. Will taking these two medications together affect the absorption rate of either drug? Explain your answer.
2. What side effects and adverse reactions should Mrs. Jones watch for with ibuprofen?
3. What are some of the age-related polypharmacy problems associated with chronic pain control?

DRUG CALCULATIONS

1. Dose ordered: Tylenol 650 mg po stat and q4-6h prn pain
   Available medication:

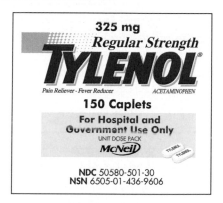

   Interpret the order: _____
   _____
   Dose to be given: _____
   _____

2. Demerol 75 mg stat and then 50 mg q4-6h prn pain
   Available medication: _____

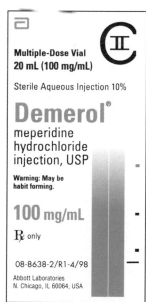

   Show the dose to be given on the syringe.

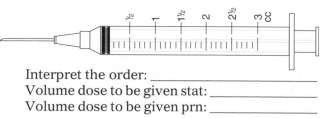

   Interpret the order: _____
   Volume dose to be given stat: _____
   Volume dose to be given prn: _____

REVIEW QUESTIONS

1. What family of drugs are Schedule II medications? What is the difference between an opioid and an opiate? _____

    _____

    _____

2. What is an analgesic? What is an antipyretic medication? What is an antiinflammatory agent? Give examples of each. _____

    _____

    _____

3. When are coanalgesics used? Name two drugs that are used as coanalgesics. _____

    _____

    _____

4. Why are salicylates not administered to children with viral diseases, especially chickenpox and influenza? _____

    _____

    _____

5. Why are opioids, opiates, and other Schedule II analgesics used for short-term acute pain rather than long-term chronic pain except in the terminally ill patient? _____

    _____

    _____

6. Name salicylates, acetaminophen, and NSAIDs commonly used as analgesics, antipyretics, or antiinflammatory agents. _____

    _____

    _____

7. Why are adjuvant medications given with analgesics? _____

    _____

    _____

8. Describe the routes of administration of the various analgesics, giving the advantages and disadvantages of each. _____

    _____

    _____

CHAPTER 17

Immunizations and the Immune System

OBJECTIVES

After studying this chapter, you should be capable of doing the following:

- Defining the various types of agents used in active and passive immunity, appropriate routes of administration, and injection sites for immunizations.
- Describing the public health guidelines for immunizations, indications for administering the agents, and contraindications to each medication.
- Discussing the agents that provide passive immunity.
- Describing the use of Rh-O immunoglobulins following the Rh-O–incompatible birth of mother and child.
- Describing why immunosuppressants are necessary following transplantation of organs and for autoimmune and allergic conditions.
- Discussing the medical needs for immunostimulants.

Michelle is an allied health professional in a pediatric setting. Dr. Jones has ordered DTP, MMR, and IPV vaccines for an 18-month-old child to provide immunity on the accepted schedule.

    Are all immunizations that are appropriate for a child this age being administered?

    What information does Michelle need to document in the chart both before Dr. Jones decides in favor of giving the immunizations and after the immunizations have been administered?

    What law requires this documentation?

KEY TERMS

Acquired immunity	Carcinogenic	Natural immunity
Active immunity	Endogenous	Naturally acquired active immunity
Antibody	Genetic immunity (inborn or natural immunity)	Naturally acquired passive immunity
Antibody titer		
Antigen	Immunity	
Antigen-antibody response	Immunodeficiency	Passive immunity
Antiserum	Immunoglobulins or immune globulins	Serum
Antitoxin		Teratogenic
Artificially acquired active immunity	Immunostimulant	Toxoid
	Immunosuppressant	Vaccination
Artificially acquired passive immunity	Killed vaccines	Vaccine
	Live vaccines	Virulence
Attenuated	Macrophage	
Avirulent	Mutagenic	

EASY WORKING KNOWLEDGE OF INDICATIONS AND SIDE EFFECTS

Common Indications for Immunizations
Initial immunizations in children
Booster immunizations as indicated
Passive immunization for those who cannot take
    active immunizations at the present time
Passive immunization in illnesses where active
    immunization is not available or applicable

Common Indications for Immunosuppressants
Organ transplantation

Common Indications for Immunostimulants
Cancer
Acquired immunodeficiency syndrome

Common Side Effects of Immunizations
Tenderness at the injection site
Fever
Erythema and induration at the injection site
Arthralgia, myalgia

**Common Side Effects of Immunosuppressants
and Immunostimulants**
Nausea, vomiting, diarrhea
Insomnia
Fever
Arthralgia
Increased susceptibility to infections
    (immunosuppressants only)

Easy Working Knowledge of Medications Used in Immunology

DRUG CLASS	PRESCRIPTION	OTC	PREGNANCY CATEGORY	MAJOR INDICATIONS
Active immunizing agents (e.g., toxoids, vaccines)	Yes; administered by physician's order or by state guidelines	No	Rubella, rubeola, mumps, and varicella vaccine; should not be given to pregnant women or those who might become pregnant within 3 months	Active immunization against specific diseases
Passive immunizing agents (e.g., immune globulins, antitoxins)	Yes; administered by physician's order	No	Used with pregnant women who have been exposed to certain viral diseases such as measles	Used in immunosuppressive conditions to achieve passive immunity over a short period of time to reduce or prevent disease processes
Immunosuppressants	Yes	No	C, D, X	Organ transplantation; immunosuppression
Immunostimulants	Yes	No	C, D	Stimulation of immune response

The immune system is a set of cells, factors, and responses, all of which work together to either destroy microorganisms by cell-mediated mechanisms or be the mechanism to produce antibodies to neutralize or destroy invading microorganisms, a significant factor in immunity following immunizations. Antibodies are gamma-globulins found in plasma that are the body's defense system against invaders. The term immunity, denoting protection against disease, is selective—a person immune to one disease may not be immune to another. Immunity may be either inborn or acquired. In the case of acquired immunity, a substance must be delivered into the body to produce the immunity. Natural immunity is inborn due to genetic factors and is species specific. Acquired immunity may be obtained by natural or artificial means, such as immunizations or immune serums, and may be active or passive (Figure 17-1 and Table 17-1).

Remarkable advances in disease prevention have been made with the development of vaccines, which provide a form of acquired immunity. Dreaded diseases of even 50 years ago such as influenza, polio, and diphtheria have been banished from industrialized nations, and ongoing work on vaccines offers hope for treating new diseases as they emerge, as well as the new vaccines for shingles, human papillomavirus, and AIDS. The widespread use of immunizations has had a great impact on the health of people in the United States by reducing many severe infections by 99% at the beginning of the twenty-first century. Two diseases that have been dramatically decreased through vaccinations are polio, which has been virtually eliminated from the Western Hemisphere, and smallpox, which has been successfully eliminated from most of the world, although bioterrorism has raised the awareness of this disease again. Through increased parental

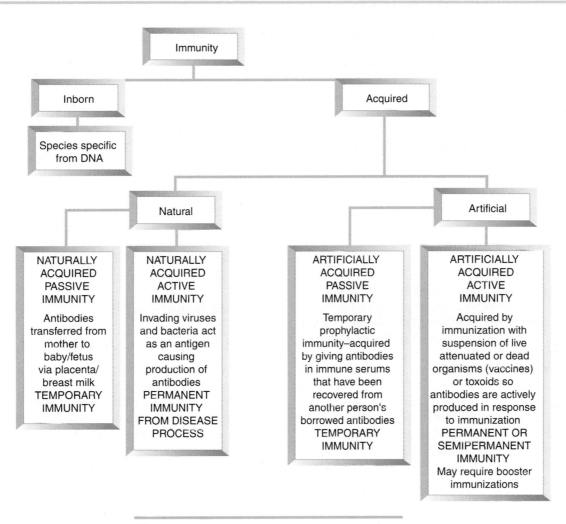

Figure 17-1 The types and extents of immunity.

TABLE 17-1 *Comparison of Active and Passive Immunity*

CATEGORY	ACTIVE IMMUNITY	PASSIVE IMMUNITY
Purpose	Disease prevention	Disease prevention and therapeutics
Source	Individually produced/various sources—self-produced immunity	Other immune humans or animals—immunity from another source
Effectiveness	High	Low to moderate
Method of administration	1. Contraction of the disease	1. From mother to fetus or baby
	2. Immunization with toxoid or vaccine	2. Administration of antibody by injection
Response time	5-21 days	Immediate
Duration	Long term, up to a lifetime	Short term, days to a few months
Ease of reactivation	Booster dose	New administration; anaphylaxis possible, can be dangerous

education and community participation, the goal of immunizing all susceptible populations and the elimination of immunizable diseases would become more of a reality. Providing safe vaccines through a simple delivery system and at low cost is a goal to assure compliance with immunizations in the future.

Role of Lymphocytes in Immunity

Lymphocytes are found in the lymphoid tissue and in circulating blood. Once the body has produced a specific antibody in the lymphoid tissue of the spleen, tonsils, lymph nodes, thymus, or in the reticuloendothelial system, the antibodies circulate throughout the body and attach to the foreign antigens, labeling these for destruction. The T-cells and B-cells respond to the antigens. T-cells and **macrophages** respond to the antigen as foreign material to produce antibodies of a cell-mediated immune-type response. Other macrophages, T-cells, and B-cells are involved in humoral immunity that increases the population of antigen-sensitive memory cells, which will respond if further contact with the same antigen occurs. The second exposure to the antigen will elicit a more powerful response from the T-cell than the first exposure.

T-Cells

T-cells are responsible for cell-mediated immunity by directly attacking the invading antigen found with viral infections, cancer cells, foreign tissue cells, fungi, and protozoa. Thus T-cells are involved with whether organ or tissue transplantation is accepted or rejected. Macrophages work with T-cells to recognize "self" from "nonself" and to boost the immune system. Killer T-cells directly destroy the cells of the antigen, whereas helper T-cells secrete substances that stimulate B-cells to form an immune response. Suppressor T-cells inhibit the B-cells and thus the immune response. The helper cells and suppressor T-cells are the control system for the immune system. With HIV, the helper T-cells decrease in number as the disease progresses and the B-cells are unable to respond to the invading disease. T-cells also act by releasing substances that stimulate other lymphocytes or macrophages to destroy antigens. The final action of T-cells is their role in suppression of the immune response.

B-Cells

B-cells, or B-lymphocytes, are responsible for antibody-mediated immunity (humoral immunity) and are dormant in the lymphoid tissue until a foreign antigen appears. Exposure to specific antigens stimulates the B-cells to multiply rapidly and produce immunity by producing antibodies that circulate in body fluids. The first response of a B-cell may be slow, weak, and of short duration. The second and subsequent responses will be more rapid, more potent, and more prolonged, allowing antibodies to specific antigens to be formed over a period of months. For example, immunizations with several doses provide the initial response to an antigen and provide a stronger reaction with the secondary response. The prolonged immunity

formation is effective in providing immunity to specific disease processes.

Antibodies

Specific antibodies are formed in response to specific antigens. The shape of the antibody that circulates in the bloodstream matches the shape of the antigen, and they bind together, destroying or inactivating the antigen. This is called the **antigen-antibody response** and is present in some way from birth until death. This immunity protects the person from the foreign substances that invade the body, or self, while not overreacting and damaging the body itself under normal circumstances.

Types of Immunity

Inborn versus Acquired Immunity

Inborn immunity is due to inherited factors that make a human immune to diseases found in animals, such as distemper, and may be called species, natural, or inherited immunity. Another form of inborn immunity is racial immunity. Some ethnic groups appear to have a greater immunity to certain diseases than other groups. As an example, groups in which the sickle cell trait is prevalent are resistant to malaria. Individual immunity in the case of a person who lives a long life or seems resistant to certain diseases is also considered inborn. Individual immunity may respond to a person's genetic makeup that prevents the person from responding to antigens giving immunity toward certain diseases or conditions such as hypertension or hyperlipidemia.

Acquired immunity develops during a lifetime as the person encounters various agents that may be disease causing. This immunity is based on the formation of antibodies to the **antigen** that enters the body to produce an immune response. Antigens are found on the surface of pathogenic organisms and on red blood cells, or with allergens, toxins, or foods that may enter the body (Box 17-1).

Acquired Immunity

In **acquired immunity,** antibodies are produced by cell stimulation to phagocytize invading organisms or foreign substances. A specific antigen provides immunity by the custom-made gamma-globulins developed in a person's immune system with naturally acquired immunity and from other sources for artificially acquired immunity. These are

BOX 17-1 TYPES OF IMMUNITY

Inborn Immunity

Inborn immunity results from the genetic makeup of an individual, an ethnic group, or a species.

Acquired Immunity

Acquired immunity results from the introduction into the body of substances (e.g., antigens) that prompt the immune system to produce antibodies or that already contain antibodies (e.g., mother's milk, immune serum from another person).

- Artificially acquired immunity—Acquired by exogenous immunization
  - Artificially acquired active immunity—Acquired by immunization with vaccines or toxoids; antibodies are actively produced in response to presence of a foreign antigen (semipermanent to permanent immunity)
  - Artificially acquired passive immunity—Acquired by immunization with serum from another person that contains antibodies (temporary immunity)
- Naturally acquired immunity—No vaccines or toxoids are involved; process is largely endogenous
  - Naturally acquired active immunity—Acquired by exposure to invading pathogens (viruses, bacteria) that act as antigens and activate the immune system to produce antibodies; an example is an unvaccinated person who is exposed to a seasonal flu virus, gets sick, produces antibodies to the virus, and is immune when exposed again to the same viral strain (permanent immunity)
  - Naturally acquired passive immunity—Immunity acquired by the fetus or infant on transfer of maternal antibodies through the placenta or breast milk (temporary immunity)

acquired by the host over a length of time and will become more potent with each exposure to the antigen (Figure 17-2).

Naturally Acquired Passive Immunity When antibodies come from sources other than the individual's own body, the immunity is called **passive immunity. Naturally acquired passive immunity,** the transfer of antibodies from mother to baby through the placenta or breast milk, especially in colostrum, is the only example of this type of immunity. Because the antibodies come from an outside source, they do not last as long as antibodies produced as a response to specific antigens by the infant, but this does provide protection for an infant until his or her own immune system can work, at approximately 6 months to 1 year of age (see Figure 17-1).

Naturally Acquired Active Immunity Naturally acquired active immunity is permanent immunity gained by having the disease itself. Antigens that force the body to make antibodies to counteract or fight the disease process remain in the body after the disease has subsided (Figure 17-3). Each time the person is invaded by the antigens, the body will produce adequate antibodies to fight the infection. Naturally acquired active immunity may last for years or even for a lifetime. The host is responsible for and engaged in the formation of antibodies in response to a disease or toxic process. Even if the infection is subclinical or mild, the host's cells are stimulated to form antibodies for active immunity. If sufficient antibodies are produced, the person will not contract the disease if further contact should occur. The disadvantage of this type of immunity is that the person must have the disease to form antibodies. (Note: It takes several weeks to produce a naturally acquired active immunity following a disease and even longer to produce an artificially acquired active immunity because the organism has been attenuated in vaccines or immunizations.)

Artificially Acquired Active Immunity With active immunity, an antigen is introduced into the body to stimulate the production of antibodies when the person has not had the disease process and immunity is desired. The antigen may be introduced by artificial means, such as immunization, to produce **artificially acquired active immunity.** The introduction of the antigen forces the person's body to produce the antibodies for fighting the specific disease. Rather than introducing the virulent agent that might be pathogenic, the **virulence** is reduced, or **attenuated,** for administration. This allows the body to produce antibodies without causing the person to have a serious illness. Most immunity found within the wellness concept of medical practice is artificially acquired active immunity—a purposefully initiated immunity for protection of a susceptible person to a specific disease. The process of **immunization** may also be called **vaccination** because the agent used is usually a vaccine. In most instances the administration of a vaccine is a preventive medical measure designed to provide protection in anticipation of possible contact with the bacterial and viral pathogen in the future.

Artificially Acquired Passive Immunity A person with no immunity who has a large exposure to a virulent organism is at danger for contracting the disease. To prevent the disease process, the person needs borrowed or "ready-made" antibodies found in immune sera to counteract the virulent microorganisms and give short-term immunity rapidly.

The process of providing a person with antibodies from another source is **artificially acquired passive immunity.** Through the use of immune

Natural   Artificial

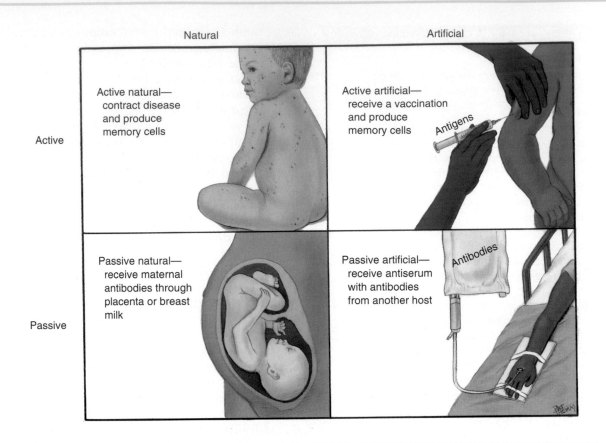

Active
Active natural—
contract disease
and produce
memory cells

Active artificial—
receive a vaccination
and produce
memory cells
Antigens

Passive
Passive natural—
receive maternal
antibodies through
placenta or breast
milk

Passive artificial—
receive antiserum
with antibodies
from another host
Antibodies

Figure 17-2   Types of active and natural immunity. (From Applegate E: *The anatomy and physiology learning system*, ed 3, St Louis, 2006, Saunders.)

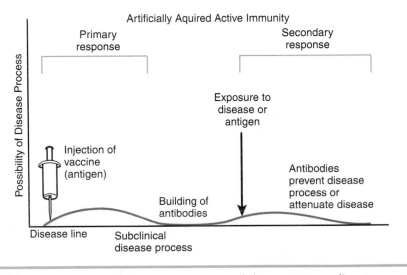

Artificially Aquired Active Immunity

Primary   Secondary
response   response

Possibility of Disease Process

Exposure to
disease or
antigen

Injection of
vaccine
(antigen)

Antibodies
prevent disease
process or
attenuate disease

Building of
antibodies

Disease line   Subclinical
disease process

Figure 17-3   Artificially acquired active immunity and the response to disease processes.

serum globulins (or antiserum) found in the blood from another source, the immunity is immediate and effective but short lived (Figure 17-4).

The **sera** prepared for immune purposes in emergency situations are often derived from animal sources. Immunization with the immune sera, either animal, such as horses, or human, is used when there is no time to wait for the body to develop its own antibodies or when the disease process would cause imminent danger, as with rubella in a pregnant woman. Use of animal antibodies may produce a sensitivity reaction called serum sickness; the

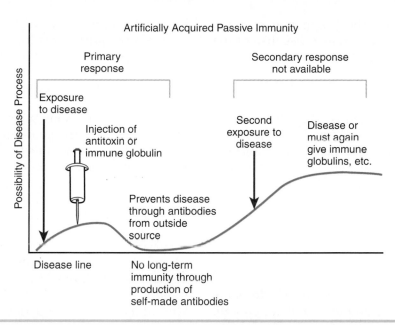

Figure 17-4 Artificially acquired passive immunity and the response to disease processes.

patient should be skin tested for hypersensitivity prior to administration of the serum. This reaction is not likely to occur if human gamma-globulins are used.

Some immune sera contain antibodies known as **antitoxins.** Antitoxins neutralize toxins from the organisms but do not act on the microorganisms themselves (Box 17-2). Antibodies do attach directly on antigens to mediate phagocytosis of the antigen by the macrophages.

Types of Active and Passive Immunizing Agents

To discuss immunizations, the terminology pertaining to their administration must be understood. As a review, remember that vaccines and toxoids are available to provide artificially acquired active immunity. Blood derivatives and antitoxins provide artificially acquired passive immunity.

Vaccines

A **vaccine** is a preparation containing a suspension of whole or fractionated microorganisms that, on administration, causes the recipient's immune system to establish a resistance to the infectious disease. The recipient's body produces antibodies toward the antigen or microbe found in the vaccine. Two major types of vaccines, killed and live attenuated, exist:

BOX 17-2	SOURCES OF IMMUNE GLOBULINS OR SERA

1. Diphtheria antitoxin, used for diphtheria, is obtained from immunized horses.
2. Tetanus immune globulin, used in preventing tetanus or lockjaw, is from human sources.
3. Immune globulins from human plasma are used for hepatitis A, measles, polio, or chickenpox.
4. Human hepatitis B immune globulins may be used to supply immunity to infants born to mothers who have hepatitis B.
5. Rabies antiserum may be obtained from either humans or horses and is the only antitoxin that is given to treat victims of bites from rabid animals.
6. Botulism antitoxin, obtained from horses, must be used soon after exposure for victims of botulism to be effective.
7. Anti-snakebite serum is an antivenom for a specific use to combat the effects of bites from poisonous snakes such as rattlesnakes.

- **Killed vaccines** are made of the whole killed microbe or some of its components such as those vaccines for pertussis or rabies.
- **Live** or **live attenuated vaccines** are composed of live microbes that have been weakened or rendered **avirulent;** examples are the vaccines for polio and for measles, mumps, and rubella combined (MMR). Immunocompromised individuals may be unable to fight the live or attenuated vaccine; therefore an immunocompromised patient may not be able to receive these vaccines. For a pregnant woman, the viral vaccines such as MMR and varicella should

not be given during the pregnancy or for 3 months prior to the pregnancy because of the danger of fetal malformation.

Toxoids

Toxoids are bacterial toxins that have been changed to a nontoxic state. After receiving a toxoid, the recipient's immune system forms antitoxins or antibodies against the natural bacterial toxin. The toxicity of the bacterial toxin has been weakened to the point that it does not cause the disease, but the toxin is still capable of stimulating the body to form antibodies.

Immune Globulins

Serum or plasma derivatives, or specific **immune globulins** (also called **immunoglobulins**), contain large concentrations of antibodies to specific antigens or diseases. These preparations are made from blood products and provide immediate short-term passive immunity. Immune globulins are used in diseases such as hepatitis B and rabies.

Antitoxins

Antitoxins are antibodies that are produced in response to a specific toxin and when administered have the ability to neutralize that toxin (e.g., diphtheria, tetanus) in a person at high risk for the disease or condition. Antitoxins are also used for short-term prophylaxis in a person who has been exposed to a specific toxin but does not have current acquired active immunity.

Who Should Be Immunized?

In today's health care, immunizations are a routine part of patient care. The critical period for immunization is from birth through school entry, with continuation through the school years and into adulthood. The required immunizations are suggested by the Centers for Disease Control and Prevention (CDC), and the various state immunization requirements are based on age groups. On entry into the school system of the United States, the child must meet the criteria set by the state and by local schools. Adults should continue to receive certain immunizations such as diphtheria-tetanus toxoid every 10 years and influenza yearly.

Certain populations have been found to be at high risk for contracting immunizable diseases:

- Adolescents, because of the declining immunization requirements for school attendance
- New parents who have allowed their immunity to wane and who are now exposed to childhood diseases because their children have the disease
- Debilitated persons, whether from physical disabilities or from age-related problems, who are now more susceptible to illness
- Migrant workers and new immigrants, who may not have been immunized at all or not adequately immunized
- Health care workers, who are exposed to diseases

In other patients who have been exposed to a disease, an **antibody titer** may be used to determine a person's immunity. The antibody titer, a laboratory test for evaluation of the antibodies circulating in the bloodstream, determines the immune state of a person to a specific disease. Persons intending to travel to areas where a disease is endemic should obtain the required and recommended immunizations before traveling. The local health department, in cooperation with the CDC, can provide a list of needed immunizations.

Patient Education for Compliance

The need to be current with immunizations as a means of disease prevention is obvious. Vaccinations do carry some risks, but the more serious risk is contracting a disease for which a vaccine is available. An example of the future hazards from disease processes that appear in adults is chickenpox leading to shingles later in life or mumps being associated with diabetes. Concerns about vaccines causing autism, hyperactivity attention deficit disorder, diabetes, and sudden infant death syndrome have caused parents to question immunizing children. However, vaccines have reduced and even eliminated many diseases that killed or severely disabled persons just several generations ago.

 CLINICAL TIP

If a patient has sustained a wound, especially a puncture wound, information concerning the level of immunity should be obtained including when the patient last received immunization against tetanus. If the patient does not remember or the record is unavailable, the health care provider will usually give a booster of tetanus toxoid.

IMPORTANT FACTS ABOUT IMMUNIZATIONS

- Immunizations are vital to the maintenance of public health and have changed the status of disease outbreaks in the world and increased the overall quality of life.
- Vaccines promote the production of antibodies against bacteria and viruses; toxoids promote the building of antibodies against bacterial toxins, not the bacteria themselves.
- Killed vaccines are made of whole killed microbes or their components. Live vaccines are made from attenuated or weakened live microbes that have been rendered avirulent in most persons.

Indications for Immunizations

The allied health professional has a definite role to play in helping the health care provider determine when a patient can safely receive an immunization. The professional should make an initial assessment of the patient's history and any symptoms of possible infection present. Any findings should be documented in the medical record for the health care provider to evaluate prior to ordering the administration of the vaccine.

- Vaccines may be safely administered, after authorization by a health care provider, to a person with a mild acute illness with or without fever unless chest congestion is present. Care should be taken that immunizations are not needlessly postponed because of mild to moderate symptoms.
- Mild to moderate local reactions from previous immunizations such as soreness, erythema, or swelling are not contraindications to further immunization.
- Taking antimicrobials, recovering from disease processes, and recent exposure to an infectious disease do not preclude the administration of the vaccines.
- A fever, even a high fever, is no longer considered an advised reason for not giving an immunization.

Contraindications to Immunizations

- Live vaccines should not be given to the following patients:
  - Those receiving steroids, radiation therapy, or antineoplastics.
  - Those who are immunosuppressed or have a current moderate to severe infection. These conditions suppress the immune system, and even the attenuated antigen, although it has been weakened, may still be sufficiently potent to produce the disease in the immunosuppressed patient.
  - Those who have received immune serum within the past 3 months because the immune serum may prevent the production of antibodies.
- Care must also be taken to assure that those who are immunized cannot harm susceptible persons in their home or work environment. Live vaccines take up to 30 days to be shed from the body, so the immunosuppressed person must be protected during this time. An example is the immunized child who is living in a home with a chronically ill grandparent or in a home where someone is undergoing chemotherapy.

Vaccines should not be administered to persons who are allergic to the substance or to any component used in manufacturing the vaccine. Giving an immunization to a patient who is allergic to a component of the vaccine could result in anaphylaxis.

- Some vaccines have egg as a component, others are made with preservatives such as mercury, and some vaccines contain antibiotics such as neomycin or polymyxin-B that were used to attenuate the microorganisms. Careful histories of possible allergic reactions should be taken with all patients to assure the immunization is not contraindicated because of components used in the manufacturing.
- Rubella and varicella vaccines are contraindicated in pregnancy because of teratogenicity to the developing fetus.
- Moderate or severe illness with fever is a contraindication to immunizations because of the danger that the patient may have an already compromised immune system.
- Other symptoms to defer immunizations are diarrhea, vomiting, and otitis.
- The health care provider should be consulted for closer evaluation if the person gives a history of seizures or high-pitched screams over a prolonged time following the administration of vaccines. These could be reasons for the nonadministration of the same immunization.

If a question exists concerning the administration of the vaccine or not, the physician will make a decision by weighing the potential for benefit against the potential for risks and provide sufficient information for parents to make informed decisions about immunizations.

Adverse Reactions to Immunizations

The importance of immunizations as a method of protection from infectious diseases cannot be stressed enough, but immunizations also have associated risks. The side effects are usually mild and transient, with such symptoms as a slight fever, minor rashes, or soreness at the injection site. Joint pain and malaise may be found with live and inactivated vaccines. The minor expected reactions such as a mild fever can be controlled by such measures as acetaminophen and sponge baths. Though these effects of immunization are common and uncomfortable, the need to give the vaccines to prevent diseases may tip the balance in favor of giving the immunization, even with risks.

Some people have unusual and severe reactions. This information is monitored by the Food and Drug Administration (FDA) and CDC. Any serious problem encountered with a vaccine must have the data sent to Vaccine Adverse Event Reporting System (VAERS). Monitoring any adverse reactions is part of the surveillance program that is in place to detect uncommon, severe, previously unseen, or rare reactions to immunizations. Some of these rare reactions have included Guillain-Barré syndrome with influenza vaccines, encephalitis with measles vaccine, or peripheral neuropathy with rubella vaccine.

Anaphylactic reactions are a possibility with immunizations, as they are with any medication. The person should be skin tested prior to the administration of antitoxins if there is any suspicion of sensitivity as this precaution will decrease the possibility of unexpected severe reactions (Box 17-3).

Because of the many advantages to the patient who receives immunotherapy, immunizations are encouraged and even required for most citizens in the United States. The advantages of immunity far outweigh the dangers of the medications in most instances. Health care professionals should encourage parents to immunize their children. Adults should also be reminded of the need for proper immunization on a regular basis because immunizations of all citizens protect public and personal health.

BOX 17-3	TYPICAL SIDE EFFECTS AND ADVERSE REACTIONS FROM SELECTED VACCINES OR TOXOIDS
VACCINE OR TOXOID	**SERIOUS SIDE EFFECTS**
Measles, mumps, rubella	Anaphylaxis, thrombocytopenia, dangers of teratogenicity in pregnancy, encephalitis
Diphtheria, tetanus, pertussis	Encephalopathy, convulsions, shocklike states
Polio (OPV)	Vaccine-associated poliomyelitis (OPV)
Hepatitis B	Anaphylaxis
Varicella	Anaphylaxis
Influenza	Guillain-Barré syndrome

DID YOU KNOW?

In early 2006 outbreaks of mumps and pertussis were both documented, although both diseases had been thought to be virtually eradicated in the United States. The pathogens were thought to have been brought to the country by world travelers who had visited countries where immunizations are not enforced and were passed to persons whose antibody levels were not sufficient to prevent the diseases, especially in adults who had not been sufficiently immunized.

Documentation of Immunizations

The National Childhood Vaccine Injury Act of 1986 provided for the compilation of Vaccine Information Statements (VIS) by the CDC for certain immunizations. These documents are available from the CDC's website (www.cdc.gov/vaccines/pubs/vis), or a set may be ordered by calling the CDC Immunization Hotline at 800-232-2522. Further requirements of the statute include the following:

- A parent or legal guardian of a child, or the adult vaccinee, must be provided with a copy of the Vaccine Information Statement (VIS) before the administration of vaccines, showing the risks and benefits of a vaccine. The medical office may add an identifier for the office on the VIS, but the CDC must approve any other change.
- A permanent record of each mandated vaccination must be given to a patient.
- VIS must be provided on: DTaP, DTP, Td, MMR, varicella, polio, Hib, or hepatitis B vaccines.

- VIS is not required but is recommended for influenza, pneumococcal, and hepatitis A vaccines.
- The patient or parent must have time to read the information prior to administration of the medication.
- The medical record must show documentation that the VIS was given and the publication date of the VIS, because revisions occur from time to time. The date appears under the CDC logo.
- From a legal standpoint, the immunization should always be recorded in the patient's medical record to show that the medication has been given. The following data must be included:
  - Date of vaccination
  - Route and site of vaccination
  - Vaccine type, manufacturer, lot number, and expiration date
  - Name, address, and title of person administering the vaccine
  - Delivery of VIS to appropriate person and the date of VIS publication
  - Signing of permission to give medication by parent/guardian prior to administration

Several reasons for keeping these records exist. First, they ensure that the person, especially a child, receives the appropriate immunization. Second, the chance of overvaccination is reduced, as is the risk of possible hypersensitivity reactions. Another reason for reporting adverse reactions to the CDC by vaccine, lot number, manufacturer, and so on is for tracking possible links to adverse reactions. Finally, the condition of the patient following the injection should be documented.

Agents for Artificially Acquired Active Immunity

Higher levels of immunity are produced and immunizations are not needed as often with artificially acquired active immunity. Live attenuated viruses give the person a mild, subclinical form of the disease to produce immunity. Inactivated bacteriologic agents are safer but shorter acting and require revaccination for continued protection.

Vaccines for Diphtheria, Tetanus, and Pertussis (DTaP, Tdap, Td)

The vaccine protects against the three diseases named in the vaccine.

- DTaP (Diphtheria, tetanus, and acellular pertussis) vaccine is for pediatric patients younger than the age of 7. DTaP contains acellular pertussis, a form less likely to cause adverse reactions.
- Tdap (tetanus, diphtheria, and acellular pertussis) is the adolescent preparation that should be used for ages 10 to 19.
- The tetanus-diphtheria vaccine (Td) is the adult version for ages older than 20 because adults are not susceptible to pertussis (whooping cough). This immunization should be administered every 10 years throughout the adult years.
- Acetaminophen given in appropriate doses before and after immunization will reduce discomfort and side effects.
- This vaccine should be withheld in a child with high fever, chest congestion, and uncontrolled seizures.
- DTaP, 0.5 mL is recommended at 2 months, 4 months, 6 months, and 15 to 18 months of age. A booster is given before the child starts school at 4 to 6 years of age. If the series is interrupted, it is not necessary to restart the series.

Tetanus Toxoid (TT)

Tetanus toxoid is given to persons who have not had the disease or whose antibody titer shows insufficient numbers of antibodies for immunity to the disease to be present.

Tetanus toxoid should be given to:

- The person with less than three doses of the vaccine at any time.
- The person with a wound who has had the proper schedule of three or more doses of the vaccine but has not had a booster in more than 10 years.
- The person, including children, who has a severe or dirty wound and who has not had a tetanus immunization in 5 years.

Vaccines for Measles (Rubeola), Mumps, and Rubella (MMR)

The MMR vaccine is a live virus vaccine that immunizes against the three diseases and is given at ages 12 to 15 months and 4 to 6 years. The two doses must be at least 4 weeks apart. It is given to persons who have not had the diseases or whose antibody titer shows insufficient numbers of antibodies for immunity to the disease to be present.

- Pregnant women, breastfeeding women, and persons with active tuberculosis should not be given this vaccine.

- Women who might become pregnant within 3 months should not receive this immunization.
- It must be reconstituted using a fluid containing no antibacterial or bacteriostatic additives.

DID YOU KNOW?

Some states now require a rubella antibody titer on all women of childbearing age to show their immune state to rubella prior to issuing a marriage license.

Poliomyelitis Vaccines (IPV, OPV)

Polio vaccines have been available for immunization against poliomyelitis as IPV (inactivated poliovirus vaccine or Salk vaccine) and OPV (oral poliovirus vaccine or Sabin vaccine). The CDC recommends the use of IPV because of adverse reactions of acquiring polio as a disease from OPV. Therefore the use of OPV is no longer recommended for routine use in the United States.

- The series of 1-mL immunizations of IPV is given at 6- to 8-week intervals in the first year of life, at 2, 4, and 6 months. A booster is given at 15 to 18 months, followed by another at 4 to 6 years.
- This vaccine is generally not given to adults older than the age of 18 unless they have not been vaccinated and are traveling to an endemic area.

Vaccine for *Haemophilus Influenzae* Type B

Haemophilus influenzae type B (Hib) vaccine is used to provide protection against the virus that is a common cause of meningitis in young children.

- The immunosuppressed child and the child allergic to diphtheria toxoid should not be given Hib.
- The Hib vaccine is given IM with a dose of 0.5 mL at 2, 4, 6, and 12 to 15 months of age.

Vaccines for Hepatitis

Hepatitis B

Hepatitis B vaccine (Hep B) is an attenuated virus vaccine that provides immunity against hepatitis B only. It is required in many states for child care facilities and school attendance.

- Hep B vaccine is recommended for health care workers, patients on hemodialysis or who receive blood products, persons at high risk for sexually transmitted diseases, drug users, and persons in contact with hepatitis B, as well as infants.
- Hep B is now given to infants beginning with the first dose either at birth or at 1 month of age and then at 2 and 4 months with the fourth injection between 6 and 18 months of age.
- The dose is 0.25 mL in the vastus lateralis muscle for infants or 1 mL in the deltoid for adults. The second of the three-immunization series is given 1 month after the first, and not later than 2 months after the initial injection. The third dose is given 6 months after the first for adults and in 2 months for children.
- The immunization may be delayed if the patient has an infection.

Hepatitis A

Hepatitis A vaccine (Havrix) is provided to persons who are traveling to areas where hepatitis A is endemic and to all children 1 year of age with a second dose in 6 months.

- Persons with chronic liver disease or those with employment that puts the individual at risk, such as health care workers, may be given the vaccine prophylactically.
- The length of protection is unknown but is believed to be up to 10 years.
- The vaccine is only given intramuscularly.

Vaccine for Chickenpox

Varicella virus vaccine (Varivax) is recommended at age 12 months of age and is a requirement in some states for admission to school.

- The length of immunity for this live, attenuated varicella virus for prophylaxis against chickenpox has not been confirmed, but studies indicate that immunity lasts for at least 6 years.
- The subcutaneous immunization of 0.5 mL should be given at 12 months of age. For the child younger than 12 years old who did not receive the vaccine and has not had the disease, the same dose may be given. For persons 13 years old and older, two doses of 0.5 mL each should be given 4 to 8 weeks apart.

- The need for a booster has not been established.
- All adults with no evidence of immunity to varicella should receive two doses of varicella vaccine 4 weeks apart.
- Varivax should not be given to the following persons: those who are hypersensitive to components of the vaccine; immunosuppressed patients; those with active untreated tuberculosis; those with febrile infections; and persons with neoplasms of the bone marrow or lymphatic system. Nor should this vaccine be given to pregnant women or those who may be pregnant within 3 months because it is an attenuated viral vaccine.

Vaccines for Respiratory Conditions

Influenza Vaccines

Influenza vaccines including the injectable and intranasal types produce immunity to only those strains of influenza viruses that are expected to cause disease in the United States in a given year.

- Immunizations are recommended yearly for all persons older than 6 months. Those who have a special need for immunization are: persons older than 65 years old; those with chronic medical conditions; those in long-term care facilities; people with chronic pulmonary or cardiovascular conditions or with chronic metabolic, renal, immunosuppressive, or hematopoietic blood diseases; children 6 months to 18 years of age on aspirin therapy (to reduce the chance of Reye's syndrome); and health care workers or household members of patients who are at high risk.
- People allergic to eggs, chickens, feathers, chicken dander, or neomycin may be allergic to the vaccine.
- A person with fever or anyone who has received the pertussis vaccine within the previous 3 days should delay taking this vaccine.
- Because the components of the vaccine change yearly, 0.5 mL IM should be given each year, preferably in October or November before the peak influenza season. Children younger than age 3 should receive 2 doses of 0.25 mL 1 month apart, whereas children ages 3 to 9 receive the 0.5 mL dose as a single dose or as 2 doses 1 month apart at the health care provider's discretion. All children younger than years of age 9 should receive both doses before November 1.

- For nonpregnant persons under 2 years and between ages 5 to 49 without severe medical conditions, an acceptable alternative to parenteral immunization is FluMist (LAIV), a live attenuated influenza vaccine that is administered intranasally.

Pneumococcal Vaccine

Two types of pneumococcal vaccine are available—one for children and the other for adults.

- Pneumococcal conjugated vaccine (PCV) is recommended for all children ages 2 to 23 months and some children between 24 and 50 months. A final dose should be given at 12 years of age for children.
- Persons with chronic disorders should receive the pneumococcal polysaccharide (PPV) vaccine.
- Adults between 19 and 64 should receive the PPV vaccine with a revaccination after the age of 65.
- Persons over 65 should be revaccinated with PPV if the initial vaccination was more than 5 years prior and the person was younger than 65 when the initial vaccine was administered.
- The dose is 0.5 mL subcutaneously or 1 mL intramuscularly.
- The vaccine should be delayed in people with fever.
- Side effects include local reactions, rash, arthritis, arthralgia, myalgia, swollen lymph glands, and malaise.

BCG Vaccine

Bacille Calmette-Guérin vaccine (BCG) is used to immunize against tuberculosis (TB).

- The vaccine is not commonly used but persons at high risk for exposure to tuberculosis, such as those traveling to areas with high incidence of TB, persons with family members with active TB, or health care workers who are routinely exposed to the disease, may be advised to take the vaccine.
- BCG vaccine is given percutaneously by rubbing 0.2 to 0.3 mL of the vaccine on the skin and then making small punctures in that area. The area should be kept dry for 24 hours without a dressing.
- The person receiving the medication should be aware that any subsequent tuberculin skin tests should show positive results and a radiograph will be necessary for further testing for tuberculosis.

Other Vaccines

Rotavirus Vaccine

The vaccine contains five strains of rotavirus, a common cause of diarrhea in children younger than 3 years of age.

- Rotavirus vaccine (Rotateq) is given orally at 2, 4, and 6 months of age.
- Rotateq may be administered with other vaccines for infants.

Meningococcal Vaccine

Meningococcal vaccine is available in two forms—one that contains inactivated bacteria (MPSV4) and one that is a bacterial conjugate (MCV4).

The meningococcal conjugate vaccine protects against four different strains of the causative bacteria for meningitis, *Neisseria meningitides*.

- The MCV4 vaccine is to be administered to 11- to 55-year-olds, but especially to college students living in dormitories or other persons at risk because of travel or working conditions.
- MPSV4 is an acceptable alternative for children and adolescents.
- Usually one dose of vaccine is adequate, but a second dose 5 years later may be indicated in persons at high risk for contracting the disease.
- Some colleges now require that all freshmen be immunized prior to admission to prevent outbreaks of the disease.
- The vaccine may be administered to anyone who has been exposed during an outbreak.
- The medication is to be administered intramuscularly for MCV4 and subcutaneously for MPSV4. Only one dose of the vaccine is recommended.
- The vaccines are safe and may be given to pregnant women.

Human Papillomavirus Vaccine

Human papillomavirus (HPV) vaccine (Gardasil) has been developed to prevent cervical cancer, precancerous genital lesions, and genital warts caused by HPV.

- The CDC recommends routine HPV vaccination for girls 11 to 12 years of age and for women up to 26 years of age given as 3 doses with the second dose 2 months following the initial immunization and the third dose at 6 months after the initial immunization.

- The immunization should not be given during pregnancy.
- The vaccine is 70% effective for cervical cancer and 90% effective for genital warts.
- The length of immunity is unknown at present but is at least 5 years.

Zoster Vaccine (Shingles Vaccine)

The zoster vaccine provides protection against shingles and the associated chronic pain.

- In October 2006 the CDC recommended that zoster vaccine (Zostavax) be administered to all people age 60 and older including those who have previously had shingles.
- Only one dose is necessary at present.
- The vaccine is not a substitute for Varivax (herpes zoster vaccine for chickenpox) in children

"Supershots"

Researchers are testing what will be called "supershots"—combinations of vaccines that give a child protection from more diseases with fewer injections. Children now receive a total of 16 immunizations in the first 2 years of life, and the new combination immunizations will reduce this number. By combining vaccines, it is hoped that the likelihood of the completion of the immunization schedule will be increased and the pain and suffering for children and parents will be reduced (Table 17-2).

- One of the most important developments is the single immunization for diphtheria, tetanus, pertussis, hepatitis B, and polio.
- Another vaccine that has been introduced is the pneumococcal conjugant-7 vaccine (Prevnar) for very young infants for protection against invasive disease caused by *Streptococcus pneumoniae*. The vaccine provides protection from meningitis, pneumonia, and other serious infections, as well as some protection from recurrent otitis media (middle ear) infections.
- Another approved supershot is the MMR vaccine with varicella vaccine.
- Pentavac (a combination of DTaP, IPV, MMR, Hib, and Hep B) and Hexavac (a combination of MMR, DTaP, Hib, IPV, Hep B, and Hepatitis) are available to further increase the number of "supershots" and to decrease the number of injections needed in children.

TABLE 17-2 *Select Agents That Provide Active Immunity*

IMMUNIZING AGENT	TRADE NAME	DOSAGE, ROUTE, SITE OF ADMINISTRATION	INDICATIONS FOR PROTECTION	SIDE EFFECTS
DTP-DTwP (inactivated whole cell bacteria)	Generic	0.5 mL IM q4-8 wk × 3 doses beginning at 2 mo, with boosters at 4-8 yr; deltoid or mediolateral thigh	Diphtheria, tetanus, pertussis, ages >2 mo to <7 yr	Swelling, local reactions, fever, irritability, crying, drowsiness, anorexia
DTaP (inactivated bacterial components)	Tri-Immunol	Same as for DTP-DTwP		
DT; Td	Generic	0.5 mL IM q10 yr; deltoid or mediolateral thigh	Diphtheria, tetanus in children >7 through adulthood; may be used with children who have contraindications to pertussis vaccine	Local reactions, headaches, myalgia, hypotension, joint pain, stuffiness
Tetanus, reduced diphtheria, acellular pertussis (adult Tdap)	Adacel	0.5 mL IM × 1 dose for persons ages 11-64	Tetanus, diphtheria, and pertussis in adults	Same as other TD listed earlier
MMR (Note: These come in individual doses, and the monovalent measles vaccine may be given at 6 mo of age.)	MMR-II	1 dose SC in outer aspect of upper arm	Rubeola, mumps, rubella after 12-15 mo, with booster at 4-6 yr	Fever, rash, jaw pain, headache, myalgia, sore throat
Rubella vaccine (Rubella vaccine should not be given to pregnant women.)	Attenuvax	1 dose SC in outer aspect of upper arm	Same as MMR	Same as MMR except jaw pain and sore throat
Polio vaccine IPV (Salk)	Generic or IPOL	0.5 mL IM × 3 doses at 4-8 wk intervals beginning at 2 mo with booster at 12-15 mo, then 1 booster at 4-6 yr	Polio (in children or adults)	Tenderness at injection site, fever, erythema
OPV (Sabin) TOPV Trivalent OPV (ACIP suggests OPV be used only in special circumstances.)	Orimune	Doses of OPV may be given for fourth and booster doses of polio vaccine, but first series of three doses should be IPV For adults and children over 2 years of age, 0.5 mL po q8wk × 2 doses, then 0.5 mL po 6 mo-1 year after dose 2	Polio in children up to 18 yr	Diarrhea, rare vaccine-associated paralysis
Haemophilus influenza B (Hib) vaccine	HibTITER (4 doses) Pedvax HIB (3 doses)	0.5 mL IM at 2, 4, and 6 mo with booster at 12-15 mo 0.5 mL IM at 2 and 4 mo; booster at 12-18 mos	Diseases caused by *Haemophilus influenzae* B such as sepsis, osteomyelitis, septic arthritis, bacterial meningitis, pneumonia	Redness at injection site, fever, vomiting, diarrhea
DTwP + Hib	Tetramune	0.5 mL IM at 2, 4, and 6 mo with a booster at 15-18 mo and 4-6 yr	Same as for DTwP and Hib separately	Same as for DTwP and Hib

(continued)

TABLE 17-2 *Select Agents That Provide Active Immunity—cont'd*

IMMUNIZING AGENT	TRADE NAME	DOSAGE, ROUTE, SITE OF ADMINISTRATION	INDICATIONS FOR PROTECTION	SIDE EFFECTS
Hepatitis B vaccine	Recombivax HB, Engerix B	See package for amounts (amounts vary with brand/age) IM deltoid or anterolateral thigh	Given to children and adults for hepatitis B protection	Redness at injection site, headache, nausea, myalgia, jaw pain, fever
Varicella vaccine (Note: should not be given to pregnant women)	Varivax	0.5 mL > 12 mo of age Adults: 0.5 mL with 2nd dose in 4-8 wk	Varicella	Local reaction at injection site, rash, fever
Tetanus toxoid (TT)	Generic	0.5 mL SC 1-12 yr 1 dose after 12 mo of age 12 yr to adults: 0.5 mL SC followed by a second dose in 4-8 wk, then every 10 yr or as needed	Tetanus used with injury-related possible infection and for prophylaxis	Local reactions, fever, chills, malaise, myalgia
Influenza vaccine Influenza vaccine A and B, live	Generic Fluogen, Fluzone	Adults: 0.5 mL IM as single dose 3-9 yr: 0.5 mL doses 1 or 2 mo apart 6 mo to 3 yr: 0.25 mL doses, 2 mo apart	Annual vaccination for influenza, especially indicated for those susceptible to URI infections	Local redness, fever, myalgia, malaise
	FluMist	0.5 mL intranasal	For use with healthy persons ages < 2 and 5-49	Runny nose, nasal congestion, cough, sore throat, low-grade fever, myalgia, chills, headache, lethargy
Pneumococcal vaccine	Pneumovax, Pnu-Immune	0.5 mL SC/IM as single dose	Pneumococcal pneumonia and bacteremia, adults and children > 2 yr	Local reaction, fever, arthralgia, myalgia, rash
BCG (bacilli Calmette-Guérin) vaccine	Generic, TICE	0.2-0.3 mL percutaneously by small puncture wounds	Tuberculosis if person is at high risk	Swollen lymph nodes
Pneumococcal 7-valent conjugate vaccine	Prevnar	0.5 mL IM infants: 4 doses at 2, 4, 6, and 15 mo; 7-11 mo: 3 doses; 12-23 mo: 2 doses; 24 mo to 9 yr: 1 dose	Invasive pneumococcal infections in infants and toddlers	Local reaction, irritability, restless sleep, drowsiness, decreased appetite
Hepatitis A vaccine	Havrix	1440 EL Units for adults >18; 720 EL Units for 2-18 yr old	Hepatitis A	Local side effects, fever, malaise, anorexia, headache, nausea
Hepatitis A and B vaccine	Twinrix	1 mL IM—3 doses with the second dose scheduled 1 mo following the first and the third dose 6 mo after the first dose for ages <18	Hepatitis A and B	Pain, redness and swelling at injection site, headache, lethargy, loss of appetite, fever, and GI symptoms
Meningococcal vaccine	MPSV4 MCV4	0.5 mL SC 0.5 mL IM	Meningitis	Fever, rash
Lyme vaccine	LYMErix	0.5 mL IM in deltoid muscle	Lyme disease	Local reaction, arthralgia, myalgia
Human papillomavirus (HPV) recombinant vaccine	Gardasil	0.5 mL IM for each dose; first dose followed by second dose 2 mo later and third dose 6 mo after first dose	Women ages 11-26 for HPV, a cause of cervical cancer	Pain, itching, swelling, and redness at injection site; fever, nausea, dizziness

TABLE 17-2 *Select Agents That Provide Active Immunity—cont'd*

IMMUNIZING AGENT	TRADE NAME	DOSAGE, ROUTE, SITE OF ADMINISTRATION	INDICATIONS FOR PROTECTION	SIDE EFFECTS
SUPERSHOTS				
Diphtheria/tetanus toxoids, DaPT, Hepatitis B vaccine, IPV vaccine	Pediarix	0.5 mL IM at 2, 4, and 6 mo	Diphtheria, tetanus, pertussis, hepatitis B, poliomyelitis	Same as with the individual vaccines listed earlier
MMR and varicella vaccine	ProQuad	0.5 mL SC at 12 mo and 12 yr	Rubeola, rubella, mumps, and chickenpox	Same as with the individual vaccines listed earlier
Meningococcal polysaccharide, diphtheria, tetanus conjugate vaccine	Menactra	0.5 mL IM	Meningitis, diphtheria, and tetanus in persons ages 11-55	Same as with individual vaccines listed earlier

GI, Gastrointestinal; *IM*, intramuscular; *IPV*, inactivated poliomyelitis vaccine; *MMR*, measles, mumps, rubella; *SC*, subcutaneous; *URI*, upper respiratory infection.

Vaccines for Specific Populations

Vaccine for Lyme Disease

Lyme vaccine (LYMErix) is specifically for individuals at risk of being bitten by tick vectors that carry Lyme disease.

• The selection of individuals to receive the immunization is based on geographic area, which can vary within counties and towns.
• The recommendations for vaccination are for 15- to 70-year-olds who reside, work, or recreate in areas of high to moderate risk for deer ticks.
• The vaccine is expensive and is not recommended for persons at low risk.
• The administration of LYMErix is a dose of 0.5 mL IM in the deltoid muscle, followed by a second dose 1 month later. A third dose should be given 1 year later before the beginning of the season for the transmission of Lyme disease, usually in April. This vaccine is not recommended for pregnant women, children younger than 15, or adults older than 70.

Rabies Vaccine

Rabies vaccine is an exception to the rule of immunization because the vaccine is given after the invasion of the disease organism.

• Rabies is slow to develop, and the affected persons may be vaccinated after transmission of the organism and still have sufficient time to build antibodies against the invading organisms and provide active immunity.
• The vaccine is a killed virus vaccine and may be given prophylactically to persons who are in routine contact with animals and to anyone bitten by a suspected rabid animal.

Patient Safety with Agents for Active Immunization

With all immunizations, the patient should remain in the office for 15 to 30 minutes to observe for adverse reactions such as shortness of breath, wheezing, or a drop in blood pressure. If the patient does not remain, this should be documented along with the time that the immunization was given, for the legal protection of the health care provider. Because adverse reactions are often not reported until the next appointment, the patient or parent should be told to immediately report reactions such as high fever (>104° F to 105° F), collapse, persistent cough (in excess of 3 hours), and seizures to the medical office.

The practitioner should not combine separate vaccines into the same syringe for administration unless the health professional approves and the package insert states approval by the FDA. Each vaccine should be given as a single medication to prevent adverse reactions and possible interactions between the active immunization components. Table 17-2 lists the more commonly administered immunizations for artificially acquired active immunity including those used in special populations who may be exposed to disease because of travel or special circumstances. Table 17-3 gives the recommended schedule of immunizations for children and adults and Box 17-4 gives a quick reference of the proper route of administration for selected vaccines.

Safety with Vaccines

The CDC, as a means of providing continued safety with vaccines, has supplied information to the immunization provider for storage and maintenance of vaccines for patient safety. Box 17-5 provides some of the safety tips related to vaccines. Others may be found at the CDC website (www.cdc.gov).

IMPORTANT FACTS ABOUT AGENTS FOR ARTIFICIALLY ACQUIRED ACTIVE IMMUNITY

- Immunizations provide antibody-antigen reactions for long-term immunity, whereas immune globulins and antitoxins provide antibodies for short-term immunity.
- Acquired active immunity provides long-term disease protection, with the person making the antibodies to the disease process, whereas passive immunity provides short-term disease prevention, with immunity being provided by antibodies from other sources.
- Vaccines contain a suspension of whole or fractionated microorganisms. Toxoids are bacterial toxins that have been changed to a nontoxic state.
- Immunizations are the administration of vaccines or toxoids. These produce artificially acquired active immunity, with antibodies developing over a period of time, providing immunity for years.
- Vaccines are safe, although mild reactions are fairly common. Serious adverse effects rarely occur.
- Live vaccines should not be given to immunocompromised patients.
- The MMR vaccine is composed of three live viruses and is contraindicated in pregnancy and in people with allergies to eggs, gelatin, or neomycin.
- Two DTP vaccines offer protection against diphtheria, tetanus, and pertussis: DTaP, or inactivated bacteria (acellular) for young children, and Tdap for the adolescent.
- Two poliovirus vaccines exist: oral poliovirus vaccine (OPV), or Sabin vaccine, which contains live attenuated viruses; and injectable inactivated poliovirus vaccine (IPV), or Salk vaccine. OPV is not recommended for use in the United States.

IMPORTANT FACTS ABOUT AGENTS FOR ARTIFICIALLY ACQUIRED ACTIVE IMMUNITY—*Cont'd*

- Varicella vaccine, a live attenuated vaccine, provides complete protection against chickenpox in most children. For those who acquire the disease after vaccination the course is usually milder. The vaccine is safe but is contraindicated in pregnant women, people with hypersensitivities, and immunocompromised people.
- Hepatitis B vaccine promotes synthesis of specific antibodies for the hepatitis B virus. It is one of the safest vaccines; all health care professionals at risk should take this vaccine.
- Two new vaccines—HPV vaccine and a vaccine for shingles—have been recently recommended for use by the CDC.
- The CDC issues the recommended vaccines yearly. These should be checked on a regular basis to ensure the proper vaccination of patients.
- Other diseases have specific vaccines, and the routine for administration of these should be obtained from the CDC to ensure safety in travel to areas of susceptibility, exposure to disease, or specific circumstances that indicate these vaccines.

DID YOU KNOW?

The vaccines of the future include those for cytomegalovirus, respiratory syncytial virus, human immunodeficiency virus (HIV), herpes simplex virus, *Staphylococcus aureus*, Group B streptococcus, malaria, and a new one for *Mycobacterium tuberculosis*.

 CLINICAL TIP

To lessen the pain of vaccines with older children, one technique is to have children blow on a feather to blow away the pain. Blowing lessens the pain perceived. Another technique is to swab the forearm with alcohol and have the child blow on the alcohol. The person cannot perceive the cold of blowing and the pain from the immunization at the same time.

Agents for Artificially Acquired Passive Immunity

Passive immunity occurs when antibodies are injected into the body for an immediate, rapid but short-lived type of immunity that lasts for only a few weeks or months.

- The agents are antitoxins—an immune agent produced in response to an antigen and capable of neutralizing toxins.

TABLE 17-3 *Recommended Immunization Schedule*

VACCINE/TOXOID	BIRTH	1 MO	2 MO	4 MO	6 MO	12 MO	15 MO	18 MO	4-6 YR	11-12 YR	14-16 YR	ADULT
Hepatitis B vaccine	Dose 1	Dose 2			Dose 3					a		Hepatitis B in adolescents or adults: 3 doses, first followed by the second in 1 mo and the third 5 mo after the second
Diphtheria, tetanus toxoids, pertussis vaccine			Dose 1	Dose 2	Dose 3		Dose 4		Dose 5		b	Use Td in unvaccinated adolescents or adults: first dose, second dose 1-2 mo later, third dose 6-12 mo after second dose, then every 10 yr
Haemophilus influenza type B vaccine			Dose 1	Dose 2	Dose 3c	Dose 4						
Poliovirus vaccine, IPV			Dose 1	Dose 2		Dose 3			Dose 4			OPV is used only in special circumstances, often with travel
Measles, mumps, rubella vaccine						Dose 1			Dose 2	(or) Dose 2d		First dose followed by second dose 28 days or more later (may be 1 or 2 doses)
Varicella vaccine						One dose only				e	f	Varicella vaccine: first dose followed by second dose 1-2 mo later
Pneumococcal vaccine												g
Influenza vaccine												h
Meningococcal Vaccine												11-Adult: 1 dose

From the Centers for Disease Control and Prevention, Atlanta.

a Children not vaccinated should have the initial series at 11 or 12 yr.

b Tetanus/diphtheria booster should be given every 10 yr unless otherwise indicated.

c If Pedavax HIB is administered, the 6-mo immunization is not required.

d Dose 2 is recommended at either 4-6 yr or 11-12 yr, both doses before 12 yr of age.

e Unvaccinated children with history of disease may be vaccinated at 11-12 yr with 1 dose.

f Unvaccinated children older than 13 should receive 2 doses at least 1 mo apart.

g A one-time vaccination for those older than 50 or at high risk for the disease.

h Yearly injection is recommended for all ages.

BOX 17-4	PROPER ADMINISTRATION ROUTES FOR IMMUNIZATIONS	
SUBCUTANEOUS	**INTRAMUSCULAR**	**ORAL**
MMR	DTaP, DT, Td	Rotateq
IPV	Hepatitis B	
Pneumococcal polysaccharide	Hib	
Varicella	IPV	
Meningococcal polysaccharide	Meningococcal conjugate	
Pneumococcal conjugate	Tetanus toxoid	
Hepatitis A	**INTRANASAL**	
	Flumist	

BOX 17-5   SAFE STORAGE OF VACCINES

- Inspect vaccines on delivery and monitor refrigerator and freezer temperatures to assure maintenance of the proper temperature chain during delivery.
- Vaccines are fragile and must be kept at recommended temperatures at all times.
- Rotate vaccine stock so that the oldest vaccines are used first.
- Administer vaccines within the prescribed time period following reconstitution.
- Wait to draw vaccines into syringes until immediately prior to administration.
- It is better to not vaccinate than to administer a dose of vaccine that has been mishandled.
- Anyone who received compromised vaccine will have to be revaccinated, making parents unhappy that a child must receive repeat doses of vaccines.
- If errors in vaccine storage and administration occur, take corrective action immediately to prevent recurrence and notify public health authorities.

- Antitoxins from human and animal sources are used for prophylactic and therapeutic purposes for specific toxins.
- Immune globulins are antibodies found in serum that are used in the prevention of diseases such as hepatitis B, tetanus, and rabies.
- The patient should be skin tested prior to administration of the antitoxin to protect the person from anaphylaxis caused by allergies.
- Care should also be taken so that active immunizing agents are not administered at the same time as immune globulins as the immune globulins may stop the actions of the immunizing agents.

Immune Globulins

Rho(D) immune human globulin (RhoGAM) is an antibody preparation used to desensitize Rh-negative mothers after delivery (Figure 17-5).

The sensitization of the mother occurs when any of the blood cells of the Rh-positive infant enter the bloodstream of the mother, usually at birth, causing an antibody formation in the mother. If that mother has a subsequent Rh-positive infant, the produced antibodies may cause erythroblastosis fetalis in the second infant. RhoGAM must be administered within 72 hours after delivery to diminish antibody formation by the mother.

Other selected agents for artificially acquired passive immunity are found in Table 17-4.

Patient Education

In today's world many childhood diseases that were fatal several generations ago are now almost eradicated in the United States because of immunizations. Parents must understand the need for immunizing children. State and federal laws require immunizations for school, although some parents may refuse to immunize the child because of cultural or religious beliefs. For the child to obtain the maximum effect from immunizations, spacing of the immunizations must be at the CDC-suggested time intervals. Immunizations and vaccines are monitored by the CDC for safety and to minimize vaccine-related injuries. Although time intervals longer than those recommended may be acceptable in some cases, shorter intervals for obtaining the immunizations required by law are unacceptable. The child who has not been properly immunized during the first year and a half of life and whose parents then wait until school age will not be allowed to attend school until the immunizations have been administered. Administering multiple vaccines over a short period of time puts the child at greater risk for adverse reactions.

Adults have a higher incidence of noncompliance than children. The allied health professional should assist the adult patient in keeping current with vaccines such as diphtheria-tetanus (Td) vaccine. The at-risk patient should be encouraged to have influenza immunizations yearly and the pneumococcal vaccine as recommended. As new vaccines are available for artificially acquired active immunity such as HPV and shingles vaccines, adults and children should be encouraged to avail themselves of this protection.

Immunizations save in direct medical costs and indirect societal costs. Parents must do their part to make sure their children are immunized with current vaccines and new immunizations as

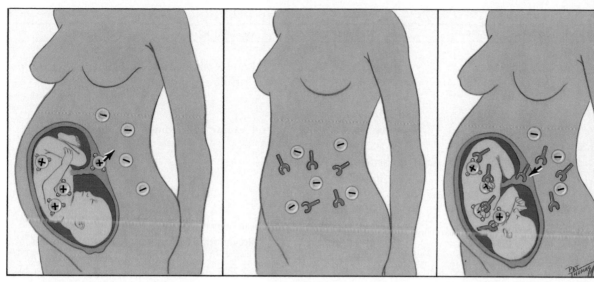

First pregnancy Rh⁻ mother exposed to Rh⁺ agglutinogens.

After exposure, Rh⁻ mother produces anti-Rh agglutinins.

Second pregnancy with Rh⁺ fetus. Anti-Rh agglutinins cause agglutination of fetal red blood cells.

Figure 17-5 RhoGAM is necessary to prevent hemolytic disease in an infant whose mother has been exposed to an Rh-positive fetus. (From Applegate E: *The anatomy and physiology learning system*, ed 3, St Louis, 2006, Saunders.)

they become available. Although 95% of all school children have been vaccinated, parents and children of migrant workers, new immigrants, and others who may not be aware of the need for and the benefits from immunization must be educated. The risk of acquiring the disease is much greater than the risk associated with the vaccines. When large numbers of a population are not immunized, the chances of exposure to infectious diseases are increased.

Persons traveling to foreign countries should contact their health care provider or local health department well in advance of the departure date for the needed (either required or suggested) immunizations. These immunizations must be given in advance to produce adequate immunity before leaving the country (Table 17-5).

IMPORTANT FACTS ABOUT PATIENT EDUCATION FOR IMMUNIZATIONS

- The CDC sets requirements to meet the needs of public health.
- Educating parents about the need for immunizations for children is an important role for the allied health professional. Continued immune states in adult patients should be checked and proper immunizations given as indicated.

IMPORTANT FACTS ABOUT PATIENT EDUCATION FOR IMMUNIZATIONS—*Cont'd*

- If a question of whether to administer an immunization or not exists, the potential for benefit must be weighed against the potential for risks.
- Documentation of immunizations is specific, and the National Childhood Vaccine Act of 1986 provides the guidelines for charting.

Immunosuppressants

With the advent of transplantation of body organs such as liver, heart, or kidney transplants, a new drug category was necessary to decrease or prevent the normal immune response of the body. This new group of drugs, known as **immunosuppressants,** is used mainly in transplantation but has other uses such as in autoimmune diseases and severe allergic reactions. When a foreign substance or organ is transplanted into the body, the immune response of antigen-antibodies is activated to process the transplanted matter as a foreign substance. Without these agents, tissue destruction and rejection of the transplanted organs would certainly occur.

TABLE 17-4 *Select Agents for Artificially Acquired Passive Immunity*

IMMUNIZING AGENT	TRADE NAME	DOSAGE, ROUTE, SITE	INDICATIONS	SIDE EFFECTS
ANTITOXINS				
Diphtheria antitoxin	Generic	Prophylactic: 10,000 U IM Therapeutic: 20,000-120,000 U IM/IV	Prevention or treatment of diphtheria	Redness at injection site
Tetanus antitoxin (from horses, so must skin test for allergies)	Generic	Prophylactic: 1500-5000 U IM/SC Therapeutic: 50,000-100,000 U IM skin test for allergies) and IV (part given IV remainder IM)	Prevention of tetanus	Tenderness at injection site
Botulism antitoxin	Generic	See package insert	Prevention of botulism	Given IV with the resultant side effects and dangers
SERUMS				
Rabies immune globulin	Imogam	20 U/kg IM (½ of dose may be used to infiltrate the wound)	Exposure to rabies	Fever, soreness at injection site
Antirabies	Generic	See package insert	Suspected exposure to rabies	Serum sickness, local pain, erythema, urticaria
Tetanus immune human globulin	Generic; Hypertet	Prophylactic: 250 U IM (children based on weight) Therapeutic: 300-600 U	Passive immunization to tetanus	Tenderness and muscle stiffness
Pertussis immune human globulin	Generic	Prophylactic: 1.25-2.5 mL, repeated in 1-2 wk Therapeutic: 1.25 mL q24-48h	Passive immunity to pertussis	Local reaction
Mumps immune human globulin	Generic	Prophylactic: 3-4.5 mL IM Therapeutic: 15-20 mL	Passive immunity to mumps	Local reaction
Hepatitis B immune globulin (H-BIG)	H-BIG, Hep-B-Gammagee	0.06 mL/kg within 7 days of exposure	Postexposure prophylaxis to hepatitis B	Local reaction, fever, urticaria
Immune human serum globulin	IV: Gamimune Gammagard IM: Gamastan Gammar	100-200 mg/kg IV q mo 200-400 mg/kg IV q mo 0.02-1.3 mL/kg IM (1.3-2 mL/kg for adults) depending on reason for use	Passive immunity for rubeola, hepatitis A, varicella, etc. IV use for immunodeficiency syndrome	Local reaction, fever, urticaria
Respiratory syncytial immune globulin	RespiGam	750 mg/kg IV	Reduce lower respiratory tract infections from RSV	Fever, diarrhea, vomiting, wheezing

IM, Intramuscular; IV, intravenous; RSV, respiratory syncytial virus; SC, subcutaneous.

TABLE 17-5 *Immunizations for Travel to Foreign Countries or for Specific Situations*

IMMUNIZING AGENT	TRADE NAME	DOSAGE , ROUTE, SITE OF ADMINISTRATION	INDICATIONS FOR PROTECTION	SIDE EFFECTS
Cholera	Generic	0.5 mL SC/IM 2 doses 1 wk to 1 mo apart	Cholera for travelers in areas of high risk	Local reaction, fever, malaise, headache
Plague	Generic	First dose: 1 mL IM; second dose: 0.2 mL IM 2-3 mo following first dose and again at 6 mos, followed by 0.1 to 0.2 mL boosters q 6 mos while in the endemic region	Plague for those at risk for exposure	Malaise, headache, local erythema
Rabies	Imovax Rabies vaccine, Imovax Rabies ID vaccine	See package insert. 3 doses, second dose 7 days after first, third dose 3-4 wk after first	Rabies: preexposure and postexposure for those at risk; only vaccine for preexposure and postexposure	Local reactions, nausea, headache, myalgia, abdominal pain
Typhoid Parenteral	Generic	0.5 mL SC with booster in 4 wk or more. Children <10: 0.25 mL, booster 0.5 mL SC or 0.1 mL ID q3 yr	Typhoid: travelers who will be in countries where typhoid is endemic	Local reactions, malaise, myalgia, fever
Oral	Vivotif Berna Vaccine	i cap 1 hr ac × 4 doses (at least 1 week before potential exposure) with booster in 5 years		GI symptoms, rash

- The dangers of using immunosuppressive medications are that these agents lower the body's ability to fight diseases, the patient is more susceptible to infections, infectious diseases, and the possibility of malignancies and the inherent side effects of each medication.
- Immunosuppression may also be the result of genetic or acquired disorders of the immune system and may occur anytime throughout life, but many are apparent at birth or shortly thereafter.
- Corticosteroids have the ability to suppress immune responses and are used to produce potent antiinflammatory and antiallergic effects by causing the lymphocytes in the blood to be redistributed in the bone marrow, lowering the number of lymphocytes in the blood. Corticosteroids are most frequently used in conjunction with other immunosuppressive agents.

Other immunosuppressive agents are used, such as the following:

- Azathioprine (Imuran), a derivative of the antineoplastic mercaptopurine, suppresses the formation of new B- and T-cells by suppressing DNA and RNA synthesis. Azathioprine is **mutagenic, teratogenic,** and **carcinogenic.**

- Cyclosporine (Sandimmune), a metabolite produced by a fungus, is a potent immunosuppressive agent but is not cytotoxic. It suppresses T-cell function, especially that of helper T-cells, thus depressing the immune response. When this medication is discontinued, normal T-cell function resumes. Administered along with corticosteroids, cyclosporine is used to prevent organ rejection following transplantation.
- Mycophenolate mofetil (CellCept) inhibits the activity of T-cells and B-cells to reduce the effectiveness of the immune system. The primary use of CellCept is to prevent the rejection in renal transplantation (Table 17-6).

Immunostimulants

Drugs to increase the immune system to treat cancer and AIDS by stimulating the immune system are called **immunostimulants.** The first agents, which became available in the 1980s with the advent of DNA technology, are used to stimulate the immune system when deficiencies exist. The acquired **immunodeficiency** may be caused by medications such as chemotherapy or it may be acquired through viral infections such as AIDS.

TABLE 17-6 *Selected Agents of Immunotherapy*

DRUG: GENERIC	TRADE NAME	USUAL ADULT DOSE, ROUTE OF ADMINISTRATION, AND FREQUENCY OF ADMINISTRATION	MAJOR SIDE EFFECTS	INDICATIONS FOR USE	DRUG INTERACTIONS
IMMUNOSUPPRESSANTS			Nausea, vomiting, decrease in blood cells, depression of bone marrow		
azathioprine	Imuran	3-5 mg/kg/day po, IV initially; 1-3 mg/kg/day as maintenance dose		Kidney and liver transplantation	Allopurinol, live virus vaccines, other immunosuppressants
cyclosporine	Sandimmune	10-14 mg/day po, IV for 1-2 wk; then taper to maintenance dose of 5-10 mg/kg/day	Renal damage	Prevention of allograft rejection	Same as azathioprine, plus cimetidine, danazol, diltiazem, ACE inhibitors, K-sparing diuretics, erythromycin, K supplements, ketoconazole
mycophenolate mofetil	CellCept	2 g/day po in 2 doses (to be given with corticosteroids and cyclosporine)	Renal damage, insomnia, dysrhythmias, arthralgia	Kidney transplantation	Acyclovir, ganciclovir, antacids, probenecid, cholestyramine, other immunosuppressants, live virus vaccines
sirolimus	Rapamune	6 mg po stat, then 2 mg/day po		Prophylaxis of organ rejection	None given
thalidomide	Thalomid	100-200 mg/day, po		Leprosy, wasting syndrome of HIV or cancer	Class X drug for pregnancy
IMMUNOSTIMULANTS			Fever, flulike symptoms, nausea, diarrhea		
alpha-interferon	Roferon-A	Varies among patients; IM, IV, SC		AIDS-related Kaposi's sarcoma, other malignancies	aminophylline, zidovudine
levamisole	Ergamisol	50 mg q8h × 3 days po		Increase T-cells in colon cancer	alcohol, phenytoin, warfarin

Immunostimulants are expected to provide control of pain and suffering found with many illnesses and are entering the market rapidly. Alpha-interferon and interleukin-2 (Proleukin) are two of the earliest medications to stimulate the production of B-cells and killer T-cells. By increasing the numbers of killer T-cells, it is thought that these drugs provide the needed T-cells to attack and destroy infections in the immunodeficient person. Many of these drugs are also used as antineoplastics (see Chapter 19). (See Table 17-6 for some of these agents.)

Patient Education for Compliance

1. A person taking immunosuppressant drugs is susceptible to infectious disease because these agents lower the body's immune response.
2. No immunizations with live virus vaccines should be administered to people taking immunosuppressants.
3. Report unusual bleeding or bruising to the health care provider, as well as sore throat and mouth sores.
4. Women of childbearing age should not take these medications; pregnancy must be avoided.
5. Avoid grapefruit juice and grapefruit when taking cyclosporine.
6. Cyclosporine should be taken at the same time each day with meals.
7. Maintain good dental hygiene.

IMPORTANT FACTS ABOUT IMMUNOSUPPRESSANTS AND IMMUNOSTIMULANTS

- Immunosuppressants are used to prevent organ rejection following transplants and to treat autoimmune diseases such as rheumatoid arthritis.
- Immunosuppressants increase the risk of infections and lymphomas.
- Cyclosporine is one of the most effective immunosuppressants available.
- Corticosteroids are often given as adjunct medications with other immunosuppressants.
- Azathioprine and other cytotoxic drugs suppress immune responses by B- and T-lymphocytes.
- Immunostimulants are a rapidly increasing field because of their use in the treatment of AIDS.
- Many immunosuppressants are also used as antineoplastic agents.

Summary

Vaccines are one of the greatest achievements in the medical field in the twentieth century. Immunizations have altered the way Americans look at quality of life, from childhood through adolescence into aging. Vicious diseases, such as smallpox, have been virtually wiped out, and polio is expected to be eradicated early in the twenty-first century.

Immunizations may provide artificially acquired active immunity in which the body builds its own antibodies to foreign antigens. This immunity is usually long acting, sometimes lasting a lifetime. Artificially acquired active immunity begins at birth and continues throughout life. Parents must be taught the dangers of not immunizing children and the importance of the laws that require certain vaccines being administered prior to attending school.

Artificially acquired passive immunity, short-term immunity, is introduced through antitoxins from human or animal sources such as immune globulins in immune serum. Passive immunity is effective immediately as the serum/antitoxin contains the needed antibodies to fight disease.

Immunizations are indicated in lifelong medical care from new infants obtaining hepatitis B vaccine to chronically ill older adults who receive influenza and pneumonia vaccines. To achieve the full potential of vaccines, adults must recognize that vaccines mobilize the body's natural defenses and they should seek vaccinations for themselves and their children. Health care workers are susceptible to many disease processes and should avail themselves of the needed immunizations for protection against pathogens found in medical settings. The vaccine delivery must be extended to adolescents and adults to assure that they are protected from such diseases as tetanus, influenza, hepatitis B, or pneumococcal disease.

Immunosuppressants are used to prevent tissue rejection by the antibody-antigen reaction when foreign tissue is introduced into the body, such as with organ transplants. AIDS, cancers, and other autoimmune diseases respond to immunostimulants or agents that increase the activity of the immune system. Immunotherapy is a relatively new area of medicine coming into the forefront with the treatment of AIDS and with organ transplants.

Critical Thinking Exercises

SCENARIO
Previc Wadhwa, who has an Rh-negative blood type, has just given birth to Jason, who is Rh-positive.

1. What medication is indicated for Mrs. Wadhwa to prevent erythroblastosis fetalis if she should become pregnant again?
2. What is the time limit for giving this medication following childbirth?
3. Would Mrs. Wadhwa need the medication if Jason had been an Rh-negative infant? Why or why not?
4. Does this medication pose a danger to Jason or to any future pregnancies? Defend your answer.
5. What would you tell Mrs. Wadhwa if she asked about the dangers of RhoGAM immunization?
6. How would you answer if she asked about the source of the medication?

◼ DRUG CALCULATIONS

1. Drug ordered: CellCept 500 mg
    Available medication:

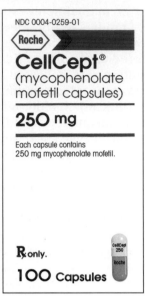

    Dose to be administered: _____

2. Drug ordered: Imuran 4 mg/kg/d po for a person who weighs 165 lb
    Available medication: azathioprine 50 mg/tab
    Dose to be administered: _____
    _____

REVIEW QUESTIONS

1. What is naturally acquired passive immunity? Naturally acquired active immunity? Artificially acquired passive immunity? Artificially acquired active immunity? _____
    _____
    _____

2. Which of the above types of immunity uses vaccines and toxoids? Which uses antitoxins and serum? Which lasts longer in the body? Why? _____
    _____
    _____

3. Discuss incidences when immunizations would be contraindicated. Do contraindications always prevent the administration of an immunization? How are the circumstances evaluated? _____
    _____
    _____

4. List the data required to be included in documentation of immunizations, mandated by the National Childhood Vaccine Act of 1986. _____
    _____
    _____

5. Adults have a higher incidence of nonconformance of immunizations. What can the allied health professional do to lower the incidence of nonimmunization? _____
    _____

6. What is the main indication for using immunosuppressants? _____
    _____

7. What is an immunostimulant? _____
    _____

CHAPTER 18

Antimicrobials, Antifungals, and Antivirals

OBJECTIVES

After studying this chapter, you should be capable of doing the following:

- Explaining the difference between pathogenic and nonpathogenic bacteria.
- Describing the various forms of bacteria that are pathogenic in the body.
- Describing factors that are important in choosing an antibiotic or antimicrobial agent.
- Explaining the difference between *bacteriostatic* and *bactericidal* agents.
- Explaining how humans can acquire drug resistance to specific antibiotics.
- Knowing why antibiotics, antimicrobials, antivirals, and antifungals may be used prophylactically and when prophylactic use is inappropriate.
- Explaining why some infections are best treated with a multidrug regimen.
- Identifying and classifying by family the antibiotics, antimicrobials, antivirals, and antifungals commonly used today.

Richard is seen in Dr. Merry's office with an infected lesion on his leg. Dr. Merry examines Richard and gives him a prescription for a topical antibiotic to be applied to the lesion three times a day. Richard is concerned because Dr. Merry did not give him an antibiotic to take orally.

  What is your response?

  In the past, Richard has taken multiple antibiotics for illnesses. How might this affect the effectiveness of antibiotics he takes in the future?

  Why is a topical antibiotic more likely to be used for localized infections? When is a systemic antibiotic more likely to be indicated?

KEY TERMS

Aerobic bacteria	Fungicidal	Pathogen
Anaerobic bacteria	Fungistatic	Photosensitivity
Antibacterial drugs	Fungus (fungi, *plural*)	Protozoa (protozoan, *singular*)
Antibiotic	Germicide	Sanitization
Antimicrobial	Germistatic agent	Semi-synthetic
Antiseptic	Helminths	Spore
Bacteria (bacterium, *singular*)	Host	Sterilization
Bactericidal	Microbe	Superinfection
Bacteriostatic	Microbiology	Synthetic
Broad-spectrum antibiotic	Narrow-spectrum antibiotic	Vector
Disinfectant/germicidal agent	Normal flora	Virus
Endemic	Opportunistic infection	
Facultative	Parasite	

Easy Working Knowledge of Antimicrobials, Antifungals, and Antivirals

DRUG CLASS	PRESCRIPTION	OTC	PREGNANCY CATEGORY	MAJOR INDICATIONS
Antibacterials (penicillins, cephalosporins, macrolides, tetracyclines, aminoglycosides, chloramphenicol, quinolone antimicrobials)	Yes	Some topical ointments and creams	B and C for most antibiotics; D for amino glycosides and tetracycline	Bacterial infections
Sulfonamides	Yes	No	B and C; D near term	Bacterial infections, especially urinary tract infections
Urinary tract antiseptics	Yes	Yes	B in last 2 trimesters	Urinary tract infections
Antitubercular drugs	Yes	No	B, C	Tuberculosis
Antifungal drugs	Yes	Yes (topical)	B, C (nystatin is preferred)	Fungal infections
Antiviral drugs	Yes	No	B, C, X	Viral infections, including HIV
Antimalarial drugs	Yes	Yes (quinine)	B, C, X	Malaria
Antiseptics, disinfectants, and germicides	Yes, including pHisoHex in some states	Yes	N/A	Cleaning and sanitizing animate and inanimate objects to remove microbes

With the discovery of sulfonamides in the 1930s and the availability of penicillin in the 1940s, a new era in the treatment of infections began. Since then, many drugs have been produced to either kill or inhibit the growth of bacteria, fungi, and viruses. These drugs have cured diseases such as tuberculosis and some types of pneumonia that until the 1950s were permanently debilitating to fatal. The average human life span in developed countries lengthened greatly, and fewer years of life are lost to devastating disease.

Antimicrobial drug therapy became a pharmacologic entity when Alexander Fleming discovered that when mold fell on a Petri dish containing *Staphylococcus*, growth of the bacteria was inhibited by the mold. Some penicillins today are still made from the same molds found by Fleming in his laboratory.

In the 1940s, during World War II, the U.S. government secretly researched penicillin to treat infections among the servicemen fighting the war. With the advent of antimicrobials, the patient could be given nontoxic medications to control infections until the body's immune system could fight the infection. Today, these medicines come from plants, animals, or chemical synthesis.

Because pathogens are multitudinous and common, affect all body systems, and spare no one, health care professionals in all fields can expect to spend time administering, documenting, and providing patient education about antibiotics as a normal part of their employment. The Centers for Disease Control and Prevention (CDC) is a reliable source of information on infectious diseases and the use of antibiotics.

What Is an Antibiotic?

The term **antibiotic** (*anti*, against + Greek *bios*, life; hence, "against life") is used to describe a group of diverse chemicals produced from natural substances including molds, bacteria, and fungi. These chemicals inhibit the growth of or kill other microorganisms when given in low concentrations. Major antibiotic families were discovered before 1955 by screening thousands of cultures from a variety of sources. For example, cephalosporins were derived from the mold *Cephalosporium*, found in the ocean near sewage outflow; streptomycin was derived from *Streptomyces*, a fungus obtained from soil that had contaminated the throat of a chicken; and lincomycin, produced by a variant of *Streptomyces lincolnensis*, came from the soil in Lincoln, Nebraska. Bacteria and fungi have been mutated, either spontaneously or by being induced to do so by ultraviolet light, to produce chemical variants of the antibiotics. Chemists using artificial means have produced other drugs resulting in the creation of families of antibiotics. Each antibiotic in a family is similar to the original chemical, with various properties that makes it useful for treating different kinds of infections. Antibiotics that contain the antibiotic molecule from a microorganism but are synthesized by a chemist are called **semisynthetics;** an example is penicillin V. Those completely synthesized in a laboratory are called **synthetics;** an example is the cephalosporins.

Antibiotics are also classified according to the spectrum of microorganisms against which they are effective. Each antibacterial agent is generally effective against only limited families of bacteria. The susceptible bacteria form the *antibacterial spectrum* of that drug.

- Some drugs, called **broad-spectrum antibiotics,** have a wide range of effectiveness against both gram-positive and gram-negative bacteria. Broad-spectrum antibiotics are widely used because of their effectiveness against many different kinds of bacteria; thus it is possible to eliminate pathogens without doing laboratory tests to identify the exact pathogen involved.
- Others, effective against a few or specific bacteria, are called **narrow-spectrum antibiotics.**

Morphologic Classification of Microorganisms

Microbiology is the study of microscopic organisms, or **microbes** ("small life"), from plantlike sources, such as fungi and molds, and the animal kingdom such as bacteria and protozoa. Viruses are not truly living microorganisms but are classified as microorganisms when discussing antibiotics.

- **Bacteria** are one-celled organisms and are found everywhere.

- **Viruses,** minute cell particles, are so small that they are only visible through an electron microscope. Viruses are actually small amounts of genetic material wrapped in a protein coat that are **parasitic** on their **hosts** for nutrition, metabolism, and reproduction. Some can mutate quickly in their hosts, causing difficulty with disease treatment.
- **Fungi** are parasitic plantlike substances that may grow as a single cell such as yeast or in colonies such as mushrooms or molds.
- **Protozoa** are unicellular, but they may colonize and become pathogenic in susceptible persons.
- Microorganisms live freely in soil and water, where they are relatively harmless. When these microorganisms leave their free environment and enter a susceptible host, they can become **pathogenic.**
- **Normal flora** are the many microorganisms normally living on our skin or in our bodies, with beneficial relationships for our bodies. Examples are certain strains of *Escherichia coli* that exist in the gastrointestinal (GI) tract to assist with digestion of food.
- **Parasites** do not live freely; they require interaction with other organisms and live on their hosts. Fungi and viruses are parasitic, as are lice and helminths.
- Some researchers consider viruses to be parasitic particles; others consider them to be primitive organisms. Of importance in the medical field is the high dependency of the parasite on the host cell for its livelihood.

Identification of Microorganisms

If the effectiveness of the drug is to be ascertained, the microorganism should be identified, and its susceptibility to the candidate drug known. Several ways to identify microorganisms follow.

Shape

- *Cocci* are round or spherical-shaped bacteria and are further subdivided by the way they combine in groups:
  - *Diplococci*—Cocci in pairs
  - *Streptococci*—Cocci in chains
  - *Staphylococci*—Clusters of cocci looking much like bunches of grapes
- *Bacilli*—Rod-shaped bacteria
- *Spirilla*—Spiral-shaped bacteria

Gram Stains

Gram staining, a quick test for narrowing the classification of bacteria, entails applying crystal violet and iodine, followed by an agent that decolorizes the stain.

- Gram-positive bacteria stain purple.
- Gram-negative bacteria do not keep the stain.
- The shape of the bacteria and the Gram stain results contribute to further specificity in identifying microorganisms.

Examples of testing bacteria by Gram stain and shape follow:

- Gram-positive cocci in clusters are staphylococci.
- Gram-positive cocci in chains are streptococci.
- Gram-positive bacilli include *Clostridium*.
- Gram-negative diplococci include *Neisseria*.

Microorganisms may also be classified according to their need for oxygen.

- **Aerobic bacteria** require oxygen to live.
- **Anaerobic bacteria** require an oxygen-free environment. Anaerobic organisms, which thrive in the oxygen-free interior of the body, tend to produce virulent infection and may be difficult to eradicate.
- **Facultative bacteria** can survive in either environment.

When our bodies are in homeostasis, the chance of normal flora becoming pathogenic or microorganisms entering the body as disease-producing bacteria, viruses, fungi, and protozoa is reduced.

Antimicrobials versus Antibiotics

Antimicrobials and antibiotics both have the capability to kill or suppress the growth of microorganisms. They are distinguished by their origins.

- Antibiotics are enhanced natural substances or synthetically formed substances originally obtained from organic sources such as plants and animals; each antibiotic bears a resemblance to the chemical that was originally obtained from the organism.
- **Antimicrobials** are a broader class including antibiotics, antifungals, antiparasitics, and drugs

like sulfa and mercury. The first antimicrobials were the sulfonamides; the second group consisted of true antibiotics such as the penicillins.

The goal of therapy with antimicrobials or antibiotics is to destroy or suppress the growth of the infecting organism for sufficient time to allow normal host defenses to control the infection and to provide a resultant cure.

- Antimicrobial medications can help cure or control most infections caused by microorganisms, but they cannot always produce a cure by themselves.
- They may be used in conjunction with surgical procedures such as incision and drainage, débridement of wounds, and excision of infected tissue.
- Antimicrobials reach target cells either through absorption of the drug at the site of application or through systemic distribution of the drug by way of the circulatory system.
- Local applications such as topical, otic, or sterile ophthalmic preparations are preferable if possible and appropriate.
- Drugs absorbed systemically can upset the balance of normal body flora, eradicating some and allowing overgrowth of others that can result in a second round of infection at a different site from the original infection and with a different causative organism—necessitating treating the new infection with another drug.

Bactericidal versus Bacteriostatic

Antimicrobials may function as **bacteriostatic agents** or as **bactericidal agents.** By inhibiting the growth of bacteria, bacteriostatic agents allow the body's defense mechanisms extra time to remove the microorganisms. **Bactericidal agents** either cause death of the bacterial cell or destruction of the cell. The antimicrobial action of bacteriostatic and bactericidal agents is not firm because the dosage of the drug, concentration of the drug at the site of infection, and virulence of the microorganism all contribute to whether the cell is destroyed outright or simply inhibited in its growth. Thus the same agent may be either bacteriostatic or bactericidal against the same microorganism.

Bacteriostatic and bactericidal agents produce their effects by the following ways:

- Bactericidal agents cause destruction (lysis) of the cell by weakening the cell wall, and bacteriostatic agents cause body fluids that are not isotonic to result in killing of bacteria. Examples are the penicillins and the cephalosporins.

- Disrupting or altering the permeability of the cell membrane, resulting in leakage of essential metabolic substances of bacteria. Drugs with this mechanism of action are *bactericidal* (e.g., polymyxin).
- Inhibiting protein building by forming defective protein molecules. These *bacteriostatic* drugs include griseofulvin, erythromycin, and tetracycline.
- Inhibiting the synthesis of metabolites essential to bacteria—a mechanism of action that is generally *bacteriostatic*. Examples include the sulfonamides, ethambutol, and isoniazid.

Factors in the Choice of Antibiotics

When treating infections the goal is to achieve the maximal antimicrobial effect while causing minimal harm to the patient. Antimicrobial therapy tries to "match the bug and the drug" while considering the physical condition of the patient, including chronic diseases and possible allergies. The appropriate antibiotic must be chosen for each individual on the basis of the causative organism, the organism's drug sensitivity, and the host factors present. In ideal medical treatment, culture and sensitivity testing to match the antimicrobial to the microbe should be done for all infections. The best antimicrobial therapy occurs when the infecting organism has been identified and is known to be sensitive to the drug selected. However, in some cases, a broad-spectrum medication may be prescribed prior to obtaining results of sensitivity testing to begin treatment. The antibiotic may be changed after testing results are available.

Drug Sensitivity

Most antimicrobial agents are effective against specific groups of microorganisms; therefore the likely microorganism should be considered when selecting a medication.

- If a tentative identification of the infective organism is difficult to make, a broad-spectrum antibiotic can be prescribed, or several antibiotics may be prescribed to be taken concurrently.
- Another indication for using more than one antibiotic is to delay the rapid increase in bacterial resistance to one drug.

- To reduce the incidence or intensity of adverse reactions for potentially toxic drugs, the dose may be decreased.
- If a potentially toxic antibiotic is necessary, a second antibiotic with the same or broader spectrum may be added to the therapy to reduce the amount of toxic medication necessary for treatment.
- In severe infections, there may be insufficient time to do sensitivity testing, and a broad-spectrum antimicrobial may have to be given for initial treatment while waiting for the test results.

A certain medication may be preferred for reasons such as greater efficacy, less toxicity, or greater sensitivity to the medication of the microorganisms involved. Alternative agents may have to be chosen if the patient is allergic to the drug of choice or if the drug has toxic effects.

CLINICAL TIP

If therapy must be started before culture and sensitivity results are available, specimens for culture should be obtained before therapy begins. If the laboratory sample is obtained after the patient has started antibiotics, the infecting agents may be suppressed and their identification impeded. Laboratory results may indicate the need for a change in the antibiotic being used.

MEDICATION ALERT

The goal of antibiotic therapy is not to kill all the infecting organisms; rather, the goal is to suppress the growth of the microorganisms to allow the host's immune system to subdue the infection.

Patient Factors

Patient factors may influence the choice of drug, route of administration, or dosage.

- The patient's immune system plays an important role in the selection of antibiotics.
- In the immunosuppressed individual, the immune system is compromised and the drug alone cannot suppress diseases.
- The antibiotic must achieve minimum concentration at the site of the infection to be effective.
- Pacemakers, prosthetic joints, and other foreign objects may cause the immune system to attack healthy cells at the site of implantation

of the object, requiring the use of antibiotics at these sites to prevent an infection that may necessitate removal of the prosthesis.

- Infants and the elderly are more susceptible to drug toxicity than the average adult because of poor metabolism and excretion, which can lead to drug accumulation and toxic levels in the blood.
- Pregnancy and lactation pose specific problems in antibiotic treatment. Some drugs can cross the placenta and into breast milk.
- Severe allergic reactions are more common with antibiotics, especially penicillin, than with any other family of drugs. The general rule is that a person who has had an allergic reaction to penicillin should not receive it again. Symptoms of hypersensitivity to antibiotics range from a rash, fever, and urticaria with pruritus to generalized erythema or anaphylaxis.

DID YOU KNOW?

A person can become sensitized to a drug even through indirect exposure such as by eating beef or chicken from animals given antimicrobials. Sensitization may also be caused by a previous use of topical antibiotics.

Acquired Antibiotic Resistance

Much has been discovered in recent years about antibiotics and the growing resistance of many microorganisms to these drugs. The trivial or inappropriate use of antimicrobials has led to microorganisms mutating, or changing their genetic structure, so that the currently available medications are no longer effective. To further complicate the antibiotic-resistant microorganism problems, pharmaceutical companies have decreased the development of new antibiotics in recent years. Such environmental factors as overcrowding and poor sanitation may play a role in microorganisms' developing antibiotic resistance because of repeated infections and repeated use of antimicrobials to fight these infections in these conditions.

Acquired resistance is of great concern because it can render the currently effective antibiotics useless. Several bacteria—*Staphylococcus aureus*, *E. coli*, and *Mycobacterium tuberculosis*—are now serious clinical problems because of drug resistance.

As a rule, microorganisms that have become resistant to a certain drug will tend to be resistant to other chemically related antimicrobials, a phe-

nomenon known as *cross-resistance. The person does not become resistant to the antibiotic; the microbe becomes resistant to the drug*. When the microbe itself becomes drug resistant, any person who gets a disease from that microbe is affected. The microorganism may become a disease-causing, more resistant microbe that can grow in the environment because of the ineffectiveness of drugs.

The main reason for the development of drug-resistant bacteria is the inappropriate use of antibiotics. The more an antibiotic is used, the faster resistant microorganisms emerge. Inept prescribing and inappropriate use of medications increase the resistance of normal flora, turning them into possible pathogens. Patients contribute to this problem by failing to take the full prescribed course of an antibiotic; the abbreviated course of treatment kills off only the more susceptible organisms, allowing more resistant ones—those that need to be eradicated—to grow with less competition in the environment. Every effort should be made to avoid the indiscriminate use of antibiotics in individuals and for infections such as viruses that do not respond to these medications.

Superinfection and Antibiotic Use

A **superinfection** is a new infection that appears during the course of treatment for a primary infection, such as a yeast infection that arises during the course of treatment with penicillin for bacterial pneumonia. Superinfection may occur via the following:

- If the antibiotic dosage was too large for the patient's size
- By the drug's inhibiting or altering the balance of normal flora within the body, thereby allowing a secondary infection to occur.

Broad-spectrum antibiotics such as the tetracyclines and ampicillin tend to kill off more normal flora and thus provoke more superinfections. Superinfections are difficult to treat because they are usually caused by drug-resistant microbes. Drugs that change the body's immune responses such as corticosteroids and immunosuppressive drugs may also permit the emergence of superinfections.

Prophylactic Use of Antibiotics

Between 30% and 50% of antibiotics prescribed in the United States are used for prophylactic reasons, to prevent an infection, rather than to treat an infection already in place. A recent example is the use of ciprofloxacin for those persons who have been exposed to anthrax.

- Much of this prophylactic drug use is not necessary, but in some situations it is appropriate and effective.
- The risk of toxic effects, superinfections, and other adverse reactions should be weighed against the advantages before using prophylactic drugs.
- People with congenital or valvular heart disease or who have had rheumatic fever may need prophylactic antibiotics before surgery or dental procedures to decrease normal flora, reducing the chance of endocarditis and bacteria.
- Neutropenia (low neutrophil counts) that increases the risk for infections may be another indication for prophylactic use.
- Finally, antimicrobial agents may be given prophylactically in single large doses to effectively treat persons who have been exposed to sexually transmitted diseases but have not yet shown signs of infection.

Misuse of Antibiotics

Antibiotics are among the most commonly prescribed medications and some of the most incorrectly used medications. Patients who are given clear explanations of why an antibiotic is prescribed are more likely to complete the full course of therapy and do not seek unneeded medications.

- Antibiotics are usually given for 5 to 14 days, with the most commonly ordered duration being 10 days. The danger of taking antimicrobial medications for too brief a time is the potential development of drug-resistant microorganisms and relapse of the disease.
- Antibiotics *can* be used, either preventatively or therapeutically, to treat the secondary infections that may occur with viral disease.
- When drug therapy is begun for most viral infections, the patient is exposed to all of the risks of the drug without receiving benefits because a virus is not a viable microorganism susceptible to antibiotics.
- For antibiotics to be most effective, they should be taken at evenly spaced intervals. If the order reads three times a day, the medicine should be taken every 8 hours and the like. This scheduling will maintain a therapeutic blood level throughout the 24-hour period.

Not taking medications because of sleep or other activities causes erratic dosing and fluctuations in blood levels, making the antibiotic less effective.

- "Saving" unused medications until another illness occurs at a later date is another misuse of antibiotics. Even though a patient may no longer be experiencing the symptoms that invoked the prescribing of an antibiotic, the medication may not have had time to kill the more virulent microorganisms. The remaining microbes will grow, and the patient will feel that the medicine "didn't work."
- Taking medications prescribed for another person without obtaining medical care is another frequent misuse, abuse, or both.
- Fever is a symptom of more diseases than just a bacterial infection; therefore giving antibiotics because someone has a fever is inappropriate. The one situation in which fever alone is an indication for antibiotics is in the immunosuppressed patient (Box 18-1).

 CLINICAL TIP
Culture and sensitivity testing should be done if possible before any antibiotic therapy is initiated, but especially in children, who may develop sensitivities to antibiotics.

PATIENT ALERT
1. Antibiotics should be taken for the full prescribed course to ensure the suppression and destruction of all pathogens, not just the weak microorganisms, to lower the incidence of drug-resistant microbes.
2. The disappearance of symptoms does not indicate an infection has been adequately treated. Medications should be continued until the prescribed course has been completed.

Patient Education for Compliance

1. Misuse of antibiotics is common and should be discouraged. Fever is only a symptom and is not an indication to begin antibiotic therapy.
2. Antibiotics are ineffective for the treatment of viral infections. Antibiotics may be used with viral diseases when secondary infections are present.

1. The selected antibiotic should be known to be effective against the common organisms isolated from the infection site.
2. The minimum number of drugs necessary to treat the infection should be used.
3. The drug of first choice should be used unless it is contraindicated. In children and the elderly, the dosage should take into account body surface area, organ function, and any concurrent diseases.
4. Unless the benefit outweighs the risk, a drug should not be used when previous allergic or adverse reactions to that drug have occurred.
5. Antibiotic therapy should be continued as long as the infection is present but should not exceed the usual treatment time for the suspected infective organisms.

IMPORTANT FACTS ABOUT ANTIBIOTICS

- Antibiotics should be carefully chosen on the basis of the sensitivity of the infecting organisms.
- Antibiotics may be given preventatively for surgery or if exposure to an unusual disease such as anthrax or malaria is likely.
- Narrow-spectrum antibiotics are effective against a few microorganisms. Broad-spectrum antibiotics are active against a wide range of microbes.
- The emergence of drug-resistant microorganisms is a major concern in antibiotic therapy. Therefore antibiotics should be prescribed only when indicated by the disease process.
- *Bactericidal* drugs kill microorganisms. *Bacteriostatic* drugs suppress bacterial growth until the person's immune system can effectively bring the body into homeostasis.

Antibacterial Drugs

Several categories of **antibacterial** drugs are effective against bacterial infections. This section discusses each family and use of individual drugs such as penicillins, cephalosporins, macrolides, tetracyclines, aminoglycosides, and miscellaneous antibiotics.

Penicillins

Penicillin, the first of the true antibiotics, has been derived from a number of strains of common molds found on bread and fruit. Natural and semi-synthetic penicillins and their related antibi-

otics remain the most effective and least toxic of the available antimicrobials. These substances act by inhibiting bacterial cell-wall synthesis, causing death of the bacterium by lysis, an action that makes most penicillins *bactericidal* agents, although in low doses they may be *bacteriostatic*. Adverse reactions generally are in the form of allergic reactions that tend to precipitate more frequently and severely than with other medications.

Generally, penicillins are categorized by their antimicrobial spectrum. This classification has four major groups: (1) narrow-spectrum penicillins, (2) narrow-spectrum antistaphylococcal penicillins, (3) broad-spectrum penicillins, and (4) extended-spectrum penicillins.

DID YOU KNOW?
Most generic names for penicillins end in -cillin, whereas many trade names have pen in their names. As an example, penicillin V (generic name) is known as Pen-VEE-K by trade name.

Narrow-Spectrum Penicillins

Penicillin G was the first penicillin developed and is still the drug of choice for treating many infections such as gonorrhea and streptococcal infections. The narrow-spectrum penicillins are considered to be first-generation penicillins. In general, penicillins are effective against (1) many gram-positive organisms such as streptococci and staphylococci; (2) gram-negative bacteria such as *Neisseria* and *E. coli;* (3) spirochetes; and (4) some anaerobic bacteria. The microbes susceptible to penicillin cause such infections as pneumonia, throat and ear infections, gonorrhea, and syphilis (Table 18-1).

Narrow-Spectrum Antistaphylococcal Penicillins

The antistaphylococcal penicillins have a narrow spectrum of action being specific for staphylococcal infections. They are used for infections caused by drug-resistant staphylococci strains (see Table 18-1).

Broad-Spectrum Penicillins

By altering the naturally occurring types of semi-synthetic broad-spectrum penicillins, second-generation penicillins are effective against a broader spectrum of microorganisms and are associated with fewer allergic reactions. Many are available in oral preparations; examples are ampicillin and amoxicillin (see Table 18-1).

TABLE 18-1 *Common Penicillins*

GENERIC NAME	TRADE NAME	USUAL ADULT DOSE, ROUTE, AND FREQUENCY OF ADMINISTRATION	INDICATIONS FOR USE	DRUG INTERACTIONS
NARROW SPECTRUM *(First Generation)*				
penicillin G*	Many trade names (Duracillin, Pentids, etc.)	600,000-4,000,000 U IM, IV, rarely po q6h	*Type of bacteria:* gram-positive and gram-negative bacteria, gram-positive aerobic cocci, gram-positive aerobic and anaerobic bacilli, spirochetes	Probenecid increases and prolongs penicillin levels in the blood
penicillin V*	Pen-VEE-K, Veetids, V-cillin	250-500 mg po q6h	*Type of infection:* upper respiratory tract infections, pneumonia, dental prophylaxis, urinary tract infections	
NARROW SPECTRUM *Antistaphylococcal*				
methicillin	Staphcillin	1-2 g IM, IV q4-6h	*Type of bacteria:* staphylococci	Probenecid increases and prolongs penicillin levels in the blood
nafcillin	Nafcil, Unipen	250 mg-1 g po, IM, IV q4-6h	*Type of infection:* Staphylococcal	
oxacillin	Bactocill, Prostaphlin	250-500 mg po, IM, IV q4-6h	infections	
cloxacillin	Cloxapen, Tegopen	250 mg-1 g po, IM, IV q4-6h	Staphylococcal infections of respiratory tract and soft	
dicloxacillin	Dynapen, Dycill	250-500 mg po, IM, IV q4-6h	tissue infections	
BROAD SPECTRUM *(Second Generation)*				
ampicillin*	Principen, Omnipen, Polycillin	500 mg-2 g po, IM, IV qid	*Type of bacteria:* gram-positive and gram-negative bacteria, gram-positive aerobic cocci, gram-positive aerobic and anaerobic bacilli, spirochetes	No significant interaction
amoxicillin*	Amoxil, Trimox, Polymox	250-500 mg po tid or 875 mg bid		
amoxicillin-clavulanate	Augmentin	250-500 mg tid or 875 mg po bid	*Type of infection:*	
bacampicillin	Spectrobid	400-800 mg po bid	Respiratory tract infections, urinary tract infections, otitis media	
EXTENDED SPECTRUM *(Third Generation)*				
carbenicillin	Geocillin	1 g po, IM, IV q4-6h	*Type of bacteria:* Pseudomonas	No significant interaction
piperacillin	Pipracil	1.5-4 g IM, IV q6-12h	*Type of infection: Pseudomonas* infections	
(Fourth Generation)				
mezlocillin	Mezlin	4-8 g IM, IV q4-6h	*Type of bacteria:* gram-positive cocci	↓ oral contraceptives
azlocillin	Azlin	200-300 mg/kg/day in divided doses IV	*Types of infection:* streptococci, Clostridium, Neisseria	

MAJOR SIDE EFFECTS OF PENICILLINS: Nausea and vomiting, diarrhea, sore mouth, hives, itching anaphylaxis

IM, Intramuscular; *IV,* intravenous.
*The effectiveness of oral contraceptives may be reduced with these penicillins.

Extended-Spectrum Penicillins

Third-generation penicillins, also known as extended-spectrum penicillins, have a wider antimicrobial action than second-generation penicillins. These medications are used for the more serious urinary tract and respiratory tract infections and for bacteremia caused by *Pseudomonas* and *Proteus* infections (see Table 18-1).

Fourth-generation penicillins are also extended-spectrum antimicrobials and are used for the most serious infections that are difficult to treat. Often these penicillins are given parenterally in combination therapy with other antimicrobials.

CLINICAL TIP

A *person allergic to one penicillin should be considered allergic to all penicillins*. If a question arises about the possibility of allergic reactions to penicillin, the person should be considered allergic.

PATIENT ALERT

- Patients should be asked about allergies each time they are seen in medical settings.
- Health care professionals should be told of any possible allergic reactions to any medication, especially penicillin, such as rashes, hives, and itching.
- Patients with penicillin allergies should wear a form of identification so that they are not inadvertently given penicillin in an emergency situation.

Patient Education for Compliance

1. Penicillin should be taken with a full glass of water 1 hour before meals or 2 hours after meals.
2. Women taking ampicillin, amoxicillin, or penicillins G and V and who are also taking estrogen-containing contraceptives should use a different form of contraception while taking these antibiotics. The effectiveness of birth control pills decreases when the specified penicillin derivatives are used concurrently.

IMPORTANT FACTS ABOUT PENICILLINS

- Penicillins weaken cell walls, causing lysis and cell death. These actions make them bactericidal.
- Gram-negative bacteria are resistant to most penicillins.

IMPORTANT FACTS ABOUT PENICILLINS—*Cont'd*

- Penicillins are the safest antibiotics available, although the medications have a high incidence of allergic reactions.
- A patient allergic to one penicillin should be considered allergic to all penicillins. Even mild reactions should be considered an allergic reaction.
- The principal differences among the penicillins are their spectrum of antibacterial action, their stability in stomach acids, and their duration of action.
- Narrow-spectrum penicillin G and V are naturally occurring substances. Penicillin-G is administered by injection because it is not stable in gastric acids. However, large doses of Penicillin-V can be administered orally.
- Some penicillins are specific for staphylococcal infections that are difficult to manage, whereas others are for *Pseudomonas* infections.

Cephalosporins

Like penicillins, cephalosporins were originally derived from a mold and are structurally related to the penicillins. Cephalosporins weaken the bacterial cell wall, resulting in lysis and death of the cell; thus they are bactericidal. The cephalosporins are active against a broad spectrum of pathogens. Because of the chemical relationship of cephalosporins to penicillin, patients who are allergic to penicillin should be given cephalosporins with caution, especially if the patient has had an anaphylactic reaction to penicillin.

DID YOU KNOW?

Cephalosporins have the prefix ceph- or cef- in their name. An example is cefadroxil (generic name), which is Duricef by trade name.

Classified in four generations, cephalosporins are used as substitutes for penicillins in persons with drug-resistant bacteria and in the treatment of certain gram-negative infections.

- First-generation cephalosporins are primarily active against gram-positive bacteria.
- Second-generation drugs have increased effectiveness against gram-negative microorganisms.
- Third and fourth generations are more active against gram-negative microbes, with the third generation not as effective against gram-positive cocci. Cefepime (Maxipime), the first drug

in the fourth generation, is used only when lower generations of cephalosporins are ineffective.

- Fourth-generation drugs are more resistant to the inactivating intestinal enzymes that cause other antibiotics to be ineffective.

Because of the expense of the first- and second-generation cephalosporins, these medications are rarely the drug of choice for treating most infections. Other antibiotics are as effective and less expensive (Box 18-2 and Table 18-2).

PATIENT ALERT

Patients with diabetes mellitus should keep a close check on blood sugar because cephalosporins tend to raise blood glucose levels. Report any excessive bruising or diarrhea.

Patient Education for Compliance

1. Cephalosporins should be taken with food if gastric upset occurs.
2. Cephalosporin suspensions should be refrigerated.
3. Some cephalosporins cannot be combined with alcohol. Individuals who are taking these medications should not consume alcohol.
4. Cephalosporins tend to intensify bleeding tendencies. Individuals who take cephalosporin should be careful with taking aspirin, other nonsteroidal antiinflammatory drugs (NSAIDs), and anticoagulants.

IMPORTANT FACTS ABOUT CEPHALOSPORINS

- Cephalosporins weaken the cell wall, causing death to bacteria.
- Cephalosporins are closely related to penicillins in their chemical structure.

IMPORTANT FACTS ABOUT CEPHALOSPORINS— *Cont'd*

- Cephalosporins are grouped into four generations. As drugs progress through the generations from one to four, there is increased activity against gram-negative bacteria.
- The most common adverse reactions to penicillins and cephalosporins are allergic reactions. Persons allergic to penicillin should be watched carefully when administered cephalosporins because up to 10% to 15% of people allergic to penicillin will also prove to be allergic to cephalosporin.

Macrolides

The macrolide antibiotics, called *macro* because of the large size of the chemical compounds, are broad-spectrum antimicrobials that act by inhibiting protein synthesis in bacteria. These drugs are bacteriostatic, but they may be bactericidal in large doses, having a unique role in treating atypical pneumonia, Legionnaires' disease, and chlamydia infections.

Erythromycin was the first macrolide and is the key drug in this group. The newer macrolides include azithromycin and clarithromycin. These drugs may cause GI symptoms, as well as headaches and dizziness (Table 18-3).

 CLINICAL TIP

Erythromycin is most effective if taken on an empty stomach, but it may be given with food if GI upset occurs.

DID YOU KNOW?

The names of macrolide drugs typically end in -mycin. The same suffix is also used in naming some aminoglycosides (e.g., erythromycin, a macrolide, and neomycin, a member of the aminoglycoside family).

IMPORTANT FACTS ABOUT MACROLIDES

- Erythromycin is the prototype of macrolides and is bacteriostatic in its mechanism of action.
- Erythromycin is active against the basic spectrum of microbes and is used for patients with penicillin allergies.

TABLE 18-2 *Select Cephalosporins*

GENERIC NAME	TRADE NAME	USUAL ADULT DOSE, ROUTE, AND FREQUENCY OF ADMINISTRATION	INDICATIONS FOR USE	DRUG INTERACTIONS
FIRST GENERATION				
cefazolin	Duricef	250 mg-1.5 g po, IM, IV q6h	*Type of bacteria:* streptococci and some staphylococci	Interact with aminoglycoside, polymyxin B, vancomycin
cefadroxil	Ancef	500 mg-1 g po q12h	*Type of infection:* staphylococcal	Probenecid increases the activity
cephalexin	Keflex, Keftab	250-500 mg po q6h	and streptococcal infections, some urinary tract infections,	of some cephalosporins
cephapirin	Cefadyl	500 mg-1 g IM, IV q6h	bone and joint diseases, upper	Some cephalosporins cause Antabuse-like reactions
cephradine	Anspor, Velosef	po: 250 mg q6h IM/IV: 500 mg q12h	respiratory tract infection	Cephalosporins decrease the effectiveness of oral contraceptives
SECOND GENERATION				
cefaclor	Ceclor	250-500 mg po q8h	Same as for first generation,	*cefamandole/ceforanide:*
cefamandole	Mandol	500 mg-1 g IM, IV q4-8h	plus *Hemophilus influenzae* and *Neisseria gonorrhoeae*	Aspirin, anticoagulants, NSAIDS (because medication
ceforanide	Precef	500 mg-4 g IM, IV q12h		may promote bleeding)
cefotetan	Cefotan	1-2 g IM, IV q12h		
cefoxitin	Mefoxin	1-2 g IM, IV q6-8h		
cefuroxime	Ceftin	50-100 mg/kg/day IM/IV 250-500 mg po tid		
cefpodoxime	Vantin	100-500 mg po q12h		
cefprozil	Cefzil	250-500 mg po 12h		
loracarbef	Lorabid	200-800 mg po qd		
cefmetazole	Zefazone	2 g qd IV in divided doses		
THIRD GENERATION				
cefdinir	Omnicef	300 mg po bid	*Type of bacteria:* Less effective	No significant interactions
cefixime	Suprax	400 mg/day in 1-2 doses po	against streptococci and pneumococci; more effective	
ceftibuten	Cedex	400 mg po qd	against gram-negative bacteria	
cefotaxime	Claforan	1-2 g IM, IV q6-8h	of gastrointestinal and	
ceftazidime	Fortaz, Tazidime	1-2 g IM, IV q8-12h	genitourinary tracts; generally used with serious infections	
ceftriaxone	Rocephin	1-2 g/day in 1-2 divided doses IM, IV		
FOURTH GENERATION				
cefepime	Maxipime	0.5-2 g IM, IV q12h	*Type of infection:* urinary tract, respiratory tract, and integumentary infections	Aspirin, other NSAIDs, anticoagulants, alcohol

MAJOR SIDE EFFECTS OF CEPHALOSPORINS: Headache, dizziness, weakness, fever, diarrhea, anorexia, nephrotoxicity, rash dyspnea, blood dyscrasias

IM, Intramuscular; *IV,* intravenous; *NSAIDs,* nonsteroidal anti-inflammatory drugs.

Tetracyclines

The tetracyclines, medications that are bacteriostatic and bactericidal, were the first group of broad-spectrum antibiotics. They are used to treat many infections such as acne, Rocky Mountain spotted fever, Lyme disease, urinary tract infections, and bronchitis. Some bacteria have become resistant to tetracyclines. Milk should not be used for administration of tetracyclines. When milk has been ingested, a 3-hour wait is recommended prior to administration of tetracyclines. If its expiration date has passed, tetracycline is dangerous (Table 18-4).

TABLE 18-3 *Selected Macrolides*

GENERIC NAME	TRADE NAME	USUAL ADULT DOSE, ROUTE, AND FREQUENCY OF ADMINISTRATION	INDICATIONS FOR USE	DRUG INTERACTIONS
ERYTHROMYCINS*				
erythromycin	Erythrocin	250-500 mg po, IV q6h	*Type of bacteria:* gram-positive and some gram-negative microorganisms *Type of infection:* illnesses of respiratory tract, gastrointestinal tract, skin, and soft tissue; drugs of choice for Legionnaires' disease	Affects effectiveness or absorption of carbamazepine, cyclosporine, digitalis, methyl-prednisolone, theophylline, and anticoagulants
erythromycin estolate	Ilosone	250-500 mg po q6h		
erythromycin succinate	EES, Ery-Ped	400 mg po bid		

MAJOR SIDE EFFECTS OF ERYTHROMYCINS: Abdominal cramping, diarrhea, oral/vaginal candidiasis, hearing loss, headache, dizziness

GENERIC NAME	TRADE NAME	USUAL ADULT DOSE, ROUTE, AND FREQUENCY	INDICATIONS FOR USE	DRUG INTERACTIONS
ERYTHROMYCIN DERIVATIVES				
azithromycin	Zithromax	250-500 mg/day po	*Type of bacteria:* gram-negative organisms and anaerobic organisms *Type of infection: H. influenzae,* Legionnaire's disease, *Chlamydia,* Lyme disease	Aluminum, magnesium antacids, theophylline, Coumadin, carbamaze-pine
clarithromycin	Biaxin	250-500 mg/day po		
dirithromycin	Dynabac	500 mg/day; po qday; ↑ absorption with food	Soft tissue infections by *Streptococcus pneumonia* and *Staphylococcus aureus;* Legionnaires' disease	

MAJOR SIDE EFFECTS OF ERYTHROMYCIN DERIVATIVES: Same as for erythromycins, plus change in taste sensation

GENERIC NAME	TRADE NAME	USUAL ADULT DOSE, ROUTE, AND FREQUENCY	INDICATIONS FOR USE	DRUG INTERACTIONS
KETOLIDES				
telithromycin	Ketek	800 mg/d × 5 days po	Bronchitis, sinusitis, pneumonia	Same and phenobarbital, phenytoin

MAJOR SIDE EFFECTS OF KELTOLIDES: Nausea, vomiting diarrhea

EES, Erythromycin ethylsuccinate; *IV,* intravenous.
*Also available as topical and ophthalmic preparations.

PATIENT ALERT

- The patient should be told to avoid the sun because of the danger of sunburning rapidly; therefore care should be used in prescribing tetracycline for teenagers with acne because teens like to sunbathe. The use of sunscreens is necessary. These medications also cannot be used in children younger than 8 years old or in pregnant women because of the permanent discoloration of developing teeth.
- Superinfections of the bowels occur with all antibiotics, but especially with tetracyclines, so significant diarrhea should be reported, as should vaginal and rectal itching or a black, furry appearance of the tongue. These are signs of fungal superinfections.

DID YOU KNOW?

The suffix -cycline is found with the tetracyclines such as doxycycline and minocycline.

Patient Education for Compliance

1. Tetracyclines should not be taken with milk products, iron supplements, or antacids.
2. Tetracyclines should be taken on an empty stomach.
3. Tetracyclines can cause GI distress, which can be reduced by taking the medication with meals, but only if absolutely necessary. Doxycycline and minocycline may be given with foods other than dairy products, as necessary.

TABLE 18-4 *Select Tetracyclines*

GENERIC NAME	TRADE NAME	USUAL ADULT DOSE, ROUTE, AND FREQUENCY OF ADMINISTRATION	INDICATIONS FOR USE	DRUG INTERACTIONS
SHORT-ACTING				
chlortetracycline	Aureomycin	250-500 mg po q6h	*Type of bacteria:*	Pregnancy category D
tetracycline	Achromycin, Sumycin	250-500 mg po q6h	Rickettsiae, *Mycoplasma pneumoniae*	Decreases effectiveness of contraceptives, antacids,
	Panmycin, Steclin	100 mg IM bid-tid	*Type of infection:* Cholera, *Chlamydia* Lyme disease, acne	calcium supplements, iron supplements, magnesium laxatives, milk products
oxytetracycline	Terramycin	Same as for tetracycline		
LONG-ACTING				
doxycycline	Vibramycin	100-200 mg po initially, then 100 mg bid	Same as short-acting plus gastrointestinal diseases	
minocycline	Minocin	200 mg po, IV initially, then 100 mg bid	Same as short-acting plus acne	

MAJOR SIDE EFFECTS OF TETRACYCLINES: Photosensitivity, permanent stains in developing teeth in fetus and in children <8 yr of age

IM, Intramuscular; *IV,* intravenous.

IMPORTANT FACTS ABOUT TETRACYCLINES
- Because of their broad spectrum of action, the use of tetracyclines can result in superinfections.
- Tetracyclines should not be given with calcium supplements, milk products, iron supplements, magnesium-containing laxatives, and most antacids.

IMPORTANT FACTS ABOUT AMINOGLYCOSIDES
- Aminoglycosides are narrow-spectrum antibiotics that are bacteriocidal and are used against gram-negative bacilli.
- Aminoglycosides are nephrotoxic and ototoxic.
- The topical use of aminoglycosides is relatively safe, even for OTC topicals, but some adverse reactions are possible.

Aminoglycosides

The aminoglycosides are a group of potent bactericidal agents that inhibit protein synthesis and are usually reserved for serious or life-threatening infections. Generally, the main spectrum sensitive to these drugs are gram-positive bacilli, but gram-positive microbes may also be affected. Aminoglycosides may be used with cephalosporins or vancomycin for synergistic effects and with penicillin with certain conditions such as neonatal sepsis. Topical, ophthalmic, and otic use of aminoglycosides is relatively safe, with few side effects. Some aminoglycosides have been found to have dangerous adverse reactions and are classified as Category D with pregnancy (Table 18-5).

PATIENT ALERT
The patient should be watched closely for tinnitus, vertigo, weakness, and changes in respiration, as well as for scant urinary output and albuminuria.

Quinolone Antimicrobials

Fluoroquinolones are broad-spectrum antimicrobials and bactericidals with mild side effects. These medications act by inhibiting enzymes needed for the bacteria's DNA. Easily absorbed on oral administration, these antimicrobials are used to treat bone and joint infections, urinary tract infections, prostatitis, gonorrhea, pneumonia, and other infections caused by susceptible microorganisms. Antacids decrease the absorption of these drugs and should not be given for 2 hours following the administration of the antibiotic. Ciprofloxacin is generally contraindicated in children younger than 16 to 18 years old because of cartilage damage, although cartilage and ligament damage can also occur in adults (Table 18-6).

Patient Education for Compliance

Ciprofloxacin should not be taken with milk or milk products, antacids, iron supplements, or magnesium laxatives.

TABLE 18-5 *Aminoglycosides*

GENERIC NAME	TRADE NAME	USUAL ADULT DOSE, ROUTE, AND FREQUENCY OF ADMINISTRATION	INDICATIONS FOR USE	DRUG INTERACTIONS
amikacin	Amikin	15 mg/kg/day in 2-3 divided doses IM, IV	*Type of bacteria*: Serious gram-negative and some gram-positive organisms	Extended-spectrum penicillins inactivate aminoglycosides, increase action of some muscle relaxants and anticoagulants, decrease effectiveness of digitalis
gentamicin	Garamycin	3-5 mg/kg/day in 2-3 divided doses IM, IV or ophthalmologic, topical	*Type of infection*: Those caused by above bacteria, plus tuberculosis (Kantrex)	
kanamycin	Kantrex	15 mg/kg/day in 2-3 divided doses po, IM, IV		
neomycin*	Neobiotic	Usually topical; nebulizer	Skin and ocular infections; used prior to GI surgery	Danger with loop diuretics and dimenhydrinate (Dramamine)
streptomycin		0.5-1 g po; IM q12-24h (not for long-term therapy)	Tuberculosis, plague, tularemia	
tobramycin	Nebcin, Tobrex	3-5 mg/kg/day in divided doses IM, IV, and ophthalmic	*Pseudomonas aeruginosa*, plus other gram-negative infections	

MAJOR SIDE EFFECTS OF AMINOGLYCOSIDES: Ototoxicity, blood dyscrasias nephrotoxicity, nausea, vomiting, and anorexia

GI, Gastrointestinal; *IM*, intramuscular; *IV*, intravenous.

> **IMPORTANT FACTS ABOUT FLUOROQUINOLONES**
> - Fluoroquinolones are broad-spectrum antibiotics.
> - The absorption of ciprofloxacin may be reduced by ingestion of milk, antacids, and iron supplements.

Other Antibiotics

Chloramphenicol

Chloramphenicol, a broad-spectrum antibacterial and antirickettsial agent, is bacteriostatic to a wide variety of gram-positive and gram-negative organisms, but it may be bactericidal in large doses. Bone marrow toxicity is a major drawback to its use. Chloramphenicol is used to treat forms of meningitis, paratyphoid and typhoid fever, typhus, Rocky Mountain spotted fever, and bacterial sepsis. It is not recommended for use in pregnant or breastfeeding women (Table 18-7).

Lincomycin

The various lincomycins are primarily bacteriostatic, although they may be bactericidal in high doses with select microorganisms. Clindamycin (Cleocin) is a semi-synthetic derivative of lincomycin used for bone and joint diseases, gynecologic diseases, skin and soft tissue infections, and septicemia. It may be administered either systemically or topically. Lincocin, a natural antibiotic, is used to treat serious streptococcal, pneumococcal, and staphylococcal infections (see Table 18-7).

Spectinomycin

Spectinomycin suppresses protein synthesis in gram-negative bacteria, especially *Neisseria gonorrhoeae*. It is administered only by intramuscular injection because it is not absorbed in the GI tract. It is usually administered as a single injection providing the full dosage. This drug is generally well tolerated (see Table 18-7).

Vancomycin

A bactericidal, vancomycin is usually the drug of last resort and should be reserved for severe infections caused by drug-resistant *Staphylococcus* and *Clostridium* infections (see Table 18-7).

Metronidazole

Metronidazole (Flagyl) is a short-acting bactericidal agent that is toxic to cells. It is used to treat infections caused by anaerobic bacteria and protozoa.

TABLE 18-6 *Fluoroquinolones (Quinolone Antimicrobials)*

GENERIC NAME	TRADE NAME	USUAL ADULT DOSE, ROUTE, AND FREQUENCY OF ADMINISTRATION	INDICATIONS FOR USE	DRUG INTERACTIONS
ciprofloxacin	Cipro	500-750 mg po q12h 400 mg IV q12h	*Type of bacteria:* gram-positive and gram-negative microorganism; drug of choice for anthrax infection or prophylaxis for anthrax infection *Type of infection:* wide variety	Increases effect of anticoagulants, caffeine; causes photosensitivity; should not be used in children and infants
enoxacin	Penetrex	200-400 mg po q12h for 1-2 wk	Urinary tract infections, gonorrhea	
lomefloxacin	Maxaquin	400 mg/day po for 2 wk	Upper respiratory and urinary tract infections	
levofloxacin	Levaquin	250-500 mg po, IV daily	Bronchitis, urinary tract infections, upper respiratory infections, skin infections, pneumonia	
norfloxacin	Noroxin	400 mg q12h for 3 days po and ophthalmic	Urinary tract infections and sexually transmitted diseases	
ofloxacin	Floxin	200-400 mg po, IV q12h	Upper respiratory infections, urinary tract infections, gonorrhea, prostate infections	
gatifloxacin	Tequin	400 mg/day po, IV for 7-14 days	Same as ofloxacin, plus gram-positive upper respiratory infections	
gemifloxacin	Factive	320 mg po qd	Same as above	
moxifloxacin	Avelox	400 mg/day po for 5-10 days	Gram-positive upper respiratory infections	

MAJOR SIDE EFFECTS OF FLUOROQUINOLONES: Dizziness, drowsiness, restlessness, rashes, nephrotoxicity, GI symptoms; with caffeine, ligament and cartilage damage, hypersensitivity and insomnia; additionally ototoxicity with norfloxacin.

GI, Gastrointestinal; *IV,* intravenous.

The patient may experience a metallic taste and diarrhea (see Table 18-7).

 PATIENT ALERT
Alcohol and Antabuse should be avoided by patients taking metronidazole.

Patient Education for Compliance

Clindamycin should be taken with a full glass of water.

OTC Antibiotics

Many antibiotics are found in OTC preparations for topical use. Perhaps the most common is Neosporin, a combination of polymyxin B, neomycin, and bacitracin.

- These OTC antibiotics are first-aid remedies that are applied to the skin either prophylactically or therapeutically.
- Bacitracin is used for the topical treatment of bacterial infections such as staphylococcal and group A streptococcal infections.

TABLE 18-7 *Miscellaneous Antibiotics*

GENERIC NAME	TRADE NAME	USUAL ADULT DOSE, ROUTE, AND FREQUENCY OF ADMINISTRATION	INDICATIONS FOR USE	DRUG INTERACTIONS
chloramphenicol	Chloromycetin	12.5 mg/kg po, IV q12h	*Type of bacteria:* gram-negative aerobic organisms *Type of infection:* meningitis, Rocky Mountain spotted fever, paratyphoid fever, typhoid fever, bacterial sepsis, typhus fever	Decreased antidiabetic agents and increased blood glucose levels, increased barbiturates, phenytoin Decreased by erythromycin lincomycin, and Cleocin
metronidazole	Flagyl	1 dose of 2 g, or 500 mg bid po for 7 days	*Type of infection:* Trichomoniasis, giardiasis, amebiasis	alcohol, Antabuse; increases effectiveness of anticoagulants

MAJOR SIDE EFFECTS: chloramphenicol: blood dyscrasias, nausea, diarrhea, dizziness, depression; **metronidazole:** dizziness, headache, GI disturbances, CNS toxicity, candidiasis

LINCOMYCINS

GENERIC NAME	TRADE NAME	USUAL ADULT DOSE, ROUTE, AND FREQUENCY OF ADMINISTRATION	INDICATIONS FOR USE	DRUG INTERACTIONS
clindamycin	Cleocin	100-300 mg po, IM, IV q6h	*Type of infection:* streptococcal, pneumococcal, and staphylococcal	erythromycin and chloramphenicol, antidiarrheals
lincomycin	Lincocin	500 mg po tid 600 mg q12h IM, IV		
vancomycin	Vancocin	125-500 mg po q6h 1 g q12h IV	*Type of infection:* severe septicemia, meningitis, pseudomembranous colitis	aspirin, furosemide, aminoglycosides, and other antibiotics because increases likelihood of ototoxicity and nephrotoxicity

MAJOR SIDE EFFECTS OF LYNCOMYCINS: clindamycin, lincomycin: GI disturbances and candidiasis; **vancomycin:** ototoxicity

GENERIC NAME	TRADE NAME	USUAL ADULT DOSE, ROUTE, AND FREQUENCY OF ADMINISTRATION	INDICATIONS FOR USE	DRUG INTERACTIONS
TOPICAL ANTIBIOTICS	Neosporin (contains bacitracin and polymyxin B)	Apply locally several times a day topically	Dermatologic infections	No significant interactions

CNS, Central nervous system; *GI,* gastrointestinal; *IM,* intramuscular; *IV,* intravenous.

- Polymyxin B is a bactericidal agent with a broad spectrum of action against aerobic gram-negative bacilli and as a sterile topical treatment of eye (by prescription), ear, and skin infections. Polymyxin B is not systemically absorbed, so systemic effects, such as neurotoxicity and nephrotoxicity, do not occur.
- Neomycin, found in triple antibiotic preparations, is a member of the aminoglycoside family of antibiotics. It is antimicrobial in these topical preparations.

IMPORTANT FACTS ABOUT MISCELLANEOUS ANTIBIOTICS

- Vancomycin is a toxic drug that is reserved for treating serious infections in patients allergic to penicillin.
- Chloramphenicol causes serious blood dyscrasias and should be used only when clearly indicated. Chloramphenicol should be taken on an empty stomach but may be taken with food if GI symptoms occur.
- Metronidazole is used against protozoa and anaerobic bacteria.
- Clindamycin should be taken with a full glass of water.

Sulfonamides (Sulfa Drugs)

Sulfonamides, or sulfa drugs, are not antibiotics— the drugs did not originate in a microorganism— but are *antibacterials* used to combat infection by slowing the growth of bacteria while the body builds its own defenses. Most of the sulfonamides are synthetically produced and bacteriostatic, but some are bactericidal. These agents are used in areas of the body where fluids can flush away the wastes of infection such as the eyes, urinary tract, and sinuses and for pneumonia and soft tissue infections.

Sulfonamides were discovered in the 1930s as a byproduct of the dye industry. They were initially effective against gram-positive and gram-negative microorganisms. However long-term use of these drugs has led to an increased bacterial resistance and antibiotics have proven to have a faster action than sulfonamides.

Sulfonamides are subdivided into two groups on the basis of their duration of action—short-acting and intermediate-acting agents.

- Because sulfonamides are rapidly excreted, high doses given at short intervals are necessary to maintain effective blood levels.
- The major indication for the sulfonamides are urinary tract infections (UTIs), but these medications are also used for chancroid, toxoplasmosis, malaria, meningococcal meningitis, *Hemophilus influenzae* infection, topically for burns, and in colitis of the lower GI tract for the antiinflammatory action.
- The effectiveness is increased because the drug leaves a residue in the urinary tract for long-term distribution in UTIs.

Sulfonamides in Combinations

Sulfonamides are combined with each other or with other medications such as trimethoprim to increase the antimicrobial action and the spectrum of action. These combinations are used for urinary tract infections, otitis media, bronchitis, shigellosis, and *Pneumocystis carinii* infections. The combination

drugs are generally well tolerated, and toxic effects are rare. The drug forms of tablets, suspensions, and intravenous solutions consist of one part trimethoprim to five parts sulfamethoxazole.

Topical Sulfonamide Preparations

Topical preparations of sulfonamides are available in several forms. Ocular preparations such as sulfacetamide (Sulamyd) are used for conjunctivitis and corneal ulcers. Skin lotions are used for seborrheic dermatitis, acne vulgaris, and skin infections. Other topical preparations such as powders and ointments are used to treat burns. These topical preparations do have some systemic absorption (Table 18-8).

PATIENT ALERT

While taking sulfonamides, the patient must take large quantities of fluids to prevent crystallization of the drug in the kidneys. This danger is minimal if the urine is kept dilute.

Patient Education for Compliance

1. Oral sulfonamides should be taken with a full glass of water on an empty stomach. Persons taking oral sulfonamides should drink 8 to 10 glasses of water a day to prevent crystallization of the sulfa in the kidneys.
2. Sulfonamides may cause photosensitivity reactions, so protective clothing should be worn and sunscreen used when in the sun.
3. The urine should be acidic for sulfonamides to have optimum effectiveness. Prunes and cranberries in any form result in acid urine. Carbonated beverages and citrus fruits should be avoided when taking sulfonamides because they produce alkaline urine.
4. Medications for urinary tract infections should be taken for 10 days to 2 weeks to prevent the development of subsequent, more resistant infections.

IMPORTANT FACTS ABOUT SULFONAMIDES

- Sulfonamides are used primarily to treat urinary tract infections and are used in combination therapy with other antiinfectives for otitis media.
- Combinations of trimethoprim-sulfamethoxazole inhibit bacteria in sequential steps, making these drugs more powerful than when used alone.
- E. coli, the most common cause of uncomplicated urinary tract infections, is susceptible to sulfonamides.

TABLE 18-8 *Select Sulfonamides*

GENERIC NAME	TRADE NAME	USUAL ADULT DOSE, ROUTE, AND FREQUENCY OF ADMINISTRATION	INDICATIONS FOR USE	DRUG INTERACTIONS
SHORT-ACTING				
sulfisoxazole	Gantrisin	1 g po q12h	*Type of infection*: urinary tract and GI tract infections; may be combined with penicillin and erythromycin for otitis media	Increase the action of anticoagulants and oral hypoglycemics; decrease the effectiveness of oral contraceptives
INTERMEDIATE-ACTING				
sulfamethoxazole	Gantanol	2 g initially, then 1 g bid po	Same as for the short-acting sulfonamides	
LONG-ACTING				
sulfasalazine	Azulfidine	3-4 g/day po in divided doses	*Type of infection*: ulcerative colitis, Crohn's disease, juvenile rheumatoid arthritis	
COMBINATION SULFONAMIDES				
trisulfapyrimidines (sulfadiazine, sulfamerazine, sulfamethazine)	Triple Sulfa	0.5-1 g qid po 1 vag tab bid × 10	*Type of infection*: urinary tract infections, otitis media, vaginal	
Trimethoprim sulfamethoxazole	Bactrim, Septra, Cotrim	80 mg TMP/400 mg SMZ po, IV q12h		
Double-strength TMP	Bactrim DS, Septra DS	160 mg TMP/800 mg SMZ po q12h		
erythromycin-sulfisoxazole	Pediazole	200-600 mg po tid	Otitis media	

MAJOR SIDE EFFECTS OF SULFONAMIDES: GI disturbances, kidney damage, drug-induced fever, diarrhea, headache, rashes, pruritus when taken po or by parenteral routes

TOPICAL PREPARATIONS				
Sulfacetamide ophthalmic ointment/solution	Sulamyd	As directed, usually 1 drop in eye tid for 7-10 days	*Type of infection*: ophthalmologic infection	
silver sulfadiazine	Silvadene Cream	Apply topically to affected area bid-qid for 7-10 days	Burns and skin infections	

GI, Gastrointestinal.

Drugs to Treat Urinary Tract Infections

Urinary tract antiseptics are restricted to the treatment of urinary tract infections. **Antiseptics** are agents that reduce microbial flora by inhibiting the growth and development of microorganisms without necessarily killing them. Three drugs are found in this category: nitrofurantoin, methenamine, and cinoxacin.

- Urinary tract antiseptics do not achieve effective concentrations in the blood or tissues to be antibacterial in these locations, and they cannot be used outside the urinary tract.
- Antiseptic drugs are usually the drugs of second choice; the preferred drugs are antibiotics or sulfonamides.
- Urinary tract antiseptics concentrate in the urine and are active against the pathogens commonly found in the urinary tract. The concurrent use of phenazopyridine (Pyridium) with these medications may mask the symptoms of infection.
- These drugs may discolor urine.

Nitrofurantoin is a broad-spectrum antibacterial that is bacteriostatic in low concentrations and bactericidal in high doses.

Methenamine decomposes into ammonia and formaldehyde. Virtually all bacteria are susceptible to formaldehyde, and resistance does not exist. Methenamine is used for treatment and prevention of recurrent and chronic urinary tract infections and is not used for acute urinary tract infections.

Cinoxacin is a close relative of nalidixic acid, with the same spectrum of action, same action in the urinary tract, and same side effects (Table 18-9).

Drugs to Treat Tuberculosis

With the emergence of multidrug-resistant mycobacteria associated with AIDS, tuberculosis has become a global public health problem. *Mycobacterium tuberculosis*, the bacterium that causes tuberculosis, is most often found in the lungs, but it may infect other body areas where the bacillus can grow in a high oxygen level. The bacilli may be dormant in the body for years and reemerge when the immune system has a lowered ability to fight disease and the person is more susceptible to the drug-resistant microorganism. Multidrug resistance has been a recent development, and resistance to isoniazid and rifampin, the two mainstays of tuberculosis therapy, has caused particular concern.

In general, antitubercular drugs can be divided into two groups:

- In the first group are medications that are fairly effective and not too toxic.
- The second-line drugs are more toxic and should be used only as necessary.
- As preventive medicine for tuberculosis, a single drug is usually recommended—most frequently isoniazid (INH), with rifampin the second choice.
- For the treatment of tuberculosis, two or more drugs to which the microorganism is sensitive should be used. The combination of medications not only decreases the risk of resistance but also reduces the chance of a relapse of the disease in the patient.
- Drug therapy may even include three or more medications given for prolonged periods of time.

TABLE 18-9 *Urinary Tract Antiseptics*

GENERIC NAME	TRADE NAME	USUAL ADULT DOSE, ROUTE, AND FREQUENCY OF ADMINISTRATION	INDICATIONS FOR USE	DRUG INTERACTIONS
nitrofurantoin	Furadantin, Macrodantin Macrobid	50 mg po tid-qid therapeutically; 50-100 mg po hs prophylactically	*Type of infection:* urinary tract infections	No significant interactions
methenamine	Mandelamine, Hiprex	0.5-1 g po qid 1 g po bid		Not given with sulfonamides
cinoxacin	Cinobac	1 g/day po in 2-4 divided doses		No significant interactions

MAJOR SIDE EFFECTS OF URINARY TRACT ANTISEPTICS: nitrofurantoin: GI disturbances, headaches, vertigo, drowsiness; **methenamine:** GI disturbances; **cinoxacin:** GI disturbances, rashes, visual disturbances, photosensitivity

GI, Gastrointestinal.

TABLE 18-10 *Select Antituberculosis Drugs*

GENERIC NAME	TRADE NAME	USUAL ADULT DOSE, ROUTE, AND FREQUENCY OF ADMINISTRATION	INDICATIONS FOR USE	DRUG INTERACTIONS
FIRST-LINE DRUGS				
isoniazid	INH, Laniazid	5-10 mg/kg/day po (usually 300 mg)	Preventive therapy for contacts of persons with tuberculosis and as treatment for those whose skin tests have recently converted from negative to positive	Increased absorption with alcohol intake Decreased Dilantin metabolism Increased hepatotoxicity when combined with drugs causing hepatotoxic effects
rifampin	Rimactane, Rifadin	600 mg/day po	Prophylactic treatment for tuberculosis	Increased absorption with alcohol intake Decreased Dilantin metabolism Increased hypotoxicity when combined with drugs causing hepatotoxic effects Increased metabolism of antidiabetic medications
rifampin-isoniazid	Rifamate	600 mg/day po	Preventive therapy for tuberculosis and treatment of active tuberculosis	
pyrazinamide	PZA	15-30 mg/kg/day po	Therapy for active tuberculosis	
ethambutol	Myambutol	15-25 mg/kg/day, po usually 1000 mg qd		
Streptomycin (see aminoglycosides)		0.5-1 g qid IM		

MAJOR SIDE EFFECTS OF FIRST-LINE DRUGS: Hepatotoxicity, neurotoxicity. Additionally, ocular toxicity with rifampin; arthritis, gout, arthritis-like reactions with pyrazinamide

SECOND-LINE DRUGS				
kanamycin (see aminoglycosides)			Therapy for active tuberculosis	
cycloserine	Seromycin	250 mg q12h po for 2 wk, then 250 mg po q6-8h		Increased absorption with alcohol intake
p-aminosalicylic acid	PAS	3-4 g po q8h		

IM, Intramuscular.

- Some drugs, such as INH and rifampin, are most effective against rapidly dividing bacilli, whereas others such as pyrazinamide are active against intracellular activity.
- The four recommended drugs that will provide the best treatment in combinations are INH, rifampin, pyrazinamide, and either ethambutol or streptomycin, given over prolonged periods of time, often a year or more.
- Vitamin B$_6$ (pyridoxine) may be added to prevent the neuropathies.
- Pyrazinamide (PZA) is a bactericidal that is most often used for active tuberculosis but may be used in combination with rifampin or rifabutin as a prophylactic medication for INH-resistant infections.
- Ethambutol should always be given in combination with other medications (Table 18-10).

Patient Education for Compliance

1. With medications for tuberculosis, the patient must be taught the reason for prolonged multidrug therapy. The length of therapy may make compliance a significant problem.
2. Isoniazid (INH) and rifampin should be taken on an empty stomach unless GI upset occurs, in which case it may be taken with meals.
3. Any changes in vision while taking ethambutol should be reported because of the possibility of ocular toxicity.

IMPORTANT FACTS ABOUT DRUGS TO TREAT TUBERCULOSIS

- The principal cause of drug resistance with tuberculosis is inadequate drug therapy resulting in drug-resistant strains. The prolonged use of multiple medications to treat tuberculosis contributes to lapses in medication therapy.
- To prevent drug resistance, tuberculosis should always be treated with at least two drugs to which the microorganism is sensitive.
- First-line drugs for treating tuberculosis are isoniazid, rifampin, pyrazinamide, ethambutol, and streptomycin. The usual four-drug regimen includes isoniazid, rifampin, pyrazinamide, and either ethambutol or streptomycin. This regimen can be used in all areas of tuberculosis treatment including drug-resistant tuberculosis.
- Isoniazid is the only drug that has been proved effective in preventing tuberculosis.

Drugs to Treat Fungal Infections

Fungi, including yeasts and molds, are spore-forming, plantlike, colorless microorganisms that are more complex than viruses or bacteria and thrive on dead plants and animals. Fungi produce many irritating symptoms because they cover the entire body, eating dead tissue from the skin, hair, and nails. Fungi are also found in soil, air, and contaminated food. Bacteria and the immune system keep fungi under control, but in susceptible persons, including pregnant women, fungi can multiply and become pathogenic.

Fungal, or *mycotic*, systemic infections can occur throughout the body. These systemic infections are in two categories: (1) **opportunistic infections** of resident flora, which occur in debilitated or immunosuppressed patients, and (2) nonopportunistic infections, which can occur in any host. Systemic fungal infections are dangerous in the chronically ill or immunosuppressed person.

- Long-term antibiotic therapy or radiation therapy can create an environment conducive to rapid fungal growth by altering the balance of normal flora or suppressing the immune system.
- The topical infections, with symptoms such as intense itching, discolored scaling of the skin, loss of hair and skin pigmentation, and blistered or broken skin between the toes, are more annoying than serious.
- Two of the most common fungal infections are ringworm infections (tinea corporis or tinea capitis) and athlete's foot (tinea pedis). Undecylenic acid is active against tinea infections, or dermatophytes, as a topical agent for superficial mycoses. The major indication is tinea pedis.
- *Candida albicans* causes thrush in the mouth and candidiasis in the vagina.
- Antifungal drugs, both systemic and topical, can be fungicidal or fungistatic based on their concentration in the body tissues.
- Therapy for systemic and topical fungal infections is usually prolonged, taking several weeks. Many mycoses resist treatment, and toxic effects from treatment may occur before a cure is achieved. The drugs are fairly specific for the disease processes (Table 18-11).
- Fungal cell membranes have little resemblance to bacterial cells; therefore antibiotics are ineffective. (The drugs used to treat topical fungal infections are discussed in Chapter 23.)
- Systemic medications must be given in high concentrations to achieve antifungal chemotherapy with resultant significant side effects. However, the benefits of treatment outweigh the risks involved. High doses are not tolerated by human hosts, so they are used only as needed.

TABLE 18-11 *Select Antifungal Drugs*

GENERIC NAME	TRADE NAME	USUAL ADULT DOSE, ROUTE, AND FREQUENCY OF ADMINISTRATION	INDICATIONS FOR USE	DRUG INTERACTIONS
SYSTEMIC DRUGS				
amphotericin B	Fungizone	0.25-1.5 mg/kg/day, IV, topical	Aspergillosis, candidiasis, coccidioidomycosis, blastomycosis	Increased potential for digitalis toxicity
micafungin sodium	Mycamine	50-150 mg IV qd	Esophageal candidiasis	

MAJOR SIDE EFFECTS OF SYSTEMIC DRUGS: Headache, anemia; GI disturbances; blurred vision, confusion, hallucinations; bone marrow suppression

GENERIC NAME	TRADE NAME	USUAL ADULT DOSE, ROUTE, AND FREQUENCY OF ADMINISTRATION	INDICATIONS FOR USE	DRUG INTERACTIONS
AZOLE ANTIFUNGALS				
fluconazole	Diflucan	100-200 mg/day, po, IV	Same as for amphotericin B, plus candidiasis, onychomycosis, cryptococcal infections, histoplasmosis	Increased liver toxicity with alcohol, increased oral hypoglycemics, and phenytoin
itraconazole	Sporanox	200 mg/day to bid po	Same as for amphotericin B	No significant interactions
ketoconazole	Nizoral	200-400 mg/day po	Same as for amphotericin B	Increased anticoagulants
griseofulvin	Grisactin Fulvicin	500 mg/day po 500 mg po bid	Tinea infections Tinea pedis, onychomycosis	Decreased anticoagulant therapy such as Coumadin and oral contraceptives
micafungin sodium	Mycamine	50-150 mg IV qd	Esophageal candidiasis	
nystatin	Mycostatin, Nilstat	400,000-600,000 mg po qid, 500,000-1,000,000 mg po bid as lozenge, suspension, tablets	*Monilia*, candidiasis	No significant interactions
posaconazole	Noxafil	200 mg po tid	Prophylaxis for *Aspergillus* and *Candida* infections in immunosuppressed individuals	cyclosporine, tacrolimus, sirolimus, cimetidine, and others
terbinafine	Lamisil	250 mg/day po and topical × 6 wk for fingernails, × 12 wk for toenails	Onychomycosis	No significant interactions
TOPICAL ANTIFUNGALS				
ciclopirox olamine	Loprox*	Apply as directed for all local antifungals; topical	Broad-spectrum antifungal	No significant interactions on local antifungals

(continued)

TABLE 18-11 *Select Antifungal Drugs—cont'd*

GENERIC NAME	TRADE NAME	USUAL ADULT DOSE, ROUTE, AND FREQUENCY OF ADMINISTRATION	INDICATIONS FOR USE	DRUG INTERACTIONS
clioquinol	Vioform[†]	Topical	Antibacterial/ antifungal	No significant interactions on local antifungals
clotrimazole	Lotrimin,[†] Gyne-Lotrimin,[†] Mycelex*,[†]	Several topical forms	Broad-spectrum antifungal	
econazole	Spectazole*	Topical	Broad-spectrum antifungal	
haloprogin	Halotex*	Topical	Broad-spectrum synthetic antifungal	
ketoconazole	Nizoral*	Topical	Tinea infections	
miconazole	Micatin,[†] Monistat*,[†]	Topical, lotion Vaginal	Tinea infections, candidiasis	
tolnaftate	Tinactin,[†] Aftate,[†] Cruex[†]	Multiple topical forms	Antifungal/ antibacterial, diaper rash	
terbinafine	Lamisil[†]	Topical		
butenafine gentian violet	Mentax*	Topical	Athlete's foot	
naftifine	Naftin*	Topical cream, gel	Candidiasis, superficial fungi	
tioconazole	Vagistat[†]	Vaginal cream	Candidiasis, vulvovaginal moniliasis	
triacetin	Fungoid,[†] Ony-Clear Nails[†]	Topical	Onychomycosis	
terconazole	Terazol*	Vaginal cream or suppository	Candidiasis	
undecylenic acid	Desenex[†]	Topical forms	Tinea infections	
sertaconazole	Ertaczo	Topical	Tinea pedis	
oxiconazole	Oxistat	Topical	Tinea infections	

MAJOR SIDE EFFECTS OF TOPICAL ANTIFUNGALS: Burning, irritation, pruritus, urticaria, local skin reactions

* Requires prescription.
[†] OTC medication.

PATIENT ALERT
• The underwear worn over moist areas should be cotton, and light-colored or white socks should be worn during treatment of fungal infections of the feet. Women should always wear underwear with a cotton crotch. Men should not wear polyester briefs. Athletic shoes and loafers should be worn with socks.

PATIENT ALERT—*Cont'd*
• Topical medications should be applied with a finger cot or gloves to prevent transfer of the pathogen to other body sites or people. For patients who are self-medicating, hands should be washed immediately after application.

Patient Education for Compliance

1. Undecylenic acid is not effective against candidiasis but is used for dermatophytes.
2. Feet, the crotch, and the underarm areas are more moist than other areas of the skin and may require the use of powders for the topical treatment of fungal infections, rather than creams or lotions, because powders tend to absorb the moisture.

IMPORTANT FACTS ABOUT ANTIFUNGALS

- Antifungals may be either fungicidal or fungistatic.
- Antifungals occur as prescription and OTC preparations. Most of the topical medications are available OTC.
- Antifungals are designed to be used for 4 weeks unless they are being used on nails. However, the agent and organism may require a time variance.
- Vulvovaginal candidiasis may be treated with a single oral dose of fluconazole.

Drugs to Treat Viral Infections

Viruses are strands of genetic material wrapped in a protein coating that prevents the ability of the virus to sustain itself independently. Viruses are parasitic on host cells, allowing the virus to reproduce. Not all viruses are harmful. Those that are range from the viruses that cause the common cold to those that cause devastating illnesses such as AIDS.

To multiply, the virus must attach to the outer membrane of the cell, then enter the cell nucleus, where there is DNA or RNA covered with a protein capsule. HIV virus is a retrovirus that attaches to the RNA and replicates on DNA causing new viruses to be placed in circulation.

The drug treatment of viral infections is problematic. By the time signs and symptoms of infection appear, replication of the virus is complete and the course of the disease has been determined. To be effective for all viral diseases, antivirals would need to be given prophylactically, which is neither practical nor safe. Another factor is the true parasitic nature of viruses, which could cause disturbances to the host cell and be toxic for the patient. Compared with the dramatic advances in antibacterials over the past 50 years, efforts to develop effective antiviral treatments have been much less successful. Most antiviral drugs work against the virus by preventing the virus from entering the host's cell or by interrupting replication of the virus.

Classification of Antiviral Drugs

The antiviral drugs, classified according to their use for either non-HIV infections or HIV, are prescribed after the virus has been identified. Drugs for HIV infection are also called *antiretroviral drugs*. The drugs for non-HIV infections are active against a narrow spectrum of viruses, and their use is limited to only a few viruses.

HIV Antivirals

Although no cure for HIV infection has been found, the advances in drug treatment have been dramatic. The trend in treating HIV infections is for once-daily dosing using antiretroviral medications. Patients prefer fewer tablets, less frequent dosing, and no food restrictions.

- The medications for HIV, which have been rapidly approved by the FDA, act to reduce HIV levels in plasma, thereby slowing the loss of immune function, preserving health, and prolonging life.
- These drugs require a triple-drug regimen, often known as a *cocktail.*
- Nucleoside/nucleotide reverse transcriptase inhibitors (NRTIs), also known as *"nukes,"* are the prime focus for once-a-day therapies and are the backbone for most current regimens by preventing healthy T-cells in the body from becoming infected with HIV.
  - The NRTIs are chemical relatives of the nucleosides in DNA; thus the medication suppresses the viral DNA and prevents HIV's reverse transcriptase enzyme from converting RNA to DNA in the infected T-cells.
  - The newer NRTIs such as tenofovir and emtricitabine have longer plasma half-lives and longer intracellular half-lives to provide longer exposure and longer periods of pharmacologic activity.
- The benefits of the antivirals for HIV are complex, the cost is high, and the toxicity is great. The HIV antivirals exhibit multiple drug interactions and cause side effects.
- The treatment does not eliminate the HIV virus, but the drugs reduce the levels of the virus, sometimes to the point of being undetectable.
- Stopping treatment may produce drug-resistant viruses.
- Routine hematology and blood chemistry studies are indicated for HIV patients taking antiviral drugs.

- The only absolute contraindication to the use of an HIV antiviral drug is hypersensitivity to the medication or concurrent conditions or drug therapy that prevent the use of the drug.
- Because HIV is treated with combinations of antivirals with antivirals or antifungals, the possibility of nephrotoxicity is very real (Table 18-12).

PATIENT ALERT

To be effective, antivirals for AIDS and AIDS-related diseases must be administered continuously for life.

Non-HIV Antivirals

The non-HIV systemic antiviral agents for herpes simplex viruses and the varicella-zoster virus include several drugs that range from basically nontoxic to highly toxic. Some antivirals, especially amantadine and rimantadine, should be used with care in the elderly (see Table 18-12).

Patient Education for Compliance

1. Drugs, especially acyclovir and valacyclovir, decrease symptoms of genital herpes simplex infection, but they do not produce a cure. If lesions are present, the disease is communicable.
2. Persons with HIV should adhere closely to prescribed dosage schedules.

IMPORTANT FACTS ABOUT ANTIVIRAL MEDICATIONS

- Viruses live on host cells, so it is difficult to suppress viral reproduction because the host's body cells would be harmed as well.
- Acyclovir and valacyclovir are the drugs of choice for herpes simplex and varicella-zoster viral infections.
- Acyclovir will reduce the symptoms of genital herpes but does not produce a cure or prevent the transmission of the disease to sexual partners if lesions are present.
- Amantadine is used for the prophylaxis and treatment of influenza A infections but not for influenza B infections.
- Resistance to antiviral drugs is a major problem. To reduce the emergence of resistant strains, drugs for HIV should be given in combination with other drugs.
- New drugs given to HIV patients should be agents that the patient has not taken before and that are not cross-resistant with drugs previously taken by the patient.

Drugs to Treat Malaria

Malaria is characterized by high fever with recurrent chills, severe sweating, and jaundice brought about by the involvement of the liver in the disease process due to microbes entering the liver. The mosquito acts as a **vector** to transmit the disease to the next human it bites.

Antimalarial drugs are administered prior to infection for prophylaxis and during exposure to prevent the development of the disease. The prophylaxis should begin 1 to 2 weeks prior to travel to an area where malaria is **endemic** and should continue for 6 weeks after the individual leaves the area. Short-term travelers may be required to take tetracycline prior to and for 4 weeks after travel. The drugs used during an acute attack of malaria selectively stop the multiplication of microorganisms and arrest the disease.

The choice of medications for the treatment of malaria is based on the strain of malaria involved and the stage in the life cycle of the organism. Travelers to areas where malaria is endemic should contact the CDC for the prophylaxis requirements. The contraindications to use are related to hypersensitivity to the medication. Quinine and its derivatives are pregnancy category X medications (Table 18-13).

DID YOU KNOW?

Quinine, a major ingredient in antimalarial medications, is readily available OTC for use with leg cramps, although this is not an FDA-approved use. It decreases muscle excitability by affecting calcium ions, which are necessary for skeletal muscles to contract. Quinine also depresses cardioconduction and acts as an oxytocic (causing contraction of the muscle) on the uterus—the reason why it is a category X drug for pregnant women. Quinidine, a related drug, is actually used to treat cardiac dysrhythmias.

IMPORTANT FACTS ABOUT MEDICATIONS FOR MALARIA

- Chloroquine is the drug of choice for the prevention and treatment of malaria.
- Quinine with adjunctive drugs is used to treat chloroquine-resistant microbes.

Drugs Used as Antiseptics and Germicides/Disinfectants

Microorganisms are everywhere. They migrate on skin, hair, furniture, and even in the air currents. Given an optimal environment, microorganisms

TABLE 18-12 *Antiviral Drugs*

GENERIC NAME	TRADE NAME	USUAL ADULT DOSE, ROUTE, AND FREQUENCY OF ADMINISTRATION	INDICATIONS FOR USE	DRUG INTERACTIONS
NON-HIV ANTIVIRALS				
amantadine	Symmetrel	200 mg/day po × 10 days	Influenza A	alcohol, CNS stimulants
rimantadine	Flumadine	100 mg bid po × 7 days	Influenza A	No significant interactions
cidofovir	Vistide	5 mg/kg IV q weekly × 2	Cytomegalovirus, retinitis	No significant interactions
ganciclovir	Cytovene	5 mg/kg IV q12h, 1000 mg po tid	Cytomegalovirus	zidovudine (AZT)
ribavirin	Virazole	20 mg/mL po q12-18h/day inhalation	Lower respiratory tract, respiratory syncytial virus	
acyclovir	Zovirax	200 mg po q4h × 10 days 500 mg/kg po tid	Herpes viruses types 1 and 2, and zoster	No significant interactions
famciclovir-penciclovir	Famvir	125 mg po bid × 5 days, 500 mg po q8h × 7 days	Genital herpes Herpes zoster	No significant interactions
penciclovir	Denavir	Apply locally q2h while awake	Herpes simplex	No significant interactions
idoxuridine	Herplex	1 drop topically in eye q1h	Herpes simplex, keratitis	No significant interactions
trifluridine	Viroptic	1 drop topically in eye q2h, up to 9 drops/day	Herpes simplex 1 and 2, keratitis	No significant interactions
vidarabine	Vira-A	0.5 in. topically in eye q3h	Herpes simplex keratitis	No significant interactions
zanamivir	Relenza Rotadisk	10 mg inhaled bid	Influenza A, B	No significant interactions
valacyclovir	Valtrex	500 mg po bid × 5 days	Genital herpes, herpes zoster	No significant interactions
foscarnet	Foscavir	60 mg/kg IV q8h	Herpes viruses, cytomegalovirus, Epstein-Barr virus, varicella-zoster	No significant interactions

MAJOR SIDE EFFECTS OF NON-HIV ANTIVIRALS: GI distress, dizziness, tinnitus, unpleasant taste; may be toxic as nephrotoxicity, hepatic dysfunction, blood dyscrasias

GENERIC NAME	TRADE NAME	USUAL ADULT DOSE, ROUTE, AND FREQUENCY OF ADMINISTRATION	INDICATIONS FOR USE	DRUG INTERACTIONS
HIV ANTIVIRALS				
abacavir	Ziagen	300 mg po bid	HIV	alcohol, St. John's wort
didanosine	Videx, ddI	200 mg po bid	Advanced HIV	Care with antituberculosis drugs, alcohol, furosemide, estrogens, tetracyclines, nitrofurantoin, diuretics
delavirdine	Rescriptor*	400 mg po tid	Advanced HIV	
indinavir	Crixivan	800 mg po q8h	HIV infection	cisapride, midazolam, triazolam, rifampin, Rescriptor, ketoconazole
lamivudine	Epivir*	150 mg po bid	HIV	Same as indinavir
nelfinavir	Viracept	750 mg po tid × 24 wk	HIV	Same as indinavir
nevirapine	Viramune*	200 mg po bid	HIV	Same as indinavir Numerous life-threatening (see literature)
ritonavir	Norvir	600 mg po bid	HIV	Antianxiety agents, cisapride, meperidine, piroxicam, propoxyphene

(continued)

TABLE 18-12 *Antiviral Drugs—cont'd*

GENERIC NAME	TRADE NAME	USUAL ADULT DOSE, ROUTE, AND FREQUENCY OF ADMINISTRATION	INDICATIONS FOR USE	DRUG INTERACTIONS
saquinavir	Invirase*	600 mg po tid	Advanced HIV	Antituberculosis drugs, Dilantin, nonsedating antihistamines
stavudine	Zerit	40 mg po q12h	Advanced HIV	zidovudine
zalcitabine	Hivid	0.75 mg po q8h	HIV	probenecid, cimetidine, Maalox, metoclopramide, didanosine
zidovudine	Retrovir	100 mg po q4h	HIV with impaired immunity	ganciclovir
amprenavir	Agenerase	1200 mg po bid	HIV	amiodarone, lidocaine, quinidine, warfarin, tricyclines

MAJOR SIDE EFFECTS OF HIV ANTIVIRALS: Nephrotoxicity, nausea, vomiting, anorexia, renal failure, diarrhea, headache, blood dyscrasias; additionally paresthesia with amprenavir

COMBINATION MEDICATIONS

zidovudine-lamivudine	Combivir	One tab po bid	HIV	Other HIV drugs, interferon, alpha fluconazole, probenecid

CNS, Central nervous system; *GI*, gastrointestinal; *HIV*, human immunodeficiency virus; *IV*, intravenous.
*Used in combination with other antivirals.

TABLE 18-13 *Antimalarials*

GENERIC NAME	TRADE NAME	USUAL ADULT DOSE, ROUTE, AND FREQUENCY OF ADMINISTRATION	INDICATIONS FOR USE	DRUG INTERACTIONS
chloroquine	Aralen	300-700 mg/wk po 2 wk prior to exposure and for up to 4 wk after leaving endemic area	Acute malaria and prophylaxis	No significant interactions
hydroxychloroquine	Plaquenil	400 mg/wk po	Acute attacks and prophylaxis	No significant interactions
mefloquine	Lariam	5 tabs po with water, then 250 mg weekly, then every other week	Same as Plaquenil	quinine, beta-blockers, calcium channel blockers
primaquine		15 mg po qd × 14 days	Prophylaxis and to prevent relapses of malaria	quinacrine
quinine		250-650 po mg q8h × 6-12 days	Acute attacks, either separately or with sulfonamides or tetracycline	mefloquine
pyrimethamine	Daraprim	25 mg po once a week up to 10 wk	Prophylaxis	No significant interactions
pyrimethamine with sulfadoxine	Fansidar	2-3 tabs/day po	Acute attack for chloroquine-resistant disease	No significant interactions
doxycycline* (tetracycline)	Vibramycin	100 mg/day po for 1-2 days before travel, continuously throughout travel, and 4 wk after travel	Prophylaxis	See interactions for tetracyclines in Table 18-4

MAJOR SIDE EFFECTS OF ANTIMALARIALS: Nausea, diarrhea, headaches, blurred vision, vertigo, rashes

*See antibiotics.

can produce infection. Pasteur began the practice of antiseptic technique in the nineteenth century, and the medicinal choices for antisepsis with less toxicity have increased over the years. Antiseptics and disinfectants are used to reduce microbial growth, wound contamination, and ultimately the risk of wound infection. The terms *antiseptic* and *germicidal/disinfectant* are not interchangeable, although both types of agents are used to control and prevent infection.

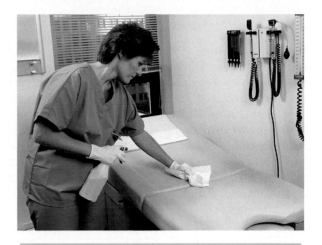

Figure 18-1 Disinfectants are used to clean rooms.

Antiseptics versus Disinfectants

Antiseptics are agents applied to living tissue to clean wounds or to prepare skin for surgery or injections.

- The objective of antiseptic therapy is to decrease the number of bacteria and allow normal body defense mechanisms to work.
- Antiseptics are used to eliminate disease or as prophylactic agents for activities such as hand washing.

Disinfectants are applied to inanimate objects to reduce the bacterial growth (Figure 18-1). **Germicides,** which kill microorganisms, may be used on either living or nonliving objects.

- As a rule, disinfectants are too harsh for living tissue, but they are used to disinfect surgical instruments and to clean rooms.
- Germicides may be further subdivided into bactericides, fungicides, virucides, and amebicides. Some drugs are **germistatic** and may be used for **sanitization,** but these drugs do not kill the microbes.
- Disinfectants may not kill all types of microorganisms, especially spores, viruses, and fungi.

The sensitivity of a microorganism to a disinfectant and an antiseptic varies and depends on factors such as the microorganism's ability to form spores. If the cell cannot be penetrated, the bacterium is resistant to drugs. In actual clinical use, the effectiveness of antiseptics and disinfectants is extremely variable, depending on the product, how it is applied, and the situation in which it is used. The ability of the agent's ingredients to dissolve, work, and mix in the presence of organic matter affects the agent's effectiveness, with the results being difficult to evaluate. Antiseptic and disinfectant solutions vary in their antimicrobial potency, their spectrum of activity, and the time they take to act, as well as their duration of action. The toxicity to the microorganisms is determined in part by the duration of exposure to the chemicals. Seventy percent ethanol reduces the bacteria on the skin by 50% in 36 seconds, whereas benzalkonium chloride 1:1000 requires 7 minutes of exposure to achieve the same effect.

- Some of the chemicals are broad spectrum or nonselective in their action, such as formaldehyde, glutaraldehyde, and iodine.
- Hexachlorophene and benzalkonium chloride are primarily effective against both gram-positive and gram-negative bacteria.
- Alcohol is bactericidal to vegetative forms of both gram-positive and gram-negative bacteria.

When properly used, antiseptics have limited use in treating local infections, but they are effective in preventing microorganisms from entering the body and decreasing possible microbial contamination.

The complete removal of all pathogenic microorganisms is accomplished by using disinfectants in such areas as surfaces in operating rooms and patient rooms. Dirt and organic materials should first be removed from the area by sanitization, and then the surface is treated with phenols, iodophors, or isopropyl alcohol, which should be allowed to air dry. These products may be used in combination with alcohol to increase the overall ability to kill germs.

 CLINICAL TIP

After sanitizing instruments, the allied health professional should be sure that the instrument is dry before placing it in the disinfectant to prevent diluting the disinfecting solution and decreasing its effectiveness.

Iodine Preparations

Iodine preparations (iodophors) are rapid-acting, potent germicides that are superior for effectively removing microorganisms such as bacteria, viruses, and protozoa from the skin. Tincture of iodine is especially effective, but it causes residual staining of the skin and also local stinging because of its alcohol base. Iodine preparations such as Betadine are used to disinfect the skin prior to surgery. Allergic reactions to iodine are common and should be evaluated because the resultant stain may mask the redness and swelling.

CLINICAL TIP

A patient allergic to seafood may be allergic to iodine preparations. Ask prior to using odophors.

Alcohol

Alcohol preparations can be used as antiseptics and can be used alone or in combination with other topical agents to prepare the skin for surgery or injection. Ethyl alcohol is effective in concentrations of less than 70%; isopropyl alcohol is bactericidal in concentrations between 50% and 90%, with 70% being the desired concentration. Alcohol is added to other antiseptics to increase the antiseptic effect, but this additive may cause skin irritation. The swabs or prep wipes for giving injections contain isopropyl alcohol for its bactericidal effects. The area should be air-dried for ultimate cleaning.

Hexachlorophene

Hexachlorophene is used as a surgical scrub or skin cleanser. It is effective against gram-positive microorganisms, which are the usual bacteria found on the skin. With repeated use, the hexachlorophene accumulates on the skin to maintain antibacterial activity.

Hydrogen Peroxide

Hydrogen peroxide has limited usefulness because it does not penetrate skin and breaks down rapidly into molecular oxygen and water. Its effervescence may facilitate mechanical cleaning of debris from a wound, whereas its effectiveness at killing microbes is limited. Hydrogen peroxide is damaging to new tissue, causing the forming tissues to slough.

Silver Preparations

Silver preparations are antiseptics. Silver nitrate is used as an ophthalmic antiseptic in the eyes of newborns to prevent gonococcal infections. Silver sulfadiazine (Silvadene) is used for burns because of its ability to better penetrate wounds.

Mercury Preparations

The bacteriostatic mercurial preparation thiomersal is not as effective as other antiseptics but is a popular OTC first-aid preparation. It is also used as a preservative in contact lens solutions to reduce microflora growth and replication in the eye.

PATIENT ALERT

People wearing contact lenses who are allergic to thiomersal should take care in choosing eye preparations. Mercury is the usual antiseptic used in lens solutions.

Other Disinfectants and Antiseptics

Antiseptics and disinfectants should not be taken orally because they are toxic when ingested or absorbed through the skin.

- Weakened sodium hypochlorite (10%) may be used as an antiseptic to irrigate a wound. It is also used as a disinfectant on countertops, floors, and other surfaces as a virucide.
- Boric acid is a mild bacteriostatic and fungicidal that is used as an eyewash or irrigant. It is also a first-aid treatment for dry or chapped skin, minor rashes, and insect bites. Boric acid is considered to be nontoxic (Table 18-14).

CLINICAL TIP

Any dilute hypochlorite solution made in the office should be made daily because it remains fully potent for only 24 to 36 hours. The dilution should be 1:10 to be effective. Care must be taken to dilute the sodium hypochlorite solution so that it will not discolor surfaces or clothing. Some facilities purchase a prediluted product because of convenience and stability of the solution.

TABLE 18-14 *Antiseptics and Disinfectants/Germicidals**

GENERIC NAME	TRADE NAME OR COMMON NAME	PRIMARY ANTIMICROBIAL USE	ANTISEPTIC	DISINFECTANT
ALCOHOLS				
ethanol	ethyl alcohol	Vegetative bacteria	X	
isopropyl (70%)	rubbing alcohol		X	
ALDEHYDES				
formaldehyde (10%-37%)		Bacterial spores, viruses, fungi		X
glutaraldehyde (2%)	Cidex			X
IODINE PREPARATIONS				
povidone iodine (0.5%-10%)	Betadine, Iodine	Vegetative microorganisms and spores	X	X
iodine solution (2%)			X	
tincture of iodine (2%)		Bacteria, spores, fungi, viruses	X	
CHLORINE COMPOUNDS				
sodium hypochlorite 10%—disinfectant 0.15%-0.5%—antiseptic	Clorox	Bacteria, spores, fungi, viruses	X	X
oxychlorosene	Clorpactin	Useful with local infections that are drug resistant	X	
PHENOL COMPOUNDS				
hexachlorophene	Dial soap, pHisoHex (℞)	Vegetative gram-positive bacteria	X	
OTHERS				
chlorhexidine 1%	Exidine cleanser, Hibiclens	Spores, bacteria, fungi, viruses	X	
boric acid		Bacteria, fungi	X	
thiomersal (0.1%)/ thimerosal	Merthiolate	Vegetative bacteria and fungi	X	
gentian violet		Yeast infections	X	
hydrogen peroxide (1.5%)		Vegetative microorganisms		X
benzalkonium chloride (0.02%-0.5%)	Zephiran	Vegetative gram-positive bacteria	X	X
silver nitrate (0.1%-0.5%)		Vegetative bacteria and fungi	X	
silver sulfadiazine (1%)	Silvadene ℞	Vegetative bacteria and fungi	X	

*Antiseptics and germicidals/disinfectants may cause such side effects as skin irritation, rashes, and skin dryness.

Disinfectants

Disinfectants are used to clean and store surgical instruments, disinfect operating rooms, and **sterilize** objects that cannot be sterilized by exposing them to high temperatures. Formaldehyde and glutaraldehyde are irritating to the skin and should be used only on inanimate objects. Other common disinfectants are sodium hypochlorite (bleach) and alcohol.

IMPORTANT FACTS ABOUT ANTISEPTICS AND DISINFECTANTS
- *Antiseptics* are used on living tissue, and *disinfectants* are used on inanimate objects. *Germicides* may be used on either animate or inanimate objects.

Summary

With the advent of penicillin and sulfonamides, a new era in health care was launched. From the time penicillin was first used in the early 1940s, antimicrobials have been used in medical offices on a daily basis. As bacteria, fungi, and viruses become resistant to one type of antimicrobial agent, new agents must be found to replace the one that is no longer effective. The FDA approves new antimicrobials many times a year, with special rapidity for approving agents used to treat debilitating diseases such as AIDS.

Patient education in the use of antimicrobials is a major responsibility of the allied health professional. If the drug is not taken for the prescribed time, drug-resistant bacteria become the victors in the battle against disease. (Two of the major strains of drug-resistant bacteria are those that cause tuberculosis and those that cause staphylococcal infections.) To limit the possibility of drug-resistant bacteria developing, patients taking antimicrobials must follow the routine for the prescribed time so that more virulent bacteria are killed or controlled while the body's own defense system suppresses any remaining microorganisms. Without the body's defense system, antibiotic therapy would rarely be successful. *People do not become drug resistant; the microorganism becomes drug resistant, and the microbes will continue to multiply in a drug-resistant state.*

The key to treating infection is to match the medication to the microorganism. Some antimicrobials are effective against a broad spectrum of organisms; others are specific and effective against a narrow spectrum. The best match can be obtained by performing culture and sensitivity testing. The effectiveness of the antibiotic depends on its ability to concentrate at the site of the infection and to distinguish infection-producing foreign materials such as debris from other foreign objects such as prostheses and pacemakers in the body. Superinfections also can become a problem with antibiotic therapy, especially when treatment is over a prolonged period of time.

Patients should also be instructed not to "save" medications but to complete the full prescription. Microbes grow when the full treatment has not been taken, and a microorganism's susceptibility to the same drug administered at a later date may be decreased.

Antibiotics are available in several categories such as penicillins, cephalosporins, macrolides, tetracyclines, aminoglycosides, and some miscellaneous groups. Antibiotics are found in many OTC preparations for topical use. These preparations are first-aid medications that may be used therapeutically or prophylactically with lacerations, abrasions, insect bites, and so on. The same antibiotics are found in ophthalmic and otic preparations.

Sulfonamides are not antibiotics but are antibacterials used to treat an infection while the body responds with its own defense mechanisms. Urinary tract antiseptics are used to treat pathogen-caused infections of the urinary tract by concentrating the drug in the urine. Tuberculosis has traditionally been treated with rifampin and isoniazid, but as the causative organism is becoming resistant to these drugs, new drugs are being introduced. Medications for tuberculosis must be given in combination to prevent the development of drug-resistant bacteria, to effectively eradicate organisms, and for their synergistic effects.

Medications for fungal infections may be either topical or systemic. Fungal infections are difficult to cure because fungi live on the dead skin of the body or within body tissues. Long-term antibiotic therapy or radiation therapy allows the naturally occurring fungi on the skin to grow, leading to superinfections.

Viruses do not respond to antibiotics, and antibiotics should be administered in viral infections only if there is a secondary microbial infection. The problem with developing antiviral medications is that often the virus is virulent within the body before signs and symptoms of the disease are evident.

Drugs for malaria may be given prophylactically prior to travel to regions where malaria is endemic and therapeutically for the treatment of active malaria.

Antiseptics, disinfectants, and germicidals are mainstays of the physician's office. Antiseptics are used on living tissue, disinfectants on inanimate objects, and germicides on both. The agent should be chosen to match the medical use. Disinfectants include sodium hypochlorite, used to decontaminate surfaces where body fluids may be found. Sodium hypochlorite is an excellent virucide, but care must be taken to avoid discoloration of surfaces where it is used.

Care must be taken in treating individuals who might have had allergic reactions to antibiotics in the past. Care must also be taken not to use medications when they are not indicated because of the danger of drug-resistant microorganisms developing.

Critical Thinking Exercises

SCENARIO

Janie comes to the office complaining of a sore throat, hoarseness, cough, and runny nose. Dr. Merry has examined Janie and told her that she has a virus. Janie tells you as she leaves the office that she just does not understand why Dr. Merry did not give her an antibiotic. Janie's health history is nonsignificant except for the symptoms of the present respiratory tract infection.

1. What reason do you give Janie to explain why Dr. Merry did not prescribe an antibiotic?
2. What do you tell Janie about the misuse of antibiotics?
3. Is a prophylactic prescription for an antibiotic indicated in this case?

DRUG CALCULATIONS

1. Order: Cefadyl 500 mg IM stat
   Available medication:

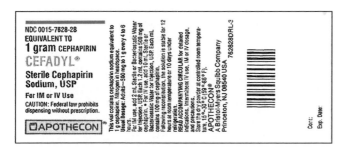

What diluent and what volume of diluent should be added to the vial? _____
_____
What volume of medication should be administered for the order? _____

Show on the syringe the amount of cefadyl that should be administered.

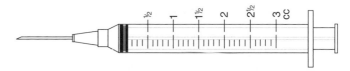

2. Order: clindamycin palmitrate oral solution 150 mg q8h
   Available medication:

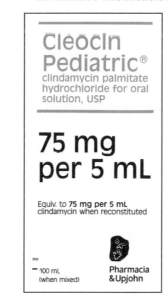

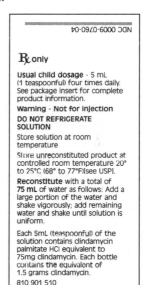

What volume of medication should be administered with each dose? _____
How can this medication be administered using a household measurement? _____
_____

Show on the utensil the amount of medication that should be given to the child.

REVIEW QUESTIONS

1. Why are antibiotics effective against bacteria but not viruses? _____
_____
_____

2. What is acquired antibiotic resistance? How does a bacterium become drug resistant? _____
_____
_____

3. What spectrums are used to classify penicillins? Name a commonly used medication in each spectrum. _____
_____
_____

4. What is meant by *generation* when discussing penicillin? _____
_____
_____

5. What is the main indication for the use of sulfonamides? Are these drugs bacteriostatic or bactericidal? What does the patient need to be told concerning fluid intake? _____
_____
_____

6. What is the difference in use between an antiseptic and a disinfectant? _____
_____
_____

7. What are the uses of antiseptics in the medical office? _____
_____
_____

8. How do disinfectants work? _____
_____
_____

CHAPTER 19

Antineoplastic Agents

OBJECTIVES

After studying this chapter, you should be capable of doing the following:
- Defining antineoplastic medications.
- Explaining the difference between curative and palliative uses of chemotherapeutic drugs.
- Classifying tumors by the tissues in which they originate.
- Describing the role of the allied health professional in chemotherapy.
- Describing how to safely handle and administer antineoplastics.
- Identifying and classifying the various chemotherapeutic medications.

Jack has cancer of the esophagus and is undergoing chemotherapy for it. After chemotherapy treatments, Jack has nausea and anorexia. His tongue is red, swollen, and sore.
  Is this an expected effect of antineoplastics? Why or why not?
  What suggestions do you have to help with the dietary intake?
  Can Jack expect alopecia from all types of chemotherapy? Why or why not?
  How would you explain to Jack what stage II carcinoma is.

KEY TERMS

Alkylating agent	Cell cycle phase	Neoplasm
Alopecia	Chemotherapy	Nystagmus
Antimetabolite	Cytotoxic agent	Plant alkaloids
Antineoplastic agent	Extravasation	Proliferation
Ascites	Malignant	Radioisotope
Ataxia	Metastasis	Stomatitis
Benign	Mitotic alkaloids	Teratogenic
Biotherapy	Morbidity	Tumor
Cancer	Mortality	
Carcinogenic agent	Mutagenic	

EASY WORKING KNOWLEDGE OF INDICATIONS AND SIDE EFFECTS

Seven Warning Signs of Cancer
Change in bowel or bladder habits
A sore that will not heal
Unusual bleeding or discharge
Thickening or a lump in the breast or elsewhere
Indigestion or difficulty swallowing
Obvious change in a wart or mole
Nagging cough or hoarseness

Common Side Effects of Antineoplastic Medications
Stomatitis
Nausea and vomiting
Diarrhea
Alopecia
Local tissue injury
Suppression of blood elements

365

Easy Working Knowledge of Antineoplastics

DRUG CLASS	PRESCRIPTION	OTC	PREGNANCY CATEGORY	MAJOR INDICATIONS
Alkylating agents	Yes	No	C, D, X (especially in first trimester)	Carcinomas, sarcomas, lymphomas, leukemias, and polycythemia vera
Antimetabolites	Yes	No	D	Carcinomas, trophoblastic tumors, osteogenic sarcomas
Antibiotics/antitumor	Yes	No	C, D	Carcinomas, sarcomas, lymphomas, leukemias
Mitotic inhibitors (plant alkaloids)	Yes	No	D	Carcinomas, leukemias, Hodgkin's disease, Ewing's sarcoma
Hormone therapy	Yes	No	C, D, X	Prostate cancer, breast cancer, endometrial cancer, adrenal cancer
Immunosuppressants	Yes	No	C, D	Kaposi's sarcoma, leukemias
Radioisotopes	Yes	No	C, D	Thyroid cancer, polycythemia vera, metastatic cancer

A neoplasm (neo-, *new*, plus Greek plasma, meaning *formation*) is any new or unusual growth of tissue in plants or animals. Neoplasms are also called tumors. If the tumor has uncontrolled growth and spread of the abnormal cells, it is known as *cancer*. Neoplasms, named for site of origin, may be benign or malignant. Figure 19-1 shows the appearance and characteristics of benign and malignant neoplasms. Neoplasms are named by the tissue where the lesion originates. Benign neoplasms are named by the site plus the suffix "oma." For example, lipoma is a benign neoplasm originating in fat tissue. (Note: Some malignant tumors also end with -oma.) Malignant neoplasms are characterized by the names ending in sarcoma, from connective tissue; carcinoma and melanoma, from epithelial tissue; lymphoma, from blood-forming tissue; and blastoma, from nerve tissue (Table 19-1).

The drug treatment of tumors and malignancies, or **chemotherapy,** is increasingly important as an adjunct to surgery and radiation therapy. Chemotherapy is performed using **antineoplastic agents** that do not directly kill cancer cells; rather, they interfere with cell reproduction and growth, thus causing death to the cells. Because cancer cells tend to **proliferate** rapidly, they are more vulnerable to chemotherapy than healthy, noncancerous cells are. Nevertheless, many healthy cells die in the course of chemotherapy, and the individual undergoing such therapy can expect significant side effects from the toxic drugs used in chemotherapy. With the **morbidity** and **mortality** from cancer continuing to pose a major public health problem in the United States, the search for better treatment including better chemotherapeutic regimens is an ongoing quest.

What Is Cancer?

Cancer is not a single disease; more than 100 different types of cancer have been identified. All have the uncontrolled division of abnormal cells in common with cancer cells reproducing faster than normal cells.

- Cancer is a mass of cells that has no useful function but can cause dysfunction and structural alterations in surrounding cells.
- As the tumor increases in size, normal cells do not receive the necessary nutrition or blood supply and decrease in number, causing loss of normal body functions, especially in the late stages of the disease.
- The incidence of cancer increases with age, although young children can have malignancies.

The original site of a tumor is called the *primary site*. As the tumor **metastasizes** to new locations in the body, each new site is referred to as a *secondary site*. Malignant cells may spread in several ways.

- First, the cells may directly extend, or metastasize, to the neighboring tissue. This occurs as the ulceration or hemorrhagic masses produce local infiltration and distortion of the structures.
- Second, the detached cells may move along lymphatic vessels or as an embolism of the lymphatic vessels to the regional lymph nodes or

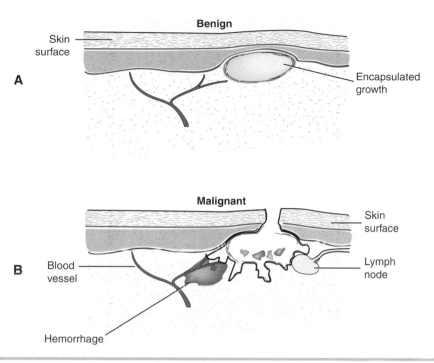

Figure 19-1 **A,** Benign neoplasms remain localized, are smooth and freely movable, compress local tissue, and do not break the skin. **B,** Malignant neoplasms metastasize to new and distant tissues through the lymph system and blood vessels, causing hemorrhage. They also have an irregular shape, invade local tissue, and often ulcerate through the skin.

TABLE 19-1 *Examples of Benign and Malignant Neoplasms by Tissue of Origin*

TISSUE OF ORIGIN	BENIGN (SITE + "-OMA")	MALIGNANT
Connective, nerve, and muscle tissue	Lipoma, a benign neoplasm of adipose tissue	*Sarcoma* (liposarcoma = malignant neoplasm of adipose tissue)
Epithelial tissue	Adenoma, a benign neoplasm of glands	*Carcinoma* (adenocarcinoma = malignant neoplasm of glands)
	Nevus, a neoplasm of pigmented cells	*Melanoma* (malignant neoplasm of pigmented cells)
Blood-forming tissue including lymphoid tissue, plasma cells, and bone marrow	Lymphangioma, a benign neoplasm of lymph vessels	*Lymphoma* (lymphangiosarcoma = malignant neoplasm of lymph vessels; leukemias)
Nerve tissue ganglion cells	Ganglioneuroma, a benign neoplasm of nerve ganglion cells	*Blastoma* (neuroblastoma = malignant neoplasm of ganglion cells)

Note: The headings "Benign" and "Malignant" are not all-inclusive but are examples of the naming of tumors. Entities in *italics* are names indicative of malignant neoplasms.

invade the lymph nodes; thus, the lymphatic tissue is the usual site for the invasion and spread of the tumor or abnormal cells.
- Cells may also form an embolus that moves through blood vessels to organs throughout the body. Tumors in venous blood tend to travel to the lungs, whereas those in the arterial system tend to form secondary neoplasms in the bone and brain. Primary gastrointestinal (GI) neoplasms tend to metastasize to the liver.

- Finally, cells may invade a body cavity by diffusion.

Metastatic tumors mimic the primary tumor, making diagnosis of the primary site possible by cell morphology. Specific cancers tend to metastasize to specific secondary sites by traveling through the circulatory or lymphatic systems to grow, but, because of the travel of the cancerous cells, the secondary sites may be some distance from the primary site. The secondary tumors tend to resemble the cells at the primary site and are so named such as lymphoma for tumors originally found in the lymphatic system or melanoma for tumors from melanocytes in skin pigment (see Table 19-1).

Classifying Tumors

Tumors are *classified* by stage of invasion and degree of metastasis (grade), from stage I to stage IV. The overall treatment of a neoplasm is based on stage and grade.

Malignant lesions are classified by grade and stage to show the extent of the spread of the disease. Grade 0 is normal tissue. Grade 1 tumor is the most differentiated, looking more like the parent tissue, and is least malignant. Grade 2 is moderately well differentiated with some structural change from normal tissue. Grade 3 is poorly differentiated and has extensive change from normal tissue. Grade 4 has no resemblance to the tissue of origin and is anaplastic (has loss of cell differentiation).

The stages of tumors show the extent of the spread of the cancer. These are used in the planning of antineoplastic treatment. Stage 0 is cancer in situ, or cancer only at the localized site, without invasion of surrounding tissue. Stage 1 is a tumor limited to its site of origin. Stage 2 is cancer with only local spread. Stage 3 has extensive local spread and regional spread. Stage 4 has widespread metastasis throughout the body.

Antineoplastic Agents

Antineoplastic agents, also called *chemotherapeutic agents*, kill tumor cells directly and also interrupt cell replication of normal and abnormal cells to shrink the tumor and provide palliation and cure. Figure 19-2 shows how malignant cells respond to chemotherapy. When antineoplastic agents are prescribed and administered for malignant tumors, the size, site, grade, and stage of the tumor are considered. Chemotherapy may be the primary treatment or may be used in combination with surgical removal of the tumor and radiation. If the tumor is extensive, chemotherapy may be used to reduce the size of the tumor followed by the surgical procedure and further use of chemotherapeutic regimens. In other cases the tumor may be excised followed by chemotherapy and

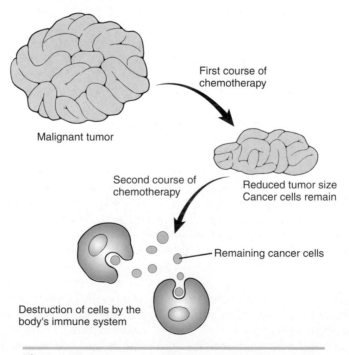

Figure 19-2 A cancer cell's response to chemotherapy.

radiation. The second course of chemotherapy is aimed at destroying the cancer cells that are not destroyed by the body's immune system.

Each antineoplastic agent has a specific point of action in cell replication or mitosis where it is effective (Figure 19-3). Chemotherapeutics have the ability to interrupt cell growth or replication of normal and malignant cells as they go through the various phases of cell replication. **Antimetabolites** interfere with DNA synthesis, whereas the plant alkaloids, or mitotic inhibitors, interfere with cell reproduction in the metaphase. Some drugs such as the alkylating agents, antibiotics, and hormones are active in several stages of the cell cycle and not specific to a single phase. The goal of combination therapy for chemotherapy is to destroy cancer cells at various stages of the cell replication process. Cancers with a fast growth factor and short cell replication cycles are the most vulnerable to chemotherapeutic agents.

Antineoplastic agents are most frequently given in combinations of two or more at a time. Some of these combinations are used for **palliative** effect. Other medications that are **cytotoxic** are used in the long-term treatment of malignancies in the hope of either curing the disease or placing it in remission. The metabolic rate of a malignant tumor cell is more rapid than that of a normal cell, causing malignant cells to be more sensitive to products that interfere with cell growth.

Many antineoplastic medications also have immunosuppressive properties that decrease the patient's ability to produce antibodies to attack infecting organisms. Because of the immune system suppression, the patient is susceptible to infections.

Understanding Side Effects of Antineoplastic Agents

The most serious cell destruction from antineoplastics occurs in the bone marrow, epithelium of the GI tract, hair follicle, and sperm-forming cells. Cells in these areas normally replicate rapidly (as cancer cells do), making them susceptible to killing by anticancer drugs.

- Bone marrow suppression with chemotherapy leads to infection, bleeding, and anemia.

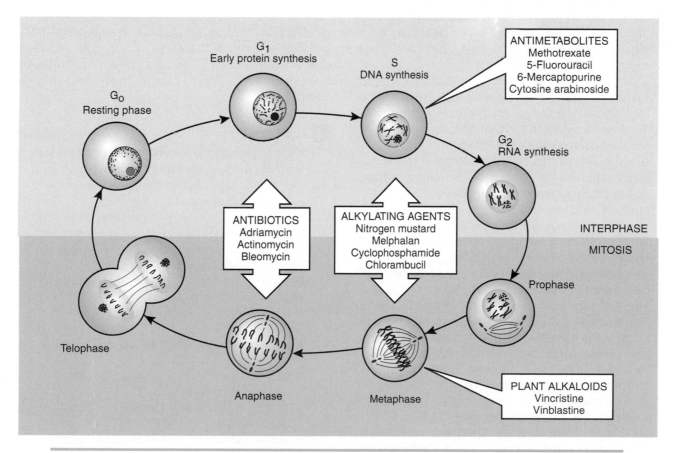

Figure 19-3 Phases of the cell replication cycle, showing where chemotherapeutic medications exert their effects.

TABLE 19-2 *Antiemetics Commonly Used with Antineoplastic Therapy*

GENERIC NAME	TRADE NAME
prochlorperazine	Compazine
trimethobenzamide	Tigan
metoclopramide	Reglan
lorazepam	Ativan
polonosetron HCl	Aloxi
ondansetron	Zofran

- The digestive tract epithelium is especially sensitive to cytotoxic drugs, leading to **stomatitis** that begins within a few days of the onset of therapy and persists for several weeks following the end of treatment. The other common effect in the intestinal tract is diarrhea because the loss of epithelial cells prevents fluids from being absorbed in the intestines. Patients at risk for diarrhea should be told to eat a high-fiber diet, to give the stools a firmer consistency, and to eat constipating foods such as cheese. However, fiber from fresh fruits and vegetables should be avoided.
- **Alopecia** results from injury to the hair follicles and begins 7 to 10 days after treatments are started. Regeneration usually begins 1 to 2 months following the last treatment.
- Cytotoxic effects in the reproductive system include teratogenic effects on the growing fetus and on the germinal epithelium of the testes. Women undergoing chemotherapy should be advised not to become pregnant because of the danger of fetal malformations. Male patients should be told that anticancer drugs might cause irreversible sterility.
- Nausea and vomiting from chemotherapy is usually more severe than nausea and vomiting from most medications. Premedication with a combination of antiemetics based on the type of chemotherapy prescribed may reduce the nausea and vomiting (Table 19-2).
- Weight loss and a resultant malnutrition in the patient taking chemotherapeutic agents occurs. Because the patient has many GI symptoms including anorexia, a diet high in proteins and calories should be consumed. Nutritional supplements may be used to increase calories and to prevent excessive weight loss. Sweets and fatty foods should be decreased, and fluids should be taken at times other than with meals. Clear, cool, unsweetened liquids are best tolerated. Consuming food at room temperature may help manage nausea and vomiting.

BOX 19-1   SYMPTOMS OF ORGAN TOXIC EFFECTS FROM ANTINEOPLASTICS

Cardiac Toxic Effects
Congestive heart failure
Changes in S-T waves
Angina while receiving medication
Ventricular fibrillation; death

Nephrologic Toxic Effects
Weight gain
Change in vital signs
Fluid overload

Neurologic Toxic Effects
Change in cognitive abilities
Nystagmus
Ataxia
Dizziness, difficulty changing positions
(cerebellar dysfunction)

Hepatic Toxic Effects
Bleeding disorders, pruritus
Jaundice
Nausea and vomiting
Ascites

Certain chemotherapeutic agents have dose-limiting effects in the form of adverse reactions that occur when the maximum permissible dose has been given to the individual patient (Box 19-1).

PATIENT ALERT

- If hair loss is expected and the patient desires to wear a hairpiece, the hairpiece should be selected before treatment is begun so that hair color and style will look as normal as possible.
- Patients undergoing chemotherapy should avoid highly seasoned foods and foods with strong odors. Eating small, frequent meals of complex carbohydrates and drinking liquids 30 to 60 minutes before meals will help manage the nausea. The sensation of taste is altered while taking antineoplastics. Eating tart foods that are either cold or at room temperature enhances food intake.
- Any of the following should be reported to the physician:
  - Rashes
  - Loss of taste
  - Tingling in face, fingers, and toes (peripheral neurotoxicity)
  - Dizziness, headache, confusion, slurred speech, convulsions (central nervous system neurotoxicity)

PATIENT ALERT—Cont'd

- Unusual bleeding, bruising, fever, sore throat, mouth sores (bone marrow dysfunction)
- Yellowing of eyes or body, clay-colored stools, dark urine (hepatotoxicity)
- Cough, shortness of breath, weight gain, fluid retention (pulmonary fibrosis or cardiotoxicity)
- Because of immune system compromise from chemotherapy, patients should avoid contact with persons with communicable diseases and should have limited contact with persons who may have a subclinical illness such as children who have fever or signs of possible disease.

IMPORTANT FACTS ABOUT ANTINEOPLASTIC AGENTS IN GENERAL

- Cancer cells are characterized by proliferation, invasion into normal tissue, and metastasis.
- Neoplasms may be either benign or malignant. Antineoplastic agents are used most often for malignant growths.
- Cancer treatment may entail any single or combination of surgery, radiation therapy, and chemotherapy. Surgery and radiation therapy are the treatments of choice for solid tumors.
- Antineoplastic agents are the treatment of choice for cancers that are found in several sites throughout the body.
- Most antineoplastic drugs work best on tumors formed of cells that multiply rapidly, rather than on slow-growing tumors.
- Anticancer drugs are more effective when used as combination therapy rather than single-drug therapy because the cancer cells are less likely to mutate and become drug resistant.
- Toxic effects on normal cells are a major obstacle to successful chemotherapy.
- Antineoplastics must have one of three possible benefits to be used: cure, palliation, or prolongation of life.

Patient Education for Compliance

1. Because anxiety is an expected response, cancer patients should be made aware of the fact that they will need emotional support for themselves and their families.
2. Good nutrition is essential during chemotherapy. The patient should follow instructions about specific nutritional needs.

Patient Education for Compliance—cont'd

3. The patient should be prepared for rapid hair loss (alopecia) when the side effect is to be expected from the specific chemotherapy regimen used. Be sure the patient knows that all body hair may also be lost. Advise the patient that the hair will grow back when therapy is terminated. The new hair may not have the same texture or thickness as prior to chemotherapy.
4. Lesions in the mouth and bleeding gums are common with chemotherapy. Good oral hygiene is essential.
5. Cool, sweetened beverages are best tolerated.
6. Fever, sore throat, infections, and blood dyscrasias are common side effects of chemotherapy.
7. Sedatives and antiemetics may be given prior to administration of antineoplastics to minimize nausea and vomiting.

Selecting Patients for Chemotherapy

Allied health professionals are not directly involved in selecting patients for chemotherapy or chemotherapy for patients. Because patient discussions may be held in facilities where allied health professionals work, this section is included for a better understanding of the entire treatment process.

Not all patients or types of cancer are candidates for chemotherapy. The decision to institute treatment is made on an individual basis after the patient has been informed of possible risks and benefits of therapy, and informed consent has been obtained. The patient should not be put at great risk with little to gain. What is unacceptable to one patient might be eagerly pursued by another, depending on a variety of life factors.

Some cancers respond better to chemotherapy than others. The patient with a highly responsive type of cancer should be reasonably treated. Those with a minimal chance of response probably would be better off not taking on the dangers and discomforts of treatment.

The following facts are known about cancer chemotherapy:

1. Cancer chemotherapy is most effective against small tumors because they have a more efficient blood supply and the drug is delivered to the cancer site more efficiently.
2. Small tumors have a higher percentage of fast-growing cells, so cytotoxic medications result in a higher cell destruction.

3. Chemotherapy helps eradicate the micrometastases that may remain after surgery or radiation therapy of the tumor mass.

4. In general, a combination of chemotherapeutic agents has a higher success rate than single-drug chemotherapy. Each drug must be effective as a single agent and must work synergistically with other drugs to address different stages of the cell cycle.

5. Chemotherapy is directed toward controlling abnormal cell growth and reducing the number of actively dividing cells. In high doses, chemotherapy will destroy a higher percentage of cancer cells. Healthy cells will also be destroyed, but these healthy cells will repair themselves quickly and regenerate to normal numbers faster than cancer cells.

Classes of Antineoplastic Agents

Antineoplastic agents are divided into various classes on the basis of their probable mechanism of action in the cell (see Figure 19-3).

Alkylating or Alkylating-Like Agents

Some of the earliest agents used to treat neoplasms were alkylating agents, which poison cancer cells. During World War I, chemical warfare was introduced using nitrogen mustard. Alkylating agents were observed to inhibit cell growth, and so were investigated for their ability to inhibit the growth of malignant cells, inhibiting cell reproduction by irreversible binding to DNA. Eventually the cell dies from inability to maintain cell metabolism (Table 19-3).

The alkylating medications are highly toxic compounds and are used to treat metastatic ovarian, testicular, and bladder cancer and for the palliative treatment of undesirable symptoms of other cancers. The newer drugs in this category are the lipid-soluble nitrosoureas used in treating brain tumors and testicular or ovarian cancers.

Antimetabolites

Antimetabolites are only effective against cells that actively participate in cell metabolism. They interfere with the synthesis phase of metabolism, blocking the chemical reactions necessary for normal cell growth and reproduction.

The antimetabolites are divided into three classes:

1. *Folic acid antagonists*, which act by preventing folic acid from achieving its active form needed for DNA replication.
2. *Pyrimidine antagonists*, which inhibit the normal synthesis and replication of DNA.
3. *Purine antagonists* are effective against the purine-based proteins, adenine and guanine, essential for DNA synthesis.

Certain antimetabolites such as mercaptopurine (Purinethol) are also used in immunosuppressive therapy (such as for organ transplantation), antiviral medications, and in the treatment of gout (see Table 19-3).

Mitotic Inhibitors (Plant Alkaloids)

The primary **mitotic inhibitors** are vinblastine (Velban), vincristine (Oncovin), and vinorelbine (Navelbine), derived from the periwinkle plant, and etoposide (Toposar), derived from the May apple. Thus these medications as a group are known as **plant alkaloids** or **mitotic alkaloids.** They prevent the chromosomes from dividing and migrating to the end of the cells to stop further cell replication or mitosis. If **extravasation** occurs with these medications, tissue injury is expected. Alopecia is not as common as with the other cytotoxic drugs (see Table 19-3).

> **DID YOU KNOW?**
> Vinca, the periwinkle plant, is an evergreen ground cover. It takes more than 6 tons of the leaves to produce 1 oz of the drug.

Hormones and Hormone Antagonists

Hormones and **hormone antagonists,** the least toxic of the anticancer medications, have various uses in the treatment of malignant diseases. These drugs act on specific hormone receptors or target lesions, making their action on malignant cells highly selective.

Adrenocorticosteroids—hormones (or steroids) naturally found in the adrenal cortex—produce remission in certain malignancies by retarding the proliferation of lymphocytes. They are especially useful in treating acute lymphocytic leukemia. Often these hormones are used in conjunction with radiation therapy to decrease radiation edema. A major group of adrenocorticosteroids used in cancer therapy is the glucocorticoids.

Sex hormones are used for palliation and for some cures in carcinomas of the reproductive tract. Estrogens may be administered to relieve symptoms of prostate cancer and with breast cancer in postmenopausal women. Androgens, male hormones, are used in premenopausal women with breast cancers.

Antiestrogens such as tamoxifen (Nolvadex) and antiandrogens are used to inhibit hormone production in advanced stages of cancer. Tamoxifen, used for breast cancer, increases the risk of endometrial cancer and must be used with caution. Antiandrogens reduce the stimulation of androgen production in prostate cells (see Table 19-3).

Antitumor Antibiotics

Antitumor antibiotics bind to DNA, thereby inhibiting DNA and RNA synthesis. Antitumor antibiotics are used only to treat cancer; they are not used to treat infections. Antitumor antibiotics are poorly absorbed through the GI tract and therefore are given parenterally, usually intravenously (see Table 19-3).

Immunosuppressants

Immunosuppressants such as interferon may be produced naturally by white blood cells or synthetically using recombinant DNA techniques. Interferon exerts a variety of effects on tumor cells, with an antiproliferative action. The antiproliferative and cytotoxic actions stop rapid cell production and increase the efficacy of antineoplastic drugs. Some immunosuppressants can even render cancer cells nonmalignant. The exact action of these drugs is unknown, but cancer research is exploring the potential for immunotherapy to bring about cures (see Table 19-3).

Radioisotopes

Radioactive isotopes, or **radioisotopes,** are used to treat many types of cancer. The isotopes may be inserted locally as pellets, administered as radiation therapy, or administered systemically as capsules or solutions. Radium 426 needles and iridium 192 needles are used for intrauterine carcinoma. Cobalt 60 is used for a wide variety of tumors. Aurum (gold) 198 is used for intracavitary administration, particularly to treat pleural and peritoneal effusions. The patient and family *must* be made aware that these treatments cause exposure to ionizing radiation (see Table 19-3).

▪ PATIENT ALERT

Care must be taken by all persons working with radioisotopes to keep exposure to radiation to a minimum. Excretions from patients being treated with radioactive isotopes are considered radioactive.

Newer Drugs and Drug Delivery Systems

Many new drugs are being studied to treat AIDS-associated cancers and to improve the treatment and survival of cancer patients. New medications that have been approved address different cell-type malignancies occurring in specific body organs. A promising area of study is the use of liposomes as a delivery system for lipid-soluble drugs. Being used for solid tumors, especially breast and lung cancer and Kaposi's sarcoma, liposomes are used to carry cytotoxic medications so that they come in direct contact with the tumor. By attaching to liposomes, the drugs become "smart bombs" that target the tumor cells but not normal cells.

Drugs to treat or slow the progression of breast cancer are another area of intense research interest. The cancer gene *HER-2/neu* produces a protein that alters genes. This causes slowing of the progression of breast cancer.

IMPORTANT FACTS ABOUT SPECIFIC ANTINEOPLASTIC AGENTS

- Certain anticancer drugs are effective only in specific phases of the cell cycle. These medications must be in place when the cells enter the phase in which the medication works. Hormones and hormone antagonists are not specific to any phase in the cell cycle.
- Alkylating agents injure cells by binding to DNA and inhibiting DNA and RNA synthesis.
- Antimetabolites are similar to natural metabolites and are able to disrupt metabolic processes by damaging the DNA template by acting on the folic acid needed for cell metabolism.
- Antitumor antibiotics are used to treat malignancies, not infections. Many antitumor antibiotics are cardiotoxic.
- Hormonal anticancer drugs act through specific hormone receptors on target cells and are highly selective in their action.
- Glucocorticoids, a subset of hormonal anticancer drugs, are toxic to malignancies of lymphoid organs such as leukemias and lymphomas.
- Tamoxifen is an antiestrogen used in the adjuvant treatment of breast cancer following surgery. Tamoxifen seems to increase the risk of endometrial cancer, so it should be used with care.
- Prostate cancers are treated with gonadotropin-releasing hormone agonists and androgen suppressants, which reduce the stimulation of prostate cells by androgens.

Text continued on page 379

TABLE 19-3 Select Medications Used as Antineoplastic Agents*

GENERIC NAME	TRADE NAME	USUAL ADULT DOSE, ROUTE, AND FREQUENCY OF ADMINISTRATION	MAJOR SIDE EFFECTS	INDICATIONS FOR USE	DRUG INTERACTIONS
ALKYLATING AND ALKYLATING-LIKE DRUGS					
nitrogen mustard (mechlorethamine)	Mustargen	0.4 mg/kg IV as single dose or in divided doses	Nausea, vomiting, bone marrow suppression, diarrhea, dermatitis, hepatic/renal toxicity, alopecia, myalgia, fever, malaise	Lymphosarcoma, Hodgkin's disease	No immunizations, alcohol
cyclophosphamide	Cytoxan Neosar	1-5 mg/kg po; 40-50 mg/kg IV qd in divided doses for 2-5 days		Broad spectrum of neoplasms	Antigout medications
chlorambucil	Leukeran	4-10 mg/day po		Leukemias, malignancies of the lymphatic system	Antigout medications and live virus vaccines
melphalan	Alkeran	6 mg daily po for 2-3 weeks, no medication for 4-5 weeks, then 2 mg daily as maintenance dose		Multiple myeloma, carcinoma of breast and ovary, lymphocytic leukemia, lymphomas, mycotic fungus, polycythemia vera	Antigout medications
busulfan	Myleran	4-8 mg/day po		Chronic myelocytic leukemia, malignancies of blood-forming organs	Alcohol, anticoagulants, phenytoin, live vaccines
uracil mustard		0.5 mg/kg po qwk for 4 wk		See nitrogen mustard	See nitrogen mustard
ifosfamide	Ifex	1.2 g/m² BSA/day IV		Cancer of testes	None identified
NITROSOUREAS					
temozolomide	Temodar	150 mg/m² BSA/day po		Astrocytoma	None identified
carmustine	BiCNU	150-200 mg/m² BSA IV q6wk		Brain tumors, multiple myelomas, Hodgkin's disease	cimetidine
lomustine	CCNU	130 mg/m² BSA po, topical as single dose; repeat in 6 wk		Brain and GI tumors, mycotic fungoids, psoriasis	Live virus vaccines
cisplatin	Platinol	IV; varies with neoplasm		Metastatic testicular and ovarian cancers, bladder cancer	Antigout medications
carboplatin	Paraplatin	300-400 mg/m² BSA IV		Ovarian carcinoma	Live virus vaccines
ANTIMETABOLITES			Severe bone marrow suppression, mouth/stomach ulcers, anorexia, diarrhea, nausea, vomiting, chills/fever, alopecia		

Generic name (class)	Trade names	Usual dose	Common side effects	Uses	Drug interactions
methotrexate (folic acid analogue)	Amethopterin, Mexate, Rheumatrex, MTX	2.5-30 mg/day po, IM, IV; 10-25 mg/wk for psoriasis		Acute lymphocytic leukemia in children, psoriasis, uterine choriocarcinomas, lymphosarcomas	Alcohol, NSAIDs, probenecid, salicylates, live virus vaccines
leucovorin (folic acid analogue)	Wellcovorin	10 mg/m² BSA po, IM, IV q6h		Megaloblastic anemia; to prevent and treat toxicity induced by folic acid antagonists	None
mercaptopurine (purine analogue)	Purinethol, 6-MP	2.5 mg/kg/day po		Acute lymphocytic leukemias; Hodgkin's disease; tumors of the lymphatic system; carcinomas of the reproductive tract, liver, pancreas, GI tract, and breast; actinic keratosis	Antigout medications
fluorouracil (pyrimidine analogue)	5-FU, Efudex, Adrucil	12 mg/kg/day IV × 4 days, then 6 mg/kg IV qod × 4 doses	Hematologic side effects, GI symptoms, dermatitis	Acute myelocytic leukemias	
cytarabine (pyrimidine analogue)	Cytosar	2 mg/kg/day IV × 10 days	Same as above	Tumors of the head, neck, brain, liver, gallbladder, and bile ducts	Same as for methotrexate and other antimetabolites plus cyclophosphamide
capecitabine (pyrimidine analogue)	Xeloda	2500 mg/m² BSA/day po	Stomatitis	Breast and colon cancer	leucovorin, phenytoin, warfarin, antacids
MITOTIC INHIBITORS (PLANT ALKALOIDS)					
vincristine	Oncovin	0.5-1.5 mg/kg/wk IV	Peripheral neurotoxic effects	Acute leukemia	Antigout medications, live virus vaccines, doxorubicin
vinblastine	Velban, Velsar	0.1-0.5 mg/kg/wk IV	Bone marrow suppression, nausea and vomiting	Hodgkin's disease, lymphosarcomas, choriocarcinoma	Antigout medications, live virus vaccines
vinorelbine	Navelbine	30 mg/m² BSA/wk IV		Lung, breast, and ovarian cancers; Hodgkin's disease	Live virus vaccines

*Medications used as antineoplastics have highly individualized doses based on the BSA of the patient and the neoplasm being treated. The dosages in this table are provided as typical doses only.

(continued)

TABLE 19-3 *Select Medications Used as Antineoplastic Agents—cont'd*

GENERIC NAME	TRADE NAME	USUAL ADULT DOSE, ROUTE, AND FREQUENCY OF ADMINISTRATION	MAJOR SIDE EFFECTS	INDICATIONS FOR USE	DRUG INTERACTIONS
HORMONE THERAPY					
estrogen			Feminization in males, blood clots		
estramustine	Emcyt	14 mg/kg/day po		Prostate cancer	Dairy products
diethylstilbestrol (DES)	Stilphostrol	50 mg tid, po, IV up to 200 mg tid		Prostate cancer and breast cancer	Oral anticoagulants
androgen		100 mg IM 3 × per wk	Masculinization of females	Breast cancer in pre-menopausal women	
testolactone	Teslac	50 mg tid po		Same as above	
calusterone	Methosarb	150-300 mg/day po		Breast cancer in post-menopausal women	
fluoxymesterone	Halotestin	10-40 mg/day po		Metastatic breast cancer	Hypoglycemics, cephalosporins, anticoagulants
antiestrogens			Hot flashes and weight gain in females		
tamoxifen	Nolvadex	20-40 mg/day po		Treatment and prevention of breast cancer	Estrogens
anastrozole	Arimidex	1 mg/day po		Breast cancer	None
raloxifene	Evista	60 mg/day po		Breast cancer	None
antiandrogens			Impotence in males		
bicalutamide	Casodex	50 mg/day po		Prostate cancer	Warfarin sodium
flutamide	Eulexin	250 mg tid po		Prostate cancer	None
goserelin	Zoladex	1 implant q28d		Metastatic prostate cancer	None
progestins					
megestrol	Megace	40 mg/day po		Endometrial and breast cancer	None
gonadotropin-releasing hormone	Lupron	1 mg/d SC or 2.5 mg IM qmo	GI bleeding, myocardial infarction, edema, hot flashes, impotence	Prostate cancer, endometriosis	None
ANTITUMOR ANTIBIOTICS			Nausea, vomiting, anorexia, alopecia, dermatitis, hepatotoxicity, cardiotoxicity, nephrotoxicity, blood dyscrasias		
dactinomycin	Actinomycin D, Cosmegen	500 mcg/day IV × 5 days		Testicular cancer, Wilms' tumor, lymphoma	Antigout medications, live virus vaccines
bleomycin	Blenoxane	10-20 U/m² BSA IM, IV, SC 1-2 × per wk		Hodgkin's disease, squamous cell carcinoma	None
doxorubicin	Adriamycin	60-75 mg/m² BSA IV @ 21-day intervals		Same as for bleomycin and brain tumors	Antigout medications, live virus vaccines

Generic	Trade	Dosage	Uses	Side effects	Drug interactions
methotrexate	Trexall	Various doses either po, IM, or IV depending on disease process	Leukemia, lymphoma, breast cancer, osteosarcoma		digoxin, vaccines, NSAIDs, alcohol, penicillins
mithramycin/ plicamycin	Mithracin	25-30 mcg/kg/day IV × 8-10 days	Testicular tumors		Oral anticoagulants, calcium medications, live virus vaccines, aspirin, NSAIDs
mitomycin	Mutamycin	20 mg/m² BSA IV	Adenocarcinomas, squamous cell carcinomas, malignant melanomas		None
daunorubicin	Cerubidine	30-60 mg/m² BSA IV × 3-5 days	Leukemias	Hematuria, gum hyperplasia, tremors, headaches, nausea, vomiting, hematologic dangers	Antigout medications, live virus vaccines
IMMUNOSUPPRESSANTS/ BIOLOGICAL RESPONSE MODIFIERS					
interferon alfa-2a	Roferon	Various, IM, IV, SC	Chronic hepatitis C, malignant melanomas, Kaposi's sarcoma, leukemias		Glucocorticoids, thiazide diuretics, alcohol
interferon alfa-2b	Intron	2,000,000 IU/m² BSA × 3/wk	Leukemia, Kaposi's sarcoma		Antihypertensives
aldesleukin interleukin 2	Proleukin	600,000 IU/kg IV q8h × 14 doses	Renal cell cancers		None
levamisole	Ergamisol	50 mg po q8h × 3 days	Colon cancer		None identified
BCG (Bacillus Calmette-Guérin) vaccine	TheraCys	3 vials instilled in bladder intravesically	Bladder cancer		
tacrolimus	Prograf	0.05-0.1 mg/kg/day po, IV	Transplants		Numerous
LIPOSOME PRODUCTS					
doxorubicin	Adriamycin, Doxil	20-75 mg/m² qd-qwk, IV	Metastatic breast cancer		
tretinoin	Antragen	45 mg/m²/day po	Kaposi's sarcoma		
MISCELLANEOUS ANTINEOPLASTICS					
asparaginase	Elspar	200 U/kg/day IM, IV × 28 days	Acute lymphocytic leukemias	Hepatotoxicity, pancreatitis, thrombocytopenia, anemia	Steroids, vincristine, antigout medications, methotrexate, live virus vaccines

(continued)

TABLE 19-3 *Select Medications Used as Antineoplastic Agents—cont'd*

GENERIC NAME	TRADE NAME	USUAL ADULT DOSE, ROUTE, AND FREQUENCY OF ADMINISTRATION	MAJOR SIDE EFFECTS	INDICATIONS FOR USE	DRUG INTERACTIONS
anastrozole	Arimidex	1 mg po qd	Hot flashes, headaches, depression, nausea, vomiting, leukopenia	Breast cancer	None
cladribine	Leustatin	0.09 mg/kg/day IV × 7 days		Leukemias	Live virus vaccines
dacarbazine	DTIC–Dome	Dose varies IV	Hepatotoxicity, thrombocytopenia, seizures	Malignant melanoma, Hodgkin's disease	Live virus vaccines
docetaxel	Taxotere	60-100 mg/m^2 BSA IV q3wk	Same as dacarbazine	Breast cancer	Cyclosporine, terfenadine, erythromycin, troleandomycin
erlotinib	Tarceva	150 mg po qd	GI symptoms, rash, eye pain, fatigue, mouth ulcers	Lung cancer	None
exemestane	Aromasin	25 mg po daily		Breast and prostate cancer	None identified
gemcitabine	Gemzar	1000 mg/m^2 BSA/wk IV	Lung disease	Pancreatic cancer	Live virus vaccines
hydroxyurea	Hydrea	20-30 mg/kg po every third day	Leukopenia, anemia, thrombocytopenia	Head, neck, and ovarian cancer, myelocytic leukemia, malignant melanoma	Antigout medications, live virus vaccines
irinotecan	Camptosar	125 mg/m^2 BSA/wk IV × 4 wk	Severe diarrhea, hepatotoxicity	Colorectal cancer	Laxatives, diuretics, live virus vaccines
mitotane	Lysodren	2-6 g/day po		Adrenocortical carcinomas	CNS depressants
paclitaxel	Taxol	175 mg/m^2 BSA IV q3wk	anemia, leukopenia	Ovarian and breast cancer	Live virus vaccines
procarbazine	Matulane	2-4 mg/kg/day po	anemia, bleeding tendency	Hodgkin's disease	Alcohol, antihistamines, anticholinergics, tricyclic antidepressants, medications containing caffeine, monoamine oxidase inhibitors, CNS depressants, meperidine

BSA, Body surface area; *CNS,* central nervous system; *GI,* gastrointestinal; *IM,* intramuscular; *IV,* intravenous; *NSAIDs,* nonsteroidal antiinflammatory drugs; *SC,* subcutaneous.

BOX 19-2   PRECAUTIONS IN HANDLING ANTINEOPLASTIC AGENTS

- Follow OSHA and U.S. Pharmacopeia 797 guidelines.
- Follow written guidelines for handling antineoplastic drugs.
- Protect and secure packages of hazardous drugs.
- Educate all people who are handling hazardous drugs—the patient, the family, and other health care workers—in procedures needed for safely handling hazardous drugs. Be sure that drugs do not escape from containers while being prepared and administered.
- Maintain a register of the staff who administer the drugs.
- Women of childbearing age should not reconstitute cytotoxic drugs.
- Use a biologic safety cabinet with a laminar air flow hood.
- Medications should be prepared in a closed room with excellent ventilation and with equipment for irrigating the skin and eyes in case of spills. An OSHA spill kit should be available.
- Biohazard wastes should be disposed of properly.
- Use personal protective equipment including long-sleeved clothing, a plastic apron, gloves, safety glasses, and a face mask when working with chemotherapeutic agents.
- Reconstituted medications must not be sprayed into the atmosphere. Diluents must be allowed to slowly run down the sides of the ampules to prevent back spray. Air in the syringe must be expelled into sterile cotton or gauze to prevent spray. Powders must be reconstituted so that no excess pressure in the vial would allow the medication to spray through the needle hole. The syringes, intravenous sets, and needles should have locked fittings, and all fittings should be secure.
- All materials used in preparing and administering chemotherapy should be disposed of in leakproof, puncture-resistant containers marked "BIOHAZARD."
- Because of the teratogenicity of antineoplastics, health care workers who are pregnant, breastfeeding, or trying to conceive a child should not handle cytotoxic medications or provide direct care for patients who are receiving cytotoxic medications.
- These precautions should also be used with patients receiving radioisotopes, to prevent unnecessary exposure to radiation.

Handling and Administering Antineoplastic Agents

In 2004, USP 797, a regulation developed by the U.S. Pharmacopoeia, was initiated to provide safety in preparing toxic drugs. The Food and Drug Administration has the responsibility of enforcing the standards of this edict in facilities where sterile products are prepared or where manipulations are performed during the compounding of sterile products. Products that are covered may be biologics, diagnostics, drugs, and radio-pharmaceutics including cytotoxics. The monitoring of the environment of the facility is also included to enhance patient safety and the decrease in the chance for cross contamination of sterile preparations.

Cytotoxic medications are usually given via parenteral routes—intramuscularly, subcutaneously, intravenously, intrathecally, and so on. Oral medications that are no less toxic are available for use at home.

Most antineoplastics cause tissue damage if given subcutaneously or intramuscularly. For medications given by either of these routes, the medication should be drawn and then the needle should be changed to the smallest possible gauge to prevent damage to normal tissue as the drug is injected. The most reliable and most commonly used route of administration is the intravenous route.

Special precautions are necessary when using cytotoxic medications to obtain the best outcome for the patient and to protect the staff who administer the medications. The Occupational Safety and Health Administration (OSHA) has identified safety precautions, which include wearing personal protective equipment and using special exhaust systems when preparing and administering antineoplastic medications. The goal is to prevent unwanted exposure in the allied health professional to drugs that disrupt natural biologic processes. The exact protocol for administering antineoplastic medications will vary with the medical setting, but as a general guideline, the allied health professional should use strict aseptic technique, follow all safety measures, and stay within the scope of practice. The complexity of chemotherapeutics and the hazards associated with their administration require administration under the direct supervision of a specialist. Although allied health professionals would infrequently, if ever, be asked to administer antineoplastics, these drugs may be found in their practice setting. They should appreciate the poisonous nature of these drugs, practice personal safety measures, and follow precautions for handling these medications.

The drugs to treat cancer are **mutagenic, teratogenic,** and **carcinogenic** when absorbed through the skin, lungs, or GI tract. Because of these characteristics, direct contact of the drug with the skin, eyes, and mucous membranes can cause local injury to the patient or health care professional administering the medication. Personnel must observe regulations to prevent chronic exposure to cytotoxic drugs. Box 19-2 outlines precautions requiring written policies and procedures.

Because antineoplastic agents are toxic, hematologic testing and blood chemistry studies may be done to monitor renal and hepatic function. Testing is begun before the first treatment and is repeated throughout the course of chemotherapy and during follow-up. Dosage may be based on either body weight or body surface area, so the exact amount of the drug needed is administered. Use of a nomogram is the best means of dosage calculation because body surface area—weight and height—is considered in dosage.

Summary

Rapid changes are occurring in the area of antineoplastics. Investigational medications are being used to prolong the lives of patients who might otherwise have died. New categories of medications have been shown to be effective and are being used to alter DNA and RNA to prevent abnormal cell mitosis.

Antineoplastic medications are classified according to their effect on specific phases in a cell's cycle of reproduction or replication. According to their potential mechanism of action, these medications are divided into antimetabolites, alkylating agents, mitotic inhibitors, antitumor antibiotics, hormones, immunosuppressants, and radioactive agents. Most forms of malignancy are treated by some combination of surgery, chemotherapy, and radiation therapy. A fourth modality, use of liposomes, may also be used.

Antineoplastic agents are nonselective in their actions, affecting both normal, healthy cells and cancerous cells. Cells that replicate quickly are more susceptible to the agents used in chemotherapy than cells with a slower rate of growth. Most side effects of antineoplastic therapy occur in the bone marrow, GI tract, and hair follicles because these organ systems are dominated by cells that grow and reproduce quickly. Patients should be educated about these side effects because patients who know what to expect in advance will be more compliant with treatment. Knowledge of expected side effects, possible adverse reactions, their symptoms, and the improvement of those symptoms promotes patient safety when antineoplastics are part of the treatment program.

Review of Precautions and Responsibilities in Handling Antineoplastic Medications

Because of the toxic effects of chemotherapeutic agents, health professionals working with these drugs must also use extreme care and follow all precautions for their own safety. Instructions for using and administering anticancer medications should be written, as should safety precautions. Pregnant women must avoid contact with these medications because of possible harm to the fetus.

Health care professionals who prepare or administer cytotoxic medications or who care for patients receiving these medications should be aware of the dangers involved. Cytotoxic drugs are poisons, and exposure to these drugs creates a health hazard for the professional. The exposure may be through unintentional ingestion of the drug on food, through inhalation of drug dust or aerosolized droplets, or through direct skin contact (see Box 19-2).

Critical Thinking Exercises

SCENARIO

Jane has been diagnosed with carcinoma of the breast. She has undergone a mastectomy and is now scheduled to undergo chemotherapy that will cause alopecia. She tells you she is afraid of hair loss, nausea, and vomiting. Her friends have told her these are the worst problems associated with chemotherapy.

1. How do you help Jane prepare for alopecia?
2. How do you help her prepare for nausea and vomiting?
3. What do you tell Jane about her dietary needs while she is receiving chemotherapy?
4. What should Jane be taught about contact with people with infectious diseases?

DRUG CALCULATIONS

1. Order: doxorubicin hydrochloride 20 mg/m^2 for a person who is 5'4" tall and weighs 125 lb
   Dose to be given: _____

2. Order: vincristine 1.2 mg/m^2 for a person who is 73" tall and weighs 185 lb
   Dose to be given: _____

REVIEW QUESTIONS

1. Define antineoplastic medications and their general mode of action. _____
   _____
   _____

2. What is an immunosuppressant? Why are these agents beneficial in treating malignancies but harmful to the patient?_____
   _____
   _____

3. Describe the more common side effects that patients receiving chemotherapy might expect. _____
   _____
   _____

4. List the precautions necessary when preparing and administering cytotoxic medications. _____
   _____
   _____

5. Why should patients expecting alopecia buy hairpieces prior to beginning chemotherapy? _____
   _____
   _____

6. How can the patient taking chemotherapy have some relief of nausea and vomiting without taking medications? _____
   _____
   _____

CHAPTER 20

Nutritional Supplements and Alternative Medicines

OBJECTIVES

After studying this chapter, you should be capable of doing the following:

- Discussing the medical indications for nutritional supplements.
- Identifying the vitamins that are fat soluble and water soluble for use by the body.
- Identifying the minerals that are used as supplements and for electrolyte replacement in the body.
- Discussing common home remedies that are used as alternative medicinal forms to gain an appreciation of patients' use of these remedies.
- Describing the use of herbal medicines.
- Understanding over-the-counter (OTC) nutritional supplements and their interactions with the therapeutic medications prescribed by a health care provider.
- Describing cultural differences in the use of herbals and alternative medicines.

Carol has a long history of severe arthritis in her knees. She is on a limited income and cannot afford to buy prescription items for her arthritis. She drinks milk to which vitamin D has been added.

    Why is this important to Carol?

    If Carol is allergic to milk, what OTC preparations other than calcium tablets may be used to provide calcium?

    If Carol has a history of epigastric burning, what OTC preparation could she use to enhance her calcium intake and also help her epigastric discomfort?

    What are the implications of using glucosamine?

KEY TERMS

Acid	Hypervitaminosis	Solute
Alkaline	Inorganic	Solvent
Alternative medicine	Ion	Teratogenic
Avitaminosis	Isotonic	Tetany
Base	Mineral	Vitamin
Complementary medicine	Nutrient	
Electrolyte	Osteomalacia	
Folk medicine	Paresthesia	
Hemoglobinuria	Pellagra	
Home remedy	Salt	

EASY WORKING KNOWLEDGE OF INDICATIONS AND SIDE EFFECTS

Common Signs and Symptoms of Nutritional Imbalance	Common Side Effects of Vitamins, Minerals, and Herbs
Nonspecific complaints	Irritability
Abnormal bone formation	Anorexia
Neurologic damage	Headaches, flushing
Inability to build and repair tissue	Indigestion, nausea, diarrhea, constipation
Change in energy levels	Abdominal cramping and pain
Intellectual impairment	Discolored stools
Muscle wasting	Insomnia
Obesity, emaciation	Hypotension
Loss of hair	
Delayed healing of wounds	

Easy Working Knowledge of Nutritional Supplements and Alternative Medicines

DRUG CLASS	PRESCRIPTION	OTC	PREGNANCY CATEGORY	MAJOR INDICATIONS
Vitamins	Yes	Yes	A, C, X (retinol A)	Supplement food sources of vitamins
Minerals	Yes	Yes	None	Supplement food sources of minerals
ALTERNATIVE MEDICINES				
Home remedies	No	Yes	None	Folk medicine (to treat disease by folklore)
Herbals/plants	No	Yes (regulated by U.S. Dept. of Agriculture)	None, regulated by USDA under the Dietary Supplements Heath Education Act (DHSEA)	Alternative medicine (to treat disease by herbals)

itamins and minerals are essential compounds for specific body functions such as growth, maintenance, and reproduction—the vital body functions. These compounds are normally obtained from the plant and animal products and fluids we ingest. Microorganisms require few raw materials from their environment. As life forms become more sophisticated, with highly specialized cells and organs, the ability to synthesize necessary nutrients is lost. Thus the human body must depend on exogenous sources for nourishment, especially for vitamins.

The OTC market for nutrition supplements in the United States is one of the largest in the pharmaceutical field, with more than half of U.S. citizens taking vitamins, minerals, and herbal preparations without a prescription. The allied health professional needs a working knowledge of vitamins and minerals, their sources, the symptoms of vitamin deficiencies, and possible toxic effects from overdose. Signs of vitamin deficiencies and excesses are listed in Table 20-1.

Vitamins

Vitamins have no energy value but are required for the metabolism of fats, carbohydrates, and proteins. These organic compounds, or **nutrients,** regulate body functions and are necessary in trace amounts to the body for growth and health.

- The needed amount varies somewhat over the life cycle; growing children, the elderly, and pregnant or lactating women have increased needs.
- A vitamin deficiency produces certain symptoms, just as excessive supplementation produces symptoms (in this case, toxic effects).
- Exactly how vitamins work, the indications for their use, and how the body uses vitamins are not completely understood, but we do know that a vitamin deficiency may result in compromise of homeostasis and thus deficiency-related diseases.
- Although vitamins are not themselves a source of energy, they are essential for energy

TABLE 20-1 *Signs of Vitamin Deficiencies and Excesses*

VITAMIN	SIGNS OF DEFICIENCY	SIGNS OF EXCESS
FAT-SOLUBLE		
A	Night blindness, skin lesions, dryness of conjunctiva, softening of cornea in children	Acute confusion, irritation, diarrhea, dizziness, peeling of skin, severe vomiting
D	Bone and muscle pain, weakness, softening of bone	*Early:* Diarrhea, headache, increased thirst and urination, nausea and vomiting *Late:* Bone and muscle pain, increased blood pressure, pruritus, lethargy, mood alterations, pancreatitis
E	Decreased reflexes, loss of muscle coordination, loss of muscle mass, anemia	*Acute:* Visual disturbances, headaches, nausea, stomach pain, weakness *Chronic:* Increased bleeding tendencies, impaired sexual function, altered thyroid metabolism
K	Bleeding	Flushing, dyspnea, chest pain, alterations in taste
WATER-SOLUBLE		
B$_1$ (thiamine)	Peripheral neuritis, loss of muscle strength, depression, memory loss, anorexia, dyspnea	Very little toxicity when taken by mouth
B$_2$ (riboflavin)	Sore throat and mouth, swollen tongue, anemia, dermatitis of face	Low toxicity levels
B$_3$ (niacin)	Skin eruptions, sore mouth, diarrhea, headache, dizziness, insomnia, impaired memory, dementia	Flushing, pruritus, dizziness, dysrhythmias, muscle pain, nausea, vomiting, diarrhea, dry skin
B$_6$ (pyridoxine)	Seborrheic-like lesions of skin, sore mouth, seizures, peripheral neuritis	Low toxicity except in chronic overuse; then neurotoxicity such as lack of muscle coordination, clumsiness, numbness
B$_9$ (folic acid)	Megaloblastic anemia	Allergic reactions, redness of skin, fever, rashes, pruritus
B$_{12}$ (cyanocobalamin)	Nervous system damage, memory loss, confusion, dementia, abnormal blood cell production	No toxic effects
C (ascorbic acid)	Gingivitis, scurvy, anemia	Kidney stones, dizziness High doses—diarrhea, redness of skin, nausea and vomiting

production and for the regulation of metabolic processes.

- Some vitamins occur in usable form in the diet; others are inactive in their natural form but are converted to active chemical compounds within the body. Bacteria in the gastrointestinal (GI) tract form vitamin K, vitamin D is synthesized in the body on exposure to sunlight, and vitamin B is manufactured in small amounts in the GI tract.
- Vitamins are important as the enzyme system breaks down food sources during the metabolic process.
- Insufficient intake of vitamins may be caused by inadequate diet as a result of cultural, religious, or personal preferences, fad dieting, alcoholism, poverty, lack of food, or ignorance.

- The signs of vitamin deficiency are abnormal tiredness, aches, pains, and general malaise. In the United States, the severe **avitaminosis** that produces diseases such as beriberi, pellagra, rickets, or scurvy is rarely seen.
- An adequate diet of food prepared to retain vitamins is the best way to prevent vitamin deficiency.

Some experts believe that the average American diet contains adequate vitamins and that vitamin supplements are not necessary to meet the U.S. Recommended Daily Allowance (RDA) set by the Food and Nutrition Board of the National Academy of Sciences. The RDA should not be considered the minimum daily requirement for persons at risk for deficiencies because RDA applies to people in good health. The ill, the elderly, teen-agers, pregnant and nursing women, and people who smoke may need supplements to compensate for deficiencies in the diet. Although the practice of taking vitamins is widespread, in most cases vita-min supplementation is not necessary and excessive consumption can be harmful. Sources of vitamins are listed in Table 20-2.

Vitamins are divided into two major groups, fat-soluble and water-soluble.

- The fat-soluble vitamins are A, D, E, and K.
  - The fat-soluble vitamins are stored in the liver and fatty tissues.
  - A deficiency of these vitamins would occur only after a long period of deprivation, either from lack of food intake or from a disease that prevents absorption.
  - Because of the prolonged storage time of fat-soluble vitamins, excessive intake may lead to toxic effects.
- The water-soluble vitamins are the B complex vitamins—B_1 (thiamine), B_2 (riboflavin), B_3 (niacin), B_5 (pantothenic acid), B_6 (pyridoxine), B_9 (folic acid), and B_{12} (cyanocobalamin)—and vitamin C.
  - The water-soluble vitamins are not stored in the body in large amounts, and even a brief period of deprivation can lead to deficiency.
  - Toxic effects of water-soluble vitamins are rare because excess amounts are excreted, not stored in the body.

DID YOU KNOW?

Successive letters of the alphabet were assigned as new vitamins were isolated, with some letters being assigned out of order. Because vitamin K is necessary for blood clotting, it was named for the word Koagulation. Later it became evident that vitamin B was not a single vita-min but actually a group of vitamins. Subscript numbers were then added. The numbers now seen as missing had been assigned to fractions of the group that were later found to be identical to an already named segment. In fact, all of the vitamins but C are actually groups of related substances to which subscript numbers are assigned (e.g., B_1, B_2, B_3).

Many vitamin preparations with varying ingredients are on the market today, both as prescriptions and as OTC medications, varying from a single vitamin to multivitamin capsules and tablets. The most popular OTC multivitamin preparations contain all of the vitamins needed to meet daily requirement without regard to the vitamin content of the person's diet. Extra-strength or high-potency vitamins are rarely necessary, and many contain chemicals not associated with needs for deficiency states.

Vitamin preparations are also included in the Food and Drug Administration's (FDA's) pregnancy categories. The pregnancy classification for the major vitamins is found in Table 20-3.

Patient Education for Compliance

1. Vitamins taken in addition to dietary sources are called vitamin supplements. Specific vitamin supplements may be useful at designated times in the life cycle.
2. Healthy, nonsmoking, nonpregnant adults who eat a well-rounded diet should not need vitamin supplements.
3. Foods with synthetic vitamins added during processing are labeled "fortified" or "enriched."
4. Vitamins that are purchased OTC generally have lower vitamin content than prescription medications, especially the fat-soluble vitamins.
5. To prevent vitamin loss, vegetables should be cooked in a minimal amount of water for the shortest time necessary to obtain the desired doneness.

Fat-Soluble Vitamins

Because fat-soluble vitamins are stored for long periods of time, medications containing fat-soluble vitamins—vitamins A, D, E, and K—should be used only when a medical condition has been found for which a particular vitamin is needed. Fat-soluble vitamins are of clinical importance because persons who have diseases that interfere with the absorption of fats will eventually develop fat-soluble vitamin deficiencies. For sources of fat-soluble vitamins see Table 20-2.

1. **Vitamin A**, also known as retinol.
   - The functions of Vitamin A include:
     - Eyesight and visual adaptation to light including night adaptation—retinol is part of rhodopsin, a retinal pigment needed for vision by the rods in the eyes. Often the first sign of vitamin A deficiency is night blindness.
     - Needed for the structural and functional integrity of the skin and mucous membranes causing skin lesions and dysfunctions of the mucous membranes with deficiencies.
     - Promote normal growth and development of teeth and bones.
   - Relatively safe when given at the RDA recommended dosage.

TABLE 20-2 *Sources of Vitamins and Minerals*

VITAMIN	SOURCE
FAT-SOLUBLE VITAMINS	
A	Fish oils, butter, yellow fruits and vegetables, milk, cheese, liver
D	Fortified cereals, dairy products, candy, liver, eggs, fish
E	Wheat germ oil, vegetable oils, leafy vegetables
K	Green vegetables, cabbage, cauliflower, fish liver oils, eggs, milk, meat
WATER-SOLUBLE VITAMINS	
B_1 (thiamine)	Pork products
B_2 (riboflavin)	Milk and milk products, meats, grains
B_3 (niacin)	Meats, legumes, enriched grains, peanuts
B_6 (pyridoxine)	Chicken, fish, eggs, whole grains
B_9 (folic acid)	Green leafy vegetables, milk, eggs, yeast
B_{12} (cyanocobalamin)	Fresh shrimp, oysters, milk, eggs, cheese
B_5 (pantothenic acid)	Wide variety of foods
B_7 (biotin)	Wide variety of foods
C (ascorbic acid)	Citrus fruits, tomatoes, melons, cabbage, strawberries, broccoli
MINERALS	
Iron	Lean red meat, whole grains, egg yolks, legumes, raisins, prunes, apricots
Calcium	Milk, sardines, cheese, salmon, green leafy vegetables, whole grains
Phosphorus	Fish, beef, pork, cheese, milk, legumes, carbonated beverages, processed meat, foods prepared using phosphoric acid
Magnesium	Green leafy vegetables, whole grains, legumes
Sodium	Table salt, milk, meat, processed foods, carrots, celery
Potassium	Oranges, bananas, prunes, red meats, vegetables, milk and milk products, yams, coffee
Chloride	Table salt, milk, meat, processed foods
Zinc	Meats, oysters, eggs, milk, whole grains
Fluorine/fluoride	Fluorinated water, tea, seafood

- Deficiencies of vitamin A may lead to skin lesions and dysfunction of mucous membranes.
- Increased dosages are highly **teratogenic** and may cause birth defects when taken during pregnancy.
- Excessive amounts lead to alopecia, headache, and lip cracking.

2. **Vitamin D,** or calciferol, is a group of sterols that are synthesized in the body when a person is exposed to sunlight or artificial ultraviolet light.
   - Vitamin D is necessary for the absorption of calcium and phosphorus in the intestines and for the calcification of bone.
   - A deficiency in vitamin D leads to rickets, osteomalacia, and osteoporosis. Hypoparathyroidism may also occur because calcium cannot be absorbed for use by the body without vitamin D.
   - Because of the relationship among vitamin D, calcium, and nerve and muscle conduction, a deficiency in vitamin D also mani-

TABLE 20-3 *Food and Drug Administration Pregnancy Categories for Vitamins*

PREGNANCY CLASSIFICATION	VITAMIN
A	B_1 (thiamine), B_6 (pyridoxine), B_9 (folic acid)
C	D, B_{12} (cyanocobalamin), C (ascorbic acid)
X	A
Unclassified	B_3 (niacin), B_2 (riboflavin), K, E

fests as impaired nerve responses and **tetany** resulting from hypocalcemia.

- Vitamin D supplements are necessary for patients who have malabsorptive diseases, those who are housebound, patients on dialysis, and individuals who are not exposed to sunlight on a daily basis because of the need for sunlight for synthesis. (The sunlight exposure need only be 10 minutes over the course of a day.)

- Excessive doses of vitamin D may lead to renal calculi and cardiovascular disease with the early signs of excessive amounts being weakness, lethargy, anorexia, bone pain, and nausea and vomiting.

3. **Vitamin E,** or alpha-tocopherol, has antioxidant properties and seems to protect red blood cells from hemolysis.
   - Vitamin E is essential for health, but its role in human nutrition is not clearly understood.
   - This vitamin is absorbed by the intestines in the presence of bile salts.
   - It has been associated with a decrease in the risk of death from coronary artery disease when foods high in vitamin E are eaten.
   - Postmenopausal women not taking estrogen need vitamin E.
   - Topical application for temporary relief of minor burns and chapped skin.
   - Excessive amounts of vitamin E alter hormone metabolism with resultant symptoms.

4. **Vitamin K** is required for the synthesis of blood clotting factor, prothrombin, in the liver.
   - The lack of vitamin K can lead to bleeding and hemorrhage. The human requirements are not precisely known.
   - Vitamin K is used to prevent hemorrhagic disease of newborns and to treat toxicity of oral anticoagulants such as warfarin sodium.
   - The primary source of this vitamin is bacterial synthesis by normal intestinal flora using bile salts.
   - Malabsorption syndrome of the intestinal tract may lead to a deficiency. Because infants do not have the necessary bacteria in the GI tract, the newborn may be given an injection of vitamin K to prevent excessive bleeding.
   - Antibiotic therapy may impair or eliminate the bacteria needed for vitamin K synthesis.
   - Excessive amounts lead to brain damage, hepatic disease, and hemoglobinuria (see Table 20-4 for fat-soluable vitamins).

Water-Soluble Vitamins

The water-soluble vitamins are the B complex and C vitamins. The B vitamins vary in structure and function but are grouped together because they were first isolated from the same sources, yeast and liver. Water-soluble vitamins are not stored in fatty tissues and therefore are rapidly used or excreted through the urine. A daily dietary supply of these vitamins is necessary to prevent deficiency for persons needing these vitamins. Under normal circumstances, **hypervitaminosis** does not occur. The most common condition causing a deficiency in water-soluble vitamins in adults is alcoholism because of the associated anorexia, decreased food intake, and damage to the digestive and metabolic systems. Fasting, metabolic diseases, and anorexia nervosa may also lead to a deficiency, as may excessive cooking and boiling of foods. When food is heated, the water-soluble vitamins break down and dissolve into the water, only to be washed away. As a rule, any condition that predisposes a person to a water-soluble vitamin deficiency will reduce the levels of multiple B vitamins at the same time. See for Table 20-2 sources of water-soluble vitamins.

1. **Vitamin B$_1$,** or thiamine, is essential to normal functioning of the nervous system.
   - A deficiency produces beriberi, in which the symptoms of weakness, **paresthesia,** and sensory and motor dysfunction can progress to severe psychosis, ataxia, and cardiovascular damage.
   - Large doses may cause warmth, sweating, urticaria, tightness in the throat, and GI tract bleeding.

2. **Vitamin B$_2$,** or riboflavin, promotes the metabolism of carbohydrates, fats, and proteins and the synthesis of DNA.
   - The absence of riboflavin will change the cornea of the eye, causing symptoms such as burning, itching, and photophobia. Other symptoms may include glossitis and seborrheic dermatitis. Riboflavin has no known toxic effects, but the medication may color urine orange.

3. **Vitamin B$_3$**—niacin or nicotinic acid—is also necessary for the metabolism of food products, along with riboflavin.
   - Niacin also aids in building tissue proteins.
   - Pellagra is a disease caused by a deficiency of niacin.
   - Other symptoms of deficiency include anorexia, apathy, weakness, dermatitis, diarrhea, and dementia.
   - Niacin excess may manifest as flushing of the skin, itching, hypotension, tachycardia, and decreased glucose tolerance.

4. **Vitamin B$_6$,** or pyridoxine, is necessary for the metabolism of amino acids, formation of blood, and maintenance of nervous tissue.
   - Depression, abnormal brain waves, seizures, and anemia are symptoms of vitamin B$_6$ deficiency.
   - Toxic effects from pyridoxine include clumsiness and nerve degeneration.

TABLE 20-4 *Vitamins*

GENERIC NAME	TRADE NAME	ROUTE OF ADMINISTRATION	USUAL ADULT DOSE AND FREQUENCY OF ADMINISTRATION	INDICATIONS FOR USE	DRUG INTERACTIONS
FAT-SOLUBLE					
Vitamin A (retinol)	Aquasol A	po, IM	4000-5000 IU/day	Malabsorption syndrome deficiencies due to GI diseases	Antilipemics, laxatives, mineral oil, oral contraceptives
tretinoin	Retin A		Apply daily hs	Facial wrinkles, diaper rash, acne	Medicated soaps, shampoos, cologne
isotretinoin	Renova	topical			
Vitamin D	Accutane A & D ointment	po topical	0.5-2 mg/kg/day	Acne, antineoplastic Diaper rash, chafed skin	Tetracycline
Calciferol	Calderol	po	25 mcg-1.5 mg/day	Metabolic bone disorders	Antacids, thiazide diuretics, cardiac glycosides, calcium-containing preparations
Calcitriol	Rocaltrol	po	0.25 mcg/day	Hypocalcemia in dialysis patients	
ergocalciferol	Calciferol, Drisdol	po, IM	10,000-80,000 mcg/day	Hypoparathyroidism	
Vitamin E	Aquasol E Vite E cream	po topical	Individualized prn	Vitamin E deficiency Chafed, chapped skin, diaper rash	Oral anticoagulants, iron, antilipemics, mineral oil
Vitamin K	Mephyton	po	5-25 mg	Hypoprothrombinemia	Antilipemics, oil preparations, antiseizure drugs, oral anticoagulants, anti-infectives, salicylates
	Aqua-MEPHYTON	IM	0.5-1 mg first hour after birth	Hemorrhagic disease of newborn	
WATER-SOLUBLE					
Vitamin B_1 (thiamine)	Betalin, Biamine	po	10-20 mg/day	Malabsorption and metabolic disorders, thiamine deficiency	Neuromuscular blockers
Vitamin B_2 (riboflavin)		po	5-30 mg/day	Riboflavin deficiency	Phenothiazines, alcohol, tricyclic depressants, probenecid
Vitamin B_3 (niacin)					
nicotinic acid	Nicobid, Niaspan	po, IM	100 mg tid 10-20 mg/day	Hyperlipoproteinemia; dietary supplement	Lovastatin, probenecid, sulfinpyrazone
Vitamin B_6 (pyridoxine)		po, IM, IV, SC	Varies with age, gender use	Pyridoxine deficiency, INH poisoning	INH, alcohol, hydralazine, penicillamine, chloramphenicol, estrogens, oral contraceptives, immunosuppressants
Vitamin B_9 (folic acid)	Folvite	po, IM, IV, SC	Same as B_6	Megaloblastic and macrocytic anemia	Sulfonamides, triamterene, alcohol, methotrexate, steroids, estrogens, phenytoin, oral contraceptives

TABLE 20-4 *Vitamins—cont'd*

GENERIC NAME	TRADE NAME	ROUTE OF ADMINISTRATION	USUAL ADULT DOSE AND FREQUENCY OF ADMINISTRATION	INDICATIONS FOR USE	DRUG INTERACTIONS
Vitamin B_{12} (cyanocobalamin)	Rubramin PC, Crysti-12, Cyanoject	IM, SC	Varies	Pernicious anemia, B_{12} deficiency	Chloramphenicol, antineoplastics, aminoglycosides, colchicine, K supplements, alcohol, vitamin C, cimetidine
	Nascobal	Nasal spray	1 spray of 500 mcg/wk		
hydroxocobalamin	Hydrobexan	IM, SC	Varies		
Vitamin C (ascorbic acid)	Cecon	po, IM, IV, SC	70-500 mg/day	Scurvy, vitamin C deficiency, burn patients, and those who need wound healing treatment	Salicylates, primidone, iron supplements, folic acid supplements, anticoagulants, B_{12}

Note: Vitamin and mineral dosages depend on age, gender, and medical condition of the person.
IM, Intramuscular; *IV,* intravenous; *SC,* subtucaneous.

5. **Vitamin B_9,** or folic acid, is necessary for the synthesis of DNA and RNA.
   - Folic acid also promotes amino acid metabolism and the formation of red and white blood cells.
   - The symptoms of deficiency include macrocytic anemia, glossitis, and diarrhea.
   - The March of Dimes organization suggests that all women of childbearing age take folic acid supplements, at least 400 mcg/day, to prevent neural tube defects in the developing fetus.
6. **Vitamin B_{12},** or cyanocobalamin, promotes normal function of all cells, especially those of the nervous system.
   - It assists with blood formation and the metabolism of carbohydrates, fats, proteins, and folates, while also assisting in the synthesis of RNA and DNA.
   - Its metabolism is connected with that of folic acid (vitamin B_9).
   - A deficiency in vitamin B_{12} causes pernicious anemia.
   - Symptoms include anorexia, indigestion, paresthesia of the hands and feet, poor coordination, and depression.
   - Many people are given regular injections of vitamin B_{12} to provide a feeling of wellbeing.
7. **Vitamin B_5,** also known as *pantothenic acid* or *coenzyme A,* is present in many foods, and deficiencies and toxicities rarely occur.

   - Pantothenic acid is necessary for glucose synthesis in the intermediate metabolism of carbohydrates and for the synthesis of steroid hormones and acetylcholine.
   - Found in multivitamins in a dose between 10 and 24 mg/dosage form.
8. **Vitamin B_7,** also called *vitamin H* or *biotin,* is a cofactor in the metabolism of fats and carbohydrates.
   - Biotin is synthesized by the intestinal bacteria in sufficient amounts.
   - In experiments, symptoms of deficiency included fatigue, depression, anorexia, myalgia, and dermatitis. This cofactor causes no toxic effects.
9. **Vitamin C,** ascorbic acid, is necessary for building and maintaining strong tissues for wound healing, resistance to infections, and enhanced iron absorption.
   - A deficiency in vitamin C causes scurvy.
   - Symptoms of deficiency include easy bruising, delayed wound healing, swollen and inflamed gums, and secondary infections.
   - In larger doses (>1000 mg), nausea, diarrhea, and overabsorption of iron may occur.
   - Doses up to 10 mg/day have been given prophylactically for the common cold, to promote wound healing, and as adjunct therapy in cancer treatment.
   - The most toxic effects are diarrhea and the production of kidney stones in those who are so prone (see Table 20-4).

Some lifestyle choices such as alcoholism, tobacco use, and eating disorders are important in vitamin absorption. The allied health professional should be aware of possible needs for vitamin supplements (Table 20-5).

Vitamins and Supplements for the Elderly

As individuals age, their nutritional needs change and the need for dietary supplements increases. Older persons cannot absorb and store nutrients as easily as when they were younger. Many elderly do not eat adequate foods containing sufficient calories to obtain the nutrients as needed. The goal for these persons is to boost energy and strength, provide nutrition for weight gain as needed, aid in the recovery from illnesses, and provide extra minerals to maintain health. Many formulations of vitamins and supplements are available in liquid and solid forms for persons older than 50 years of age. The multivitamins used with younger adults may not contain adequate supplements for the geriatric patient. Drug companies have formulated many products to meet specific needs such as cardiovascular health, prostate health, and protection against osteoporosis in postmenopausal women. Supplements such as vitamins and minerals may even contain the wording for ages "50+" to indicate products for the older adult.

DID YOU KNOW?
Recent research has shown the possibility that vitamins C and E, used with ibuprofen, will decrease one's chances of getting Alzheimer's disease.

Patient Education for Compliance

1. Vitamins should not be taken on an empty stomach.
2. Riboflavin (B_2) may change the color of urine to dark orange-yellow.
3. Niacin (B_3) may cause flushing and a sensation of warmth around the neck and face, with tingling and itching that may be reduced by taking aspirin 325 mg 30 minutes prior to taking niacin. These side effects usually subside when the drug is taken for about 2 weeks.
4. Vitamin B_{12} is not readily absorbed through the GI tract. This vitamin should be given by injection for better absorption.
5. Excessive doses of vitamin C may cause diarrhea and kidney stones.
6. Vitamins may change the color of urine and stools.

TABLE 20-5 *Lifestyle Choices and Vitamin Supplements*

LIFESTYLE CHOICE	VITAMIN SUPPLEMENT NEEDED
Restricted diet	B_{12}
Extensive exercise	B_2
Oral contraceptives	B_3, B_6, B_9, B_{12}, C
Smoking	C
Alcohol	B_1, B_9, B complex
Caffeine	B complex, C
Excessive stress	B complex

IMPORTANT FACTS ABOUT VITAMINS
- Vitamins are compounds that are required in minute amounts for growth and the maintenance of health.
- Vitamins participate in energy transformation and metabolism of food products but do not actually provide energy.
- For most people, diet alone will supply the necessary vitamins.
- Vitamins are divided into two groups, the fat-soluble vitamins (A, D, E, and K) and the water-soluble vitamins (B complex and C).
- Fat-soluble vitamins are stored in the body and do not require daily replenishment. Water-soluble vitamins not immediately used by the body are excreted in urine and must be replenished on a daily basis.

Minerals

Minerals are inorganic solid substances, usually occurring as part of the earth's crust.

- Minerals are important parts of body composition and are necessary in small amounts for the body to function normally.
- Humans obtain minerals by eating plants grown in mineral-rich soil or from food products obtained from animals that have eaten these plants.
- Like vitamins, minerals have no energy value but are necessary to regulate body processes and serve as structural components of cells, accounting for approximately 4% of body weight.
- The body uses minerals found in all body fluids and tissues to make vitamins, maintain blood pressure, and maintain both intracellular and extracellular fluid balance.
- As minerals dissolve in body fluids, they exist as **acids, bases,** and **salts.** The dissolved minerals are called **electrolytes** because they have the

ability to form charged particles called **ions.** Water is the **solvent,** and electrolytes are the **solutes.** Together they form normal salt concentrations found in the body fluid. This 0.9% concentration of sodium chloride is **isotonic.** Changes in this concentration as a consequence of either raising or lowering the percentage of the salt in the solution will destroy body cells.

- Most minerals in foods occur as salts, which are soluble in water. The minerals leave the food and remain in the cooking water; therefore food should be cooked in as little water as possible and for the briefest time needed.
- The major electrolytes in the body are sodium, chloride, potassium, calcium, phosphate, and magnesium.
- Mineral supplements may be necessary during periods of rapid growth and in some clinical situations; an example is iron for anemia.
- People taking potassium-depleting diuretics may need potassium supplementation.
- The health of the absorbing tissue and the amount of the mineral in the food being eaten, as well as the mineral needs of the person, will also influence absorption of minerals.
- Minerals are subdivided into two classes; major elements (macronutrients) and trace elements (micronutrients). This classification is based on body needs and not on importance.
- Calcium accounts for about one half of the minerals in the body; another one quarter is phosphorus. Sources of minerals are found in Table 20-2, and the medications for minerals are found in Table 20-6.

1. **Iron (Fe⁺),** stored in the body, most notably in the bone marrow, is an essential component of blood hemoglobin and is also used in antibody formation. A dietary deficiency or malabsorption produces an iron-deficiency anemia. Young children, teenagers, and pregnant women most frequently need iron supplements. Men usually do not need iron supplements and should avoid OTC medications that contain iron to avoid the risk of iron toxicity.
   - Ferrous sulfate is the drug of choice for those needing supplementary iron.
   - Coffee and tea interfere with iron absorption.
   - To avoid gastric upset, iron should be taken with meals. For patients with severe gastric disturbances, alternative iron products such as ferrous gluconates are available.
   - Iron supplements tend to cause constipation.
   - Iron ingested in large amounts is toxic and may cause poisoning. Death from iron poisoning is possible but is more common in young children than in adults. The FDA has placed a warning box on iron products used with children because of the danger of iron poisoning.
   - Iron dextran is used for patients who find oral iron either ineffective or intolerable. This medication should be given by deep intramuscular injection by the Z-track method to prevent discoloration of the skin. Iron dextran may cause side effects such as shock, seizures, and chest pain.
   - Iron sucrose is administered intravenously.

2. **Calcium (Ca⁺)** deficiency is usually caused by metabolic rather than nutritional deficits
   - Calcium is necessary for the following:
     - Bone and tooth formation
     - Proper functioning of the body
     - Contraction and relaxation of muscles including the heart
     - Blood clotting
     - Nervous system transmission including to and from the brain
     - Secretion of insulin
   - Calcium absorption is dependent on vitamin D. Bone deformities such as rickets, osteomalacia, and osteoporosis occur with a deficit of calcium.
   - Calcium may be deposited in joints and soft tissues, causing limitation of movement or pain.
   - Calcium may inhibit iron and zinc absorption.
   - Diseases such as hyperthyroidism and malignancies may cause hypercalcemia.
   - The latest pharmacologic suggestions for postmenopausal women not taking estrogen are to include vitamin E and calcium supplements in their dietary intake to slow the development of osteoporosis. The calcium requirement for a premenopausal woman is 1000 mg/day. The postmenopausal woman not taking estrogen needs 1500 mg/day.
   - Calcium carbonate (Tums) and calcium chews are good sources of replacement calcium for the postmenopausal woman.
   - Signs of hypercalcemia are confusion, headache, nausea and vomiting, and coma.

3. **Phosphorus (P⁺),** is also necessary for bone and tooth formation, as well as for energy. Inadequate nutrition is the main cause of deficiency.
   - Through regulation of acid-base balance, phosphorus maintains the normal intact structure of the cell membranes and is part of nucleic acids.

TABLE 20-6 *Minerals*

GENERIC NAME	TRADE NAME	ROUTE OF ADMINISTRATION	USUAL ADULT DOSE AND FREQUENCY OF ADMINISTRATION	INDICATIONS FOR USE	DRUG INTERACTIONS
IRON					
ferrous sulfate	Feosol, Slow Fe	po	325 mg tid	Iron deficiency anemia	antacids, tetracycline, calcium supplements
ferrous gluconate	Fergon	po	325-600 mg qd to qid		
ferrous fumarate	Feostat	po	200 mg qd to qid		pancreatin, ascorbic acid
iron dextran	Imferon, INFeD	IM (Z-track method)	Individually calculated		
iron sucrose	Venofer	IV	100 mg/dialysis treatment	Iron deficiency with dialysis	oral iron preparations
CALCIUM					
calcium acetate	Phos-Ex, Phos-Lo	po	Varies	Nutritional supplement	dairy products, digoxin, tetracyclines, phenytoin
calcium citrate	Citracal	po			
calcium glubionate	Neo-Calglucon	po			
calcium gluconate		IV		Nutritional supplement and hypocalcemic tetany	
calcium carbonate	Os-Cal, Titralac, Tums, Viactiv	po chewable			nutritional supplement and antacid
PHOSPHORUS					
potassium phosphate	Neutra-Phos, K-Phosphate	po, IV	Varies	Nutritional supplement	antacids, glucocorticoids, NSAIDs, ACE inhibitors, salicylates, K supplements, antihypertensives, K-sparing diuretics
sodium phosphate	Nu-phosphate	IV		Urinary acidifiers	
MAGNESIUM					
magnesium chloride	Slow Mag	po	Varies	Antacid, laxative, dietary supplement	tetracyclines
magnesium citrate	Citroma, Citro-Nesia	po			
magnesium hydroxide	MOM	po			
magnesium oxide	Epsom salts	po			
magnesium sulfate	Mag sulfate	IV		Anticonvulsant	
SODIUM					
sodium chloride	Salinex, Ocean Mist Normal saline Sodium chloride for injection	Ophthalmic, po, nasal solution, injection	Varies	Flushing, hydration, fluid-electrolyte balance, acid-base balance	oxytocin

TABLE 20-6 *Minerals—cont'd*

GENERIC NAME	TRADE NAME	ROUTE OF ADMINISTRATION	USUAL ADULT DOSE AND FREQUENCY OF ADMINISTRATION	INDICATIONS FOR USE	DRUG INTERACTIONS
POTASSIUM					
potassium acetate			Varies	Vitamin K deficiency, acid-base balance	ACE inhibitors, NSAIDs, beta-blockers,
potassium citrate/ bicarbonate	K-Lyte	IV, po			
potassium chloride	K-Lor, K-Dur, Klor-Con, Slow-K, Micro-K	po, IV			K-sparing diuretics, heparin, salt substitutes
potassium gluconate	KAON	po			
potassium sulfate		IV			
CHLORINE		⟵ IN COMBINATION WITH OTHER ELECTROLYTES ⟶			
ZINC					
zinc acetate	Galzin	po	25 mg tid	Wilson's disease	
FLUORIDE	Fluorotab, Luride	po	Varies	Dietary supplement, osteoporosis, treatment and prevention of dental caries	aluminum hydroxide, milk and dairy products

ACE, Angiotensin-converting enzyme; *NSAIDs,* nonsteroidal antiinflammatory drugs.

- The storage of fats and metabolism of other nutrients depend on this mineral.
- Phosphorus supplements also contain potassium, calcium, and sodium and can cause GI upsets, electrolyte imbalances, and bone or joint pain.
- A deficiency in phosphorus manifests with confusion, anemia, weakness, and bone brittleness.
- The toxic effects of increased phosphorus include low blood levels of calcium and kidney stones.

4. **Magnesium (Mg^+)** and calcium are interdependent.
   - Magnesium is required for the following:
     - Synthesizing proteins
     - Stimulating muscle contraction and nerve transmission
     - Activating enzymes
     - Aiding in bone formation
   - Supplemental magnesium is provided in combinations with other minerals such as aluminum, simethicone, and calcium, as found in antacids.
   - An excess or deficit in magnesium results in spasms, convulsions, and tetany, similar to what is seen in calcium deficiency.

- Insufficient amounts of magnesium cause muscle contractility and diarrhea; excessive intake causes CNS depression, coma, and hypotension.

5. **Sodium (Na^+)** is the major electrolyte in extracellular fluid.
   - The sodium content in the body is regulated by dietary intake and excretion by the kidneys.
   - Sodium helps regulate body fluid balance and acid-base balance and regulates nerve transmission and cell membrane irritability.
   - Signs of sodium deficiency are nausea, headache, mental confusion, hypotension, weakness, anxiety, and muscle spasms.
   - Edema, hypertension, and cardiovascular disturbances are signs of excess sodium.
   - Sodium is only as far away as table salt—the primary source of the electrolyte.

6. **Potassium (K^+)**, is a major electrolyte of intracellular fluid.
   - Potassium is necessary for:
     - Maintaining cell structure
     - Vital in regulating muscle function, especially cardiac muscle
     - Aids in protein synthesis and carbohydrate metabolism

- Tissue breakdown and acid-base imbalances occur with deficiencies.
- Hypokalemia can produce loss of muscle tone, weakness, paralysis, cardiac arrhythmias, and digitalis toxicity in the person taking digitalis
- Hyperkalemia is manifest with lethargy, confusion, diarrhea, nausea and vomiting, and decreased urinary output.

7. **Chlorine (Cl⁻)** is a major electrolyte, along with sodium, in extracellular fluid.
   - It serves as a buffer, an enzyme activator, and a component of gastric hydrochloric acid.
   - A deficiency in chlorine is rare except in patients taking medications that cause loss of NA and Cl on a long-term basis.
   - Toxic levels do not occur.
8. **Zinc (Zn⁺)** is a component of DNA and RNA.
   - It is essential for sexual development, aids in wound healing, and helps ensure normal taste and smell.
   - Deficiency of zinc is indicated by skin lesions.
   - The toxic effects are poor muscle coordination, vomiting, diarrhea, and renal failure.
9. **Fluorine/fluorides (Fl⁻)** protect against dental caries and contribute to bone formation and integrity.
   - The sign of excessive fluoride treatment is mottled stains on the teeth.
   - Fluoride supplements may be useful for children living in areas where the water supply is not fluorinated.

Use of Mineral Supplements

Mineral supplements should be used with care because excessive amounts can be hazardous to one's health. A healthy person who eats a balanced diet will obtain sufficient minerals to counteract normal losses of minerals through perspiration, saliva, urine, and feces. When excessive concentrated forms of minerals are taken on a regular basis over a period of time, the mineral levels become more than the body needs and can cause toxic effects. Excessive quantities of minerals can cause hair loss and changes in blood, muscles, blood vessels—in fact, changes in almost all tissues. Mineral supplements should be taken only on the advice of a health care provider.

IMPORTANT FACTS ABOUT MINERALS
- Minerals are essential for normal body function.
- The minerals called *electrolytes* are essential for homeostasis.

Patient Education for Compliance

1. The pharmacist is an excellent source of information on possible side effects of vitamin and mineral supplements such as staining of the teeth and GI upsets. The patient should pay attention to any special labels on the medicine bottles.
2. Minerals that are not necessary should not be taken because of the danger of changing electrolyte balances.
3. Liquid preparations of iron should be taken with a dropper or straw to prevent staining of the teeth and mucous membranes. Solutions should be dropped on the back of tongue, and the mouth should be rinsed following administration.
4. Iron should be taken on an empty stomach, but it may be taken with food if GI upset occurs.
5. Iron supplements may cause constipation.
6. Antacids and iron should not be taken at the same time.
7. Calcium carbonate (e.g., Tums) is a good replacement for calcium in postmenopausal women who have GI upset from taking calcium tablets. Postmenopausal women need vitamin D (synthesized on exposure to sunlight) for effective absorption. Some calcium tablets are formulated with vitamin D added.
8. Fluoride drops should not be taken with milk or dairy products. Rinses and drops should be used at bedtime to ensure that nothing is eaten after use. Water should not be taken after fluoride use to prevent diluting the drops.

Alternative Medications

Over the past 20 to 30 years, the use of **alternative medicine** is an approach to illness that has increased rapidly in the United States. This interest has been prevalent worldwide for many years, especially in countries without access to modern medicines. Use of plant and animal substances for treatment often lack scientific evidence of safety and efficacy. Herbal therapy, however, is at the root of pharmacology—herbs and natural medicines were used before manufactured medications were available.

One of the most rapidly growing types of alternative therapy is the treatment of osteoarthritis using such medications as glucosamine or chondroitin. These are nutritional supplements, and some research supports the fact that glucosamine aids in the repair and formation of cartilage.

Chondroitin is a protein that allows for the elasticity of the cartilage.

The term **complementary medicine** indicates that scientific research has been conducted and the practice is accepted by mainstream medicine. Complementary therapies include diet, exercise, counseling, biofeedback, massage therapy, relaxation techniques, and hypnosis, which generally are not invasive. Home remedies and folk remedies are still popular in many cultures (Table 20-7) and may coexist with modern pharmocologic therapy.

Cultural Differences in Using Alternative Medicine

The first alternative medicines were home remedies. How the ancient remedies were used is unknown, but we can reasonably assume they were used for medical, social, and psychologic purposes—to clean a wound or ease childbirth, restore harmony between the spirit world and humans, increase sexual prowess or attract a mate, or treat depression. In today's world, many **folk** or **home remedies** are used on a daily basis. Each culture has its primary medical providers who provide folk remedies. In the United States, most cultural groups use some form of complementary or alternative therapies, using both medicinal treatments and social or psychic adjustments.

Among Native Americans, medicine men and women used plants and herbs blessed for medicinal use. Remedies included herbal drinks, which produced cures when used with prayers, rituals, and healing ceremonies. Illness was prevented through prayer, charms, and the use of objects with power to protect the owner. Some of these forms of healing and health maintenance continue today.

Historically, certain African and Latin American cultures have attributed disease to disharmony in relationships between humans and supernatural forces. Discord may occur between the person and ancestral spirits, evil spirits, or living relatives. Treatments are provided by trained, culturally accepted healers, who may be elderly women healers ("Grannies"), shamans, or root doctors. Herbs, roots, and oils are used for healing. Talismans are worn to ward off evil spirits. Religious rituals such as the laying on of hands are used to treat disease.

TABLE 20-7 *Examples of Home and Folk Remedies*

REMEDY	USED FOR	ADMINISTRATION METHOD
Hot chicken soup	Fever, cold, flu	Ingested
Lemon in water	Cold and congestion	Ingested
Potato juice	Arthritis	Ingested
Orange juice and gelatin	Arthritis	Ingested
Onions	Fever	Slices placed on feet
	Cold	Ingested in water
	Congestion	Onion vapors inhaled
	Earache	Boiled as hot pack and applied to affected area
	Headache	Placed raw on neck or soles of feet
	Stomach or intestinal distress	Ingested
	Blood clotting disorders	Ingested
	Heart disease	Ingested
Vinegar	Sore throat	Gargled
	Sunburned skin	Applied topically
	Pruritus, contact dermatitis	Applied topically
	Chronic fatigue syndrome	Ingested
Dandelion tea	Urinary tract infections	Ingested
Gelatin	Diarrhea	Ingested
Garlic	Antiseptic	Applied topically or ingested
	Antibiotic, coronary heart disease, decrease blood cholesterol, hypertension, antitumor agent	Ingested

Some Latin American populations including those who have emigrated to the United States practice a fusion medicine. Illness is viewed as having a natural cause, as an act of God, as punishment, or as the result of witchcraft or a curse. The healers are *curanderos* (native healers), *yerberos* (herbalists), *espiritualistas* (spiritualists), or *brujos* (those who use witchcraft or magic). Hot and cold foods such as herbal teas are used to treat some conditions. Massage may be used, and religious medals may be worn. Some Hispanic Americans wear an *azabache*, a black stone, to ward off the evil eye that causes disease.

In Eastern (Asian) medicine, the objective is to keep the body in balance between the opposing forces of yin (cold) and yang (hot) for the maintenance of good health. Illness occurs when the body is out of balance. The Chinese physician prescribes a variety of therapies including herbs, acupuncture, diet changes, exercise, meditation, or the services of spiritual healers. Herbs may be applied externally or taken orally to correct physical disorders. Herbs are given in combinations for the person who needs to strengthen body energy. Herbs, soups, meditation, acupressure, acupuncture, and liniments such as tiger balm may be used to maintain health. In Eastern medicine the goal is health promotion and stabilization.

In Western medicine such as is found in North America, the scientific-medical paradigm of illness and treatment predominates. Western-trained physicians identify illness as a physical, chemical, or physiologic disturbance in the body from normal (even when they say, "It's all in your head"), and they focus on interventions, often invasive in some manner, to correct the disturbances. Aggressive treatment of symptoms and their causes has been the norm; however, alternative therapies such as massage, acupuncture, yoga, and dietary changes are increasingly accepted.

Federal Regulation of Herbal Supplements

Herbal supplements are minimally regulated by the FDA, and the U.S. Department of Agriculture and the FDA regulate these as food supplements. They must be labeled by content but not by medicinal uses, doses, and dangers. In 1994 Congress passed the Dietary Supplement Health and Education Act, which defined herbal supplements such as vitamins, minerals, amino acids, and herbs. Minimal quality control exists, and false claims are numerous. The maker of the herbal supplement must only prove that it is a "food substance" and label it as a dietary supplement.

These products are not subject to the stringent rules and testing required for pharmaceuticals. The FDA must prove that a supplement is unsafe before it can legally remove the supplement from the market. Because many patients do not have complete knowledge about the interactions of pharmaceutical products and herbal products, physicians and allied health professionals should interview the patient about all medications and supplements being taken, whether prescription or OTC. Patients should be encouraged to discuss the use of herbal preparations without reproach and understand that the physician is interested in discussing herbal supplement use to prevent drug/herb interactions.

Commonly Used Herbal Supplements and Their Sources

The most commonly used herbal supplements are Saint John's wort, for depression; melatonin, for sleep; *Echinacea*, for immune system support and stimulation; *ginseng*, for energy; *Gingko*, to improve memory; feverfew, for migraines; saw palmetto, for prostate disease; *ephedra* (*Ma-huang*), as a bronchodilator and stimulant; and *valerian*, as a tranquilizer. Herbs are sometimes called "nature's medicine chest," for good reason (Table 20-8).

Different parts of the herb—blossoms, seeds, stems, and roots—may be used for medicinal purposes. The flowers found in many seasonal gardens are used for medicinal uses; in colonial New England, the herb garden was necessary for every self-sufficient household. The leading uses of herbal products are listed in Box 20-1.

Safety with Herbal Supplement Use

The health care professional and the consumer should be aware that "natural" does not necessarily mean "safe." Some herbal supplements can be harmful because of the herb itself, the amount consumed, the part of the plant used, or from contaminants that have entered during the growing or processing of the herb. Important considerations with herbal supplements include:

- Interactions between prescribed medications and supplements being taken OTC
- Mistaken identification of allergic responses to the supplements
- Possibility of the patient being treated with herbal supplements and forgoing a medical diagnosis and treatment until the disease has become too advanced to treat

TABLE 20-8 *Select Herbs Used for Medicinal Therapy*

HERB	ACTION	USES
Echinacea (caution during pregnancy and lactation)	May have antibiotic action	*Internal:* Colds, influenza, URIs, ear infections, septicemia, bladder infections *External:* Cuts, boils, abscesses, wounds, hives, eczema, insect bites, herpes
Garlic	Strengthens cardiovascular system, decreases cholesterol, decreases blood pressure (BP)	*Internal:* Digestive disorders, diarrhea, liver and gallbladder problems, URI, influenza, rheumatoid arthritis, bladder infection *External:* Hookworm, roundworm, ringworm, athlete's foot, swelling, minor skin infections
Gingko (not during pregnancy or lactation)	Vasodilation, improves blood circulation, decreases blood clots, decreases retinal damage from macular degeneration	*Internal:* Vertigo, Alzheimer's disease, tinnitus, phlebitis, leg ulcers, peripheral vascular disease, cerebral atherosclerosis, headaches, depression, strokes, heart attacks, lack of concentration
Golden seal (not during pregnancy or in young children)	Dries secretions, reduces inflammation, mild antimicrobial, aids in digestion	*Internal:* Diarrhea, irritable bowel syndrome, colitis, ulcers, gastritis, gingivitis, vaginal yeast infections, otitis
Saw palmetto	Reduces size of prostate gland; dries secretions; aids with digestion, sleep, and coughs	*Internal:* Benign prostatic hypertrophy, nasal congestion, asthma, bronchitis, URIs, sinusitis, sedative, diuretic, expectorant, bladder infections *External:* Antiseptic
Aloe	Decreases pain of burns and skin irritations, antihistamine, laxative	*Internal:* Digestive disorders, gastric ulcer, laxative *External:* Burns, wound infections, insect bites, skin irritations, chickenpox, acne, poison ivy
Panax ginseng (may cause asthma attacks, increases BP, heart palpitations, postmenopausal bleeding)	Calms stomach, stimulates vital organs	*Internal:* Depression, fatigue, stress, URIs, influenza, inflammation, respiratory tract disorders
Astragalus	Strengthens body, speeds metabolism, promotes tissue regeneration, increases energy	*Internal:* General weakness or fatigue, loss of appetite, diarrhea, blood abnormalities, URIs, AIDS, cancer, chronic fatigue
Cayenne	Stimulates heart, increases circulation, improves digestion, boosts energy	*Internal:* Poor circulation, indigestion, physical or mental exhaustion, lowered energy *External:* Pain, arthritis, strains, sore muscles and joints, increases blood flow, stops external bleeding
Siberian ginseng (may cause asthma, increases BP, heart palpitations, postmenopausal bleeding)	Increases immune system; increases resistance to disease, stress, and fatigue	*Internal:* Depression, fatigue, stress, URIs, influenza, respiratory problems, damaged immune system

(continued)

TABLE 20-8 *Select Herbs Used for Medicinal Therapy—cont'd*

HERB	ACTION	USES
Bilberry (cannot be used for long period of time)	To treat eye problems like glaucoma and cataracts, decreases plaque in arteries, diarrhea, decreases blood sugar	*Internal:* Eye strain, cataracts, glaucoma, night blindness, nearsightedness, diarrhea, constipation, stomach cramps *External:* Spider veins, varicose veins, hemorrhoids, burns, skin disorders
Dong quai	Gynecologic complaints	*Internal:* Menstrual irregularity, stabbing pain, poor circulation, carbuncles, palpitations, blurred vision, lightheadedness
Saint John's wort (headaches, increases BP, photosensitivity, multiple drug interactions)	Germicidal, antiinflammatory, antidepressant	*Internal:* Depression *External:* Wounds, scar tissue
Valerian	Mild tranquilizer, improves sleep	*Internal:* Insomnia, anxiety, nervousness, anxiety-induced palpitations, headaches, intestinal pain, menstrual cramps
Feverfew (may alter clotting times)	Blocks inflammatory substances in blood	*Internal:* Migraine headaches
Ginger	Motion sickness, digestion, dizziness, burns, may prevent heart disease and strokes by decreasing BP and internal clotting	*Internal:* Vomiting, abdominal cramping, cough, menstrual irregularities, motion sickness, morning sickness, colds, flu, arthritis, increases BP and cholesterol
Kava kava	Antidepressant, diuresis, antiseptic/antiinflammatory agent for urinary tract	*Internal:* Urinary tract disorders, prostate inflammation, gout, rheumatism, insomnia, depression, muscle spasms
Ephedra (similar to ephedrine)	Bronchial decongestant, CNS stimulant, increases heart rate, increases BP	*Internal:* Fever, coughing, wheezing, nasal or chest congestion, indigestion, asthma, obesity
Alfalfa	Nutritional supplement, body cleanser	*Internal:* Inflammation of bladder, diuresis, indigestion, constipation, halitosis
Kelp	Goiter remedy, thyroid disorders (iodine-rich)	*Internal:* Hypothyroidism, goiter
Parsley	Expectorant, diuretic, laxative	*Internal:* Indigestion, congestion, asthma, irregular menstrual periods, PMS, increases BP, congestive heart failure
Rose hip	Nasal and chest congestion	*Internal:* Colds and flu
Tea tree oil	Skin disorders	*External:* Cuts, abrasions, insect bites, acne, fungal infections, flea shampoo for pets
Melatonin	Tranquilizer, sedative	Sleep

BP, Blood pressure; *PMS,* premenstrual syndrome.

BOX 20-1   LEADING USES OF HERBAL PRODUCTS

DISORDER	HERB COMMONLY USED
Upper respiratory infection	*Echinacea*, elderberry, *Astragalus*
Burns	Calendula, tea tree, *Aloe*, lavender oil
Headaches	Feverfew, black cohosh
Allergies	Freeze-dried nettle leaf, *Coleus*, grape seed
Rashes	Calendula, tea tree, flaxseed oil
Insomnia and stress	Valerian, passion flower, kava
Premenstrual syndrome	Vitax, black cohosh, dong quai
Depression	Saint John's wort, *Gingko*, kava, SAM-e
Diarrhea	Blueberry leaf, bilberry
Menopause	Black cohosh, Vitax, evening primrose oil
Nausea	Peppermint, ginger
Urinary tract irritability	Cranberry
Cholesterol and lipid control	Flax seed oil
Prostate health	Saw palmetto
Memory enhancement	Ginseng

Some serious problems such as toxic effects on the liver and heart, fetal malformations, and the production of abnormal cells leading to cancer have been reported with the indiscriminate use of herbal supplements. Adverse reactions to these supplements cannot be determined very well because they are not reportable by law. Herbal products with the potential to cause toxic effects and the interactions with certain drugs are listed in Table 20-9.

It is difficult to evaluate the safety of herbs because herbal supplements may contain a mixture of plants and other materials. When potent herbs are compared with equally potent medications, the side effects are comparable or more severe. To date no study has shown herbs to be more effective than the chemicals purified from them, and the safety of these products cannot be proven because the chemicals have not been tested for purity. Prescription medications from herbs produce essentially the same actions as quantities of herbs themselves and have a higher safety factor because of the quality standards required for medication approval.

Herbal supplements should always be used with caution.

TABLE 20-9   *Herbs with a Potential for Toxic Effects*

HERB	EFFECT
Echinacea	Immunosuppression with long-term use
Garlic	Not used with anticoagulants; has hypoglycemic effects, so may affect insulin
Gingko	Not used with anticoagulants
Goldenseal, *Cunica* flowers, wolfsbane (*Aconitum vulparia*), mountain tobacco	Affect heart and vascular system; *Cunica* can induce toxic gastroenteritis, nervous system disturbances, muscle weakness, and death
Wormwood, absinthe, mugwort, madwort (*Alyssum*)	Narcotic poison (oil of wormwood) can damage nervous system and cause mental impairment
Belladonna, deadly nightshade (*Solanum*)	Toxic alkaloids of atropine and hyoscyamine can cause anticholinergic symptoms ranging from blurred vision, mydriasis, dry mouth, and inability to urinate to unusual behavior and hallucinations
Buckeye, horse chestnut (*Aesculus hippocastanum*)	Contains coumadin glycoside, which may interfere with blood clotting
Hemlock (*Conium*), spotted parsley, Saint Bennett's herb, spotted cowbane, fool's parsley	Contains toxic alkaloid conium and other related alkaloids
Lobelia, Indian tobacco, wild tobacco, asthma weed, emetic weed	Excessive use produces severe vomiting, pain, sweating, paralysis, decreased body temperature, coma, and death
Ephedra	Contains ephedrine, pseudoephedrine, sympathomimetic-like to give actions of epinephrine, increase BP, increase heart rate; used to make methamphetamine (also called herbal Fen-Phen, which has FDA warnings)
Periwinkle, *Vinca*	Alkaloids that are cytotoxic may cause liver, kidney, and neurologic damage; base for antineoplastic agents

- Special care should be taken by patients with allergies, those sensitive to medications, those taking medicines for chronic illnesses, and those older than 65 years of age or younger than 12 years of age.
- The lowest possible dose should be taken to protect against adverse reactions. Herbal supplements are best absorbed on an empty stomach, but they should be discontinued if nausea consistently develops within 2 hours after ingestion.
- Herbal supplements interact with many drugs, and the health care professional should document all herbal products being used by a patient.
- Pregnant or lactating women are advised not to take herbal products without a physician's advice.
- It is safer to buy herbs than to grow them at home, although the safety factor cannot be proven even with purchased supplements.
- Herbals should be bought from a reputable source because toxic contaminants such as pesticides and heavy metals may be found in some herbal products.

Patient Education for Compliance

1. Herbs are not regulated as strictly as medications by the FDA but are sold as food supplements. Herbal supplements, if used, should be purchased from a reputable source.
2. Patients should be careful about taking prescription medications and herbal supplements together.
3. Physicians should be informed of any herbal supplements being used so that drug interactions can be prevented.
4. Before taking herbals, the consumer should acquire as much information as possible about the products.

IMPORTANT FACTS ABOUT ALTERNATIVE MEDICINES

- Alternative medicines include treatments for which scientific evidence of safety and usefulness is lacking. These are popular in many cultures.
- Complementary medicine includes those treatments for which a scientific basis has been found and the treatment is used in mainstream medicine.
- Herbs are considered a dietary supplement and therefore are regulated as food supplements by the Department of Agriculture and FDA rather than under the strict regulations as medications under the FDA.

Summary

Vitamins and minerals are essential compounds needed to keep the body in homeostasis. If adequate diets are consumed, most people will not need vitamin and mineral supplements. The FDA considers vitamins and minerals to be medications, and the government regulates their production and use. Young children and the elderly, pregnant or lactating women, and patients undergoing chemotherapy generally need to take vitamin and mineral supplements. Absorption disorders and immune system deficiencies may also require the daily intake of additional vitamins. Some diseases are the result of insufficient vitamins or minerals such as scurvy and beriberi, or the disease processes such as osteoporosis and anemias may be improved by supplementation.

Vitamins are divided into two groups. The fat-soluble vitamins—A, D, E, and K—are absorbed and stored by the body and do not require replacement on a daily basis. Vitamin B complex and vitamin C, water-soluble vitamins, are not stored, and the excess is excreted in the urine. A well-balanced diet is essential for a continuing supply of the water-soluble vitamins. Hypervitaminosis is usually not a health problem with the water-soluble vitamins, but an excess of fat-soluble vitamins may cause acute and chronic detrimental conditions. Some OTC supplements are formulated as vitamin and mineral combinations. Minerals, like vitamins, usually occur in adequate amounts in foods. Iron supplements are given for anemias, whereas calcium supplements are used to prevent osteoporosis in postmenopausal women. The minerals absorbed from supplements depend on the needs of the body.

Complementary medicines are used to supplement traditional professional medical care, whereas alternative medicines are practices that either are unfounded or are not based on scientific research related to traditional medical care. Folk medicines and home remedies that are based on herbs have been used throughout history, with some cultures having deeper roots in these traditions than others. Many alternative therapies and folk medicines depend on herbs as the basis of treatment.

Herbal supplements are from a variety of plant materials, contain many biologically active ingredients, and are used primarily for the treatment of mild or chronic illnesses. Many pharmaceuticals contain these same ingredients but in a purified form. The danger with herbal supplements, which are considered food supplements, is that they are not subject to the strict supervision by the FDA.

As well, many of their interactions with prescription medicines are unknown or just coming to light. The dangers of using herbal supplements are not fully known, but documentation of all herbal supplements being used by a patient is essential.

Critical Thinking Exercises

SCENARIO

Kim is in good health and eats a well-balanced diet. She has heard that taking vitamins may make her feel better, and she is considering taking multivitamins that contain water-soluble and fat-soluble components.

1. What do you tell her about excessive water- and fat-soluble vitamins? Should she need vitamins?
2. What can Kim expect to gain by using these vitamins?
3. What risks will she be taking?
4. Kim says that when she was pregnant she had to take vitamins. Why were vitamins important then and not necessary now?

DRUG CALCULATIONS

1. Order: Potassium chloride 80 mEq
   Available medication:

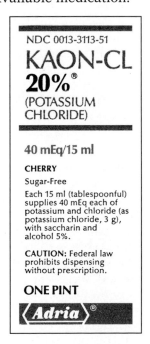

Dose to be given: 30 mL
How many ounces of medication would be given to the patient? _____

Draw the dose to be given on the medicine cup.

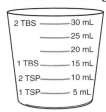

2. Order: Vitamin B_{12} 1500 mg twice a week
   Available medication: cyanocobalamin 1000 mg/mL
   What dose should be administered? _____

   Show the amount of medication on the syringe below.

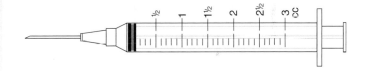

REVIEW QUESTIONS

1. Name three groups of people who might need vitamin supplements. _____
   _____

2. What are vitamins? Minerals? Electrolytes? _____
   _____
   _____

3. Which vitamins are water-soluble? Fat-soluble? _____
   _____
   _____

4. Why is toxicity with fat-soluble vitamins a possibility? Why is toxicity not as likely with water-
   soluble vitamins? _____
   _____

5. What vitamin is necessary for calcium to be effective? What are two sources of this vitamin?
   _____
   _____

Medications Related to Body Systems

CHAPTER 21
Endocrine System Disorders, 404

CHAPTER 22
Eye and Ear Disorders, 435

CHAPTER 23
Skin Condition Disorders, 455

CHAPTER 24
Musculoskeletal System Disorders, 475

CHAPTER 25
Gastrointestinal System Disorders, 493

CHAPTER 26
Respiratory System Disorders, 523

CHAPTER 27
Circulatory System Disorders, 546

CHAPTER 28
Urinary System Disorders, 583

CHAPTER 29
Reproductive System Disorders, 593

CHAPTER 30
Neurologic System Disorders, 620

CHAPTER 31
Drugs for Mental Health and Behavioral Disorders, 656

CHAPTER 32
Drugs of Abuse and Misuse, 680

CHAPTER 21

Endocrine System Disorders

OBJECTIVES

After studying this chapter, you should be capable of doing the following:

- Defining hormones and their functions.
- Explaining how hormones secreted by the anterior and posterior pituitary glands affect diseases and their treatment.
- Describing the role of the thyroid gland and its replacements and the antagonistic medications.
- Discussing the forms of steroids/corticosteroids and their role in treating disease processes.
- Describing the role of hypoglycemic and adjunctive agents in treating diabetes mellitus (DM).
- Describing the role of glucose and glycogen in homeostasis.

Dianne, age 45, has recently been diagnosed as having type 2 DM. She had no idea that she had any medical problems until she went to her physician and her blood glucose test was elevated above 300 and the HgA$_{1C}$ above 15.

What symptoms do you think may have been present that she might not have realized were important?

What role will exercise and diet play in the control of the glucose levels with this type of diabetes? What is the role of weight loss with type 2 DM?

Can Dianne expect to take insulin for this type of illness? Why or why not?

If not insulin, what classes of medications might be used?

Can these oral medications be used during pregnancy for gestational diabetes? Why or why not?

KEY TERMS

Action onset	Hormone	Osteoporosis
Action peak	Hyperglycemia	Polydipsia
Bolus	Hypoglycemia	Polyphagia
Endogenous	Hypothalamus	Polyuria
Exogenous	Islet of Langerhans	Replacement therapy
Glucocorticoid	Lipodystrophy	Steroid
Goiter	Mineralocorticoid	Target organ
Growth hormone	Negative feedback	Tropic hormone

EASY WORKING KNOWLEDGE OF INDICATIONS AND SIDE EFFECTS

Common Symptoms of Endocrine Diseases

Mental deviations

Exceptional changes in energy levels

Growth abnormalities

Skin, hair, and nail changes

Weakness and atrophy of muscles

Emotional disturbances or psychologic disorders

Edema

Changes in blood pressure with heart irregularities

Sexual irregularities

Changes in urinary output

Common Side Effects of Medications for Endocrine Diseases

Corticosteroids:

Short-term—increased appetite and swelling; long-term—Cushingoid syndrome

Thyroid preparations: palpitations, tremors, nervousness, tachycardia, increased blood pressure, headache, exophthalmus, weight loss, and irritability

Hypoglycemics: hypoglycemia, nausea, heartburn, diarrhea, headache, weight gain

Easy Working Knowledge of Drugs Used in the Endocrine System

DRUG CLASS	PRESCRIPTION	OTC	PREGNANCY CATEGORY	MAJOR INDICATIONS
Anterior pituitary hormones	Yes	No	B, C	Growth stimulants, thyroid-stimulating hormone, adrenocorticotropin, gonadotropin
Posterior pituitary hormones	Yes	No	C	Antidiuretic hormone, oxytocin
Thyroid hormones				
Triiodothyronine (T$_3$), Thyroxine (T$_4$)	Yes	No	A, C	Hypothyroidism
Calcitonin	Yes	No	C	Osteoporosis
Thyroid inhibiting preparations	Yes	No	D, X (I-131)	Thyroid malignancies, hyperthyroidism
Steroids/corticosteroids				
Glucocorticoids	Yes	Yes-topical	C	Chronic inflammations, allergies
Mineralocorticoids	Yes	No	C	Antiinflammatory, Addison's disease
Corticosteroid inhibiting agents	Yes	No	C, D	Cushing's disease, malignancies of adrenal glands
Hypoglycemics				
Insulin	Yes	Yes (except lispro)	B, C	Type 1 diabetes mellitus
Oral hypoglycemics	Yes	No	B, C, (should not be used in pregnancy)	Type 2 diabetes mellitus
Hyperglycemics				
Glucagon	Yes	No	B	Hypoglycemia

The endocrine system is a network of internal glands that are without ducts secreting hormones directly into the bloodstream. Hormones are carried by the blood or the lymphatic system to tissues or other glands throughout the body (Figure 21-1). Adequate hormones are necessary for vital functions in the body. Hormones stimulate various tissues throughout the body to increase their activity. The action of hormones is slower in onset and of longer duration than stimulation of the body systems by the nervous system. Some hormones are effective only in certain types of tissue or an organ, called the target organ. Target hormones have specific receptors on the membrane of the target organ. As the hormone attaches to this receptor site, it acts as a key, releasing the hormone to produce its effect. Hormone specificity and the cellular receptor sites together form a complex regulatory system to ensure homeostasis. Only specific receptor material binds a hormone so that it may begin its activity when the cell or site recognizes the hormone. Therefore, hormones have no effect on tissues that do not carry the specific receptors for the particular hormones (Figure 21-2).

The **hypothalamus,** located in the brain, regulates hormone secretions, much as a thermostat regulates temperature in a heating-cooling system. The hypothalamus is influenced by the body itself and by environmental factors. These cause the hypothalamus to produce releasing hormones that are received in the pituitary gland to maintain homeostasis. The hypothalamus also responds to the internal environment to control this release by **negative feedback,** a physiologic response that inhibits further secretions of a hormone. Similarly, increased hormone secretions may cause cessation of the external stimuli, ending the secretion response internally (Figure 21-3).

What Are Hormones?

Some hormones regulate the activity of other hormones and have a specific physiologic effect on metabolism including substances that cause the anterior and posterior pituitary gland to release tropic or stimulating hormones for the other glands of the endocrine system. These integrated relationships are between the activities

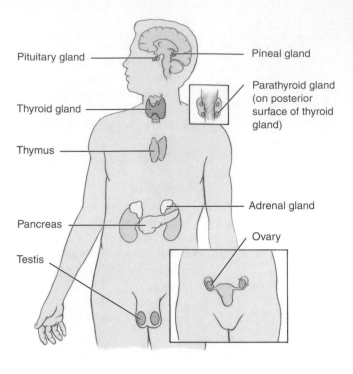

Figure 21-1 The major endocrine glands of the body. (From Applegate E: *The anatomy and physiology learning system*, ed 3, Philadelphia, 2006, Saunders.)

of the different endocrine system glands (Figure 21-4).

Hormones are substances from steroids or are nonsteroidal amino acid derived.

Steroid hormones are characterized by the following:

- Manufactured from cholesterol by endocrine cells and are lipid soluble
- Chemicals that act as messenger agents to regulate the inner environment of the body in cooperation with the nervous system
- Secreted by the adrenal glands and sex glands
- Transported in the plasma

Nonsteroid hormones, synthesized from amino acids, are characterized by the following:

- Protein hormones such as insulin and glucagons, parathyroid hormones, calcitonin, **growth hormones** (GHs), and adrenocorticotropin hormone
- Glycoproteins including follicle stimulating hormone, luteinizing hormone, thyroid-stimulating hormone, and chorionic gonadotropin
- Peptides such as antidiuretic hormone, oxytocin, and releasing hormones
- Amino-acid derivatives that include epinephrine, norepinephrine, melatonin, thyroxine, and triiodothyronine

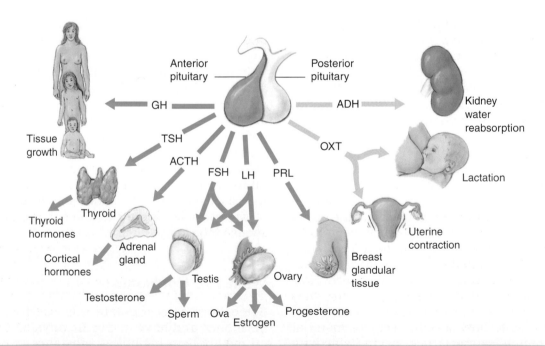

Figure 21-2 Hormone-receptor action of hormones in the body. *GH*, Growth hormone; *TSH*, thyroid stimulating hormone; *ACTH*, adrenocorticotropin; *FSH*, follicle stimulating hormone; *LH*, luteinizing hormone; *PRL*, prolactin; *OXT*, oxytocin; *ADH*, antidiuretic hormone. (From Applegate E: *The anatomy and physiology learning system*, ed 3, Philadelphia, 2006, Saunders.)

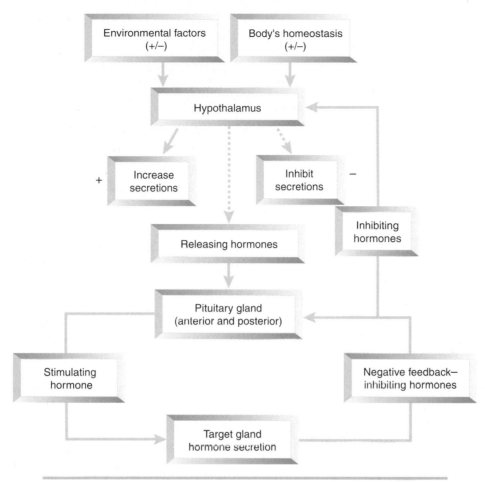

Figure 21-3 The relationship between negative feedback and homeostasis.

Hormones are necessary substances for the following:

- Regulation of vital processes such as the secretion of gastric enzymes and fluids and the motor activities of the digestive tract
- Production of energy
- The composition and volume of extracellular fluid
- Adaptation of the body, through immunity or accommodation, to the external environment
- Growth and development
- Reproduction and lactation

Hormones that are not used completely must be inactivated or excreted from the internal environment for the body to stay in homeostasis. Inactivation occurs by enzymes in the blood or in intracellular spaces, liver, kidneys, or target organs. Excretion is primarily in the urine, but to some extent waste is found in bile. Most hormones have short half-lives of 10 to 20 minutes, reflecting their rapid use or excretion. Some hormones exert their effect immediately, as the hormone leaves the bloodstream to access the target organs, whereas the effects of others persist for hours, resulting in prolonged stimulation of an organ, contributing to the extensive flexibility of the endocrine system.

Two major therapeutic uses of hormones exist. First, in case of a deficiency, the needed hormone is administered as **replacement therapy.** Second, in certain diseases, large doses of hormones may be given therapeutically to produce beneficial results, such as corticosteroids for inflammation or arthritis. Hormones may also be used for endocrine diagnostic testing such as adrenocorticotropin hormone for adrenal insufficiency testing. When used either therapeutically or diagnostically, as in the situations cited, the hormone becomes a pharmacologic agent.

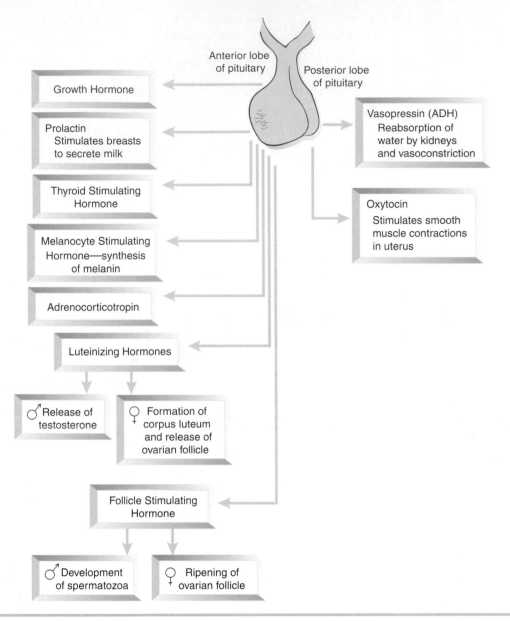

Figure 21-4 The relationship between the pituitary gland and other glands of the endocrine system.

Pituitary Gland Hormones

The pituitary gland is located below the hypothalamus and is about the size of a pea. Called "the master gland," it regulates the endocrine system. The hormones of the pituitary exert a distinctive effect: They regulate the secretion of hormones from other endocrine glands. The anterior lobe of the pituitary secretes the **tropic hormones**, named for the gland they affect such as thyrotropin, which affects the thyroid, or adrenocorticotropin, which affects the adrenal glands. Responding to the neurohormones or hypothalamic-releasing factors, these hormones cause the endocrine glands to secrete their specific hormones.

Anterior Pituitary Gland

The anterior pituitary gland communicates with the hypothalamus by releasing regulating factors that are delivered through blood vessels; the posterior pituitary gland has only neuronal stimulation, with no direct contact through blood vessels. The anterior pituitary gland secretes six major hormones that are controlled by the hypothalamus (see Figure 21-4):

1. GH—stimulates the growth of almost all tissues and organs.
2. Adrenocorticotropic hormone (ACTH), or adrenocorticotropin—acts on the adrenal cortex

to promote the synthesis and release of adrenocortical hormones.

3. Thyrotropin (TSH or thyroid-stimulating hormone)—acts on the thyroid gland to promote the synthesis and release of thyroid hormones.
4. Prolactin—stimulates milk production and secretion in women.
5. Follicle-stimulating hormone (FSH)—promotes follicular growth in the ovary and spermatogenesis in the testes.
6. Luteinizing hormone (LH)—promotes ovulation and the development of the corpus luteum in the female and acts on the testes to promote androgen production in the male.

The anterior pituitary hormones are used therapeutically as follows:

- *Somatotropin*, or GH, is produced by the anterior pituitary gland to help in the regulation of growth. Absence of this hormone during childhood results in most cases of dwarfism. Excessive production of GH in the adult causes *acromegaly*, whereas if this excessive stimulation occurs before epiphyseal lines are closed, the result is *gigantism*.
  - The main replacement of GH is for children who have growth failure because of the body's lack of production of **endogenous** somatotropin. Some people develop antibodies to the treatment, but these rarely decrease the effectiveness of the treatment, which is expensive (in the neighborhood of $2000 per year). Treatment is prolonged and may result in as much as a 6-inch growth in height. The efficacy of GH replacement therapy declines as the person grows older and is usually lost by age 20 to 24 years (Table 21-1).
  - Octreotide, a GH inhibitor, is used to lower blood GH levels (see Table 21-1).
- *Adrenocorticotropic hormone* (ACTH) is used primarily for diagnostic testing and is rarely used therapeutically because its effects are highly variable. It cannot be given orally, and it can produce undesired side effects because it stimulates the production of other hormones (see Table 21-1).
- *Thyroid-stimulating hormone (TSH, thyrotropin)* stimulates thyroid gland function by increasing the uptake of iodine, increasing the synthesis and release of thyroid hormones, and promoting thyroid growth (Figure 21-5). It is used diagnostically to differentiate pri-

mary hypothyroidism from secondary hypothyroidism, and it may also be used to test for anterior pituitary gland deficiencies (see Table 21-1).

Posterior Pituitary Gland

The posterior pituitary gland produces two hormones: oxytocin, active on the reproductive system, and antidiuretic hormone (ADH or vasopressin), active on the urinary system. Oxytocin and ADH are synthesized in the neurosecretory cells of the hypothalamus. ADH promotes renal conservation of water, whereas oxytocin functions during labor and delivery. (Oxytocin is not discussed in this book because it is not routinely used in ambulatory care.) Hypofunction of the posterior pituitary gland results in diabetes insipidus, causing the person to void profuse amounts of dilute urine, leading to dehydration. The patient should be taught the importance of recording intake and output and reporting chest pain, shortness of breath, or headaches (see Table 21-1).

Those pituitary hormones related to the reproductive system are discussed in Chapter 29.

Patient Education for Compliance

1. When taking somatotropin (growth hormone) therapy, regularly scheduled visits to the health care provider are important to measure height and weight.
2. When taking ACTH, notify the physician of any signs of infection.
3. Do not stop taking ACTH abruptly; it must be tapered off.
4. Patients taking ADH should monitor fluid intake and output, as well as weight, as indications of dehydration.
5. Report shortness of breath, chest pain, or headaches with ADH therapy.

IMPORTANT FACTS ABOUT PITUITARY HORMONES

- Release of hormones from the anterior pituitary gland is influenced by the hypothalamus and is inhibited by negative feedback.
- GH deficiency results in dwarfism.
  Excessive amounts of GH cause gigantism in children and acromegaly in adults.
- GH replacement therapy is indicated only for children deficient in GH. It is not indicated for children who are simply short.
- GHs can elevate blood glucose levels in children with diabetes.

TABLE 21-1 *Select Drugs Used as Agents of the Pituitary Gland*

GENERIC NAME	TRADE NAME	USUAL ADULT DOSE, ROUTE, AND FREQUENCY OF ADMINISTRATION	INDICATIONS FOR USE	MAJOR SIDE EFFECTS	DRUG INTERACTIONS
ANTERIOR PITUITARY GLAND					
Growth Hormone					
somatrem	Protropin	0.1 mg/kg IM/SC 3 × per wk	Deficiency of growth hormone in children Prader-Willi syndrome	Changes in blood sugar levels, headache, muscle weakness, transient edema	ACTH, glucocorticoids, adrenocorticoids
somatropin (DNA recombinant)	Humatrope Genotropin Omnitrope	0.06 mg/kg IM/SC 3 × per wk Varies	Pediatric patients with growth failure		insulin
sermorelin	Geref	0.03 mg/kg SC hs daily	Deficiency of growth hormone		None indicated
Growth Hormone Inhibitor					
octreotide	Sandostatin	50 mcg tid SC, IV	Inhibit rapid or excessive growth	Sinus bradycardia, diarrhea, headache, cardiac dysrhythmias, changes in blood glucose levels	sulfonylurea, antidiabetic medications, insulin, glucagon
Adrenocortical Hormones					
corticotropin	Acthar, ACTH	Varies with patient IM, SC, IV	Diagnostic testing	Insomnia, acne, abdominal stress, delayed wound healing, increased susceptibility to infection	amphotericin, insulin, oral hypoglycemics, digoxin, diuretics, potassium supplements, live virus vaccines
cosyntropin	Cortrosyn	Varies with patient IM, IV			
Thyroid-Stimulating Hormone					
thyrotropin alfa	Thyrogen, Thyropar	4-14 IU/day, SC or IM	Diagnostic testing and treatment of thyroid cancer	Headache, nausea, bradycardia, CHF, menstrual irregularities, anaphylaxis	No major interactions
POSTERIOR PITUITARY GLAND					
Antidiuretic Hormone					
vasopressin	Pitressin	Varies SC, IM, IV, intranasally	Diabetes insipidus, acute massive hemorrhage	Abdominal pain and distress, nausea and vomiting, headache, chest pain, confusion	carbamazepine, lithium, chlorpropamide, clofibrate, norepinephrine
desmopressin	DDAVP	Varies po, nasal spray	Diabetes insipidus, primary nocturnal enuresis		None noted
lypressin	Diapid	1-2 sprays in each nostril qid	Diabetes insipidus, primary nocturnal enuresis		None noted

ACTH, Adrenocorticotropic hormone; *CHF*, congestive heart failure; *IM*, intramuscular; *IV*, intravenous; *SC*, subcutaneous.

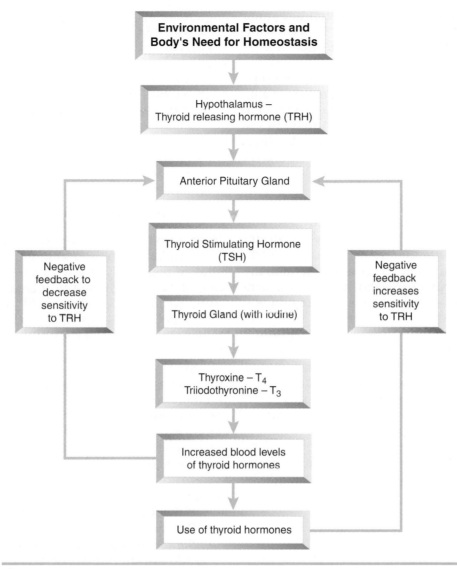

Figure 21-5 The relationship between the thyroid gland hormones and homeostasis.

Thyroid Gland Hormones

The thyroid gland, located in the anterior neck, is the largest of the glands consisting of two lobes on either side of the larynx. TSH (thyroid-stimulating hormone), secreted by the anterior pituitary gland, controls the secretion of T_3 and T_4. The three hormones secreted are (1) thyroxine (T_4), (2) triiodothyronine (T_3), and (3) calcitonin (see Figure 21-5).

T_3 and T_4 do the following:

- Stimulate protein synthesis.
- Increase blood sugar levels.
- Decrease serum cholesterol levels.
- Increase metabolism for the production of heat and energy.
- Enable normal mental development and normal growth.

- Require iodine for production. Diets deficient in iodine lead to **goiter,** as the thyroid gland enlarges to try to adjust to the lack of iodine.

Hyposecretion may be caused by glandular destruction from radiation therapy, lack of iodine, surgical removal of the thyroid, or pituitary dysfunction. The signs of hyposecretion of T_3 and T_4 are weight gain, slowed metabolism, sluggishness, constantly feeling cold, and loss of concentration. When hormone secretions are suppressed, cretinism, found in infants and children, and myxedema in adults occurs. Cretinism can be avoided by testing infants for thyroid function.

Oral thyroid replacements may be extracted from the endocrine glands of animals or be synthetically prepared. The two hormones, T_3 and T_4, or a combination of the two, may be used with the dose gradually adjusted for the individual's needs for lifelong therapy.

Thyroid hormones are approved for supplemental or replacement needs of hypothyroidism. These medications are not indicated or approved for the treatment of obesity, although they do affect metabolism. Doses that would be necessary for weight reduction could produce life-threatening cardiovascular effects.

- Thyroid hormones are usually initiated in small doses and are individualized until adequate response is reached. The physiologic effect of overdose is hyperthyroidism, with symptoms of psychotic behavior, diarrhea, increased blood pressure and heart rates, and cardiovascular reactions such as angina attacks.
- Long-term overuse of thyroxine has been associated with **osteoporosis** in postmenopausal women. Thyroxine is contraindicated in patients who have had a myocardial infarction.
- Thyroid replacement therapy may exacerbate DM, leading to an increased requirement for insulin or oral hypoglycemics.
- Thyroid replacement medications do not readily cross the placenta, so their use in pregnancy does not affect fetal development (Table 21-2).

 CLINICAL TIP

Patients with diabetes taking thyroid medications and insulin/oral hypoglycemics should be watched closely. Discontinuing thyroid medication when taking hypoglycemics may lead to severe hypoglycemic reactions because thyroid replacement medications tend to increase blood sugar levels.

Estrogen therapy may increase the amount of thyroid hormone needed because estrogens increase the binding proteins that tie up circulating hormones, thereby decreasing the amount available at the target tissues.

Patient Education for Compliance

1. Thyroid replacement therapy is lifelong therapy. The patient should not discontinue the medication without consulting a physician.
2. When counseling patients who are beginning thyroid replacement therapy, inform them that it should be

Patient Education for Compliance—cont'd

taken in the morning (on an empty stomach) to avoid insomnia resulting from the increased metabolism.
3. Palpitations, nervousness, and headaches may be signs of toxicity.
4. Iodized salt is an excellent source of the iodine needed for proper thyroid function.

Antithyroid Medications

Hypersecretion of thyroid hormones may be the result of tumors or autoimmune diseases such as Graves' disease. Excessive secretions and circulation of T_3 and T_4 result in increased cell metabolism, weakness, anxiety, and heat production. Treatment is with antithyroid medications, irradiation of the thyroid gland, or surgical removal of the tissue.

Antithyroid medications interfere with the synthesis of thyroid hormones. Iodine or iodide ions, radioactive iodine, and thionamide derivatives are the drugs of choice for antithyroid therapy. These agents will cross the placenta and stop fetal thyroid development and cross into breast milk to affect the infant.

- Iodine medications may be given to inhibit thyroid hormones by saturating the thyroid gland. This decreases the vascularity of the thyroid gland and is often used as preoperative preparation to thyroid surgery to decrease the risk of hemorrhage.
- Radioactive iodine, iodine 131 (^{131}I), may be used to treat thyroid hypersecretion because it destroys the tissue of the thyroid gland (see Table 21-2).

Patient Education for Compliance

1. Patients receiving radioactive iodine should be taught the necessary precautions for radioactive isotopes and their dangers.
2. Propylthiouracil should be taken at regular intervals around the clock.
3. Iodine solutions should be diluted in fruit juices or beverages to make them palatable.
4. A brassy taste, a burning sensation in the mouth, and soreness of gums and teeth are signs of excessive iodine and should be reported to the physician immediately.

TABLE 21-2 Select Drugs Used as Agents of the Thyroid and Parathyroid Glands

GENERIC NAME	TRADE NAME	USUAL ADULT DOSE, ROUTE, AND FREQUENCY OF ADMINISTRATION	INDICATIONS FOR USE	MAJOR SIDE EFFECTS	DRUG INTERACTIONS
SYNTHETIC THYROID REPLACEMENT†					
levothyroxine (T₄)	Levothroid	0.1-0.2 mg/day po	Hypothyroidism	Weight loss, tremors, nervousness, headaches, sweating, exophthalmos, insomnia	cholestyramine, lithium, chlorpromazine, imipramine, anticoagulants
liothyronine (T₃)	Cytomel, Synthroid, Euthroid	0.25-1 mg/day po			
liotrix (T₃, T₄)	Thyrolar	60-120 mg/day po			
thyroglobulin (T₃, T₄)	Proloid	60-120 mg/day po			
NATURAL THYROID REPLACEMENT					
desiccated thyroid (T₃, T₄)	Armour thyroid	60-120 mg/day po	Hypothyroidism		Same as for synthetic thyroid
ANTITHYROID PREPARATIONS					
thionamide derivatives, propylthiouracil	Propyl-Thyracil	300-400 mg/day po initial; 100-150 mg/day po maintenance	Hyperthyroidism	Rashes, nauseas and vomiting, myalgia, stomach pain, fever, increased bleeding tendencies	anticoagulants, digitalis, ¹³¹I
methimazole	Tapazole	15-60 mg/day po initial; 5-15 mg/day po maintenance			Same as above
¹³¹I—RAI	Iodotope	4-10 millicuries po, IV			Same except ¹³¹I
CALCITONIN					
calcitonin salmon	Calcimar, Miacalcin	IM/SC nasal spray	100 U/day IM/SC; 1 spray/day in alternating nostrils	Basically no side effects and no interactions	
PARATHYROID GLAND MEDICATIONS					
teriparatide	Forteo	20 mcg/day SC	Osteoporosis, for those at high risk for fractures	Dizziness, headache, depression, hypertension, arthralgia, nausea/vomiting, diarrhea	digoxin

IM, Intramuscular; IV, intravenous; SC, subcutaneous.

Calcitonin

Calcitonin is secreted by the thyroid gland, but calcium levels in the blood are also regulated by parathyroid hormone. Calcitonin and parathyroid hormone work together to ensure an adequate supply of calcium for neuromuscular and endocrine function. Calcitonin salmon, while not preventing osteoporosis, has the same effects as human calcitonin and is safer for the treatment of osteoporosis in postmenopausal women. Calcium and vitamin D intake must be adequate for calcitonin salmon to be effective. Calcitonin salmon is administered by a nasal spray with a metered dose application. No interactions with other medications occur (see Table 21-2).

Patient Education for Compliance

Teach patients how to activate the metered dose pump for the nasal spray of calcitonin salmon. The spray should be refrigerated between uses.

Parathyroid Hormone

The parathyroid secretes parathyroid hormone (PTH), which in cooperation with calcitonin regulates calcium levels in the blood. When the blood levels of calcium decrease, PTH acts on the bone and kidney cells to release calcium. New bone cell development is reduced, and old bone is dissolved to maintain calcium homeostasis. One drug, teriparatide (Forteo), which is a parathyroid hormone, is used with postmenopausal women and men with osteoporosis who are at high risk for fractures (see Table 21-2).

Corticosteroids/Steroids

The adrenal glands are located directly over each kidney and are composed of two parts: an outer portion called the *cortex* that secretes a number of hormones that are essential for life including cortisone, hydrocortisone, aldosterone, and deoxycorticosterone. An inner portion, called the *medulla* (see Figure 21-1), secretes epinephrine and norepinephrine and is considered part of the sympathetic nervous system. The hormones of the adrenal cortex are activated by adrenocorticotropic hormone from the anterior pituitary gland. The most important function of the adrenal cortex hormones is the regulation of water and salt metabolism, regulation of carbohydrate metabolism, and production of antiinflammatory effects. The terms *adrenocorticosteroids, corticosteroids,* and *steroids* all refer to the same natural or synthetic substances that may be grouped as mineralocorticoids, glucocorticoids, or mixed steroids.

Adrenal Cortex Hormones

The adrenal cortex has three levels. The outer level secretes **mineralocorticoids,** and the middle level secretes **glucocorticoids.** (The inner layer secretes small amounts of male and female sex hormones). Like all tropic hormones, ACTH is regulated by the hypothalamus, which is influenced by the sleep-wake cycle, negative feedback, and stress. More corticotropin is available during the wake period to regulate body metabolism. Negative feedback inhibits the release of corticotropin, keeping cortisol levels relatively constant day to day. As stress rises in the body, corticotropin stimulates the secretion of cortisol to increase the body's ability to cope with stress from exercise, infections, anxiety, surgery, and so on.

Glucocorticoids regulate the metabolism of proteins and carbohydrates, particularly when the body is under stress.

- With therapeutic use, the glucocorticoids cause retention of sodium, which leads to water retention throughout the body and possible hypertension.

- Glucocorticoids are potent antiinflammatory agents and are used in acute and chronic inflammatory processes including organ transplants.
- The steroids are also used for collagen disorders, dermatologic conditions, and hematologic, ophthalmic, respiratory, and rheumatic disorders.
- Glucocorticoids may be administered orally, intramuscularly, intraarticularly, intravenously, topically, or by inhalation, for either local or systemic effect. Preparations for intramuscular use have repository actions that allow the drug to be released slowly from the muscle for a longer duration of action. Therapeutic doses vary widely and must be adjusted to meet the needs of each patient.
- The adverse effects include damage to joint tissue when used intraarticularly too often.
- Long-term use will lead to cushingoid symptoms such as fatigue, weakness, edema, "moon face," "pot belly," "buffalo hump," and excessive hair growth.
- After long-term or high-dose steroid therapy, cessation of steroid use must be done slowly and in small decrements.
- Steroids are used with caution in patients with gastrointestinal ulcers or colitis, renal disease, herpes simplex, and emotional instability and are contraindicated in patients with systemic fungal infections, tuberculosis, and local viral infections.
- Ocular use over long periods of time may lead to glaucoma and cataracts.
- Live virus vaccines may not be effective while the patient is taking steroids and could even put the patient at risk for developing infections.
- Infections and infectious diseases may advance at an alarming rate because steroids suppress the inflammatory response in the body.
- The drug interactions are numerous and are listed in Table 21-3.

Administration of Steroids

Steroids are given in two unique ways:

1. Alternate-day therapy (ADT) is used to reduce or eliminate the adverse reactions of the drug. The short-acting medicine is given every other day in the morning, with its effects persisting into the second day, when the body's adrenal gland functions by negative feedback. On the following day, the medication is given again. This

TABLE 21-3 *Common Drug Interactions Associated with Glucocorticoids*

INTERACTIVE MEDICATIONS	POSSIBLE RESPONSE
amphotericin B	Potentiates hypokalemia
digitalis	Possible digitalis toxicity
diuretics	Potential for hypokalemia, decreased therapeutic effect of diuretics
antibiotics, macrolides	Increased clearance of drug from bloodstream
anticoagulants	Increased chance of thrombosis by inhibiting anticoagulants
insulin, oral hypoglycemics	Increased requirements of medication for diabetes mellitus, increased blood glucose levels
isoniazid	Increased doses of isoniazid
oral contraceptive, estrogen	Increase steroids, drugs inhibit the steroid metabolism
phenobarbital, phenytoin, rifampin	Increase steroids due to the enhanced metabolism of steroids
antacids	Decreased steroid absorption

routine allows the person's adrenal gland to function, and there are fewer adverse reactions.
2. Declining or decreasing dosage so that the body receives a therapeutic dose more rapidly, and then the amount is tapered off. Usually the drug is given in 2-day increments, although this may change, with individual dosing for specific conditions. Depending on the increments and the total dosage, the dosage declines by a tablet per day or so until the total dose has been given.

Table 21-4 lists typical steroid/corticosteroid medications and their drug form. Topical steroids used for dermatologic conditions are found in Table 21-5. Over-the-counter (OTC) glucocorticoid preparations for topical use usually contain 0.5% to 1% hydrocortisone.

Mineralocorticoids regulate blood levels of sodium and potassium.

- These drugs increase the rate of sodium and reabsorption by the kidney causing sodium and water retention and loss of potassium.
- The most important mineralocorticoid is aldosterone, which acts on the distal tubules of the nephrons of the kidneys.
- Mineralocorticoids are usually administered in conjunction with glucocorticosteroids for

TABLE 21-4 *Select Drugs Used as Steroids/Corticosteroids*

GENERIC NAME	TRADE NAME	USUAL ADULT DOSE, ROUTE, AND FREQUENCY OF ADMINISTRATION	INDICATIONS FOR USE	MAJOR SIDE EFFECTS	DRUG INTERACTIONS
GLUCOSTEROIDS					
cortisone acetate	Cortistan, Cortone	Varies; individualized doses po, IM	Allergies, body stress, replacement therapy, antiinflammatory agents, leukemia, pruritus	Insomnia, mood changes, personality changes	See Table 21-3
hydrocortisone	Cortisol, Cortef	Varies po, topical, IM, IV, enema			
hydrocortisone sodium succinate	Solu-Cortef	Varies IM, IV			
prednisolone	Cortolone, Delta Cortef	Varies po			
	Orapred	Oral disintegrating tablet	Use with pediatric patients		
methylprednisolone	Medrol	Varies po			
methylprednisolone acetate	Depo-Medrol	Varies IM	Same as above and bursitis		
methylprednisolone sodium succinate	Solu-Medrol	Varies IM, IV			
paramethasone	Haldrone	Varies po			
betamethasone	Celestone	Varies po			
dexamethasone	Decadron	Varies po, IM, IV	Same as above and prior to radiation, chemotherapy		
prednisone	Deltasone	Varies po	Same as indication above for glucosteroids and multiple sclerosis		
prednisone acetate	Predcor	Varies, po			

Generic	Trade	Route/Dosage	Use	Adverse Reactions	Interactions
prednicarbate	Dermatop	Topical	Contact dermatitis		
triamcinolone	Aristocort, Kenacort	po, topical, gingival	Same as oral lesions		
fluocinolone	Synalar	Topical	Contact dermatitis		
flurandrenolide ointment	Cordran	Topical			
clobetasol	Olux-E Foam	Topical	Antiinflammatory, antipruritic in topical dermatitis except rosacea or perioral dermatitis		
desonide	Verdeso Foam, Desonate Gel	Topical	Mild to moderate atopic dermatitis		
beclomethasone	Flovent, Vanceril, Beclovent, Azmacort	Inhaled	Asthma, bronchitis		
fluticasone	Flonase, Beconase		Rhinitis		
MINERALOCORTICOIDS					
deoxycorticosterone acetate	DOCA acetate, Percorten acetate	Varies IM	edema, weakness, hypertension		digitalis, diuretics
fludrocortisone	Florinef	Varies po	Addison's disease		
INHIBITORS OF CORTICOSTEROIDS					
aminoglutethimide	Cytadren	250 mg bid-tid po	Cushing's syndrome	Nausea, headache, fever, drowsiness, dizziness, muscle pain	dexamethasone
trilostane	Modrastane	30 mg qid po			

TABLE 21-5 *Examples of Over-the-Counter Steroid Preparations*

NAME OF PRODUCT	FORM OF MEDICATION
Cortaid	Cream, ointment, lotion, spray
Preparation H with hydrocortisone	Cream
Lanacort	Cream, ointment
Aloe Gel HC (*Aloe vera* and hydrocortisone)	Gel
Caldecort	Ointment, spray, rectal foam
Gynecort, Cortef Feminine	Cream
Bactine HC	Cream

replacement therapy in adrenocortical insufficiency with resulting Addison's disease.

- One of the main uses of steroids is long-term replacement therapy for the hormone-deficient patient (see Table 21-4).
- *Adrenal steroid inhibitors* suppress adrenal cortex function in malignancies of the adrenal gland or other adrenal hyperplasias. The preferred therapy is irradiation of the pituitary gland; the medications are used temporarily until the radiation therapy is effective. The adverse reactions are cardiovascular irregularities and liver dysfunction. Precocious sexual development occurs in males, and females acquire masculine features (see Table 21-4).

Patient Education for Compliance

1. Before medical or dental procedures, the health care professional should be informed that steroids are being taken because of bleeding, altered healing processes, and altered response to infection.
2. Watch for salt and water retention such as weight gain and edema of the feet and lower legs when taking steroids.
3. Do not stop taking steroid medications abruptly unless directed by the prescriber.
4. Reduce the intake of sodium-rich foods and increase the intake of potassium-rich foods when using steroid preparations.
5. Nonprescription medications should not be taken with steroids without consulting a physician or pharmacist because of the numerous drug interactions.
6. Topical steroid preparations should be used only on affected areas and sparingly to minimize possible systemic absorption.

IMPORTANT FACTS ABOUT CORTICOSTEROIDS/ STEROIDS

- Steroids may be administered orally, parenterally, topically, by inhalation, or by local injection.
- Glucocorticoids influence the metabolism of fats, carbohydrates, and proteins and affect skeletal muscles, the cardiovascular system, the immune system, and the central nervous system.
- Aldosterone, the major mineralocorticoid, acts on the kidney to promote the retention of sodium and water and allows the excretion of potassium.
- Excessive doses of steroids can cause cushingoid symptoms and Cushing's disease.
- Adrenal insufficiency is known as *Addison's disease.*
- When used in low doses for replacement therapy, steroids are therapeutic. Conversely, when used chronically for pharmacologic needs in nonendocrine diseases, the drugs have severe adverse effects.
- Glucocorticoids are used to reduce inflammatory and immune system responses such as arthritis, allergic disorders, asthma, cancer, and suppression of organ transplant rejection.
- When used with NSAIDs, steroids increase the risk of peptic ulcers.
- Steroids can increase the risk of toxic effects from digoxin.

Drugs Used as Hypoglycemics

The pancreas secretes two hormones, insulin and glucagon, that regulate the metabolism of protein, fat, and especially carbohydrates. A cluster of cells known as the **islet of Langerhans** produces insulin, which acts as the key to open body cells to glucose. Insulin and glucagon allow cells to receive an adequate supply of glucose for body fuel by regulating the blood glucose level. Insulin has three distinct purposes: (1) It aids in the utilization of glucose as energy; (2) it prompts the storage of excess glucose as glycogen in the liver; and (3) it is responsible for the conversion of glucose to fat. Insulin decreases blood glucose levels, but when the level becomes too low, glucagon stimulates the breakdown of glycogen to increase the circulating glucose.

Diabetes Mellitus

The most common disease involving the pancreas as an endocrine gland is DM. This disease is the sixth leading cause of death in the United States, affecting about 16 million Americans with between 90% and 95% of cases of diabetes having adult onset. The person with DM has a disorder of carbohydrate metabolism that involves insulin deficiency, insulin resistance, or both. These three metabolic disorders lead to hyperglycemia. Most authorities today believe that any abnormal level of pancreatic function may lead to DM, either type 1 (T1DM) or type 2 (T2DM) (Table 21-6). Patients with T1DM diabetes have very little or no endogenous insulin and require exogenous insulin for survival. With T1DM, the person seems to have a genetic abnormality with autoimmune destruction of the beta cells of the islet of Langerhans. T2DM diabetes usually is maturity onset, although recent research shows a rise in the disease in obese children. The patient has some insulin function with the production being low or the secretions of the beta cells insufficient to meet the needs of the individual. T2DM may be the result of aging, improper diet, or genetic factors that lead to insulin resistance. The classic signs of T1DM and T2DM are hyperglycemia, **polydipsia, polyphagia,** and **polyuria.**

Those obese persons with insulin resistance may be prone to metabolic syndrome, a cluster of conditions that occur together increasing the risk for heart disease, stroke, and diabetes. Having one of the four conditions found in the syndrome - obesity around the waist, hypertension, hyperglycemia, and hyperlipidemia - increases the risk for serious disease. In combination, the risk is even greater and the person having one of the factors is more likely to have the others. A family history of T2DM with insulin resistance or a history of gestational diabetes increases the likelihood of the disease.

Insulin resistance is the loss of insulin activity as a result of either a defect in the insulin receptor site or of failure of insulin receptor-directed metabolism. Insulin resistance is often a precursor to full-blown DM. The body keeps secreting more and more insulin that is not used, until finally the pancreas ceases production and the person has diabetes.

Another concern is that certain medications increase blood glucose levels and cause hyperglycemia in the prediabetic person. These drugs include glucocorticoids such as prednisone, thiazide diuretics such as hydrochlorthiazide (Hydro-Diuril), and epinephrine.

Treatment of Diabetes Mellitus

Treatment for DM includes dietary adjustment to limit carbohydrates ingested and the control of the use of glucose by consistent exercise and drug control. The drugs for DM are in three categories: insulins, oral hypoglycemics, and drugs that affect glucose absorption or production including new drugs for adjunct therapy. The adjunct medications increase the effectiveness of other hypoglycemic agents. The insulins and sulfonylureas are hypoglycemic medications that decrease blood glucose levels. The antidiabetic medications delay absorption of glucose in the diet and inhibit glucose produced in the liver

TABLE 21-6 *Comparison of Types 1 and 2 Diabetes Mellitus*

	TYPE 1 (T1DM)	TYPE 2 (T1DM)
Former name	IDDM, juvenile-onset diabetes, Type 1 DM	NIDDM, adult-onset diabetes, Type 2 DM
Usual age of onset	Childhood/adolescence	Usually >40 yr
Onset speed	Rapid	Gradual
Family history	Usually negative	Frequently positive
Predominance	5%-10% of people with diabetes	90%-95% of people with diabetes
Etiology	Autoimmune process	Unknown; strongly familial
Primary cause	Loss of insulin secretion	Insulin resistance or decreased insulin
Insulin secreted	None in later stages	Levels may be low, normal, or high (resistance)
Ketosis	Common	Uncommon
Symptoms	Polyuria, polyphagia, polydipsia, weight loss	May be asymptomatic
Body	Thin/undernourished	Frequently obese
Blood glucose levels	Fluctuate in response to body activities and illness	More stable
Treatment	Insulin replacement, diet, and exercise	Exercise and reduced caloric intake; in some cases, oral hypoglycemics or even insulin

IDDM, Insulin-dependent diabetes mellitus; *NIDDM,* non-insulin-dependent diabetes mellitus.

to lower blood glucose levels, especially the post-prandial blood glucose levels. Persons with T1DM must administer exogenous insulin for life and must adjust their diets and exercise. Patients with T2DM secrete some endogenous insulin, and diet alone may control the elevated serum glucose levels. Many do not adhere to the dietary controls, or diet alone may be insufficient; for those persons with T2DM, an oral hypoglycemic or an antidiabetic drug may be ordered.

When too much insulin secreted or sufficient glucagon is not available, the body cells will use the available glucose and the serum glucose level drops, precipitating a hypoglycemic reaction. Table 21-7 compares the signs and symptoms of hypoglycemia and hyperglycemia, important factors in patient teaching.

TABLE 21-7 *Comparison of Signs and Symptoms of Hypoglycemia and Hyperglycemia*

	HYPOGLYCEMIA/ INSULIN SHOCK	HYPERGLYCEMIA/ DIABETIC COMA
Onset	Sudden	Gradual
Skin	Pale, moist	Flushed, dry
Tongue	Moist	Dry
Breath	No change	Fruity odor (acetone smell)
Thirst	None	Intense
Respirations	Shallow	Deep
Vomiting	Rare	Common
Pulse	Fast, bounding	Fast, weak
Urine	No glucose/acetone	Positive for glucose/ acetone
Serum glucose	↓ 50 mg/dL	↑ 200 mg/dL
Blood pressure	Normal	Low
Abdominal pain	Common. acute	None

Administration of Insulin in Type 1 Diabetes Mellitus

One function of the allied health professional who works with persons with diabetes may be teaching self-administration of insulin. Teaching good aseptic techniques and how to administer the exact amount of insulin to be given according to the physician's orders is an important function in this area. The allied health professional has a responsibility to ensure the patient can effectively administer insulin as ordered. (See Chapter 15 for the parenteral administration of medications.)

T1DM requires insulin to be replaced by injection because insulin is inactivated in the digestive tract when taken by mouth. The forms of insulin differ with respect to their time and course of action, route of administration, and source. Insulin is usually given by subcutaneous or intramuscular injection using an insulin syringe (Figure 21-6). Regular insulin may be administered intravenously in emergencies or illnesses in which immediate insulin action is necessary. Illnesses, trauma, and stress increase blood glucose levels, and thus higher doses of insulin may be required to keep the person in homeostasis. The dosage of insulin is individualized and may change over time depending on changes in the person's life.

Human recombinant insulin is less antigenic than animal insulins used in the past and is the preferred insulin medication today. Because of the protein differences in the types of insulin, changing from one insulin preparation to another requires dosage adjustments. Patients should be sure that they do not interchange the types. The terms *Iletin* and *purified* indicate an animal derivative, whereas *Humulin*, *Novolin*, and *Lantus* are DNA recombinant derivatives. *Humalog* is a modified human derivative.

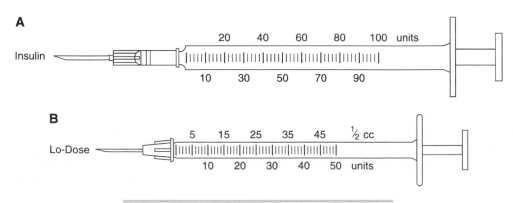

Figure 21-6 **A,** U100 syringe. **B,** Lo-Dose syringe.

The commercial insulin preparations produce similar effects in the body but vary in time for **action onset,** time to **action peak,** and **duration.** The six types of insulin are (1) lispro (Humalog) and glulisine (Apidra), (2) regular, (3) isophane (NPH), (4) Lente, (5) Ultralente, and (6) glargine (Lantus) and detemir (Levimir) insulins (Table 21-8) (Figure 21-7).

Two processes have been used to prolong insulin's effects: adding a protein to natural insulin and altering natural insulin by adding zinc. A graph of action has been added to assist with understanding how the types of insulin interact throughout the day (Figure 21-8).

- *Lispro* (Humalog) and *glulisine* (Apidra) insulin are rapid-acting insulins with effects beginning within 5 minutes of administration and lasting 2 to 4 hours.
  - This type of insulin is administered just before eating.
  - The person must eat within 15 minutes of taking lispro insulin or be in danger of a hypoglycemic reaction.
  - With glulisine, the medication may be taken 15 minutes prior to eating or 20 minutes after starting a meal.
  - Another important action of these medications is that it better prevents the rapid elevation in blood glucose levels immediately after eating.
  - Unlike other insulins, lispro is not available OTC but requires a prescription.
- *Regular* (insulin R) insulin is a clear solution that may be given intravenously in an emergency or subcutaneously or intramuscularly on a regular basis.
  - It has a rapid onset (30 to 60 minutes) and a short duration of action.
  - Regular insulin is stable for 2 to 4 weeks at room temperature and does not have to be refrigerated if used in that time period.
  - Exposure of the medication to sunlight or heat must be avoided.
- *Isophane* (NPH; insulin N) insulin has the addition of a large protamine molecule to decrease the solubility of the insulin and prolong its absorption time.
  - The action is delayed, and the duration of action is extended, so the drug is given one to two times daily.
  - Because protamine is a foreign protein, allergic reactions to the medication are possible.
  - This medication is a suspension that requires the particles to be mixed with the solvent prior to administration.
- *Lantus* (glargine) and *detemir* (Levemir) insulins are synthetic, long-acting 24-hour insulins

TABLE 21-8 *Course of Action of Insulin Preparations*

INSULIN TYPE	LETTER/BOTTLE	ONSET	PEAK	DURATION
QUICK-ACTING				
Lispro-Humalog	Lispro H	5 min	½-1 hr	2-4 hr
glulisine	Apidra			
SHORT-ACTING				
Regular insulin	R	½-1 hr	2-4 hr	5-7 hr
INTERMEDIATE-ACTING				
isophane insulin (NPH)	N	1-2 hr	6-12 hr	18-24 hr
Lente insulin	L	1-2 hr	6-12 hr	18-24 hr
LONG-ACTING				
Ultralente insulin	U	4-6 hr	16-18 hr	20-36 hr
Lantus		Lasts for 24 hr with no evident peak and duration to last to next injection; a once-per-day insulin preparation		
detemir, DNA	Levemir	Lasts up to 24 hr		
COMBINATIONS				
NPH/regular mixtures, 70/30, 50/50, 75/25		½ hr	7-12 hr	16-24 hr

NPH, Neutral protamine Hagedorn.

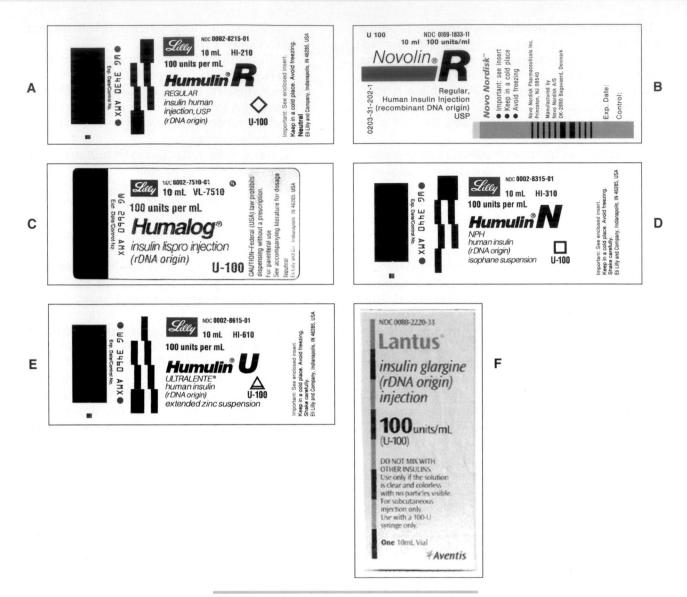

Figure 21-7 Labels for different types of insulin.

that do not show an evident peak but maintain continuous hypoglycemic action for persons with T1DM and some T2DM when given every 24 hours.

- Lantus insulin should be clear and should be discarded if cloudiness appears.
- Neither of these insulins should be mixed with any other type of insulin.
- This medication should be taken daily at bedtime with recent literature stating it may require twice-daily dosing.
- Insulin detemir should be discarded if it appears cloudy.
- The chance of nocturnal hypoglycemia is less with detemir than with NPH insulin.

- **Lente and Ultralente insulins** are prepared by adding zinc to regular insulin to prolong the action.
  - Ultralente insulin has large insulin crystals that dissolve slowly, giving Ultralente a long duration of action.
  - Lente insulin is composed of 70% Ultralente and 30% Semilente insulin. This compound has an intermediate duration of action.
  - The Lente insulins are relatively allergy-free because no protein has been added.

Table 21-9 lists the drugs commonly used as hypoglycemics, including the new insulin products

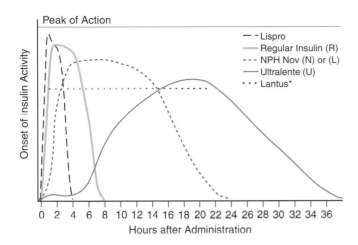

Figure 21-8 Peak times of various types of insulin.

that are inhaled. Boxes 21-1 and 21-2 list drug interactions with insulin and oral hypoglycemic agents.

Mixing Insulins for Treatment

Many times treatment for the person with diabetes requires the mixing of two different insulin preparations such as regular insulin with NPH insulin. It is preferable to mix the solutions rather than inject the two medications separately. Specific guidelines are used for mixing the insulins:

- Regular insulin can be used with any insulin but Lispro. When drawing two types of insulin, regular insulin should be drawn into the syringe first to avoid the possibility of contaminating the regular insulin with other types.
- Lispro insulin is made by Eli Lilly Company, and it may be mixed with other Lilly products such as Humulin-U or Humulin-N. As with regular insulin, lispro insulin should be drawn into the syringe first.
  - Insulin detemir should not be mixed with any other insulins or solutions.
  - Isophane insulin is compatible with regular insulin and with lispro when mixed with the Lilly products.
  - Some insulins come premixed, or the person may prepare the mixture. Mixtures of regular and isophane insulin such as 70/30 (70% isophane [NPH] and 30% regular insulin) are relatively stable (Figure 21-9).
  - Premixed lispro insulin (Humalog) and regular insulin (Humulin R) based on specific percentage of 75/25 is available and is stable at room temperature.
- Lente insulins may be mixed with each other or with regular insulin. When mixed together, no change in time of onset or duration occurs. When Lente is mixed with regular insulin, the zinc alters the regular insulin, delaying and prolonging its actions. These combinations should be injected immediately.
- Lantus insulin may not be mixed with any other solutions or types of insulin.

Insulin Delivery Systems

New methods of insulin delivery have been introduced as an alternative to the traditional syringe-plus-needle delivery system. Insulin pens, the size of a large fountain pen (Figure 21-10), are convenient and flexible but more expensive than the traditional syringe and vial. They incorporate a cartridge of insulin containing 300 units rather than using a vial; some pens are completely disposable. The pens are simple to use: dial the dose for a quick, easy, and accurate amount of insulin. The problem with this method is that the patient must take two injections if the needed dosage is not available as premixed percentages. The pen is pressed against the skin at the injection site, and the insulin is administered by pressing the button on the top of the pen.

Jet injectors deliver insulin by creating enough pressure to "spray" the insulin through the skin into the subcutaneous tissue without using a needle. These injectors are expensive and cause stinging and pain. Bruising may occur in people with little subcutaneous tissue such as children, thin adults, and the elderly.

Portable insulin pumps, approximately the size of a pager or cell phone (Figure 21-11), are computerized devices that deliver a continuous, regulated dose of insulin. Insulin is delivered under the skin through a tiny needle or cannula in the abdomen; the needle should be replaced and moved to a new site every 1 to 3 days. The pump delivers a continuous insulin trickle—an amount that mimics the secretions of the pancreas. The patient may also self-administer **boluses** of insulin before meals to cover the food eaten. External pumps cost about $3000 to $5000, with another $300 per month for supplies, making them too expensive for most people.

Implantable insulin pumps are surgically implanted into the abdomen, usually on the left side, to deliver insulin either intraperitoneally or intravenously. Like the external pump, it delivers

Text continued on page 427

TABLE 21-9 Drugs Used as Hypoglycemics and Hyperglycemics

GENERIC NAME	TRADE NAME	USUAL ADULT DOSE, ROUTE, AND FREQUENCY OF ADMINISTRATION	INDICATIONS	DRUG INTERACTIONS
INJECTABLE INSULIN			T1DM, and some T2DM that is resistant to oral hypoglycemics	Box 21-1
				Not to be used with smokers, asthma, COPD
Short-Acting				
lispro	Humalog, Novalog	Individualized, SC, 15 min prior to meal		
glulisine	Apidra	Individualized, SC, 15 min ac or 20 min after starting meal		
regular insulin	Iletin I (beef/pork), Iletin II (pork). Humulin R (human), Novolin R (human)	IM, IV; 30-60 min prior to meals		
Intermediate-Acting				
isophane (NPH) insulin	Humulin N (human), Novolin N (human)	Daily, SC, individualized		
lente insulin	Humulin L (human), Novolin L (human)	Daily, SC, individualized		
Long-Acting				
ultralente insulin	Humulin U, Ultralente	Daily, individualized, SC		
glargine insulin	Lantus	Individualized up to bid, SC; if qd take in pm	T1DM and T2DM, long-acting insulin	
detemir insulin	Leremir			
Mixtures				
NPH/R 70/30 insulin	Humulin 70/30, Novolin 70/30	Daily, individualized, SC		
NPH/R 50/50 insulin	Humulin 50/50 Pen	SC		
NPH/R 75/25 insulin	Novolin 75/25 Pen	SC		
lispro/regular 75/25	Humalog/Humulin R 75/25	SC		

MAJOR SIDE EFFECTS OF INJECTABLE INSULIN: Hypoglycemia.

GENERIC NAME	TRADE NAME	USUAL ADULT DOSE, ROUTE, AND FREQUENCY OF ADMINISTRATION	INDICATIONS	DRUG INTERACTIONS
INHALED INSULIN				
Rapid-Acting–(r-DNA)	Exubera	ī to īī puffs 10 min ac	T1DM or T2DM	Same as with injectable insulin

MAJOR SIDE EFFECTS OF INHALED INSULIN: Coughing, SOB, sore throat, dry mouth.

ORAL ANTIDIABETIC MEDICATIONS

Sulfonylureas				
First-Generation			T2DM	See Box 21-2
tolbutamide	Orinase	250-2000 mg/day, po		
acetohexamide	Dymelor	250-750 mg/day, po		
tolazamide	Tolinase	250-500 mg qAM, po		
Second-Generation				
glipizide	Glucotrol-standard	5-40 mg 30 min ac, po		
	Glucotrol XL	5-20 mg qAM, po		
glyburide nonmicronized	DiaBeta, Micronase	1.25-20 mg/day, po		
micronized	Glynase PresTab	0.75-12 mg/day, po		
glimepiride	Amaryl	1-2 mg, po with breakfast		
Alpha-Glucosidase Inhibitors				
acarbose	Precose	50-100 mg, po with meals		
miglitol	Glyset	25-100 mg po tid		
Biguanides			Some T1DM	Iodine dyes, alcohol, acarbose
metformin	Glucophage	500-1000 mg po qd-tid		
with glyburide	Glucomet	ī-īī tab po qd-bid		
Thiazolidinediones (glitiazones)				Oral contraceptives are reduced by 30% with loss of contraception
rosiglitazone	Avandia	4 mg/day, po		
pioglitazone	Actos	15-30 mg/day, po without regard to meals		
Meglitinides			T2DM diabetes; not for use with T1DM	Large doses of aspirin and ibuprofen; sulfonamides, warfarin, MAOIs, probenecid, oral contraceptives, thyroid preparations, TB medications
nateglinide	Starlix	60-120 mg ac each meal		

(continued)

TABLE 21-9 Drugs Used as Hypoglycemics and Hyperglycemics—cont'd

GENERIC NAME	TRADE NAME	USUAL ADULT DOSE, ROUTE, AND FREQUENCY OF ADMINISTRATION	INDICATIONS	DRUG INTERACTIONS
DPP-4 Inhibitors				
sitagliptin	Januvia	50 mg po bid	TIIDM with diet and exercise	Lanoxin and other oral hypoglycemics except metformin and thiazolidinediones
sitagliptin + metformin	Janumet	50 mg sitagliptin and 500 mg metformin po bid		

MAJOR SIDE EFFECTS OF ORAL ANTIDIABETIC MEDICATIONS: Sulfonylureas: GI irritation, nausea, vomiting, weakness, fatigue, dizziness; **Alpha-Glucosidase Inhibitors:** Flatulence, abdominal distention, diarrhea; **Biguanides:** anorexia and nausea; **Meglitinides:** Hypoglycemia, nausea, vomiting, diarrhea, myalgia, respiratory symptoms, headaches, arthralgia, back pain; **DPP-4 inhibitors:** hypoglycemia, nausea, vomiting, diarrhea, myalgia, respiratory symptoms, headaches, arthralgia, back pain, and respiratory symptoms.

GENERIC NAME	TRADE NAME	USUAL ADULT DOSE, ROUTE, AND FREQUENCY OF ADMINISTRATION	INDICATIONS	DRUG INTERACTIONS
AMYLIN GLP-1 ANALOGS				
Incretin Mimetic				
exenatide	Byetta	5-10 mcg bid SC	Improve glycemic control with T2DM	acetimnophen, ACE inhibitors, digoxin. lovastatin, erythromycin, estrogens, MAOIs, corticosteroids
Synthetic Human Amylin				
pramlintide acetate	Symlin	30-60 mcg qd SC	Improve glycemic control with T1DM and T2DM	Same as for exenatide

MAJOR SIDE EFFECTS OF AMYLIN GLP-1 ANALOGS: Nausea, vomiting, diarrhea, jitteriness, headache, dyspepsia, ↓ appetite.

GENERIC NAME	TRADE NAME	USUAL ADULT DOSE, ROUTE, AND FREQUENCY OF ADMINISTRATION	INDICATIONS	DRUG INTERACTIONS
HYPERGLYCEMICS				
glucagon		0.5-1 mg, SC, IV, IM	Hypoglycemia	diazoxide
diazoxide	Proglycem	1 mg/kg po q8h	Hypoglycemia from hyperinsulinism of pancreatic cancer	Anticoagulants
glucose	Glutose	10-20 g po		Antiepileptics, medications that are used as hypotensives

MAJOR SIDE EFFECTS OF HYPERGLYCEMICS: Constipation, anorexia, nausea, vomiting, abdominal pain, heart conditions.

DM, Diabetes mellitus; IM, intramuscular; IV, intravenous; NPH, Neutral protamine Hagedorn; SC, subcutaneous.

BOX 21-1	DRUGS THAT INTERACT WITH INSULIN

ANTAGONISTIC EFFECT	POTENTIATION
acetazolamide	alcohol
AIDS antivirus	ACE inhibitors
chlorpromazine	anabolic steroids
diazoxide	oral anticoagulants
diltiazem	beta-blockers, propranolol
niacin	chloroquine
nicotine	clofibrate
oral contraceptives	diazoxide
rifampin	fenfluramine
sympathomimetics	lithium
thiazide diuretics	monoamine oxidase (MAO) inhibitors
	metoprolol
Hormones	pantamide
corticotrophin	pyridoxine
estrogens	salicylates
glucagons	tetracyclines
glucocorticoids	sulfinpyrazone
growth hormones	
progestins	
thyroid hormones	

BOX 21-2	DRUGS THAT INTERACT WITH ORAL HYPOGLYCEMIC AGENTS

Antagonists to Sulfonylureas
adrenergic-blocking agent
diazoxide
insulin
monoamine oxidase inhibitors (MAOIs)
alcohol
oral anticoagulants
ranitidine
salicylates
cimetidine
sympatholytics
probenecid
clofibrate
ethacrynic acid
sulfonamides

Antagonists to Carbohydrate Inhibitors
charcoal
digestive enzymes
corticosteroids
alcohol

Potentiators of Sulfonylureas
beta-blocking agents
calcium channel blockers
hormones
steroids
isoniazid
sympathomimetics
alcohol
phenothiazine
phenobarbital
phenytoin
rifampin

Potentiators of Meglitinides
NSAIDs
Sulfonamides
Warfarin sodium
Probenecid
MAOIs
Beta blockers

Antagonists to Meglitinides (especially nateglinide)
Thyroid hormones
Thiazide diuretics
Corticosteroids
Sympathomimetics

a maintenance dose of insulin continuously and boluses may be added as needed. An external telemetry device adjusts insulin delivery. The advantage of this method is that, like the insulin produced naturally in the body by the pancreas, the insulin from the pump goes directly to the liver to prevent excess sugar production. The patient has less hypoglycemia, less weight gain, and an improved quality of life.

An inhaled or pulmonary insulin delivery system is a human form of insulin that is to be used just prior to ingestion of meals for short or rapid-action. Intranasal insulin is a spray, whereas insulin powders are inhaled through the mouth into the lungs, where both rapidly enter the bloodstream. Absorption is similar to or faster than regular insulin, and the duration is longer, although the bioavailability is approximately 10% to 30% of that by injection. Because only 10% of the insulin is absorbed, large doses are required. These systems cannot be used to meet base insulin needs. Longer-acting insulin delivered by injection may still be necessary. The oral powder administration container is approximately the size of a flashlight. These expensive medications given through nasal pathways are irritating to the mucous membranes and cannot be used by smokers or those who have smoked within the past 6 months because of the danger of overdose of insulin. The new medication, Exubera, is approved for adults with either T1DM or T2DM but it is relatively short lived. Recent research has been directed toward long-acting inhaled insulins.

Other clinical research is toward buccal, nasal, and oral insulins. Oralgen will be delivered buccally, and RapidMist with an aerosol delivery system goes directly onto the buccal mucosa. Oral insulin has been difficult to produce because of the breakdown by digestion. The research is based

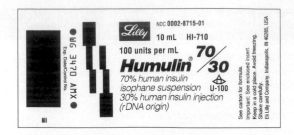

Figure 21-9 Humulin 70/30.

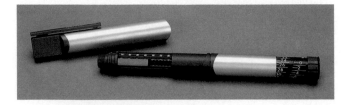

Figure 21-10 Insulin pen.

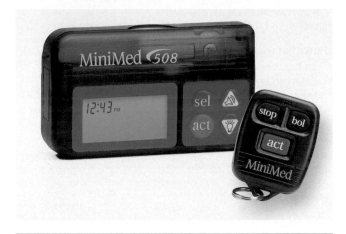

Figure 21-11 Insulin pump. (Courtesy MiniMed Inc., Sylmar, Calif.)

on coating the medication to have increased absorption to provide bioavailability.

The insulin patch is a delivery method under experimentation. Placed on the skin, the patch would provide a continuous low dose of insulin. The patient can adjust the insulin to meet needs at mealtime by pulling a tab to release more insulin. The problems with this system are that insulin is not readily absorbed through the skin and the absorption rate of transdermal medications varies greatly.

Adverse Reactions to Insulin

Insulin is usually well tolerated, although some patients may have allergic reactions. Switching to a different insulin product will usually eliminate this problem.

- Some reactions such as **lipodystrophy** occur at the injection site if the patient does not keep the injection sites rotated.
- Weight gain is a common side effect with insulin administration.
- Blurred vision and hypoglycemia are the more common side effects. The person with diabetes should be taught to recognize the signs of hypoglycemia and should have readily absorbed sugar and a fat product such as peanut butter available (see Table 21-7).
- Smoking delays the absorption of insulin, and people needing insulin should not smoke for 30 minutes following the injection.
- Pregnancy dramatically increases the requirements for insulin.
- Illness may require an increased need for insulin.
- Skipping meals may result in hypoglycemia.
- Sudden increases in exercise may cause hypoglycemic episodes.
- Amounts of insulin should not be adjusted without the knowledge of the physician.
- The person with diabetes should wear medical identification so that, in case of emergency, behavioral changes can be evaluated for hyperglycemia or hypoglycemia. This person should also monitor blood glucose levels on a regular basis.
- Care should be used when taking OTC preparations because of the sugar content of some medications. As OTC drugs are occasionally reformulated, labels should be read before each purchase. Reading labels and checking with the pharmacist are important steps in medication safety for the person with diabetes.

Drugs Used as Oral Antidiabetic/ Hypoglycemic Agents

The oral antidiabetic drugs are in six families: sulfonylureas, biguanides, alpha-glucosidase inhibitors, thiazolidinediones, metglitinides, and amylin/GLP-1 analogs. These agents are used for T2DM diabetes and should be used only after exercise and diet have not controlled the elevated blood sugar values. The patient with T2DM who loses weight may be able to discontinue the use of oral hypoglycemic agents.

- *Sulfonylureas*, derivatives of sulfonamide antibiotics but without the antibiotic activity, were the first oral hypoglycemic agents and are in two groups, first-generation and second-generation medications.

- The second-generation agents are the most potent and produce therapeutic effects in lower doses with a longer duration of action, allowing for once-daily administration. Table 21-10 gives the onset and duration of action of these medications.
- Sulfonylureas such as glipizide (Glucotrol) or glimepiride (Amaryl) enter the beta cells of the pancreas, causing the release of insulin from the pancreas, with a subsequent lowering of blood glucose levels.
- These drugs have no true insulin-like activity but do increase insulin secretions.
- Sulfonylureas have no value in the treatment of T1DM.
- The drugs are absorbed by the intestines and transported to the pancreas, causing a delay from administration to action.
- Sulfonylureas produce hypoglycemia that is more severe in patients who are elderly, debilitated, or malnourished.
- Because the medications vary in onset and duration of action, the patient must adhere to a strict diet time and well-balanced meals.
- Hypersensitivity reactions such as photosensitivity, jaundice, rashes, and blood dyscrasias have occurred with oral hypoglycemics.
- These medications are contraindicated with T1DM and liver and renal disease and should not be used during pregnancy.

TABLE 21-10 *Duration of Action of the Sulfonylureas*

GENERIC NAME	TRADE NAME	ONSET OF ACTION	DURATION OF ACTION
FIRST-GENERATION AGENTS			
tolbutamide	Orinase	1 hr	6-12 hr
acetohexamide	Dymelor	1 hr	12-24 hr
tolazamide	Tolinase	4-6 hr	12-24 hr
chlorpropamide	Diabinese	1 hr	24-72 hr
SECOND-GENERATION AGENTS			
glipizide			
standard	Glucotrol	1-1.5 hr	12-24 hr
sustained-release	Glucotrol XL	1-1.5 hr	24 hr
glyburide			
nonmicronized	DiaBeta, Micronase	2-4 hr	12-24 hr
micronized	Glynase PresTab	1 hr	24 hr
glimepiride	Amaryl	1 hr	24 hr

- Sulfonylureas become less effective after 10 years of use (see Table 21-9).
- *Glucose absorption inhibitors* include the alpha-glucosidase inhibitors acarbose (Precose) and miglitol (Glyset), which delay the absorption of carbohydrates by slowing the absorption of glucose in the small intestines.
  - Alpha-glucosidase is the enzyme that breaks down carbohydrates to monosaccharides; thus this group of drugs works by inhibiting the enzyme and reducing the postprandial rise in glucose.
  - Medications in this group can be used alone or in combination with insulin, metformin, or sulfonylureas.
  - These medications have early side effects of flatulence, diarrhea, and abdominal pain that subside with continued use (see Table 21-9).
- *Biguanides* act by lowering cellular resistance to insulin.
  - Metformin (Glucophage), the drug in this category, decreases the production of glucose by the liver but does not release insulin from the pancreas and thus does not cause hypoglycemia. It reduces blood glucose levels in patients who no longer produce insulin in sufficient quantities to prevent hyperglycemia.
  - The medication is recommended only for patients with good kidney function.
  - Metformin is used for T1DM and T2DM.
  - Metformin is not recommended for use by the elderly (see Table 21-9).
- *Thiazolidinediones*, or glitazones, are a class of antihyperglycemic medications that are not related to any of the other oral medications for T2DM.
  - The glitazones such as rosiglitazone (Avandia) are effective in persons with insulin resistance, even those who no longer respond to sulfonylureas. These medications decrease insulin resistance and improve blood glucose control.
  - Their action is to increase insulin sensitivity in adipose tissue, muscles, and the liver.
  - These medications may be used alone or in combination with metformin or sulfonylureas.
  - No evidence indicates that the medications cause liver failure, as other oral hypoglycemics do (see Table 21-9).
- *Meglitinides*, repaglinide (Prandin) and nateglinide (Starlix), are used to stimulate the beta

cells to release insulin in an action similar to the sulfonylureas.

- These short-acting medications can be used alone or in combination with metformin for patients with T2DM.
- These medications are also called *rapid insulin releasers*.
- Persons who eat carbohydrates with a following blood sugar spike can most likely benefit from these medications.
- Repaglinide and nateglinide should be taken 10 to 15 minutes before meals and do not need to be taken if the meal is skipped.
- These medications can be used with injected long-acting insulin therapy to provide blood glucose control.
- *DPP-4 (dipeptidyl peptidase-4) inhibitors* are the newest addition to the oral hypoglycemic agents for treating T2DM. At present the only drug in this class is sitagliptin (Januvia).
  - It may be used alone or in combination with metformin or a thiazolidinedione.
  - Less weight gain and fewer incidences of hypoglycemia occur with this drug.
  - It works to reduce the release of glucagon and increase the release of insulin to restore blood glucose levels toward normal after eating.
  - Sitagliptin has a fixed dose of 50 mg bid.

New Medications Used as Hypoglycemics

Two new groups of injectable medications, called amylin GLP-1 analogs, have been recently introduced. Both of these injectable medications stimulate secretion of insulin in the beta cells when large amounts of glucose are found in the bloodstream and actually seem to promote beta cell regeneration. The drugs, which curb the appetite, control blood glucose levels while minimizing the chance of hypoglycemia by delaying gastric emptying, thus lowering high postprandial blood glucose levels. These drugs may also be used in patients who have undergone islet transplantation.

- *Incretin mimetics* are a new class of hypoglycemics used for treating T2DM.
  - Medications in this group are given subcutaneously to persons whose diabetes cannot be controlled with oral hypoglycemics.

- This group of drugs may be used for stand-alone therapy with T2DM.
- The medication is administered twice a day before the morning and evening meal.
- Exenatide (Byetta) is the first drug in the new class
- Exenatide is available in 5 mcg and 10 mcg per dose prefilled pen-injector devices.
- Long-term use of exenatide seems to cause weight loss
- *Synthetic human amylin* may be used as adjunct therapy with insulin for uncontrolled T1DM and T2DM.
  - The first medication in this class is pramlintide (Symlin) that is available in vials for injection.
  - The usual dose is injected SC before meals and before snacks of 30 g of carbohydrates or more.
  - Pramlintide should not be mixed in the same syringe with insulin preparations. Two separate syringes for insulin and pramlintide should be used and the injection sites must be at least 2 inches away from each other. Always use a new syringe and needle with pramlintide.
  - Side effects include decrease in appetite with the resultant decrease in caloric intake and weight loss.

Patient Education for Compliance

1. Insulin pens should be agitated by rolling in the hands.
2. The person taking insulin should not smoke for 30 minutes after taking insulin because nicotine produces vasoconstriction and slows the circulation of insulin.
3. Diet and exercise are important in the control of diabetes. The person taking insulin should not skip meals and must exercise routinely. If the meal is skipped, the insulin should not be injected.
4. Blood glucose levels should be monitored on a routine basis.
5. Persons with diabetes should wear medical ID at all times.
6. When using lispro insulin, the patient must eat within 15 minutes of drug administration.
7. Suspensions of insulin should be gently rolled between the hands to dispense the ingredients into the liquid. Vigorous agitation makes the drug frothy, causing an inaccurate dose.
8. Regular and lispro insulin are clear, not suspensions.
9. Injection sites should be rotated using each site once a week.

Patient Education for Compliance—cont'd

10. Unopened vials of insulin should be stored in the refrigerator but not frozen. Vials in current use can be stored at room temperature for up to 1 month but must be kept out of heat or direct sunlight.

11. Persons with diabetes should always read labels of OTC medications or check with a pharmacist before buying these medications. The sugar content of OTC medications changes frequently, so the patient should check each time the medication is purchased.

12. Inform patients that reduced food intake, vomiting, diarrhea, excessive alcohol consumption, and excessive exercise may cause hypoglycemia.

13. Teach patients the signs of hypoglycemia—tachycardia, palpitations, sweating, nervousness, headache, confusion, and fatigue.

14. Persons with diabetes should always carry oral carbohydrates to counteract the hypoglycemic reaction, preferably an easily synthesized carbohydrate such as sugar, nondiet soda, or juice. A carbohydrate that is slower in digestion such as peanut butter or fruit should immediately follow the rapid digested carbohydrate.

15. Patients using Exubera should be taught the correct administration techniques to prevent hypoglycemic reactions.

16. Patients using Exubera should not smoke and should not use the medication if they have smoked in the past 6 months.

IMPORTANT FACTS ABOUT HYPOGLYCEMICS

- DM is characterized by sustained hyperglycemia. Type 1 is insulin-dependent, whereas type 2 is non-insulin-dependent DM.
- T1DM, an autoimmune disease, represents a complete absence of insulin and must be treated with insulin. T2DM results from a cellular resistance to insulin and may be treated with oral hypoglycemics and/or insulin, but diet and exercise must be used in conjunction with medications.
- Six forms of injectable insulin are used in the United States: lispro, regular, isophane, Lente, Ultralente, and Lantus. One form of inhaled insulin, Exubera, is available.
  - Lispro insulin has a rapid onset (15 minutes) and short duration of action.
  - Regular insulin has a rapid onset (30 minutes) and short duration of action.
  - Isophane and Lente insulin have intermediate onset and duration of action.

IMPORTANT FACTS ABOUT HYPOGLYCEMICS—*Cont'd*

- - Ultralente has a prolonged onset and prolonged duration of action.
  - Lantus provides a continuous 24-hour supply of insulin, with no plasma peak.
- All insulins should be given subcutaneously, but regular insulin may be administered intramuscularly or intravenously if necessary.
- Insulin suspensions (isophane, Lente, Ultralente) should be rolled in the hands prior to use to mix the suspended ingredients in the liquid. Insulin solutions (lispro, regular, and Lantus) do not require blending.
- Many new insulin delivery systems such as internal pumps and nasal sprays are available. Oral administration and insulin patches are being investigated.
- Patients taking hypoglycemics should wear medical identification at all times.
- Patients with T2DM may not need oral hypoglycemics following weight reduction and exercise programs.
- Oral hypoglycemics are used for patients with T2DM who do not respond to diet and exercise changes.
- T2DM requires a change in lifestyle for quality of life in the person who is diagnosed with this type DM. Patients must become experts in controlling their diabetes.
- The new hypoglycemics—alpha-glucosidase inhibitors, biguanides, glitizones, meglitinides and amylin/GLP-1 analogs—do not cause hypoglycemia.
- Oral hypoglycemics must be evaluated for use in pregnancy and lactation as they cross the placenta and are found in breast milk.
- Sulfonylureas should not be used with alcohol.

Hyperglycemic Agents

Hyperglycemic medications that elevate the blood sugar level are antagonists to insulin. These medications may be used to treat hypoglycemic reactions or the hypersecretion of insulin from the pancreas in diseases such as pancreatic cancer.

Glucagon is produced in the alpha cells of the pancreatic islets, where insulin decreases the blood glucose levels. This agent stimulates the breakdown of glycogen and increases the body's use of glucose, causing blood sugar levels to rise. Glucagon is given parenterally for an insulin overdose found with T1DM diabetes. It is not effective in starvation-caused hypoglycemia because starvation depletes glycogen storage, and glucagons must have glycogen to work. Glucagon may also be used with barium in gastrointestinal radiography to relax the gastrointestinal tract.

Diazoxide is an oral preparation that produces a prompt increase in blood glucose levels by inhibiting pancreatic insulin release. It is used in patients with inoperable pancreatic cancers. Glucose tablets and gels in tubes are available for use in persons with hypoglycemic reactions. These agents are monosaccharide tablets that can be carried for emergency use. Glucose tablets are especially effective for emergency use in children (see Table 21-9).

Summary

The endocrine system has no concrete hands-on physiology because the hormones may be either endogenous or exogenous. The hormones are transported mainly in the bloodstream to the target cells where the response occurs, and their action is inhibited by negative feedback to the organ of origin. The endocrine system integrates and regulates body function through the hormones. Pathologic conditions result from underproduction or overproduction of the hormones. For underproduction, replacement therapy is usually prescribed. For overproduction, medications, surgery, or irradiation may be used.

Medications for the pituitary gland are used for replacement therapy related to specific disorders such as GH for children who fail to grow and growth-inhibiting hormone for children with gigantism or adults with acromegaly. Hormones from the posterior pituitary gland are used to treat diabetes insipidus.

The thyroid gland secretes three hormones: thyroxine (T_4), triiodothyronine (T_3), and calcitonin. T_3 and T_4 affect all body cells by increasing metabolism, whereas calcitonin regulates calcium levels in the body. Replacement therapy is necessary for hypothyroidism to increase the circulating hormone. Medications are also used in hyperthyroidism to block the synthesis of thyroid hormone.

The corticosteroids—glucocorticoids and mineralocorticoids—originate in the adrenal cortex. These steroids have many pharmacologic effects including antiinflammatory action; metabolism of carbohydrates, fats, and proteins; as immunosuppressants for organ transplants; and for physiologic and psychologic response to stress. Steroids are given by mouth, parenterally, topically, and other routes. Some topical preparations are available OTC.

The primary hormones of the pancreas are insulin and glucagon. When insulin causes blood glucose levels to decrease, glucagon is released. This allows the use of glycogen stored in the liver, which again increases blood glucose levels. The negative feedback allows more insulin to be released, which maintains the homeostasis of carbohydrate metabolism.

The relative absence or deficiency of insulin secretions is the cause of DM, either from insufficient secretions or resistance of the body to insulin, or both. DM is of two types: T1DM that is insulin-dependent, and T2DM that is considered non-insulin-dependent although insulin may be needed in some cases of T2DM. Insulins come in several types, depending on their onset and duration of action. Several novel delivery devices are on the market or are in experimental use for the administration of insulin. Different types of injectable insulin may be mixed to provide adequate coverage throughout the day, but the dosages of each must be individualized to each patient's needs and physical condition. T2DM is usually treated with dietary management, weight reduction, exercise, and oral hypoglycemics if necessary.

The oral hypoglycemics are used by the millions of Americans with T2DM. Some act by increasing insulin secretion by the pancreas; others inhibit carbohydrate metabolism. The newer medications act by increasing the function of glucose metabolism in the body cells when diabetes is caused by insulin resistance.

The newer medications for treating DM may be injected as primary medications, such as pramlintide, or used as adjuvant medications for T2DM such as exenatide. Both of these medications decrease the classic symptoms of DM and also lower the A_{1c}.

Critical Thinking Exercises

SCENARIO

Josie has been taking steroids for a prolonged period of time as treatment for rheumatoid arthritis. She has gained weight, especially in her face, and notices that her skin is thin and bleeds easily.

1. What do you need to tell Josie about salt and water intake?
2. What about the chance of menstrual irregularities?
3. She is concerned about the increased hair on her face and body. How can you explain this to her?

4. What other symptoms can she expect?
5. After you talk with her, she says she is going to stop taking the medicine at once because she is afraid of the side effects. What do you tell her about abruptly discontinuing these medications?

DOSAGE CALCULATIONS

1. Order: Humulin R 25 U and Humulin N 30 U
   Available medication:

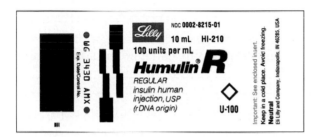

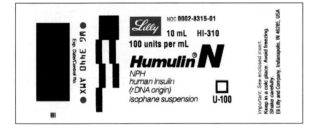

2. Order: Synthroid 0.1 mg
   Available medication:

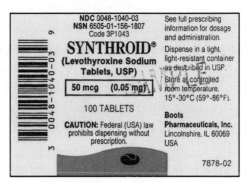

Dose to be given: _____

Show the correct amount of insulin on the marked syringes.

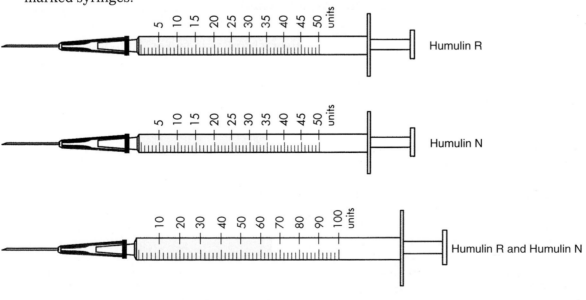

Humulin R

Humulin N

Humulin R and Humulin N

REVIEW QUESTIONS

1. What is a hormone and what is its function? _____
_____

2. What are the two major therapeutic uses of hormones? _____
_____

3. What hormones are secreted by the thyroid gland? _____
_____

4. What is an adrenocorticoid? A glucocorticoid? A mineralocorticoid? A steroid? _____
_____

5. What are the two unique ways that steroids are ordered? _____
_____

6. What is the only drug for type 1 diabetes? How is it administered? Why can it not be administered by mouth? _____
_____

7. What are the sources for insulin replacement? Which source is most like the body's insulin? _____
_____

8. What is the time to onset, peak time, and time of duration of the different insulin types? Describe these in terms of lispro, regular, isophane, Lente, Ultralente, and Lantus insulins. _____
_____
_____
_____

9. What are some of the newest forms of insulin administration techniques being developed to avoid the regular injections? _____
_____

10. How do the sulfonylureas work? Do they produce hypoglycemia? _____
_____

11. How do the biguanides work? Do they cause hypoglycemia? _____
_____

12. Why would insulin need to be administered to a patient who is taking an oral hypoglycemic? _____
_____

CHAPTER 22

Eye and Ear Disorders

OBJECTIVES

After studying this chapter, you should be capable of doing the following:

- Describing the anatomy of the eye and ear.
- Explaining the difference between ophthalmic and otic preparations.
- Recognizing ophthalmic and otic medications and their uses.
- Describing the drugs used in the treatment of vertigo.
- Describing how to store ophthalmic and otic preparations to prevent their being inadvertently interchanged.

Gene has an inflammation of the cornea of his left eye. He has been prescribed an antiinflammatory solution to use in his eye three times a day. Gene tells you that in the past, Dr. Merry has prescribed the same medication for use in his ears for an infection. The expiration date on the old medication has not passed.

    Can Gene use the otic solution rather than buy the new ophthalmic medicine?
    Why can Gene expect some blurring of vision after instilling the drops?
    Where should Gene instill the drops in his eyes?

KEY TERMS

Accommodation	Conjunctivitis	Otitis media
Adrenergic agonist	Cycloplegia	Ototoxicity
Anticholinergic agent	Glaucoma	Paresthesia
Ataxia	Hordeolum	Photophobia
Auditory ossicles	Keratitis	Presbyopia
Auralgia	Miosis	Sympathomimetic agent
Blepharitis	Miotic	Tinnitus
Cataract	Mydriasis	Tonometry
Cerumen	Myopia	Tympanic membrane
Chalazion	Nystagmus	Uveitis
Cholinergic agent (or	Open-angle glaucoma	Vasocongestion
parasympathomimetic)	Ophthalmic preparations	Vertigo
Closed-angle glaucoma	Otic preparations	

EASY WORKING KNOWLEDGE OF INDICATIONS AND SIDE EFFECTS

Common Symptoms of Ear and Eye Disorders
Eyes
Visual disturbances
Eye redness
Pain or burning in or around the eye
Ears
Loss of hearing
Vertigo or dizziness
Tinnitus
Earache and increased pressure in the ear

Common Side Effects of Medications
Ophthalmic
Changes in intraocular pressure
Burning, stinging, or pain on administration
Blurred vision or diplopia
Photophobia
Headache
Increased tears
Otic
Tinnitus
Burning or itching of ear canal
Dizziness

Easy Working Knowledge of Drugs Used for Ear and Eye Disorders

DRUG CLASS	PRESCRIPTION	OTC	PREGNANCY CATEGORY	MAJOR INDICATIONS
OPHTHALMIC				
Antiinfective	Yes	Yes (boric acid)	B, C	Eye infections
Antiinflammatory/ corticosteroids	Yes	No	C	Eye inflammation
Irrigating solutions	Yes	Yes	B	Foreign bodies
Antiglaucoma	Yes	No	C, X	Glaucoma
Mydriatics, cycloplegics	Yes	No	B, C	Diagnostic studies
Local anesthetics	Yes	No	C	Eye irritation
Immunomodulators	Yes	No	C	Dry eyes
Artificial tears, lubricants	Yes	Yes	N/A	Replace tears
Antiallergics	Yes	Yes	B	Eye allergies
Diagnostic aids	Yes	No	C	Diagnostic studies
OTIC				
Antiinfectives, antibiotics	Yes	No	C	Middle ear and external canal infections
Antiinflammatory/ corticosteroids	Yes	No	C	Ear inflammation
Combination preparations	Yes	No	B, C	Infections, inflammations
Ceruminolytics	Yes	Yes	B	Soften ear wax
Ear analgesics	Yes	Yes	B, C	
DRUGS FOR VERTIGO	Yes	Yes	B, C	Vertigo and motion sickness

Eye

The eye is one of the most delicate yet most valuable of the sense organs. The eye captures light and transforms it into images in the brain, but any impairment of sight results in visual disorders (Figure 22-1).

- The protective outer layer of the eye consists of the cornea and the sclera.

- The cornea is the transparent anterior covering of the middle layer of the eye that allows the entrance of light. It has no blood vessels and receives nourishment by diffusion of nutrients from the aqueous humor and oxygen from the air and surrounding structures. The eye surface has a thin layer of epithelial cells called the *conjunctiva* that is resistant to infection.

- The sclera, a continuation of the cornea, is not transparent but is a white fibrous

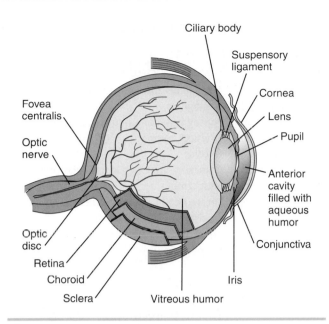

Figure 22-1 Anatomy of the eye. (From Young AP, Proctor DB: *Kinn's the medical assistant: an applied learning approach,* ed 10, St Louis, 2007, Saunders.)

covering that maintains the shape of the eyeball.

- The middle layer of the eye consists of the iris, choroid, and ciliary body.
  - The iris gives the eye its color and surrounds the pupil, an opening that is surrounded by muscle to alter its size. The nervous system causes the relaxing and constricting of the iris to control the amount of light that enters the eye. Constriction of the pupil is **miosis;** dilation of the pupil is **mydriasis.** Drugs may be used to produce either of these conditions, for ocular examinations or to treat eye diseases.
  - The lens is a transparent mass of fibers that lies behind the iris, ensuring a clear image in sharp focus and strong signals for interpretation on the retina. On each side of the lens is a ciliary body that contains muscles to change the shape of the lens for **accommodation.** Accommodation occurs readily in young people, but as the lens loses elasticity with age, the ability to focus on near objects is lost, and the point at which an object is in focus recedes—this condition, known as **presbyopia,** usually starts at approximately age 40 to 45. If the lens loses its transparency and becomes cloudy, the condition is called a **cataract.** The ciliary muscles contract to accommodate the eye; a paralysis of the ciliary muscle is called **cycloplegia.**

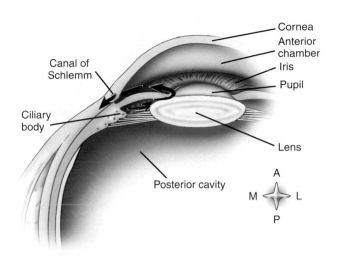

Figure 22-2 Aqueous humor passes into the anterior chamber through the pupil, where it is drained away by the ring-shaped canal of Schlemm. (From Thibodeau GA, Patton KT: *Anthony's textbook of anatomy and physiology,* ed 17, St Louis, 2003, Mosby.)

- The third layer of the eye consists of two distinct chambers, anterior and posterior.
  - The anterior chamber is the space between the cornea and the lens and is occupied by a fluid called the *aqueous humor* that is formed to bathe the lens, iris, and posterior cornea. The fluid flows forward between the lens and the iris into the anterior chamber to help maintain the shape of the anterior eye before being drained from the eye through the canals of Schlemm (Figure 22-2). The balance between production and absorption of aqueous humor helps maintain proper pressure within the eye.
  - The posterior chamber lies between the lens and retina and is filled with the colorless, transparent, gel-like *vitreous humor* that holds the retina firmly against the wall of the eye and helps maintain the shape of the eye.
  - The retina has visual sensory receptors called cones and rods and is connected to the brain by the optic nerve (see Figure 22-1).
- The eye is protected by the following:
  - Eyelashes to catch foreign materials
  - Blinking to keep the corneal surface free of mucus and moistened by the tears secreted by the lacrimal glands

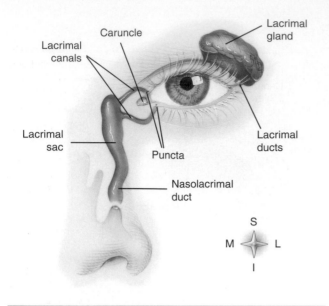

Figure 22-3 Lacrimal apparatus of the eye. (From Thibodeau GA, Patton KT: *Anthony's textbook of anatomy and physiology*, ed 17, St Louis, 2003, Mosby.)

- Tears that are bactericidal, preventing infections and draining into the inner corners of the eyelid into the nasolacrimal ducts (Figure 22-3)

Medications and the Eye

Medications specifically formulated for use in the eye are called **ophthalmic preparations.** Medications given for systemic diseases may cause ocular side effects (Table 22-1). Similarly, medications given for eye conditions may cause systemic effects and variations in homeostasis (Table 22-2).

Antiinfective and Antiinflammatory Agents

Like other infections, ocular infections should be cultured to determine the antibiotic of choice. In many cases, however, treatment is started before the culture results are available to limit the severity of the infection. Sometimes systemic medications are used with ocular medications.

Most antiinfective agents do not readily penetrate the eye, although some topical agents are absorbed when the mucous membrane has been injured or inflamed.

- Such ocular infections as **conjunctivitis, hordeolum, chalazion, blepharitis, keratitis,** and

TABLE 22-1 *Ocular Side Effects from Systemic Medications*

DRUG	POSSIBLE SIDE EFFECTS
aspirin	Allergic keratitis and conjunctivitis
barbiturates	Nystagmus
marijuana	Nystagmus, conjunctivitis, double vision, miosis
clonidine	Miosis
corticosteroids	Cataracts, increased intraocular pressure
ethyl alcohol	Nystagmus
ibuprofen	Altered color vision, blurred vision
indomethacin	Mydriasis
isoniazid	Optic neuritis
lithium	Exophthalmos
opiates	Miosis
phenothiazine	Cataracts
phenytoin	Nystagmus
thiazide diuretics	Transient myopia, yellow color to vision

Modified from Salerno X: *Pharmacology for health professionals*, St Louis, 1999, Mosby.

uveitis are treated with topical antiinfective and antiinflammatory agents.
- To avoid possible sensitization to systemic antiinfectives and to discourage drug-resistant strains, the antibiotic that is prescribed for ophthalmic symptoms is usually administered locally.
- Ophthalmic antiviral medications are available for viral eye conditions such as viral conjunctivitis caused by the common cold.
- In some instances, especially with viral infections, both eyes are treated to prevent spread of the infection (Table 22-3).

 CLINICAL TIP

Specific precautionary measures for antiinflammatory and antiinfective ophthalmic preparations follow:
- Only ophthalmic preparations should be used in the eye.
- Ophthalmic preparations are sterile when opened, and care must be taken to prevent contamination of the container.
- Care must be taken prior to administration to ensure that sulfa preparations have not darkened from their normal light yellow color.
- The action of sulfonamides is inhibited by ophthalmic anesthetics, and the two agents should be administered 30 to 60 minutes apart.
- Sulfonamides are incompatible with thimerosal (a mercurial antiseptic) and silver preparations.

TABLE 22-2 *Ophthalmic Medications with Adverse Systemic Effects*

DRUG AND CLASS	ADVERSE EFFECTS
ANTIMICROBIAL	
chloramphenicol	Aplastic anemia
ANTICHOLINERGICS	
atropine	Increased temperature, tachycardia, delirium
cyclopentolate	Convulsions, hallucinations
scopolamine drops	Acute psychosis
ANTIGLAUCOMA MEDICATIONS	
Beta-blocking agents	Bradycardia, syncope, decreased blood pressure, asthma, congestive heart failure, nausea, hallucinations, anorexia, headaches, weakness, depression
Cholinergic agents	Salivation, nausea and vomiting, asthma attacks, low blood pressure
Carbonic anhydrase inhibitors	Diarrhea, headache, nervousness, nausea and vomiting, diuresis, anorexia, parenthesis, weight loss, photosensitivity
Prostaglandin agonists	Upper respiratory tract infection; muscle, back, joint, and chest pain; angina, rash
Osmotic diuretics	Nausea and vomiting, headache, increased thirst, dry mouth, diarrhea, confusion
Anticholinergics	Sweating, flushing, tachycardia respiratory depression, mental pattern

CLINICAL TIP—*Cont'd*

- Silver nitrate, used for gonococcal infections at birth, comes in a collapsible capsule containing five drops. Each capsule to be used should be tested with one drop to ensure a liquid state prior to administration.
- When irrigating the eye, turn the patient's head toward the affected side to prevent cross-contamination of the unaffected eye.
- Ophthalmic corticosteroids may have systemic effect if used over a prolonged time.
- Contact lens, especially soft lens, should be removed prior to administration of ophthalmic preparations to prevent absorption of the medication by the lens.
- A good rule for administration of ophthalmic topical medications is to allow time (15 minutes to 1 hour) between administration of different ophthalmic medications unless prescribed otherwise.

Agents for Glaucoma

Glaucoma is the name for a group of diseases characterized by increased intraocular pressure (IOP) as a result of excessive production of aqueous humor or diminished ocular fluid outflow (Figure 22-4). Several terms are used to describe glaucoma—primary or secondary, acute or chronic, and open- or closed-angle glaucoma. If the pressure is persistently high, blindness may occur secondary to optic nerve damage. Primary medications used to treat glaucoma include beta-adrenergic-receptor-blocking agents, cholinergics, and sympathomimetics. The aim of treatment for glaucoma is to decrease IOP, thus decreasing damage to the optic nerve.

- *Beta-adrenergic-receptor blockers* (beta-blockers) when used with glaucoma decrease the production of aqueous humor, thus reducing IOP (Table 22-4).
- **Cholinergic agents** or **miotics** cause pupils to constrict or contract, causing **myopia.** Miotics open the spaces for the outflow of aqueous humor. Because the pupil cannot accommodate to changes in illumination caused by medications, end-of-day and nighttime activities are particularly hazardous for these individuals. Other miotics are *cholinesterase inhibitors,* which inhibit the enzyme destruction of acetylcholine. Cholinesterase inhibitors are usually reserved for people who had no response to other antiglaucoma agents (see Table 22-4).
- **Sympathomimetic agents** mimic the sympathetic nervous system to dilate the pupils with open-angle glaucoma. Dipivefrin is converted to epinephrine to lower the IOP by decreasing aqueous humor production and increasing its outflow (see Table 22-4).
- Oral *carbonic anhydrase inhibitors* are used to lower IOP. They decrease the aqueous production by reducing the volume of aqueous humor more than 50%. (Diuretics are discussed in Chapters 27 and 28.) These oral medications are used for open-angle, secondary, and angle-closure glaucoma (see Table 22-4).
- *Prostaglandin agonists* approved for the topical treatment of open-angle glaucoma and ocular hypertension are considered as effective as beta-blockers with fewer side effects. Now considered the first-line medications for glaucoma, these agents reduce IOP by increasing aqueous humor outflow. These medications are usually well tolerated with the major side effect being irreversible browning of the pigment of the iris (see Table 22-4).

TABLE 22-3 Select Drugs Used as Ophthalmic Agents

GENERIC NAME	TRADE NAME	USUAL ADULT DOSE, ROUTE,* AND FREQUENCY OF ADMINISTRATION	MAJOR SIDE EFFECTS	INDICATIONS FOR USE	DRUG INTERACTIONS
ANTIINFECTANTS/ANTIINFLAMMATORY AGENTS					
triple antibiotic	Neosporin Ophthalmic Ointment	Small amount in conjunctival sac q3-4h	Stinging, irritation, tearing	Broad-spectrum antibacterial for superficial ocular infections and gram-positive infections	None identified
	Mycitracin Ophthalmic Ointment	Same as above			
ciprofloxacin	Ciloxan solution	gtt ïï q4h prior to surgery			None identified
polymyxin B	Polysporin ophthalmic Ointment or Solution	Small amount in conjunctival sac or gtt ï-ïïï in eye			None identified
bacitracin	Baciguent Ointment	Small amount in conjunctival sac several times a day			None identified
chloramphenicol	Chloromycetin Ophthalmic Solution	gtt ïï in eye qid		Gram-positive and gram-negative organisms; superficial intraocular infections	None identified
erythromycin	Ilotycin Ointment	Small amount in conjunctival sac up to 6 times per day		Bacteriostatic, neonatal conjunctivitis	None identified
gentamicin	Genoptic, Garamycin Ointment or Solution	2-3 times per day; gtt ï q4h		Gram-positive and gram-negative organisms that are drug resistant	None identified
tobramycin	Tobrex Solution, Ointment	gtt ï or ïï q4h ¼ to ½ inch in conjunctival sac q8h		Same as gentamicin	Care with systemic aminoglycosides
with dexamethasone	TobraDex Solution	gtt ï or ïï qid or q6h		Same as gentamicin	
sulfacetamide	Bleph-10, Sulamyd Solution	gtt ï or ïï q1-3h		Same as gentamicin	Must be given 30 minutes after ocular anesthetics
sulfisoxazole	Gantrisin Solution	gtt ï or ïï q1-3h		Same as gentamicin	
ANTISEPTICS					
benzalkonium chloride 1:5000	Zephiran	Irrigation		Prophylaxis; treatment of eye infections; many are over-the-counter preparations	None identified
boric acid	Blinx, Collyrium	2% solution prn 5%-10% ointment			
silver nitrate 1%		Solution; gtt ïï OU at birth		Neonates after birth for prophylaxis of gonococci	

ANTIFUNGALS				
natamycin	Natacyn, Nalcon-A solution	Individualized, usually gtt ii q6h	Fungal blepharitis, conjunctivitis, or keratitis	Not systemically absorbed
ANTIVIRALS				
idoxuridine	Dendrid, Herplex Solution, Ointment	gtt i q1h in day and q2h at night; ointment q4-5h	Viral infections of eye, herpes simplex, keratitis	None identified
trifluridine	Viroptic Solution	gtt i q1h, up to 9 drops/day		
vidarabine	Vira-A Ointment	½ inch of ointment in eye q 3h		Specific for this: photosensitivity, sensation of foreign body in eye, swelling of eye, eye irritation
CORTICOSTEROIDS				
dexamethasone	Maxidex Suspension, Decadron Solution, Ointment	Varies with patient and condition	Allergic or inflammatory disorders; used in combinations with antibiotics and mydriatics such as Isopto-Cetapred, Medrapred, and Optimyd	May have systemic effects over prolonged periods of use (see discussion of corticosteroids in Chapter 21)
polyvinyl alcohol hydrocortisone	Liquifilm Tears/Forte Hydrocortone	gtt i or ii prn; gtt i-iii q1h while awake, q2h at night tid-qid	Burning, tearing, blurred vision, headache, pain	
acetate	Cortamed Ointment			
prednisolone sodium phosphate	Inflamase, Inflamase Forte, Pred Forte as suspensions and solutions	Varies		
NONSTEROIDAL ANTIINFLAMMATORY				
flurbiprofen	OcuFen Solution	Used prior to ophthalmic surgery as ordered	Inhibits intraocular miosis	None identified
suprofen	Profaned Solution	Same		
ketorolac	Acular Solution	gtt i qid	Prophylaxis; treatment of ocular inflammation	Nore identified

*The route of administration in this table is topical unless otherwise stated.

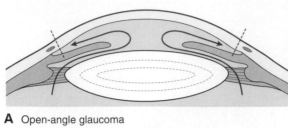

A Open-angle glaucoma

B Closed-angle glaucoma

Figure 22-4 A and **B,** Flow of aqueous humor causing an increase in intraocular pressure in glaucoma. (From Damjanov I: *Pathology for the health professions*, ed 3, St Louis, 2006, Saunders.)

- *Osmotic diuretics* are used to reduce IOP following surgery or in the treatment of acute glaucoma. These oral agents are glycerin (Osmoglyn) and isosorbide (Isordil) (see Tables 22-2 and 22-4).

Mydriatics and Cycloplegics

Mydriatics and cycloplegics are used to dilate the pupil for ophthalmologic testing and other ophthalmologic conditions.

- **Adrenergic agonists** that mimic the sympathetic nervous system may bring about pupillary dilation, or **mydriasis,** whereas **cycloplegic** agents cause paralysis of the ciliary muscles, or prevent accommodation. These agents, used primarily in the diagnosis of ophthalmologic disorders, cause dilation of the iris opening, leading to its relaxation and a possible increase in IOP. For this reason, patients receiving these medications should be watched for the abrupt onset of acute glaucoma. Applied topically, these drugs cause vasoconstriction, pupillary dilation, an increase in the outflow of aqueous humor, a decrease in the production of aqueous humor, and relaxation of the ciliary muscles. The inherent danger is that many of these agents are available over the counter (OTC) to reduce redness in the eyes caused by **vasocon-**

gestion. Prescription medications are used to treat wide-angle glaucoma and secondary glaucoma, produce mydriasis for ocular examinations, and relieve ocular vasocongestion (Table 22-5).

- **Anticholinergic agents** that block the parasympathetic nervous system cause dilation and are used to relax the inflamed intraocular muscles to relieve pain with uveitis. Other uses are for the accurate measurement of refractive errors and before and after intraocular surgery. Some of these medications are administered in combinations to produce greater mydriasis (see Table 22-5).

Local Ophthalmic Anesthetic Agents

Local ophthalmic anesthetic agents are used to eliminate the blink reflex and pain associated with ophthalmic procedures. These agents may also be used for **tonometry,** removal of foreign objects, suturing or removal of sutures, and radial keratotomy. The eye should be protected until the anesthesia wears off because of loss of the blink reflex (Table 22-6).

Immunomodulators

An emulsion medication to increase tear production, cyclosporine (Restasis) is considered as an immunomodulator or as an immunosuppressant. Available only as a prescription medication, cyclosporine should not be administered in a person wearing contact lens nor should it be administered with other topical ophthalmic medications. Prior to administration the medication should be inverted several times to place the medication back into the emulsion (Table 22-7).

Artificial Tears and Lubricants

Artificial tear solutions or lubricants are demulcents used to produce eye lubrication when tear production is decreased, lubricate artificial eyes, moisten contact lens, and remove debris from the eye. The products are normal saline with agents added to extend eye contact time. These products are usually used three to four times a day. An artificial tear insert (Lacrisert) and ointment preparations are used for prolonged effect. The ointments are also used to protect the eyes of patients with impaired blink reflexes and in persons who need lubrication at night (see Table 22-7).

Text continued on page 447

TABLE 22-4 *Drugs Used to Treat Glaucoma*

GENERIC NAME	TRADE NAME	USUAL ADULT DOSE, ROUTE, AND FREQUENCY OF ADMINISTRATION	MAJOR SIDE EFFECTS	INDICATIONS FOR USE	DRUG INTERACTIONS
BETA-ADRENERGIC-BLOCKING AGENTS			Local burning, stinging, eye irritation, visual disturbance, pruritus	Glaucoma	Systemic—bradycardia/tachycardia, confusion, insomnia, weakness, respiratory symptoms, GI disturbances
betaxolol	Betoptic Solution	0.25% gtt ī bid			
carteolol	Ocupress Solution	gtt ī̄ bid			
levobunolol	Betagan Solution	0.25% gtt ī bid; 0.5% gtt ī daily			
metipranolol	Optipranolol 0.3% Solution	gtt i bid			
timolol	Timoptic Solution	gtt ī 1-2 × per day			
CHOLINERGIC (MIOTICS) DIRECT-ACTING AGENTS			Local—blurred vision, myopia, eye irritation, headaches; no systemic side effects		
carbachol	Carboptic Solution	gtt ī tid			None identified
pilocarpine	Isoptocarpine Solution	gtt ī bid			None identified
	Pilomiotin Ocusert	Insert disk in eye q7 days			None identified
CHOLINESTERASE INHIBITORS					
demecarium	Humorsol Solution	gtt ī qd or bid			None identified
isoflurophate	Floropryl Ointment	Thin ribbon application ¼ inch tid-qd-q3d			
SYMPATHOMIMETICS			Local—same as cholinergic agents; Systemic—see Table 22-2		
dipivefrin	Propine Solution	gtt ī qd-bid			None identified

(continued)

TABLE 22-4 Drugs Used to Treat Glaucoma—cont'd

GENERIC NAME	TRADE NAME	USUAL ADULT DOSE, ROUTE, AND FREQUENCY OF ADMINISTRATION	MAJOR SIDE EFFECTS	INDICATIONS FOR USE	DRUG INTERACTIONS
CARBONIC ANHYDRASE INHIBITORS					
acetazolamide	Diamox	500 mg tab bid po			Amphetamines, quinidine, methamine
dichlorphenamide	Daranide	25-50 mg tab qd-tid po			
methazolamide	Neptazane	50-100 mg tab bid-tid po			
dorzolamide (drops)	Trusopt 2% Solution	gtt ī bid-tid			
PROSTAGLANDIN INHIBITORS			Local—blurred vision, burning, stinging, photophobia, ↑ brown pigmentation; systemic—see Table 22-2		None identified
latanoprost	Xalatan Solution	gtt ī daily HS			
unoprostone	Rescula Solution	gtt ī bid			
travoprost	Travatan 0.005% Solution	gtt ī qd			
bimatoprost	Lumigan 0.03% Solution	gtt ī bid			
OSMOTIC DIURETICS				Glaucoma, increased intraocular pressure	Amphetamines, quinidine
glycerin	Osmoglyn Ophthalgan Solution	1-1.5 g/kg/day po gtt ī-īī in eye q3-4h			
isosorbide	Isonate	1.5 g/kg/day po			
MISCELLANEOUS				Glaucoma to reduce aqueous humor production	No significant interactions identified
apraclonidine	Iopidine 0.5% Solution	gtt ī or īī in eye 3 × a day			
brimonidine	Alphagan Solution	gtt ī q8 hr			

TABLE 22-5 Drugs Used as Mydriatics or Cycloplegics

GENERIC NAME	TRADE NAME	USUAL ADULT DOSE, ROUTE, AND FREQUENCY OF ADMINISTRATION	MAJOR SIDE EFFECTS	INDICATIONS FOR USE	DRUG INTERACTIONS
MYDRIATICS/CYCLOPLEGICS					
atropine	IsoptoAtropine Solution 0.125%-4% / Ointment 0.5%-1%	gtt ī-īī bid-tid / Small amt bid-tid	Burning, itching, blurred vision	Glaucoma; mydriasis for ocular surgery	No significant interactions identified
cyclopentolate	Cyclogyl 0.5%-1% Solution	gtt ī			
homatropine	Isopto Homatropine Solution 2%-5%	gtt ī-īī			
scopolamine	Isopto Hyoscine Solution 1%	gtt ī-īī bid-tid			
tropicamide	Opticyl, Tropicacyl Solutions 0.5%-1%	gtt ī			
ADRENERGIC AGONISTS/ANTICHOLINERGICS					
epinephrine	Epifrin, Glaucon* 0.5%-2% Solution	gtt ī daily-bid	Burning and stinging on initial application	Mydriasis, decreases eye redness	No significant interactions identified
hydroxyamphetamine	Paredrine* 1% Solution	gtt ī-īī as mydriatic			
naphazoline	Albalon, Vasocon* 0.1% Solution / Allerest, VasoClear† 0.012%-0.03% Solution	gtt ī q3-4h / gtt ī up to qid			
oxymetazoline	OcuClear† 0.025% Solution	gtt ī q6h			
phenylephrine	Neo-Synephrine* 2.5%-10% Solution / Prefrin, AK-Nefrin† 0.12% Solution	gtt ī prn / gtt ī or īī up to qid			
tetrahydrozoline	Murine Plus, Visine† 0.05% Solution	gtt ī or īī up to qid			

*Prescription medications.
†Over-the-counter medications.

TABLE 22-6 Drugs Used as Ocular Anesthetics

GENERIC NAME	TRADE NAME	USUAL ADULT DOSE, ROUTE, AND FREQUENCY OF ADMINISTRATION	MAJOR SIDE EFFECTS	INDICATIONS FOR USE	DRUG INTERACTIONS
tetracaine	Pontocaine 0.5% Solution	gtt ī-īi immediately prior to surgical procedure and for anesthetic action in eye injuries	Burning on initial administration	Anesthetizing the eye for ophthalmologic procedure and for eye trauma	No significant interactions identified
proparacaine	Ophthaine, Ophthetic 0.5% Solution	Same as for tetracaine	Same as for tetracaine	Same as for tetracaine	No significant interactions identified

TABLE 22-7 Drugs Used as Eye Lubricants

GENERIC NAME	TRADE NAME	USUAL ADULT DOSE, ROUTE, AND FREQUENCY OF ADMINISTRATION	MAJOR SIDE EFFECTS	INDICATIONS FOR USE	DRUG INTERACTIONS
ARTIFICIAL TEARS/LUBRICANTS					
Most of these agents are over-the-counter medications, with a base of normal saline. A few examples are provided	Lacrisert Ophthalmic Insert Lacri-Lube Ointment Duratears Solution, HypoTears, Tearisol	1-2 inserts daily topically As needed at night topically As needed topically	No major side effects because of saline base	Artificial tears, eye lubricants	No significant interactions identified
IMMUNOMODULATORS*					
cyclosporine	Restasis 0.05% emulsion	One vial applied topically q12h	Do not use with contact lens in place Discard any medication left in vial	Increase tear production	

*Do not use immunomodulators with contact lens in place and discard any medication left in vial.

Ophthalmic Antiallergic and Decongestant Agents

Three agents are used for allergic eye disorders. Cromolyn sodium prevents histamines from producing allergic reactions and relieves the tearing, itching, redness, and discharges related to allergic eye conditions. It may be used with corticosteroids. Levocabastine (Livostin) is used for allergic conjunctivitis. Lodoxamide ophthalmic is used to treat vernal (spring) conjunctivitis and keratitis (Table 22-8). OTC medications are to be used for the short term only.

Decongestant agents are weak adrenergic agents that reduce eye redness by acting as topical vasoconstrictors to constrict blood vessels in the conjunctiva. Most of these medications are available OTC (see Table 22-8).

Ophthalmic Staining Agents

Fluorescein sodium is a nontoxic, water-soluble dye used to diagnose corneal epithelial defects caused by injury or infection and to locate foreign bodies in the eye. When applied to the cornea, fluorescein stains corneal lesions green and foreign bodies have a green ring surrounding them. The agent is also used in the fitting of hard contact lens, as a dye for retinal studies, and for ophthalmic angiography (Table 22-9).

Patient Education for Compliance

1. Care should be taken when using ophthalmic preparations to prevent contamination of the medications by touching the applicator to the eye.
2. Wear dark glasses with medications that cause photosensitivity as some medications cause photophobia in bright lights.
3. Consult a physician if the eyes do not show improvement after using ophthalmic antifungals for 7 to 10 days.
4. Treatment with antivirals should continue for 3 to 5 days after healing.
5. Corticosteroids should be used for only a limited time because systemic effects may occur with long-term use.
6. When using corticosteroids in patients with diabetes, blood glucose levels should be monitored closely for hyperglycemia.
7. Ophthalmic suspensions and emulsions should be placed back into solution by agitation or inversion prior to administration.

Patient Education for Compliance— cont'd

8. When using anticholinergics, be careful to illuminate dark areas because of visual difficulty in dim light.
9. When using anticholinergics, use care in driving and other hazardous activities because of the lack of eye accommodation. Close-up visual acuity will be greatly diminished, making reading and other close-up activities difficult.
10. When using ophthalmic anticholinergics, protect the eyes by dimming lights and wearing dark glasses in the sunshine.
11. Take carbonic anhydrase inhibitors early in the day for maximum benefit.

IMPORTANT FACTS ABOUT OPHTHALMIC AGENTS

- Most ophthalmic antiinfective agents do not readily penetrate the eyes but are effective when the mucous membranes are inflamed or injured.
- Many ophthalmic solutions cause burning or stinging on application and cause headaches.
- Before administering topical ophthalmic medications, removal of contact lens is recommended except with wetting and lubricants especially manufactured for contact lens. The lens should not be reinserted for 15 to 30 minutes following administration, depending on the medication.
- Ophthalmic medications cause systemic effects if used over prolonged time periods, particularly corticosteroids, beta-adrenergic blockers, and cholinergic agents.
- Glaucoma is characterized by an increase in intraocular pressure caused by either excessive production of aqueous humor or diminished outflow of ocular fluids.
- Sympathomimetic agents are used to treat open-angle glaucoma by decreasing aqueous humor production and increasing its outflow.
- Mydriatics and cycloplegics paralyze ciliary muscles and are used as diagnostic aids. Mydriatics dilate the pupil. Miotics constrict the pupil.
- Anticholinergic agents are used to treat inflamed intraocular muscles during procedures to measure refractive errors and before and after intraocular surgery.
- Many adrenergic agents that mimic epinephrine are available OTC and act by causing vasoconstriction and pupillary dilation to reduce redness in the eye. These agents must be used with care with glaucoma.
- Local ophthalmic anesthetics are used to reduce the blink reflex and eliminate the pain associated with ophthalmic procedures.

TABLE 22-8 Drugs Used as Ophthalmic Antiallergic and Decongestant Agents*

GENERIC NAME	TRADE NAME	USUAL ADULT DOSE, ROUTE, AND FREQUENCY OF ADMINISTRATION	MAJOR SIDE EFFECTS	INDICATIONS FOR USE	DRUG INTERACTIONS
ANTIALLERGENIC AGENTS					
cromolyn sodium[†]	Opticrom Solution	gtt ï in eye 4-6 × per day	Burning, and stinging	Ophthalmic allergies and allergic conjunctivitis	No significant interactions identified
levocabastine	Livostin Solution	gtt ï in eye qid	Stinging, redness of eye, headache		
lodoxamide	Alomide Solution	Varies with age	Burning, blurred vision, tearing, itching		
ketotifen 0.025%[†]	Zaditor solution	Varies		Allergic conjunctivitis	No contact lens wear
olopatadine	Patanol solution	gtt ï-ïï bid		Allergic conjunctivitis	None
pemirolast 1%	Alamast solution	gtt ï in eye tid		Allergic conjunctivitis	No contact lens wear
epinastine	Elestat solution	gtt ï in eye bid			No contact lens wear
OCULAR DECONGESTANTS					
phenylephrine	AK Nefrin Solution	gtt ï or ïï qid	↑ocular pressure	Ophthalmic vascular congestion	
naphazoline[†]	Clear-Eyes Solution	Same as above			
oxymetazoline[†]	Visine, Ocu-Clear Solutions	Same as above			
tetrahydrozoline[†]	Visine Allergy Relief Solution	Same as above		Relief of allergies	

*These medications are applied topically unless otherwise indicated.
[†] OTC medications.

TABLE 22-9 *Drugs Used as Ophthalmic Diagnostic Aids*

GENERIC NAME	TRADE NAME	USUAL ADULT DOSE, ROUTE, AND FREQUENCY OF ADMINISTRATION	INDICATIONS FOR USE	DRUG INTERACTIONS
fluorescein	Fluorescite Solution	gtt i̅ to i̅i̅ in eye	Diagnosis of corneal epithelial defects, fittings of contact lens, ophthalmic angiography	Should not be used with soft contact lenses
	Fluor-I-Strip Chemical Strip	Application of strip to eye		

MAJOR SIDE EFFECTS: Burning, stinging, staining of contact lens.

*These medications are used topically.

IMPORTANT FACTS ABOUT OPHTHALMIC AGENTS—Cont'd

- Artificial tears or lubricants are basically normal saline solutions to which buffers have been added to prolong their contact with the eye, and thus their effectiveness. Most are OTC preparations and are used with contact lens.
- Antiallergic agents are used for allergies that affect the eyes. These agents reduce the itching and redness associated with allergic reactions.

Ear

The ear, the sensory organ of hearing and equilibrium, has three major parts: the external ear, middle ear, and inner ear (Figure 22-5).

- The external ear has two main parts, the auricle and the external auditory canal. The **tympanic membrane,** or eardrum, separates the middle ear and outer ear.
  - Because the ear canal is a dark, moist channel near the eardrum, bacteria can travel down the canal and cause infection such as swimmer's ear.
  - Bacterial and fungal infections of the canal are fairly common, especially in children, as the ear canal is shorter and straighter than in adults.
- The middle ear contains three bones, the **auditory ossicles**—stapes, incus, and malleus—which vibrate to transmit sound waves to the inner ear.
  - The eustachian tube connects the middle ear cavity to the pharynx to equalize pressure on both sides of the tympanic membrane.
  - Chewing gum, yawning, and swallowing will help to equalize the pressure when a sudden change in elevation causes the ears to feel as if they are obstructed.

- Microorganisms can travel up the eustachian tube from the pharynx to cause **otitis media,** especially in children.
- The inner ear communicates sound waves to the acoustic nerve through the bony labyrinth to transmit sound waves to the sacs and tubes filled with fluid and hairlike nerve receptors.
  - The cochlea of the bony labyrinth is the primary organ of hearing, and the fluids in the vestibule maintain equilibrium and balance.

Individuals with ear disorders may have **auralgia, vertigo,** and **ataxia.** The ear is an important sensory organ that carries countless clues about the environment to the brain. Infections in the inner ear cause hearing impairment and imbalance.

Typical Ear Conditions

External ear conditions seen in ambulatory care include infections, ear wax accumulation, and minor trauma. Many ear disorders are minor and easily treated with OTC medications; some are self-limiting. Sometimes hair follicles become infected, causing furuncles. Seborrheic dermatitis, psoriasis, and contact dermatitis may also cause ear inflammation. Pain, fever, malaise, pressure, and a sensation of fullness in the ear, with some hearing loss, are common symptoms of ear disorders.

Otic Preparations

Ear conditions are treated with systemic medications such as antibiotics, but this section discusses medications that are instilled into the external ear to treat bacterial or fungal infections and are labeled **otic.**

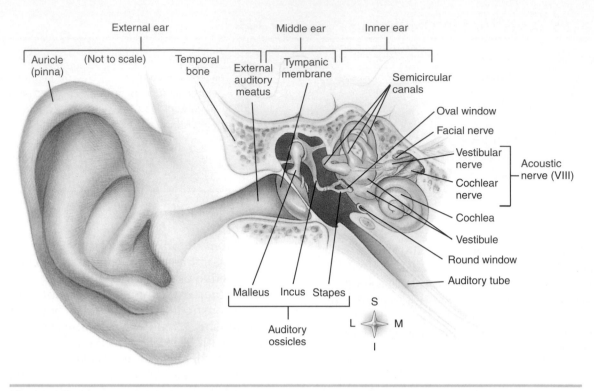

Figure 22-5   Anatomy of the ear. (From Thibodeau GA, Patton KT: *Anthony's textbook of anatomy and physiology*, ed 17, St Louis, 2003, Mosby.)

- *Drying agents* used in the external auditory canal are usually combinations of alcohol, boric acid, and hydrogen peroxide to dry the canal and prevent outer ear infections following activities such as swimming.
- *Antiinfective* ear preparations may be either instillations or irrigations. These agents inhibit growth of or kill bacteria, thus reducing swelling, relieving pruritus, and promoting drainage of external ear infections (Table 22-10).
- *Corticosteroids*, used to suppress the uncomfortable symptoms associated with ear inflammation, also reduce edema and pruritus in the ear. Corticosteroids should not be used to treat viral or fungal infections, or in someone with a perforated eardrum.
- Otic preparations are often found in combinations to treat more than one symptom or condition at the same time. Combination medications may contain two or more antibiotics, an antibiotic-benzocaine combination, or an antibiotic-corticosteroid combination (see Table 22-10).
- *Ceruminolytics* soften hardened **cerumen** that has blocked the external ear canal, a condition common with people wearing hearing aids. The hardened wax can interfere with hearing and block the actions of medications instilled into

the ear canal. A ceruminolytic is often ordered to soften the wax prior to ear irrigations. Many of these preparations can be bought OTC (Table 22-11).
- Ear analgesics can be warmed mineral oil, sweet oil, or glycerin used to relieve pain. Medications with a benzocaine base may be prescribed for auralgia (see Table 22-11).

Signs of Ototoxicity

Some patients may think they have ear infections or vertigo when they are actually experiencing **ototoxicity**—a detrimental effect on cranial nerve VIII or the organ of hearing—from medications. Ototoxicity can affect the hearing, balance, or both. The most common signs are **tinnitus,** vertigo, and difficulty with equilibrium. When ototoxicity occurs, the causative medication should be discontinued. Box 22-1 lists some of the more common medications that cause ototoxicity.

Patients with Ménière's disease present with many of the same symptoms as ototoxicity. The patient feels that the room is in motion and has a sensation of pressure or fullness in the ear (Table 22-12). The drug of choice to reduce the symptoms of ototoxicity is meclizine (Antivert or Bonine).

TABLE 22-10 *Drugs Used as Otic Antiinfectives*

GENERIC NAME	TRADE NAME	USUAL ADULT DOSE, ROUTE, AND FREQUENCY OF ADMINISTRATION	MAJOR SIDE EFFECTS	INDICATIONS FOR USE	DRUG INTERACTIONS
DRYING AGENTS					
acetic acid solutions	Vo-Sol*	gtt iv-vi tid-qid as instillation, irrigation	Irritation, swelling, urticaria, overgrowth of nonsusceptible microorganisms	To treat external ear infections, and to dry ear after contact with water	No significant interactions identified
boric acid solutions	Ear Dry, SwimEar†, AuraDry†	Fill ear with solution tid-qid			
isopropyl alcohol		Same			
ANTIBIOTICS					
chloramphenicol otic	Chloromycetin Otic Solution*	gtt ii-iii tid-qid	Same side effects		No significant interactions identified
ofloxacin	Floxin Otic Solution*	gtt v-x bid			
CORTICOSTEROIDS					
dexamethasone	Decadron Solution*	gtt i-iii in ear canal tid-qid			No significant interactions identified
hydrocortisone	Otall Solution*	gtt iii-v in ear canal tid-qid			
COMBINATION PRODUCTS					
hydrocortisone-acetic acid	Acetasol Solution*	gtt iii-v q4-6h			No significant interactions identified
Above + alcohol	EarSol HC Solution*	gtt i-ii qid			
celestin, neomycin, hydrocortisone, thonzonium	Coly-Mycin S Otic Solution*	gtt iii-v in ear canal tid-qid			
oxytetracycline, polymyxin B, hydrocortisone	Cortisporin Otic Solution*	gtt ii-iii in ear canal tid-qid			
boric acid, isopropyl alcohol	Aurocaine Z Solution†	gtt ii-iii tid-qid			
isopropyl alcohol, glycerin	SwimEar Drops†	gtt iii-iv in ear after swimming			
acetic acid, boric acid, benzalkonium, aluminum acetate	Burrow's Solution†	Varies with use as irrigation or instillation			

* Prescription medications.
† Over-the-counter medications.

TABLE 22-11 *Drugs Used as Ceruminolytics or Ear Analgesics**

GENERIC NAME	TRADE NAME	USUAL ADULT DOSE, ROUTE, AND FREQUENCY OF ADMINISTRATION	INDICATIONS FOR USE	DRUG INTERACTIONS
CERUMENOLYTICS				
carbamide peroxide	Debrox, Murine Ear Drops, Auro Ear Drops[†]	gtt v-x in ear canal bid × 3-4 days	Softening and removal of cerumen	No significant interactions identified
EAR ANALGESICS				
glycerin, mineral oil, sweet oil	None	Fill ear canal with warm solution	Relieve itching and burning in ear	No significant interactions identified
benzocaine-antipyrine	Auralgan, Auroto[‡] Solution	gtt ii q4-6h in ear	Analgesic	
Above + phenylephrine	Tympagesic[‡] Solution	gtt ii q4-6h in ear	Analgesic, antihistamine	

*These medications are applied topically unless otherwise stated.
[†] Over-the-counter medications.
[‡] Prescription medications.

CLINICAL TIPS

- To instill medications in a child's ear, gently pull the auricle down and back; in an adult or older child, pull the auricle up and back.
- Ear medications should be warmed to room temperature before instillation. Cold medications may cause otalgia and vertigo. (See Chapter 14 for the correct technique for instilling otic and ophthalmic medications.)
- Otic medications should never be used in the eye. Any medications used in the eye should be labeled "ophthalmic." In an emergency, ophthalmic medications may be used in the ear with the physician's permission.

Patient Education for Compliance

1. If the ear is draining, medications should not be instilled in the ear without consulting a physician.
2. Never occlude the external ear with a tight-fitting plug of any type after instillation of a medication because the occlusion may cause the eardrum to rupture due to increased pressure in the ear canal. Cotton plugs may be used because these do not increase pressure but allow air to pass through the fibers.

IMPORTANT FACTS ABOUT OTIC MEDICATIONS

- Many external ear conditions include infections and ear wax accumulations and are minor. These conditions are easily treated or are self-limiting.
- Pain, fever, malaise, increased pressure, and a feeling of fullness in the ear with hearing loss are common signs of middle ear infections.

BOX 22-1   SOME MEDICATIONS THAT CAUSE OTOTOXICITY

Antibiotics
amikacin (Aminkin)
streptomycin
neomycin
gentamicin (Garamycin)
erythromycin (E-mycin, Eryc)
kanamycin (Kantrex)
tobramycin (Nebcin)
vancomycin (Vancocin)

Diuretics
acetazolamide (Diamox)
furosemide (Lasix)
bumetanide (Bumex)
ethacrynic acid (Edecrine)

Antineoplastic Medications
cisplatin (Platinol AQ)
bleomycin (Blenoxabe)
vincristine (Oncovin)
There are many more medications that cause ototoxicity but those listed are the more damaging.

IMPORTANT FACTS ABOUT OTIC MEDICATIONS— *Cont'd*

- Children often have middle ear infections that accompany pharyngitis because of the angle of the eustachian tube relative to the pharynx.
- Ototoxicity may occur from systemic medications. The symptoms include tinnitus, loss of balance, and vertigo.

TABLE 22-12 *Drugs Used for Vertigo*

GENERIC DRUG	TRADE NAME	USUAL ADULT DOSE, ROUTE, AND FREQUENCY OF ADMINISTRATION	INDICATIONS FOR USE	DRUG INTERACTIONS
meclizine	Anti-Vert,* Bonine[†]	12.5-50 mg/day po in divided doses	Vertigo, motion sickness	No significant interactions identified
diphenhydramine	Benadryl[†]	15 50 mg q4h po, IM, IV		
dimenhydrinate	Dramamine[†] Calm X[†] Chewable Tablet	50-100 mg q4-6h po, IM As directed by manufacturer		
scopolamine	Transderm-Scop* Transdermal Patch	Apply patch behind ear as needed		

MAJOR SIDE EFFECTS OF DRUGS USED FOR VERTIGO: Drowsiness, except with scopolamine

*Prescription medications.
[†] Over-the-counter medications.

Storage of Eye and Ear Preparations

Ophthalmic and otic liquid preparations are packaged in containers that are easily confused. Ophthalmic medications are sterile and are manufactured to be safe when used on the thin membrane of the eye, whereas otic medications do not require sterility and are administered in a nonsterile ear canal. The small bottles are similar in shape, and many of the names are the same for the otic and ophthalmic drugs. Because of these similarities, ophthalmic and otic medications should not be stored in the same area. One way of preventing this potential medication confusion is to place ophthalmic medications on one shelf and otic medications on another. The allied health professional must be extremely careful to return medications to their correct place. A good rule of thumb in a workplace where ophthalmic and otic preparations are stored in close proximity is to check the name of the medication and route of administration more than the usual three times to ensure that the correct medication has been chosen. While checking the accuracy of the preparation, make sure the expiration date has not passed; this is especially important with ophthalmic preparations because of the delicate tissue on the surface of the eye. When ototoxicity is drug induced, the causative medication should be discontinued.

Summary

Preparations to treat ophthalmic disorders are divided into specific categories. Medications used in the eyes should be labeled "ophthalmic" to ensure proper strength and sterility. Many medications used in the eye cause stinging or burning on instillation. Some are systemically absorbed, and the patient should be aware of the effects of these medications.

Otic medications are agents used to treat ear disorders. Medications are available by prescription and OTC to treat many ear infections and ototoxicity.

Critical Thinking Exercises

SCENARIO

Jimmy's mother asks why every time Jimmy, age 2, has a sore throat, he seems to have an earache.
1. What do you expect Dr. Merry to tell her?
2. She wants to know if she should use the ear drops cold to relieve the earache. What is the best answer?
3. Can she buy any of the otic drops OTC that will relieve the minor pain of an earache and remove the excess wax found in Jimmy's ear? If so, which preparations?

DOSAGE CALCULATIONS

1. Order: Pontocaine Ophth Sol 0.5% gtt ii OU stat and q4h until scratching sensation disappears
Interpret the order:
What is the indication for this medication?

_____

_____

_____

2. Order: Debrox gtt v AD bid × 4 d
Interpret the order:
What is the indication for this medication?

_____

_____

_____

REVIEW QUESTIONS

1.   What does a cycloplegic do? _____
_____

2.   Why is it important to know the systemic medications that may cause ophthalmic side effects?
_____
_____

     How would this knowledge be used in prescribing ophthalmic medications? _____
_____

3.   What kind of systemic reactions can occur from the use of ophthalmic medications? What is the role of the allied health professional in watching for these reactions? _____
_____
_____

4.   Why must any medication used in the eye be labeled "ophthalmic"? _____
_____
_____

5.   What do miotics do? What is their use in glaucoma? _____
_____

6.   How does fluorescein demonstrate corneal defects from injury and foreign bodies on the cornea?
_____
_____

7.   What is a ceruminolytic? _____
_____

CHAPTER 23

Skin Conditions

OBJECTIVES

After studying this chapter, you should be capable of doing the following:
- Describing how topical medications are absorbed into the skin.
- Explaining why topical medications may have systemic effects.
- Discussing the various classes of medications that are used to treat dermatologic conditions.
- Describing the general properties of dermatologic preparations, both legend and over the counter (OTC), and their indications.
- Defining and naming typical topical keratolytics, acne preparations, ectoparasiticidal agents, and agents for alopecia.

Johnny fell off his bicycle and skinned his knee. His mother has cleansed the wound with soap and water.
- Why is this step in treatment important, other than to remove bacteria?
- Dr. Merry wants the medication to go into the deeper crevices of the abrasion. Would you expect him to prescribe an ointment or a cream? Why?
- How often do you think the bandage will be changed using a regular antibiotic dressing?
- What should you tell Johnny's mother about keeping the bandage dry?
- Why is it important to obtain a health history of possible allergies even when applying a topical medication?
- If Dr. Merry orders an occlusive dressing, what would you expect to place on the abrasion?

KEY TERMS

Acne	Emollient	Papule
Actinic keratosis	Eschar	Pediculicide
Antiseptic	Furuncle	Psoriasis
Bactericidal agent	Hives	Pustule
Bacteriostatic agent	Impetigo	Rubs
Bath	Keratin	Scabicide
Carbuncle	Keratolytic agent	Seborrheic dermatitis
Comedo/comedones	Liniment	Sebum
Disinfectant/germicidal agent	Lotion	Skin cleanser
Eczema	Nits	Ulceration
Edema	Occlusive dressing	Vehicle

EASY WORKING KNOWLEDGE OF INDICATIONS AND SIDE EFFECTS

Common Symptoms of Skin Disorders	Common Side Effects of Medications for Skin Disorders
Dermatologic lesions or eruptions	Burning
Pruritus and hives	Pruritus
Inflammation	Skin dryness
Edema	Rashes
Discomfort	Thinning of skin
Erythema	Irritation of skin

Easy Working Knowledge of Drugs Used for Skin Conditions

DRUG CLASS	PRESCRIPTION	OTC	PREGNANCY CATEGORY	MAJOR INDICATIONS
ANTIINFECTIVES				
Antibiotic	Yes	Yes	B, C	Skin infections
Antiviral	Yes	Yes	B, C	Herpetic infections, viral infections
Antiinflammatory/ corticosteroids	Yes	Yes	C	Inflammatory responses
Antifungal	Yes	Yes	B, C	Candida/tinea infections
Acne preparations	Yes	Yes	B, C, D (tetracyclines), X (tazarotene, isotretinoin)	Acne vulgaris
Keratolytics	Yes	Yes	C, X (podophyllum)	Hyperkeratotic skin lesions
Shampoos	Yes	Yes	C	Seborrheic dermatitis
Topical anesthetics	Yes	Yes	B, C	Pain, itching
Topical antipruritics	No	Yes	B	Itching
Sulfonamides	Yes	No	B, C	Burns and minor bacterial wound infections
Proteolytic enzymes	Yes	No		Débridement of wounds
PROPHYLACTIC AGENTS				
Sunscreens	No	Yes		Prevent sunburns
Protectives	No	Yes		Protects skin from irritants
Scabicides/pediculicides	Yes	Yes	B	Skin parasites
MISCELLANEOUS				
minoxidil	Yes	Yes	C	Alopecia
fluorouracil	Yes	No	D	Actinic keratosis, superficial basal cell carcinomas

Skin, the body's largest organ, is a complex structure that is divided into three main layers—the epidermis composed of a thin layer of epithelial cells that are continuously sloughed and replaced; the dense, fibrous dermis that contains blood vessels, nerve endings, and gland openings within connective tissue; and the subcutaneous layer that consists mainly of loose connective tissue and adipose (fat) tissue such as nail beds, sweat and oil glands, and elastic and fibrous tissues. The subcutaneous level acts to connect the dermis to the muscle layer (Figure 23-1).

The skin has six functions:

1. Protect the deeper tissues from drying
2. Provide a mechanical barrier against bacteria that may cause infection
3. Regulate body temperature by allowing heat to spread into the atmosphere and the loss of heat through perspiration
4. Interact with the environment through the nerve endings of pain, touch, pressure, and temperature to respond to factors in the surroundings to ensure safety
5. Excrete minerals and water through sweat glands
6. Prevent absorption of toxic substances while having the ability to absorb substances in desired instances (the function of importance pharmacologically)

Medications may be absorbed through the skin for local effect or they may be slowly absorbed in sufficient quantities for systemic effect. Some medications may be injected into the upper layers of the skin (intradermally) or into the subcutaneous (SC) tissues for a release into the bloodstream for transport throughout the body. (See Chapter 15 for parenteral medication administration.)

Classification of Dermatologic Preparations

Several kinds of medications, such as antiinfective agents, antiinflammatory agents, enzymatic preparations, and antinauseant medications, have systemic effect on the body when applied to the

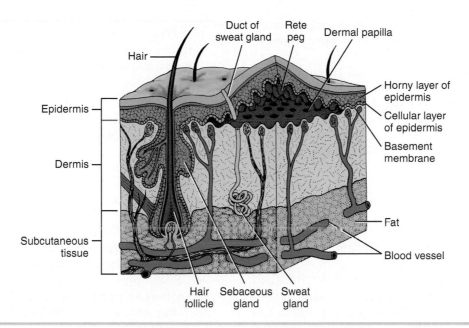

Figure 23-1 Structure of the skin. Medications are absorbed through the epidermis to the dermis and then absorbed into the bloodstream, as well as for local response to pain by nerve fibers. (From Young AP, Proctor DB: *Kinn's The Medical Assistant: an applied learning approach*, ed 10, St Louis, 2007, Saunders.)

skin. The rate of absorption of the medication depends on the form of the drug, size of the molecules (the smaller the molecule, the more rapidly the drug is absorbed), and the base of the medication (oil or the more readily absorbed water bases). Such medications as hormones, antianginals, antihypertensives, analgesics, and antihistamines may be specifically applied transdermally for prolonged release in systemic therapy. The general goals of therapy are to remove the cause of the skin disorders, find measures to restore and maintain normal function of the skin, and relieve symptoms such as itching, dryness, pain, or inflammation. These medications are discussed in the appropriate chapters for their medicinal use. (Chapter 14 describes the proper administration of transdermal medications.)

Some systemic medications cause skin diseases such as exfoliative dermatitis and scaling of skin that will eventually slough. The patient taking any medications should be evaluated for the possibility of adverse skin reactions. Box 23-1 lists the types of medications that may produce reactions from erythema to life-threatening responses.

Dermatologic Preparations and Absorption

Many forms of dermatologic preparations, such as liquids, ointments, gels, beads, pastes, plasters, creams, powders, and sprays, are available to treat

BOX 23-1	MEDICATIONS THAT CAUSE SKIN DISORDERS
Erythemas	**Lupuslike Erythemas**
barbiturates	hydantoins
carbamazepine	hydralazine
furosemide	isoniazid
gold	procainamide
griseofulvin	quinidine
penicillin	trimethadione
phenothiazines	
phenytoin	
sulfonamides	
tetracyclines	

various skin disorders. The selected form depends on the desired therapeutic effect and the ability of the skin to absorb the medication. **Keratin** of the skin, when moisturized, provides a waterproof barrier to the body; therefore water-based medications are absorbed through hydrated skin.

- Some drugs are placed in dressings to trap the perspiration of the skin and prevent water loss to assist with hydration and absorption.
- Water-soluble drugs are more readily absorbed and excreted, whereas fat-soluble drugs have slower excretion rates.
- In some areas of the body, such as behind the ear or on the eyelids, the thinness of the skin allows rapid absorption of medication, whereas

areas like the palms of the hands and the soles of the feet are so thick as to be almost impenetrable by any medications.

- Some products contain lanolin to smooth the skin and apply moisture in a lipid-soluble base. Other products are in an alcohol base to dry the skin. The product use dictates the base needed for the medication, its method and site of application, and its ability to be absorbed.

Just as with medications taken by other routes, the patient's medical record should be checked for allergies to topical medications. The skin should be clean and dry for optimal absorption.

- If the medication is for a specific site, such as a topical antiinfectant for an infected wound, the drug should be applied to the specific site without spreading to the surrounding tissues.
- If patches are used for systemic medications, the sites should be rotated to avoid irritation to the skin and prevent decreased absorption that may occur because of sensitization of the skin to the medication.

Types of Preparations for the Skin

Preparations for the skin come in many different forms, their use dependent on the exact condition being treated.

- **Baths** are used to cleanse skin, to lower body temperature, or for the application of medications.
    - Usually baths are taken with soap or cleansing gels and water, but in some skin conditions even water may not be tolerated.
    - Persons with dry skin should bathe less frequently than those with oily skin and should use an oily lotion rather than one with an alcohol base to hydrate the skin.
    - Baths for soothing irritated skin conditions may have gelatin, oatmeal (Aveeno), or starch added to the water.
    - Oils added to these products or used by themselves such as Alpha-Keri or oilated oatmeal (Aveeno Oilated Oatmeal) may be added to a tub of water to prevent drying.
    - A lubricating medication or topical product should be applied immediately after a bath while the skin is moist to increase absorption and hydration.

DID YOU KNOW?

Soaps are made by splitting fats with alkalis, making a glycerol and the alkali salt of the fatty acid, or soap. Soaps are made from different oils such as olive oil (to make castile soaps), coconut oil, and animal fats.

- *Soaps* are relatively alkaline and can irritate the skin.
    - Because of the friction needed to cleanse skin with soap, the soap becomes a mechanical **antiseptic,** whereas other soaps may have medications added to make them chemical antiseptics also.
    - Some products that are called soaps are actually **disinfectants/germicidal agents.**
    - Soap and water promote healthy skin, whereas perfumed or medicated products may cause irritation in a person with hypersensitive skin.
    - Soap should be adequately rinsed off and not left on the skin because of its drying effect.
- *Gels* are found in an alcohol base and are drying; therefore gels are appropriate for use on oily skin and weepy or vesicular lesions.
- *Skin cleansers* are usually free of soap or are modified soap products that are used with persons who have sensitive, dry, or irritated skin or those who have had an allergic reaction to soap products.
    - Cleansers are less irritating, may contain an **emollient** to smooth the skin, and may have a slightly acidic to neutral pH. Examples are Neutrogena Bars and Aveeno Cleansing Bars.
- **Emollients** are fatty or oily substances that smooth or soften irritated skin and mucous membranes and may be used as a vehicle to apply medications. Examples of emollients are: lanolin; petroleum jelly; vitamins A, D, and E ointments; creams for burns and chafing such as A & D ointment or cream; and cold creams such as Nivea skin products, Noxzema, and Lubriderm.
- *Skin protectants* coat minor skin irritations and are used to protect the skin from chemical irritants such as benzoin and benzoin compounds. Sween's Cream is used to protect skin in colostomy and ileostomy patients and to protect the skin of bedridden persons at pressure points.
- **Lotions** are liquids that have an insoluble powder or suspension.
    - These products may be mildly acid or alkaline and are used for dressings. Others,

such as calamine or Caladryl lotion, may be used for their soothing effect in contact dermatitis, insect bites, or prickly heat.

- **Rubs** and **liniments** are indicated for the relief of pain on *intact* skin such as the pain associated with muscle aches, neuralgia, rheumatism, arthritis, and sprains or strains.
  - These medications produce heat to relieve aches and pains.
  - Because of the danger of burning the skin or causing severe irritation, external heat such as a heating pad or hot water bottle should not be used with liniments and rubs unless prescribed by a physician.
  - The ingredients may include counterirritants such as camphor or methylsalicylate or analgesics such as salicylate substances that have the potential to burn or irritate the skin.
  - Local anesthetics and antiseptics may also be added to these products for relief of pain.

IMPORTANT FACTS ABOUT THE TYPES OF SKIN PREPARATIONS

- Skin preparations are used on a daily basis. They include soaps, gels, disinfectants, baths, lotions, and sunscreens.
- Soaps and baths are drying to the skin.
- Skin protectants should be used to protect the skin around pressure ulcers or ostomies to prevent further trauma.
- Rubs and liniments tend to produce vasodilation and heat. External heat should not be applied to skin after a liniment or rub has been applied because of the chance of burning the skin.

Antiinfective/Antiinflammatory Topicals

The skin is subject to infections by bacteria, fungi, and viruses. Topical antiinfectives may be used alone as therapy in superficial wounds. Where wounds have deep penetration of infection, systemic antiinfectives may be indicated.

Topical Antibiotics

Topical antibiotics, much like systemic antibiotics, are used for the most common organisms found in skin infections—*Streptococcus pyrogenes* and *Staphylococcus aureus.* These organisms cause infections such as folliculitis, **impetigo, furuncles, carbuncles,** and cellulitis. (Figure 23-2 shows characteristics of various skin lesions.)

Antiinfectives may be **bacteriostatic agents, bactericidal agents,** germicides, disinfectants, or antiseptics.

Antiinfectives such as isopropyl alcohol, hexachlorophene, iodine, Lysol, and benzalkonium chloride were discussed in Chapter 18. Table 23-1 lists typical topical antibiotics, both OTC and legend medications.

CLINICAL TIP

If culture and sensitivity testing is to be performed on skin wounds, this should be done before applying topical antiinfective medications or administering systemic antiinfectives to prevent antibiotic resistance.

Patient Education for Compliance

1. Topical medications should be applied at regular intervals throughout the day.
2. Cleanse the area prior to applying the topical medication.

IMPORTANT FACTS ABOUT TOPICAL ANTIINFECTIVE/ANTIINFLAMMATORY AGENTS

- Topical antibiotics may be used to help clear mild to moderate acne.
- Topical antibiotics are available OTC (e.g., Neosporin Cream) and are used for minor trauma. These agents are found in first-aid kits.

Topical Antivirals

Antivirals are applied several times a day to skin lesions such as herpes and herpes zoster.

- Acyclovir is applied six times a day for 7 days.
- Multiple OTC preparations are available for treating such viral disorders as cold sores (herpes simplex). Table 23-2 lists the prescription medications used topically for viral infections.

Patient Education for Compliance

1. Use gloves or other protective equipment when applying antiviral medications to herpes infections to prevent the spread of the viral infection.
2. Avoid eye contact with antivirals.

PRIMARY LESIONS

MACULE
Flat area of color change (no elevation or depression)

Example: Freckles

PAPULE
Solid elevation less than 0.5 cm in diameter

Example: Allergic eczema

NODULE
Solid elevation 0.5 to 1 cm in diameter. Extends deeper into dermis than papule

Example: Mole

TUMOR
Solid mass—larger than 1 cm

Example: Squamous cell carcinoma

PLAQUE
Flat elevated surface found on skin or mucous membrane

Example: Thrush

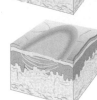

WHEAL
Type of plaque. Result is transient edema in dermis

Example: Intradermal skin test

VESICLE
Small blister—fluid within or under epidermis

Example: Herpesvirus infection

BULLA
Large blister (greater than 0.5 cm)

Example: Burn

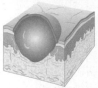

PUSTULE
Vesicle filled with pus

Example: Acne

SECONDARY LESIONS

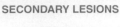

SCALES
Flakes of cornified skin layer

Example: Psoriasis

CRUST
Dried exudate on skin

Example: Impetigo

FISSURE
Cracks in skin

Example: Athlete's foot

ULCER
Area of destruction of entire epidermis

Example: Decubitus (pressure sore)

SCAR
Excess collagen production after injury

Example: Surgical healing

ATROPHY
Loss of some portion of the skin

Example: Paralysis

Figure 23-2 Characteristics of skin lesions. (From Young AP, Proctor DB: *Kinn's The Medical Assistant: an applied learning approach,* ed 10, St Louis, 2007, Saunders.)

TABLE 23-1 *Select Topical Antiinfectives**

GENERIC NAME	TRADE NAME	USUAL ADULT DOSE, ROUTE, AND FREQUENCY OF ADMINISTRATION	INDICATIONS FOR USE
mupirocin	Bactroban† ointment and cream, 2%	Apply tid	Skin infections, broad spectrum
bacitracin	Baciguent‡ Bacitin† ointment, powder, and cream	Apply qid	Gram-negative bacteria
gentamicin	Garamycin† cream, ointment	Apply qid	Broad spectrum
neomycin	Myciguent† cream, ointment	Apply qid	Broad spectrum
neo-lycin, polymyxin B, gramicidin	Triple Antibiotic‡ Neosporin‡ cream, ointment	Apply qid	Broad spectrum
nitrofurazone	Furacin† soluble dressing	Apply tid-qid	Burns, ulcers, infections
hexachlorophene	Dial soap‡	As soap for bathing	Soap; do not use on infants

SIDE EFFECTS OF TOPICAL ANTIINFECTIVES: mupirocin: local irritation and burning; **nitrofurazone:** pruritus, burning, ulceration; **hexachlorophene:** kills normal bacterial flora; **bacitracin, gentamicin, neomycin, neo-polycin, polymyxin B, gramicidin:** allergic dermatitis; **nitrofurazone:** pruritus, burning, ulceration; **hexachlorophene:** kills normal bacterial flora.

* Topical antiinfectives have no major drug interactions.
† Prescription medications.
‡ Over-the-counter medications.

TABLE 23-2 *Select Topical Antivirals*

GENERIC NAME	TRADE NAME	USUAL ADULT DOSE, ROUTE, AND FREQUENCY OF ADMINISTRATION	INDICATIONS FOR USE	DRUG INTERACTIONS
acyclovir	Zovirax 5%* ointment, powder	Topically 5× per day	Herpetic lesions and other dermatologic viral conditions	
penciclovir	Denavir* ointment	Topically q2h × 4 days	Herpetic lesions	
vidarabine	Vira-A* ointment	Topically 5 × per day	Herpes simplex of and around the eyes	
idoxuridine	Herplex* solution	Apply gtt † qh during day; q2h at night	Herpetic lesions	Iodine
	HESper-L† gel	Apply locally 5× per day		
docosanol	Abreva† cream 10%	Apply to lesions 5× per day; up to 10 days	Cold sores, herpes simplex	

MAJOR SIDE EFFECTS OF TOPICAL ANTIVIRALS: acyclovir: local pain, rash, pruritus, burning; **penciclovir:** headache, Pruritus, rash; **vidarabine:** irritation, rash.

* Prescription medication.
† Over-the-counter medication.

IMPORTANT FACT ABOUT TOPICAL ANTIVIRALS
- Care should be taken when applying topical antivirals to prevent spread of the virus.

Topical Corticosteroids

Topical corticosteroids are used to relieve the inflammation and pruritus of contact dermatitis, insect bites, minor burns, seborrheic dermatitis, **psoriasis,** and **eczema.**

- These medications are usually found in creams, ointments, lotions, and gels to facilitate absorption at the site of action.
- The **vehicle** for topical corticosteroids may be an emollient or a drying agent.
- Absorption is high in areas of thin skin, but penetration is poor with thick skin.
- These preparations vary widely in strength, with those available OTC being of low potency.

TABLE 23-3 *Select Topical Antiinflammatory/Corticosteroid Agents*

GENERIC NAME	TRADE NAME	USUAL ADULT DOSE, ROUTE, AND FREQUENCY OF ADMINISTRATION	INDICATIONS FOR USE	DRUG INTERACTIONS
betamethasone	Diprolene 0.05%* cream, ointment	Apply locally bid-tid	Inflamed tissue, psoriasis, rashes, insect bites, eczema	Usually none with topical antiinflam- matory agents
	Diprosone 0.025%-0.05%* cream, ointment, lotion, gel			
	Uticort 0.025%* lotion	Same		
	Valisone 0.1%* cream, lotion, ointment	Same		
clobetasol	Temovate 0.05%* cream, ointment	Apply locally bid		
diflorasone	Psorcon,* ointment	Same		
	Maxiflor 0.05%* ointment	Same		
amcinonide	Cyclocort 0.1%* cream, ointment, lotion	Apply locally tid		
desoximetasone	Topicort 0.05%-0.25%* cream, ointment	Apply locally bid-tid		
fluocinonide	Fluonex* cream, ointment	Same		
	Lidex 0.05%* gel	Same		
halcinonide	Halog 0.025%-0.1%* cream, ointment	Same		
triamcinolone	Aristocort 0.1%* cream, ointment, lotion	Same		
	Kenalog 0.1%* and others in the same forms			
hydrocortisone	Westcort 0.2%* cream, ointment	Same		
	Cortizone 10† cream, ointment	Same		
	Hycort 1%† lotion	Same		
	Cortaid† and other preparations in cream, ointment, 0.5%†	Apply locally tid-qid		
desonide	DesOwen* cream	Apply locally tid		
	Tridesilon 0.05%* cream	Same		
dexamethasone	Decaspray 0.04%* aerosol spray	Same		
	Decadron 0.1%* cream	Same		
fluocinolone	Flurosyn,* Synalar 0.01%-0.2%* cream, solution	Apply locally tid-qid		
mometasone	Elocon 0.1% cream, ointment	Apply locally bid-tid		
prednicarbate	Dermatop 0.1%* cream	Sparingly 2-4 × daily		

*Prescription medication.
† Over-the-counter medication.
‡No major side effects are found with topical antiinflammatory agents.

- Systemic toxicity may be a side effect with long-term therapy using high-potency topical corticosteroids.
- Apply in a thin film and gently rub into the skin; gels and lotions are used in hairy areas. The site of application influences the choice of the form of steroid.
- Creams rub easily into the tissue if needed for weepy, wet tissue lesions.
- Ointments are more moisturizing because of the lipid base and are best for application on dry or scaly areas.
- Ointments are more occlusive to the skin; creams and lotions are less occlusive.

Chapter 21 discusses systemic corticosteroids. For select legend and OTC topical corticosteroid medications, see Table 23-3.

Patient Education for Compliance

1. Apply a thin film of medication.
2. Cleanse the skin and then apply medication; the best time is after a shower, for better absorption. The skin should be dried prior to application.
3. Do not cover corticosteroid preparations with occlusive clothing or dressings unless directed.
4. Avoid sunlight on treated areas.
5. Avoid prolonged use of corticosteroids.
6. Do not apply to weeping or denuded areas unless specifically prescribed by the physician.
7. Use only on prescribed areas.
8. Avoid contact with the eyes.
9. Do not use tight diapers, diaper covers, or plastic pants when applying corticosteroids to infants.

Topical Antifungals

Topical antifungal medications, such as clotrimazole (Desenex, Cruex) and tolnaftate (Tinactin), are used to treat fungal infections of the hair, nails, or skin. Because of the dampness and warmth of some body areas such as the feet, axilla, perineal area, and under the breasts, fungal infections seem to thrive in these areas.

- Most antifungals change the integrity of the cell membrane of the fungus, making the medication either fungistatic or fungicidal.
- Topical antifungals are generally used to treat *Candida* and tinea infections. The common forms of tinea include tinea pedis (athlete's foot), tinea corporis (ringworm of the body), tinea cruris ("jock itch"), tinea capitis (ringworm of the head), and tinea versicolor (infection of skin, with yellow or tan-colored branlike patches). Fungal infections of the nails, or onychomycosis (tinea unguium), are difficult to treat and require prolonged therapy with oral and topical medications.
- *Candida* infections include vulvovaginal candidiasis, which is common in women of reproductive age.
- The topical antifungal preparations come in sprays, lotions, creams, ointments, and powders and are available as both prescription and OTC medications.
- Some are combined with corticosteroids; an example is Lotrisone.
- Fungal medications should not come in contact with the eye or delicate mucous membranes.

- For topical antifungals to be effective, the skin should be clean and dry prior to application.
- If no improvement occurs with OTC medications in 2 to 3 weeks, the patient should see a physician (Table 23-4).

Patient Education for Compliance

1. Cleanse the skin with soap and water and dry it before applying medications.
2. If the condition persists or worsens, contact a physician.
3. Use the full treatment, even if symptoms improve, because therapy is long term for fungal infections.
4. Do not use occlusive dressings because they tend to hold perspiration and allow for growth of fungi. The skin should remain dry.

IMPORTANT FACTS ABOUT TOPICAL ANTIFUNGAL MEDICATIONS

- Topical antifungals are available in many forms for fungal and candidal infections.
- Many fungal infections, but especially those of the nails, are difficult to treat and may require prolonged therapy.

Acne Preparations

Acne vulgaris is a skin disease with increased **sebum** and oil production and increased formation of keratin, usually on the face, chest, back, and neck. Acne appears as **papules, pustules,** and **comedo/comedones.** The treatment includes the reduction of sebum and bacteria. Many preparations are available OTC; other preparations require a prescription.

Antibiotics such as tetracycline and erythromycin are used for treatment for acne. However, a drug specific for the condition is isotretinoin (Accutane), a derivative of vitamin A. This medication is considered as pregnancy category X with many teratogenic effects. Because of the severe side effects that may be caused by isotretinoin, it is reserved for severe disfiguring cases of acne. Those physicians prescribing and the persons taking the drug must enroll in S.M.A.R.T. (System to Manage Accutane-Related Teratoxicity) program to ensure no woman beginning the therapy is pregnant nor becomes pregnant while taking the drug. A prescription written for isotretinoin must have a special sticker applied by the physician before it can be filled.

TABLE 23-4 Select Antifungals for Use in Dermatologic Conditions[‡]

GENERIC NAME	TRADE NAME	USUAL ADULT DOSE, ROUTE, AND FREQUENCY OF ADMINISTRATION	INDICATIONS FOR USE	MAJOR SIDE EFFECTS	DRUG INTERACTIONS
clotrimazole	Mycelex,* Mycelex G,* Lotrimin,[†] Gyne-Lotrimin[†]	Vaginal tablets and cream use hs; topical cream, troches, solution, ointment use bid	Candidiasis and tinea infections	Local irritation, pruritus, burning sensation, scaling, dryness, erythema, blistering, peeling, stinging, urticaria	
econazole	Spectazole* cream	Apply topically daily to bid	Tinea		
haloprogin	Halotex[†]	Apply topically daily to bid	Tinea		
itraconazole	Sporanox* 100 mg cap	1 cap daily po	Tinea		
	Sporanox lotion	Apply topically bid			
ketoconazole	Nizoral 2% cream	Apply topically daily or bid	Tinea capitis and seborrheic dermatitis		H₂ blockers, anticholinergics
	Nizoral AD 1% shampoo	Shampoo 2× week			
	Nizoral 200 mg tab	1 to 2 tabs po daily			
miconazole	Micatin[†] Monistat Derm 1%*[†] topical cream, spray	Apply topically bid	Candidiasis and tinea infections		
	Monistat[†] vaginal suppository/cream	Insert vaginally hs			
	Metrazol powder	Apply topically bid			
miconazole, zinc oxide, petroleum	Vusion ointment	Apply topically after each diaper change × 7 days	Complicated candidiasis of diaper rash		
oxiconazole	Oxistat* cream, lotion	Apply topically daily for 2-4 wk	Candidiasis and tinea infections		
sertaconazole	Ertaczo	Apply topically daily	Tinea only		
undecylenic acid	Desenex, Cruex,[†] Caldesene[†], Fungoid[†] in cream, ointment, powder, solution, soap, spray	Apply topically bid	Candidiasis and tinea infections and diaper rash		
ciclopirox	Loprox* cream, lotion	Apply topically bid	Tinea only		
haloprogin	Halotex* cream, solution	Apply topically bid	Tinea only		
tolnaftate	Tinactin[†] powder, cream, solution, spray, gel Absorbine[†] solution Aftate, NP-27[†] cream, ointment	Apply topically bid	Tinea only		

Drug	Formulation	Directions	Indication
terbinafine	Lamisil 250 mg po cream, solution†	1 tab po daily / Apply topically qd to bid	Tinea only
naftifine	Naftin† cream, gel	Apply topically daily	Tinea only
butenafine	Lotrimin Ultra cream, Mentax* cream 1%	Apply topically bid / Apply topically daily for 4 wk	Tinea pedis
nystatin	Mycostatin* tab suspension troche / Powder, cream, ointment / Vaginal tablets	1 tab po bid; Swish and swallow / Dissolve in mouth qid / Apply topically bid-tid × 14 days / 1 tab vaginally hs	Candidiasis, diaper rash
Nystatin/ triamcinolone	Mycolog* cream, ointment	Use topically tid-qid	Candidiasis
amphotericin B	Fungizone†	Apply topically bid	Tinea infestations
ciclopirox	Loprox, Rentax Nail Lacquer	Apply topically as directed	Tinea infestations

* Prescription medication.
† OTC medication.
‡ No major side effects are found with topical antifungal agents. However, gastrointestinal disturbances may occur with large oral dosages.

Two combination oral contraceptives (Estrostep and Ortho Tri-Cyclin) have been approved for treating women at least 15 years of age who have reached menarche and have not responded to topical medications for acne. The benefits are from the estrogen that suppresses and inactivates sebum production.

Only a few of the available topical preparations for acne are discussed here.

- **Benzoyl peroxide** is the ingredient in many OTC preparations such as Acnomel, Acne-10, Benoxyl, Clearasil, Dryox, Fostex, Neutrogena, and Oxyderm. Benzoyl peroxide is also found in prescription medications. It promotes peeling of the skin and suppresses the growth of bacteria by releasing active oxygen.
- **Topical and systemic antibiotics** are used to treat acne. The oral antibiotic of choice is usually tetracycline. The most commonly prescribed topical antibiotics prescribed for mild to moderate acne are erythromycin and clindamycin. These two agents work by decreasing sebaceous fatty acid by-products and preventing the formation of new acne lesions. (Oral antibiotics are discussed in Chapter 25.)
- **Tretinoin** (Retin-A), an irritant, stimulates the rapid turnover of epithelial cells followed by skin peeling. It reduces the fatty acids within the comedones and causes the comedones to be removed, finally suppressing the formation of new plugs. This drug is a category X preparation and should not be used in pregnant women or those who may become pregnant. Tretinoin is applied to the face once a day for peeling. This preparation is also used to remove fine wrinkles caused by aging or sun. The patient should be instructed to wash hands after application to avoid exposure of the drug to sensitive tissues such as the eyes and mucous membranes.
  - Tretinoin (Renova) is used for fine wrinkle removal on the face.
- **Keratolytic agents** increase the effectiveness of skin peeling agents.
- **Adapalene** (Differin) reduces the formation of comedones and may even appear to exacerbate the acne prior to becoming effective. Adapalene is not systemically absorbed. The risk of sunburn is also increased with this agent, but this tends to subside as therapy continues.
- **Azelaic acid** (Azelex) is used for mild to moderate acne and acts by suppressing the growth of bacteria that are the underlying cause of acne.

- **Tazarotene** (Tazorac) is a vitamin A derivative that has been classified as pregnancy category X and should not be used during pregnancy. Tazarotene is used for acne and psoriasis (Table 23-5).

Patient Education for Compliance

1. Keep acne preparations away from eyes, mouth, and other mucous membranes.
2. Expect dryness and peeling of skin with most acne preparations; discontinue with rash or irritations.
3. Water-based cosmetics should be used with acne preparations. Do not counter-treat the desired dryness of these preparations with emollients.
4. After applying topical erythromycin, wait 1 hour before applying any other topical medication or cosmetics.
5. The skin may turn yellow with topical tetracycline.
6. Topical tetracyclines may stain fabrics.
7. Persons using tretinoin are susceptible to sunburn and should wear sunscreen (SPF 15 or greater) and protective clothing. If sunburned, do not apply tretinoin to the skin.
8. When using tretinoin, the skin should be washed and dried 15 to 30 minutes prior to application. Contact with the eyes, nose, or mouth should be avoided.
9. Before using Renova, cosmetics should be removed. Up to 6 months of treatment may be needed to see a response for the treatment.

IMPORTANT FACTS ABOUT ACNE PREPARATIONS
- Acne preparations contain benzoyl peroxide, which is drying to the skin. Oil-based creams and cosmetics should not be used following application of these medications.
- Some of the acne preparations are applied to the skin to cause peeling. Care should be taken in the sun to prevent burning.
- Vitamin A preparations should not be used during pregnancy.

Keratolytic Agents

Keratolytic agents or keratin dissolvers are used to promote shedding of the horny layer of skin and to soften scales with effects ranging from peeling to extensive desquamation of the skin.

- Salicylic acid, resorcinol, and sulfur are the drugs of choice, but benzoyl peroxide may be used for this therapy.

TABLE 23-5 Select Medications for Acne and Psoriasis

GENERIC NAME	TRADE NAME	USUAL ADULT DOSE, ROUTE, AND FREQUENCY OF ADMINISTRATION	INDICATIONS FOR USE	MAJOR SIDE EFFECTS	DRUG INTERACTIONS
ACNE PREPARATIONS					
benzoyl peroxide 2.5%-10%	Pan-Oxyl, Desquam, Benzox, Persa-Gel, Benzagel† as soap, cream, gel, liquid, lotion, mask	Apply topically daily to tid	Acne	Dryness of skin	Usually none with topicals.
ANTIBIOTICS					
clindamycin	Cleocin T* solution	Apply topically bid		Dryness, scaling, peeling of skin, stinging and burning, itching tenderness	
erythromycin with benzoyl peroxide	EryDerm, A/T/S, T-Stat* solution Benzamycin* cream	Apply topically bid Apply topically daily		Same as above	
tetracycline	Topicycline* solution or ointment	Apply topically bid			
clindamycin 1.2%/tretinoin 0.025% gel	Ziana gel	Apply topically daily		Inflammation of throat/nose, dry skin,	No abrasive soaps/cleansers, sun exposure
doxycycline	Oracea 40 mg delayed-release capsule	1 cap daily	Pustules/papules of rosacea	Headaches, dizziness, blurred vision; flulike symptoms; loss of appetite	See doxycycline in Chapter 18
minocycline	Solodyn Extended-release tab	1 mg/kg/day	Inflammatory lesions of acne	Lightheadedness, dizziness; do not use before age 12 because it will darken teeth	See minocycline in Chapter 18
OTHERS					
tretinoin (retinoic acid)	Retin-A* Renova‡ Cream, gel, liquid, emollient Avista	Apply topically daily Apply topically daily hs	Acne Fine facial wrinkles	Redness, edematous blisters, crusting stinging	
adapalene	Differin* gel, cream	Apply topically daily		Burning, pruritus, erythema, dryness, scaling	
azelaic acid	Azelex* cream	Apply topically bid		Same as above with tingling and depigmentation	
tazarotene	Tazorac*‡ gel	Apply topically hs	Acne and psoriasis		
isotretinoin	Accutane*‡ po	0.5-2 mg/kg/day × 15-20 wk	Acne	Hives, swelling of lips, mouth, face; difficulty breathing	carbamazepine
calcipotriene/betamethasone	Taclonex ointment	Apply topically daily			

* Prescription medication.
† Over-the-counter medication.
‡ Pregnancy category X drug.

- The medications are used to treat dandruff, **seborrheic dermatitis,** acne, and psoriasis, as well as warts and corns.
- Salicylic acid, podophyllum resin, and cantharidin may be used for common warts, as well as for venereal warts.
- Podophyllum is teratogenic and also has the potential for systemic reactions. Podophyllum is not particularly effective against common warts. These resins should be applied, then washed off in 1 to 6 hours. They should be used at weekly intervals for 4 weeks.
- Cantharidin (Cantharone) is used to remove common warts. This agent is harmful to normal skin, so the skin should be cleaned immediately with acetone or alcohol in the event it accidentally touches normal skin (Table 23-6).

Patient Education for Compliance

1. Keratolytic agents are for external use only. Avoid contact with the face, eyes, mucous membranes, and normal skin around warts.
2. Soaking the area in warm water for 5 minutes prior to application may enhance the effect of the medication.

IMPORTANT FACT ABOUT KEROLYTIC AGENTS

- Keratolytic agents promote shedding of the horny layer of the skin such as warts, calluses, and corns.

Treatments for Seborrheic Dermatitis

Shampoos for seborrheic dermatitis are available OTC and by prescription. Seborrheic dermatitis is characterized by inflammation and scaling of the face or scalp and may be found under arms, on the chest, and in the anogenital region. Seborrheic dermatitis begins on the scalp and is characterized by yellowish, brownish-gray greasy scales. Ketoconazole, an antifungal, may be used as a shampoo. Other medications such as pyrithione zinc or selenium sulfide are available OTC (Selsun Blue, Head and Shoulders) and by prescription (Selsun, Exsel) because of the stronger strength. These agents may cause skin irritation, alopecia, and discoloration of the hair.

Topical Anesthesia and Antipruritics

Topical anesthetics such as lidocaine (Solarcaine, Anbesol) and dibucaine (Nupercainal) are used for itching of the skin or mucous membranes and for desensitizing the skin to painful stimuli. These medications are available as OTC preparations (see earlier) and are available for prescription use as tetracaine (Pontocaine) and lidocaine (Xylocaine) (Table 23-7).

Dilute solutions of phenol have been used for anesthesia and pruritus. Lotions of calamine or phenolated calamine are often used for pruritus. A cream with diphenhydramine (Benadryl) alone or with calamine (Caladryl) may be bought OTC for relief of pruritus. These medications for itching may be used three to four times a day without side effects or adverse reactions. Cornstarch and oatmeal baths (Aveeno) are also used, especially for children with chickenpox (see Table 23-7).

CLINICAL TIP
Calamine lotion should be used with chickenpox. The use of Caladryl lotion is not recommended because it contains an antihistamine that is contraindicated for the relief of pruritus of chickenpox. When an oral antihistamine is prescribed, calamine lotion (without diphenhydramine) should be used.

IMPORTANT FACTS ABOUT TOPICAL ANESTHETICS

- Topical anesthetics come in many forms to relieve the pain of insect bites, abrasions, minor burns, and wounds. The topical anesthetics are used for such conditions as sunburns and hemorrhoids.
- Antipruritics are applied topically for itching.

Topical Treatment of Burns

Burn treatment is dependent on the type of burn and its depth, as well as the percentage of the body area that has been burned (Figure 23-3). Types of burns include thermal, chemical, and electrical burns, as well as inhalation of smoke. Emergency treatment may be accomplished by using dressings such as Duoderm or OpSite. Topical antiinfective agents may also be indicated. Two **sulfonamides** are frequently used because of their broad spectrum of action against gram-positive and gram-negative bacteria.

Silver sulfadiazine (Silvadene) is used with second- and third-degree burns for the prevention of infections and to soften **eschar** and facilitate its removal. Silvadene, the preferred antiinfective agent used in most burn centers, is available in a 1% cream and is used on burns continuously after cleansing and débriding.

TABLE 23-6 *Select Keratolytics*

GENERIC NAME	TRADE NAME	USUAL ADULT DOSE, ROUTE, AND FREQUENCY OF ADMINISTRATION	INDICATIONS FOR USE	DRUG INTERACTIONS
salicylic acid	Compound W, Wart-Off, Mediplast, Sal-Plast[†] as gels, plasters, adhesives, cream solutions, lotions, ointments, shampoo	Lotion—apply topically qd-bid Plasters—apply topically, leave in place 48 hr Shampoo— topically qd-qod Solution, creams— topically qd	Hyperkeratotic skin conditions, common/plantar warts, psoriasis, calluses, corns, dandruff	Usually none with topical preparations
with podophyllum	Verrex[‡], Podofin[‡], Podocon-25* liquid, powder	Topically qd-q wk	Venereal warts	
resorcinol 1%-10%	Found in many OTC and ℞ in shampoos, ointments, lotions, creams	Apply topically daily	Acne, eczema, psoriasis, seborrheic dermatitis	
sulfur 2%-10%	Found in many OTC and ℞ in lotions, gels, shampoos	Apply topically daily	Acne, eczema, psoriasis, seborrheic dermatitis	
cantharidin	Cantharone, Verr-Canth* Powder	Apply topically and cover with tape for 24 hr; then remove	Common warts and virally induced skin diseases	
imiquimod	Aldara* cream	Apply topically daily × 7 days or 3 × weekly	Venereal warts	
ammonium lactate	Lac-Hydrin lotion, cream	Apply topically bid	Acne, eczema, psoriasis, seborrheic dermatitis	

MAJOR SIDE EFFECTS OF KERATOLYTICS: Local—burning, irritation; Systemic—tinnitus, dizziness, ototoxicity, headaches.

* Prescription medication.
[†] OTC medication.
[‡] Used by medical professionals only; not dispensed.

 CLINICAL TIP
Before using sulfadiazine, be sure the patient is not allergic to either of the active ingredients, silver and sulfa.

- Mafenide (Sulfamylon) is also a broad-spectrum bacteriostatic agent that penetrates eschar, even in the presence of pus and serum. This agent rapidly diffuses through burns and is effective against bacterial invasion into the wound. For this reason, this agent is used frequently for second- and third-degree burns. Mafenide is relatively nontoxic, but some burning, stinging, or pain may occur on application (Table 23-8).

Proteolytic enzymes are used to clean and débride tissues of debris and exudates by dissolving the protein of the necrotic tissue. Some of these medications are combined with antibiotics to add bactericidal action (see Table 23-8).

Patient Education for Compliance

1. Burns should be cleaned and débrided before sulfonamides are applied.
2. Burns should be continuously covered with sulfonamides to soften eschar.

TABLE 23-7 *Select Topical Anesthetics and Antipruretics*[‡]

GENERIC NAME	TRADE NAME	USUAL ADULT DOSE, ROUTE, AND FREQUENCY OF ADMINISTRATION	INDICATIONS FOR USE	DRUG INTERACTIONS
TOPICAL ANESTHETICS				
benzocaine	Benzocaine,* Anbesol, Boil-Eze, Oragel, Diet Ayds, Solarcaine, Dermoplast[†] as cream, liquid, gel, ointment, spray, aerosol[†]; also available in otic drops	As needed topically	Anesthesia	None noted
lidocaine	Xylocaine, Anestacon* Derma Flex[†] as gel, ointment, solution, aerosol spray	As needed topically	Anesthesia	None noted
lidocaine with prilocaine	EMLA Gel	As needed topically prior to venipuncture	For site anesthesia	None noted
tetracaine	Pontocaine[†] solution, cream, ointment	As needed topically	Toothache, sunburn, pruritus, oral pain	None noted
dibucaine	Nupercainal[†] cream, ointment	As needed topically	Sunburn, rectal pain, pruritus	None noted
ethyl chloride 2%	ethyl chloride spray	As needed topically	Freezing prior to minor surgical procedures, sprains, strains	None noted
ANTIPRURETICS				
Calamine	Calamine lotion	Apply topically as needed		
with diphenhydramine	Caladryl cream, lotion			
oleated oatmeal	Aveeno powder	Mix with bath water as needed for itching		

* Prescription medication.
[†] OTC medication.
[‡] No major side effects are found with topical anesthetics and antipruritics.

IMPORTANT FACTS ABOUT BURN MEDICATIONS
- Burns are classified by type, degree, and amount of the body burned. Sulfonamides are often used for second- and third-degree burns.
- Proteolytic enzymes are used to débride and clean tissues of debris and exudate.

Prophylactic Agents

Sunscreens are used when extended exposure to the sun may lead to premature aging of the skin or to sunburn during leisure activities or occupations that require outdoor exposure. Some chemicals and medications such as tetracyclines, sulfonamides, thiazides, phenothiazines, tricyclic antidepressants, and antineoplastic agents, as well as cosmetics, may increase the chance of **photosensitivity.** Tissue aging occurs when ultraviolet-absorbing waves are present in sufficient amounts to cause destruction of tissue. The skin becomes red and painful, and it burns, with the peak reaction occurring 24 to 48 hours after exposure. The result may be skin damage that may result in precancerous or cancerous tissues.

Sunscreens either absorb or reflect harmful rays from the sun. Absorbing agents are chemicals that absorb harmful rays into the skin to prevent erythema, burns, and other harmful effects. Those that reflect the rays are opaque, like pastes, and must be applied heavily to be effective; examples are zinc oxide and titanium dioxide.

The Food and Drug Administration (FDA) has classified sun products by their sun protection factor (SPF). The SPF is the ratio between the exposure of ultraviolet radiation (UVR) waves and the time required to cause erythema with or without sunscreen, or the minimum erythema dose (MED). The best way to choose a sunscreen is by the type of skin and the length of time in the sun. Generally the recommendation as required by some

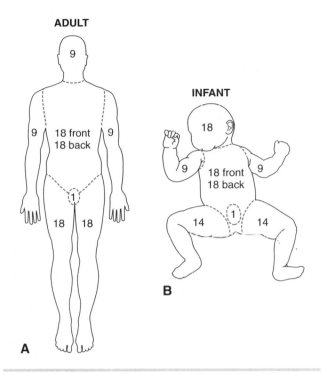

ADULT

INFANT

A

B

Figure 23-3 "Rule of Nines" used to evaluate burns. **A**, Adult. **B**, Child.

medications is a minimum SPF of 15. In the tropics, an SPF of 30 is recommended when a person is in the sun for even a brief period of time.

The efficacy of a sunscreen is related to its ability to stay on the skin through exercise, sweating, and swimming. Some sunscreens are water resistant, whereas others are classified as very water resistant or waterproof. Water-resistant sunscreens should remain on the skin for 40 minutes in water; waterproof sunscreens should remain on the skin twice as long. Some protectants have dual sun protection factors on the label, one for dry conditions and one for use in water.

Skin Protectives

Protectives form a film on the skin to prevent maceration of the skin and prevent drying of the skin. These products will also keep out light, air, and dust. Nonabsorbable powders may not be useful as protectants because they tend to stick to wet surfaces and are difficult to remove. These nonabsorbable powders include zinc oxide, zinc stearate, bismuth preparations, and talcum powder. Collodion (a mixture of alcohol, ether, and pyroxylin) is applied for protection; the ether in alcohol evaporates, leaving a thin, transparent film on the skin. Flexible collodion is collodion mixed with

TABLE 23-8 *Medications Used for Burns and Débridement**

GENERIC NAME	TRADE NAME	USUAL ADULT DOSE, ROUTE, AND FREQUENCY OF ADMINISTRATION	INDICATIONS FOR USE	DRUG INTERACTIONS
SULFONAMIDES				
silver sulfadiazine*	Silvadene cream	Apply topically tid- qid with continuous coverage	Second- and third-degree burns	Proteolytic enzymes
mafenide*	Sulfamylon cream	Apply topically daily to bid		
MAJOR SIDE EFFECTS OF SULFONAMIDES: Erythema, rash.				
PROTEOLYTIC (DÉBRIDING AGENTS)—ENZYMES				
collagenase	Santyl, Biozyme C ointment	Apply topically daily	Débride wounds	Cleansing agents
sutilains	Travase ointment	Apply topically daily		
trypsin	Granulex crystals	Sprinkle in wound bid-tid		
fibrinolysin/ desoxyribonuclease	Elase ointment	Apply topically daily		
OTHER PROTEOLYTIC (DÉBRIDING) AGENTS				
dextranomer	Debrisan Hydrophilic beads	Once a day or as indicated by change in bead color		
flexible hydroactive dressing and granules	Duo-Derm granule dressing	Use topically daily		

*Prescription medication.

TABLE 23-9 *Scabicides/Pediculicides*

GENERIC NAME	TRADE NAME	USUAL ADULT DOSE AND FREQUENCY OF ADMINISTRATION	INDICATIONS FOR USE	DRUG INTERACTIONS
Lindane	Kwell* cream, lotion,	As directed	Scabies/	Usually none
permethrin	shampoo	One application	pediculosis	with topical
malathion	Nix,† Elimite* shampoo	One application,	Head lice,	preparations
	Ovide,* lotion	followed by another	scabies	used as
	A-200,† Rid-X†	application in 10-14 days	Lice	directed

MAJOR SIDE EFFECTS OF SCABICIDES/PEDICULICIDES: All: Rash; **permethrin, malathion:** pruritus, irritation, burning, and erythema.

* Prescription medication.
† OTC medication.

camphor and castor oil to make an elastic, flexible film. Styptic collodion contains tannic acid as an astringent, as well as a protectant. All of these agents protect the skin, allowing the stimulation of healing to occur and preventing further trauma.

Medications for Scabies and Pediculosis

Scabicides and **pediculicides** are used against animal parasites. Pediculosis is an infestation of lice on the skin of humans—pediculosis pubis (pubic lice), pediculosis corporis (body lice), or pediculosis capitis (head lice).

- Pediculosis corporis is usually found around the waist, collar, or axillary area because after biting the individual the parasite is absent from the body but is found hiding in the clothing worn. The drug for pediculosis is lindane (Kwell). The topical creams and lotions are applied to the affected area and left on for 12 hours, then thoroughly washed off. The shampoo is worked into the scalp for 4 minutes, shampooed, and then rinsed. Finally, the **nits** are combed from the hair shafts. Repeated applications of lindane, a strong insecticide, may cause central nervous system toxicity, especially in children. To prevent repeated infection, patients should practice good hygiene techniques.
- Scabies are small parasites that bore into the horny layer of the skin, causing irritation and pruritus. Itching most frequently occurs at night. A month after the mites burrow under the skin, symptoms such as watery blisters between the fingers appear. The infestation then spreads

around the wrists and elbows and onto the buttocks. Lindane lotion used with scabies is left on the entire body for 8 hours. Other medications such as crotamiton (Eurax), permethrin (Nix, Elimite), and malathion (Ovide) are applied to the infested areas. Elimite, the prescription drug for scabies, is applied from the neck down over the body and is left on for 12 hours before washing off. This may be repeated in 7 to 10 days if needed. Clothing and bed linens must be treated at the same time the skin is treated to destroy the mites (Table 23-9).

Patient Education for Compliance

1. Do not apply scabicides and pediculicides to the face unless specifically instructed to do so by a physician.
2. Wear gloves for application.
3. Do not apply conditioners to hair following use of medications for lice.
4. Treat all household and sexual contacts concurrently.
5. Avoid open flames around Ovide and other malathion derivatives because they are flammable. Do not use hairdryers, and do not smoke.

IMPORTANT FACTS ABOUT SCABICIDES AND PEDICULICIDES

- Medications for scabies and pediculosis are found in prescription and OTC forms.
- Malathion and lindane can be absorbed into the body, causing systemic reactions if used too often.

Miscellaneous Items

- Minoxidil (Rogaine) in different strengths may be used for alopecia in men and women by

TABLE 23-10 *Miscellaneous Dermatologic Preparations*

GENERIC NAME	TRADE NAME	USUAL ADULT DOSE, ROUTE, AND FREQUENCY OF ADMINISTRATION	INDICATIONS FOR USE	DRUG INTERACTIONS
minoxidil	Rogaine topical solution	Apply 1 mL of 2% solution to affected area of scalp daily	Baldness	Usually none with topical preparations
finasteride	Propecia	1 mg po qd	Baldness	
coal tar*,†	Various OTC as shampoo and soaps	As directed topically	Psoriasis, seborrheic dermatitis	
fluorouracil	Efudex* cream, solution	Apply topically bid for disintegration of tissues; may take 2-6 wk	Actinic keratosis, superficial basal cell carcinomas	
mexoryl SX	Anthelios SX moisturizing cream	Apply topically qd	Sunscreen	

MAJOR SIDE EFFECTS: coal tar: skin irritation; **fluorouracil:** itching, burning, rash, increased sensitivity to sunlight.

* Prescription medication.
† OTC medication.

applying 1 mL of solution to thinning areas of the hair twice a day. This medication was originally produced as an antihypertensive, but excessive hair growth was seen to be a persistent side effect, and the FDA approved its use for baldness as well.

- Another hair stimulant for use in men is finasteride (Propecia), an androgen inhibitor. As a category X medication in women, handling of the medication or contact with semen may be teratogenic to the male fetus.
- Psoriasis is a dermatitis identified by red, raised lesions covered with dry silvery scales. Coal tars, used for psoriasis, are found in shampoos, lotions, and creams. Pine tar shampoo and soaps are the most common and may be used daily. In severe cases, chemotherapeutic agents such as methotrexate may be used.
- Alefacept (Amevive) is the first biologic therapy for psoriasis. This medication, given by injection, is expensive (approximately $1000 per month) and inconvenient but produces prolonged remission. Long-term use may result in malignancies.
- Fluorouracil (Efudex) is used for **actinic keratosis** and superficial basal cell carcinoma. The agent works by causing a mild inflammation that progresses to severe inflammation with burning, stinging, and vesicle formation. This is followed by tissue disintegration, necrosis, erosion, **ulceration,** and finally healing (Table 23-10).

Patient Education for Compliance

1. Use gloves or a cotton-tip applicator when applying fluorouracil, and apply only to affected areas.
2. Areas where medications have been applied to cause sloughing of skin may be unsightly for several weeks after therapy.
3. When applying fluorouracil, the skin surrounding the lesion may be protected by encircling the lesion with Vaseline.

Summary

Many preparations for treating skin disorders exist. They may be bought OTC and may be the same medications as prescription drugs but of weaker strength. Many topical preparations such as soaps, baths, and skin protectants are used on a daily basis.

Antiinfectives and antiinflammatories are some of the same medications with the same indications as described in Chapter 18 but are in topical bases for dermatologic uses. Antiinfectives used topically do not have the systemic effect or the dangers of drug resistance found with systemic preparations. Dermatologic therapeutic agents cover a wide range of medications, from antiinfectives and antiinflammatories to preparations for acne, burns, baldness, itching, and parasites.

Many patients use OTC medications for warts, contact dermatitis, itching, sunburn, or lesions caused by diseases such as chickenpox. Protective agents such as sunscreens and skin protectants around colostomies or pressure sores are important in the prophylaxis of skin trauma.

Critical Thinking Exercises

SCENARIO

James plays football and has a problem with athlete's foot. He does not want to go to the dermatologist with the problem but wants to use a product that can be bought OTC.

1. Is an OTC product a possible answer for his problem? Explain.
2. What forms of medication can be obtained OTC for fungal infections?
3. What OTC medication would you think that James might try?

4. James also wants to know how long he can use this medicine if it does not seem to help his fungal infection before he must see a physician. How would you answer?

DRUG CALCULATIONS

1. Order: Tetracycline 250 mg qid
   Available medication: Tetracycline 0.25 g caps
   Dose to be administered: _____
   _____
   _____

2. Order: Kwell Shampoo, Wash hair hs and rep in 1 wk. Comb hair p̄ washing
   Interpret the order: _____
   _____
   _____
   _____

REVIEW QUESTIONS

1. How are the form and size of the molecule related to absorption of medications through the skin?
   _____
   _____

2. What is the difference between a soap and a cleanser? _____
   _____
   _____

3. How are topical antiinfectives used for such conditions as impetigo, carbuncles, and furuncles?
   _____
   _____

4. What are indications for topical corticosteroids? _____
   _____
   _____

5. What are the many forms of antifungals? Why are all of these forms necessary? _____
   _____
   _____

6. What is the leading ingredient in acne preparations, and how does it act on the skin?
   _____
   _____

7. How are topical anesthetics used? _____
   _____
   _____

8. What antiinfective class of medications is used for burns? How do these preparations facilitate burn treatment? _____
   _____

CHAPTER 24

Musculoskeletal System Disorders

OBJECTIVES

After studying this chapter, you should be capable of doing the following:

- Describing the causes and symptoms of joint and muscle pain.
- Discussing therapy for osteoporosis.
- Explaining the classes of medications used to treat musculoskeletal conditions.
- Describing how muscle relaxants affect the body.
- Explaining appropriate patient education for patients taking skeletal muscle relaxants.
- Identifying the medications used for arthritis.

Ms. Werner is approaching menopause and cannot drink milk because of allergies. She comes to Dr. Merry for a regular office visit and asks if she needs to be concerned about her lack of calcium intake. Dr. Merry suggests that Ms. Werner use Tums as a calcium substitute. As she is leaving the office, Ms. Werner questions the use of an over-the-counter (OTC) preparation.

What is your response concerning the use of Tums?

A few weeks later Ms. Werner calls to say that she has heard of an OTC product for calcium that is eaten as candy.

What would be your response if she asks for the name of the product?

Should she use Tums with this candylike preparation?

KEYWORDS

Ankylosing spondylitis
Ankylosis
Arthritis
Articulate
Crepitus
Disease-modifying antirheumatic
    drug (DMARD)
Enteric-coated tablet
Exacerbate

Fibromyalgia
Fusion
Hyperuricemia
Immunosuppressant
Kyphosis
Muscle spasm
Muscle spasticity
Myasthenia gravis
Nonsalicylate

Nonsteroidal antiinflammatory
    drug (NSAID)
Ossification
Osteoarthritis
Osteoporosis
Pannus
Purine
Salicylate
Tinnitus

EASY WORKING KNOWLEDGE OF INDICATIONS AND SIDE EFFECTS

Common Symptoms of Musculoskeletal Disorders	Common Side Effects of Medications Used for Musculoskeletal Disorders
Joint stiffness, pain, inflammation, swelling	Nausea and vomiting
Weight loss	Pain in abdomen
Bone mass loss, deformation of bones	Drowsiness, dizziness, orthostatic hypotension
Fatigue, malaise, weakness, fever	Headache
Tenderness and swelling of joints and bones	Constipation and diarrhea
Loss of motion, immobility	Visual changes

Easy Working Knowledge of Drugs Used for Musculoskeletal Conditions

DRUG CLASS	PRESCRIPTION	OTC	PREGNANCY CATEGORY	MAJOR INDICATIONS
OSTEOPOROTIC MEDICATIONS				Prevention/treatment of osteoporosis
Bisphosphonates	Yes	No	C	
Bone resorptive inhibitors	Yes	No	X	
Calcitonin	Yes	No	C	
Calcium carbonate	Yes	Yes		
Parathyroid hormone	Yes	No	C	
ANTIRHEUMATIC/ANTIARTHRITIC MEDICATIONS				
Nonsteroidal Antiinflammatory Drugs				
Salicylates	Yes	Yes	C	Antiinflammatory agents/analgesics
Nonsalicylates	Yes	Yes	B, C, D	
Disease-Modifying Antirheumatic Drugs				
Immunosuppressants	Yes	No	D	Relieve symptoms of rheumatoid arthritis
Gold salts	Yes	No	C, D	
Others	Yes	No	B, C, D	
Antigout medications	Yes	No	C, D	Relieve symptoms of gouty arthritis
Skeletal muscle relaxants	Yes	No	B, C	Reduce muscle spasms and spasticity
anticholinesterase agents	Yes	No	C	Increase muscle tone

The musculoskeletal system is really two different systems that work closely together for the body to be held erect and to be mobile. The two systems include a sturdy collection of connective tissue, muscles, and bones that allow change of position and give the human height and form (Figures 24-1 and 24-2).

The muscular system includes muscles, which are slightly contracted at all times, and specialized connective tissue such as tendons and ligaments. Tendons connect muscle to bone, whereas ligaments are strong fibrous tissues that bond bones together to facilitate motion. Muscles require electrical impulses from nerves for stimulation. These nerve impulses stimulate muscle contraction and relaxation to produce movement. These physiologic actions are the basis for muscle relaxants to work on the peripheral and central nervous systems. Muscle relaxants relieve pain of muscle spasms by relaxing muscle contractions. Several disease processes, among them myasthenia gravis, fibromyalgia, muscle spasticity, multiple sclerosis, and spinal cord diseases or injuries, result in inability of the muscles to contract and relax properly.

The skeletal system consists of bones and the joints where bones meet. Bones **articulate** in joints to allow the body to be mobile and flexible. The articulation sites are covered with cartilage. The capsule surrounding the joint is lined with a synovial membrane and filled with synovial fluid, called a *bursa*. Diseases of the joints are considered **arthritis,** of which there are many different types. A reduction in bone mass is called **osteoporosis.**

Osteoporosis and Medications for Treatment

Osteoporosis is a metabolic musculoskeletal disease characterized by a porous appearance of bone mass. In older adults the resorption of existing bone begins to exceed the formation of new bone, and deterioration in bone mass and bone density occurs. Women with diminished estrogen have increased bone loss. In the presence of decreased calcium intake and decreased physical activity, fractures occur from softening of the bone or an increase in bone formation that is more porous than normal. Usually, the patient is not aware of the loss of bone mass. The first signs may be fractures without causative trauma. Most fractures occur in the

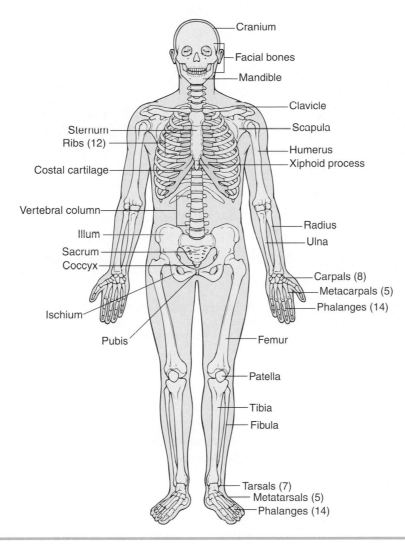

Cranium
Facial bones
Mandible
Clavicle
Scapula
Sternum
Ribs (12)
Humerus
Xiphoid process
Costal cartilage
Vertebral column
Radius
Illum
Ulna
Sacrum
Coccyx
Carpals (8)
Metacarpals (5)
Phalanges (14)
Ischium
Pubis
Femur
Patella
Tibia
Fibula
Tarsals (7)
Metatarsals (5)
Phalanges (14)

Figure 24-1   The skeletal system. (From Frazier MS, Drzymkowski JW: *Essentials of human diseases and conditions*, ed 4, St Louis, 2008, Saunders.)

vertebrae, hip, and wrist with dorsal and lumbar vertebral fractures being the most common, causing loss of height, chronic back pain, and spinal deformities such as kyphosis. Bone mass in both men and women changes across the life span, with the peak amount of bone mass occurring in the third decade of life; a loss begins after that time. In women, bone loss accelerates at menopause and for several years thereafter.

- To prevent osteoporosis, adults need to maximize bone strength by ensuring sufficient intake of calcium and vitamin D throughout life and by promoting lifestyle measures such as regular exercise.
- Calcium may be obtained from milk and milk products or through calcium carbonate supplements such as Tums.

- Viactiv, an OTC chewable supplement in a candylike form, is used for calcium replacement.
- Products containing calcium and vitamin D are also available and even preferable in the prevention of osteoporosis.

Medications Used to Treat Osteoporosis

The medications for women include agents that decrease bone resorption and those that promote bone formation. The antisorptives include bisphosphonates and calcitonin—the mainstays of osteoporotic treatment—and estrogen therapy when needed. Biphosphates are the preferred treatment choice with calcitonin prescribed for persons unable to tolerate biphosphates (Table 24-1).

- Biphosphates such as alendronate (Fosamax), risedronate (Actonel), and ibandronate (Boniva)

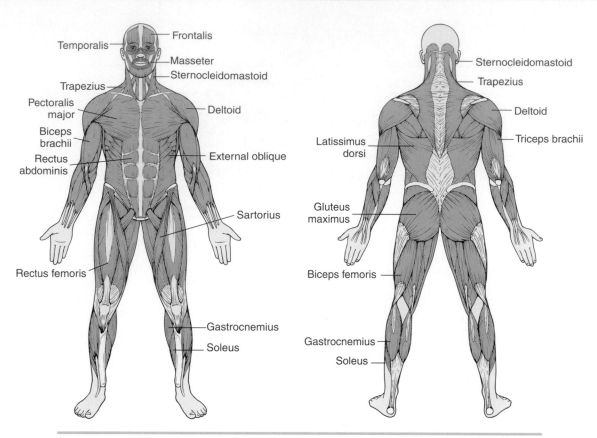

Figure 24-2 Muscles of the body. (From Frazier MS, Drzymkowski JW: *Essentials of human diseases and conditions*, ed 4, St Louis, 2008, Saunders.)

are approved for osteoporosis and are safe for prevention of fractures. Alendronate and risedronate are available in a weekly dosing for the patient with osteoporosis, whereas ibandronate is a monthly dosing. For these medications to be effective, the patient must also have an adequate intake of calcium and vitamin D. Biphosphates should be taken on an empty stomach upon arising, with 6 to 8 oz of plain water. Patients should be instructed not to lie down or eat for 30 to 60 minutes after dosing.

- To decrease resorption of bone, raloxifene (Evista) is prescribed to both prevent and treat osteoporosis in postmenopausal women. This drug is a pregnancy category X. It can be taken without regard to meals.
- Calcitonin salmon nasal spray (Miacalcin), for the treatment of osteoporosis and not a prophylactic agent, inhibits bone resorption and decreases bone loss and the chance of resultant fractures. Calcitonin salmon is a safe drug when sprayed into alternating nostrils daily.
- Teriparatide (Forteo) is a parathyroid hormone that has been approved to stimulate new bone formation (see Chapter 21).

- Men are also treated for osteoporosis, but not as frequently as women. The decline in bone mass in men begins at approximately age 50, followed by the same rate as in women. The exception with women is the accelerated rate of bone loss during menopause. The drugs used for treatment are the same as in women, except that testosterone is substituted for the estrogen (see Table 24-1).

Patient Education for Compliance

1. Calcium preparations must be accompanied by vitamin D (from sunlight or other sources) to be effective.
2. Biphosphates must be taken on an empty stomach at least 30 to 60 minutes before breakfast to be effective.
3. Biphosphates may cause esophagitis if they become lodged in the esophagus; therefore these should be taken with a full 8-oz glass of water, and the patient should remain in an upright position for at least 30 to 60 minutes after taking the medication.

TABLE 24-1 *Medications Used to Prevent and Treat Osteoporosis*

GENERIC NAME	TRADE NAME	USUAL ADULT DOSE, ROUTE, AND FREQUENCY OF ADMINISTRATION	INDICATIONS FOR USE	DRUG INTERACTIONS
BISPHOSPHONATES			Osteoporosis	
teriparatide acetate	Forteo	200 mcg/dose SC		digoxin
Biphosphates				
alendronate	Fosamax*	5-10 mg/day po		Basically none
with vitamin D	Fosamax 70-D	† tab per week po		
	Fosamax-70*	70 mg once a week po		Basically none
risedronate	Actonel	5 mg po qd or 35 mg po q week		Antacids, NSAIDs
ibandronate	Boniva	150 mg po q mo		Dietary supplements, antacids, NSAIDs

MAJOR SIDE EFFECTS OF BISPHOSPHONATES: alendronate: headache, GI symptoms; **risedronate:** arthralgia, rash; ***ibandronate:*** dysphagia, bone pain, heartburn, gastric ulcers, dyspepsia, chest pain, myalgia, numbness; **teriparatide acetate:** leg cramps, nausea, dizziness, headaches, orthostatic hypotension, tachycardia.

CALCITONIN			Osteoporosis	
calcitonin salmon	Miacalcin*	1 nasal spray/day		
calcium carbonate	Tums, Vivactil Chewable, Os-Cal-D†	i-ii tab po daily		
BONE RESORPTIVE INHIBITORS			Prevention of osteoporosis	
raloxifene	Evista	60 mg/day po		ampicillin, estrogen replacement preparations, anticoagulants

MAJOR SIDE EFFECTS OF BONE RESORPTIVE INHIBITORS: Hot flashes, flulike symptoms, arthralgia, sinusitis, insomnia with raloxifene.

GI, Gastrointestinal; *NSAIDs,* nonsteroidal antiinflammatory drugs; *SC,* subcutaneous.
*Prescription medication.
†OTC medication.

Patient Education for Compliance—cont'd

4. Calcium carbonate should be taken with or after meals to promote absorption.
5. Calcium carbonate with vitamin D preparations are available and preferable for prevention of osteoporosis.
6. Calcium and tetracycline should be taken at least 1 hour apart.
7. Nostrils should be alternated on a daily basis when using intranasal calcitonin salmon.

IMPORTANT FACTS ABOUT DRUGS FOR OSTEOPOROSIS

- Calcium is necessary for musculoskeletal health.

IMPORTANT FACTS ABOUT DRUGS FOR OSTEOPOROSIS—*Cont'd*

- The preferred drugs for osteoporosis prevention are the biphosphates.
- Calcitonin salmon inhibits bone resorption and is a safe medication for osteoporosis and bone growth because it mimics body chemicals.
- Bisphosphonates are used for the prevention and treatment of osteoporosis by suppressing bone resorption.
- Biphosphates should be taken on an empty stomach with 6 to 8 oz of water. A full stomach essentially ceases the effects of the medication.
- Calcitonin is the safest drug for osteoporosis but is not as effective as estrogen or biphosphates.

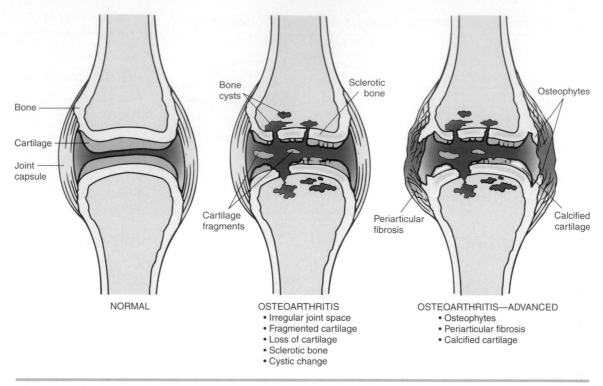

Figure 24-3 Degeneration of joints and cartilage with sclerotic and cystic changes due to osteoarthritis. (From Damjanov I: *Pathology for the health professions*, ed 3, St Louis, 2006, Saunders.)

Joint Diseases and Their Treatment

Arthritis is characterized by joint pain and limitation of movement in the joint.

- The most common type of arthritis is **osteoarthritis,** a degenerative noninflammatory disease causing destruction of bones and joints because of constant wear and tear. It has an insidious onset in the large weightbearing joints because the cartilage in the joint gradually becomes thinner as the body loses its ability to keep pace with the need for replacement. Osteoarthritis is characterized by dull, aching pain and joint soreness and stiffness with little limitation of movement. As the disease progresses, deformity may occur and **crepitus** may occur in the joints on movement. The disease usually progresses to loss of joint stability, decreased range of motion, and an increase in pain because the bone enlarges and deforms the joint, leading to joint replacement surgery (Figure 24-3).

- Another form of arthritis, *rheumatoid arthritis,* can manifest in numerous forms. Considered an autoimmune disease, it can be found in all age groups but usually peaks between 20 and 50. Joints are red, swollen, tender, and warm, with considerable pain and limitation of movement. Rheumatoid arthritis is a progressive disease that begins with stiffness and fatigue and progresses to **ankylosis** or permanent **fusion** of the joint. Synovitis with resultant **pannus** formation also occurs, and this permits the overgrowth of tissue, which eventually converts to scar tissue, causing the joint to become stiff. With prolonged illness, the scar tissue replaces bony tissue and further ankylosis occurs. Replacement surgery may also be done in rheumatoid arthritis when the joints are sufficiently deformed to prevent movement (Figure 24-4).

- *Bursitis* is an inflammation of the *bursa,* a small, enclosed space in joints that contains small amounts of synovial fluid. It may occur when the joint is traumatized, overused, or infected, or when deposits of calcium accumulate in it. The shoulder, knee, and elbow are the common sites of bursitis. The common signs are tenderness on movement and inability to flex or extend the joint. With chronic inflammation, calcification may occur in the affected joint.

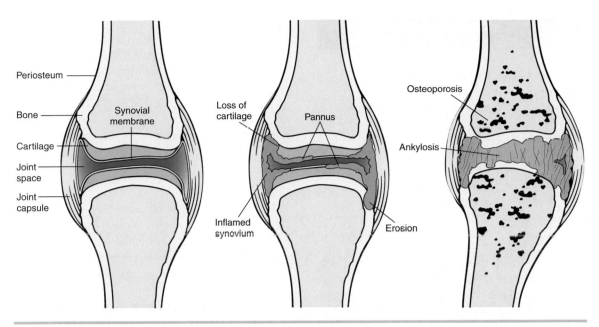

Figure 24-4 Pathologic changes in rheumatoid arthritis. The first joint illustrates a typical joint. The second joint shows synovitis and loss of articular space due to pannus formation. The third joint is ankylosed due to rheumatoid arthritis and osteoporosis. (From Damjanov I: *Pathology for the health professions*, ed 3, St Louis, 2006, Saunders.)

Medications for Arthritis and Arthritis-Like Conditions

No cure for arthritis currently exists, just alleviation of symptoms. The goals of treatment for arthritis therapy are threefold: (1) to relieve pain, inflammation, and stiffness; (2) to maintain joint function and range of motion; and (3) to prevent joint deformity. These objectives are achieved through physical therapy, surgery, and pharmacotherapy. Patient education concerning excessive rest of a joint or excessive use of the joint—too much rest will cause stiffness, and too much exercise will intensify the inflammation and pain—must be stressed. The patient must understand that medications are only part of the necessary treatment.

General Characteristics of Arthritis Medications

Antiarthritic medications are used to treat all rheumatoid conditions and may be used for conditions such as osteoarthritis, inflammatory conditions, and other joint diseases. Some of these medications have already been discussed in the section on analgesics in Chapter 16 and in the section on corticosteroids in Chapter 21. The more commonly used **salicylates** and **nonsteroidal antiinflammatory drugs** (NSAIDs) are briefly discussed here to assist in understanding their use as musculoskeletal agents. Antiarthritic medica-

tions are used for symptomatic relief, but many produce short-term remission of the disease in certain cases. Rarely does remission continue, and the disease **exacerbates,** with further progression of symptoms and increased debilitation. Drug therapy, therefore, is long term and requires full cooperation of the patient.

Antiarthritic medications usually fall into three categories: NSAIDs, **disease-modifying antirheumatic drugs** (DMARDs), and glucocorticosteroids.

- NSAIDs may be further subdivided into **salicylate** and **nonsalicylate** medications. Safer than the other two types of medications, these drugs give rapid relief of symptoms but do not prevent the progression of the disease.
- DMARDs are more toxic and have a slower onset of action. These agents require regular monitoring of the patient, but they do delay the progression of the disease.
- Glucocorticosteroids provide rapid relief of symptoms, do not prevent the progression of the disease, and are toxic with long-term use. Therefore steroids should be used only for short-term, acute therapy.

The needed medications are selected according to the severity of the symptoms, how the patient responds to treatment, and the patient's ability to tolerate the side effects of the medications.

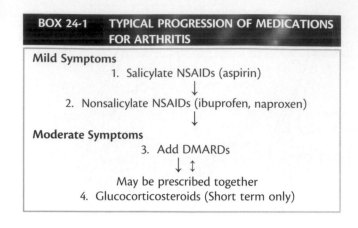

BOX 24-1   TYPICAL PROGRESSION OF MEDICATIONS FOR ARTHRITIS

Mild Symptoms

1. Salicylate NSAIDs (aspirin)
   ↓
2. Nonsalicylate NSAIDs (ibuprofen, naproxen)
   ↓

Moderate Symptoms

3. Add DMARDs
   ↓ ↕
May be prescribed together
4. Glucocorticosteroids (Short term only)

The agents for initial therapy are NSAIDs (Box 24-1). If the arthritis cannot be controlled with NSAIDs, DMARDs may be added. DMARDs are more toxic and could take several months to become effective. Glucocorticosteroids are used on a short-term basis to provide symptomatic relief until DMARDs become effective. Some physicians use NSAIDs and DMARDs at the same time in an effort to delay joint degeneration.

- *Salicylate NSAIDs* are effective, fast-acting, and, considering their ability to relieve symptoms, inexpensive. Their actions are generally antiinflammatory to give relief, but these agents also provide analgesia. **Enteric-coated medications** may be used to reduce the chance of gastric symptoms and gastric bleeding. A sign of salicylate toxicity is **tinnitus.** Compliance with these medications may be difficult to achieve because the patient may not believe that aspirin and other OTC salicylates can be effective for arthritic symptoms (Table 24-2).
- *Nonsalicylate NSAIDs* are also effective as antiinflammatory and analgesic agents. These medications act much as the salicylate medications do; patients who do not respond to salicylates may respond to nonsalicylates and may respond better to one nonsalicylate than to another. These drugs are more expensive but tend to cause less gastrointestinal (GI) disturbance and tinnitus. However, when used for long-term therapy, nonsalicylate NSAIDs may cause GI ulceration. Therefore these medications should be taken with meals or food. At present, many of these medications are on the market to treat not only arthritis but also other musculoskeletal conditions such as bursitis and tendonitis. Patients who are hypersensitive to aspirin may be hypersensitive to these aspirin-like medications. Contrary to some patients' beliefs,

acetaminophen (Tylenol), an analgesic, is *not* effective for inflammatory or arthritis-like symptoms. Meloxicam (Mobic) is an antiinflammatory, analgesic, antipyretic that is specific for osteoarthritis and should not be taken with other NSAIDs (see Table 24-2).

Patient Education for Compliance

1. Salicylates may cause asthma attacks in susceptible persons.
2. Persons taking salicylates should notify the physician immediately if ringing in the ears occurs.
3. Salicylates should not be used by children.
4. Aspirin preparations that smell like vinegar should be discarded. The smell is a sign of disintegration of acetylsalicylic acid.
5. Patients taking diclofenac (Voltaren) should have liver function tests regularly and should report any signs of jaundice, nausea, or fatigue.
6. Many nonsalicylate NSAIDs may not be taken with aspirin because of the similarity of the drug following metabolism. The patient should be told which drugs may or may not be taken together.
7. NSAIDs may mask signs of infection because of their antiinflammatory or analgesic properties.
8. Ibuprofen (Motrin) may cause visual problems including diminished vision and changes in visual color.
9. NSAIDs should be taken with food, milk, or a full glass of water to reduce gastric upset.
10. Alcohol should not be consumed with NSAIDs because of the increased risk of GI bleeding.

IMPORTANT FACTS ABOUT JOINT DISEASES AND THEIR TREATMENTS

- Because they cause gastric irritation and bleeding, NSAIDs should be used with care in people with peptic and gastric ulcer disease or bleeding disorders.
- NSAIDs suppress inflammation and relieve the mild to moderate pain found with rheumatoid disease.
- The three objectives of arthritis therapy are to reduce pain, inflammation, and stiffness; to prevent joint deformity; and to maintain joint function.
- Three classes of drugs are used to treat rheumatoid conditions: NSAIDs, DMARDs, and glucorticosteroids.
- NSAIDs and steroids quickly relieve the symptoms of arthritis, whereas DMARDs take longer to relieve symptoms.
- NSAIDs and steroids do not slow the progression of rheumatoid diseases, but DMARDs slow the progression of rheumatoid arthritis.

TABLE 24-2 *Antiinflammatory/Analgesic Agents (NSAIDs)*

GENERIC NAME	TRADE NAME	USUAL ADULT DOSE, ROUTE, AND FREQUENCY OF ADMINISTRATION	INDICATIONS FOR USE	DRUG INTERACTIONS
SALICYLATES			Antiinflammatory/ analgesic agents	Antacids, corticosteroids, ACE inhibitors, beta blockers, methotrexate, anticoagulants, probenecid, sulfinpyrazone, sulfonylurea, alcohol, penicillin, naproxen, valproic acid, oral hypoglycemics
aspirin	Ecotrin, Bayer, Bufferin[†]	2.6-5.2 g/day po		
choline salicylate	Arthropan*	ʒ i-ii qid po		
choline magnesium salicylate	Trilisate[†]	tab ii tid-qid po		
magnesium salicylate	Magan, Mobidin, Doan's Pills[†]	tab ii tid-qid po tab ii tid po		
salsalate	Disalcid, Salsitab, Mono-Gesic, Arthra-G*	tab/gelcap ii tid po		
sodium salicylate		3.6-5.4 g/day in divided doses po		

MAJOR SIDE EFFECTS OF SALICYLATES: GI symptoms, bleeding tendencies.

GENERIC NAME	TRADE NAME	USUAL ADULT DOSE, ROUTE, AND FREQUENCY OF ADMINISTRATION	INDICATIONS FOR USE	DRUG INTERACTIONS
NONSALICYLATES			Analgesic, arthritis, antiinflammatory	
diclofenac with misoprostol	Voltaren, Cataflam Arthrotec	25-100 mg/day bid po 50-75 mg po bid		ACE inhibitors, lithium, warfarin, aminoglycosides
diflunisal	Dolobid	500-1000 mg/day po in divided doses		digoxin, furosemide, methotrexate, warfarin
etodolac		Lodine	800-1200 mg/day po in divided doses	
fenoprofen	Nalfon	300-600 mg po tid-qid		
flurbiprofen	Ansaid	200-300 mg/day po in 2-4 divided doses		
ibuprofen	Motrin,* Rufen, Advil[†]	600-800 mg po tid-qid		
indomethacin	Indocin	25-50 mg po tid	Gout and arthritic conditions	Not for use by children younger than 14 or pregnant or lactating women
ketoprofen	Orudis (plain and extended-release)	150-300 mg/day po in divided doses	Analgesic, anti-inflammatory, arthritis	See all above
meclofenamate	Meclomen	200-400 mg/day po in divided doses		

(continued)

TABLE 24-2 *Antiinflammatory/Analgesic Agents (NSAIDs)—cont'd*

GENERIC NAME	TRADE NAME	USUAL ADULT DOSE, ROUTE, AND FREQUENCY OF ADMINISTRATION	INDICATIONS FOR USE	DRUG INTERACTIONS
meloxicam	Mobic	7.5-15 mg po daily		
nabumetone	Relafen	1000-2000 mg/day po in divided doses with food		
naproxen	Naprosyn*	250-500 mg po bid		
naproxen sodium	Anaprox, Aleve†	275-550 mg po bid 220-440 mg/day po in divided doses		
oxaprozin	Daypro	600-1200 mg/day po in divided doses		
piroxicam	Feldene	20 mg po qd		
sulindac	Clinoril	150-200 mg po bid		
tolmetin	Tolectin	200-400 mg po tid		

MAJOR SIDE EFFECTS OF NONSALICYLATES: GI symptoms, bleeding tendencies.

COX INHIBITORS			Antiinflammatory/ analgesic for arthritis	
celecoxib	Celebrex	100-200 mg bid or 200 mg/day po		lithium, cannot be used by persons allergic to sulfa medications
DMARDs				
methotrexate	Rheumatrex	7.5-20 mg qwk po, IM, IA, IV	Immunosuppressant	Vaccines, NSAIDs, probenecid, sulfinpyrazone, trimethoprim-sulfamethoxazole
azathioprine	Imuran	1-2.5 mg/kg/day po		Allopurinol
abatacept	Orencia	750 mg IV	Antirheumatic agent	Vaccines, corticosteroids,
adalimumab	Humira	40 mg SC q2wk	Moderate to severe rheumatoid arthritis	Live virus vaccines
etanercept	Enbrel	25 mg IM twice weekly	Osteoarthritis, RA	None

MAJOR SIDE EFFECTS OF DMARDs: methotrexate: hepatotoxicity, bone marrow suppression; **azathioprine:** GI disturbances, blood dyscrasias; **abatacept:** headache, cough, URI, hypotension, hypertension; **adalimumab:** injection site erythema, pain, pruritus, headache; **etanercept:** headache, cough, dizziness, dyspepsia, abdominal pain.

GOLD SALTS				
gold sodium thiomalate	Myochrysine	10-50 mg IM q week in increasing increments	Antirheumatic, antiinflammatory	None noted
aurothioglucose	Solganal	25-50 mg IM q2-3wk		
auranofin	Ridaura	6 mg po qd		

MAJOR SIDE EFFECTS OF GOLD SALTS: Pruritus, rashes, stomatitis, renal toxicity, blood dyscrasias.

TABLE 24-2 *Antiinflammatory/Analgesic Agents (NSAIDs)—cont'd*

GENERIC NAME	TRADE NAME	USUAL ADULT DOSE, ROUTE, AND FREQUENCY OF ADMINISTRATION	INDICATIONS FOR USE	DRUG INTERACTIONS
MISCELLANEOUS				
glucosamine chondroitin		1200-1500 mg qd po	Natural supplement for arthritis	Possibly heparin
hydroxy-chloroquine	Plaquenil	400-600 mg/day po	RA	None noted
sulfasalazine	Azulfidine	2 g/day po in divided doses	(Not FDA approved for RA use)	
penicillamine	Cuprimine, Depen	125-250 mg/day po		
sodium hyaluronate	Hyalgan	Weekly × 3 or 5 IA	Osteoarthritis of knee	No other meds in knee
anakinra	Kineret	100 mg SC qd	Moderate to severe RA	None
infliximab	Remicade	3-5 mg/kg IV q2wk	RA	None
leflunomide	Arava	20 mg po qd	RA	methotrexate, rifampin

MAJOR SIDE EFFECTS OF MISCELLANEOUS ANTIINFLAMMATORY/ANALGESIC AGENTS: glucosamine chondroitin: flatulence, rash; **hydroxychloroquine:** visual damage; **penicillamine:** bone marrow depression, autoimmune disorders; **anakinra:** headache, GI symptoms, sinusitis; **infliximab:** respiratory infections, coughing, stomach pain; **leflunomide:** headache, nausea, vomiting, anorexia, constipation, flatulence, diarrhea.

ACE, Angiotensin-converting enzyme; *DMARD,* Disease-modifying antirheumatic drug; *FDA,* Food and Drug Administration; *GI,* gastrointestinal; *IA,* intraarticular; *IM,* intramuscular; *IV,* intravenous; *NSAIDs,* nonsteroidal antiinflammatory drugs; *RA,* rheumatoid arthritis; *SC,* subcutaneous.
*Prescription medication.
†OTC medication.
‡Can be used with anticoagulants.

IMPORTANT FACTS ABOUT JOINT DISEASES AND THEIR TREATMENTS—*Cont'd*

- Aspirin is the least expensive treatment for arthritis, but it is associated with GI distress when taken over a prolonged period of time.
- Nonsalicylate NSAIDs are more expensive than salicylates, but the GI distress caused by these medications is decreased.

- *Cox-2 inhibitors* are used to suppress inflammation while causing minimal side effects. Celecoxib (Celebrex) is indicated for osteoarthritis and rheumatoid arthritis. It should not be used by people with sulfa allergies (see Table 24-2). The other Cox-2 inhibitors have been removed from the market due to the toxic effects to the circulatory system.
- *Glucocorticosteroids* are powerful medications that reduce inflammatory responses and therefore are useful in treating inflammatory joint disease. These medications palliate arthritis but do not provide remission or halt the progression of the disease. For people with several joints involved, oral steroids may be prescribed, whereas for those with only one or two joints involved, intraarticular medications may be given with less toxicity, a higher effectiveness, and more dramatic mobility (Figure 24-5). With steroids, joints that were previously immobile may become mobile but these medications should be reserved for short-term therapy in patients who have not responded to other medications or for treatment of an exacerbation of the disease. The oral steroids most frequently used are prednisone and prednisolone. Betamethasone (Celestone), dexamethasone (Decadron), methylprednisolone (Depo-Medrol), and triamcinolone (Aristocort) may be used intraarticularly or parenterally. (See Chapter 21 for additional information on corticosteroids.)
- **Immunosuppressants** may be used for treating rheumatoid conditions by reducing the body's own autoimmune response to its own tissues

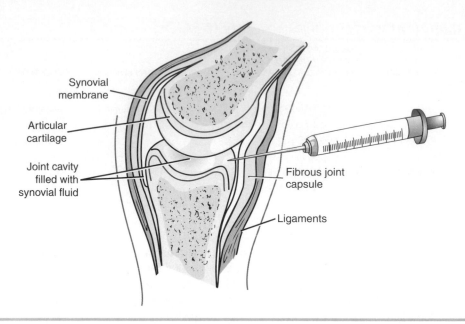

Figure 24-5 Intraarticular injections of glucocorticosteroids may be used with patients suffering from inflammatory joint disease.

to provide a therapeutic effect. These DMARD agents include gold salts, penicillamine (Cuprimine), cyclosporine (Neoral), hydroxychloroquine (Plaquenil), and sulfasalazine (Azulfidine). All of these agents have to be taken therapeutically for several weeks to be effective against the rheumatoid conditions.

- Methotrexate (Rheumatrex), also used as a chemotherapeutic agent (see Chapter 19), is the fastest acting of the DMARDs and is the first choice in this group. Patients taking methotrexate should take folic acid concurrently.
- Azathioprine (Imuran) is an antimetabolite and may be used orally or intravenously.
- Gold salts are expensive but seem to reduce the synovitis that is seen with rheumatoid diseases. These medications have been used since 1930 to relieve joint stiffness and pain and may even halt the progression of joint degeneration. The medications do not reverse any joint damage that has previously occurred. Oral gold preparations cause fewer toxic effects, but when taken orally, gold preparations cause GI distress (see Table 24-2).
- DMARDs that are used with moderate to severe rheumatoid arthritis include adalimumb (Humira), abatacept (Orencia), anakinbra (Kineret), and etanercept (Embral). This medication may be administered in conjunction with other DMARDs and may be self-administered (see Table 24-2).

- Hydroxychloroquine (Plaquenil), an antimalarial medication, may produce remission of rheumatoid arthritis. This drug is usually reserved for patients who have not responded to other antiarthritic treatment. Several months may be required to produce a therapeutic effect, and NSAIDs should be used during this interval.
- Penicillamine (Cuprimine) can produce remission of rheumatoid arthritis. It should not be used unless the arthritis does not respond to more conventional therapy. This drug has a slow onset of action and may not produce therapeutic effects for several months.
- Infliximab (Remicade), an antineoplastic agent, is administered intravenously with methotrexate for rheumatoid arthritis.
- Glucosamine chondroitin, a combination of glucosamine (a form of amino sugar) and chondroitin (a large protein molecule), is typically used with joint conditions such as osteoarthritis. Glucosamine is extracted from crab, lobster, and shrimp shells, whereas chondroitin is from animal cartilage. This therapy is not by prescription but is rather considered a nutritional supplement. The effectiveness has not been determined, although studies have shown the pain relief at the same level as NSAIDs. The cartilage damage from osteoarthritis may be slowed. Because glucosamine is an amino sugar, persons with diabetes mellitus should check

TABLE 24-3 *Antigout Agents*

GENERIC NAME	TRADE NAME	USUAL ADULT DOSE, ROUTE, AND FREQUENCY OF ADMINISTRATION	INDICATIONS FOR USE	DRUG INTERACTIONS
colchicine		0.5-0.6 mg/day po, IV prophylactically; 0.5-1.2 mg po q1-2h for acute attack	Gout	None noted
allopurinol	Zyloprim	200-800 mg/day po		Anticoagulants
probenecid	Benemid	250-500 mg po bid		Indomethacin and other NSAIDS, aspirin and other salicylates, heparin
sulfinpyrazone	Anturane	100-400 mg/day po		Anticoagulants, salicylates, antineoplastics, cefotetan, cefamandole, cefoperazone, plicamycin, nitrofurantoin

MAJOR SIDE EFFECTS OF ANTIGOUT AGENTS: colchicine: GI disturbance, diarrhea, nausea, abdominal pain; **allopurinol:** Skin reaction, alopecia, GI distress, bone marrow suppression, liver toxicity; **probenecid:** Headache, anorexia, sore gums, urinary tract discomfort; **sulfinpyrazone:** GI distress, dermatitis.

GI, Gastrointestinal; *IV,* intravenous; *NSAIDs,* nonsteroidal antiinflammatory drugs.

blood sugar levels more frequently. Combined with anticoagulant agents, chondroitin may cause bleeding in some persons because this supplement is similar in chemical structure to heparin (see Table 24-2).

Gouty Arthritis

Gouty arthritis, or gout, is associated with an inborn error in uric acid metabolism causing **hyperuricemia.** Uric acid is a byproduct of purine metabolism. With gout, it accumulates and crystals are deposited in tissues and joints. Factors that increase the risk for gout include obesity, alcohol use, hypertension, and exposure to lead. The onset usually occurs in middle age in both genders, but women are often not affected until postmenopause.

Gouty arthritis produces acute pain, swelling, redness, warmth, and tenderness of joints, especially of the big toe, ankle, instep, knee, and elbow. The patient may have an elevated temperature and may have uric acid crystals on the skin. The treatment goals are to end the attack as soon as possible, prevent recurrence of the acute condition, and decrease the possibility of complications from deposits of uric acid. Patient education includes giving the patient specific information about avoiding foods high in purines, such as oat-

meal, cheese, red meat, tomatoes, alcohol, shellfish, and fatty foods (Figure 24-6).

Medications for Gout

The medications used to treat acute gout include colchicine, NSAIDs, and corticosteroids. A derivative of the autumn crocus, colchicine is an antiinflammatory agent, not an analgesic, and is specific for gout. Colchicine is ineffective for any other disease.

- The drug may be used to treat acute gouty attacks, to reduce the incidence of attacks in chronic gout, and to abort a possible attack. The medication works by decreasing the migration of neutrophils to the joint, thus decreasing joint inflammation. Colchicine should be used with care by elderly patients because of the dangers of GI, renal, hepatitic, and cardiac diseases.
- Allopurinol (Aloprim or Zyloprim), probenecid (Benemid), and sulfinpyrazone (Anturane) decrease the production of uric acid. These drugs are indicated in the prophylaxis and treatment of chronic gouty arthritis.
- Probenecid has no antiinflammatory or analgesic effects and cannot be given during an acute attack of gout. It may even precipitate an acute attack at the initiation of the medication.

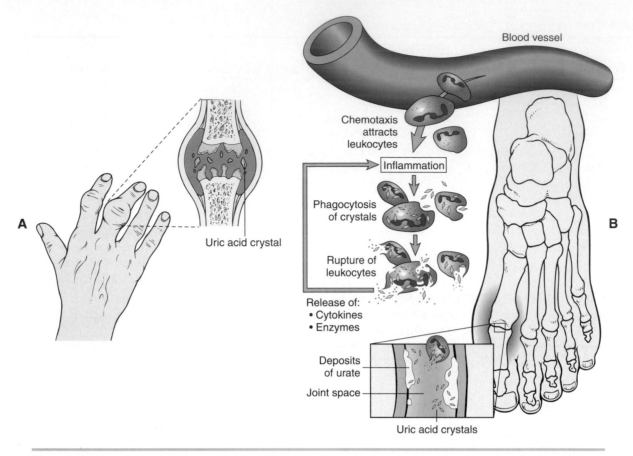

Figure 24-6 **A,** Gout. **B,** Gouty arthritis. Uric acid crystals are deposited in the connective tissue and joints. It is most often found in the joint of the great toe. (**A** from Frazier MS, Drzymkowski JW: *Essentials of human diseases and conditions,* ed 4, St Louis, 2008, Saunders; **B** from Damjanov I: *Pathology for the health professions,* ed 3, St Louis, 2006, Saunders.)

- Sulfinpyrazone is used for chronic gout attacks (Table 24-3).

IMPORTANT FACTS ABOUT MEDICATIONS FOR GOUT

- Colchicine is an antiinflammatory specific for gout. It is not an analgesic, and it does not relieve the pain of gout.
- Allopurinol reduces the uric acid levels in blood and may be used as prophylaxis for gout.
- Probenecid is used for relief of symptoms from chronic gouty arthritis conditions.

Diseases Involving Muscles

When the neuromuscular junction of the central nervous system does not function in homeostasis, skeletal **muscle spasms** and **muscle spasticity** occur.

Skeletal muscle spasms cause pain and a decreased level of functioning and use. Most muscle spasms are caused by local injury. Others may result from mineral deficiencies or diseases that cause seizures. Each type of spasm must be treated by its cause. Skeletal muscle injuries are usually self-limiting and are treated with rest, physical therapy, and possibly antiinflammatory medications. Centrally acting skeletal muscle relaxants are used for spasms that do not respond quickly to other therapy. These medications are not always effective.

The exact way the centrally acting skeletal muscle relaxants such as carisoprodol (Soma), methocarbamol (Robaxin), and tizanidine (Zanaflex) work is not completely understood, but they are used to treat localized spasms resulting from muscle injury.

- These drugs decrease local pain and tenderness, increase range of motion, and cause sedation.
- No studies have shown that one medication is better than others or whether these muscle relaxants are more effective than NSAIDs and other analgesic antiinflammatory agents. The choice

TABLE 24-4 *Medications Used to Treat Muscle Spasms and Spasticity*

GENERIC NAME	TRADE NAME	USUAL ADULT DOSE, ROUTE, AND FREQUENCY OF ADMINISTRATION	INDICATIONS FOR USE	DRUG INTERACTIONS
CENTRALLY ACTING MUSCLE RELAXANTS			Muscle spasms and muscle spasticity	Other CNS
baclofen	Lioresal	15-20 mg po tid-qid		depressants and MAO inhibitors
carisoprodol	Soma	350 mg po qid		
chlorzoxazone	Paraflex, Parafon Forte, Remular-S	250-500 mg po tid-qid		
cyclobenzaprine	Flexeril	10 mg po tid		
diazepam	Valium, Zetran	2-10 mg tid-qid po, IM, IV	(May also be used as a peripheral muscle relaxant)	
metaxalone	Skelaxin	800 mg po tid-qid		
methocarbamol	Robaxin	1000 mg po qid		
tizanidine	Zanaflex	4-8 mg po bid-tid		CNS depressants, phenytoin, alcohol, antihypertensives
orphenadrine	Norflex	60 mg q12h IM		
	Banflex, Anteflex,	100 mg po q AM and PM		
	Myolin, Norgesic,	1 to 2 tab q4-6 h		
	Norgesic Forte	1 tab q4-6h		

MAJOR SIDE EFFECTS OF CENTRALLY ACTING MUSCLE RELAXANTS: Drowsiness, lightheadedness, dizziness, may cause physical dependence when used over prolonged periods of time; additionally dry mouth and heartburn with tizanidine.

PERIPHERALLY ACTING MUSCLE RELAXANT				
dantrolene	Dantrium	25-100 mg bid-tid po, IV		

CNS, Central nervous system; *IM,* intramuscular; *IV,* intravenous; *MAO,* monoamine oxidase.

of a skeletal muscle relaxant is usually determined by the preference of the physician and the response of the patient to the medication.

- Because of the central nervous system depression, the patient should be warned about driving or participating in other hazardous activities until the effects of this medication are known.
- Diazepam (Valium) and baclofen (Lioresal) are the only medications that are effective as central muscle relaxants and for muscle spasticity caused by neuromuscular disorders (Table 24-4).

Patient Education for Compliance

1. Skeletal muscle relaxants cause central nervous system depression, and hazardous activities such as driving should be avoided until the patient can evaluate the effects of the medication.

Patient Education for Compliance—cont'd

2. The effects of opioids and other analgesics are intensified by skeletal muscle relaxants.
3. Alcohol should be avoided when taking skeletal muscle relaxants because of the synergistic action of the two agents.

IMPORTANT FACTS ABOUT SKELETAL MUSCLE RELAXANTS

- Skeletal muscle relaxants give relief for muscle injuries, but a side effect is depression of the central nervous system. Patients should avoid hazardous activities until the effects of the medication can be evaluated.

TABLE 24-5 *Medications Used for Myasthenia Gravis*

GENERIC NAME	TRADE NAME	USUAL ADULT DOSE, ROUTE, AND FREQUENCY OF ADMINISTRATION	INDICATIONS FOR USE	DRUG INTERACTIONS
ambenonium neostigmin	Mytelase Prostigmin	5 mg po q3-4h 150 mg/day po, may be increased	Relieve symptoms of myasthenia gravis	Aminoglycosides, cholinesterase inhibitors
pyridostigmine	Mestinon, Regonol	60-1500 mg/day po, IM, IV		
MAJOR SIDE EFFECTS: GI symptoms, sweating, pinpoint pupils, watery eyes, increased respiratory secretions.				

GI, Gastrointestinal; *IM,* intramuscular; *IV,* intravenous.

IMPORTANT FACTS ABOUT SKELETAL MUSCLE RELAXANTS—*Cont'd*

- Skeletal muscle relaxants are chosen by the preference of the physician and the response of the patient. These drugs all seem to have the same effectiveness.
- Diazepam (Valium) and baclofen (Lioresal) are the only centrally acting muscle relaxants that are also useful with spasticity and other muscular conditions.
- Localized muscle spasms may be treated with centrally acting muscle relaxants or NSAIDs.

Diseases with Muscle Spasticity

Muscle spasticity is caused by muscle stimulation from either the spinal cord or the brain found with patients with central nervous system injuries or strokes, as well as in diseases such as multiple sclerosis and cerebral palsy.

- Centrally acting and direct-acting muscle relaxants are the drugs of choice for muscle spasticity.
- Physical therapy accompanies medication therapy for the relief of spasticity.
- Diazepam (Valium) and dantrolene (Dantrium) are the drugs of choice in peripheral action or direct-acting skeletal muscle relaxants (see Table 24-4).

Myasthenia gravis is a progressive, incurable autoimmune disease characterized by skeletal muscle weakness and fatigue caused by loss of acetylcholine receptors.

- Cholinesterase-inhibiting agents such as neostigmine (Prostigmine) and pyridostigmine

(Mestinon) block cholinesterase and allow acetylcholine to accumulate to increase muscle strength and function.
- These drugs block the nerve stimulation from the spinal cord to prevent the muscle from overresponding to the stimulus.
- The dosages of these medications vary greatly with the severity of the disease (Table 24-5).

Patient Education for Compliance

1. For evaluation of the drug's effectiveness as treatment progresses, patients taking medications for myasthenia gravis should record the time the medications are taken and when signs and symptoms recur following medication administration, for evaluation of the drug's effectiveness as treatment progresses.
2. Cholinesterase inhibitor dosage is variable. Patients must be taught to recognize the need for more or less medication and to adjust the dosage as needed.
3. Treatment for myasthenia gravis is lifelong.

IMPORTANT FACTS ABOUT MEDICATIONS FOR MUSCLE SPASTICITY

- Spasticity is treated with four medications: baclofen (Lioresal), diazepam (Valium), tizanidine (Zanaflex), or dantrolene (Dantrium).
- Myasthenia gravis is treated with cholinesterase inhibitors to increase muscle strength.

Fibromyalgia

Fibromyalgia is a painful, debilitating syndrome that causes chronic pain in the muscles and soft tissues surrounding the joints. Symptoms include aching of muscles throughout the body, stiffness, fatigue, disturbed sleep, and depression. Overreaction to bright lights, odors, and loud noises makes the symptoms worse. The patient has specific tender points that are indicative of fibromyalgia. The treatment is NSAIDs and physical therapy (see Table 24-2).

Summary

The musculoskeletal system is composed of two distinct systems. These systems are often discussed together because they work together to keep the body upright and provide mobility. Daily wear and tear on these systems takes its toll, and disease processes such as arthritis and muscle injuries become more prevalent with aging. Also, softening and decrease in bone mass (osteoporosis) may occur, especially in postmenopausal women. The treatment of osteoporosis centers on increasing the bone mass. Biphoshates are drugs that are specific for osteoporosis. For therapy to be successful, vitamin D and calcium must also be present.

Pain is a common symptom of all musculoskeletal conditions; it is treated on a short-term basis for acute conditions or on a long-term basis for the person with chronic lifelong arthritic conditions. NSAIDs and DMARDs are used to treat arthritic conditions. NSAIDs may be changed as the patient becomes tolerant of one. DMARDs are more toxic and are used as the rheumatoid symptoms increase, although some therapeutic protocols suggest using these medications early in the disease process to prevent deformities of joints. The natural supplements glucosamine and chondroitin are used for osteoarthritis.

Gout is a painful inflammatory condition of joints due to hyperuricemia. Colchicine is specific for acute gout attacks; other medications may be given for the long-term decrease in the production of uric acid. All antigout medications tend to cause GI distress.

Skeletal muscle spasms and spasticity may occur from muscle injury or from such diseases as multiple sclerosis, strokes, or cerebral palsy. These conditions may be treated with centrally acting or peripherally acting muscle relaxants, which tend to decrease pain and tenderness and increase the range of motion of the body part. Patients taking muscle relaxants should be warned against engaging in hazardous activities because of the central nervous system depression that accompanies these medications.

Myasthenia gravis is a progressive, incurable disease related to the diminished release of acetylcholine or the excessive release of cholinesterase. It is treated with neuromuscular blocking agents or cholinesterase inhibitors. These drugs increase muscle strength and reduce muscle flaccidity. The dosage of these drugs varies greatly and depends on the state of the disease.

Critical Thinking Exercises

SCENARIO

Mr. Quan has been diagnosed with osteoarthritis and has been taking aspirin, but he believes there must be a better product for his condition and the pain.

1. What do you tell him?
2. Mr. Quan returns to the office 2 months later complaining of ringing in his ears and stomach pain. What suspicions come to mind?
3. What suggestions can you give Mr. Quan to relieve his stomach discomforts with the NSAID that is now prescribed?
4. If he wants to take aspirin now that the ringing has stopped, what type of aspirin would you expect the physician to suggest?

▮ DRUG CALCULATIONS

1. Order: dexamethasone 6 mg IM
   Available medication:

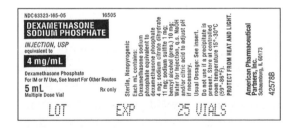

Dose to be given: _____

Show the amount on the syringe below.

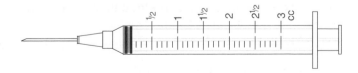

2. Order: indomethacin 50 mg
    Available medication:

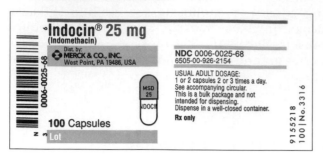

    Dose to be given:_____

REVIEW QUESTIONS

1. What drugs are specific for osteoporosis? Gouty arthritis? _____
    _____
    _____

2. What are the three types of medications used to treat arthritic symptoms? Which are usually used
    first? Which are fast acting? Which are the slowest? _____
    _____
    _____

2. What are the three types of medications used to treat arthritic symptoms? Which are usually used
    first? Which are fast acting? Which are the slowest? _____
    _____
    _____

3. What are some of the side effects of aspirin or salicylate therapy? _____
    _____
    _____

4. Why is it safer to use steroid preparations intra-articularly than systemically? _____
    _____
    _____

5. How do immunosuppressants work in the treatment of arthritis? What are their dangers?
    _____
    _____

6. How do the gold preparations have therapeutic effect in arthritis therapy? _____
    _____
    _____

7. Why would a medication for hyperuricemia be important in the treatment of gout? _____
    _____
    _____

8. What symptoms do skeletal muscle relaxants relieve? _____
    _____
    _____

CHAPTER 25

Gastrointestinal System Disorders

OBJECTIVES

After studying this chapter, you should be capable of doing the following:

- Describing how medications move through the gastrointestinal (GI) tract to be absorbed for use throughout the body.
- Discussing the medications used for prophylaxis in mouth and tooth disorders and as therapeutics for mouth diseases.
- Explaining the actions of medications used for stomach and gallbladder conditions.
- Describing the actions of pancreatic enzymes, antiflatulents, antidiarrheals, carminatives, cathartics, and laxatives.
- Describing how antiinflammatory agents are used with large bowel conditions.
- Discussing preparations used for anorectal disorders.
- Explaining the proper choice and use of medications for intestinal parasites including the needed prophylaxis to prevent recurrence.
- Discussing drugs used for appetite suppressants and their side effects.

Kim is flying to Europe in 2 weeks. She has had motion sickness on previous air trips and does not want to be nauseated on this long trip. She asks Dr. Merry if there is any medication she can take to prevent air sickness.
- What medications could Dr. Merry prescribe?
- Can Kim expect these drugs to make her sleepy?
- Are all these medications taken by mouth, or are other methods available? (Do not consider injections.)

KEY TERMS

Acid rebound	Caries	Halitosis
Adsorbent	Carminative	Laxative
Anorectal	Cathartics	Mastication
Anthelmintics	Cholelithiasis	Palliative
Anticholinergics	Defecation	Peristalsis
Antidiarrheal	Dentifrice	Prokinetic agent
Antiemetic	Diaphoresis	Regurgitation
Antiflatulent	Effervescence	Stomatitis
Anticaries agent	Emesis	Ulcer
Antisecretory agent	Emetic	Viscosity
Antiseptic	Expectorate	Xerostomia
Antispasmodics	Gastroesophageal reflux disease	
Antiviral	(GERD)	
Astringent	Gingivitis	

EASY WORKING KNOWLEDGE OF INDICATIONS AND SIDE EFFECTS

Common Symptoms of Gastrointestinal Disorders

Loss of appetite and weight loss
Abdominal pain
Nausea and vomiting
Change in bowel habits (diarrhea, constipation)
Flatulence
Blood or mucus in feces
Fever
Heartburn, indigestion, difficulty swallowing
Diaphoresis

Common Side Effects of Gastrointestinal Medications

Antacids
Constipation or diarrhea
Electrolyte imbalances
Laxatives
Electrolyte imbalances
Habituation
Other Gastrointestinal Medications
Headache, dizziness, confusion, vertigo, drowsiness
Rash
Abdominal pain or cramping
Diarrhea or constipation
Blurred vision
Dry mouth

Easy Working Knowledge of Drugs Used for Gastrointestinal Conditions

DRUG CLASS	PRESCRIPTION	OTC	PREGNANCY CATEGORY	MAJOR INDICATIONS
Oral Preparations				
Mouthwashes/gargles	No	Yes		Antiseptic and anesthetic
Fluoride preparations	Yes	Yes		Fluoridating agents
Oral antifungals	Yes	No	B, C	Oropharyngeal candidiasis
Saliva substitutes	No	Yes		Replace salivary secretions
Oral antiviral agents	Yes	Yes	B, C	Herpes simplex infections
Oral topical anesthetics	Yes	Yes	C	Mouth lesions and irritations
Antacids and Related Drugs	Yes	Yes	B (sucralfate), C	Reduce gastric acids
Antiulcer and GERD Agents				
Antibiotics	Yes	No	B	Treat *Helicobacter pylori*
Antisecretory agents				
H₂-receptor blockers	Yes	Yes	B, C	Treat ulcers and GERD by blocking histamines
Proton or gastric pump inhibitors	Yes	No	B, C	Inhibit production of HCl with ulcers and GERD
Prostaglandins	Yes	No	X	Inhibit gastric secretions and protect gastric mucosa
Antispasmodics	Yes	No	B, C	Reduce gastric spasm and slow gastric motility
Prokinetic agents	Yes	No	C	GI stimulant
Pancreatic Enzymes	Yes	No	C	Pancreatic enzyme replacement
Gallstone Solubilizing Agent	Yes	No	B (ursodiol) X (chenodiol)	Dissolves gallstones
Antiemetics	Yes	Yes	B, C	Stop vomiting
Agents for Large Intestines				
Antiflatulents	No	Yes	C	Relief of GI gas
Laxatives/cathartics	Yes	Yes	C, X (castor oil)	Relief of constipation, and in preparation for gastric diagnostic testing
Antidiarrheals	Yes	Yes	B, C, D (Pepto-Bismol)	Relieve symptoms of diarrhea
GI antiinflammatory	Yes	No	B, C	Inflammatory and irritative colon disorders
Anorectal preparations	Yes	Yes	C	Rectal fissures and hemorrhoids
Antiinfective, Anthelmintic	Yes	Yes	C	Intestinal parasites
Anorexiants	Yes	Yes	B, C, X	Appetite suppression and weight loss

Many medications discussed in this chapter are over-the-counter (OTC) drugs used daily for such common disorders as gastritis, indigestion, or constipation. Many of the drugs relieve symptoms rather than control or cure diseases or disorders of the gastrointestinal (GI) tract. The same medications may cause electrolyte imbalances when they are absorbed systemically.

Gastrointestinal System and How Drugs Act

Primary digestion, the process of converting food into chemical substances that can be used by the body, begins with the intake of food that is chewed and broken down by saliva in the mouth and then swallowed into the stomach. It ends with the absorption of nutrients by cells in the intestines and the excretion of waste products at the anus. The biliary system and pancreas assist with the digestion of food (Figure 25-1). The processes that occur are digestion and absorption. As the large food particles are chewed into smaller particles by the teeth, the enzymes of saliva begin the breakdown of complex molecules to molecules that can be absorbed and utilized by the body. After **mastication** has been completed, the food is swallowed from the mouth through the pharynx into the esophagus and finally into the stomach. In the stomach the bolus of food mixes with enzymes and other fluids from the gastric mucosa and is further broken down by churning action into a semisolid mixture called chyme. **Peristalsis** moves the chyme through the stomach toward the pyloric sphincter. If the mixture passes through the stomach too slowly, the rate at which nutrients are digested and absorbed is diminished; if the mixture passes too rapidly, the gastric juices are not allowed to mix and the ability of the food to be absorbed is decreased. The pyloric sphincter allows the passage of the chyme from the stomach into the small intestines for absorption by the villi. The accessory organs—gallbladder, liver, and pancreas—add secretions of mucus and enzymes into the small intestine to aid in the further breakdown of food substances for use by the body. Residue from the digestion in the small intestine passes into the large intestine, where digestion does not continue; rather it absorbs electrolytes and excess fluids to maintain fluid balance. The remaining residue from the chyme becomes fecal material that is pushed through the large intestine to the rectum for expulsion from the body. This process of diges-

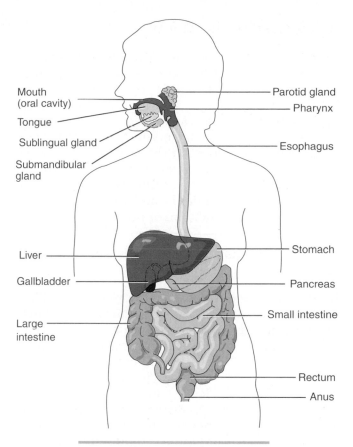

Figure 25-1 The digestive system.

tion is also important for the breakdown and absorption of medications.

Many of the drugs for GI disorders work in three ways on muscular tissue and glandular tissue, either directly on the tissues or through the influence of the autonomic nervous system. The drugs may do the following:

1. Increase or decrease the function of the GI tract by changing muscle tone, and change the secretions of or into the GI tract
2. Increase or decrease emptying time as food passes through the stomach, or change the rate of peristalsis in the stomach and intestines
3. Replace enzyme deficiencies

Through these actions, medications counteract hyperacidity or flatulence, induce or prevent vomiting, and help diagnose disorders of the GI tract (e.g., agents used in radiology). GI medications are also used for parasites, antibiotics, anesthetics, and oral conditions.

Drugs Used in the Mouth

Trauma, nutritional deficiencies, and dental disorders may cause mouth disorders, and systemic diseases may cause **stomatitis.** Symptoms such as blistering of the tongue and mucous membranes of the mouth and gums, as well as pain and inflammation in the mouth, may occur. Medications generally have little effect in the mouth but may be administered by buccal application or through the mucous membranes of the oral cavity. Good oral hygiene is essential in maintaining the body in good physical condition, or homeostasis.

Agents Used as Mouthwashes and Local Anesthetics

Most of the medications for the mouth are OTC preparations such as mouthwashes, lip balms, and agents to treat toothaches, **gingivitis,** or irritation of gums from dental appliances. Mouthwashes and gargles are dilute aromatic solutions with a sweetener added. Commercial mouth products such as Cepacol, Scope, and Listerine contain one or more active ingredients, either an **antiseptic** such as alcohol or phenol; an anesthetic such as eugenol or clove oil; an **astringent** such as zinc chloride; or an **anticaries** agent such as fluoride. A detergent product (Plax) is also available to help maintain good oral hygiene. Other OTC mouth preparations include antiseptic and anesthetic mouthwashes with phenol or phenol-like compound bases. These compounds temporarily relieve sore gums and remove plaque buildup. All of these products should only be used as adjunctive care to proper brushing and flossing of teeth.

 CLINICAL TIP

Mouthwashes have a high alcohol content, up to 27%, and should not be used by young children, who tend to swallow these products. Mouthwashes should not be used by persons taking disulfiram (Antabuse) for alcoholism.

The American Dental Association classifies mouth rinses by the following:

1. Anesthetic use such as Chloraseptic or antibacterial use such as Peridex (to be used twice a day)
2. Cosmetics such as Lavoris and Scope (used as often as needed to mask mouth odors)
3. Fluorides such as Reach with fluoride (should be used daily to prevent caries)
4. Oxygenating agents such as Permax and Peroxyl (used to loosen debris in inaccessible areas of the mouth)
5. Phenolic compounds such as Listerine that are antibacterial, and prebrushing rinses such as Plax to aid in the removal of plaque

- *Mouthwashes,* such as those containing alcohol (Cepacol and Listermint), are used for **halitosis** and as gargles for sore throats. Gum and mouth diseases, the most common cause of halitosis, cannot be treated with mouthwashes. Sore throats are usually caused by bacterial or viral infections in the throat, and gargling with mouthwash cannot reach the site of the infection, which is most often deep in the throat. OTC lozenges and sprays such as benzocaine (Chloraseptic or Spec T) containing anesthetics may also be used for pain and discomfort in the mouth and for sore throats.

- *Topical anesthetic agents* may be used for temporary relief of oral lesions caused by medications, antineoplastic treatment, poor dental care, or systemic disease while proper treatment for the disease or condition becomes effective. Adults who have gum irritation caused by dental appliances and teething infants may use these phenol or topical anesthetic preparations for relief. These topical anesthetics come in gels, ointments, aerosol sprays, and rinses. Lozenges, pastes, and film-forming gels are formulated for prolonged pain relief.

- *Hydrogen peroxide,* an oxygenating agent, is used as a weak antibacterial agent in the mouth. It works by **effervescence** of the oxygen in the mouth, loosening tissue debris and reducing bacteria in the mouth. Rinses such as Oxygel rinse are available to be used for irritations in the mouth, and a gel (Peroxyl) is available for minor mouth irritation. The gel is applied, allowed to work, and then **expectorated** after use; these agents should not be swallowed.

- *Fluoride products* are available as mouthwashes, toothpaste, tablets, and solutions for the prevention of dental caries by hardening tooth enamel. The mouthwashes should be used for a 1-minute gargle once a day after brushing teeth. Then nothing should be taken by mouth for 30 minutes. Fluoride products also come as tablets and drops to be used by children for the prevention of dental caries in areas where the water is not adequately fluorinated. These drops are generally well tolerated (Table 25-1).

- **Dentifrices,** or toothpastes, are aids to cleaning teeth and will reduce most plaque buildup if used daily. These agents contain mild abrasives with a foaming agent and flavorings, either in a paste, gel, or powder form. Many types of toothpaste have fluoride added for daily tooth contact of fluorine. Some dentifrices such as Sensodyne and Promise contain desensitizing ingredients such as potassium nitrate for hypersensitive teeth to reduce the pain associated with heat or cold. Other pastes claim to have whitening agents that whiten teeth either by abrasion or with hydrogen peroxide.

- **Whitening agents** containing carbamide peroxide (Rembrandt Blocking Gel and Colgate Tooth Whitener) are OTC products used to bleach teeth discolored by tobacco, coffee, tea, alcohol, and the like. These agents should be used according to directions to prevent permanent tooth damage.

- *Oral antifungals* such as clotrimazole (Mycelex lozenges) and ketoconazole (Nizoral) are used for candidiasis (thrush) in the oropharyngeal area. The lozenges should be dissolved, not chewed, to ensure coverage of the affected area during a 15- to 30-minute period. These medications bind to the oral mucosa and remain for therapeutic action for up to 3 hours. Most of the medication passes through the body without being absorbed and is excreted in feces.

- When saliva is absent or secretions are minimal, *saliva replacement* is a natural therapeutic. Water is frequently used but is a poor substitute because it lacks the ions and the lubrications needed. Artificial saliva products such as Entertainer's Secret or Salivart are similar in the chemical and physical properties of saliva and are cellulose derivatives with flavoring agents and antibacterials included to increase **viscosity.** Indicated for the symptomatic relief of dry mouth and throat, the OTC products may be used as desired throughout the day. Most saliva products come in sprays, although lozenges are available. Quickly swallowed, these agents must be administered repeatedly throughout the day to be effective. Most of the products are particularly useful as replacements for relieving

dry mouth found with speaking, eating, and other daily activities, but they may be used therapeutically in chronically ill persons who need mouth moisture, such as persons with cancer or stroke victims, those persons recovering from removal of the parotid glands, and with mouth breathers. A prescription medication, cevimeline (Evoxac), is available for treating **xerostomia.**

- *Antivirals* may be prescribed as either systemic or local agents for viral infections that occur in the mouth. The treatment is **palliative** when treating herpes zoster and herpes simplex infections, varicella, and HIV lesions. One topical medication, docosanol (Abreva), has been approved by the Food and Drug Administration for OTC use. Acyclovir (Zovirax) is used for the symptomatic relief of shedding of the oral mucosa, local pain, and encrusted lesions caused by the disease process. Care should be taken to prevent contact with the lesions while treatment is in progress (see Table 25-1).

Patient Education for Compliance

1. Care should be taken with oral topical anesthetics to prevent injury to local tissues because of loss of sensation. Patients using topical oral anesthetics should not eat or drink while the mouth and throat have decreased sensations.
2. Local topical anesthetics are only temporary agents for the relief of toothaches, lesions from ill-fitting dentures, or disease. Professional dental care should be obtained for prolonged symptoms.
3. Fluoride drops may cause etching of glass if stored in a glass container.
4. Food and drink should be avoided for 30 minutes following the use of fluoride products.
5. Dentifrices, if used once a day, should be used at night to reduce the buildup of plaque.
6. Dentifrices with fluoride added will be helpful in the prevention of caries.
7. Directions on whitening agents should be followed to prevent tooth damage.

IMPORTANT FACTS ABOUT ORAL PREPARATIONS
- Many of the oral preparations are OTC medications that are used to relieve mouth lesions caused by local or systemic diseases.
- Good oral hygiene is essential to prevent oral lesions.

TABLE 25-1 *Oral Preparations*

GENERIC NAME	TRADE NAME	USUAL ADULT DOSE, ROUTE, AND FREQUENCY OF ADMINISTRATION	INDICATIONS FOR USE	SIDE EFFECTS	DRUG INTERACTIONS
TOPICAL ANESTHETICS			Mouth lesions and irritations	Mouth irritation, drying of mucosa, sloughing of tissue, changes in taste	Usually none
benzocaine[†]	Hurricaine Aerosol Oragel, Numzit Gel	1 spray tid-qid Apply gel to area tid-qid			
	Chloraseptic, Spec T Lozenges	Dissolve 1 lozenge po q2h			
	Chloraseptic Spray Benzodent Ointment	1 spray q2-4h Apply ointment locally tid-qid			
lidocaine	Xylocaine* (ointment, or spray)	Apply or spray q2-3h			
ORAL ANTISEPTICS			Antiseptic, anesthetic, anticaries		Must not be used by young children, who might swallow, or by alcoholics taking Antabuse
Mouthwashes[†]	Cepacol, Listerine, Scope, Lavoris	Swish as directed or desired			
hydrogen peroxide	Paramax[†], Peridex* as mouthwash Peroxyl[†] mouthwash or gel	Apply or swish bid	Relieves mouth irritation and removes debris		Usually none
FLUORIDE PREPARATIONS*	Fluor-A-Day tablets, Luride drops	0.25-1 mg/day po	Prevent dental caries		Usually none

Drug	Trade Name	Dosage	Use	Side Effects	Drug Interactions
ORAL ANTIFUNGALS*					
clotrimazole	Mycelex lozenges	Dissolve 10 mg po 5× daily	Oropharyngeal candidiasis		None indicated
ketoconazole	Nizoral	200-400 mg/day po		Stomach cramping, nausea, vomiting, diarrhea	astemizole, terfenadine
nystatin	Mycostatin/Nilstat lozenges/suspension	Dissolve 1-2 lozenges 4-5 × per day; 4 mL suspension qid, swish and swallow			None indicated
SALIVA SUBSTITUTES					
Selected saliva substitutes†	Entertainer's Secret, Moi-Stir, Swabsticks, Salivart, Salix	Spray as desired Lozenges as desired	Replace saliva	None	None
Cholinergic agonist					
cevimeline*	Evoxac	30 mg po 3×/day	Increases saliva output		None
ORAL ANTIVIRALS*					
acyclovir	Zovirax* tablet ointment	200 mg po q4h Apply locally q3h	Herpes lesions and varicella lesions of mouth		Usually none
penciclovir	Denavir*	Apply locally q2h for 4 days			
docosanol	Abreva†	Apply topically 5 × daily			

Note: A prescription is required for all oral antifungals except docosanol.
* Prescription medication.
† Over-the-counter medication.

Drugs Used for Gastric Conditions

As food enters the stomach, it is mixed with hydrochloric acid and the enzymes pepsin, rennin, and lipase. The acidic environment of the stomach is necessary for enzymes to work and to inhibit or kill the microorganisms found in food or other materials that are ingested. Sometimes, however, the acid becomes so strong that it actually eats away at the stomach wall. The stomach usually has a mucin, or mucous, covering, but when excessive secretions occur the gastric surface may break down. Worry and stress seem to increase the secretions of the stomach, making the wall more sensitive to the acid, causing **ulcers** and sloughing of the gastric tissue. The terms *gastric ulcer, peptic ulcer,* and *stomach ulcer* are used interchangeably for this condition. If the lesion is found at the junction of the stomach and duodenum, *duodenal ulcer* is the term that applies.

The antiulcer medications fall into five distinct categories: antacids; mucosal protectants (forming barriers to ulcers; e.g., sucralfate); antibiotics; **antisecretory agents,** which enhance mucosal defenses; and **antispasmodics.** These drug groups work together to eradicate the microorganism *Helicobacter pylori* and to reestablish an intact lining of the stomach through neutralization of hydrochloric acid.

OTC medications are often used as the first therapeutic agents for gastric conditions because they are readily available. These agents relieve the burning sensation that occurs with the acid reflux into the esophagus causing heartburn. Some antisecretory agents are also available OTC and may be used by the patient prior to seeing the physician. If the patient does not receive therapy during the early stages of gastric discomfort, peptic ulcers may occur, and the treatment is more difficult.

- *Antacids,* alkaline compounds used to neutralize hydrochloric acid in the stomach, are indicated for peptic ulcer disease. Newer medications are replacing these as mainstays of ulcer therapy. The medications are used as prophylaxis for stress-induced ulcers and to relieve symptoms of **GERD (gastroesophageal reflux disease).** By neutralizing acid, these drugs protect the intestinal mucosa. With the exception of sodium bicarbonate (baking soda), these agents are poorly absorbed and do not alter systemic pH when used as directed. However, overuse of the antacids may actually interfere with proper digestion.

- To be most effective, antacids should be taken on a regular basis, not just when there is discomfort to relieve pain. The usual dosage is seven times a day: before meals, 1 to 2 hours after meals, and at bedtime. Because these medications are inconvenient to take so frequently and tend to have an unpleasant taste, compliance usually follows pain rather than as scheduled dosages.

- The medications come in liquids (which must be shaken back into a suspension before administration) and chewable tablets (which should be followed by a glass of water after chewing thoroughly).

- The effectiveness of antacids is limited by their short duration of action, approximately 30 minutes on an empty stomach. Food acts as a buffer for antacids, continuing their activity for 2 to 3 hours. The chronic use of antacids produces **acid rebound** to neutralize antacids.

- The families of antacids are classified by their formulation as aluminum compounds, magnesium compounds, calcium compounds, and sodium compounds. Each has a different effect on the bowels and the systemic pH (Table 25-2).

- Sodium bicarbonate is a household chemical that is indiscriminately used as an antacid. *The indiscriminate use of sodium bicarbonate as an antacid is very dangerous because the chemical is absorbed systemically, changing the acid-base balance of the entire body.*

- Aluminum and magnesium salts are mixed to form magaldrate compounds, which are used to prevent the diarrhea and constipation that occur with the exclusive use of aluminum or magnesium. These agents may have added ingredients such as simethicone, which is an **antiflatulent** (e.g., Gelusil, Maalox-Plus, Mylanta) or mineral oil (Haley's MO). Some also have saccharin or sorbitol (an osmotic laxative) added.

TABLE 25-2 *Properties of Antacid Families*

ANTACID	CONSTIPATION	DIARRHEA	CHANGE SYSTEMIC PH
Aluminum compounds	Yes	No	No
Magnesium compounds	No	Yes	No
Calcium compounds	Yes	No	No
Sodium compounds*	No	No	Yes

*Should not be used routinely.

- Other uses of antacids include replacement therapy for some needed minerals.
  - Aluminum carbonate may be used for hyperphosphatemia.
  - Calcium carbonate is used for osteoporosis in postmenopausal women.
  - Magnesium deficiency from alcoholism and other conditions may be treated with magnesium hydroxide.

Thus antacids must be chosen with care to suit the needs of each patient and should not be taken for prolonged periods of time. Relief of the acute symptoms of GERD, heartburn, and hyperactivity is the indication for continued use (Table 25-3).

Patient Education for Compliance

1. Alcohol consumption exacerbates ulcer symptoms.
2. Patients should be aware that dark, tarry stools and "coffee-ground" vomitus are signs of GI bleeding.
3. Certain foods such as colas, acid juices, coffee, chocolate, and spices aggravate stomach and gallbladder conditions.
4. Chewable antacids should be taken seven times a day followed with a glass of water or milk to improve absorption.
5. Liquid suspensions need shaking prior to administration and should not be followed by any liquids that will dilute the antacid.
6. Antacids and H_2-receptor blockers should be taken at least an hour apart, with antacids taken first.
7. Antacids should not be taken routinely with other medications because the acid content of the stomach may be necessary for absorption of some drugs.

IMPORTANT FACTS ABOUT ANTACIDS
- Because antacids interfere with the absorption of many medications, especially antibiotics, other medications should not be given with antacids.
- The ideal time to give antacids is 2 hours after meals, when acid rebound occurs.

Other Medications for Peptic Ulcers

The goal of ulcer treatment should be to alleviate symptoms, promote healing of the ulcer, prevent complications (such as hemorrhagic obstruction), and prevent recurrence of the ulcer. *H. pylori* has been found in 90% of cases of peptic ulcer disease and is believed to be an opportunistic infection at the site of the ulcer. Optimal antiulcer therapy requires drug therapy and changes in lifestyle (Box 25-1). Diet itself plays only a minor role in the treatment of ulcers, but eating five or six small meals will be helpful in treatment by reducing fluctuations in stomach acidity to facilitate healing. Smoking retards disease recovery, and aspirin and other nonsteroidal antiinflammatory drugs (NSAIDs) may irritate the stomach.

- *Mucosal protectants* include the following (Table 25-4):
  - sucralfate (Carafate), a complex of aluminum hydroxide and sulfated sucrose, used to promote the healing of peptic ulcers by adhering to the gastric ulcer, forming a mechanical protectant against hydrochloric acid and digestive enzymes. It is nonsystemic in nature and has its soothing effect locally in the GI tract like antacids. But, unlike antacids, it does not have the potential for altering pH. To be effective, sucralfate should be administered on an empty stomach. When used over prolonged periods of time, sucralfate may cause deficiencies in fat-soluble vitamins.
  - misoprostol (Cytotec) inhibits gastric secretions and protects the gastric mucosa from the irritant effects of certain medications. This medication is not for the treatment of gastric or duodenal ulcers but is for use as a protectant for those who are susceptible to medication-induced gastric irritation. It should be taken on an empty stomach because foods and antacids decrease the rate of absorption.

TABLE 25-3 *Antacids and Related Drugs*

GENERIC NAME	TRADE NAME	USUAL ADULT DOSE, ROUTE, AND FREQUENCY OF ADMINISTRATION	INDICATIONS FOR USE	DRUG INTERACTIONS
SELECTED ANTACIDS*			Reduce stomach acid	tetracyclines, quinidine, morphine, penicillin, pseudoephedrine, INH, aspirin, dicumarol, digoxin, allopurinol, anticholinergics, corticosteroids, H$_2$-receptor antagonists, thyroid hormones, salicylates, corticosteroids, chlorpromazine
Sodium compounds				
sodium bicarbonate, baking soda		Not advised, but indiscriminately used at home		
with acetaminophen as effervescent tablets/powders	Bromo-Seltzer	1 tablet or packet po q4-6h		
with aspirin as effervescent powders/tablets	Alka-Seltzer	1 tab or packet po q4-6h		
Aluminum compounds				
aluminum carbonate	Basaljel tablets/ suspension	3-6 doses po per day		
aluminum hydroxide	AlternaGEL, Amphojel	3-6 doses po per day		
*Magnesium compounds**				
magnesium hydroxide*	Phillips Chewable tablets	1 or 2 chewable tablets po prn		
	Milk of Magnesia	3-6 doses po per day as suspension		
Calcium compounds			Also used with prevention of osteoporosis	
calcium carbonate*	Tums, Titralac, Rolaids	3-6 doses po per day		
calcium magaldrate*	Riopan, Gaviscon, Aludrox, D-Gel, Gelusil, Maalox	3-6 doses po per day as tablets/liquids		

MAJOR SIDE EFFECTS OF ANTACIDS: Constipation.

Note that medications under drug interactions apply to the entire table.
* OTC medication.

- *Antisecretory agents* decrease the secretion of gastric fluids. H$_2$-receptor antagonists, cimetidine (Tagamet) and ranitidine (Zantac), inhibit the interaction of histamine (H$_2$) at the H$_2$ receptors. Histamine receptors in the gastric mucosa mediate the secretion of gastric acid and pepsin that increase the volume and strength of acid secretions on stimulation. The H$_2$-receptor antagonists work directly to inhibit the acid secretions. These medications are not affected by food, so they may be taken with meals. Antacids and H$_2$-receptor antagonists should not be taken at the same time. These medications are well tolerated in the short term and for chronic maintenance therapy. These antagonists are also used for GERD (see Table 25-4).

- *Proton pump inhibitors* (PPIs) (also called gastric pump inhibitors) work by inhibiting the chemicals that are essential to the production of hydrochloric acid. Omeprazole (Prilosec), lansoprazole (Prevacid), esomeprazole (Nexium), and rabeprazole (AcipHex) are the chief medications in the class. These agents, for the short-term treatment of benign gastric ulcers and GERD, are effective when used in combination with antibiotics for *H. pylori* to promote ulcer healing and prevent recurrence. All gastric pump inhibitors should be used only for *confirmed* active duodenal ulcers and erosive esophagitis or for pathologic hypersecretory conditions. Prolonged use of gastric pump inhibitors for benign disease will lead to the drying of body fluids (see Table 25-4).

TABLE 25-4 *Antiulcer Medications*

GENERIC NAME	TRADE NAME	USUAL ADULT DOSE, ROUTE, AND FREQUENCY OF ADMINISTRATION	INDICATIONS FOR USE	DRUG INTERACTIONS
PROTECTIVE BARRIERS FOR GASTRIC ULCERS			Protect the stomach against formation of ulcers	
sucralfate*	Carafate	1 g po qid	Protect gastric mucosa	Magnesium antacids
misoprostol*	Cytotec	200 mcg po qid	Prevention of NSAID-induced gastric ulcers	Same

MAJOR SIDE EFFECTS OF PROTECTIVE BARRIERS FOR GASTRIC ULCERS: sucralfate: constipation; **misoprostol:** diarrhea, nausea, abdominal pain.

GENERIC NAME	TRADE NAME	USUAL ADULT DOSE, ROUTE, AND FREQUENCY OF ADMINISTRATION	INDICATIONS FOR USE	DRUG INTERACTIONS
COMBINATION MEDICATIONS			Treatment of *Helicobacter pylori*	
bismuth/tetracycline/ metronidazole	Helidac	1 blister pack po/day × 14 days		Antacids, ketoconazole
amoxicillin/ clarithromycin/ lansoprazole	Prevpac	1 pk po qAM and qPM × 14 days		
ANTISECRETORY/ H$_2$-RECEPTOR ANTAGONISTS			Reduce histamine secretions in stomach	caffeine, antacids, calcium channel blockers, cisapride, carbamazepine, and many others
cimetidine	Tagamet,* Tagamet-HB†	800 mg/day po in divided doses		
famotidine	Pepcid,* Pepcid AC†	20-40 mg/day po as single hs dose or in divided doses		
ranitidine	Zantac*†	300 mg/day po as hs dose or 150-300 mg bid		
nizatidine	Axid*†	300 mg po hs or in 2 divided doses per day		

MAJOR SIDE EFFECTS OF ANTISECRETORY/H$_2$-RECEPTOR ANTAGONISTS: Headaches, constipation.

(continued)

TABLE 25-4 *Antiulcer Medications—cont'd*

GENERIC NAME	TRADE NAME	USUAL ADULT DOSE, ROUTE, AND FREQUENCY OF ADMINISTRATION	INDICATIONS FOR USE	DRUG INTERACTIONS
PROTON PUMP INHIBITORS*			Short-term treatment of ulcers and GERD; reduce gastric acid production	
Omeprazole	Prilosec*†	20-40mg/day po	Above plus erosive esophagitis	Oral anticoagulants, diazepam, phenytoin
with sodium bicarbonate	Zegerid	20-40 mg packet mixed in water po qd		
with sodium bicarbonate and magnesium hydroxide	Zegerid with magnesium hydroxide	Chew 20-40 mg tab qd	Same	
lansoprazole	Prevacid*	15-30mg/day po		ketoconazole, iron salts, ampicillin, digoxin, sucralfate
rabeprazole	AcipHex*	20 mg/day po (must be swallowed whole)		
esomeprazole	Nexium*	20-40 mg/day po (must be swallowed whole)		ampicillin, clarithromycin
pantoprazole	Protonix*	40 mg/day po		No significant interactions noted

MAJOR SIDE EFFECTS OF PROTON PUMP INHIBITORS: Headaches, abdominal pain, diarrhea, nausea, constipation, plus rash with omeprazole.

GERD, Gastroesophageal reflux disease; *NSAID,* nonsteroidal antiinflammatory drug.

* Prescription medication.

†Over-the-counter medication.

Patient Education for Compliance

1. Sucralfate should be taken on an empty stomach 1 hour before meals and not within 2 hours of any other medication.
2. Patients with peptic ulcer disease should eat five or six small meals a day to decrease the fluctuation of gastric acidity throughout the day.
3. H_2-receptor antagonists may be taken once a day (at bedtime), twice a day, or four times a day, without regard to meals. Acid secretions peak during sleeping hours, so H_2-receptor blockers should always be administered at bedtime, although other times for dosages may be desired.
4. Cigarette smoking decreases the effects of H_2-receptor blockers because smoke increases the amount of acid produced by the stomach.

- *Antispasmodics* such as belladonna alkaloids (Bellergal) are actually **anticholinergics** that decrease secretions and slow peristalsis with irritable bowel syndrome, ulcerative colitis, diverticulitis, ulcers, and biliary spasm. Oral agents should be administered 30 minutes before meals and at bedtime to reduce the frequency of heartburn and allow healing of the irritated tissue. The medications do not cause central nervous system symptoms, but they may cause visual disturbances, increased confusion in demented patients, and changes in heart rhythm; therefore these medications should not be used by patients with glaucoma, urinary retention, or obstructive bowel syndrome (Table 25-5).
- *Antibiotics* are the common therapy for *H. pylori* with the use of two antibiotics (to reduce the risk of drug resistance) in combination with bismuth salts (Pepto-Bismol) to prevent the bacteria from attacking the stomach wall. Antibiotics of choice are amoxicillin, tetracycline, metronidazole (Flagyl), and clarithromycin (Biaxin) (Table 25-6). Some physicians prefer to add a PPI or an antisecretory agent to the regimen (see Table 25-4). Some medications come in blister packs containing bismuth

TABLE 25-5 *Drugs to Treat Gastrointestinal Ulcers and Spasms*

GENERIC NAME	TRADE NAME	USUAL ADULT DOSE, ROUTE AND FREQUENCY OF ADMINISTRATION	INDICATIONS FOR USE	DRUG INTERACTIONS
SELECTED ANTISPASMODICS			Peptic ulcers, spasms, intestinal and biliary colic	Usually none
belladonna	Bellafoline	1-2 tab po tid-qid		
with phenobarbital	Donnatal	1-2 tab po tid-qid		
with ergotamine and phenobarbital	Bellergal S	1-2 tab po tid-qid		
hyoscyamine	Anaspaz, Levsin, Levsinex	0.125-0.25 mg po tid-qid; 0.375 mg po q12h (timed-release)		
clidinium	Quarzan	2.5-5 mg po tid-qid ac and hs		levodopa, cardiac glycosides, antihistamines
glycopyrrolate	Robinul	1-2 mg po bid-tid		
methscopolamine	Pamine	2.5-5 mg po qid		
propantheline	Pro-Banthine	15 mg tid and 30 mg hs po		
dicyclomine	Bentyl, Di-Spaz	10-20 mg po qid		None indicated

MAJOR SIDE EFFECTS: Dizziness, headache, insomnia, drowsiness, visual disturbances, changes in heart rhythm.

Note: All of the drugs listed in this table require a prescription.

salicylate tablets, metronidazole tablets, and antibiotics, with a dose of one or two blister packs per day. (see Table 25-4).

- *Prokinetic agents* are used to stimulate GI motility by lowering esophageal sphincter pressure and accelerating gastric emptying and movement of food through the intestines. These agents are used to treat the symptoms of GERD when lifestyle changes and diet do not relieve the symptoms. Metoclopramide (Reglan) is also used for vomiting associated with cancer chemotherapy (Table 25-7).

IMPORTANT FACTS ABOUT MEDICATIONS TO TREAT PEPTIC ULCERS

- Sucralfate creates a protective barrier in the stomach against acids and pepsin.
- Misoprostol is used to prevent gastric ulcers caused by taking NSAIDs.
- The goals of peptic ulcer disease therapy are to alleviate symptoms, promote healing of the ulcer, prevent complications, and prevent recurrence of the disease process.
- Lifestyle changes concerning smoking, alcohol, and carbonated beverages may be required when treating GI symptoms. Stress relief and dietary changes are essential in ulcer treatment.

TABLE 25-6 *Treatment for Helicobacter pylori*

MEDICATION	DOSE
SHORT-TERM THERAPY	
Helidac (bismuth subsalicylate with metronidazole and tetracycline)	1 pack per day
or	
Tritec (Ranitidine with bismuth citrate)	400 mg bid 1 tablet pc
omeprazole (Prilosec)	40 mg per day
clarithromycin (Biaxin)	500 mg tid
LONG-TERM THERAPY	
Prevpac	
lansoprazole (Prevacid)	2 × 30-mg capsule bid
amoxicillin (Trimox)	4 × 500-mg capsule bid
clarithromycin (Biaxin)	2 × 500-mg tablet bid

IMPORTANT FACTS ABOUT MEDICATIONS TO TREAT PEPTIC ULCERS—*Cont'd*

- H_2-receptor antagonists suppress secretion of gastric acid by blocking gastric H_2.
- PPIs, or gastric pump inhibitors, inhibit H^+ and K^+ ions, which generate gastric acids.

TABLE 25-7 *Prokinetic Agents*

GENERIC NAME	TRADE NAME	USUAL ADULT DOSE, ROUTE, AND FREQUENCY OF ADMINISTRATION	INDICATIONS FOR USE	DRUG INTERACTIONS
PROKINETIC AGENTS				
metoclopramide*	Reglan	10-15 mg po, IV qid	GERD plus may be used for vomiting with chemotherapy for cancer	alcohol

MAJOR SIDE EFFECTS: Diarrhea, abdominal pain, headache, restlessness, drowsiness, fatigue, insomnia, headaches, dizziness.

Note: Requires a prescription.
GERD, Gastroesophageal reflux disease.

TABLE 25-8 *Drugs Used as Pancreatic Enzymes*

GENERIC NAME	TRADE NAME	USUAL ADULT DOSE, ROUTE, AND FREQUENCY OF ADMINISTRATION	INDICATIONS FOR USE	DRUG INTERACTIONS
			Pancreatic enzyme replacement to aid in digestion	Antacids, iron supplements
pancreatin	Pancreatin	2 ×500 mg po tid before meals, 1-3 caps with snacks		
pancrelipase	Cotazym, Creon, Pancrease, Ultrase, Viokase	900 mg po with meals and 300 mg with snacks		

Note: All of the drugs listed in this table require a prescription.

Drugs Used as Pancreatic Enzyme Replacements

The pancreas produces four main digestive enzymes—lipase, amylase, chymotrypsin, and trypsin—to aid in the digestion of fats, carbohydrates, and proteins. Pancreatic enzyme replacements are available in two basic preparations—pancreatin (Pancreatin) and pancrelipase (Cotazym, Pancrease MT)—that are from animal sources. The capsules contain enteric-coated microspheres and antacids to protect them from inactivation by gastric juices may be prescribed to accompany these medications. The dosage is individualized, but the enzymes must be taken with every food intake (Table 25-8).

Drugs Used with Gallbladder Disease

The gallbladder is the only site from which cholesterol is excreted from the body. Most stones found with **cholelithiasis** are from cholesterol alone and cannot be seen on radiographs, whereas stones from calcium are observable on radiographs. When symptoms of cholelithiasis occur, oral radiopaque drugs such as Telepaque or Bilopaque may be given to the patient prior to having radiographic gallbladder studies to aid visualization of the gall-bladder. The number of tablets is based on the weight of the patient. Following a low-fat evening meal, the tablets are taken at 5-minute intervals until all ordered tablets have been taken; then the patient should take nothing by mouth including water until the test has been performed.

In patients who are asymptomatic but have been shown to have gallstones, medications to dissolve gallstones may be used.

- Chenodiol (Chenix) is a naturally occurring bile acid that reduces the production of cholesterol and assists in dissolving cholesterol-based stones. The best results occur in women with small stones with therapy taking as long as 2 years.
- The preferred medication, because it is well tolerated, is ursodiol (Actigall), for reducing cholesterol in bile. The usual prolonged treatment is one tablet in the morning and one tablet in the evening, every 12 hours (Table 25-9).

Drugs for Emesis

Antiemetics are used to suppress nausea and vomiting. **Emesis,** or **regurgitation,** may caused by activation of the vomiting reflex by either (1) signals

TABLE 25-9 *Drugs Used to Treat Gallbladder Disease*

GENERIC NAME	TRADE NAME	USUAL ADULT DOSE, ROUTE, AND FREQUENCY OF ADMINISTRATION	INDICATIONS FOR USE	DRUG INTERACTIONS
			Dissolve gallstones	
chenodiol	Chenix	250 mg po bid for 2 weeks, then increased		Usually none
ursodiol	Actigall, URSO	8-10 mg/kg/day po q12h		aluminum antacids, cholestyramine, colestipol, oral contraceptives, estrogens

MAJOR SIDE EFFECTS: Absence of taste, biliary pain, diarrhea, nausea, vomiting with chenodiol.

Note: All of the drugs listed in this table require a prescription.

from the stomach or small intestines or (2) the direct action of compounds that cause vomiting such as anticancer medications, ipecac, or opiates used for pain (see Box 25-2 for an explanation of emesis occurring with chemotherapy).

The antiemetic drugs are separated into several classes, depending on how they work on the body (Table 25-10).

1. *Serotonin antagonists* are the most effective drugs for suppressing nausea and vomiting caused by antineoplastic medications. The side effects include diarrhea and headache. The two drugs are ondansetron hydrochloride (Zofran) and granisetron (Kytril).
2. *Dopamine antagonists* are a major category of antiemetics. The group is divided into three groups: phenothiazines, butyrophenones, and a group of other medications. These medications suppress vomiting by blocking dopamine-2 receptors. Phenothiazines such as promethazine (Phenergan) are used orally, parenterally, or rectally, or any of the three, for the nausea and vomiting of chemotherapy, surgery, and toxic poisoning. These medications are also used with psychiatric disorders.
3. *Benzodiazepines* such as lorazepam (Ativan) and diazepam (Valium) are also given for chemotherapy patients. Both provide sedation and suppress the anticipation of emesis while producing some amnesia of the emesis. These medications are discussed in Chapter 31.
4. *Anticholinergics* block acetylcholine and histamine and are used to treat motion sickness. Scopolamine is also a cholinergic antagonist used for prevention and treatment of motion sickness through oral, subcutaneous, or transdermal administration (see Box 25-3 for an explanation of vomiting from motion sickness).

BOX 25-2 VOMITING FROM CHEMOTHERAPY

Chemotherapy may cause severe nausea and vomiting, and these side effects may even be the reason why patients discontinue chemotherapy. Vomiting may be anticipatory emesis (occurring prior to receiving anticancer drugs and triggered by memories of previous severe nausea and vomiting), acute emesis (occurring shortly after chemotherapy is administered), or delayed emesis (occurring a day or two after chemotherapy). For emesis prevention, a medication may be administered prior to the chemotherapy. For the patient receiving chemotherapy that causes emesis, a combination of medications may be required using several of the antiemetic classes to be effective.

5. *Phosphorated carbohydrate solution* (Emetrol) contains dextrose, fructose, and phosphoric acid. It works immediately by reducing the hyperactivity of the smooth muscle of the gastric wall. Because of its sugar base and its availability OTC, patient education for persons with diabetes mellitus should include the danger of using the medication.
6. A popular antiemetic, trimethobenzamide hydrochloride (Tigan), may be administered by mouth, injection, or rectal suppository. Painful when given parenterally, the Z-track method is the preferred route for intramuscular injection of the medication (see Chapter 15 for the methodology of Z-track) (see Table 25-10).

Patient Education for Compliance

1. Medications for motion sickness should be taken 30 to 60 minutes prior to travel.
2. Transdermal scopolamine is a 72-hour patch that is placed behind the ear.

TABLE 25-10 Medications Related to Emesis

GENERIC NAME	TRADE NAME	USUAL ADULT DOSE, ROUTE, AND FREQUENCY OF ADMINISTRATION	INDICATIONS FOR USE	MAJOR SIDE EFFECTS	DRUG INTERACTIONS
SEROTONIN ANTAGONISTS*					
ondansetron	Zofran	4-8 mg tid po, IV	Postchemotherapy nausea	Diarrhea, headache	Usually none
granisetron	Kytril	1 mg po, IV 1 hr prior to chemotherapy			
DOPAMINE ANTAGONISTS*			Nausea and vomiting of various causes, including motion sickness	Dizziness, dry mouth, headache, restlessness, hypotension	alcohol, lithium, tricyclic antidepressants, monoamine oxidase inhibitors, hypotensive agents, antithyroid agents
chlorpromazine	Thorazine	10-25 mg q4-6h po, IM, IV			
perphenazine	Trilafon	8-16 mg/day po, IM, IV			
prochlorperazine	Compazine	5-10 mg tid-qid po, IM, IV, rectal suppository			
promethazine	Phenergan	25 mg po, IM, IV, rectal suppository q4-6h			
thiethylperazine	Torecan	10 mg po, IM, rectal suppository 1-3 × per day			
butyrophenones (haloperidol)	Haldol	1-2 mg po, IM, IV q12h			alcohol, CNS depression, lithium
OTHER DOPAMINE ANTAGONISTS			Nausea and vomiting with chemotherapy	Dizziness, headache, restlessness, dry mouth, hypotension	
metoclopramide	Reglan	10-15 mg po qid 1-2 mg/kg IV 30 min prior to chemo and q2-4h prn			alcohol

ANTICHOLINERGICS

	Trade Name	Dosage	Common Uses	Side Effects	Drug Interactions
Antihistamines			Motion sickness, nausea and vomiting from various causes	Sedation, dry mouth, blurred vision, urinary retention	No significant interactions noted
dimenhydrinate*[†]	Dramamine	50-100 mg po, IM, IV q4-6h prn			
diphenhydramine*[†]	Benadryl	10-50 mg po, IM, IV q4-6h prn			
hydroxyzine*	Atarax, Vistaril	25-100 mg po, IM q6h prn			
meclizine*[†]	Bonine,[†] Antivert*	25-50 mg/day po 2-3 × daily			
*Other Anticholinergics**					
scopolamine	Transderm scopolamine	0.5-mg transdermal patch q3d			
MISCELLANEOUS AGENTS			Nausea and vomiting from various causes		
phosphonated carbohydrate solution[†]	Emetrol and others	15-30 mL po q1-3h prn			
trimethobenzamide*	Tigan	250 mg po, IM, tid-qid 200 mg rectal supp tid-qid		Drowsiness, dizziness, blurred vision, headache, hypotension	CNS depressant
aprepipant	Emend	250 mg po AM of chemotherapy, 80 mg po qam × 2 days following chemotherapy	Nausea and vomiting with chemotherapy	Tiredness, nausea, hiccups, constipation, diarrhea, anorexia	terfenadine, cisapride, astemizole, warfarin

CNS, Central nervous system; *IM*, intramuscular; *IV*, intravenous.
* Prescription medication.
[†] OTC medication.

IMPORTANT FACTS ABOUT DRUGS FOR EMESIS

A combination of medications may be necessary to prevent emesis from chemotherapy.

Drugs Used for Intestinal Conditions

Drugs for intestinal conditions include antiflatulents and laxatives/**cathartics.** Both groups of drugs are often used with OTC preparations and have names that are commonly recognized.

Antiflatulents

Some people have excess gas that requires relief of gastric and intestinal distention. Medications including some antacids that are used as antiflatulents or **carminatives** are bought OTC, with simethicone being the most common active ingredient (e.g., Phazyme, Gas-X, Mylanta).

- Simethicone disperses and prevents the formation of gas pockets in the GI tract.
- Antiflatulents are used to relieve gas following gastroscopy and bowel radiography.
- Patients with an excess production of gas should avoid gas-forming foods such as cabbage, onions, and beans and avoid the use of straws when drinking liquids (Table 25-11).

Bowel Function in Constipation and Diarrhea

Bowel function is a major concern in the elderly (constipation) and young children (diarrhea).

- The elderly have increased constipation that may lead to bowel obstruction or habituation of laxatives because of multiple chronic illnesses, polypharmacy, and the decline in body function.
- Health care professionals should obtain a full history of laxative use and possible misuse because these medications interfere with the absorption and metabolism of prescription items.
- Patient education may include the need for dietary change by avoiding such constipating foods as cheese and sugar, having adequate fluid intake, and eating a high-fiber diet.
- Constipation is common in children with contributing factors such as emotions, new environments, dietary changes, and fever.
  - Parents should avoid the indiscriminate use of laxatives but rather should try adding fruits, vegetables, and fluids to the diet.
  - Glycerin suppositories for children are the most appropriate treatment for constipation in children age 10 years and younger.
- Diarrhea in children may cause rapid electrolyte imbalances, and early treatment is necessary to keep the body in homeostasis.
- Some medications may alter the color of stools. Patients should be made aware of this possibility to prevent unnecessary concern if this discoloration should occur (Table 25-12).

Laxatives and Cathartics

Laxatives and **cathartics** are drugs used to induce **defecation.** Laxatives result in the leisurely production of a soft-formed stool over a period of 1 to 2 days. Cathartics produce a prompt, fast, intense fluid evacuation from the bowel and are used most often for diagnostic testing.

Laxatives

Laxatives are valuable when used properly, but many forms of these drugs are abused, especially by the elderly, who may have preconceived ideas concerning the need for daily evacuation of the bowels for good health. The indiscriminate use of laxatives leads to dependence and laxative abuse.

TABLE 25-11 *Antiflatulent*

GENERIC NAME	TRADE NAME	USUAL ADULT DOSE, ROUTE, AND FREQUENCY OF ADMINISTRATION	INDICATIONS FOR USE	DRUG INTERACTIONS
simethicone	Mylicon, Phazyme	80-160 mg po qid	Flatulence, including that caused by radiographic studies	Usually none

Note: The drug listed in this table is available over the counter.

TABLE 25-12 *Medications That May Change the Color of Stools*

DRUG	POSSIBLE COLOR CHANGE
Antacids with aluminum salts (e.g., Maalox, Mylanta)	White specks or white discoloration of stools
Anticoagulants, such as those containing warfarin	Red-orange to black due to intestinal bleeding
Bismuth or iron salts (including Pepto-Bismol)	Black
Laxatives with phenolphthalein	Red
Laxatives containing *senna*	Yellow to orange to brown
Drugs containing phenazopyridine (Pyridium)	Orange to red
rifampin	Red to orange or brown

The "normal" frequency of bowel evacuation varies from three bowel movements per day to a bowel movement once every 3 days. Constipation is related to the hardness of stools rather than to their frequency. Laxatives should be used for constipation and hard, dry stools, not for soft, hydrated stools. If a laxative is necessary, it should be only for a short time in conjunction with dietary changes and exercise. The advertising for OTC laxatives tends to encourage habitual self-medication when these agents are not actually needed. Using a laxative may perpetuate the patient's perception that a laxative is again necessary.

Excessive laxative use develops over some years, and the dependency goes unnoticed until daily use of the laxative is necessary. If laxative abuse is not discovered, permanent bowel damage such as obstruction or perforation and electrolyte imbalances may occur. By purging the intestinal tract, the patient will need 2 to 5 days to refill the bowel, during which time the habitual laxative user will take another laxative because a daily bowel movement has not occurred. Over a period of time, the body becomes reliant on the laxative for a bowel movement, leading to pathologic changes such as heart irregularities. Cardiac arrest may even occur from loss of potassium.

To bring about bowel retraining, changes in lifestyle and diets may also be necessary. Thus it is better to avoid laxative misuse than to face retraining due to indiscriminate use of laxatives and cathartics.

- Laxatives are beneficial when used appropriately for constipation, which is a side effect of many medications.
- Softening of stools will prevent painful elimination and is useful in medical conditions in which irritation and straining should be avoided.
- Laxatives can also be used with patients who have a loss of abdominal and gastric muscle tone.
- With **anthelmintic** therapy, laxatives are used to obtain stool specimens, empty the GI tract before medication administration, and expel dead parasites.
- Laxative therapy is also used to empty the intestines prior to diagnostic or surgical procedures.
- Laxatives should not be used by patients with abdominal pain, nausea, intestinal cramping, or known intestinal diseases unless specifically under a physician's order.
- These drugs are not indicated in intestinal obstructions and should never be used on a routine basis.

Types of Laxatives

Laxatives, mostly OTC preparations, are classified by their source, site of action, degree of action, or mechanism of action (Figure 25-2) (Table 25-13).

- *Osmotic saline laxatives* work by increasing the amount of water in the large intestine and thus in feces. This hydration of intestinal contents causes the fecal mass to swell, stretching the intestinal wall and increasing peristalsis. Low doses of these medications work in 6 to 12 hours, whereas large doses work in 2 to 6 hours but can cause considerable abdominal cramping.
  - Osmotic saline laxatives can cause a substantial water loss from body cells, and replacement is necessary to keep the body in homeostasis.
  - Because of the saline content and fluid retention, these laxatives should not be used with patients with hypertension, heart failure, or edema.
  - Milk of magnesia is the mildest of the saline laxatives and the preferred laxative in this category for children.
  - Cephulac, another osmotic saline laxative, contains fructose and lactose; thus it should be used with care in people with diabetes.

DID YOU KNOW?

Milk of magnesia (MOM) may be used as an antacid in low doses.

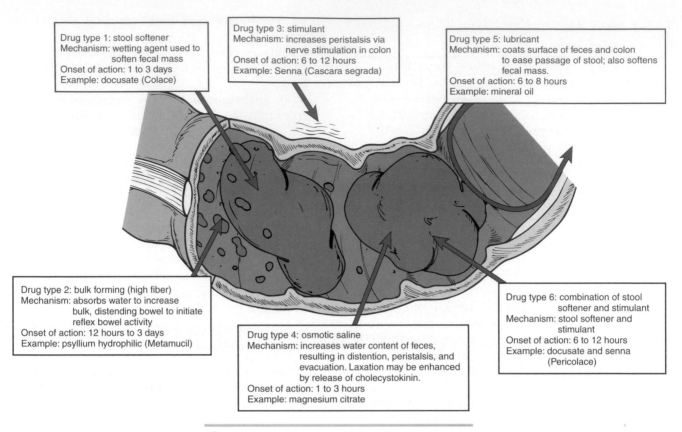

Drug type 1: stool softener
Mechanism: wetting agent used to
        soften fecal mass
Onset of action: 1 to 3 days
Example: docusate (Colace)

Drug type 3: stimulant
Mechanism: increases peristalsis via
        nerve stimulation in colon
Onset of action: 6 to 12 hours
Example: Senna (Cascara segrada)

Drug type 5: lubricant
Mechanism: coats surface of feces and colon
        to ease passage of stool; also softens
        fecal mass.
Onset of action: 6 to 8 hours
Example: mineral oil

Drug type 2: bulk forming (high fiber)
Mechanism: absorbs water to increase
        bulk, distending bowel to initiate
        reflex bowel activity
Onset of action: 12 hours to 3 days
Example: psyllium hydrophilic (Metamucil)

Drug type 4: osmotic saline
Mechanism: increases water content of feces,
        resulting in distention, peristalsis, and
        evacuation. Laxation may be enhanced
        by release of cholecystokinin.
Onset of action: 1 to 3 hours
Example: magnesium citrate

Drug type 6: combination of stool
        softener and stimulant
Mechanism: stool softener and
        stimulant
Onset of action: 6 to 12 hours
Example: docusate and senna
        (Pericolace)

Figure 25-2 Site of action for types of laxatives.

- *Bulk-forming laxatives* stimulate peristalsis by swelling, increasing bulk, and modifying the consistency of stools to stimulate the intestinal tract.
    - Natural or semisynthetic cellulose derivatives such as methylcellulose (Citrucel) and polycarbophil (Fiber-Con) are the active ingredients in bulking agents, which are among the least harmful of the laxatives.
    - The patient must take sufficient fluids for these medications to work.
    - Prunes and bran have similar effects as these laxatives.
    - The onset of action occurs in 12 hours to 3 days.
    - Bulk-forming agents are the laxatives of choice with pregnancy (see Table 25-13).
- *Stimulant laxatives* are from botanical sources except for bisacodyl (Dulcolax). These laxatives are absorbed to stimulate peristalsis, acting in 6 to 8 hours, and are habit forming. When intestinal motility is increased, water has less time for absorption in the large intestines, resulting in watery stools.
    - *Senna, cascara sagrada,* and *aloe* cross into breast milk.
- *Bisacodyl,* a relatively nontoxic agent that acts by stimulating peristalsis in the colon, is often used prior to diagnostic testing. These tablets should not be crushed or chewed because of possible irritation to the stomach, nor should the tablets be taken with milk or antacids because of interference with absorption.
- *Cascara sagrada* (Ex-Lax) is the mildest of the laxatives in this group. These medications may discolor urine to pink, red, or brown.
- *Castor oil,* obtained from the seeds of castor beans, passes rapidly through the stomach unchanged, causing irritation of the small intestines. The rapid movement into the small intestines and the colon is the basis for effectiveness. Castor oil is not recommended for pregnant or lactating women (see Table 25-13).
- *Lubricant laxatives* (mineral oil and olive oil) allow water to penetrate the fecal mass.
    - Laxatives do not increase bulk, but the oily agents coat the surface of the stool and soften the stool to ease defecation, usually acting in 6 to 8 hours.

TABLE 25-13 *Laxatives and Cathartics*

GENERIC NAME	TRADE NAME	USUAL ADULT DOSE, ROUTE, AND FREQUENCY OF ADMINISTRATION	INDICATIONS FOR USE	MAJOR SIDE EFFECTS	DRUG INTERACTIONS
OSMOTIC LAXATIVES†			Relieve constipation	Usually none except abdominal cramping	Usually none
polyethylene glycol	MiraLax	1 tbsp po in 8 oz water/day			
lubiprostone	Amitiza	24 mcg caps bid		Occasional diarrhea	None
lactulose	Cephulac, Chronulac, Kristalose	15-60 mL po, 1 package po reconstituted and taken po per day	(including chronic idiopathic constipation)		
sodium phosphate	Fleet's	1½ oz in 8 oz water po, or as an enema		Abdominal cramping	
Magnesium Compounds					
magnesium hydroxide	Milk of Magnesia, Phillip's Chewable	30-60 mL po hs Chew 300-600 mg hs			
magnesium citrate	Citrate of Magnesia, Citroma	1 8-oz glass po qd 5-10 oz qd			
magnesium sulfate	Epsom salts	15 g in 8 oz of water po			
BULK-FORMING LAXATIVES†			Constipation	Flatulence and bulky stools	
methylcellulose	Citrucel	1 tsp in 8 oz water po		Abdominal cramping, flatulence	K-sparing diuretics, salicylates, digoxin
polycarbophil	Fiber-Con, Mitrolan, Fiber-All	2 tabs po qd up to qid			
psyllium hydrophilic	Effersyllium, Perdiem, Metamucil, Serutan	1 tsp in 8 oz of water po up to qid			
STIMULANT LAXATIVES†					
bisacodyl	Dulcolax	10-15 mg diagnostic testing po or 1 rectal suppository		Abdominal cramping, nausea, diarrhea, flatulence	
cascara sagrada	Senokot, Ex-Lax, Black Draught, Fletcher's	1 tab or 1 tsp po hs			
senna castor oil	Purge	10-15 mL or 2 tabs po hs 45-60 mL po			

(continued)

TABLE 25-13 *Laxatives and Cathartics—cont'd*

GENERIC NAME	TRADE NAME	USUAL ADULT DOSE, ROUTE, AND FREQUENCY OF ADMINISTRATION	INDICATIONS FOR USE	MAJOR SIDE EFFECTS	DRUG INTERACTIONS
LUBRICANT LAXATIVES[†]					
mineral oil	Kondremul, Petrolagar	15 mL po			
olive oil		15 mL po			
STOOL SOFTENERS/ MOISTENING AGENTS					
docusate sodium	Colace	1-4 tabs/caps po			
docusate calcium	Surfak	240 mg/day po			
docusate potassium	Dialose	1-3 caps po daily			
glycerin		1 rectal suppository			
CATHARTICS/BOWEL EVACUANTS*					
polyethylene glycol electrolyte solution	GoLYTELY, Colyte, Peg Lyte, PEG-ES	4 L po (240 mL every 10 min until all consumed)		Bloating, nausea, abdominal fullness	

* Prescription medication.
[†] OTC medication.

- Large doses of these laxatives tend to cause leakage of oil from the rectum.
- Glycerin suppositories, another lubricant laxative usually effective in 15 minutes to an hour, increase peristalsis in all age groups (see Table 25-13).
- *Stool softeners*, or fecal moistening agents, decrease the consistency of stools by reducing the surface tension. These medications work by absorbing water into the stool, lubricating the rectum, and increasing stool bulk.
  - Docusate (Colace) acts as a detergent, permitting water and fatty substances to penetrate and mix with the fecal material. These medications usually take 1 to 3 days to be effective and are effective for patients who should avoid straining necessary for bowel movements. They may be combined with laxatives in such medications as Peri-Colace and Doxidan to soften stools while enhancing stool evacuation.
  - Stool softeners have a wide margin of safety and few potential adverse reactions (see Table 25-13).

Cathartics or Bowel Evacuants

Bowel evacuants (cathartics) such as polyethylene glycol (GoLYTELY) are bowel-cleansing solutions of mixtures similar to body fluids so that water and electrolytes are not absorbed.

- These agents can be used even in patients who are sensitive to electrolyte imbalance because water is not lost and electrolyte balance is maintained.
- When used prior to diagnostic testing, the patient must drink large amounts of these fluids (about a gallon) within 2 to 3 hours; bowel movements begin about an hour after starting the dosing.
- If the rectal excretions become clear, the laxative may be stopped at that point.
- Oral medications should not be given within an hour of starting the solutions because the medicine may be flushed from the GI tract with the laxative (see Table 25-13).

Patient Education for Compliance

1. Use of laxatives to force evacuation may initiate abuse of laxatives.
2. Laxatives should not be used by patients with abdominal pain, nausea, and abdominal cramping.
3. Constipation refers to the consistency of stools, not the frequency, an important fact with geriatric patients.

Patient Education for Compliance— cont'd

4. Changing the dietary consumption of fiber may be all that is necessary to reduce constipation.
5. Bulk-forming laxatives and surfactants should be taken with a full glass of water.
6. Castor oil should be mixed with juice to improve the taste and should not be administered at night or to someone who has difficulty swallowing.
7. When given in small doses, osmotic laxatives soften stools, but these agents cause watery evacuation with large doses.
8. Glycerin suppositories are the safest treatment for constipation in all age groups.

IMPORTANT FACTS ABOUT LAXATIVES AND CATHARTICS

- Laxatives promote defecation.
- Laxatives and stool softeners should be used for legitimate reasons only, such as for diagnostic tests, before surgical procedures, and for medical conditions that prevent the straining required for bowel movements.
- The elderly should be taught to avoid constipating foods such as cheese and sugar and to have adequate fluid intake and a high-fiber diet.
- Bulk-forming laxatives should be given with water.
- Stimulant laxatives should be used with discrimination.
- Suppositories may cause rectal irritation.
- Osmotic laxatives require an increased intake of fluids to prevent dehydration.
- Stimulating laxatives and osmotic laxatives should not be given at bedtime because of their rapid onset of action.

Drugs Used for Relief of Diarrhea

Antidiarrheal agents are used to treat diarrhea, a symptom of bowel disorders and not a disorder itself. Diarrhea consists of stools of excessive volume and fluidity with increased frequency of defecation and is associated with cramping pain due to rapid passage of intestinal content. The management of diarrhea depends on finding the underlying cause, replacing water and electrolytes as needed, reducing cramping, and reducing the passage of stools. Diarrhea is usually self-limiting and resolves without further effects. Chronic diarrhea needs evaluation for cause and treatment by the findings. Diarrhea in children may become a medical emergency in as little as 24 hours because of the loss of electrolytes. The antidiarrheal agents

TABLE 25-14 *Antidiarrheals*

GENERIC NAME	TRADE NAME	USUAL ADULT DOSE, ROUTE, AND FREQUENCY OF ADMINISTRATION	INDICATIONS FOR USE	DRUG INTERACTIONS
cholestyramine*	Questran	4 g po 1-2 × per day	Relieve symptoms of diarrhea	Anticoagulants, digoxin, thiazides, penicillins tetracyclines, propranolol, thyroid replacement, folic acid
bismuth subsalicylate[†]	Pepto-Bismol	15 mL po every 30-60 min or 2 tabs po every 30-60 min until diarrhea is checked		Anticoagulants, oral hypoglycemics
activated charcoal[†]	CharcoCaps	2 caps po q30-60 min until diarrhea is checked		
kaolin/pectin (attapulgite)[†]	Kaopectate	60-120 mL po after each loose stool		digoxin
OPIOIDS/SYNTHETIC OPIOIDS				
loperamide	Imodium AD[†], Imodium*	2 tabs initially, then 1 tab after each loose stool		
diphenoxylate/ atropine*	Lomotil (Schedule V)	1 tab po 4× per day		alcohol, CNS depressants, MAO inhibitors
camphorated opium tincture*	Paregoric* (Schedule III)	1-2 tsp po qid mixed with water		

MAJOR SIDE EFFECTS OF OPIOIDS/SYNTHETIC OPIOIDS: loperamide: Dizziness, dry mouth, depresses CNS; **diphenoxylate/atropine:** same as loperamide plus agitation, tachycardia, numbness of hands/feet, drowsiness.

CNS, Central nervous system; *MAO*, monoamine oxidase.
* Prescription medication.
[†] OTC medication.

may be classified as adsorbents and opioid or synthetic opioid medications (Table 25-14).

- **Adsorbents** act by coating the walls of the GI tract, absorbing the toxins or bacteria that are causing the diarrhea, and excreting these agents with the stools.
  - OTC medications include activated charcoal, bismuth salts, kaolin, pectin, attapulgite, and the prescription drug cholestyramine (Questran).
  - These medications are usually taken after each loose bowel movement until the diarrhea is controlled.
  - Constipation may follow the use of large amounts of these products.
  - Medications given during the time that adsorbents are being used may not be absorbed at expected levels.
  - Pepto-Bismol may be used as an antidiarrheal, antacid, or antiulcer medication; it absorbs irritants of the GI tract.
  - Attapulgite, a hydrated magnesium aluminum silicate, is replacing the kaolin and

pectin in Kaopectate, a commonly used adsorbent that is safe for all ages.
- *Opioid* and *synthetic opioid medications* are prescription drugs that inhibit GI motility, decrease hyperperistalsis, and slow the passage of intestinal contents to allow for the reabsorption of water and electrolytes, thus slowing stool frequencies.
  - Loperamide (Imodium) is a prescription medication but is also found as Imodium AD in an OTC preparation for acute nonspecific and chronic diarrhea.
  - Diphenoxylate and atropine (Lomotil) is a synthetic opioid. This Schedule V medication inhibits the propulsion of food through the GI tract.
  - Camphorated opium tincture (Paregoric) is a scheduled medication and requires a prescription dependent on the amount of paregoric in the drug. This agent slows the passage of food in the GI tract by slowing the contractions of the smooth muscle, prolonging the time before defecation. GI secretions are also reduced. Paregoric should

TABLE 25-15 *Gastrointestinal Antiinflammatory/Antiirritant Agents*

GENERIC NAME	TRADE NAME	USUAL ADULT DOSE, ROUTE, AND FREQUENCY OF ADMINISTRATION	INDICATIONS FOR USE	DRUG INTERACTIONS
mesalamine	Rowasa	Enema—hs; rectal	Irritable/inflammatory	Usually none
mesalamine delayed release	Lialda	suppository bid	bowel disease	
		800 mg tab po tid	Crohn's disease	
		1 tab daily	Ulcerative colitis	
sulfasalazine	Azulfidine	1 g po tid-qid		
olsalazine	Dipentum	1 g/day po in 2 doses		warfarin
balsalazide	Colazal	2.25g po 3×/day		
tegaserod maleate	Zelnorm	6 mg po bid on empty stomach	Irritable bowel disease	None
alosetron	Lotronex	0.5 mg po bid	Same	fluvoxamine

MAJOR SIDE EFFECTS: mesalamine: abdominal pain, cramping, headache, weakness, dizziness; **sulfasalazine:** nausea, fever, joint pain, rashes; **olsalazine:** abdominal cramping, diarrhea, dyspepsia, joint pain, anorexia; **tegaserod maleate:** headaches, diarrhea; **alosetron:** constipation, bloody diarrhea, heartburn, nausea and vomiting.

Note: All of the drugs in this table require a prescription.

always be diluted with water prior to administration (see Table 25-14).

Patient Education for Compliance

1. Antidiarrheals are available OTC and by prescription.
2. Pepto-Bismol, the drug of choice, acts as an antiseptic and antidiarrheal to soothe the GI tract.

Antiinflammatory Agents for the Gastrointestinal Tract

Antiinflammatory medications for ulcerative colitis are available as rectal suppositories, enemas, and oral tablets (Table 25-15).

* Mesalamine (Rowasa) is specifically for the management of ulcerative colitis and Crohn's disease. It is administered as oral tablets three times a day, suppositories twice a day, or a retention enema at bedtime to be retained for 8 hours.
* Sulfasalazine (Azulfidine) is a member of the sulfonamide family, but its only indication is for irritable bowel syndrome.
* Olsalazine (Dipentum) is a salicylate derivative used for ulcerative colitis and other chronic inflammatory bowel diseases.
* Balsalazide (Colazal), a salicylate, has the same indications for chronic inflammatory bowel disease.

IMPORTANT FACTS ABOUT ANTIINFLAMMATORY AGENTS FOR THE GI TRACT
* Medications for the lower GI tract are primarily used to restore a normal bowel pattern.
* Inflammatory bowel disease may be treated with salicylates, sulfasalazine, glucocorticoids, and immunosuppressants.

Anorectal Preparations

Anorectal preparations are used to provide symptomatic relief from the discomfort of hemorrhoids and other anorectal disorders.

* Some contain the topical anesthetics benzocaine and dibucaine such as Preparation H and Nupercainal Ointment.
* Other preparations contain hydrocortisone to reduce swelling, suppress inflammation, and relieve itching and stinging.
* Acting as emollients to lubricate the rectum and reduce irritations, some preparations contain lanolin or mineral oil.
* Astringents such as witch hazel and bismuth subgallate are used to reduce swelling, inflammation, and irritation.
* Nupercainal, Preparation H, and Anusol are some OTC names for these medications, which come in several forms: suppositories, creams, ointments, foams, and pads. In Table 25-16 Nupercainal is shown as a typical anorectal medication.

TABLE 25-16 *Anorectal Preparation*

GENERIC NAME	TRADE NAME	USUAL ADULT DOSE, ROUTE, AND FREQUENCY OF ADMINISTRATION	INDICATIONS FOR USE	DRUG INTERACTIONS
dibucaine*	Nupercainal Ointment or Suppositories	Apply topically qid	Hemorrhoids, rectal fissures	None noted

* Over-the-counter medication. Cortisone suppositories and ointments may also be used; some require a prescription, and others do not. See Chapter 21.

IMPORTANT FACTS ABOUT ANORECTAL PREPARATIONS

- Anorectal preparations containing topical anesthetics are found as OTC preparations.
- When hydrocortisones are added, many then become prescription medications.

Drugs Used for Intestinal Parasites

Anthelmintics are used to treat parasitic worms. The intestinal tract is a common site for infections with early infestation being asymptomatic and then causing severe problems as the infection progresses (Table 25-17).

- The most common types of parasitic worms are pinworms, flukes, roundworms, and tapeworms. The dosages of medications for parasites are based on weight. Allied health professionals should obtain an accurate body weight for all family members when medication is indicated.
- Mebendazole (Vermox) is relatively slow-acting for the treatment of roundworms and pinworms. With any treatment for pinworms, all household contacts of the patient should be treated at the same time. Strict hygiene is essential to prevent reinfection—disinfect toilets, launder undergarments and linens, wash hands before and after eating and using the toilet, and take showers instead of baths.
- Pyrantel (found in Antiminth, Pin X, and other anthelmintics) is an OTC preparation. Most of the dose is excreted in the feces because the drug is not absorbed in the GI tract. The medication acts by killing the parasite; therefore the entire dose must be taken at one time.
- Praziquantel (Biltricide) is absorbed by the helminth, causing the worms to detach from the host's body tissues. Transient headaches and abdominal discomfort are the most frequent reactions, but drowsiness may occur.
- Thiabendazole (Mintezol) has analgesic, antipyretic, and antiinflammatory actions, providing relief of the abdominal cramping that comes with the therapeutic treatment.
- Many of the anthelmintic agents are enhanced when given with fatty food to slow the distribution of the drug. Also, tablets may be chewed or crushed to increase their absorption. Care must be taken to prevent reinfection that occurs with poor sanitation and hygiene.

Patient Education for Compliance

1. When treating for intestinal parasites, the entire household should be treated. Linens, clothes, and so on should be disinfected.
2. Good sanitary practices are essential to prevent reinfestation of the parasites.

Drugs Used to Suppress Appetite

About 50% of Americans are obese, a state in which the individual's total body weight consists of a greater amount of fat than normal (25% over the ideal weight for men, and 35% for women). Obesity in children and teens is considered one of the leading health problems in the United States today. Genetics, anxiety, stress, and poor self-image are some of the most common reasons for this condition. Obese persons tend to have greater incidence of cardiovascular disease and a higher incidence of type 2 diabetes mellitus (T2DM). The condition is managed through diet, behavioral modification, prescription and nonprescription medications, surgical procedures, and other nondrug therapy.

Anorexiant drugs, or appetite suppressants, include a wide variety of medications that act on the brain as weak stimulators to suppress the appetite center in the hypothalamus (Table 25-18).

- Most drugs act directly to mimic the sympathetic nervous system, but the exact mechanism of action is not understood.
- Most of these prescription medications are controlled substances and are subject to the regulations governing scheduled drugs.

TABLE 25-17 *Anthelmintics*

GENERIC NAME	TRADE NAME	USUAL ADULT DOSE, ROUTE, AND FREQUENCY OF ADMINISTRATION	INDICATIONS FOR USE	DRUG INTERACTIONS
mebendazole*	Vermox	100 mg po bid for 3 days	Roundworms, pinworms	None
pyrantel*[†]	Antiminth,* Pin-Rid,[†] Pin-X[†]	po based on body weight	Roundworms, pinworms, hookworms	
praziquantel*	Biltricide	po based on body weight	Tapeworms, flukes	
thiabendazole*	Mintezol	po based on body weight	Threadworms, roundworms	
albendazole*	Albenza	po based on body weight	Pork and dog tapeworms	

MAJOR SIDE EFFECTS: mebendazole and **pyrantel:** abdominal cramping, diarrhea **praziquantel:** headaches, drowsiness, abdominal discomfort; **thiabendazole** and **albendazole:** abnormal cramping, anorexia, nausea and vomiting, dizziness, drowsiness.

*Prescription medication.
[†] OTC medication.

TABLE 25-18 *Anorexiants*

GENERIC NAME	TRADE NAME	USUAL ADULT DOSE, ROUTE, AND FREQUENCY OF ADMINISTRATION	INDICATIONS FOR USE	DRUG INTERACTIONS
NONAMPHETAMINE				
diethylpropion (Schedule IV)	Tenuate	25 mg po bid-tid ac		
	Tenuate Dospan	75 mg po in AM		
mazindol (Schedule IV)	Mazanor, Sanorex	1 mg/day po; may be increased		
phendimetrazine (Schedule III)	Adphen, Bontril, Obalan, Adipost	35 mg po bid-tid 105 mg/day po ac breakfast		
phentermine (Schedule IV)	Fastin Adipex-P	30 mg/day po 37.5 mg/day po		
orlistat	Xenical Alli (OTC)	120 mg po tid ac 60 mg po tid with meals		pravastatin
phenmetrazine	Preludin	75 mg po daily		None

MAJOR SIDE EFFECTS OF NONAMPHETAMINE ANOREXIANTS: Stimulation of CNS, dizziness, euphoria, fatigue, insomnia, palpations, hypertension, cardiac dysrhythmias, dry mouth, abdominal discomfort, constipation, nervousness; additionally flatulence, rectal incontinence with orlistat.

GENERIC NAME	TRADE NAME	USUAL ADULT DOSE, ROUTE, AND FREQUENCY OF ADMINISTRATION	INDICATIONS FOR USE	DRUG INTERACTIONS
AMPHETAMINES				
dextroamphetamine (Schedule II)	Dexedrine	5-10 mg po daily to bid	Weight loss/ obesity	MAO inhibitors
benzphetamine (Schedule III)	Didrex	25-50 mg/day po		
phentermine resin (Schedule IV)	Ionamin	15-30 mg/day po		
sibutramine (Schedule IV)	Meridia	10-15 mg/day po		

MAJOR SIDE EFFECTS OF AMPHETAMINES: Stimulation of CNS, dizziness, euphoria, fatigue, insomnia, palpations, hypertension, cardiac dysrhythmias, dry mouth, abdominal discomfort, constipation, nervousness.

Note: All of the drugs listed in this table require a prescription except Alli.
CNS, Central nervous system; *MAO,* monoamine oxidase.

- The amphetamines and amphetamine-like substances such as dextroamphetamine (Dexadrine) are Schedule II drugs because of the danger of habituation.
- Other prescription drugs that are used as anorexiants are either Schedule III, such as benzphetamine (Didrex), or Schedule IV medications, such as diethylpropion (Tenuate) and phentermine (Fastin, Adipex-P).
- Bulking agents such as methylcellulose (Fiber Trim) and psyllium hydrophilic mucilloid (Metamucil) may be used to give the patient a feeling of fullness and loss of craving for food.
- Anorexiants have a number of limitations and should be used as an adjunct to behavior modification, diet, and exercise.
  - Short-acting anorexiants usually work for 3 to 4 hours and should be taken about 30 to 60 minutes before meals.
  - Long-acting medications last for about 12 hours and should be taken 12 hours before sleep to prevent insomnia.
  - The use should be short term because tolerance may occur within just a few weeks.

IMPORTANT FACTS ABOUT ANOREXIANTS

- Anorexiants are for the short-term treatment of obesity because of the danger of habituation. Behavior modification, diet, and exercise should be added to drug therapy for the long-term treatment of obesity.
- Anorexiants that stimulate the central nervous system may cause insomnia, nervousness, and related side effects.
- Prescription anorexiants are scheduled drugs controlled by the Drug Enforcement Administration.

Summary

Many products used in the GI tract are available OTC and have easily recognizable names. Mouthwashes and gargles, as well as dentifrices that contain fluorides, are used for tooth care and to prevent caries. Dental therapeutics are important to retain teeth for chewing food and to prevent gum diseases. Fluoride replacement is especially important in children who do not live where fluorine has been added to the water.

Oral antifungals (lozenges and liquids) are used for thrush by coating the mouth.

Saliva is necessary for the lubrication of food as it passes through the mouth into the GI tract. Replacement of saliva requires multiple applications daily for needed moisture in chronically ill patients.

Antivirals, used for the symptomatic relief of herpes simplex, varicella, and HIV infections of the mouth, should be applied using techniques that will not spread lesions during the treatment. Viral lesions and lesions from dental work, antineoplastics, or disease processes may be relieved with topical anesthetics.

Gastric conditions are treated with many types of medications to relieve hyperacidity, ulcers, spasms of the GI tract, nausea, and vomiting. Digestants are used to assist with the digestion of food intake. Antacids are used either to decrease acid secretions or to neutralize the secreted hydrochloric acid when hyperacidity of the stomach occurs and the wall of the stomach may be affected by these oversecretions. Antacids have aluminum and magnesium as their bases, with each having the opposite effect on the bowels; magnesium causes diarrhea, aluminum causes constipation. To prevent either of these side effects, some antacids, known as magaldrate, now contain both of these compounds. Calcium carbonate, an antacid, is also effective as a calcium substitute in the prevention of osteoporosis. Sodium bicarbonate (baking soda), the one antacid that interacts with the body fluids to change electrolyte levels, should be avoided as a routine antacid.

Optimal antiulcer therapy requires drug and lifestyle changes. Antibiotic therapy, using two antibiotics to prevent the chance of forming drug-resistant strains of microorganisms, is used for *H. pylori* bacterial ulcers. H_2-receptor antagonists that are effective against the histamine found in the GI tract decrease acid secretions by inhibiting the histamines secreted by the gastric mucosa. When antacids and antisecretory agents are to be given therapeutically, the agents should be given at least 1 hour apart to be effective. Proton pump inhibitors decrease hydrogen and potassium, chemicals that are essential for the formation of hydrochloric acid in the stomach. Some antiulcer medications protect the gastric wall by coating the wall to reduce gastric irritations.

Symptoms of GERD may be reduced by using antispasmodics to decrease secretions and slow gastric motility. Prokinetic medications stimulate gastric motility and lower esophageal sphincter pressure. These agents are also used for the treatment of nausea caused by chemotherapy and may be used for GI disorders when lifestyle changes have not been effective.

Digestive enzyme supplements are specifically for the digestion of fat in persons who produce insufficient pancreatic enzymes. Cholesterol gallstones may be dissolved by medications, but this is a long process, taking up to 2 years to be effective.

Antiemetics work in several ways to suppress vomiting. Some are used with chemotherapy and surgery, whereas others are used to treat motion sickness or the hyperactivity of the stomach that is associated with ingestion of toxins. Some antiemetics for motion sickness are available OTC and should be taken 30 to 60 minutes prior to beginning a trip, whereas others are available by prescription for prolonged transdermal application.

Because of the ease of obtaining laxatives, these drugs may be the most misused of all medications, especially by the elderly. Rebound constipation occurs when the person depends on a laxative for bowel action. Laxatives work several ways in the body, so the chosen type should be matched to the cause of the constipation. The allied health professional should do extensive patient teaching about physiologic body function to stop the vicious circle of excessive laxative use.

Antidiarrheals, available either by prescription or OTC, are used to treat diarrhea from various causes. Some of the preparations have an opioid/synthetic opioid classification and should be taken with care. One of the most effective treatments for diarrhea is Pepto-Bismol, which coats the intestinal tract and is bacteriostatic in the stomach.

Irritable bowel syndrome is treated with salicylates and antibiotics. Some preparations are retention enemas that are used at bedtime.

Anorectal preparations—most available OTC—are used for hemorrhoids and other rectal or anal discomforts. Most are topical anesthetics, hydrocortisone, or a combination of both agents. Emollients are used to lubricate the rectum, whereas astringents are used to decrease the swelling, inflammation, and irritation.

Anthelmintics are used to treat the intestinal parasites, such as pinworms, roundworms, tapeworms, and flukes, most commonly found in the United States. Anthelmintics are enhanced when given with fatty foods. When treating one member of a family for intestinal parasites, the entire household should be treated.

Anorexiants are used for the treatment of obesity and should be used short term, with behavioral modification and diet forming the long-term treatment of obesity. These drugs cause central nervous system irritability and are scheduled medications because of their habit-forming nature.

Critical Thinking Exercises

SCENARIO
Sally comes to the medical setting stating she has heartburn on a daily basis. She states that she has also been constipated.
1. What type of antacid should she take?
2. How often and at what time of day should she take the antacid?
3. How should she space her routine medications with the antacid?
4. What suggestions would you make if Sally begins to have diarrhea?
5. What lifestyle changes might help Sally's bowel and gastric conditions?

DRUG CALCULATIONS

1. Order: Surfak 100 mg hs
   Available medication:

Dose to be given: _____

2. Order: Zantac 37.5 mL IM stat
   Available medication:

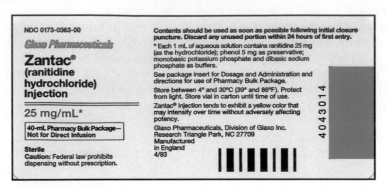

Dose to be given: _____

Show the volume of medication on the syringe provided.

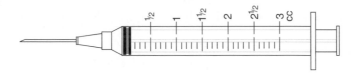

REVIEW QUESTIONS

1. What is the indication for using fluoride products? In what forms are they available?
   _____
   _____

2. What are the indications for antacids? _____
   _____
   _____

3. What bacterium has been found to cause peptic ulcers? What are two antibiotics used in the treatment of bacterial peptic ulcers? _____
   _____

4. What is an antiemetic? What are the classes of antiemetics? How do medications for motion sickness work? _____
   _____
   _____

5. What two special groups of patients must be watched closely with the use of laxatives? Why do these populations need special considerations? _____
   _____
   _____

6. Why are laxatives and cathartics used? What is the difference between laxatives and cathartics?
   _____
   _____

7. How do adsorbent antidiarrheals work? Opioid/synthetic opioid antidiarrheals? _____
   _____
   _____

8. What is the purpose of anthelmintics? What are some of their side effects? _____
   _____
   _____

CHAPTER 26

Respiratory System Disorders

OBJECTIVES

After studying this chapter, you should be capable of doing the following:

- Briefly discussing the respiratory tract as the source of oxygen intake and the exchange with carbon dioxide.
- Describing the effects of antihistamines, decongestants, and the use of nasal preparations with respiratory conditions.
- Briefly explaining the need for corticosteroids in acute and chronic disease processes of the respiratory system and the side effects of these drugs found following long-term therapy.
- Discussing mucolytics, expectorants, and antitussives and their effects on respiratory secretions.

Mac, age 3, has a cough and congestion due to an upper respiratory infection (URI). He visits Dr. Merry because he has begun to wheeze. Mac's mother is concerned that Mac might have asthma need corticosteroids. Dr. Merry checks Mac and finds that he also has otitis media.

Would you expect Mac to have an earache with a URI?

Dr. Merry prescribes a decongestant. What side effects would Dr. Merry tell Mac's mother may occur?

Why would Dr. Merry prescribe a decongestant rather than an antihistamine?

KEY TERMS

Anomaly	Epistaxis	Palliative
Antihistamine	Expectorant	Patent
Antitussive	Expectoration	Productive cough
Asonomia	Extrapyramidal symptoms	Rale
Asthma	Exudate	Rebound congestion
Bronchiectasis	Hemoptysis	Rhinitis
Coryza	Metered dose inhaler (MDI)	Rhinorrhea
Decongestant	Mucokinetic agent	Sputum
Dry powder inhaler (DPI)	Mucolytic	Stomatitis
Dysphonia	Mucus	Tenacious
Dyspnea	Nebulizer	Tenacious cough
Emphysema	Nonproductive cough	

Common Symptoms of Respiratory System Disorders	Common Side Effects of Medications for Respiratory System Conditions
Pain in respiratory tract including chest pain and sore throat	Dry mouth
Difficulty with breathing—dyspnea, wheezing, rales—leading to cyanosis	Tachycardia
Acute or chronic cough, productive or nonproductive	Sleeplessness and nervousness
Dysphonia	Nausea, vomiting, and anorexia
Fatigue and malaise	Stomatitis
Chills, fever, and headaches	Drowsiness
Hemoptysis and epistaxis	Hypotension
	Decreased coordination

Easy Working Knowledge of Drugs Used to Treat Respiratory System Disorders

DRUG CLASS	PRESCRIPTION	OTC	PREGNANCY CATEGORY	MAJOR INDICATIONS
Antihistamines	Yes	Yes	B, C	Treatment of histamine-caused allergies such as rhinitis
Decongestants	Yes	Yes	C	Relief of nasal and upper respiratory congestion including colds and influenza
Nasal sprays/drops	Yes	Yes	C	Relief of nasal membrane edema, as decongestants, and for seasonal allergic rhinitis
Combination decongestant products	Yes	Yes	C	Common cold
Antitussives	Yes	Yes	B, C	Relief of cough, especially nonproductive cough
Mucolytics	Yes	Yes	B	Decrease viscosity of respiratory secretions
Expectorants	Yes	Yes	C	Promote coughing and expectoration of mucus and sputum
Bronchodilators	Yes	Yes	B, C	Dilate bronchial tree to increase O_2-CO_2 exchange
Glucocorticoids	Yes	No	C, D	Relieve acute and chronic asthma
Asthmatic prophylactic agents	Yes	Yes	B	Prevention of an asthma attack
Influenza prophylactic agents	Yes	No	C	Prevention of influenza symptoms

The respiratory tract carries oxygen to and removes carbon dioxide from the lungs, or external respiration. The circulatory system carries the oxygen to the body cells, where it is exchanged with carbon dioxide on the cellular level—or cellular (internal) respiration. These two components of oxygen exchange maintain the body pH and homeostasis. Thus any change in the respiratory system affects all body systems. Disease processes increase the work of the respiratory system. In severe respiratory problems, impaired oxygen–carbon dioxide exchange must be treated before other body system disorders can be addressed.

How Respiration Controls Body Functions

The respiratory tract contains the nasal passages, mouth, pharynx, larynx, trachea, bronchial tree, lungs, and alveoli, as well as accessory organs such as the skeletal muscles of the chest wall and the diaphragm (Figure 26-1). As the steps to cardiopulmonary resuscitation, ABC, teach, A, or airway, and B, or breathing, are the first steps for the maintenance of life, followed by C, or circulation (cardiac function), to send the needed oxygen to the body cells for maintenance of homeostasis. Respirations regulate the functionality of body systems and adjust to any changes in the metabolic state of the person.

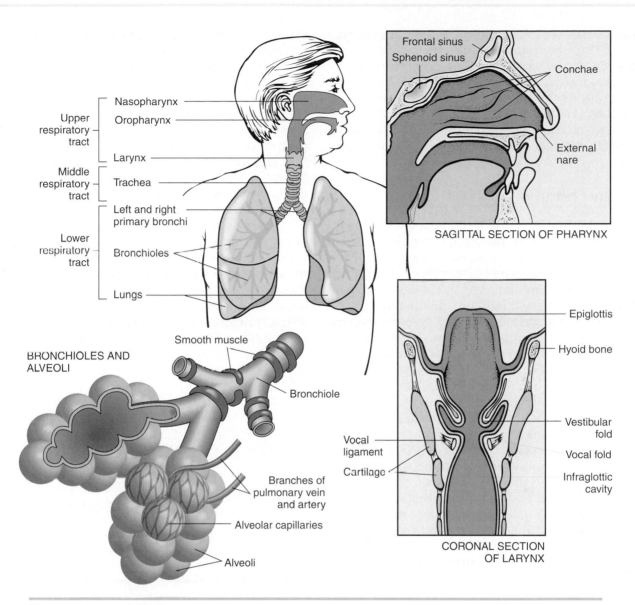

Figure 26-1 Respiratory system, showing upper, middle, and lower tracts. (From Damjanov I: *Pathology for the health professions*, ed 3, St Louis, 2006, Saunders.)

The nasal passages (cavity) warm incoming air, remove noxious substances, and moisten the air before circulation throughout the body. The **patency** of the respiratory tract and the presence of the needed secretions and their tenacity determine the efficiency of the respiratory tract. When **anomalies**, diseases, or injuries occur, medications become part of the treatment provided to ensure the air flows through the air passages and into the cells of the body for a constant supply of oxygen and continuous removal of carbon dioxide.

Respiratory tract secretions produce a thick mucus that bathes the upper tract to protect against toxins. These secretions, in addition to cilia, prevent pathogens from entering the lower respiratory tract. The watery fluids in the lower respiratory tract coat the epithelium of the lungs as protectants. When these secretions become **tenacious** during obstructive pulmonary diseases, the cilia have difficulty removing these protectants into the pharynx for expulsion. If the cilia are ineffective and the moisture in the respiratory tract is insufficient to keep secretions thin, the secretions collect to form excessive amounts of mucus, resulting in difficulty breathing.

The tracheobronchial tree is innervated by the autonomic nervous system, allowing smooth muscle to work to improve ventilation. The basic rhythm and control for inspirations and expirations comes from the medulla of the brain. The chemoreceptors and baroreceptors in the carotid and aortic blood vessels lead to the stimulation of the respiratory centers when voluntary control of breathing is necessary. Thus the respiratory centers control the pH of the blood, and vice versa. Fear, pain, stress, exercise, blood pressure, body temperature, and blood oxygen levels modify the respiratory centers and their control of the rhythm and depth of respiration. Although the respiratory system may be affected by voluntary controls, the final control is involuntary.

Oxygen Therapy

Oxygen therapy is used to treat inadequate oxygen intake resulting from pathologic conditions such as chronic obstructive pulmonary disease (COPD), pneumothorax, or other respiratory conditions that decrease pulmonary gas exchanges. Oxygen is ordered by prescription and administered by inhalation through various delivery systems such as masks or nasal cannulas (Figure 26-2). Oxygen should be available in the medical setting such as a physician's office, for use in emergency situations. The allied health professional should know the proper and competent use of the available equipment and should ensure that it is in working condition at all times.

In disease processes such as COPD, low doses of oxygen are administered to promote respiratory gas exchange. The effectiveness of oxygen therapy depends on the carbon dioxide content of the blood and the response of the involuntary respirations caused by stimulation of the medulla of the brain. Because oxygen–carbon dioxide exchange is impaired in individuals with chronic respiratory diseases, the carbon dioxide content of the blood tends to rise. Because of the chronically increased carbon dioxide levels and decreased oxygen levels in the blood with COPD, the respiratory center of the brain is relatively insensitive to carbon dioxide stimulation, decreasing the involuntary response for breathing. Therefore these patients are usually prescribed very low doses of oxygen (1-2 L/minute) to stimulate respiration. Larger doses will only further suppress the involuntary respiratory center. In patients with COPD or respiratory distress, high concentrations of oxygen cause hypoventilation and resultant anoxia.

Oxygen toxicity is difficult to recognize, but one of the first signs of too much oxygen is mental confusion. Another early sign is aching or burning in the sternal area with a dry, hacking cough. Respiratory distress, nausea, vomiting, restlessness, twitching, loss of feeling, and tremors in any order may follow. Excessive oxygen intake for a long period of time can lead to convulsions and death.

CLINICAL TIP
Everyone in the immediate vicinity of oxygen should be aware that oxygen will support combustion. No smoking, matches, or electrical equipment that might spark should be in the room with oxygen therapy.

Patient Education for Compliance

Oxygen should not be used with an open flame or when there is a possibility of sparks because of the danger of explosion.

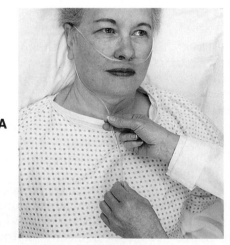
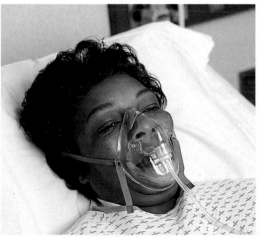

Figure 26-2 A, Nasal cannula. **B,** Simple face mask. (From Perry AG, Potter PA: *Clinical nursing skills and techniques,* ed 6, St Louis, 2006, Mosby.)

Understanding Upper Respiratory Tract Conditions

The upper respiratory tract consists of the nasal cavity, sinuses, pharynx, larynx, trachea, and mouth. The symptoms of the upper respiratory tract condition **rhinitis** are sneezing, **epistaxis,** runny nose, **dysphonia,** itching, and congestion. The congestion comes from dilation of nasal blood vessels and the resulting engorgement of these vessels. The symptoms may be related to allergies or may be nonallergic. Allergic rhinitis is caused by histamine release, whereas nonallergic rhinitis is often a symptom of the common cold.

Histamine is a chemical found in the body tissue that protects the body from factors in the environment that produce allergic and inflammatory reactions. The greatest concentration of histamine is in the skin, gastrointestinal tract, and lungs—organs most frequently exposed to environmental toxins and requiring protection from the associated damages. One class of histamines causes allergic reactions in the respiratory tract. Free histamines play a role in the inflammatory process and defend exposed tissue from injury by damaging agents. The principal action of histamine is vascular dilation and contraction of the smooth muscles of the bronchial tree and the gastrointestinal tract. For the person who is sensitized to histamine release in the respiratory tract, sneezing, increased nasal secretions, itching and watery eyes, and bronchoconstriction may result, and this may lead to dyspnea and airway obstruction.

Drugs Used for Nasal Congestion

Several classes of medications are used to treat rhinitis, among them antihistamines, decongestants, cromolyn, and intranasal glucocorticoids. All may be used to treat allergic rhinitis. Decongestants are used to treat the nonallergic rhinitis, **coryza,** or the common cold.

Antihistamines

Hypersecretion of nasal fluids due to allergies may require the use of **antihistamines** (if the secretions are related to allergies) to block the H_1 receptor sites. This action prevents the histamine from reaching the exposed tissue to cause edema, inflammation, and itching. The drugs are found in first-generation drugs such as diphenhydramine (Benadryl) and brompheniramine (Dimetane) that have been available for many years, and the newer second-generation drugs such as cetirizine (Zyrtec) and loratadine (Claritin) (Table 26-1).

- The first-generation antihistamines, or the earlier-developed antihistamines, are nonselective in their effects on peripheral and systemic histamine receptors, although these agents produce the same degree of therapeutic response to histamine. The main difference is in their degree of activity, which varies.
  - Chlorpheniramine (Chlor-Trimeton) may cause insomnia in the elderly.
  - In acute conditions, diphenhydramine (Benadryl) is still the medication of choice for allergies.
- The second-generation antihistamines, or the more recent products, are not as sedating or drying and seem to act more selectively on the peripheral histamine receptors. These agents are equal to or better in their antiallergic effects than the first-generation medications.
- Antihistamines have their greatest therapeutic effect on nasal allergic reactions.
- Antihistamines are not effective against histamines that are already attached to the receptor sites, so the antihistamine is most effective if taken before contact with the allergy-causing compounds. Therefore these medications are more likely to be effective at the beginning of the allergy season.
- Antihistamines fail to reduce the asthma that frequently accompanies the seasonal allergic responses such as hay fever.
- Antihistamines are **palliative;** they do not provide protection over a long period of time.
- Dozens of antihistamines are available for use, and tolerance to them can develop. Antihistamines may be used interchangeably to find the most effective agent to relieve the symptoms of allergies. The antihistamine must be matched to the patient. When choosing from among the available antihistamine products, factors such as potency, duration of action, and the incidence of side effects such as drowsiness must be evaluated. Often, several medications may be tried before finding the appropriate drug for the individual.
- Because histamine also causes motion sickness, antihistamines are used to relieve these symptoms, as well as vertigo, hay fever, allergic coughs, allergic rhinitis, and allergies to insect bites and contact dermatitis. Other over-the-counter (OTC) antihistamine medications are used to relieve nausea, vomiting, and motion sickness.

TABLE 26-1 *Antihistamines*

GENERIC NAME	TRADE NAME	USUAL ADULT DOSE, ROUTE, AND FREQUENCY OF ADMINISTRATION	INDICATIONS FOR USE	DRUG INTERACTIONS
FIRST-GENERATION DRUGS			Acute and chronic allergic reactions including allergic rhinitis, dermatitis, and hay fever	alcohol, anticholinergics, MAO inhibitors
azatadine*	Optimine	1-2 mg po bid		
brompheniramine[†]	Dimetane	Up to 40 mg/day po		
chlorpheniramine[†]	Chlor-Trimeton	2-4 mg po q4-6h		
clemastine*[†]	Tavist	1.34 mg po bid[†] 2.68 mg po bid*		
cyproheptadine*	Periactin	4-20 mg/day po		
dexchlorpheniramine*	Polaramine	2 mg po q4-6h		
dimenhydrinate[†]	Dramamine	50-100 mg po q4-6h		
diphenhydramine*[†]	Benadryl	25[†]-50*mg po q4-8h		
meclizine*[†]	Antivert,* Bonine	25-100 mg/day po or 12.5 mg q4-6h		
phenindamine	Nolahist	25 mg po q4-6h		
trimeprazine*	Temaril	2.5 mg po qid		
tripelennamine*	PBZ	25-50 mg po q4-6h		
triprolidine/ pseudoephedrine[†]	Actifed	tab i q4-8h		

MAJOR SIDE EFFECTS OF FIRST-GENERATION ANTIHISTAMINES: Drowsiness, sedation, dry mouth, hypotension, constipation, palpitations, anorexia, urine retention.

GENERIC NAME	TRADE NAME	DOSE	INDICATIONS	DRUG INTERACTIONS
SECOND-GENERATION DRUGS			Same	Same
cetirizine*[†]	Zyrtec	5-10 mg/day po		
fexofenadine*[†]	Allegra	60 mg po bid or 180 mg hs		
loratadine	Claritin	10 mg/day po		
desloratadine	Clarinex	5 mg/day po		
SECOND-GENERATION DRUGS WITH DECONGESTANT*			Same	Same
ceterizine/guaifenesin	Zyrtec D	5-10 mg/day po		
fexofenadine/ guaifenesin	Allegra D	tab i po bid		
loratadine/ guaifenesin	Claritin D	tab i po bid or qd, depending on release of medication		
NASAL SPRAY ANTIHISTAMINE				
azelastine	Astelin	2 sprays each nostril twice daily	Environmental irritants and seasonal allergic rhinitis	None indicated

MAJOR SIDE EFFECTS OF NASAL SPRAY ANTIHISTAMINE: Epistaxis, headache.

MAO, Monoamine oxidase.
* Prescription medication.
[†] Over-the-counter medication.

- These products are also used as sedatives because one of the major side effects is sedation. Many OTC drugs contain antihistamines as sleeping aids (e.g., Nytol).
- The oral absorption of these agents is good, and most have an onset of action time of 15 to 60 minutes.
- When antihistamines are given for the nasal secretions of a common cold, the resultant thickening of the bronchial secretions may cause airway obstruction, especially in patients with COPD.
- More antihistamines and antihistamine combinations with decongestants are being sold OTC rather than on a prescription-only basis, although the dosage may be reduced in OTC products.
- Care should be taken with patients who have glaucoma, ulcers, or urine retention because of the drying effects of antihistamines and the resultant build-up of pressure in the eye.
- **Extrapyramidal symptoms** such as tremors, dystonia, and Parkinson-like symptoms should be reported immediately.

Patient Education for Compliance

1. Care should be taken when using antihistamines and operating machinery because of the sedating effects of these medications. The patient should evaluate his or her state of alertness before operating machinery or driving a car.
2. Antihistamines are drying, and a frequent sip of water, a piece of hard candy, or chewing gum may temporarily relieve this side effect in the oral cavity.
3. When taking antihistamines for motion sickness, the dose should be taken approximately 30 minutes to 1 hour prior to travel departure.
4. Patients with benign prostatic hypertrophy or cardiovascular disease should not use antihistamines without the supervision of a physician.
5. Alcohol should not be used with antihistamines because of the synergistic effects.
6. When using medications for allergic rhinitis, allergens such as pollution and smoke should be avoided.
7. Because many cold and cough preparations contain antihistamines, the patient should not mix cold and cough preparations without professional advice. Self-medication of antihistamines may produce increased sedation.

IMPORTANT FACTS ABOUT ANTIHISTAMINES

- Allergic rhinitis, the most common of all allergic disorders, is treated with antihistamines, decongestants, and nasal preparations.
- Antihistamines are used to decrease the histamine secretions throughout the body and may cause dizziness, drowsiness, photosensitivity, and headaches.
- Antihistamines are used to relieve coughs and colds caused by allergies and to relieve motion sickness.
- Antihistamines relieve rhinorrhea, sneezing, and itching but do not relieve nasal or chest congestion.
- Sedation is a common side effect of first-generation antihistamines, but this has been reduced in second-generation agents.

Decongestants

Decongestants are used to relieve nasal congestion and are vasoconstricting agents that shrink the swollen mucous membranes of the nasal airway passage of the upper respiratory tract (Table 26-2).

- These agents come in both oral and nasal preparations.
- Most oral agents are adrenergic medications or medications that mimic the effects of the sympathetic nervous system.
- Warnings on the labels of OTC preparations instruct patients with hypertension, hyperthyroidism, diabetes mellitus, or ischemic heart disease to use this group of drugs with care. Decongestants may increase blood sugar levels in persons with diabetes mellitus.
- Decongestants and antihistamines are often combined, but care should be taken to keep the dosage within a safe range.
- Two agents, phenylephrine and pseudoephedrine, are considered safe as decongestants when used as the label indicates. Medications containing these agents cause vasoconstriction and shrinking of swollen membranes, with a resultant decrease in nasal drainage.
  - Phenylephrine is the most widely used of the decongestants. It is used topically by itself or as an active ingredient in combination with other preparations for oral and topical use.
  - Pseudoephedrine has a high incidence of central nervous system stimulation and is not as widely used as phenylephrine.

TABLE 26-2 *Decongestants*

GENERIC NAME	TRADE NAME	USUAL ADULT DOSE, ROUTE, AND FREQUENCY OF ADMINISTRATION	INDICATIONS FOR USE	DRUG INTERACTIONS
NASAL DECONGESTANTS			Nonallergic rhinitis, such as common cold	MAO inhibitors
ephedrine 0.5%	Vicks, Vatronel	2-3 gtt in nostril q8-12h		
epinephrine 0.1%	Asthma Haler Mist, Bronkaid Mist, Primatene Mist	1-2 inhalations q4-6h		
naphazoline 0.05%	Allerest	2 gtt or sprays in nostril q3h		
oxymetazoline 0.05%	Afrin 12 Hour, Dristan 12 Hour, Neo-Synephrine	2 sprays in nostril q12h 2-3 nasal sprays q12h		
phenylephrine 0.125%-1%	Neo-Synephrine, Sinex	several gtt in nostril q2-4h 1-2 nasal sprays q3-4h		
tetrahydrozoline 0.1%	Tyzine	2-4 gtt in nostril q3-4h		
xylometazoline 0.1%	Otrivin	2-3 gtt in nostril q8-10h 2-3 nasal sprays q8-10h		

MAJOR SIDE EFFECTS OF NASAL DECONGESTANTS: Elevated blood sugar, elevated blood pressure, cardiac dysrhythmias, nervousness, restlessness, dizziness, headaches, irritability.

ORAL DECONGESTANTS				
pseudoephedrine	Sudafed, Drixoral, Sudafed-SR	60 mg po q6-8h po 120 mg q12h (sustained release)		
COMBINATION DECONGESTANTS				
guaifenesin/ pseudoephedrine	Mucinex D	2 tabs q12h		
pseudoephedrine/ chlorpheramine	Sudafed Plus, Chlor-Trimeton	tab i po q12h 2-4 mg tid-bid		
pseudoephedrine (in combination with acetaminophen and dextromethorphan)	Allerest, Contac, many OTC combinations	tab i po q12h		
ZINC PREPARATIONS				
zirconium glucosamine (Note: Zicam is available in several different formulas and forms.)	Zicam Cold-Eeze	1 dose q4h as nasal spray or gel Nasal gel applied locally qid	Common cold	Usually none

Note: All of the drugs listed in this table are available OTC.
MAO, Monoamine oxidase; *OTC,* over the counter.

- When decongestants such as oxymetazoline (Afrin) and phenylephrine (Neo-Synephrine) are used topically in the nose, the action is rapid. With oral medications such as pseudoephedrine (Sudafed and Contac), the responses are delayed and prolonged.
- Persons taking ephedra as an herbal supplement should be extremely careful when using decongestants because of the synergistic action.
- Decongestants, topical and oral, are for short-term use, with **rebound congestion** occurring within just a few days of constant use. The patient may develop habituation with the use of these drugs when used on a regular basis for prolonged time.
  - With topical nasal agents, the possibility of rebound congestion becomes greater as the effect of the nasal spray wears off. To overcome this, patients tend to use larger doses of the medication more frequently. This cycle of escalating congestion followed by increased doses of medication will become progressively worse unless the patient stops using topical decongestants completely.
  - Discontinuation of the topical sprays often produces severe congestion for several days until the mucous membranes adjust to the lack of medication. Therefore topical decongestants are inappropriate for patients with chronic rhinitis symptoms.
  - Because of the danger of rebound congestion, the time limit of using topical decongestants on a regular basis should be 5 days.

IMPORTANT FACTS ABOUT DECONGESTANTS
- Decongestants should be used only on the advice of a physician for those patients with heart disease, glaucoma, and prostate cancer. Self-medication using OTC preparations should be avoided.
- Decongestants may cause tachycardia, nervousness, restlessness, insomnia, blurred vision, and nausea and vomiting.
- Overuse or continued use of nasal sprays causes rebound congestion, making the symptoms worse and bringing an inherent danger of increasing medications for relief.

IMPORTANT FACTS ABOUT DECONGESTANTS—
Cont'd
- Topical decongestants (e.g., nasal sprays) act rapidly and produce minimal systemic effects.
- Oral decongestants work slowly, producing central nervous system stimulation but no rebound congestion, and should be used for long-term therapy.

Cromolyn Sodium

Intranasal cromolyn sodium (Nasalcrom) relieves allergic rhinitis by preventing the release of histamine after the exposure to allergens (Table 26-3).

- Cromolyn provides no relief for nonallergic rhinitis but is more effective if used prior to the onset of the symptoms.
- It may take approximately a week for cromolyn to be effective, so this medication should be used throughout the allergy season. If nasal congestion is present, a topical decongestant may be used prior to the use of cromolyn.

Glucocorticoids

The nasal glucocorticoids such as fluticasone (Flonase) and triamcinolone (Nasacort) are the most effective medications for prolonged seasonal and perennial rhinitis. These agents suppress the symptoms of allergic rhinitis—congestion, **rhinorrhea,** sneezing, itching, and erythema.

- The glucocorticoids should be saved for times when conventional medications have not been effective. Different from the use of corticosteroids for other conditions, minimal systemic effects are seen with this topical nasal use.
- The use of these drugs should be limited to 1 month at a time (see Table 26-3).

IMPORTANT FACTS ABOUT CROMOLYN AND GLUCOCORTICOIDS
Of the intranasal steroids, only dexamethasone (Decadron) presents a significant risk for systemic toxicity.

Over-the-Counter Products for Upper Respiratory Conditions

Many forms of OTC medications are available for upper respiratory conditions, as shown in Tables 26-1 and 26-2. Some are combinations of

TABLE 26-3 *Miscellaneous Nasal Preparations*

GENERIC NAME	TRADE NAME	USUAL ADULT DOSE, ROUTE, AND FREQUENCY OF ADMINISTRATION	INDICATIONS FOR USE	DRUG INTERACTIONS
cromolyn sodium, intranasal	Nasalcrom, Intal	One nasal spray 3-6 × per day	Allergic rhinitis	Usually none
INTRANASAL GLUCOCORTICOIDS			Same	Same
beclomethasone	Beconase, Vancenase	1 puff in nostril bid-qid		
budesonide	Rhinocort	2 nasal puffs bid or 4 puffs qAM		
dexamethasone	Decadron, Turbinaire	2 nasal puffs bid-tid		
flunisolide	Nasalide	2 nasal puffs bid		
fluticasone	Flonase	2 nasal puffs qd		
triamcinolone	Nasacort	2-4 nasal puffs per day		
mometasone	Nasonex	One spray in nostril hs		
ciclesonide	Omnaris	2 sprays in each nostril qd		

MAJOR SIDE EFFECTS OF MISCELLANEOUS NASAL PREPARATIONS: Nasal stinging and burning; **ciclesonide:** epistaxis, headache.

Note: All of the drugs listed in this table are prescription drugs.

decongestants or antihistamines, with antitussives or analgesics. These products have many formulas and are among the most commonly purchased OTC medications. Many of these drugs have the same active ingredient as found with prescription items; however, the dosage has been reduced in many instances. Other newer OTC medications have zinc bases such as Cold-Eeze or homeopathic medications such as Airborne.

Combination Over-the-Counter Products

Combination OTC products should be carefully selected because these agents have multidrug formulas, with some containing drugs unnecessary for the specific condition. These OTC medications may contain two or more combinations of medicines such as a nasal decongestant, **antitussive,** antihistamine, caffeine, and analgesics.

- The decongestants, antitussives, and analgesics are used to relieve obvious cold symptoms, such as runny nose, cough, and fever, whereas antihistamines suppress the secretion of mucus by their anticholinergic action. Caffeine, a stimulant, may be added to counteract the sedation of the antihistamine.
- The most common need for combination preparations is the common cold, with symptoms of rhinorrhea, cough, sneezing, sore throat, headache, malaise, and aching. A cold is self-limiting because of its viral nature, but the symptoms should be addressed for patient comfort.
- Antipyretic-analgesic combinations should be avoided in most viral infections to prevent missing the diagnosis of a secondary bacterial infection that may be present.
- The disadvantages of the combination medications are the subtherapeutic levels found with some dosages and the excessive levels of other chemical agents. Because no single medication relieves all of the symptoms of a cold, the pharmaceutical industry has formulated various combination products to relieve the multiple symptoms.
- If the patient has only one symptom to relieve, then a single-entity preparation should be used. The allied health professional should encourage the patient to ask a physician or pharmacist for assistance in finding the proper medication.
- Under Food and Drug Administration regulations, a brand-name product may be reformulated and sold under the same name. Thus without being extremely careful to read the label of medications with each purchase, the patient may buy a product without the same products being in the combination as with previous purchases. The allied health professional

should be sure the patient is aware to read all labels of OTC medications before purchasing the agents to ensure the formula is the one needed or the medication contains the same ingredients.

- When several symptoms occur together, each symptom should be addressed separately. If an adverse reaction occurs when using combination medications, the offending medication may not be identified. For safety, if an analgesic-antipyretic is necessary, it should be selected and given separately.

Zinc-Based Over-the-Counter Products

In recent years, zinc-based products such as Cold-Eeze and Zicam have been used for symptoms of the common cold. Some products are available as zinc gluconate lozenges, which are not popular because of their unpleasant taste. Other items are available as zinc gluconate glycine (Zicam) as dose spoons, nasal sprays, swabs, and gels and tablets that melt in the mouth and may cause loss of smell and taste. Zinc-based chemicals are also found in combination with decongestants and antihistamines for relief of symptoms of the common cold (see Table 26-2).

Herbal Cold Prophylactic Products

Airborne is a unique blend of herbal extracts, vitamins, electrolytes, and amino acids for a boost to the immune system. It is to be used as a prophylaxis for the common cold. This product is available as an effervescent tablet and a lozenge.

INTERESTING FACTS
Airborne was created by a teacher who was constantly exposed to germs in the classroom.

Patient Education for Compliance

1. Nasal stinging and burning may occur with topical nasal products. Zinc-based sprays may cause anosmia.
2. The nasal applicators for topical decongestants (nose drops and nasal sprays) should be cleaned after each use.
3. The tip of a nasal spray should not touch the nasal mucosa, and the container of medication should not be shared with anyone.
4. Nasal drops should be administered in a lateral headlow position to allow the spread over the nasal mucosa.

Drugs Used for Coughs

U.S. citizens spend billions of dollars a year on OTC medications, with approximately one third being used for upper respiratory tract conditions such as colds, cough, allergies, and related symptoms. Table 26-4 compares the signs and symptoms of allergies, influenza, and the common cold.

Coughing is a reflex stimulated by the central nervous system, peripheral nervous system, and the respiratory muscles. A cough may be beneficial to remove foreign matter from the respiratory tract, clear airways, and remove excess secretions from the bronchial tree. Cough preparations are used to suppress the intensity and frequency of the cough while allowing the secretions to be eliminated.

- The **productive cough** from COPD should not be suppressed.
- The cough that deprives a person of sleep or causes discomfort due to upper respiratory tract infections (URI) should be treated.
- A nonproductive dry cough should be treated because it can be exhausting, painful, and detrimental to the circulatory system and the elasticity of the respiratory system.
- When coughing is prolonged or spastic, **hemoptysis** may occur.

Antitussives

The two major groups of antitussives are opioid and nonopioid. The opioid cough suppressants that contain hydrocodone require a prescription and are Schedule III medications. Codeine cough suppressants are Schedule V medications and may not require a prescription, depending on the laws of each state. Nonopioid antitussives may require a prescription; some are available OTC (Table 26-5).

Opioid Cough Suppressants

Codeine and hydrocodone are used because they elevate the cough threshold and suppress cough. Codeine and codeinelike products are the most effective cough suppressants for routine prescription use.

- Codeine decreases both the frequency and intensity of the cough.
- Given orally, the doses remain low ($\approx$ one tenth of that needed to relieve pain), so the chance

TABLE 26-4 *Differences Among Allergic Rhinitis, Colds, and Influenza*

SIGNS AND SYMPTOMS	ALLERGIC RHINITIS	COMMON COLD	INFLUENZA
Fever	No	Occasionally	Common with fever 102 °F-104 °F with sudden onset
Aching/pain	No	Very occasionally	May be severe
Sneezing	Yes	Yes	Infrequent
Itching	Yes	No	No
Cough	Occasionally	Usually	Yes
Occurrence	Seasonal	Anytime	Anytime
Headache	Maybe	Infrequent	Usually
Cause	Allergens	Viral	Viral

Modified from Salerno E: *Pharmacology for health professionals*, St Louis, 1999, Mosby.

TABLE 26-5 *Cough Suppressants*

GENERIC NAME (SCHEDULE)	TRADE NAME	USUAL ADULT DOSE, ROUTE, AND FREQUENCY OF ADMINISTRATION	INDICATIONS FOR USE	DRUG INTERACTIONS
OPIOIDS				
codeine*[†]	Various with codeine[‡]	10-20 mg po q4-6h	Suppression of dry, irritating coughs of upper respiratory diseases	See under *analgesics* in Chapter 16
hydrocodone*(III)	Hycodan, Atuss HD, Histussin	5-10 mg q4-6h		alcohol
with hydrocodone (III)	Tussionex	1-2 tsp po q12h		

MAJOR SIDE EFFECTS OF OPOIDS: Nausea, constipation, dizziness.

NONOPIOIDS			Cough suppression	MAO inhibitors
dextromethorphana[†]	Sucrets Cough	10-30 mg po q4-8h		
with guaifenesin	Robitussin DM, Romilar CF	10 mL q4-6h		
diphenhydramine[†]	Benadryl, Benylin, Nytol, Sominex	25 mg po q4-6h		Basically none
diphenhydramine/ guaifenesin	Benylin DM	10 mL q4-6h		
benzonatate*	Tessalon	100 mg cap po tid		Basically none

MAJOR SIDE EFFECTS OF NONOPOIDS: Nausea, mild dizziness, drowsiness; additionally dry mouth and constipation with diphenhydramine.

* Prescription medication.
[†] Over-the-counter (OTC) medication.
[‡] Codeine cough preparations are by prescription, although some preparations that are Schedule V drugs may be bought OTC, depending on the amount of codeine present and state regulations. Customer must sign for OTC medications to show proof of receipt.

BOX 26-1 COMMON OVER-THE-COUNTER PREPARATIONS CONTAINING DEXTROMETHORPHAN

Benylin Cough
Children's Nyquil
Cheracol D
Multisymptom Tylenol Cold
Naldecon-DX
Novahistine DMX
Nyquil Nighttime Cold Formula
Robitussin CF Liquid
Tylenol Cold Medication
Vicks Formula 44D and 44M

of physical dependence is low when taken as directed.

- Most cough mixtures are Schedule III, IV, or V medications. Some codeine preparations are Schedule V medications that may be bought OTC if the patient, in some states, signs a roster showing that he or she has received the medication.

Nonopioid Cough Suppressants

The nonopioid cough suppressants do not have the gastrointestinal side effects of the codeine preparations and are nonaddicting. Dextromethorphan and its combinations (Box 26-1) are found in OTC medications.

- Dextromethorphan is generally well absorbed and is the most effective of the nonopioid cough medicines while not suppressing respirations. Used in recommended doses, it is just as effective as codeine except for acute severe coughs. Dextromethorphan should not be taken with MAO inhibitors because of the chance of excitability, sedation, and severe hypertension.
- Diphenhydramine (Benadryl) is the active ingredient in many OTC preparations and in some prescription medications, with the antitussive dosage being 25 mg every 4 to 6 hours. The cough suppression comes with the sedation.
- Benzonatate (Tessalon) is related to tetracaine, a local anesthetic, and relieves coughing by peripherally anesthetizing the cough receptors. This medication comes in gelcaps that should be swallowed intact to prevent anesthesia in the mouth. This drug may affect the gag reflex but has no major systemic effects or interactions with other medications. The onset of action is about 15 to 20 minutes, with a duration of action of approximately 8 hours (see Table 26-5).

Patient Education for Compliance

1. If a cough produces significant amounts of sputum, care should be taken in using OTC cough medications because these medications suppress the coughing needed to expel sputum. All OTC labels should be read carefully prior to taking OTC drugs.
2. If a cough persists for more than 10 days, consult a health care provider. This precaution should also be taken if high fever or chest pain is present.
3. Antitussives should be taken only in specified dosages.
4. Avoid irritants such as smoking and dust to decrease throat irritation. This is important with throat conditions.
5. Chew gum, drink frequent sips of water, or suck on sugarless hard candy to diminish coughing. However, sugarless products may produce flatulence.

IMPORTANT FACTS ABOUT COUGH SUPPRESSANTS

- Coughing is necessary to clear secretions from the respiratory tract. Antitussives should be used when coughing is nonproductive, interrupts daily activities, or is excessive.
- Cough preparations containing codeine or codeinelike medications cause drowsiness and should be taken with care when operating machinery.
- Codeine and codeinelike preparations are the most effective cough suppressants. Only small doses are necessary for effective treatment. Many antitussives are Schedule III drugs. A few codeine combinations that are Schedule V drugs are available for OTC purchase in some states by signing an OTC narcotic register.
- Dextromethorphan is the most effective nonopioid cough suppressant available.

Understanding Lower Respiratory Tract Disorders

The lower respiratory tract consists of the bronchial tree and the lungs. These passageways must be kept patent for the flow of air, so smooth muscles regulate the size of the passage lumen and cartilage gives support to keep them open. When diseases occur in the lower respiratory tract, the exchange of oxygen and carbon dioxide cannot occur in the single-layered capillaries of the alveoli. These changes may cause serious alterations of the blood gases. Acute conditions may include pneumonia and acute asthmatic attacks. Chronic conditions such as COPD, emphysema, and chronic asthma may lead to bronchiectasis and atelectasis. Symptoms of lower respiratory diseases include dyspnea, wheezing, tenacious sputum, and chest congestion and discomfort. Treatment of these diseases includes maintenance of airways using bronchodilators, mucokinetic agents, and expectorants. Chronic conditions may be treated using corticosteroids to reduce the swelling of the bronchial tree and sympathomimetics to reduce the edema and to stimulate vasodilation and bronchodilation.

Drugs for Acute Conditions of the Lower Respiratory Tract

Mucokinetic Agents

Patients with chronic respiratory diseases have excessively thick, tenacious sputum that must be thinned for **expectoration** to promote the removal of secretions. Mucokinetic agents, or **mucolytics,** are drugs that react with mucus to make it more watery and thus make the cough more productive, making sputum easier to expectorate and preventing the retention of mucus. **Mucus** is the normal secretion from the mucous membranes of the respiratory tract, whereas **sputum** is an abnormal secretion originating in the lower respiratory tract. Sputum may contain pathologic microorganisms because thick mucus in the lower respiratory tract tends to remain longer and normal flora may become pathologic (Table 26-6).

- Hypertonic saline solution and acetylcysteine are used for their mucolytic actions.
- Hypertonic saline (1.8% sodium chloride) stimulates a cough by irritating the respiratory mucosa while attracting water to the secretions to assist with excretion.

 CLINICAL TIP

Hypertonic saline may be used for relief as a home remedy by using table salt and water as a gargle or as an inhalation through mists or in a room humidifier. If a humidifier is not available, table salt in boiling water for inhalation of vapor will assist with the removal of thick, tenacious mucus of respiratory diseases.

- Acetylcysteine (Mucomyst) is a prescription mucolytic that is used as an inhalation agent to make mucus less viscous for easier removal by coughing or suctioning. The drug itself has an unpleasant, musty odor.

Expectorants

Expectorants render coughs more productive by stimulating respiratory tract secretions, which decreases the viscosity of the mucus. These medications are available OTC and by prescription.

- The drug with greatest evidence of safety and effectiveness is guaifenesin.
- Expectorants are often added to other medications such as antihistamines, decongestants,

TABLE 26-6 *Mucolytics/Expectorants*

GENERIC NAME	TRADE NAME	USUAL ADULT DOSE, ROUTE, AND FREQUENCY OF ADMINISTRATION	INDICATIONS FOR USE	DRUG INTERACTIONS
acetylcysteine[†]	Mucomyst	3-5 mL of 20% solution; 6-10 mL of 10% solution, inhaled	Thin, viscous mucus	Usually none
guaifenesin*[†]	Hytuss,* Robitussin,[†] Dura-Tuss*	100-400 mg po q4-6h 600-1200 mg/day	Increase output of respiratory tract fluids	
	Mucinex*[†]	200-400 mg tabs po q4h		
dornase alfa*	Pulmozyme	2.5 mg/day inhaled	Expectorant for cystic fibrosis	

MAJOR SIDE EFFECTS: acetylcysteine: runny nose, throat irritation, nausea; **dornase alfa:** sore throat, laryngitis, fever, rhinitis.

* Prescription medication.
[†] Over-the-counter medication.

and antitussives to help remove mucus. Most of these have no significant contraindications.

- A specific expectorant for cystic fibrosis is dornase alfa (Pulmozyme). It digests extracellular DNA to improve pulmonary function and reduces the risk of respiratory infections. The drug works within 3 to 7 days of beginning the medication (see Table 26-6).

Drugs for Chronic Conditions of the Lower Respiratory Tract

COPD, an irreversible condition, is a common respiratory term for diseases such as emphysema, asthma, and chronic bronchitis. Cigarette smoking and toxic fumes lead to chronic irritation of the bronchial tree, causing increased and thickened pulmonary secretions that eventually lead to a gas exchange problem with a resultant chronic cough, susceptibility to infection, and difficulty in engaging in physical activity. Bronchodilators and mucolytic agents are used, along with breathing exercises and oxygen therapy, to assist in relieving the respiratory symptoms (palliative), but the damage to the lungs is irreversible.

Asthma is a condition caused by an antigen-antibody reaction that results in wheezing, shortness of breath, and a feeling of suffocation due to constriction of the bronchioles. This may be caused by many factors such as irritants (chemical and dust), exercise, infections of the respiratory tract, allergies, gastroesophageal reflux disease, and salicylates. The airway becomes inflamed with edema and mucous plugs, and hyperactivity of the bronchial tree adds to the symptoms. During asthmatic attacks, when bronchiole constriction and increased secretions are present, bronchodilators are used for relief. Antiinflammatory agents such as glucocorticoids and cromolyn are often used for symptomatic relief. Most medications for asthma are administered by inhalation. This method enhances more rapid therapeutic effects for the acute attack because the medication is delivered directly to the site where it is needed and the systemic effect is minimized.

Inhalation Medications for Chronic Pulmonary Diseases

Three devices for inhalation administration are metered dose inhalers, nebulizers, and dry powder inhalers, each of which provides a different form of medication.

- Medication administration with a **metered dose inhaler** (MDI) delivers a fine mist of medication that is usually accomplished with one or two puffs from a hand-held pressurized device. Medications delivered by this method include albuterol (Ventolin) and terbutaline (Brethaire). Approximately 10% of the medication administered by an MDI reaches the lungs. Eighty percent is swallowed in the mouth and pharynx and may cause **stomatitis** with long-term use. The patient must be taught to use this device correctly. Correct administration is difficult, but the use of a spacer will aid the patient in appropriate administration. (See Chapter 14 for proper administration of medications by inhalation.)
- **Dry powder inhalers** (DPIs) including albuterol (Ventolin) and tiotropium (Spiriva) deliver a given amount of medication in the form of dry powder into the lungs. DPIs are breath activated and easier to use than MDIs. Approximately 20% of the medicine given by a DPI reaches the lungs.
- A **nebulizer** uses a small machine that converts a solution into a mist, using such medications as epinephrine (Primatene) and isoetharine (Bronkometer). The mist droplets are inhaled either through a face mask or through a mouthpiece. The degree of effectiveness of a nebulizer depends on the size of the medication droplet as it reaches the body and the effectiveness of the patient's respiratory system.

Patient Education for Compliance

1. When the medication administered by MDI requires two puffs, a full minute should elapse between puffs.
2. Patients should gargle after the use of medications delivered by MDI and DPI to prevent throat irritation.

Epinephrine, Ephedra, and Beta-Adrenergic Drugs

The major drugs used to treat asthma and other congestive obstructions of the airways include sympathomimetic medications and xanthine derivatives (Table 26-7).

- The nonselective adrenergic medications such as epinephrine and ephedrine stimulate the cells of the body to produce vasoconstriction and the reduction of edema, whereas other medications stimulate vasodilation and bronchodilation.

TABLE 26-7 *Bronchodilators*

GENERIC NAME	TRADE NAME	USUAL ADULT DOSE, ROUTE, AND FREQUENCY OF ADMINISTRATION	INDICATIONS FOR USE	DRUG INTERACTIONS
epinephrine*†	Adrenalin,* Bronkaid,† Medihaler,† Primatene†	0.3 mg by injection 2.25% in nebulizer inhaled 10 gtts of 1% solution by inhalation q3-4h	Dilation of bronchial tree	Anesthetics, tricyclic depressants, beta-blockers, digitalis, cardiac glycosides, ergotamine and its derivatives
ephedrine†	Vicks Vatronol	25 mg po tid-qid		Same as above

MAJOR SIDE EFFECTS OF EPINEPHRINE AND EPHEDRINE: Increased heart rate, tachycardia, palpitations, muscle tremors, CNS stimulation, nervousness, anorexia, nervousness.

GENERIC NAME	TRADE NAME	USUAL ADULT DOSE, ROUTE, AND FREQUENCY OF ADMINISTRATION	INDICATIONS FOR USE	DRUG INTERACTIONS
BETA-ADRENERGIC AGENTS			Same	Same
formoterol	Foradil	1 cap inhaled (aerolizer)		
clenbuterol	Xopenex	0.63 mg-1.25 mg inhaled (nebulizer)		
isoproterenol*	Isuprel	5 mg po 3-4 × per day; 10 mg sublingual 4 × per day		β-blockers, amitriptyline
albuterol*	Proventil, Ventolin, Ventodisk	2-4 mg po tid-qid 2 puffs inhaled (MDI) q4-6h 1-2 caps inhaled (DPI) q4-6h 2.5 mg inhaled (nebulizer) tid-qid		Same as isoproterenol, plus MAO inhibitors
bitolterol*	Tornalate	2-3 puffs inhaled (MDI) q4-6h		None indicated
isoetharine†	Bronkometer	4 inhalations by nebulizer q4h		See isoproterenol
pirbuterol*	Maxair	2 puffs inhaled (MDI) q4-6h		None indicated
terbutaline*	Brethaire Brethine, Bricanyl	2-3 puffs inhaled (MDI) q4-6h 2.5 mg po tid 0.25 mg by injection SC		Albuterol
metaproterenol*	Alupent, Metaprel	2-3 inhalations q3-4h; 20 mg po tid-qid		Same as albuterol
salmeterol*	Serevent	2 inhalations (MDI) q12h		None indicated
eformoterol	Brovana	2 nebulizer doses/day	COPD, including bronchitis and emphysema	aminophylline, theophylline, diuretics

MAJOR SIDE EFFECTS OF BETA-ADRENERGIC AGENTS: Increased heart rate, tachycardia, palpitations, muscle tremors, CNS stimulation, nervousness, anorexia, nervousness **Additionally: formoterol:** tremors, muscle cramps, insomnia, headache; **eformoterol:** pain, headache, nervousness, hypokalemia.

GENERIC NAME	TRADE NAME	USUAL ADULT DOSE, ROUTE, AND FREQUENCY OF ADMINISTRATION	INDICATIONS FOR USE	DRUG INTERACTIONS
METHYLXANTHINES				Caffeine, cimetidine, fluoroquinolone, antibiotics, rifampin, phenobarbital, phenytoin
theophylline/ aminophylline*	Elixophyllin, Slo-Phyllin, Aminophylline	Varies by immediate and sustained-release factors		
oxtriphylline*	Choledyl	800-1200 mg/day in divided doses		

TABLE 26-7 *Bronchodilators—cont'd*

GENERIC NAME	TRADE NAME	USUAL ADULT DOSE, ROUTE, AND FREQUENCY OF ADMINISTRATION	INDICATIONS FOR USE	DRUG INTERACTIONS
dyphylline*	Dilor, Lufyllin	15 mg/kg po qid		
MAJOR SIDE EFFECTS OF METHYLXANTHINES: Nausea, anxiety, restlessness, gastric upset, GERD, headache, insomnia, tachycardia, nervousness.				
ANTICHOLINERGIC AGENTS			None	
ipratropium*	Atrovent	2-4 puffs inhaled (MDI) 4 × per day		
tiotropium	Spiriva	1 cap inhaled daily	same	Basically none
MAJOR SIDE EFFECTS OF ANTICHOLINERGICS: Dry mouth, plus sinusitis, UTI, dyspepsia, rhinitis with tiotropium.				
COMBINATION BRONCHODILATORS			Dilation of bronchial tree	None
fluticasone/ salmeterol	Advair disc	1 dose bid inhaled	Used in chronic asthma	
	Advair HFA aerosol	1 dose inhaled bid		
ipratropium/ albuterol*	Combivent	2-3 puffs inhaled (MDI) tid		
MAJOR SIDE EFFECTS OF COMBINATION BRONCHODILATORS: Dry mouth with fluticasone/salmeterol.				

CNS, Central nervous system; *COPD*, chronic obstructive pulmonary disease; *DPI*, dry powder inhaler; *GERD*, gastroesophageal reflux disease; *MDI*, metered dose inhaler; *UTI*, urinary tract infection.
* Prescription medication.
† Over-the-counter medication.

- Epinephrine (Adrenalin) and ephedrine are indicated in the treatment of bronchial asthma and bronchitis and to prevent bronchospasm.
- These drugs have a rapid onset of action with a duration of 1 to 3 hours when used by inhalation, or 1 to 4 hours when given parenterally.
- Ephedrine is not as potent as epinephrine but is useful when taken orally. It has a longer duration of action than epinephrine but also causes nervousness and stimulation of the heart and nervous system.
- β-Adrenergic (Beta-2) drugs such as isoproterenol (Isuprel) and albuterol work as both cardiac and respiratory agonists.
  - The main action is on the smooth muscle of the bronchial tree and on the heart. A typical medication is Isuprel, which can be taken orally and by injection.
  - β-2 receptor medications are the most effective medications to reduce acute and exercise-induced bronchospasms. The medications suppress histamine release in the lung, provide bronchodilation, and increase ciliary mobility to move mucus.
- Because β-2 agents are selective, these medications have replaced the older, less selective sympathomimetics such as epinephrine in treating asthma and other chronic pulmonary congestive conditions.
- β-2 agonists relieve ongoing asthmatic attacks, may be used prophylactically, and may be necessary for the relief of breakthrough symptoms.
- The short-acting agents begin to work almost immediately, peaking in 30 to 60 minutes and lasting for 3 to 5 hours. The long-lasting preparation (salmeterol) has a slow onset of action but persists for 12 hours. Salmeterol (Serevent) is preferred for prophylaxis but is not effective in aborting an attack because of the slowness of its action.
- Inhaled preparations have fewer side effects than systemic medications.
- All of these drugs may be administered by inhalation and may also be given orally or by injection if needed.

TABLE 26-8 *Glucocorticoids Used in Treating Asthma*

GENERIC NAME	TRADE NAME	USUAL ADULT DOSE, ROUTE, AND FREQUENCY OF ADMINISTRATION	INDICATIONS FOR USE	DRUG INTERACTIONS
beclomethasone	Beclovent, Vanceril	2 puffs (MDI) qid	Chronic or acute asthma attacks	See Chapter 21
budesonide	Pulmicort	1-4 puffs bid-qid (MDI)	Same	Same
	Pulmicort Respules	Inhaled bid	For ages 12 and younger	
dextromethasone	Decadron Respihaler	3 puffs (MDI) tid-qid		
flunisolide	AeroBid, Nasalide	2-4 puffs (MDI) bid		
fluticasone	Flovent	2-4 puffs (MDI) bid		
triamcinolone	Azmacort	2 puffs tid-qid		
prednisone	Deltasone	5-60 mg/day po		
prednisolone	Prelone	5-60 mg/day po		

MAJOR SIDE EFFECTS: beclomethasone and budesonide: oropharyngeal candidiasis; See Chapter 21 for systemic side effects.

Note: All of the drugs listed in this table are prescription medications.
MDI, Metered dose inhaler.

Xanthine Derivatives

Xanthine derivatives relax the smooth muscles of the bronchial tree and stimulate cardiac muscle and the central nervous system. They include theophylline/aminophylline (Slo-Phyllin and Elixophyllin).

- These medications are used for the prevention and treatment of bronchial asthma and for the treatment of emphysema, COPD, and bronchitis.
- Some states do not allow generic substitutions of these products. The release time for action varies between generic and trade name drugs because the base and filler have different times of release.
- Patients with heart failure, heart disease, hypothyroidism, convulsive disorders, and acute pulmonary edema cannot use these derivatives.
- Theophylline, the basic active ingredient of xanthines, is orally available in standard or sustained-release formulas with forms that are effective for up to 24 hours.
- Because theophylline has a narrow therapeutic range and because the β-2 agonists are safer and more effective, the xanthines are not used as frequently today (see Table 26-7).

Anticholinergic Medications

Anticholinergic (atropine-like) medications may be used for asthma by drying the mucous membranes and are used with patients who cannot use other bronchodilators.

- With asthma, anticholinergic medications offer some relief of the symptoms of asthma.
- Ipratropium (Atrovent) is used in patients with chronic asthma and has a rapid onset of action (30 seconds) and reaches maximum effect in 3 minutes, lasting for 6 hours (see Table 26-7).

Glucocorticoids

Glucocorticoids are effective as antiasthma medications and are usually administered by inhalation, but may be given orally or by injection (Table 26-8).

- When used for a short period of time with acute asthma or other acute pulmonary diseases, the adverse reactions of glucocorticoids are minor. However, long-term systemic use has severe adverse effects (see Chapter 21).
- When used with asthma, these medications suppress inflammation and reduce the hypersecretions of the bronchial tree.
- The prophylactic administration in chronic asthma is preferably given by inhalation to prevent systemic side effects, whereas oral use is effective in the treatment of severe asthma.
- The inhaled doses are given on a daily basis, at a lower dose, and not as needed because of the slowness in developing the needed therapeutic effects.
- Inhaled glucocorticoids are safe and highly effective.
- The inhaled glucocorticoids are dispensed by MDI and DPI. The most frequently used

TABLE 26-9 *Asthmatic Prophylactics*

GENERIC NAME	TRADE NAME	USUAL ADULT DOSE, ROUTE, AND FREQUENCY OF ADMINISTRATION	INDICATIONS FOR USE	DRUG INTERACTIONS
cromolyn	Aarane, Crolom, Intal, Nasalcrom	30 mg qid topically 2-4 puffs 4 × per day DPI, MDI, nasal spray, nebulizer	Prophylaxis in chronic asthma	None
nedocromil	Tilade	2 puffs (MDI) qid		

MAJOR SIDE EFFECTS: cromolyn: wheezing and coughing.

LEUKOTRIENE ANTAGONISTS

zafirlukast	Accolate	20 mg po bid		aspirin, warfarin, glucocorticoids, phenytoin, cyclosporine, astemizole, theophylline
zileuton	Zyflo	600 mg po qid		theophylline, warfarin, propranolol
montelukast	Singulair	5-10 mg po qd in PM		None

MAJOR SIDE EFFECTS OF LEUKOTRIENE ANTAGONISTS: zileuton: liver toxicity, dyspepsia; **montelukast:** headaches, GI symptoms.

Note: All of the drugs listed in this table are prescription medications.
GI, Gastrointestinal; *MDI,* metered dose inhaler.

oral glucocorticoids are prednisone and prednisolone on alternate days for long-term therapy.

Patient Education for Compliance

Patients using inhaled glucocorticoids should rinse their mouths after inhaling medications to prevent the possibility of oral candidiasis.

Other Medications for Asthma

Cromolyn (Intal and Nasalcrom) and nedocromil (Tilade) are used to prevent asthma attacks but are not useful for an ongoing attack (Table 26-9).

- Cromolyn suppresses inflammation but does not dilate the bronchial tree (see earlier discussion on antihistamines). It inhibits the release of histamines, so it acts as an antiallergenic. Cromolyn is the drug of choice as a prophylactic for moderate allergic asthma, especially in children, because of its safety and efficacy. It has no therapeutic effect on an acute asthma attack. It is also used to reduce the symptoms of seasonal allergic attacks. The most common side effects are wheezing and coughing on administration.

- Nedocromil is also antiinflammatory and antiallergic but has an unpleasant taste.
- Leukotrienes contribute to the inflammation associated with asthma. Leukotriene antagonists block the bronchoconstriction, mucous production, and inflammation that occur with asthma.
  - Zafirlukast (Accolate), an oral medication, was the first medication in this new antiinflammatory class. It is used as maintenance therapy for patients with chronic asthma. It has few side effects but has multiple drug interactions.
  - Zileuton (Zyflo), a medication for oral administration, is rapidly absorbed, but its place in asthma therapy is not completely understood, although it is used for prophylaxis and treatment of chronic asthma in persons older than 12 years.
  - Montelukast (Singulair) acts as a bronchodilator, respiratory stimulant, and leukotriene receptor antagonist. This medication should be given at night for maximum effectiveness. The agent cannot be used with acute asthma attacks but must be used prophylactically. If the patient needs to use short-acting bronchodilators more frequently while on montelukast, the physician should be notified.

Patient Education for Compliance

1. Cromolyn is for the prophylaxis of asthma and should be administered 30 minutes before exercise.
2. β-2 agonists taken for long-term therapy should be taken on a regular schedule and not only as needed.
3. Alternate-day dosing such as with glucocorticoids for asthma is appropriately achieved by taking one dose every other day at the same hour.
4. If symptoms of asthma become worse, the patient should not change doses or self-medicate without a physician's direction to do so.
5. A patient with thick secretions from the lung should drink six to eight glasses of water per day to decrease the viscosity of the bronchial secretions.
6. OTC and prescription medications for respiratory disorders should not be mixed because of the chance of multiple doses of similar drugs, especially sympathomimetic drugs.
7. Smoking should be avoided because this worsens breathing problems and affects the dosage of medications.
8. Colas, coffee, chocolate, and charbroiled foods should be avoided when taking xanthine preparations such as theophylline and its derivatives.

IMPORTANT FACTS ABOUT MEDICATIONS FOR ASTHMA

- Many of the β-2 agonists are inhaled forms and are delivered by MDI, DPI, or nebulizers. These medications rarely cause systemic side effects.
- Asthma and COPD are chronic inflammatory diseases that cause inflammation of the airways, hyperactivity of bronchial secretions, and bronchospasm. Allergy may be the underlying cause of asthma.
- COPD and asthma are treated with antiinflammatory agents and bronchodilators with many available as MDIs, DPIs, and nebulizers. The correct use of these devices is tricky, and patient education on their use is essential.

IMPORTANT FACTS ABOUT MEDICATIONS FOR ASTHMA—Cont'd

- Inhaled β-2 antagonists are the most effective medications to relieve acute bronchospasm and for exercise-induced acute bronchospasm attacks.
- Inhaled salmeterol has a delayed onset and extended duration of action. It is used to prevent COPD and asthma.
- Glucocorticoids are for preventive therapy in respiratory tract illnesses and should be used on a regular short-term schedule when indicated because they suppress the inflammation of asthma.
- Inhaled glucocorticoids are relatively safe, with oropharyngeal candidiasis and dysphoria being the major side effects. Using a spacer device during administration of inhaled medications and gargling after use may reduce these undesirable effects.
- Cromolyn is an inhaled antiinflammatory medication used for the prophylaxis of respiratory conditions.
- Theophylline relieves COPD and asthma by bronchodilation, but the xanthines have been replaced by newer drugs with fewer side effects.

Medications for Inhibition of Influenza

Some of the newer medications on the market are those that are used to lessen or inhibit the signs and symptoms of influenza. These products are not substitutes for the influenza vaccine administered to prevent or attenuate symptoms of the disease. Rather, they are for patients who, for medical or personal reasons, desire prophylaxis against the disease following exposure to the virus. These medications are relatively expensive and are not widely used (Table 26-10).

- Rimantadine (Flumadine), a tablet, is used in the prophylaxis and treatment of influenza A viral infections.
- Oseltamivir (Tamiflu) is indicated for the treatment of uncomplicated influenza infections

TABLE 26-10 *Drugs Used For Inhibition Of Influenza Virus*

GENERIC NAME	TRADE NAME	USUAL ADULT DOSE, ROUTE, AND FREQUENCY OF ADMINISTRATION	INDICATIONS FOR USE	DRUG INTERACTIONS
rimantadine	Flumadine	100 mg po bid	Prophylaxis of influenza	acetaminophen, aspirin, cimetidine
oseltamivir	Tamiflu	75 mg po bid × 5 days		None
zanamivir	Relenza	1 inhalation (5 mg) bid		

MAJOR SIDE EFFECTS: rimantadine: nausea, insomnia, dizziness, nervousness, anorexia, dry mouth; **oseltamivir:** nausea, vomiting, insomnia, vertigo, bronchitis; **zanamivir:** headache, dizziness, nausea, vomiting, diarrhea.

Note: All of the drugs listed in this table are prescription medications.

with symptoms for less than 2 days. This medication may be taken without regard to food.

- Zanamivir (Relenza) is another medication for the inhibition of the influenza virus. To use this drug, patients should not have had symptoms for more than 2 days. This medication is administered by oral inhalation into the respiratory tract using a Diskhaler device. The 5-mg blister pack is inhaled twice a day approximately 12 hours apart. Inhaled bronchodilators should be used to open the airways prior to using zanamivir. Safety in patients with COPD has not been established, and a question has arisen concerning safety in coronary patients.

Patient Education for Compliance

The new antiviral influenza medications must be used within 2 days of the onset of symptoms to be effective.

Summary

The respiratory tract is necessary for the inspiration of oxygen and the expiration of carbon dioxide. Through external respiration, or the exchange of oxygen and carbon dioxide in the lungs and respiratory tract, and internal respiration, or the exchange of gases at the cellular level in body tissues, oxygen is supplied to the body. The effectiveness of the respiratory system affects the body's ability to function in homeostasis.

Oxygen is essential to sustain life. Allied health professionals should expect to help patients with oxygen therapy and must be able to explain why a low dose of oxygen is most appropriate for COPD. The need for safety around flames should be explained during patient teaching.

Antihistamines are used to relieve allergic reactions throughout the body, and are also used frequently in individuals with respiratory tract disorders to relieve rhinorrhea and allergic bronchitis. The allied health professional must know the symptoms of allergic conditions versus the common cold versus influenza to be sure that an antihistamine is the correct medication. If the congestion is from colds, a decongestant is more appropriate, to relieve the thickened mucus.

Cough-suppressing preparations are indicated for dry, nonproductive coughs that interrupt daily activities. If the cough is productive, suppression is not appropriate and an expectorant may be administered to help expel the secretions. For thick phlegm or sputum, mucolytics may be prescribed to decrease the viscosity of the secretions for easier removal. Because many of these preparations are available OTC, the allied health professional should have a working knowledge of the indications for each.

Because topical nasal preparations are readily available, the allied health professional should explain the dangers of rebound congestion to all patients using these preparations. The patient should be made aware that nasal decongestants are for short-term therapy, usually no longer than a week. Cromolyn may be used prophylactically for asthma over a long period of time.

Bronchodilators induce smooth muscle relaxation, which eases breathing. These drugs are used to treat asthma, COPD, and chronic bronchitis. Some agents such as epinephrine and β-2 agonists are used in acute respiratory attacks. Others are for long-term therapy such as leukotriene agonists; albuterol, used for exercise-induced asthma; and cromolyn. Glucocorticoids are administered by inhalation and achieve local effects throughout the respiratory tract. They are relatively safe to use short term for the relief of bronchoconstriction and to liquefy thick mucous secretions.

COPD and asthma should be treated on an individualized basis, as should allergic conditions. In treating these conditions, especially with antihistamines, drug tolerance occurs and medications may need changing on a regular basis. For the person with seasonal allergies, prophylaxis by avoiding allergens is indicated; for the chronic allergic reaction, cromolyn may be indicated for long-term prophylaxis.

A group of medications to prevent or reduce the symptoms of influenza are available taken orally and as nasal preparations. Because of the expense of these medications, these drugs are not used routinely. The best prophylaxis for influenza remains the annual immunization with influenza vaccine.

Critical Thinking Exercises

SCENARIO

Smokey has COPD, and his breathing has become progressively more difficult. His physician has prescribed sympathomimetic bronchodilators for his condition. Smokey wants to know how these will help his condition when he is administering the medications by breathing them through the mouth rather than taking a tablet.

1. How would you explain the actions, safety, and prolonged use of the medicines to Smokey?
2. He also tells you that the prescribed low dose of oxygen does not seem to help him at all, and he wants to increase the flow to 6 L/minute, rather than the prescribed 2 L/minute as ordered. How would you explain the dangers of this change?
3. What questions should the allied health professional ask about bronchial secretions and the ability to expel these secretions?

▌ DRUG CALCULATIONS

1. Order: guaifenesin ER 600 mg q12h
   Available medication:

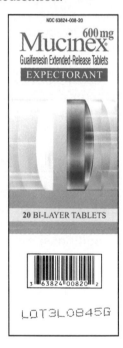

   NDC 63824-008-20
   Mucinex® 600 mg
   Guaifenesin Extended-Release Tablets
   EXPECTORANT
   20 BI-LAYER TABLETS
   3 63824 00820 2
   LOT3L0845G

   Dose to be administered: _____

   _____

2. Order: diphenhydramine 60 mg
   Available medication:

   N 0071-2220-17
   ELIXIR
   Benadryl ®
   (Diphenhydramine Hydrochloride Elixir, USP)

   Caution—Federal law prohibits dispensing without prescription.

   4 FLUIDOUNCES

   PARKE-DAVIS
   Div of Warner-Lambert Co
   Morris Plains, NJ 07950 USA

   Elixir P-D 2220 for prescription dispensing only.
   Contains—12.5 mg diphenhydramine hydrochloride in each 5 mL. Alcohol, 14%.
   Dose—Adults, 2 to 4 teaspoonfuls; children over 20 lb, 1 to 2 teaspoonfuls; three or four times daily.
   See package insert.
   Keep this and all drugs out of the reach of children.
   Store below 30°C (86°F). Protect from freezing and light.

   Exp date and lot

   2220G102

   Dose to be administered. _____

   _____

   What amount of medication would be administered in household utensils? _____

REVIEW QUESTIONS

1.   Why do we use antihistamines? Decongestants? _____
_____
_____

2.   What is the indication for topical nasal glucocorticoids? What is the safety factor in using these medications? _____
_____

3.   When would you expect the physician to order a cough suppressant? A mucolytic? An expectorant?_____
_____
_____

4.   What is the common medication found in nonopioid cough suppressants? What are the expected side effects? _____
_____

5.   What do bronchodilators do? _____
_____

6.   What are the three inhalation devices used to deliver medications as topical bronchodilators? How does each one work? _____
_____

7.   Glucocorticoids are generally discouraged for long-term oral therapy. Why are the topical agents for asthma considered reasonably safe for long-term use? _____
_____

8.   What medications are available for the prophylaxis of influenza? _____
_____
_____

9.   Why must the prophylactic agents for asthma be taken on a regular basis rather than prn?_____
_____
_____

CHAPTER 27

Circulatory System Disorders

OBJECTIVES

After studying this chapter, you should be capable of doing the following:

- Discussing how medications are used for circulatory diseases and the need for patient compliance through education.
- Describing the use of medications to relieve stable (exertional) angina and variant (vasospastic) angina.
- Explaining how cardiotonics are used in coronary disease.
- Explaining how medications are used to maintain regular and adequate cardiac rhythm.
- Explaining the objectives of antihypertensive therapy, the medications used, and how they may be individualized for patient compliance.
- Describing the prevention of atherosclerotic heart disease through the use of hypolipidemics and peripheral vasodilators.
- Discussing the role of anticoagulants and their antagonists, thrombolytics, and antiplatelet agents in heart disease.
- Describing the use of hematopoietics and erythropoietics as a means of building blood components.

Ms. Ellory, age 67, has a history of angina pectoris for which Dr. Merry has prescribed nitroglycerin patches. Ms. Ellory knows she should change the patch daily, leaving it off for several hours during the day.

What else does Ms. Ellory need to know about the placement of the patches?
What does she need to know about the administration of the nitroglycerin tablets that Dr. Merry has also prescribed?
How long can these sublingual tablets be considered effective for use after the container has been opened?
Should Ms. Ellory carry this medication with her at all times? Why or why not?
Can she put some of the tablets in another clear medicine bottle with other medications? Why or why not?

KEY TERMS

Angina pectoris	Hemostasis	Peripheral vascular resistance
Aggregation	High-density lipoprotein (HDL)	Point of maximum impulse (PMI)
Arrhythmia	Hypertension	Thromboembolism
Arteriosclerosis	Inotropic effect	Thrombus
Atherosclerosis	Intermittent claudication	Triglycerides
Automaticity	Ischemia	Vasoconstrictors
Chronotropic effect	Low-density lipoprotein (LDL)	Vasodilators
Digitalization	Myocardial infarction (MI)	Very low density lipoprotein
Dromotropic effect	Necrosis	(VLDL)
Ectopic beats	Orthostatic hypotension	
Embolus	Paresthesia	

EASY WORKING KNOWLEDGE OF INDICATIONS AND SIDE EFFECTS

Common Symptoms of Circulatory Disorders

Chest pain
Dyspnea/tachypnea
Fatigue and weakness
Palpitations/tachycardia
Bradycardia
Pallor, cyanosis
Edema
Syncope
Unusual sweating
Nausea, vomiting, anorexia
Headache
Anxiety

Common Side Effects of Circulatory Medications

Orthostatic hypotension
Urinary frequency
Headaches, dizziness, lightheadedness
Anorexia
Nausea, diarrhea, or constipation
Fatigue and weakness
Bradycardia

Easy Working Knowledge of Drugs Used to Treat Circulatory Disorders

DRUG CLASS	PRESCRIPTION	OTC	PREGNANCY CATEGORY	MAJOR INDICATIONS
Antianginal agents	Yes	No	B, C, X (amyl nitrate)	Relieve angina pectoris
Cardiac glycosides	Yes	No	C	Relieve congestive heart failure
Antiarrhythmic agents	Yes	No	B, C, D	Treat dysrhythmias and disorders of cardiac rhythm
Diuretics	Yes	Yes (caffeine, etc.)	B, C	Treat edema of congestive heart failure and hypertension
Antihypertensives	Yes	No	B, C, D (ACE inhibitors)	Hypertension
Peripheral vasodilators	Yes	No	C (cilostazol)	Peripheral vascular disease due to atherosclerosis or hyperlipidemia
Hypolipidemics	Yes	No	B, C, X (statins)	Elevated serum lipoproteins
Anticoagulants	Yes	No	B, C, X (oral anticoagulants)	Prevent venous thrombi
Thrombolytics	Yes	No	B, C	Dissolve thrombi
Antiplatelet medications	Yes	Yes	C, D (aspirin in the third trimester)	Prevents aggregation of platelets and prevents arterial thrombi
Topical hemostatics	Yes	No		Topical hemostasis
Hematopoietics/ erythropoietics	Yes	No	C	Increase the production of blood cells

According to statistics from the American Heart Association, cardiovascular disease is the leading cause of death in the United States, with one out of every five deaths directly related to this disease. More than 60 million Americans, both men and women, have some type of heart condition. Major advances have been made in the knowledge and treatment of heart disease, and with this knowledge have come major changes in the pharmacologic treatment of heart conditions.

Function of the Circulatory System

The circulatory system is composed of the heart and the blood vessels with any part having the potential to be affected by disease. The circulatory system has two primary functions: (1) the delivery of oxygen, nutrients, hormones, and other essential body substances to cells throughout the body and (2) the removal of waste products from cells. The pulmonary circulation is responsible for the exchange of oxygen and carbon dioxide by carrying blood to the lungs to receive inhaled oxygen and removing carbon dioxide by exhalation. The coronary circulation promotes the nutrition and health of heart muscle itself. The systemic circulation delivers the blood and its components to all tissues except the lungs and the myocardium.

A strong muscle about the size of a fist, the heart is in the thorax between the lungs. The two thin-walled atria are essentially receiving and holding chambers for blood before it enters the two thick-walled ventricles to be pumped to the lungs or body. The pumping of the heart forces the blood from the heart into either the pulmonary or systemic circulation. The pulse of the heart can be felt beating at the **point of maximum impulse (PMI)**. This landmark is used to take an apical pulse before cardiac medications are administered (Figure 27-1).

The myocardium, the main layer of the cardiac muscle, is supplied with nutrients by the coronary arteries that branch off the aorta just as it leaves the heart (Figure 27-2). The flow of blood through the coronary arteries systemically depends on the force of the heart contractions. When myocardial function is decreased, the ability of the heart to contract is also decreased. Drugs that work on the force of the contraction of the heart, an action referred to as **inotropic effect,** are the cardiac glycosides.

How Drugs Affect the Cardiac Electrical Conduction System

The electrical conduction system in the heart consists of various specialized tissues. The heart sets its own rhythm at the sinoatrial node, the pacemaker of the heart, found on the posterior wall of the left atrium near the entrance of the vena cava. The atrioventricular node, on the floor of the left atrium near the interarterial septum, continues the impulses to the bundle of His, or atrioventricular bundle. From this point the conduction spreads to the left and right sides of the heart through the bundle branches to the Purkinje fibers, or conduction myofibers. The contraction of the heart depends on this electrical conduction system (Figure 27-3). The conduction of the regularly spaced electrical impulses through the cardiac

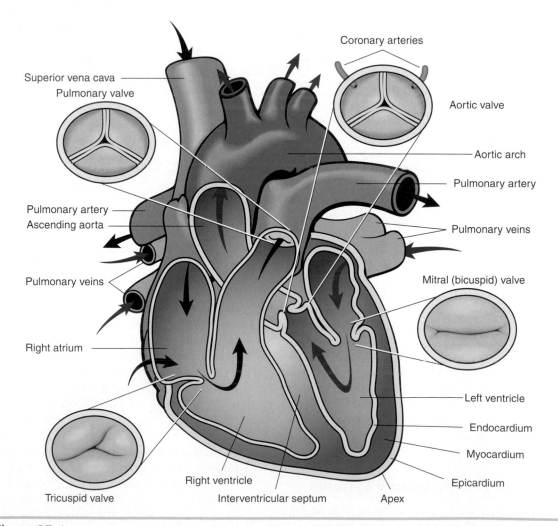

Figure 27-1 Internal view of the heart. (From Damjanov I: *Pathology for the health professions,* ed 3, St Louis, 2006, Saunders.)

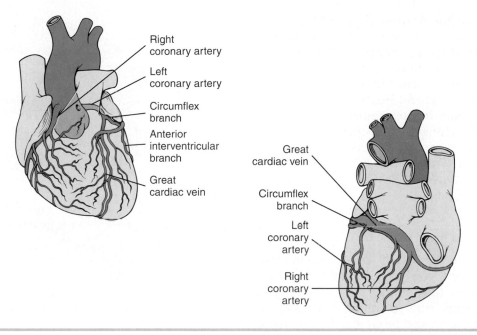

Figure 27-2 Coronary arteries that are affected by vasodilators such as nitroglycerin. (From Frazier MS, Drzymkowski JW: *Essentials of human diseases and conditions*, ed 4, St Louis, 2008, Saunders.)

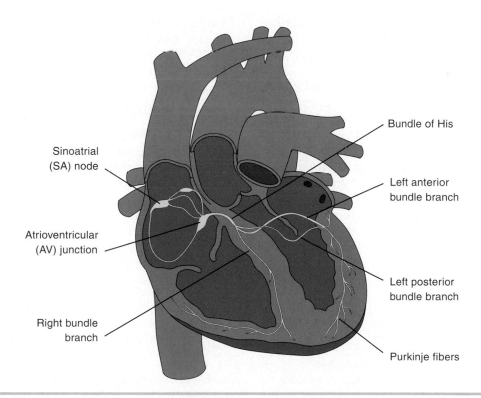

Figure 27-3 Conduction system of the heart affected by antiarrhythmic agents. (From Young AP, Proctor DB: *Kinn's the medical assistant: an applied learning approach*, ed 10, St Louis, 2008, Saunders.)

muscle produces the normal rhythm. When the heart does not beat in a regular rhythm, antidysrhythmics, or **dromotropic drugs,** may be ordered. If the heart rate is too fast or too slow, medications may be prescribed to either increase or decrease the rate, or to convert the heart to normal sinus rhythm using **chronotropic medications.** The calcium channel blockers and antianginal medications act on the coronary arteries to lessen the work of the heart. Table 27-1 summarizes the effects of different types of cardiac medications on heart action.

Diseases of the Heart and Its Vessels

Coronary artery disease (CAD) occurs when insufficient blood flows through the coronary arteries. **Arteriosclerosis** is hardening and narrowing of the arteries, mainly due to aging. It causes decreased blood flow to the heart itself. Narrowing of the arteries may also occur when plaque from fatty deposits develops in the arteries, or **atherosclerosis.** Atherosclerosis differs from arteriosclerosis because atherosclerosis contains deposits of fat (Figure 27-4).

Angina pectoris is spasms of the cardiac muscle as a result of **ischemia** to the myocardium. Drugs to dilate blood vessels, or vasodilators, are used for angina.

A **myocardial infarction** (MI), or heart attack, occurs when an area of the heart is deprived of blood supply and the result is cell **necrosis** of the myocardium because the damaged cells of the myocardium will not regenerate. Following an MI, the contractility of the myocardium is permanently reduced and, depending on the site of the infarct, the conduction system may also be affected. Medications are directed toward establishing sufficient myocardial action for adequate contractility of the heart to produce sufficient force to pump blood through the body.

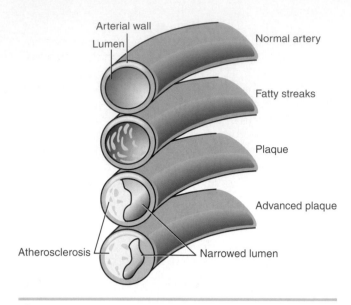

Figure 27-4 Atherosclerosis and narrowing of the lumen of an artery.

Drugs That Directly Affect the Heart

Vasodilators are used to relax or dilate vessels throughout the body. Some work on either veins or arteries; others work on both. Peripheral vasodilators are discussed later in this chapter. This section discusses coronary vasodilators for angina pectoris.

Drugs for Angina Pectoris

Angina is the temporary interference of blood, oxygen, or nutrients to the heart resulting in coronary ischemia. Drug therapy is based on relaxation of the coronary smooth muscle in an effort to bring about vasodilation and therefore improve blood flow to the heart. Coronary vasodilators are primarily nitrates that produce only temporary relief.

Stable, or *exertional, angina* is often triggered by physical activity or stress and is related

TABLE 27-1 *How Cardiac Medications Affect Heart Action*

DRUG GROUP	HEART TISSUE	PHARMACOLOGIC ACTION
A—Cardiac glycosides	Myocardium	Positive inotropic (increases force of myocardial contraction)
B—Antidysrhythmics	Cardiac conduction	Positive/negative dromotropic (increases/decreases the conduction of electrical impulses through the heart muscle)
		Positive/negative chronotropic (increases/decreases heart rate to convert to normal sinus rhythm)
C—Calcium channel blockers	Coronary arteries	Vasodilation of coronary arteries
Antianginal medications	Same	Lessens the work of the heart

to arteriosclerosis. The goal of therapy for stable angina is to reduce the intensity and frequency of anginal attacks by decreasing cardiac oxygen demand. Three types of medications are used for treating stable angina: nitrates, β-blockers, and calcium channel blockers. These drugs only relieve symptoms; they do not affect the underlying diseases.

Variant, or *vasospastic, angina* is caused by coronary artery spasms that restrict the blood flow to the myocardium. The goal of treatment of vasospastic angina is to reduce the number and severity of attacks by increasing cardiac oxygen. Calcium channel blockers and nitrates are used to dilate the vessels of the heart.

The third type of angina is *unstable angina.* This medical emergency is treated in a hospital situation and only rarely in an ambulatory care setting.

Nitrates

Nitrates, the oldest and most frequently used antianginal medications, are not true coronary artery dilators, as previously thought, because the arteries are already dilated by arteriosclerotic vascular disease. The nitrates dilate systemic vessels to reduce cardiac work and oxygen consumption. The nitrates relax vascular smooth muscle as the drug is converted into nitric oxide. A decrease in venous return to the heart causes a decrease in blood pressure. These actions reduce the workload of the heart. Nitrates are used during attacks of angina to relieve intense pain and are used prophylactically to prevent attacks. The most common route of administration is sublingual, with almost immediate onset of action (within minutes) but with a short duration of action (< 30 minutes) (Table 27-2).

- *Nitroglycerin* (NTG) is the most widely used drug among the nitrates. It is effective, fast acting, and inexpensive, acting directly on vascular smooth muscle to dilate blood vessels. Nitrate preparations decrease cardiac oxygen demand in stable angina, whereas in variant angina they relax the spasms and increase oxygen supply. The initial use produces a severe headache that can be relieved with mild analgesics such as acetaminophen. Patients on high doses of nitroglycerin or those who have continuous therapy over a length of time may develop a tolerance. To prevent the tolerance, the lowest effective doses of daily nitroglycerin preparations should be given and long-acting formulas should be used on an intermittent basis, allowing the patient to be drug free at some time during the day (usually at night). Any acquired tolerance is reversible when the nitrates are withheld for short periods of time.
- Nitroglycerin preparations are available for administration in a variety of routes producing

TABLE 27-2 *Onset and Duration of Action of Nitrates*

DRUG AND FORM	TIME TO ONSET OF ACTION	DURATION OF ACTION
NITROGLYCERIN		
Sublingual	1-3 min (R)	30-60 min (B)
Translingual spray	2-3 min (R)	30-60 min (B)
Transmucosal tablets	1-2 min (R)	3-5 hr (L)
Oral capsules/tablets SR	20-45 min (S)	3-8 hr (L)
Transdermal patches	½-1 hr (S)	24 hr (L)*
Topical ointment	½-1 hr (S)	24 hr (L)*
ISOSORBIDE MONONITRATE		
Oral tablets	½-1 hr (S)	6-10 hr (L)
Oral tablets SR	½-1 hr (S)	7-12 hr (L)
ISOSORBIDE DINITRATE		
Sublingual/chewable tablets	2-5 min (R)	1-3 hr (L)
Oral tablets	20-40 min (S)	4-6 hr (L)
Oral tablets/capsules SR	30 min (S)	6-8 hr (L)
AMYL NITRATE	30 sec (ultra R)	3-5 min (B)

B, Brief-acting; *L*, long-acting; *R*, rapid onset; *S*, slow onset.
*Should not be used for more than 12 hours, to prevent tolerance.

similar responses, but the time of onset and duration of action differ. Some preparations are rapidly effective (1 to 5 minutes) and last for about an hour, whereas for others the effect is slower in onset but lasts for several hours. Few agents have a rapid onset and long duration of action. The rapid-onset medications are used to treat an ongoing anginal attack and should be administered as soon as the pain begins. These agents may also be used prophylactically prior to anticipated exertion. Long-acting preparations are used for sustained protection against angina attacks (see Table 27-2).

- *Sublingual nitroglycerin* (Nitrostat) begins to work rapidly. It lasts for about an hour and is an ideal preparation for acute anginal pain. Administration should begin as soon as the pain begins and should not be delayed until the pain is severe. If one tablet is not sufficient, one or two additional tablets should be taken at 5-minute intervals. For persistent pain, the patient should obtain emergency medical attention because unresponsiveness to nitroglycerin may be a sign of an MI.

- *Transdermal nitroglycerin* (Transderm Nitro) is available as a patch containing a reservoir of nitroglycerin that is slowly released for absorption through the skin. These patches should be applied once a day to a hairless area of skin. The site should be rotated daily to avoid local irritation. To avoid developing tolerance to nitroglycerin, the patch should not be worn for more than 10 to 12 hours per day. The patch is usually applied in the morning and removed in the evening. The patches have a slow onset and are not effective for an ongoing anginal attack.

- *Topical ointment* (Nitroglycerin ointment) must be measured on a paper provided with the medication to ensure proper dosage. Topical ointment sites should also be rotated.

- *Nitroglycerin spray* (Nitrolingual) is especially useful in patients who have decreased dexterity. Each container holds 200 sprays that are immediately absorbed, providing quicker relief than with other forms of nitroglycerin. Like the tablets, the mist may be sprayed into the mouth every 5 minutes for 3 doses. Each spray contains 0.4 mg of nitroglycerin, and the medication in this form is not sensitive to heat, light, or moisture. Patient education for using the nitroglycerin spray should include the priming of the container by pointing the nozzle away and depressing until a click is heard. This should be repeated every 6 weeks if the container is not used. To use the spray, remove the cap and do not shake. Hold the bottle as close to the mouth as possible to release the spray into the mouth (under the tongue is not necessary). DO NOT INHALE SPRAY. No food or drink should be taken for 5 to 10 minutes following administration.

If nitroglycerin is to be discontinued, this action should take place over a period of time. Abrupt discontinuation of long-acting nitroglycerin preparations may cause angina and vasospasms (Table 27-3).

 CLINICAL TIP

The allied health professional should instruct the patient that the sublingual tablet is to remain under the tongue until it dissolves. The patient should also be taught that nitroglycerin is chemically unstable and loses its effectiveness over a period of time. The medication bottle should not be opened until it is needed, because its shelf-life is longer in a dark, tightly closed container. After the container is opened, the drug is effective for approximately 6 months and the date on which it was opened should be written on the container. Six months after the container is opened, the medication should be discarded and replaced with a new bottle.

β-Adrenergic Blockers

β-Adrenergic blockers (β-blockers) reverse sympathetic heart action caused by exercise, stress, or physical exertion. In the heart, sympathetic stimulation causes increased rate and force, as well as increased oxygen use. β-Blockers decrease the heart rate and the force of contraction, causing decreased oxygen use to prevent the development of myocardial ischemia and pain. The actions of β-blockers allow their use for the chronic management of angina by lessening the frequency of attacks or by delaying the onset of pain during exercise, allowing increased work capacity of the heart and increased exercise tolerance. (β-Blockers are discussed later in this chapter.)

Propranolol (Inderal) is often used for the treatment of angina, and it may be used in combination with nitrates for angina control. The dosing

TABLE 27-3 Antianginal Agents

GENERIC NAME	TRADE NAME	USUAL ADULT DOSE, ROUTE, AND FREQUENCY OF ADMINISTRATION	INDICATIONS FOR USE	MAJOR SIDE EFFECTS	DRUG INTERACTIONS
NITRATES					
nitroglycerin	Nitrostat	0.15-0.6 mg SL prn	Angina pectoris	Headache, hypotension, tachycardia, light-headedness, dizziness, burning sensation in mouth with spray	Use with care with hypotensives, β-blockers, verapamil, diltiazem, sildenafil, alcohol
	Nitrolingual	0.4-0.8 mg translingual spray prn			
	NitroMist	0.2-0.8 mg translingual spray prn and prophylactically			
	Nitrogard	1-2 mg transmucosal tab q3-8h			
	Nitrong SR, nitroglycerin SR	2.5-6.5 mg po tid-qid*			
	Transderm Nitro, Nitro-Dur, Nitro-Disc	1 patch daily; remove after 12-14 hr			
	Nitro-Bid IV	5 mcg/min IV			
	Nitro-Bid, Nitrol Ointment	1″-2″ q8h			
isosorbide mononitrate	ISMO, Monoket	20 mg po bid*			
	Imdur SR	30-120 mg/day po			
isosorbide dinitrate	Isordil, Sorbitrate	2.5-10 mg SL q4-6h			
	Sorbitrate	Chew 5-10 mg q2-3h			
	Isordil Titradose	5-30 mg po q6h*			
	Isordil Tembids SR, Sorbitrate SA	40 mg po q6-12h*			
	Dilatrate SR, Isotrate Timecelles	40 mg po q6-12h*			
amyl nitrate		0.18-0.3 mL inhaled			

(continued)

TABLE 27-3 *Antianginal Agents—cont'd*

GENERIC NAME	TRADE NAME	USUAL ADULT DOSE, ROUTE, AND FREQUENCY OF ADMINISTRATION	INDICATIONS FOR USE	MAJOR SIDE EFFECTS	DRUG INTERACTIONS
β-ADRENERGIC BLOCKERS					
propranolol	Inderal	10-90 mg po bid-qid	In combination with nitrates for angina pectoris	Insomnia, depression, bizarre dreams	theophylline, calcium channel blockers, reserpine, cimetidine, phenytoin, alcohol
CALCIUM CHANNEL BLOCKERS (See Table 27-5 class III and Table 27-11 for other calcium channel blockers used with angina)			Angina pectoris	Fatigue, headache, flushing, dizziness, hypotension, GI disturbances, constipation	
bepridil	Vascor	200-400 mg/day			digitalis
MISCELLANEOUS ANTIANGINAL MEDICATIONS					
ranolazine	Ranexa	500-1000 mg bid	Antianginal/anti-ischemic	GI symptoms, headache, dizziness, nausea, weakness, indigestion	quinidine, sotalol, ketoconazole, HIV medications, macrolide, antibiotics, diltiazem, verapamil, grapefruit

GI, Gastrointestinal; *IV*, intravenous; *SA*, sustained action; *SL*, sublingual; *SR*, sustained release.
*To avoid tolerance, the doses should allow the patient to be medication free at some time during the day.

goal is to reduce the pulse to 50 to 60 beats per minute at rest and 100 beats per minute during exercise. β-Blockers should be avoided with asthma and may mask hypoglycemia in patients with diabetes mellitus (see Table 27-3).

Calcium Channel Blockers

Calcium channel blockers are drugs that interfere with the movement of calcium ions through cell membranes. They are used to treat the pain of angina pectoris. Because vascular smooth muscle contraction is dependent on calcium movement from extracellular to intracellular sites, the inhibition of calcium prevents this contraction, allowing vasodilation to occur. These medications are indicated for vasospastic angina. Calcium blockers also dilate larger coronary arteries to increase the flow of blood to the heart.

- *Verapamil* (Calan) and *diltiazem* (Cardizem) have a primary use as antidysrhythmics but are used for their vasodilating properties when treating angina. These medications also decrease the heart rate and therefore decrease the heart's work.
- *Nifedipine* (Adalat), *nicardipine* (Cardene), *amlodipine* (Norvasc), *felodipine* (Plendil), and *isradipine* (DynaCirc), used as antihypertensives (see later in this chapter), are also used for angina because their properties cause vasodilation and relaxation of coronary artery spasms with minor effect on decreasing heart rate.
- *Bepridil* (Vasocon) is specifically for angina pectoris. It slows the heart rate and also has antiarrhythmic properties. This medication is limited to the patient who is unresponsive to other drug therapy (see Table 27-3).

Combining the Medications for Angina

Combinations of these medications—nitrates, β-blockers, and calcium channel blockers—may be used for the treatment of angina. The therapeutic goal in medication use is to reduce the frequency and intensity of anginal attacks without overly suppressing the cardiac action. Before administering calcium channel or β-blockers, it is important to take the patient's blood pressure and pulse to ensure both are within normal range. Patients taking these medications should move slowly from a lying position to a sitting or standing position because of the chance of **orthostatic hypotension.**

Patient Education for Compliance

1. Nitroglycerin sublingual tablets should be labeled with the date of opening.
2. Nitroglycerin sublingual tablets should be carried at all times in an easily accessible, dark container.
3. To prevent tolerance to nitroglycerin, nitroglycerin patches should be rotated on a daily basis and should not be worn more than 10 to 12 hours per day.
4. The mouth should be moist for the absorption of sublingual and buccal nitroglycerin tablets.
5. The nitroglycerin tablet should not be swallowed but should be placed under the tongue until it has fully dissolved.
6. Medical evaluation is necessary for a possible MI if acute anginal pain has not been relieved after taking three to five sublingual nitroglycerin tablets.
7. Long-acting nitroglycerin should not be discontinued abruptly because vasospasm may occur. The medication must be tapered off.
8. Nitroglycerin ointment should be measured on the supplied paper and applied in 1- to 2-inch strips as directed by the physician. This also should be removed at some point, usually at night, to prevent tolerance from occurring.
8. Transdermal nitroglycerin is for the prophylaxis of angina.
9. Changes in lifestyle—diet, smoking cessation, and weight control—are important while using medications for angina pectoris.
10. Headaches caused by nitroglycerin will gradually diminish with long-term use and may be relieved by nonsteroidal antiinflammatory drugs.
11. Patients using nitroglycerin should avoid alcohol and medications for erectile dysfunction.

IMPORTANT FACTS ABOUT MEDICATIONS FOR ANGINA PECTORIS

- Angina pectoris occurs when the oxygen supply to the heart is insufficient to meet the oxygen demands of the heart.
- Drugs that increase myocardial oxygen flow will decrease anginal pain. Cardiac oxygen needs are determined by heart rate, heart contractility, the venous return to the heart, blood pressure, and heart pressure.
- Three types of angina exist:
  - Chronic stable, or exertional, angina caused by coronary atherosclerosis

---

IMPORTANT FACTS ABOUT MEDICATIONS FOR ANGINA PECTORIS—*Cont'd*

- • Variant, or vasospastic, angina caused by coronary artery spasm
- • Unstable angina, which requires immediate medical care
- Drugs for stable angina relieve pain by decreasing venous return to lower the demand of oxygen by the heart, not by increasing the oxygen supply.
- Drugs for variant angina increase oxygen supply but do not decrease oxygen demand. NTG further dilates atherosclerotic veins to relieve stable angina.
- Three common side effects of nitroglycerin are headache, orthostatic hypotension, and tachycardia.
- The continuous use of nitroglycerin results in tolerance. To prevent tolerance, the dose should be the lowest possible effective dose and dosing should be on an intermittent schedule, with at least 8 hours of the day being drug free.
- Nitroglycerin with a rapid onset should be used for anginal attacks or for prophylaxis prior to exertion. Nitroglycerin preparations of long duration are for protection against anginal attacks and should be administered on a fixed schedule.
- β-Blockers prevent stable angina by decreasing heart rate and heart contractility, thus reducing cardiac oxygen need.
- Calcium channel blockers relieve the pain of stable angina by reducing oxygen demand to the heart.

Congestive Heart Failure and Its Treatment

Heart failure affects more than 2 million Americans, with almost half a million cases, primarily in the elderly, added each year. Patients have symptoms such as tiredness, fatigue, shortness of breath, rapid heart rate, and peripheral edema. When the contractility of the heart is decreased and the heart pumps less blood than it receives, congestive heart disease occurs, causing blood to accumulate in the heart chambers. Less blood circulates in the body, leading to retention of electrolytes including sodium in the tissues. This allows fluids to remain in the intracellular spaces, causing edema. Congestive heart failure is a progressive disease that is characterized by reduced cardiac output, ventricles that do not contract efficiently, and the accumulation of fluids or congestion in the tissues and lungs. Of all the factors, the depressed contractility of the heart is the major cause of heart failure. The principal drugs for heart failure change the force and rate of the heart. The overall goals of therapy for congestive heart failure are to correct the underlying cause and gain the patient's compliance in pharmacologic treatments and nonpharmacologic care such as decreasing the sodium in the diet, limiting alcohol, increasing exercise, and lowering stress levels.

Medications for Treating Congestive Heart Failure

The three major classes of drugs for heart failure are (1) vasodilators, which reduce symptoms; (2) diuretics, which are used to reduce the edema in the peripheral vessels and to reduce the blood volume overload; and (3) the cardiac glycosides, which are used to reduce the symptoms in chronic heart failure.

The *cardiac glycosides* (the digitalis group or Digoxin) are the oldest medicinal agents for congestive heart failure and are obtained from the plant leaves of digitalis. These drugs increase the force of myocardial contractions, decrease the size of the heart, and slow the conduction of electrical impulses. The increased force of contractions improves the efficiency and output of the heart without increasing oxygen consumption. With the reduction of edema, weight is lost and blood volume is reduced. Normal blood circulation is restored, and the kidney function is increased. Digoxin produces improvement of exercise tolerance and reduces fatigue. However, even with this improvement of symptoms of CHF, this medication does not alter the course of the disease process and does not prolong life.

After treatment with cardiac glycosides, the heart beats more forcefully within a shorter period of time to increase the amount of blood pumped from the heart, improving circulation and decreasing the congestion. Because cardiac glycosides slow the heart rate, the patient must be taught to count his or her pulse prior to taking the medication to be sure the pulse rate is above 60. If the pulse is below 60, the patient should not take the medication and should call the physician for instruction (Table 27-4).

 CLINICAL TIP

Digitalis works in the body much like the spark plug in an automobile—it makes the heart work on all cylinders.

Digitalization is the administration of glycosides at a rapid rate to produce an effective blood digitalis level. Subsequently a maintenance dose

TABLE 27-4 *Cardiac Glycosides*

GENERIC NAME	TRADE NAME	USUAL ADULT DOSE, ROUTE, AND FREQUENCY OF ADMINISTRATION	INDICATIONS FOR USE	DRUG INTERACTIONS
digoxin	Lanoxin, Lanoxicaps	0.125-0.5 mg/day po	Congestive heart failure, arrhythmias, and to control ventricular rate	See Box 27-2

MAJOR SIDE EFFECTS: Nausea, vomiting, headache, low pulse, visual disturbances, cardiac arrhythmias, ectopic heartbeats.

BOX 27-1   SIGNS AND SYMPTOMS OF DIGITALIS TOXICITY

Confusion
Loss of appetite
Headaches, malaise, fatigue
Nausea, vomiting, diarrhea
Palpitations or bradycardia
Irregular pulse
Visual changes (unusual)—halos or rings of light around objects or seeing lights or bright spots
• Changes in color perception
• Blind spots or blurred vision
Decreased urinary output
Excessive nocturnal urination
Swelling
Decreased consciousness
Difficulty breathing when lying down

---

is used to maintain a therapeutic level. Dosing with digoxin is highly individualized, and each patient should be carefully evaluated until an effective dose has been established, after which monitoring is generally not necessary. The difference in therapeutic and toxic levels is slim, and the patient must be watched closely for signs of toxicity (Box 27-1).

Patient Education for Compliance

1. Patients should be warned not to double up on missed doses of digoxin.
2. Switching between brands and formulations of digoxin may lead to altered responses, as the bioavailability differs with different brands.
3. Patients should monitor the pulse for rate and rhythm daily prior to taking digoxin. The pulse rate should be above 60 and below 90 prior to taking the medication.

BOX 27-2   DRUGS THAT INTERACT WITH DIGOXIN

Drugs That Decrease Digoxin Levels
cholestyramine
kaolin/pectin
neomycin
sulfasalazine

Drugs That Increase Digoxin Levels
aminoglycosides
antacids
colestipol
erythromycin
omeprazole
tetracycline
alprazolam
amiodarone
captopril
diltiazem
nifedipine
nitrendipine
propafenone
quinidine
verapamil

Drugs That Increase the Incidence of Dysrhythmias
Thiazide and loop diuretics
amphotericin
glucocorticoids

Drugs That Decrease Heart Rate and Contractility
β-blockers
verapamil
diltiazem

Drugs That Increase Heart Rate and Contractility
Sympathomimetics

IMPORTANT FACTS ABOUT DRUGS FOR CONGESTIVE HEART FAILURE

• Therapy for heart failure is to relieve pulmonary and peripheral edema, increase the quality of life, and prolong life expectancy.

Cardiac Dysrhythmias and Their Treatment

Medications used to treat disorders of cardiac rhythm, or **arrhythmias,** are called antidysrhythmics or antiarrhythmics. Although the term *arrhythmia*, meaning loss of rhythm, is most often used, perhaps the term *dysrhythmia* is a better way of denoting an abnormal heart rhythm. Dysrhythmia is actually a deviation from normal rhythm and may be from CAD, electrolyte imbalances, cardiac conduction abnormalities, or even thyroid disease, as well as chronic drug therapy. Some dysrhythmias may have only mild effect on cardiac output, whereas others may cause severe compromise of cardiac pumping ability.

Dysrhythmia may be caused by an alteration of the electrical impulse, and medications may be used to regulate the rhythm. Any change from the normal automatically controlled heartbeat, or normal sinus rhythm, may be caused by electrical impulses that are not interpreted into a normal heart rhythm. The cells may produce *ectopic beats*. When severe dysrhythmia occurs, especially in ventricular disorders, the patient may be having a medical emergency needing hospital care. This section focuses on medications used in an ambulatory care setting.

The therapeutic effect of antidysrhythmic medications lies in their ability to restore the ions of the heart to a normal or improved condition with an improved ability to pump blood. Antidysrhythmia medications, found in four distinct groups by their effect, do not cure the dysrhythmia, but they do attempt to restore normal cardiac function (Table 27-5).

- Class I drugs bind to the sodium channels and interfere with the sodium ion movement during heart excitation, making the heart less excitable. These medications also slow the conduction velocity, prolong the heart's refractory period, and decrease the **automaticity** of the heart's action.
  - *Quinidine* is used to treat *supraventricular arrhythmias* such as atrial flutter and atrial fibrillation and some *ventricular dysrhythmias*. It depresses the myocardium and the conduction system, decreasing the contractile force of the heart and slowing the heart rate.
  - *Procainamide* (Pronestyl or Procan-SR), related to procaine, depresses cardiac muscle excitability to electrical stimulation and slows conduction to increase the refractory period.
  - *Disopyramide* (Norpace) is another medication to decrease cardiac excitability and is a cardiac depressant.
  - *Lidocaine*, an anesthetic, is used for ventricular arrhythmias and is given parenterally as a bolus. Two medications chemically and therapeutically related to lidocaine, mexiletine (Mexitil) and tocainide (Tonocard), have been modified for oral administration for use in ambulatory care.
  - *Phenytoin* (Dilantin), a medication for epilepsy, can alter nerve functions to act as an antidysrhythmic. It is especially useful in ventricular dysrhythmias induced by the use of digitalis.
- Class II antidysrhythmic medications are the β-adrenergic blockers that increase heart rate, heart excitability, conduction velocity, and automaticity, particularly of the ventricles. These indications are discussed with the medications for the cardiac system that mimic the sympathetic nervous system.
  - *Propranolol* (Inderal) is the most common β-blocker used as an antidysrhythmic. Besides having the β-blocking effect, it also has quinidine-like depression of the excitability of the cardiac muscle to delay

TABLE 27-5 *Cardiac Antidysrhthmics*

GENERIC NAME	TRADE NAME	USUAL ADULT DOSE, ROUTE, AND FREQUENCY OF ADMINISTRATION	INDICATIONS FOR USE	MAJOR SIDE EFFECTS	DRUG INTERACTIONS
CLASS I					
quinidine	Cardioquin	200-600 mg po q2-4h	Treatment of supraventricular and ventricular dysrhythmias	Nausea, vomiting, diarrhea, fatigue, weakness, tinnitus, hypotension, severe headache, blurred vision, dizziness	β-blockers, digitalis, potassium, nifedipine, procainamide
	Quinaglute (SR)	200-400 mg/dose IV			
	Quinidex (SR)*	300-600 mg po q8h			
		324-972 mg q8-12h			
procainamide	Pronestyl	250-500 mg po q3h		Same as quinidine	pimozide, neuromuscular blockers, quinidine, alcohol, cimetidine
	Procan-SR	250-750 mg po q6h			
disopyramide	Norpace (CR) (SR)	400-800 mg/day po		Dry mouth, constipation, visual disturbances, urinary retention	pimozide, other antidysrhythmics
mexiletine	Mexitil	200 mg po q8h		GI distress, dizziness, light headiness, tremors	urinary acidifiers, metoclopramide, phenytoin, rifampin
tocainide	Tonocard	1200-1800 mg/day po		Same as above	antacids, rifampin
phenytoin	Dilantin	100 mg po q6-12h		Blurred vision, vertigo, nystagmus, hyperplasia of gingiva	glucocorticoids, CNS depressants, alcohol, antacids, others (see Table 30-7)
flecainide	Tambocor	200-400 mg/day po			Same as disopyramide
moricizine	Ethmozine	600-900 mg/day po			theophylline, cimetidine
propafenone	Rythmol	450-900 mg/day po			propranolol, digoxin, warfarin
CLASS II					
propranolol	Inderal	20-30 mg po tid-qid	Depress depolarization	Rashes, metal confusion	diuretics, NSAIDs, hypotensives, xanthines
	Inderal LA	60-100 mg po bid			
acebutolol	Sectral	600-1200 mg/day po			

(continued)

TABLE 27-5 *Cardiac Antidysrhythmics—cont'd*

GENERIC NAME	TRADE NAME	USUAL ADULT DOSE, ROUTE, AND FREQUENCY OF ADMINISTRATION	INDICATIONS FOR USE	MAJOR SIDE EFFECTS	DRUG INTERACTIONS
CLASS III				Dizziness, nausea, vomiting, anorexia, bitter taste, weight loss, paresthesia of hands and feet, weakness	
amiodarone	Cordarone	800-1600 mg po, IV bid	Life-threatening ventricular arrhythmia		cardiac glycosides, anticoagulants
sotalol	Betapace	80-320 mg/day po			antiarrhythmics, phenothiazine, digoxin, terfenadine, astemizole, sympathomimetics
dofetilide	Tikosyn	Individualized po for the elderly			None identified
CLASS IV					
verapamil	Calan, Isoptin	240-480 mg/day po in 3-4 divided doses	Dysrhythmias due to SA and AV node hyperexcitability	Headaches, dizziness, GI disturbances, constipation	β-blockers, digoxin, procainamide, quinidine, theophylline
diltiazem	Covera-HS Cardizem, Tiazac	180-480 mg po hs 240-480 mg/day po in 3-4 divided doses	Same as for verapamil		Same as for verapamil
nifedipine	Adalat, Procardia	10 mg po tid		same as for verapamil	same as for verapamil

AV, Atrioventricular; CNS, central nervous system; GI, gastrointestinal; IV, intravenous; LA, long acting; NSAIDs, nonsteroidal antiinflammatory drugs; SA, sinoatrial; SR, sustained release.

ventricular repolarization. The most common cardiovascular adverse reactions are hypertension and decreased heartbeat. This medication is most frequently given by mouth but may be given intravenously in emergency situations (see Table 27-5).

- Class III antidysrhythmic medications interfere with the outflow of potassium during repolarization to prolong the potential contraction duration of the Purkinje fibers and the muscle fibers of the ventricles. The prolonged period decreases the frequency of heart failure.
  - *Amiodarone* (Cordarone) decreases automaticity, prolongs atrioventricular (AV) conduction, and may even block the exchange of sodium and potassium. This action can cause serious side effects and is used only for life-threatening dysrhythmias that have not responded to other medications.
  - *Sotalol* (Betapace) is also used as a class III antidysrhythmic in life-threatening ventricular dysrhythmics. These medications would not be seen in most physicians' offices (see Table 27-5).
- Class IV agents are referred to as *calcium channel blockers* because they decrease the entry of calcium into the cells of the heart and blood vessels. The pacemaker cells—sinoatrial (SA) and atrioventricular (AV) nodes—require calcium for normal activity and for normal sinus rhythm. Reducing calcium decreases the rate of the SA node and the conduction velocity of the AV node and is effective in the treatment of supraventricular tachycardia. These calcium antagonists may also decrease the ability of the heart to produce forceful contractions, leading to congestive heart failure. The medications also relax smooth muscle and cause vasodilation and are therefore useful with angina and for hypertension.
  - *Verapamil* (Calan, Isoptin) works on the SA node to decrease its activity, thus decreasing the heart rate. It also decreases AV node conduction and is used for AV node dysrhythmias. Verapamil is contraindicated in patients with known SA or AV node problems or with congestive heart failure.
  - *Diltiazem* (Cardizem) is less potent than verapamil in decreasing the heart rate but is more potent as a vasodilator. It is used mainly as an antihypertensive agent but may be used for dysrhythmia (see Table 27-5). (See Table 27-11 for more calcium channel blockers.)

Patient Education for Compliance

1. Antidysrhythmic medications must be taken at prescribed levels and must not be skipped unless the patient is told to do so by a physician.
2. The patient should take no over-the-counter medications with antidysrhythmics without obtaining permission from a physician.
3. Avoid alcohol and nicotine with antidysrhythmics.

IMPORTANT FACTS ABOUT ANTIDYSRHYTHMICS

- Dysrhythmias result from alteration of the electrical impulses beginning at the SA node that regulate the cardiac rhythm. Antidysrhythmics control rhythm by correcting or compensating for the altered rhythm.
- Treatment of ventricular dysrhythmias is directed at eliminating the abnormal rhythm.
- All antidysrhythmic medications can worsen existing conditions and generate new rhythm disorders.
- Class I antidysrhythmic medications block cardiac sodium channels slowing the impulse conduction.
- Quinidine blocks sodium channels and delays ventricular repolarization.
- Propranolol and other class II medications are β-blockers that decrease SA automaticity, AV velocity, and myocardial contractility.
- Class III antidysrhythmics block potassium channels, prolonging ventricular repolarization.
- Class IV antidysrhythmics (verapamil, diltiazem) reduce the automaticity of the SA node, conduction of the AV node, and myocardial contractility, identical to the effects of β-blockers.

Hypertension and Its Treatment

Hypertension, a chronic cardiovascular disease affecting millions of Americans, is described as a silent killer because 25% of the American population has hypertension. The effects of hypertension kill 2500 Americans every day, and two out of every five deaths in the United States are related to hypertension and cardiovascular disease. In approximately 90% of cases there is no apparent cause, and more than one third of those affected have no idea they have hypertension. Hypertension with an unknown etiology is referred to as *essential* or *primary hypertension*. Generally in adults, a blood pressure above 120/80 is now considered prehypertensive with 140/90 being hypertensive. The diagnosis of hypertension should not be made on the basis of a single blood pressure reading. When either the systolic pressure, the diastolic pressure, or both are above baseline for an extended period of time, hypertension is suspected. Unless the blood pressure poses an immediate danger, readings should be done on two subsequent visits, a week to several weeks apart. Two readings should be taken at each visit and averaged.

Risk factors for hypertension include family history, stress, obesity, smoking, sedentary lifestyle, diabetes mellitus, and excessive lipid blood levels. When hypertension is not properly treated, the risk of stroke, cerebral hemorrhage, coronary heart disease, congestive heart failure, and renal failure increases. Renal failure is increased during hypertension because the flow of the blood through the kidneys is reduced.

Blood pressure is controlled by a complex interaction among the nervous, hormonal, and renal systems. When blood pressure drops, this information activates the sympathetic nervous system. Epinephrine increases the heart rate and the force of the heart contractions to elevate cardiac output and blood pressure. At the same time, the renin-angiotensin-aldosterone (RAA) mechanism helps regulate blood pressure by increasing or decreasing blood flow through the kidneys. The increase in blood volume from the retention of water and sodium causes an increase in blood pressure. The RAA system, therefore, functions to help in the maintenance of blood volume and blood pressure.

Blood pressure also responds to changes in the arterial blood flow. **Peripheral resistance** in blood vessels as well as blood volume and blood viscosity are factors in the pressure exerted on the arterial walls. Atherosclerosis, with the reduced arterial diameter, will require more force when pushing blood through the vessels—or increased blood pressure. Finally, the cardiac output and the ability of the heart to pump blood proficiently affect blood pressure.

Antihypertensive Therapy

Antihypertensive therapy is often a difficult area in which to obtain patient compliance because the patient is asked to comply with therapy for a disease that is basically asymptomatic. Long-term therapy is necessary to prevent the morbidity and mortality associated with uncontrolled hypertension. Noncompliance is associated with a poor prognosis, whereas compliance with an individualized regimen is associated with a good prognosis.

Categories of Antihypertensive Medications

Antihypertensive medications are classified into five major categories: (1) diuretics, (2) centrally and peripherally acting adrenergic inhibiting agents, (3) ACE inhibitors, (4) angiotensin II receptor antagonists, and (5) vasodilators. The adrenergic-inhibiting agents include such groups of medications as β-adrenergic blockers, rauwolfia derivatives, and α-adrenergic blockers. The types of medications used to treat hypertension are found in Box 27-3. Each medication has a specific indication for use. The choice of antihypertensives must be individualized, but treatment may become more aggressive with each level.

Antihypertensive Therapy and Lifestyle Changes

The basic approach for antihypertensive therapy begins with changes in lifestyle (Figure 27-5). If this does not produce the desired effects, medication therapy may be started to lower the blood pressure out of the hypertensive range. Treatment begins with the addition of one drug. If this drug fails to produce the desired effects, another medication

---

BOX 27-3   TYPES OF MEDICATIONS USED TO TREAT HYPERTENSION

Angiotensin-converting enzyme (ACE) inhibitors act by dilating arterial blood vessels and decreasing blood volume.

Angiotensin II receptor antagonists act by blocking angiotensin II, which causes vasoconstriction.

α/β-Adrenergic blockers dilate blood vessels by working on the α- and β- cells to decrease the formation of norepinephrine.

Antiadrenergic drugs (centrally acting) work on the α- and β-receptors of the sympathetic nervous system to dilate blood vessels.

β-Adrenergic blockers cause the heart to beat less frequently and cause dilation of the blood vessels.

Calcium channel blockers relax the smooth muscle of the blood vessels to cause dilation.

Vasodilating agents block the movement of calcium into the smooth muscle of the blood vessels to cause relaxation and dilation.

Diuretics cause the excretion of sodium and water to decrease blood volume and blood pressure.

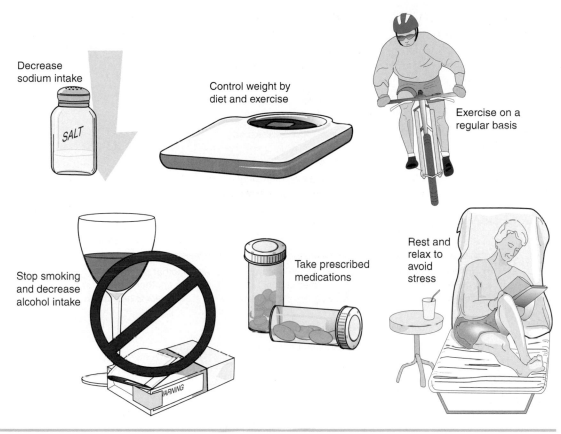

Decrease
sodium intake

SALT

Control weight by
diet and exercise

Exercise on a
regular basis

Stop smoking
and decrease
alcohol intake

WARNING

Take prescribed
medications

Rest and
relax to
avoid
stress

Figure 27-5 To treat hypertension, it is important to strive for multidisciplinary lifestyle modifications.

may be added. Before a second medication is added, the patient's compliance in taking the first medication and with lifestyle changes should be carefully evaluated and documented. This will help determine whether an adequate dosage of the first medication was prescribed. If treatment with two medications is not successful, further close evaluation for compliance should be done. If a third medication is needed, it may also be added (Figure 27-6).

Adding Medications for the Treatment of Hypertension

The initial drugs used in the treatment of hypertension are usually either diuretics or β-blockers. Alternatively, ACE inhibitors, calcium channel blockers, α-adrenergic blockers, or α/β-adrenergic blockers may be used for initial therapy as needs are determined. When supplemental medications are added, centrally acting sympatholytics, adrenergic neuron blockers, and direct-acting vasodilators are those usually considered. Because of the many undesirable side effects of the drugs used as supplemental medications, these drugs are not suitable for therapy by themselves.

When medications are added, each medication is chosen from a different class with a different mechanism of action. Multidrug therapy increases the chance of success because several receptor sites are being attacked at the same time for blood pressure control. When medications are given together, a lower dosage of each is possible than when one drug is used alone. Using multiple medications may have the positive effect of reducing the side effects and adverse reactions that occur with the use of higher doses of one medicine. Finally, medications are usually started in low doses and then gradually increased as needed for blood pressure control. Medicinal treatment for concurrent illnesses and diseases may have synergistic action for treatment of both diseases; an example is the hypertensive patient with angina who uses a calcium channel blocker to treat both conditions. However, antihypertensive medications may also have antagonistic effects on diseases.

Some ethnic and cultural groups may react in unexpected ways to the medical implications of hypertension, and their response to antihypertensives may differ from the normal expected response.

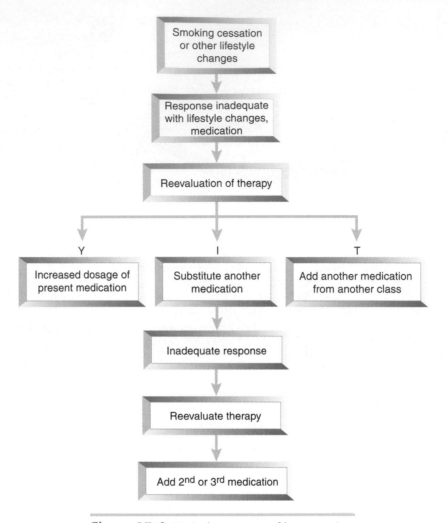

Figure 27-6 Typical treatment of hypertension.

African American patients are at increased risk for hypertension and generally have a better response to diuretics and calcium channel blockers than to ACE inhibitors and β-blockers. Hypertension is more common in women who have taken oral contraceptives for 5 years than in those who have not. Age, smoking, and estrogen replacement therapy also increase the risk of hypertension. In the elderly, a group with significant rates of hypertensive disease, medications should be started at lower doses and at less frequent intervals because of the sensitivity of the aging body to fluid depletion and because of impaired cardiovascular reflexes.

If the patient has hypertension that has been controlled for a year, the medication dose may be decreased, but all lifestyle modifications must continue. If the drug dosage is lowered slowly, the disease may be controlled with less medication. In reducing the dosage, it is important to be sure the patient continues to follow the prescribed regimen faithfully and continues regular follow-up evaluations to detect any return of a blood pressure value indicating increased blood pressure readings.

Diuretics

Diuretics block the reabsorption of sodium and chloride, allowing more water to be excreted. The increase in urinary output is directly related to the degree to which resorption of sodium and chloride is blocked. The diuretic that works early in the nephron blocks the greatest amount of sodium and chloride solutes and produces greatest diuresis with resultant acid-base imbalance and electrolyte level disturbances. The diuretics are mainstays of hypertensive therapy and may be used alone or in combination with other antihypertensives. The four major categories of diuretics are (1) high-ceiling (loop) diuretics, (2) thiazide diuretics, (3) osmotic diuretics, and (4) potassium-sparing agents.

- **High-ceiling (loop) diuretics** are the most effective diuretics available, producing greater loss of fluids and electrolytes by acting on the loop of Henle (Figure 27-7). These medications are not used routinely for hypertension but are used when diuresis is necessary to provide decreased blood pressure by reducing blood volume and promoting vasodilation. Because of the loss of electrolytes, potassium replacements are necessary with these drugs.
  - *Furosemide* (Lasix) is the most frequently prescribed loop diuretic, acting on the ascending loop of Henle. See Table 27-6 for the other loop diuretics that act in a similar manner to furosemide.
- **Thiazide diuretics,** the most commonly used as antihypertensive agents, reduce blood volume, producing an initial reduction in blood pressure and reducing arterial resistance for long-term antihypertensive effects. These agents increase the excretion of sodium, chloride, potassium, and water while raising uric acid and glucose levels, but the diuresis from thiazides is less than that found with loop diuretics. Potassium may be replaced by medication or by eating potassium-rich foods such as bananas, greens, meats, and apricots, to name a few.
  - *Hydrochlorothiazide* (HydroDIURIL) is the most widely used of the thiazide diuretics. One of the most widely prescribed medications, the thiazide diuretics work in the early segment of the distal convoluted tubules (see Figure 27-7) and are not effective in patients with impaired renal function.
  - Also included in this group of medications used for hypertension are four drugs that

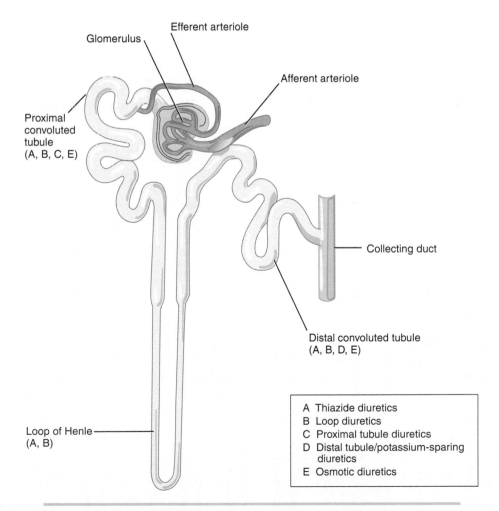

Figure 27-7 The action of a kidney nephron and its relationship to diuretics.

TABLE 27-6 Diuretics

GENERIC NAME	TRADE NAME	USUAL ADULT DOSE, ROUTE, AND FREQUENCY OF ADMINISTRATION	INDICATIONS FOR USE	MAJOR SIDE EFFECTS*	DRUG INTERACTIONS
LOOP DIURETICS				Loss of potassium, dehydration, elevated blood sugar and uric acid levels, hearing loss	
furosemide	Lasix	20-80 mg/day po, IM, IV, up to 600 mg/day	Hypertension, congestive heart failure, renal disease		digoxin, NSAIDs, aminoglycosides, potassium-sparing diuretics, lithium
torsemide	Demadex	5-20 mg/day po, IV, up to 200 mg/day			Other antihypertensives, NSAIDs, digoxin,
ethacrynic acid	Edecrin	50-100 mg/day po, IV			anticoagulants, lithium amphotericin, heparin, lithium
bumetanide	Bumex	0.5-2 mg/day po, IV			Same as ethacrynic acid
THIAZIDE DIURETICS			Hypertension, edema, diabetes insipidus	Loss of potassium, dehydration	digitalis, lithium, cholestyramine, colestipol
chlorothiazide	Diuril, Duragen	500 mg po qd-bid			
hydrochlorothiazide	HydroDIURIL, Esidrix	25-100 mg/day po			
cyclothiazide	Anhydron	2 mg/day po			
hydroflumethiazide	Diucardin, Saluron	50 mg po qd-bid			
methylclothiazide	Enduron	2.5-10 mg/day po			
polythiazide	Renese	1-4 mg/day po			
THIAZIDE-LIKE DIURETICS			Same as thiazide diuretics	Same as for thiazide diuretics	Same as thiazide diuretics
chlorthalidone	Hygroton	25-100 mg/day po			
metolazone	Zaroxolyn	5-20 mg/day po			
indapamide	Lozol	1.25-5 mg/day po			
quinethazone	Hydromox	50 mg po qd-bid			
DISTAL TUBULE/ POTASSIUM-SPARING DIURETICS			Congestive heart failure, hypertension	Nausea, vomiting, dizziness	anticoagulants, NSAIDs, lithium, ACE inhibitors, potassium-containing diuretics, potassium-containing supplements
amiloride	Midamor	5 mg/day po			
spironolactone	Aldactone	50-100 mg po bid			
triamterene	Dyrenium	50-100 mg po bid			

ACE, Angiotension-converting enzymes; *IM*, intramuscular; *IV*, intravenous; *NSAIDs*, nonsteroidal antiinflammatory drugs.
NOTE: All diuretics may cause orthostatic hypotension and dry mouth
†For combination diuretics and antihypertensives, see Table 27-7.

are not true thiazides but are similar in function and structure: *chlorthalidone* (Hygroton), *indapamide* (Lozol), *metolazone* (Zaroxolyn), and *quinethazone* (Hydromox) (see Table 27-6).

- **Potassium-sparing diuretics** produce a modest increase in urinary output and a decrease in potassium excretion. These diuretics are seldom used alone in hypertension but are frequently added to primary agents. These drugs tend to counteract the potassium loss caused by thiazide and loop diuretics, and potassium replacement is not indicated. The patient should be told to watch the diet to avoid excessive intake of potassium-rich foods.
  - *Spironolactone* (Aldactone), typical of potassium-sparing diuretics, blocks aldosterone usage in the distal nephron (see Figure 27-7). This action causes the retention of potassium and excretion of sodium. Care should be taken with ACE inhibitors (see the discussion of ACE inhibitors later in this chapter) (see Table 27-6).
- **Combination diuretics** include thiazide diuretics that are combined in single-dose medications with potassium-sparing diuretics. The fixed-dose combinations may provide diuretic activity and decrease potassium depletion. In addition, diuretics may be combined with antihypertensives to provide simple compliance by the patient after hypertension has been stabilized through a medication and lifestyle change regimen (Table 27-7).

TABLE 27-7 *Frequently Prescribed Combination Medications for Hypertension*

TRADE NAME	CONSTITUENT MEDICATIONS	
	DIURETIC	POTASSIUM-SPARING DIURETIC
Aldactazide	HCTZ	spirolactone
Dyazide, Maxzide	HCTZ	triamterene
Moduretic	HCTZ	amiloride
Micardis HCT	HCTZ	telmisartan
Vaseretic	HCTZ	enalapril
	DIURETIC	ANTIHYPERTENSIVE
Inderide	HCTZ	propranolol
Diovan HCT	HCTZ	valsartan
Lopressor HCT	HCTZ	metoprolol
Timolide	HCTZ	timolol
Ziac	HCTZ	bisoprolol
Capozide	HCTZ	captopril
Lotensin HCT	HCTZ	benazepril
Aldoril 15	HCTZ	methyldopa
Apresazide	HCTZ	hydralazine
Hydropres	HCTZ	reserpine
Avalide	HCTZ	irbesartan
Hyzaar	HCTZ	losartan
Zestoretic	HCTZ	clonidine
Prinzide	HCTZ	lisinopril
Combipres	chlorthalidone	clonidine
Tenoretic	chlorthalidone	atenolol
Lotrel	benazepril	amlodipine
Tarka	trandolapril	verapamil
Lexxel	felodipine	enalapril

HCTZ, Hydrochlorothiazide.

Patient Education for Compliance

1. Frequent sips of water or chewing gum may relieve the dry mouth that occurs with diuretics.
2. Diuretics should be taken in the mornings for once-a-day dosing and at 8 am and 2 pm for twice-a-day dosing to prevent interference of sleep for urination.
3. Furosemide should be taken with food if gastrointestinal upset occurs.
4. Postural hypotension may occur with diuretics, and positions should be changed slowly.
5. The patient should keep a record of weight by weighing himself or herself on a regular basis and at the same time of the day when taking diuretics.
6. Patients taking thiazide or loop diuretics should avoid exposure to sunlight and ultraviolet light.
7. Patients with diabetes mellitus who take loop diuretics should test their blood glucose levels on a more frequent basis.

Patient Education for Compliance—cont'd

8. Patients taking potassium-sparing diuretics should avoid foods high in potassium and salt substitutes containing potassium.
9. Patients taking diuretics, especially elderly patients, should be sure to take in adequate fluids.

IMPORTANT FACTS ABOUT DIURETICS

- Some vasodilators work on arterial blood flow, some on venous blood flow, and some on both types of vessels.
- Hypertension is systolic pressure above 140 mm Hg or diastolic pressure above 90 mm Hg, whereas a prehypertensive state is blood pressure of 120/80 or above.

Adrenergic-Inhibiting Agents

The adrenergic-inhibiting agents include groups of medications such as β-blockers, rauwolfia derivatives, and α-adrenergic agents. The heart, blood vessels, and kidneys influence arterial blood pressure by increasing heart rate and the force of myocardial contractions, by constricting of arterioles and venules, and by releasing renin in the kidneys. Adrenergic-inhibiting (sympatholytic) agents are the most effective of the antihypertensive medications in lowering blood pressure and preventing serious cardiovascular complications (Table 27-8).

- *β-Blockers* such as nadolol (Corgard) and propranolol (Inderal) decrease cardiac output, inhibit renin secretion, and interfere with the renin-angiotensin-aldosterone (RAA) system, thereby lowering blood pressure. These medications are also used with angina and acute myocardial infarctions.
- *Aldosterone receptor antagonists* such as eplerenone (Inspra) block the binding of aldosterone in the RAA absorption to lower blood pressure. These drugs may be used separately or may be given with thiazide diuretics.
- *α/β-Blockers* such as labetalol (Normodyne) are similar to β-blockers and are used for severe hypertension. α-Receptor blockade causes vas-

odilation and decreased peripheral vascular resistance that is added to the β-blocking mechanisms.
- *Centrally acting adrenergic inhibitors* such as clonidine (Catapres) are effective in the treatment of hypertension, especially when given with a diuretic. With the sympathetic nerves functioning at a higher than normal level, these medications reduce the blood pressure, pulse rate, and cardiac output.
- *Peripherally acting adrenergic inhibitors* such as doxazosin (Cardura) and reserpine (Serpasil) are powerful antihypertensives that either interfere with the release of norepinephrine from nerve endings or block receptors in the vascular smooth muscle. These agents decrease blood pressure by decreasing vascular tone, primarily in the veins, followed by effects in the arteries.
- *ACE inhibitors* such as benazepril (Lotensin) and enalapril (Vasotec) slow the formation of angiotensin II, lowering blood volume and blood pressure. They are the most frequently used drugs for congestive heart failure. ACE inhibitors are a class of medications for the treatment of severe hypertension. These drugs result in peripheral vasodilation, renal vasodilation, and suppression of aldosterone-mediated volume expansion. ACE inhibitors are usually associated with the desirable effect of increased renal blood flow. They also interfere with mental and physical performance less. Consequently, the better quality of life afforded by ACE inhibitors should lead to better compliance (Table 27-9).

Vasodilators

Vasodilators relax the smooth muscle of the peripheral arterioles, thus decreasing peripheral resistance. The medications stimulate the sympathetic nervous system to increase heart rate and cardiac output. Because of this effect, a β-blocker may also be given to inhibit the sympathetic response and a diuretic may be used to alleviate sodium and water retention. These medications may selectively dilate arterioles or may lower blood pressure through dilation of venules and secondarily arterioles. Minoxidil (Loniten) is usually given with a β-blocker to prevent reflux tachycardia (Table 27-10).

DID YOU KNOW?
A side effect of minoxidil is increased body hair growth, which has led to its primary use in treating baldness.

TABLE 27-8 *Adrenergic-Inhibiting (Sympatholytic) Agents*

GENERIC NAME	TRADE NAME	USUAL ADULT DOSE, ROUTE, AND FREQUENCY OF ADMINISTRATION	INDICATIONS FOR USE	DRUG INTERACTIONS
β-BLOCKERS			Hypertension, angina, cardiac arrhythmias, acute myocardial infarction	Diuretics, xanthines, hypoglycemics, NSAIDs, amiodarone, ampicillin antacids, digoxin epinephrine, tacrine phenylephrine sympathomimetics
acebutolol	Sectral	200-800 mg po bid	See above	
atenolol	Tenormin	25-100 mg/day po	Hypertension	
betaxolol	Kerlone	10-20 mg/day po	Hypertension	
bisoprolol	Zebeta	5 mg qd	Hypertension	
carteolol	Cartrol	2.5-10 mg/day po	Hypertension	
metoprolol	Lopressor, Toprol XL	50-450 mg/day po	All found with acebutolol	
nadolol	Corgard	40-320 mg/day po	Hypertension and angina	
penbutolol	Levatol	20-80 mg/day po	Hypertension	
pindolol	Visken	Up to 60 mg/day po	Hypertension	
propranolol	Inderal	10-240 mg/day po	As found with acebutolol and prevention of migraine headaches	
sotalol	Betapace	80-320 mg po bid (may be increased to 240-320 mg per day)	As found with acebutolol	
timolol	Blocadren	20-60 mg/day po	As found with acebutolol plus migraine headaches and myocardial infarctions	

MAJOR SIDE EFFECTS OF β-BLOCKERS: Tachycardia, dizziness, vertigo, GI discomfort, sexual dysfunction, joint pain, bronchospasm; additionally rash, flushing, hypotension, impotence with bisoprolol.

ALDOSTERONE RECEPTOR ANTAGONIST

eplerenone	Inspra	50 mg po qd		NSAIDs, lithium ACE inhibitors

MAJOR SIDE EFFECTS OF ALDOSTERONE RECEPTOR ANTAGONIST: Headache, MI, diarrhea, cough, vaginal bleeding.

α/β-BLOCKERS

labetalol	Normodyne, Trandate	100-400 mg po, IV bid	Severe hypertension	Same as beta-blockers plus MAO inhibitors
carvedilol	Coreg	12.5 mg-50 mg po qd	Hypertension	Same

MAJOR SIDE EFFECTS OF α/β-BLOCKERS: Same as β-blockers plus orthostatic hypotension, headache, bronchospasm, dyspnea.

(continued)

TABLE 27-8 *Adrenergic-Inhibiting (Sympatholytic) Agents—cont'd*

GENERIC NAME	TRADE NAME	USUAL ADULT DOSE, ROUTE, AND FREQUENCY OF ADMINISTRATION	INDICATIONS FOR USE	DRUG INTERACTIONS
CENTRALLY ACTING ADRENERGIC BLOCKERS				
clonidine	Catapres	0.1-0.8 mg bid po; apply transdermal patch q7d	Hypertension	β-blockers, tricyclic antidepressants
guanabenz	Wytensin	4-32 mg po bid		None
guanfacine	Tenex	1-3 mg po hs		None
methyldopa/ methyldopate	Aldomet	Up to 3 g/day po, IV		MAO inhibitors, sympathomimetics

MAJOR SIDE EFFECTS OF CENTRALLY ACTING ADRENERGIC BLOCKERS: Dry mouth, drowsiness, anorexia, malaise, constipation, nightmares, impotence, CHF.

GENERIC NAME	TRADE NAME	USUAL ADULT DOSE, ROUTE, AND FREQUENCY OF ADMINISTRATION	INDICATIONS FOR USE	DRUG INTERACTIONS
PERIPHERALLY ACTING ADRENERGIC BLOCKERS				
doxazosin	Cardura	1-16 mg/day po	Hypertension	NSAIDs, estrogen
guanadrel	Hylorel	10-75 mg/day po in divided doses		tricyclic antidepressants, MAO inhibitors, phenothiazines, sympathomimetics
guanethidine	Ismelin	10-50 mg/day po		Same as above, plus minoxidil
prazosin	Minipress	1-20 mg/day po in divided doses		NSAIDs, verapamil, beta-blockers
reserpine	Serpalan, Serpasil	0.1-0.25 mg/day po		MAO inhibitors
terazosin	Hytrin	1-20 mg po hs		ACE inhibitors, NSAIDs, propranolol

MAJOR SIDE EFFECTS OF PERIPHERALLY ACTING ADRENERGIC BLOCKERS: Palpitations, nausea, vomiting, dry mouth, dyspnea, depression, headache, coughing, fatigue.

GENERIC NAME	TRADE NAME	USUAL ADULT DOSE, ROUTE, AND FREQUENCY OF ADMINISTRATION	INDICATIONS FOR USE	DRUG INTERACTIONS
ANGIOTENSIN II RECEPTOR ANTAGONISTS				
losartan	Cozaar	25-50 mg po qd-bid	Hypertension, vasodilation	cimetidine, phenobarbital, rifampin, lithium,
valsartan	Diovan	80-160 mg po qd		ketoconazole, troleandomycin
irbesartan	Avapro	150-300 mg po qd		
olmesartan medoxomil	Benicar	200 mg po qd	Same	herbal supplements
eprosartan	Teveten	400-800 mg po qd	Same	Same
telmisartan	Micardis	20-80 mg po qd	Same	warfarin, digoxin

MAJOR SIDE EFFECTS OF ANGIOTENSIN II RECEPTOR ANTAGONISTS: telmisartan: URI, dizziness, back pain, diarrhea, sinusitis.

ACE, Angiotensin-converting enzyme; *IV,* intravenous; *MAO,* monoamine oxidase; *MI,* myocardial infarction; *NSAIDs,* nonsteroidal antiinflammatory drugs; *URI,* upper respiratory infection.

TABLE 27-9 *Angiotensin Converting Enzyme (ACE) Inhibitors Used for Hypertension*

GENERIC NAME	TRADE NAME	USUAL ADULT DOSE, ROUTE, AND FREQUENCY OF ADMINISTRATION	INDICATIONS FOR USE	DRUG INTERACTIONS
benazepril	Lotensin	5-40 mg/day po	Hypertension	alcohol and diuretics
captopril	Capoten	25-100 mg/day po		
enalapril	Vasotec	5-40 mg/day po		
fosinopril	Monopril	10-40 mg/day po		
lisinopril	Prinivil, Zestril	10-40 mg/day po		
moexipril	Univasc	7.5-30 mg/day po		
quinapril	Accupril	10-80 mg/day po		
ramipril	Altace	2.5-20 mg/day po		
trandolapril	Mavik	1-4 mg po qd	Same	Same
perindopril	Aceon	2-8 mg/day po	For use with thiazides	None identified

MAJOR SIDE EFFECTS: Dry nonproductive cough, headaches, diarrhea, constipation, loss of taste, weakness, dizziness, joint pain, upper respiratory infections; **trandolapril:** dyspepsia, cough, syncope, myalgia.

TABLE 27-10 *Vasodilators*

GENERIC NAME	TRADE NAME	USUAL ADULT DOSE, ROUTE, AND FREQUENCY OF ADMINISTRATION	INDICATIONS FOR USE	DRUG INTERACTIONS
hydralazine	Apresoline	10-50 mg po, IM, IV	Hypertension	diuretics
minoxidil	Loniten	Up to 100 mg/day po		NSAIDs, nitrates, guanethidine

MAJOR SIDE EFFECTS: Headaches, anorexia, constipation, dizziness, nasal congestion.

NSAIDs, Nonsteroidal antiinflammatory drugs.

Calcium Channel Blockers

Calcium channel blockers are used to treat angina, cardiac dysrhythmia, and hypertension. These medications interfere with the influx of calcium in the vascular and smooth muscles. Of most concern in the treatment of blood pressure is the action on the vascular muscle of the peripheral arterioles because peripheral vasodilation or decreased peripheral vascular resistance lowers blood pressure during rest and exercise. The calcium channel blockers approved by the FDA for the treatment of hypertension are listed in Table 27-11. Special considerations for use in the elderly are described in Box 27-4.

Patient Education for Compliance

1. Antihypertensives are lifelong medications because these agents control but do not cure hypertension.
2. Patients should report signs of peripheral edema when taking calcium channel blockers.
3. Antihypertensives may cause drowsiness, dizziness, or lightheadedness.

IMPORTANT FACTS ABOUT ANTIHYPERTENSIVES

- Lack of patient compliance is the major cause of treatment failure of antihypertensive therapy. Medication and lifestyle compliance is difficult to achieve because hypertension is a silent disease that progresses slowly but requires lifelong, expensive treatment.
- β-Blockers and diuretics are the preferred drugs for the initial therapy of hypertension.
- β-Blockers reduce blood pressure primarily by reducing peripheral vascular resistance.
- Vasodilators and calcium channel blockers reduce blood pressure by promoting dilation of arterioles.
- When a combination of drugs is used for hypertension, each drug in the combination should have a different mechanism of action.
- ACE inhibitors are used to treat hypertension, congestive heart failure, and myocardial infarctions.
- Calcium channel blockers cause vasodilation and are therefore useful in hypertension and angina.
- Calcium channel blockers and β-blockers have similar therapeutic effects.

TABLE 27-11 *Calcium Channel Blockers Used to Treat Hypertension*

GENERIC NAME	TRADE NAME	USUAL ADULT DOSE, ROUTE, AND FREQUENCY OF ADMINISTRATION	INDICATIONS FOR USE	DRUG INTERACTIONS
amlodipine with benazepril	Lotrel	2.5-10 mg/day po	Hypertension and angina pectoris	β-blockers (both systemic and ophthalmologic) digitalis, disopyramide potassium-depleting medications, quinidine procainamide
	Norvasc	2.5/10-5/20 mg po per day		
diltiazem	Cardizem, Tiazac	30-360 mg po tid-qid		
felodipine	Plendil	5-10 mg po qd		
isradipine	DynaCirc	Up to 20 mg/day po		
mibefradil	Posicor	50-100 mg/day po		
nicardipine	Cardene	20-40 mg po tid		
nifedipine	Procardia, Adalat, Cardilate	30-90 mg/day po		
nisoldipine	Sular	10-20 mg/day po		
verapamil	Calan, Isoptin	80-120 mg po tid		
	Calan SR, Isoptin SR	180-480 mg/day po		
nimodipine	Nimotop	30 mg po q4h × 21 days	Same	rifampin, erythromycin, antifungal agents, grapefruit

MAJOR SIDE EFFECTS: Nausea, headache, dizziness, swelling of ankles and feet, dry mouth, tachycardia.

BOX 27-4	SPECIAL CONSIDERATIONS FOR USE OF CALCIUM CHANNEL BLOCKERS IN THE ELDERLY

The elderly are more susceptible to calcium channel blocking agents and have an increased occurrence of side effects such as weakness, dizziness, fainting, and falls.

Nitrates may be used with these medications, but an increased frequency and intensity of anginal attacks should be reported to the physician.

Smoking and nicotine reduce the effectiveness of these medications. Smoking should be avoided.

Use of alcohol may lead to hypotensive episodes; thus alcohol consumption should be avoided.

Gradual withdrawal is recommended with calcium channel blocking agents.

Diseases of the Blood Vessels and Their Treatment

Peripheral vascular disease is common among the elderly. The extremities become cold or numb, with **intermittent claudication** and ulcers. Usually caused by either atherosclerosis or hyperlipidemia, arteriosclerosis reduces blood flow to tissues, blood viscosity is elevated due to fat content, and the flow of blood to the tissues is diminished. The red cells are less flexible, and the lack of oxygen causes limitation of blood flow and cell exchange of oxygen and carbon dioxide on exercise, resulting in intermittent claudication, with ischemia and pain. Peripheral vasodilators have a relaxing effect on the smooth muscles of peripheral arterial walls found in skeletal muscles while having little effect on cutaneous blood flow. *Isoxsuprine* (Vasodilan) may relieve the symptoms associated with the constricting of peripheral blood vessels (Table 27-12).

Hemorrheologic Agents

Hemorrheologic agents improve the flow of blood and lower the viscosity of blood in the peripheral tissues. *Pentoxifylline* (Trental) is a hemorrheologic agent used for therapy of peripheral vascular disorders. This drug improves blood flow through rigid arteriosclerotic and atherosclerotic blood vessels and improves microcirculation. *Cilostazol* (Pletal) is the second medication in this category for use to reduce intermittent claudication that comes with walking distances (see Table 27-12).

Hyperlipidemia and Its Treatment

Some cholesterol and triglycerides are necessary for the formation of cell membrane and nerve tissue, as well as being found in plasma proteins. However, excessive dietary intake of lipids is stored as fat in adipose tissue to be reserved for energy use. Cholesterol is also stored in the

TABLE 27-12 *Drugs Used with Peripheral Vascular Diseases*

GENERIC NAME	TRADE NAME	USUAL ADULT DOSE, ROUTE, AND FREQUENCY OF ADMINISTRATION	INDICATIONS FOR USE	DRUG INTERACTIONS
PERIPHERAL VASODILATORS				
cyclandelate	Cyclospasmol	10-40 mg/day C 1 wk	Peripheral vascular disease	None
isoxsuprine	Vasodilan	10-20 mg tid-qid		
bosentan	Tracleer	62.5 mg-125 mg po bid	cyclosporine, glyburide	

MAJOR SIDE EFFECTS OF PERIPHERAL VASODILATORS: Orthostatic hypotension, flushing, dizziness, weakness, nausea, palpitations, tachycardia.

GENERIC NAME	TRADE NAME	DOSE		DRUG INTERACTIONS
HEMORRHEOLOGIC AGENTS				
pentoxifylline	Trental	400 mg tid		Other antihypertensives
cilostazol	Pletal	100 mg bid		erythromycin, diltiazem, omeprazole, ketoconazole

MAJOR SIDE EFFECTS OF HEMORRHEOLOGIC AGENTS: Dizziness, headache, abdominal distress, nausea, vomiting.

gallbladder as a part of bile acids. Excessive circulation of lipids leads to hyperlipidemia with increased concentrations of cholesterol and triglycerides that are associated with atherosclerosis. This condition leads to obstruction of blood flow and to CAD. The large- and medium-sized arteries are those usually involved with these degenerative changes. The lipids do not circulate freely in the bloodstream but instead bind to plasma proteins (albumin and globulin) to form lipoproteins.

Lipoproteins are classified by their density. The three primary groups are **very low density lipoproteins (VLDLs), low-density lipoproteins (LDLs),** and **high-density lipoproteins (HDLs).** VLDL particles are secreted by the liver, becoming smaller as the triglycerides are removed. LDLs contain the major portion of blood cholesterol and are considered to be the most harmful in the individual developing atherosclerosis. HDLs are the smallest and densest of the lipoproteins. Their function is to transport cholesterol from the peripheral cells to the liver for metabolism and excretion. Because HDL is a transport aid to rid the body of lipoproteins, the higher the HDL level, the more beneficial. This transport of lipoproteins prevents the accumulation of lipids in the arterial walls.

Adults should undergo periodic (at least every 5 years) cholesterol testing because of the clear relationship between LDL and atherosclerosis with resultant CAD. An HDL level below 35 mg/dL is considered to put a person at risk for CAD. The decision to provide medications to lower blood cholesterol is based on LDL levels, with the desired levels being below 130 mg/dL. When the level is above 130 mg/dL, the person should be treated therapeutically, especially when other risk factors for CAD such as hypertension, diabetes, and low HDL levels have been found. Familial history of CAD and aging may require further interventions such as medications.

Treatment of Hyperlipidemia

The first step in treatment is diet modification and reduction of risk factors due to lifestyle—stop smoking, have a less sedentary lifestyle, and reduce obesity. Medications are used only if diet modification and exercise programs fail to reduce LDL to acceptable levels. When medications are initiated, diet therapy must continue. For optimum medication therapy, LDL levels will be reduced without reducing HDL levels. Once begun, the antihyperlipidemic agents are continued lifelong because LDL will return to high levels if these drugs are discontinued. The treatment is prophylaxis—preventing and retarding arteriosclerosis rather than causing regression of a disease process that has occurred.

Hypolipidemics or antihyperlipidemics are the group of medications used in adjuvant therapy to reduce elevated cholesterol levels in patients with hypercholesteremia and high LDL levels. Two major categories of hypolipidemics are bile acid sequestrants and HMG-CoA reductase inhibitors. Other medications are also used for various effects on lipoproteins including combinations of medications to treat more than one condition (Table 27-13).

TABLE 27-13 *Hypolipidemics*

GENERIC NAME	TRADE NAME	USUAL ADULT DOSE, ROUTE, AND FREQUENCY OF ADMINISTRATION	INDICATIONS FOR USE	DRUG INTERACTIONS
BILE ACID-BINDING RENIN				
cholestyramine	Questran, Prevalite	4-6 g/day po	Hyperlipidemia; reduction of LDL and cholesterol	anticoagulants, digoxin thiazides, penicillin propranolol, aspirin tetracyclines, folic acid thyroid hormones
colestipol	Colestid	15-30 g/day po in single or divided doses		

MAJOR SIDE EFFECTS OF BILE ACID-BINDING RENIN: Constipation, indigestion, abdominal pain, nausea/vomiting, dizziness, headache, gallstones.

GENERIC NAME	TRADE NAME	USUAL ADULT DOSE	INDICATIONS	DRUG INTERACTIONS
STATINS				alcohol, niacin cyclosporin,
atorvastatin	Lipitor	10-80 mg po qid		digitalis, erythromycin,
fluvastatin	Lescol	20-40 mg/day po		rifampin anticoagulants,
lovastatin	Mevacor	20-80 mg/day po		oral contraceptives
pravastatin	Pravachol	10-40 mg/day po		propranolol
simvastatin	Zocor	10-80 mg po hs		
resuvastatin	Crestor	5-10 mg po daily		

MAJOR SIDE EFFECTS OF STATINS: Headache, flatulence, constipation, abdominal pain, cramping, dyspepsia.

GENERIC NAME	TRADE NAME	USUAL ADULT DOSE	INDICATIONS	DRUG INTERACTIONS
MISCELLANEOUS HYPOLIPIDEMICS				
nicotinic acid (niacin)	Nicobid, Niacor	1-2 g po bid-tid	Elevated cholesterol or triglyceride levels	
gemfibrozil	Lopid	1200 mg/day po ac morning and evening meal	Elevated triglyceride levels	statins, anticoagulants
clofibrate	Atromid-S	2 g/day po in divided doses	Primary hyperlipidemia	
ezetimibe	Zetia	10 mg qd		cyclosporine, bile acid sequestrants
fenofibrate	Tricor, Lofibra	54-160 mg po qd		warfarin, bile acid sequestrants, cyclosporine

MAJOR SIDE EFFECTS OF MISCELLANEOUS HYPOLIPIDEMICS: nicotinic acid: flushing, itching, nausea/vomiting, diarrhea; **gemfibrozil:** GI symptoms, dizziness, blurred vision, muscle pain and weakness; **clofibrate:** headache, diarrhea, skin rash; **ezetimibe:** fatigue, arthralgia, myalgia, dizziness, headache, diarrhea; **fenofibrate:** fatigue, arthralgia, headache, insomnia, dyspepsia, rash, pruritus.

GENERIC NAME	TRADE NAME	USUAL ADULT DOSE	INDICATIONS	DRUG INTERACTIONS
COMBINATION HYPOLIPIDEMICS				
ezetimibe/simvastatin	Vytorin	10/10-10/80 mg po qd	Familial hyperlipidemia	Antifungals, erythromycin, clarithromycin, amiodarone, verapamil
amlodipine/ atorvastatin	Caduet	5/10-10/80 mg po qd	Hyperlipidemia, hypertension	Same as statins and as above

MAJOR SIDE EFFECTS OF COMBINATION HYPOLIPIDEMICS: Headache, gallstones, myalgia.

- *Bile acid sequestrants* such as cholestyramine (Questran) are nonabsorbable medications used for their cholesterol-lowering effect because cholesterol is the major precursor of bile acids. These medications bind bile acids to the intestine to prevent their absorption by producing an insoluble complex that is excreted in the feces, reducing LDLs and serum cholesterol. The bile acid sequestrant medications, used for primary hypercholesterolemia, must be used with care by patients with pancreatitis, hypothyroidism, gallstones, CAD, or hemorrhoids. Because of the binding and loss of fats, deficiencies in vitamins A, D, K, and E may occur.

- *HMG CoA reductase inhibitors*, or statins, are the most effective agents for lowering LDL and cholesterol levels and cause few adverse reactions. Therefore these agents such as atorvastatin (Lipitor) and simvastatin (Zocor) are the most widely used. Because this family of medications has *-statin* in the generic name, the family is described as the "statins." Statins reduce the liver enzyme HMG CoA reductase that is necessary in cholesterol production. Patient responses for lowering elevated levels of LDL cholesterol are dose dependent. Low doses provide smaller decrease, and larger doses may reduce production of the enzyme by 45%. These medications must be continued for life to reduce the progression of CAD, decrease the number of cardiac problems, and decrease mortality (see Table 27-13).

- *Nicotinic acid* (Nicobid) reduces LDL and VLDL levels and raises HDL levels, but its use is limited by side effects. Triple therapy consisting of nicotinic acid plus bile acid–binding resin and a statin may decrease LDL cholesterol levels by 70% or more. Side effects diminish after several weeks of use and can be lessened by taking aspirin 30 minutes prior to nicotinic acid administration (see Table 27-13).

- *Fibric acid derivatives* are used to lower triglycerides and raise HDL levels.
  - *Gemfibrozil* (Lopid) is a derivative of fibric acid that decreases triglyceride and VLDL levels and raises HDL levels. Inhibiting the breakdown of fats into triglycerides and decreasing the hepatic production of triglycerides make this drug the preferred product for use in patients with hypertriglyceridemia when triglyceride levels can exceed 1000 mg/dL (normal is 10 to 190 mg/dL). It may be used together with other hypolipidemic drugs (see Table 27-13).

- *Clofibrate* (Atromid-S) decreases blood levels of triglycerides and VLDL. It has failed to reduce the mortality from CAD and has a narrow window of success in most patients (see Table 27-13).

With all hypolipidemics and associated medications, patient compliance is essential. For long-term benefit of cholesterol and LDL reduction and the prevention of CAD, the dosing and scheduling of medications should be individualized to the patient because of possible adverse effects. Serum levels of lipoproteins and liver enzymes should be drawn regularly to be sure the desired effect is being obtained while the adverse effects are not.

Patient Education for Compliance

1. Diet modifications should be carefully followed before using hypolipidemics. Drug therapy alone will not significantly lower blood lipoprotein levels.
2. Cholestyramine (Questran or Prevalite) powder must be mixed with 4 to 6 oz of water or a noncarbonated beverage. The powder should not be ingested in dry form.
3. Colestipol (Colestid) granules will not dissolve in thin liquids and should be mixed with thick liquids for ingestion.

IMPORTANT FACTS ABOUT HYPOLIPIDEMICS

- LDLs transport cholesterol to the peripheral tissue; HDLs transport cholesterol to the liver.
- Diet modification is the primary method for reducing LDL and cholesterol levels. Drugs are used only if diet modification is unsuccessful.
- Statins are the most effective drugs for lowering LDL and cholesterol levels. These medications cause the least side effects.
- Bile acid–binding resins prevent the reabsorption of bile acids in the intestines. They cause constipation and other GI effects.
- Oral medications should be given 1 hour prior to bile acid-binding resins or 4 hours after, to allow for absorption without interference from the hypolipidemics.

Medications That Affect Coagulation

Clot formation to prevent further loss of blood from wounds is necessary for survival with injuries or surgery. This **hemostasis** is necessary for homeostasis. Occasionally the body will form clots or thrombi that jam blood vessels, causing **thromboembolism.** A **thrombus** is a blood clot within a blood vessel, whereas an **embolus** is a mass of undissolved matter in the vessel that moves through the circulatory system (Figure 27-8). Anticoagulants are used to prevent venous clotting in patients with thrombohemolytic disorders. Thrombolytic agents dissolve clots and are used most frequently in hospital settings. Therefore these agents are discussed only briefly here. Antiplatelet drugs are used to keep platelets from clumping (or aggregating) and are used on a regular basis in ambulatory care.

Thrombolytic medications promote the dissolution of thrombi. Anticoagulants disrupt the coagulation process and suppress the formation of fibrin. Antiplatelet drugs prevent platelets from forming a plug by inhibiting their aggregation. Antiplatelet medications are most effective in preventing the formation of arterial thrombi, whereas anticoagulants are used to prevent the formation of venous thrombi.

Anticoagulants

Anticoagulants may be given parenterally, as heparin, or orally, as warfarin (Coumadin). Heparin must be given by injection and is safe for use in pregnancy because it does not cross the placenta. Heparin has an almost immediate onset, but a short duration of action. Therefore this agent is usually used in inpatient conditions or in intravenous tubing where blood clotting is a possibility, such as dialysis.

Oral anticoagulants are used to prevent thrombosis and have a delayed onset of action. Therefore they are not appropriate in emergency situations. Rather, these agents are used prophylactically for deep vein thrombosis or to prevent thrombus formation in such diseases as atrial fibrillation or pulmonary embolus and with heart valve replacement surgery. These medications are effective when given orally, and they can be given once a day or less when the maintenance dose has been established.

DID YOU KNOW?

Warfarin was first found in spoiled silage that caused cattle to bleed. When first developed, it was used to kill rats and is still one of the most widely used products for eliminating rodents.

Warfarin

The oldest and most used anticoagulant medication is warfarin, an antagonist to vitamin K—the factor necessary for clotting factors to work. Medication levels peak a few days after initiation of treatment, and the drug remains in the body for 2 to 5 days after the drug is discontinued. A prothrombin time is necessary to evaluate the dosage of medication being administered. The patient must be carefully watched for bruising, bloody stools, bleeding gums, and blood in the urine. The long list of interactions is included in Table 27-14. An overdose is treated with vitamin K therapy.

Antiplatelet Medications

Antiplatelet drugs are used to suppress **aggregation** of platelets. The most frequently used antiplatelet medication is aspirin. It has been proved effective in preventing myocardial infarctions and strokes. The dosage is low, with increased doses offering no further therapeutic advantages.

Other medications used as antiplatelet therapy are as follows:

- *Clopidogrel* (Plavix), which is used in patients who have recently had an MI or a stroke or have established peripheral vascular disease as secondary prevention of further disease processes, complications, or deaths for those with atherosclerosis. Dentists or surgeons should be informed if the person is taking the medication to prevent excessive bleeding.
- *Ticlopidine* (Ticlid), which is more expensive than aspirin and is no more prophylactic.
- *Dipyridamole* (Persantine) also decreases platelet aggregation and is used in combination with warfarin in heart valve replacement surgery (Table 27-15).

Thrombolytic Medications

Thrombolytic medications are used to dissolve blood clots, or thrombi, that have already formed and are effective for the treatment of myocardial infarction if given within 6 hours of the onset of chest pain. Five thrombolytic drugs are available: *streptokinase* (Streptase), *alteplase* (Activase), *urokinase* (Abbokinase), *reteplase* (Retavase), and *anistreplase* (Eminase). These medications are given in a hospital setting by health care providers experienced in caring for patients with thrombi.

Topical Hemostatics

Topical hemostatics are gelatin or cellulose sponges employed to absorb excess blood and fluids and to control bleeding during oral, ophthalmic, or prostate surgery. These agents expand on

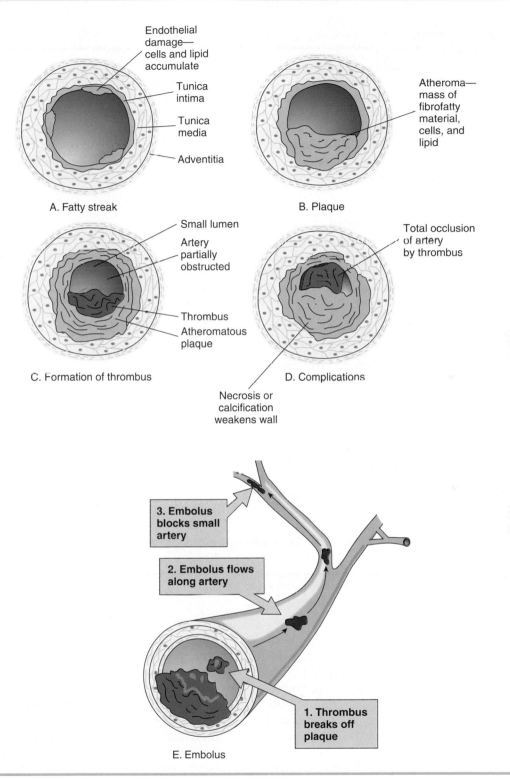

Figure 27-8   Thrombus and embolus. (From Frazier MS, Drzymkowski JW: *Essentials of human diseases and conditions*, ed 4, St Louis, 2008, Saunders.)

TABLE 27-14 *Anticoagulants*

GENERIC NAME	TRADE NAME	USUAL ADULT DOSE, ROUTE, AND FREQUENCY OF ADMINISTRATION	INDICATIONS FOR USE	DRUG INTERACTIONS
heparin		Individualized IV, deep SC	Prophylaxis of venous thrombi	antiplatelet medications
warfarin	Coumadin	2.5-10 mg/day po × 4 days, then individualized dependent on prothrombin time		NSAIDs, diuretics, thrombolytics, antacids, allopurinol, cimetidine, tricyclic antidepressants, antibiotics, estrogen, oral hypoglycemics, barbiturates
enoxaparin	Lovenox	Individualized	Same	Same

MAJOR SIDE EFFECTS: heparin: bleeding tendencies; **warfarin, enoxaparin:** excessive bleeding, alopecia, GI disturbances, dermatitis.

GI, Gastrointestinal; *IV,* intravenous; *NSAIDs,* nonsteroidal antiinflammatory drugs; *SC,* subcutaneous.

TABLE 27-15 *Antiplatelet Drugs*

GENERIC NAME	TRADE NAME	USUAL ADULT DOSE, ROUTE, AND FREQUENCY OF ADMINISTRATION	INDICATIONS FOR USE	DRUG INTERACTIONS
aspirin[†]	Bayer, etc.	325 mg/day or less po	Prevention of arterial thromboses by preventing platelet aggregation	oral anticoagulants, ACE inhibitors, diltiazem
ticlopidine*	Ticlid	250 mg po bid		None indicated
dipyridamole*	Persantine	50-100 mg po qid		
clopidogrel*	Plavix	75 mg po qd (same dosage for elderly)		NSAIDs, phenytoin, warfarin, tamoxifen, tolbutamide, torsemide

MAJOR SIDE EFFECTS: ticlopidine: GI disturbances, skin reactions, hematologic depression; **clopidogrel:** Flulike symptoms, fatigue, arthralgia.

ACE, Angiotensin-converting enzyme; *NSAIDs,* nonsteroidal antiinflammatory drugs.
* Prescription medication.
[†] OTC medication.

contact with wounds to absorb large amounts of blood and permit clotting to occur along the surfaces. These hemostatics are applied topically and are ultimately absorbed by the body. Oxidized cellulose cannot be used for permanent implants because it interferes with bone regeneration and may produce cyst formation.

- Absorbable gelatin foam (Gelfoam), absorbable gelatin film (Gelfilm), and absorbable gelatin powder (Gelfoam powder) are specially prepared nonantigenic preparations that are available in either strips or powders for complete absorption in 2 to 5 days when applied to the skin and 4 weeks to 5 months when applied to surgical wounds. These agents should be moistened with isotonic saline solutions or

thrombin solutions before being applied to a wound. The type and size of application depend on the site to be treated.

- Oxidized cellulose (Oxycel, Surgicel) is surgical gauze or cotton that exerts a hemostatic effect. The agent should not be used as a surface dressing because it inhibits the growth of epithelial tissue. No drug interactions have been reported. This dressing material is *not* premoistened. The chief uses are in removal of nasal polyps and other minor surgical procedures.
- Thrombin (Thrombinar, Thrombostat) is a sterile powder obtained from bovine prothrombin. It is used topically to treat capillary bleeding. There are no significant drug interactions.

TABLE 27-16 *Hematopoietic/Erythropoietic Stimulants*

GENERIC NAME	TRADE NAME	USUAL ADULT DOSE, ROUTE, AND FREQUENCY OF ADMINISTRATION	INDICATIONS FOR USE	DRUG INTERACTIONS
HEMATOPOIETIC AGENTS			Stimulate neutrophil production	
filgrastim	Neupogen	5 mcg/kg/d SC, IV		Concomitantly with antineoplastics
pegfilgrastim	Neulasta	6 mg SC once/ chemotherapy cycle		lithium

MAJOR SIDE EFFECTS OF HEMATOPOIETIC AGENTS: Fever, nausea/vomiting, skeletal pain.

ERYTHROPOIETIN AGENTS			Stimulate erythropoiesis, antianemic	
darbepoetin alfa	Aranesp	0.45 mg/kg SC for a single dose		androgens
epoetin	Epogen, Procrit	150 U/kg SC 3 times a week		Basically none

MAJOR SIDE EFFECTS OF ERYTHROPOIETIN AGENTS: darbepoetin alfa: Seizures, strokes, CHF, MI, diarrhea, nausea, fatigue, fever, bone pain, myalgia, dyspnea; **epoetin:** Seizures, coldness, sweating, hypertension, bone pain, headache.

CHF, Congestive heart failure; *IV*, intravenous; *MI*, myocardial infarction; *SC*, subcutaneous.

Patient Education for Compliance

1. The patient taking anticoagulants must be careful to avoid injury by using a soft toothbrush to clean the teeth and an electric razor to shave.
2. Prothrombin levels should be regularly evaluated when on anticoagulant therapy.

IMPORTANT FACTS ABOUT MEDICATIONS THAT AFFECT COAGULATION

- Hemostasis occurs with the formation of the platelet plug followed by coagulation.
- Arterial thrombi are best prevented with antiplatelet drugs; venous thrombi are prevented with anticoagulants.
- Heparin is administered subcutaneously.
- Warfarin is the prototype for oral anticoagulants. It acts by blocking the biosynthesis of vitamin K.
- Aspirin and other antiplatelet drugs suppress thrombus formation.

Medications Used as Hematopoietics and Erythropoietics

Hematopoietic stimulants are given to increase the level of white blood cells in the body, stimulating the bone marrow to produce more leukocytes, especially neutrophils. By increasing the level of neutrophils, the body is better able to fight infections following the administration of chemotherapy. On the other hand, erythropoietin stimulators cause the bone marrow to produce more erythrocytes and reduce the need for blood transfusions following hemodialysis or therapy that produces anemia. Anemia may be the result of the decrease of erythropoietin, a protein that is produced by the kidneys. These medications are administered parenterally and are expensive treatment options. Doses can be adjusted as needed to meet the needs of the patient (Table 27-16).

Summary

Cardiovascular disease is the leading cause of death in the United States. Some medications are effective on the myocardium itself, whereas others are effective on the blood vessels of the vascular system. The three actions of medications on the cardiac muscle are *inotropic* (force of myocardial contraction), *dromotropic* (conduction of the electrical impulses through the heart muscle), and *chronotropic* (the heart rate). Other medications cause vasodilation, to lessen the work of the heart. As CAD occurs (e.g., arteriosclerosis or atherosclerosis), medications are used to increase the circulation and to supply sufficient myocardial action for adequate pumping of the heart to move blood through the body.

Vasodilators such as nitrates increase the size of blood vessels to improve circulation of the blood. Nitrates are used as antianginal agents. β-Blockers and calcium channel blockers are also used in the long-term management of angina; they slow the heart and interfere with calcium movement through the cell membranes of the vascular smooth muscle. The therapeutic goal of angina treatment is to reduce the frequency and intensity of the attacks.

Cardiac glycosides, or digitalis preparations, are used to increase the force of myocardial contractions in congestive heart failure, increase the strength of contractions, slow the heart rate, and slow the conduction of electrical impulses to the heart. The efficiency of the heart is increased without increasing oxygen consumption. The glycosides tend to decrease heart rate; therefore the patient should be taught to take his or her pulse daily before taking digitalis preparations. If the pulse is below 60, the physician should be notified to decide if the patient should take the medication.

Antidysrhythmics are used to treat disorders of cardiac rhythm that occur from CAD, electrolyte imbalances, cardiac conduction abnormalities, or even from endocrine diseases such as thyroid disorders. The dysrhythmias may have little effect on cardiac output or may cause severe compromise of cardiac pumping. The medications change the electrophysiologic properties of the heart by regulating the calcium, sodium, and potassium ions that flow into the heart muscle.

Antihypertensive medications include diuretics, ACE inhibitors, β-blockers, sympatholytic agents, and vasodilators. Medications are used only when lifestyle changes have not adequately lowered elevated blood pressure. Combinations of medicines may be required, and each new drug should come from a different therapeutic category. The patient must be aware that the treatment for hypertension is lifelong therapy of lifestyle changes or medications, or both.

For diseases of the peripheral vascular system, vasodilators have a relaxing effect on the smooth muscles of the peripheral arterial walls to alleviate the symptoms of atherosclerosis or hyperlipidemia. Hemorrheologic agents are used to improve the blood flow through the rigid arteriosclerotic blood vessels and through microcirculation of the arterioles, venules, and capillaries. To reduce the circulating lipoproteins and to alleviate the hypercholesterolemia that leads to obstruction of the blood flow, hypolipidemics are used for long-term therapy along with lifestyle changes.

Anticoagulants are used to treat deep venous thrombosis by disrupting the coagulation process and the formation of fibrin. Antiplatelet medications inhibit the aggregation of platelets to prevent the formation of arterial thrombi. Aspirin is often used for its antiplatelet properties.

The hematopoietic and erythropoietic agents are used to increase the blood cells circulating in the blood when disease processes or treatment of a disease cause a drop in white or red blood cells. This treatment reduces the need for blood transfusions in persons taking chemotherapy, those on hemodialysis, or those with infections such as human immunodeficiency virus.

The many medications that affect the cardiovascular system and the blood disorders caused by thrombi formation are a major area in medical treatment today. Cardiac glycosides and nitrates are medicines that have been used for many years. The antihyperlipidemics are more recent additions for the prophylaxis of cardiac diseases. Nitrates, particularly nitroglycerin, come in various forms for use. Some are used as needed, whereas other forms are used on a daily basis, but the patient must be nitrate free at some point during the day to prevent the development of tolerance to the medication.

As more information is gathered about the leading cause of sickness and death—cardiovascular disease—the medications are changing rapidly. The lifelong need for treating hypertension continues. Vessel disease is still present, but prevention through lifestyle changes and medication will continue to improve the quality of life for those prone to cardiovascular disease in the United States.

Critical Thinking Exercises

SCENARIO

Mr. Jones has been diagnosed with essential hypertension. He asks how long he will need to take medications.

1. What do you tell him?
2. He also wants to know if there are any lifestyle changes that will help. Name several of these for Mr. Jones.
3. Given diuretics as his first medication, what foods does Mr Jones need to eat to help keep potassium at acceptable levels?
4. How often does Mr. Jones need to check his blood pressure?
5. Can other medications be added to help bring his blood pressure to within an acceptable range if diuretics alone do not accomplish this?

DRUG CALCULATIONS

1. Order: captopril 50 mg po qd in am
    Available medication:

    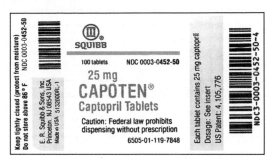

    Dose to be administered: _____

2. Order: Lanoxin 375 mcg po qam if P ↑60
    Available medication:

    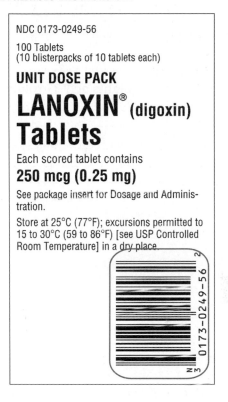

    Dose to be administered: _____

REVIEW QUESTIONS

1. How do cardiac glycosides work on heart tissue? _____
    _____
    _____

2. What chemical classification of medicines is used for anginal pain? _____
    _____
    _____

3. How do the cardiac glycosides work on the heart muscle in congestive heart failure? _____
    _____
    _____

4. What are the side effects of antidysrhythmics? _____
    _____
    _____

5. What are the five categories of medications used to treat hypertension? _____
    _____
    _____

6. What two categories of medications are used for the initial treatment of hypertension? _____
    _____
    _____

7. What is hyperlipidemia? What are the classifications of lipoproteins? _____
    _____
    _____

8. How do the statins decrease lipoprotein levels? _____
    _____
    _____

9. How do anticoagulants act? Thrombolytics? _____
    _____
    _____

10. How do antiplatelet medications stop thrombi? _____
    _____
    _____

CHAPTER 28

Urinary System Disorders

OBJECTIVES

After studying this chapter, you should be capable of doing the following:

- Discussing the need for specific electrolytes to achieve homeostasis and balance of extracellular and intracellular fluids.
- Describing how antiinfectives and antiseptics are used for urinary tract infections.
- Explaining the role of urinary tract analgesics and antispasmodics in the treatment of urinary tract conditions.
- Discussing enuresis and the medications used for its treatment.
- Discussing medications used for treating an overactive bladder (OAB).

Mrs. Smith calls to tell you that her 7-year-old son, James, is having a problem with bedwetting and she has tried withholding liquids at bedtime. This action does not seem to help James, and Dr. Merry orders DDAVP.
  What is the form of this medication?
  What side effects would be expected with this medication?
  What is the youngest age the Food and Drug Administration considers as safe for taking this medication?
  What other suggestions may be made to assist with the control of enuresis?

KEY TERMS

Anorexia	Incontinence	Pyuria
Ascites	Ion	Replacement therapy
Diuresis	Kernicterus	Solute
Dysuria	Lethargy	Solvent
Electrolyte	Oliguria	Urgency
Enuresis	Malaise	Urinary frequency
Hematuria	Nocturia	

EASY WORKING KNOWLEDGE OF INDICATIONS AND SIDE EFFECTS

Common Symptoms of Urinary System Disorders

Anorexia, nausea, vomiting
Malaise, fatigue, lethargy
Nocturia, hematuria, pyuria, proteinuria
Dysuria, urgency, frequency, incontinence
Pain in lumbar region or flank radiating into medial
  thighs, ranging from slight tenderness to intense pain
Fever
Edema and ascites
Respiratory symptoms and cardiovascular symptoms
  including hypertension and shortness of breath

Common Side Effects of Medications for Urinary System Disorders

Drying of secretions
Drowsiness and dizziness
Rash and urticaria
Gastrointestinal symptoms (nausea, vomiting, diarrhea)
Headaches
Bradycardia/tachycardia
Discolored urine

Easy Working Knowledge of Drugs for Urinary System Disorders

DRUG CLASS	PRESCRIPTION	OTC	PREGNANCY CATEGORY	MAJOR INDICATIONS
Diuretics (also see Chapter 27)	Yes	Yes	B, C	Hypertension and edema
Antiinfectives (also see Chapter 18)	Yes	No	B, C, D (sulfamethizole at term)	Urinary tract infections including pyelonephritis, cystitis, urethritis
Urinary tract antiseptics	Yes	Yes	B	Urinary tract irritation
Urinary tract antispasmodics	Yes	No	B	Genitourinary muscle relaxant
Medications for overactive bladder (OAB)	Yes	No	C	Treatment of OAB symptoms
Medications for enuresis	Yes	No	B	Enuresis in children older than 6

The urinary system is composed of organs that form and excrete urine: two kidneys, two ureters, a bladder, and a urethra. Urine is formed in the kidneys and then passes through two ureters into the urinary bladder for storage (Figure 28-1). The kidneys regulate homeostasis, maintain fluid and electrolyte balance, and eliminate bodily wastes through urine.

When the bladder is sufficiently filled (≈ 250 mL of urine), the person feels the urge to void, and urine voluntarily passes from the body through the urethra. When urine is retained for prolonged periods of time, urinary tract infections (UTIs) are more prevalent. In the male the urethra is surrounded by the prostate gland. If the prostate becomes enlarged, urine may be retained in the bladder because of constriction of the urethra. An enlarged prostate with retained urine is the main reason for bladder infections in older men. However, UTIs are more prevalent in women due to the proximity of the urethra, vagina, and anus, and the short length of the urethra. When medications have been ordered, the patient should be aware that urine can change color with the ingestion of certain drugs (Table 28-1). This is an important element in patient education with the use of urinary tract medications.

Diuretics

Diuretics (see Chapter 27 for use with cardiovascular diseases) modify kidney function to increase **diuresis.** When body fluids are lost, sodium, potassium, and chlorides are also lost. Among the most widely used of all drugs, diuretics are used to treat the edema that occurs with cirrhosis, nephrotic disease, renal failure, hypertension, and cardiovascular disease. The place of action depends on the segment of the nephron that is affected. The glomerulus filters the urine; the proximal tubule reabsorbs glucose, potassium, sodium, amino acids, water, and nutrients; and the loops of Henle reabsorb sodium and chlorides in the ascending portion. The distal tubule reabsorbs sodium and bicarbonates, with potassium, hydrogen, and ammonia being secreted (Figure 28-2). Finally, antidiuretic hormone (ADH) causes reabsorption of water in the collecting duct.

Diuretics are categorized by their site of action (see Figure 27-7). The thiazides are active in the diluting segments of the kidneys. The loop diuretics stop reabsorption of sodium and water in the loop of Henle. Distal tubule, or potassium-sparing, diuretics act at the distal renal tubules, blocking the reabsorption of sodium and the excretion of sodium and water while sparing the excretion of potassium. The osmotic diuretics help the flow of water from the body tissues to induce diuresis. (See Table 27-6 for selected diuretics and Table 27-7 for the combination medications.) These medications are included with the treatment of cardiovascular diseases because the prime agents for the treatment of hypertension and congestive heart failure are diuretics.

Fluid and Electrolyte Balance

The amount of water excreted in urine is under the direct influence of ADH and the concentration of waste products found in the urine. Approximately 60% of body weight is water as intracellular and extracellular fluids. Three fourths of body fluid is intracellular and is absolutely essential for metabolic reactions, whereas the largest portion of extracellular fluid is interstitial fluid. The intracellular fluid maintains the proper environment for homeostasis by supplying nutrients, oxygen, vitamins, and electrolytes and carrying off waste products.

- *Water* is the **solvent** in which body substances are dissolved. In infants, up to 75% of body

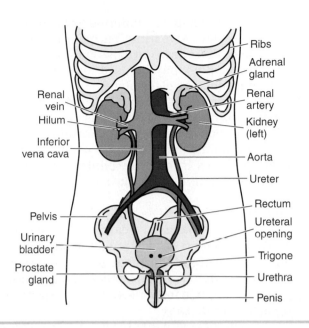

Figure 28-1 Components of the urinary system. (From Frazier MS, Drzymkowski JW: *Essentials of human diseases and conditions*, ed 4, St Louis, 2008, Saunders.)

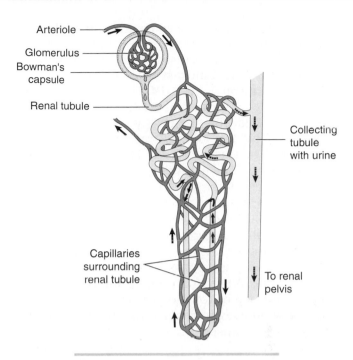

Figure 28-2 Anatomy of a nephron.

TABLE 28-1 *Medications That May Alter Urine Color*

DRUG	POSSIBLE COLOR CHANGES
amitriptyline (Elavil)	Blue-green
Anticoagulants containing warfarin	Pink, red, or dark brown (indicative of systemic bleeding)
cascara sagrada	In acidic urine, brown In alkaline urine, yellow to pink In standing urine, black
Iron salts	Brown to black
Laxatives containing senna or danthron	Pink to red to brown
Laxatives containing phenolphthalein	Pink to red
levodopa	Darkens urine and sweat
methyldopa	Pink or amber to dark urine
metronidazole	Dark urine
nitrofurantoin	Yellow to rusty brown
phenazopyridine	Orange-red urine that may stain clothes
phenytoin	Red-brown or darkened urine
phenothiazine	Pink, red, or orange urine
rifampin	Red, orange, or brown urine, saliva, sweat, or tears
Urised	blue–blue green

weight may be water; this percentage decreases with age. Infants and very young children are at greater risk for dehydration than older children and adults because of the high ratio of body surface area to body weight and immaturity of the kidneys. Obese persons also have less fluid because fat contains little water. The elderly and the obese are at risk for dehydration in situations where fluid loss occurs.

* **Electrolytes** are the substances dissolved in body fluids, called **solutes,** and are particles that develop an electrical charge when dissolved in water; examples are sodium, potassium, and chlorine. Electrolytes, or **ions,** are found inside and outside of cells. The fluids and electrolytes are acquired through food and water. Normally fluid gain is approximately equal to fluid loss. Abnormal conditions can result in loss of fluids or electrolytes, or both. This may allow for an abnormal loss of one electrolyte or excess fluids and the accumulation of another electrolyte in the body. When electrolytes or fluids are not present in normal amounts, **replacement therapy** is provided to return the body to homeostasis.

Replacement Therapy

When electrolytes are lost, replacement therapy is necessary to keep the body in fluid/electrolyte balance. Fluids and electrolytes are interdependent because as the amount of water in a body component increases, the concentration of electrolyte concentration decreases, and vice versa. To prevent loss of homeostasis, replacement therapy is indicated. The quickest way of replacement is through intravenous (IV) replacement (See Chapter 11 for information on the principles of IV therapy.) Replacement therapy may also be accomplished by oral administration, but this takes longer and is less efficient. The oral route for replacement is used in milder, chronic cases of imbalances such as diarrhea or excessive perspiration that do not require urgent and immediate treatment. Fluid and electrolyte imbalances usually occur at the same time and are corrected by giving fluids with the proper electrolytes and nutrients such as glucose, potassium, sodium, and chlorides. When oral rehydration is not practical or not efficient for the person's needs, the IV route may be used to replace the lost electrolytes and glucose because glucose aids in the absorption of electrolytes. (See Chapter 20 for a discussion of vitamins and minerals in the body and their replacement for homeostasis.) The allied health professional needs a working knowledge of the signs of electrolyte loss (Table 28-2). Electrolyte loss usu-

ally is the result of nausea, vomiting, renal disease, diarrhea, excessive sweating, burns, trauma, and the overuse of diuretics. Various fluid bases, such as water and saline, may be used for the addition of fluids, nutrients, or electrolytes.

When sodium and other electrolytes are lost during diuresis or disease conditions, fluid balance will also be affected. Sodium is the primary cation in interstitial fluids; thus when its concentration is reduced, fluid loss from extracellular sources occurs while still maintaining intracellular fluids.

- *Sodium* loss will cause the patient to experience nausea, **malaise,** weakness, headaches, and drowsiness. The usual treatment is oral administration of sodium or sodium chloride compounds. An increase in the pulse rate and blood pressure are good indications of the response to replacement therapy.

  In patients with nephrotic disease, heart failure, or cirrhosis and in patients using drugs such as corticosteroids and oral contraceptives, plasma levels of sodium may be excessive, causing edema and disease conditions such as congestive heart failure. In treating the underlying disease process, restriction of intake of salt and water is required and diuretics are given to increase the excretion of the excessive sodium and fluids.

- *Potassium* may be lost in the urine when diuretics are used, but more commonly it results from disorders of the gastrointestinal (GI) tract such as vomiting, diarrhea, or excessive use of laxatives. Respiratory or metabolic acidosis, corticosteroid therapy, and renal diseases may also lead to potassium depletion. When potassium is lost, cardiac muscle conduction and nerve impulse conduction is interrupted. As a regulator in many metabolic activities, potassium replacement is necessary to keep the body in homeostasis. Signs of potassium loss include apathy, weakness, mental disturbances, cardiac arrhythmias, and thirst. Potassium may be given through IV replacement therapy, as with sodium replacement, but oral replacement is preferred if possible. Oral preparations are less likely to cause excessive plasma levels of potassium. The preparations come in slow-release tablets, effervescent tablets, and liquid preparations. Perhaps the easiest way to replace small potassium losses is through dietary means such as by eating bananas, cabbage, dates, and raisins.

- *Calcium* deficits are associated with excessive losses from the GI tract, pancreatic diseases, and diseases of other body systems such as

TABLE 28-2 *Signs of Electrolyte Imbalances*

ELECTROLYTE	SIGNS
SODIUM	
Depletion	Lethargy, hypotension, stomach cramping, vomiting, diarrhea
Excess	Edema, hypertonicity, red flushed skin, dry mucous membranes, thirst, elevated temperature
POTASSIUM	
Depletion	Impaired skeletal muscle function, weakness, paralysis
Excess	Abdominal distention, weakness, diarrhea, paralysis
CALCIUM	
Depletion	Muscle cramping and twitching, numbness and tingling of fingers, toes, and lips
Excess	Anorexia, nausea, weakness, vomiting, coma, constipation, apathy, depression, stupor, cardiac contractility
MAGNESIUM	
Depletion	Cardiac dysrhythmias, neurotoxicity
Excess	Flushing, sweating, hypothermia, paralysis, muscle excitability, cardiac depression

parathyroid diseases. The signs are tingling of the extremities, muscle cramps, tetany, and possibly convulsions. Dietary calcium is increased, and oral calcium supplements may be added. Vitamin D therapy is frequently provided to enhance the absorption of calcium in the GI tract. A good source of calcium for elderly women is Tums or other calcium antacids. Excessive amounts of calcium caused by excessive vitamin D or calcium replacement produce **lethargy,** decreased muscle tone, and deep bone pain. The trauma patient with multiple fractures may also have an increase in calcium absorption with the same effects. Nausea, vomiting, **anorexia,** constipation, and kidney stones may result from excess calcium intake. The use of diuretics will cause calcium to be excreted from the body, resulting in decreased calcium levels in the blood. One of the signs of calcium depletion is muscle cramping for what seems to be an unknown reason.

- *Magnesium* deficits are usually the result of diet but may be caused by severe malnutrition, alcoholism, prolonged diarrhea, or intestinal malabsorption. People with magnesium deficits have neuromuscular excitability. Mild deficits are treated with the addition of foods that are rich in magnesium plus magnesium-based antacids. Excessive magnesium usually occurs in the setting of renal insufficiency. These patients must avoid antacids with a magnesium base. The signs of excessive magnesium are an increased sense of warmth, decreased deep tendon reflexes, low blood pressure, drowsiness, and lethargy. An electrocardiogram may show arrhythmias. Treatment is aimed at the cause of the excess absorption, but renal dialysis may be required.

Treating Urinary Tract Infections

Urinary tract infections (UTIs) are the most common bacterial infections reported in the United States. Between 10% and 20% of women experience a UTI during their lifetime. An upper UTI, in the kidneys and ureters, may cause pain in the lower back, flank, or stomach, with fever, sweating, headache, weakness, and nausea and vomiting. Lower UTIs in the bladder and urethra are associated with frequency, **urgency, dysuria, incontinence, hematuria,** and **oliguria.** These infections may be from cross-contamination from the GI tract, with *Escherichia coli* causing about 90% of all UTIs. Drug therapy for lower UTIs may be started before culture and sensitivity results are available because of the strong likelihood of GI contamination. If the symptoms of lower UTIs are related to dietary factors, strict adherence to a diet eliminating the irritating food should bring significant relief in a week to 10 days. (Box 28-1 lists common foods that irritate the bladder.) As the symptoms are relieved, the suspicious foods may be added back to the diet, one at a time. If the symptoms return, the patient can then identify the irritating food and avoid that food. As the foods are returned to the diet, significant amounts of water should be consumed to flush the kidneys of the irritants.

Drugs to Treat Urinary Tract Infections

Drugs used to treat UTIs and **pyuria** include antibacterials, antiseptics, and analgesics. Sulfonamides (see Chapter 18) are the most commonly prescribed antibacterial agents for UTIs. Sulfonamides suppress the synthesis of folic acid and are the drugs of choice because they have a high solubility in urine, achieve effective concentrations in the urinary tract, and are less expensive than the other antiinfectives. With recurrent infections, sulfonamides alone may not be sufficient. The systemic sulfonamides are divided into short-acting and intermediate-acting medications.

BOX 28-1   FOODS THAT IRRITATE THE BLADDER
The following foods are acidic and are considered irritants to the bladder. They should be avoided by persons who are prone to lower UTIs.
Alcoholic beverages
Guava
Apples and apple juice
Peaches
Cantaloupe
Pineapple
Carbonated beverages
Plums
Chili and other spicy foods
Strawberries
Chocolate
Sugar*
Citrus fruits
Tea
Coffee (including decaffeinated)
Tomatoes
Cranberries and cranberry juice
Vinegar
Grapes
Vitamin B complex

*Sugar seems to cause more problems in females than in males.

Short- and Intermediate-Acting Sulfonamides

The sulfonamides and TMP-SMZ (trimethoprim/ sulfamethoxazole) may be used to treat acute cystitis, acute urethral disease, acute pyelonephritis, and acute bacterial prostatitis. Long-term prophylaxis for recurrent UTIs is another use for the previously mentioned medications. Sulfonamides are used as first-line drugs in the treatment of UTIs because of lower cost. The short-acting sulfonamides, including *sulfisoxazole* (Gantrisin) and *sulfadiazine* (Microsulfon), are also included in the short-acting sulfa medications.

Intermediate-acting sulfonamides may also be used as needed depending on the extent of the infection. The only intermediate-acting sulfonamide is sulfamethoxazole (Gantanol), which has the same urinary indications for use as the short-acting medications. Because of its prolonged duration of action, it can be administered with less frequency (see Table 18-8).

Combination Sulfonamides

Trimethoprim (TMP) and sulfamethoxazole (SMZ) are marketed together as a fixed-dose combination known as TMP-SMZ (Co-Trimoxazole, Septra, Bactrim). This combination is a powerful antimicrobial and is used for uncomplicated UTIs. It is particularly useful for chronic or recurrent urinary tract infections and for prophylaxis (Table 28-3).

Other Antiinfectives

Penicillin, cephalosporins, tetracyclines, and fluoroquinolones may be added or used in conjunction with these medications for bacterial infections. (See Chapter 18 for specific discussion of the antimicrobials listed earlier.)

- Penicillins are also used against enteric-caused bacterial infections, but their usefulness is decreasing as *E. coli* strains resistant to penicillin increase.
- Cephalosporins are used for UTIs resistant to penicillin and TMP-SMZ, but these medications are relatively expensive.
- Tetracycline may be used to treat initial infections and chlamydial infections, but resistance to the tetracyclines develops rapidly. Candidal overgrowth occurs most frequently with the tetracyclines.
- Fluoroquinolones are broad-spectrum agents and are active against most organisms causing UTIs, but the cost is so expensive that it is prohibitive for some patients (see Table 28-3).

Patient Education for Compliance

1. Sulfonamides should be taken on an empty stomach with a full glass of water.
2. The entire course of treatment for a UTI should be completed, even though the symptoms may have improved.
3. Care should be taken to avoid prolonged exposure to sunlight when taking sulfonamides. If it is necessary to be in the sun, a sunscreen should be worn.
4. Drink eight to ten 8-oz glasses of water a day while taking sulfonamides.

IMPORTANT FACTS ABOUT MEDICATIONS TO TREAT URINARY TRACT INFECTIONS

- *E. coli* is the most common cause of uncomplicated UTIs.
- Most UTIs can be treated on an outpatient basis with oral medications.
- Sulfonamides are the drugs of choice for UTIs, and TMP-SMZ is the preferred medication.
- Sulfonamides should be discontinued at the first sign of a hypersensitivity reaction.
- Sulfonamides may increase the effects of warfarin and oral hypoglycemics, and a reduction in their dosage may be necessary.
- Prophylaxis for a UTI may be achieved with low doses of trimethoprim, TMP-SMZ, or urinary antiseptics.

Urinary Tract Antiseptics

The most commonly used urinary tract antiseptics are nitrofurantoin (Furadantin, Macrobid, and Macrodantin); methenamine (Mandelamine, Hiprex, Urex); and cinoxacin (Cinobac). These agents, used for prophylaxis and for treatment of upper UTIs, are medications of second choice, with their primary use being in the lower urinary tract (see Table 18-9). The urinary tract antiseptics exert antibacterial activity in the urine but have little or no systemic antibacterial effects.

- Cinoxacin (Cinobac) inhibits the replication of bacterial DNA and thus is bactericidal.

TABLE 28-3 *Drugs Used to Treat Urinary Tract Disorders*

GENERIC NAME	TRADE NAME	USUAL ADULT DOSE, ROUTE, AND FREQUENCY OF ADMINISTRATION	INDICATIONS FOR USE	DRUG INTERACTIONS
SHORT-ACTING SULFONAMIDES			Urinary tract infections	
sulfisoxazole	Gantrisin	500-1000 mg qid po, IM, SC, IV		Usually none
sulfadiazine	Microsulfon	250 mg po, IM tid		Usually none
MAJOR SIDE EFFECTS OF SHORT-ACTING SULFONAMIDES: Nausea, vomiting, rashes.				
INTERMEDIATE-ACTING SULFONAMIDES			Urinary tract infections	
sulfamethoxazole	Gantanol	1 g po bid to tid		Usually none
SULFONAMIDE COMBINATIONS			Urinary tract infections	
trimethoprim-sulfamethoxazole (TMP-MZ)	Septra, Bactrim, Cotrim	250 mg po qid		Usually none
	Septra DS, Bactrim DS	500 mg po bid		
MAJOR SIDE EFFECTS OF SULFONAMIDE COMBINATIONS: Nausea, vomiting, rashes.				
URINARY TRACT ANALGESICS				
phenazopyridine	Pyridium* AZO†	100-200 mg po tid 100 mg po tid	Urinary tract irritation	Usually none
pentosan	Elmiron	100 mg po tid	Interstitial cystitis	Usually none
DRUGS FOR OVERACTIVE BLADDER				
tolterodine	Detrol*, Detrol LA	2 mg po bid 2-4 mg po qd	Urinary antispasmodic	None
trospium	Sanctura	20 mg po bid		alcohol
solifenacin	Vesicare	5-10 mg po qd		
darifenacin	Enablex	7.5-15 mg po qd		
MAJOR SIDE EFFECTS OF DRUGS FOR OVERACTIVE BLADDER: Dry mouth, constipation, blurred vision, dyspepsia.				
URINARY TRACT ANTISPASMODICS				
flavoxate	Urispas	100-200 mg po tid	Genitourinary muscle relaxant	None
oxybutynin chloride	Ditropan	5 mg po bid–tid	Urinary antispasmodic	antihistamines
MAJOR SIDE EFFECTS OF URINARY TRACT ANTISPASMODICS: oxybutynin chloride: dry mouth, constipation.				
DRUGS TO TREAT ENURESIS				
imipramine	Tofranil*	6-12 yr: 25 mg po 1 hr prior to hs >12 yr: 75 mg po 1 hr prior to hs	Enuresis in persons older than 6 yr	alcohol, phenothiazine, cimetidine, clonidine, phenytoin
desmopressin	DDAVP*	mg po hs 10-40 mcg by nasal spray hs		carbamazepine, chlorpropamide demeclocycline
MAJOR SIDE EFFECTS OF DRUGS TO TREAT ENURESIS: imipramine: drowsiness, fatigue, dry mouth, blurred vision, constipation, impaired concentration; **desmopressin:** headaches, nosebleeds, increased blood pressure, sore throat.				

IM, Intramuscular; *IV,* intravenous; *SC,* subcutaneous.

*Prescription medication.

† OTC medication.

- Methenamine (Mandelamine, Hiprex) works by releasing formaldehyde for bactericidal or bacteriostatic effects. Because of its wide spectrum and low toxicity, methenamine is the drug of choice for long-term suppression of infections.
- Nitrofurantoin (Furadantin, Macrobid, Macrodantin) is a broad-spectrum bactericidal agent for organisms such as *E. coli, S. aureus, Proteus,* and *Enterobacter.*

Miscellaneous Urinary Tract Medications

Urinary Tract Analgesics

Urinary tract analgesia may be accomplished through topical analgesia or local anesthesia on the mucosa of the urinary tract. *Phenazopyridine* (Pyridium) is a dye that exerts a topical anesthetic effect on the lining of the urinary tract. It has no antiinfective effect but relieves the pain and burning on urination and the urinary frequency found with UTIs. Phenazopyridine has minimal side effects and is for short-term use. Patients should be advised to expect discoloration of the urine that will stain clothing (see Table 28-3).

Patient Education for Compliance

1. Pyridium may change urine to an orange-red color and may stain clothing.
2. For urinary antiseptics to be most effective, the urine should be acidic. Large doses of vitamin C, cranberries, and prunes will promote acidic urine.
3. Carbonated beverages and citrus fruits should be avoided with urinary antiseptics because they tend to make urine alkaline.
4. Fever may be a sign of a drug reaction, rather than a worsening of the infection.

IMPORTANT FACTS ABOUT URINARY TRACT ANTISEPTICS/ANALGESICS

- Urinary tract antiseptics are second-line drug choices for UTIs.
- Pyridium is a dye that can be used as an analgesic or local anesthetic on the urinary tract mucosa.
- Pyridium is used only for the symptomatic relief of burning, pain, discomfort, or urgency.

Urinary Tract Antispasmodics/Drugs for Overactive Bladder

Overactive bladder syndrome is a form of urinary incontinence found in patients of all ages, but the symptoms increase with age. The classic symptoms are urgency, frequency, and nocturia. The medications for treatment are aimed at increasing the volume of urine in the bladder, reducing the frequency of urination, and decreasing the pressure and urgency of the need to urinate. Several medications have recently been introduced for this condition (see Table 28-3).

Flavoxate (Urispas), a urinary antispasmodic, is used as a genitourinary muscle relaxant. Used to treat dysuria, urgency, nocturia, and the incontinence of cystitis and prostatitis, flavoxate is also effective for suprapubic pain. It may also be used for nocturnal **enuresis** in children older than 7 years of age. Patients with glaucoma must be closely monitored because of the possibility of increased intraocular pressure (see Table 28-3).

Oxybutynin (Ditropan) is an antispasmodic used to relieve the symptoms of urinary urgency, incontinence, frequency, and nocturia associated with neurogenic bladder conditions. The use of oxybutynin is not a cure for the neurogenic bladder or the overactive bladder but is a means for the patient to live a relatively symptom-free life.

Tolterodine (Detrol-LA) is used to relieve urinary frequency and urgency, providing relief of symptoms of the overactive bladder. The medication releases the smooth muscles of the bladder.

Trospium (Sanctura) and *darifenacin* (Enablex) are the newer medications in the group of drugs for overactive bladder. These medications work in a similar action as tolterodine.

Patient Education for Compliance

Urinary antispasmodics may cause drowsiness. Driving a car or operating machinery should be done carefully or not at all.

IMPORTANT FACTS ABOUT URINARY ANTISPASMODICS

- Urinary antispasmodics reduce the strength and frequency of urinary bladder contractions.

Drugs for Enuresis

Bedwetting, or enuresis, is fairly common in children, with the percentage of bedwetters gradually decreasing by the age of 21. Few people are still wetting at that age. Some behavioral techniques may be used with temporary improvement for those with a small or spasticlike bladder that seems to empty automatically when the bladder contains a certain volume of urine.

Imipramine (Tofranil) is an antidepressant that improves the symptoms of enuresis in some children.

Desmopressin (DDAVP) is an antidiuretic hormone that increases the reabsorption of water. This agent may be used as a nasal spray in children 6 years of age or older and in the elderly who have enuresis (see Table 28-3).

Patient Education for Compliance

Withholding fluids at bedtime is not effective in treating enuresis.

IMPORTANT FACTS
- Drugs may be used to reduce incontinence, frequency, and urgency by reducing spasms of the smooth muscles of the bladder.

Summary

The urinary system is composed of organs that are used for the excretion of body wastes. The urinary tract is also a major component in keeping the body in homeostasis and in fluid and electrolyte balance. Diuretics are grouped by the sites of action to increase the excretion of fluids, thereby reducing swelling throughout the body. Edema may be caused by several medical conditions but is most frequently associated with cardiovascular diseases. Diuretics used for cardiovascular diseases are discussed in Chapter 27.

Diuretics may cause excretion of electrolytes, and their loss may provide specific signs and symptoms. Replacement of lost electrolytes is necessary. Chronic electrolyte imbalances may be treated as an ambulatory condition as well as in an inpatient setting.

Urinary tract infections are treated with sulfonamides and their derivatives as the first choice of medications. TMP-SMZ is the best medication to

use with UTIs caused by enteric bacteria. The symptoms of UTI—urgency, frequency, dysuria, oliguria and burning on urination—are relieved by both sulfonamides and TMP-SMZ. Some foods (cranberries and cranberry juice) are indicated to treat infections, to keep the urine more acid for better effectiveness of urinary antiseptics, but they should be avoided for routine ingestion by those prone to frequent UTIs because they tend to irritate the bladder.

Urinary tract antiseptics are the second choice of medications for the prevention and treatment of UTIs. These medications have little or no systemic effect as they are urinary tract specific, and may be used for long-term therapy or prophylaxis.

Phenazopyridine is a local analgesic for UTIs, with no antiinflammatory properties. This agent does relieve the pain and burning associated with UTIs.

Urinary tract antispasmodics are used to relax the genitourinary muscles to relieve incontinence, nocturia, and dysuria. Some of the newer medications are indicated to relieve the frequency and urgency of an overactive bladder.

Enuresis is treated with medications in children older than age 6. Behavioral therapies may not be indicated, and withholding fluids at bedtime in children is not an effective treatment for the small or overactive bladder found in some children.

Critical Thinking Exercises

SCENARIO
Mary comes to see Dr. Merry complaining of urinary frequency, burning, and dysuria.
1. Should you expect to get a urine sample from Mary? Why or why not?
2. If the sample shows bacteria and Dr. Merry orders sulfonamides for Mary, what side effects should she be aware of?
3. How long should she take sulfonamide medications?
4. What food should Mary avoid to prevent irritation of the bladder?
5. Could Mary expect to take sulfonamides on a daily basis for chronic UTIs?

DRUG CALCULATIONS

1. Order: Detrol-LA 4mg po qAM
    Available medication:

NDC 0009-5191-01

Detrol® LA
tolterodine tartrate
extended release
capsules

4 mg
™

30 Capsules   **PHARMACIA**

Dose to be administered: _____
_____.

2. Order: trimethoprim/sulfamethoxazole 160/800
    mg tab i qd × 14 days
    Available medication:

100 Tablets   **NDC** 0173-0853-55

SEPTRA® DS
Double Strength
(trimethoprim and
sulfamethoxazole)

Each scored tablet contains
160 mg trimethoprim and
800 mg sulfamethoxazole.

CAUTION: Federal law prohibits
dispensing without prescription.
U.S. Patent No. 4,209,513 (Tablet)

Glaxo Wellcome Inc.
Research Triangle Park, NC 27709

595493

LOT
EXP

Store at 15° to 25°C (59° to 77°F) in a dry place.
Dispense in tight, light-resistant container as defined in the
U.S.P.
For indications, dosage, precautions, etc., see accompanying
package insert.
6505-01-016-1470

Rev. 5/96   Made in U.S.A.

NDC 0173-0853-55 4
N3 0173-0853-55 4

Dose to be administered: _____
_____

REVIEW QUESTIONS

1. What is an electrolyte? What are the four chief electrolytes? _____
    _____
    _____

2. What is replacement therapy? _____
    _____
    _____

3. What are the most commonly ordered medications for UTIs? _____
    _____
    _____

4. What is TMP-SMZ? What are the indications for this combination of medications? _____
    _____
    _____

5. How are the four urinary tract antiseptics effective in UTIs? _____
    _____
    _____

CHAPTER 29

Reproductive System Disorders

OBJECTIVES

After studying this chapter, you should be capable of doing the following:

- Discussing the sex hormones and their function in human reproduction.
- Describing the medications used in treating diseases specific to the male and female reproductive systems.
- Describing the pros and cons of different forms of contraceptive medications.
- Discussing how the medications used to treat infertility are effective.
- Providing information on medications for premenstrual syndrome and dysmenorrhea.
- Identifying medications for endometriosis.
- Discussing medications for erectile dysfunction and the dangers with nitrate medications.
- Discussing the categories of medications that impair sexual function as a side effect.

> Mr. Husain, age 65, comes to Dr. Merry worried about an inability to void that has become progressively worse. At this time, he has not voided for about 8 hours. Dr. Merry examines Mr. Husain and prescribes Proscar for him.
>
> What disease process is Proscar used for?
>
> What medications for hypertension should not be used with Proscar?
>
> If Mr. Husain were a younger man, would an enlarged prostate be as likely as it is after age 60?
>
> Mr. Husain tells you that his libido has diminished since he started taking diphenhydramine for allergies. He wants to know if there is any connection between his diminished libido and the allergy medication. What is your response?

KEY TERMS

Anabolic steroids	Depot form of medication	Negative feedback
Anabolism	Dyspareunia	Oogenisis
Androgen	Estrogen	Ovulation
Chloasma	Exogenous	Ovum
Coitus	Galactorrhea	Priapism
Contraception	Hirsutism	Progestin
Cryptorchidism	Hypogonadism	Spermatogenesis

EASY WORKING KNOWLEDGE OF INDICATIONS AND SIDE EFFECTS

Common Symptoms of Reproductive System Disorders

Sexually Transmitted Diseases (STDs)
Pelvic or genital pain
Dysuria, hematuria, purulent discharge
Burning or itching on urination
Urinary frequency or incontinence
Dyspareunia
Fever, malaise
Lesions in genital area

Infertility
Abnormal pregnancies
Endometriosis or other reproductive tract disorders including blocked fallopian tubes or tumors
Congenital malformations
Decreased sperm count

Specific to Female Reproductive System
Fever
Abnormal vaginal discharge or itching
Pain in lower abdomen or pelvic region

EASY WORKING KNOWLEDGE OF INDICATIONS AND SIDE EFFECTS—Cont'd

Specific to Female Reproductive System—cont'd
Dyspareunia or sexual dysfunction
Dysmenorrhea, amenorrhea, metrorrhagia,
    menorrhagia, or oligomenorrhea
Found with Reproductive Tract in Both Genders
Genital lesions
Breast changes (growths [benign and malignant], mastitis,
    discharge)
Psychologic response to hormone changes
Specific to Male Reproductive System
Frequency, urgency, pain, or burning on urination; oliguria
Sexual dysfunction including impotence or erectile dysfunction
Pain, swelling, or lesions of any reproductive organ

Common Side Effects of Medications for the Reproductive System
Edema and weight gain
Acne and skin discoloration, especially of face
Increased or decreased sexual stimulation or libido
Enlarged breast tissue in both sexes
Hirsutism, deepening of voice, and amenorrhea in females
Nausea and vomiting
Anxiety, depression
Headaches
Increased risk of thromboembolic disorders
Hypertension, myocardial infarction, stroke
Increased risk of cervicitis
Increased risk of gallbladder disease
Menstrual irregularities
Visual disturbances

Easy Working Knowledge of Drugs Used for Reproductive System Disorders

DRUG CLASS	PRESCRIPTION	OTC	PREGNANCY CATEGORY	MAJOR INDICATIONS
Androgens	Yes (anabolic androgens—Schedule III)	No	C, X	Hormone replacement
Benign prostatic hypertrophy agents	Yes	No	B, D, X (finasteride)	Reduce symptoms of benign prostatic hypertrophy
Estrogens/progestins	Yes	No	C, D, X	Menopause, replacement therapy, cancers in males and females
Oral and long-acting contraceptives	Yes	No	X	Prevention of pregnancy
Other contraceptives	Yes (diaphragm)	Yes	Nonapplicable	Prevention of pregnancy
Postcoital contraceptives	Yes	No	X	Prevention of pregnancy following unprotected sexual intercourse
Medications for PMS and dysmenorrhea	Yes	Yes	B, D	Relief of symptoms of PMS and menstrual cramping
Medications for infertility	Yes	No	X	Treatment of male and female infertility
Medications for erectile dysfunction	Yes	No	N/A	Treatment of erectile dysfunction

The reproductive system has been cloaked in secrecy and cultural inhibitions for centuries. Many patients are uncomfortable discussing sexual matters, especially when the patient is one gender and the physician is the other gender. Because of social perceptions about the reproductive organs and their functions, the health care professional faces challenges obtaining information concerning dysfunctions of the reproductive system. The female allied health professional plays a major role in obtaining sensitive information from a female patient who will be seen by a male physician, as does the male allied health professional with a male patient and a female physician. An open, trusting relationship between health professionals and patients is important. Medications used with the reproductive system require teaching and counseling in sensitive areas, and information must be presented and discussed with an understanding but positive approach.

The chief agents that affect the reproductive system are hormones. Some agents stimulate the secretions of hormones, whereas others block these same secretions. Medication therapy for conditions of the reproductive system can be complicated, although the names of the drugs are familiar to many people.

The structures of the female reproductive system are the ovaries, fallopian tubes, uterus, vagina, and Bartholin's glands (Figure 29-1). The ovaries respond directly to hormones secreted by the anterior pituitary to produce the female sex hormones. Beginning with puberty, females have the ability to reproduce until menopause.

In the male the urinary and reproductive systems are interrelated. The male reproductive tract consists of testes, which reside in the scrotum, the vas deferens, the prostate gland, urethra, seminal vesicles, epididymis, ejaculatory duct, and the penis (Figure 29-2). Beginning at puberty, males are capable of reproducing for the remainder of their lives.

The male and female sex hormones are necessary for the development and maintenance of secondary sex characteristics and for reproduction. The reproductive process is highly complex. It begins with the secretion of gonadotropic hormones from the anterior pituitary gland, which stimulate the development of the sex organs. Follicle-stimulating hormone (FSH) stimulates oogenesis in the ovaries and spermatogenesis in the testes. Luteinizing hormone (LH) stimulates release of an egg by the ovary and the formation of the corpus lu-

teum. In the testes, spermatogenesis and the secretion of androgens occur. The male sex hormones are called **androgens;** the female sex hormones are estrogen and progesterone (see Figure 29-1).

Influence of Hormones on the Reproductive System

In the male, FSH and interstitial cell-stimulating hormone (ICSH) stimulate the production of testosterone in the testes. Testosterone is responsible for the development of secondary sex characteristics and promotes adult male sexual behavior. Testosterone is also essential for regulating metabolism and the related growth of bone and skeletal muscles.

FSH and LH are also found in the female, where FSH stimulates growth of a graafian follicle in the ovary and the production of estrogen. During the proliferative phase of the menstrual cycle, as estrogen increases, FSH decreases, preparing the uterus to receive and nourish a fertilized **ovum.** During the proliferative phase, the endometrium, or inner glandular lining of the uterus, grows, and the endocervical glands secrete plentiful viscous mucus. This mucus nourishes sperm prior to fertilization. With increasing levels of estrogen due to maturation of the developing follicle, LH increases for ovulation at midcycle (Figure 29-3).

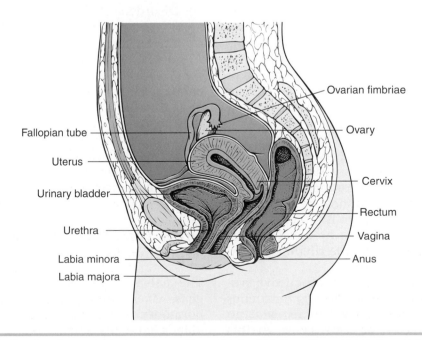

Figure 29-1 The female reproductive system. (From Frazier MS, Drzymkowski JW: *Essentials of human diseases and conditions,* ed 4, St Louis, 2008, Saunders.)

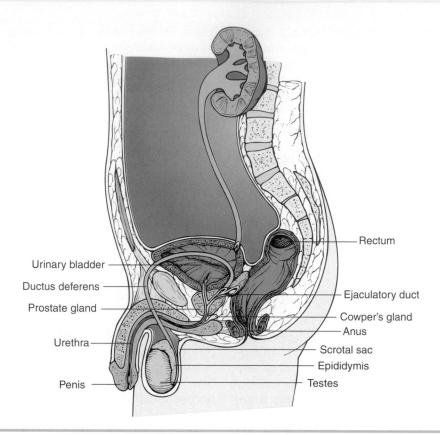

Figure 29-2   The male reproductive system. (From Frazier MS, Drzymkowski JW: *Essentials of human diseases and conditions*, ed 4, St Louis, 2008, Saunders.)

Luteinizing hormone influences the corpus luteum to form, releasing estrogen and progesterone during the secretory phase of the menstrual cycle. If the ovum is fertilized, the increased endometrial lining will support the ovum for growth and nourishment. If fertilization does not occur, the increased estrogen and progesterone decrease the release of FSH and LH by a **negative feedback** mechanism (see Chapter 21 for a discussion of negative feedback). The loss of pituitary hormone stimulation prevents the corpus luteum from producing estrogen and progesterone. Declining levels of estrogen and progesterone during the menstrual cycle cause sloughing of the endometrium, or menstruation.

Most women have variations in their menstrual cycles from month to month; therefore the time of ovulation is not always predictable. This is the physiologic reason why the rhythm method of contraception is not reliable.

Later in a woman's life, the reproductive system ceases to function at levels needed for continuation of the reproductive cycle. Women undergo the cessation of menses, or menopause. At this time, levels of estrogen decrease and women may need replacement therapy. Men also have a decrease in sex hormone production. This is sometimes called the *male climacteric*.

Disorders of the reproductive system in men and women may result in acute or chronic physical conditions and may cause emotional stress. Although the hormones are naturally produced, some disorders are indications for the use of **exogenous** male or female hormones. Such symptoms and diseases as deficiencies in hormone secretions, hypogonadism, and carcinomas of the male and female reproductive organs may be reason for hormonal treatment. Hormones are also indicated for the treatment of symptoms of menopause and for contraception.

Drugs That Affect the Male Reproductive System

The male sex hormones are referred to as *androgens*. The pituitary gland secretes stimulating hormones that travel via the blood to the target glands in the male reproductive system, the testes. ICSH, the male equivalent of LH in the female, stimulates the testes to produce testosterone.

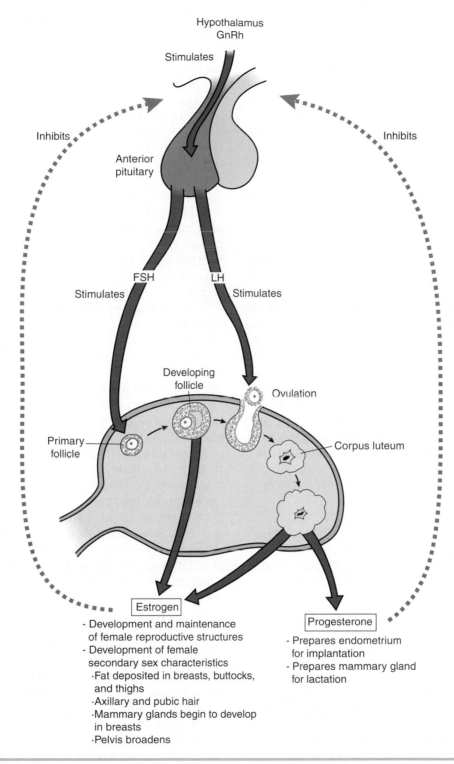

Hypothalamus
GnRh

Stimulates

Inhibits

Anterior
pituitary

Inhibits

FSH   LH

Stimulates   Stimulates

Developing
follicle

Ovulation

Primary
follicle

Corpus luteum

Estrogen

- Development and maintenance
  of female reproductive structures
- Development of female
  secondary sex characteristics
  ·Fat deposited in breasts, buttocks,
   and thighs
  ·Axillary and pubic hair
  ·Mammary glands begin to develop
   in breasts
  ·Pelvis broadens

Progesterone

- Prepares endometrium
  for implantation
- Prepares mammary gland
  for lactation

Figure 29-3   Hormone regulation of the menstrual cycle and ovarian function. (From Applegate EJ: *Anatomy and physiology learning system*, ed 3, St Louis, 2006, Saunders.)

Testosterone is the hormone responsible for producing the primary and secondary male sex characteristics. FSH from the anterior pituitary is also necessary to stimulate the production of sperm. For male hormone homeostasis, ICSH, FSH, and testosterone must be interrelated, beginning at puberty. The hormone production peaks at approximately age 20, but men continue to have significant hormone levels, some even past the age of 80.

Androgens and Anabolic Steroids

Testosterone brings about a sense of well-being and restores mental equilibrium and energy. It increases the resistance of the central nervous system to fatigue. The natural testosterone used for pharmaceutical purposes is obtained from the testes of bulls. **Anabolic steroids** may be natural or synthetically produced androgens. **Anabolism** is the constructive metabolic process by which substances are converted into other chemical components of an organism's structure. In the human male, androgens function to build new body tissue and to increase muscle strength and endurance immeasurably. (The abuse of anabolic steroids is discussed in Chapter 21.) Androgens are given to men for various conditions for therapeutic purposes. Their chief uses in males are to supplement low levels of testosterone to correct **hypogonadism** or **cryptorchidism** and to increase sperm production in cases of infertility. Androgens are also used to stimulate the production of red blood cells. An increase in red blood cells and in protein synthesis increases muscle mass, so athletes may use androgens to improve athletic performance. Anabolic steroids have serious and irreversible effects, and their use to enhance physical ability may not warrant the dangerous side effects. Because of the potential for abuse and the serious side effects, synthetically produced androgens are Schedule III medications.

Testosterone

For replacement therapy, natural testosterone is preferred to synthetic androgens. For testosterone to achieve an adequate blood level, it is given by intramuscular injection because oral testosterone is highly metabolized in the intestines and the liver before it reaches the bloodstream. The medication is available in aqueous bases for short action or oil bases or as depot medications for prolonged action of up to 4 weeks. Testosterone pellets are available for subcutaneous implantation, with an extended duration of action of 2 to 6 months. Methyltestosterone may be administered by the buccal route, whereas synthetic androgens may be effectively administered orally.

Transdermal testosterone preparations are applied in different ways. The testosterone patch, Testoderm, is applied to scrotal skin, where it is highly absorbed at a rate five times greater than at other dermal sites. The patch is left on the scrotal area for 24 hours and is changed daily for 8 weeks when used as treatment for cryptorchidism, to encourage descent of the testes into the scrotal sac. The second testosterone patch, Androderm, is applied to the back, abdomen, arms, or thighs daily, with the site of application changed every 24 hours so that no site is used more frequently than once in 7 days. Both of these patches should be applied nightly at about 10 PM so that maximum serum levels are achieved in the morning, to stimulate the normal circadian rhythm in young boys.

Androgel, a gel preparation, is applied daily to a clean, dry area on the shoulders, upper arms, or abdomen at bedtime. Buccal testosterone is placed on the gum every 12 hours in the morning and at bedtime. The site of insertion of the buccal drug should be above the incisor teeth, and the site should be rotated.

The dosage and the length of therapy depend on the diagnosis, the patient's age and gender, and the side effects or adverse reactions incurred. In the male with delayed puberty, the dose may be low initially, then gradually increased according to individual need and response. Treatment may last for several months or may continue throughout puberty if needed. When used as antineoplastic therapy, in men and women, a 3-month period is necessary to evaluate the effectiveness of treatment. During this time, women should receive a short-acting androgen because androgens may occasionally increase the extent of breast cancer. Soreness and redness at the injection site are also possible. Because of drug interactions with anticoagulants, an increase in bleeding episodes may occur. Finally, an unusual increase or decrease in libido may occur (Table 29-1).

Anabolic Steroids

Anabolic steroids, or 17-alpha-alkylated androgens, are classified as Schedule III medications because of the potential for abuse or misuse. Men who think the anabolic action will maintain strength, especially in sports, and virility into the older adult years are those who usually use these drugs. Mood, libido, and cholesterol levels may be improved, and muscle mass may increase, but the dangers of long-term use far outweigh the benefits. Therapeutically these drugs may be used to treat anemias from renal disease in both genders. For conditions characterized by a breakdown in protein metabolism, anabolic steroids may be used to promote weight gain (Table 29-2). These medications are hepatotoxic, and irreversible liver damage can occur with chronic use.

TABLE 29-1 *Androgens*

GENERIC NAME	TRADE NAME	USUAL ADULT DOSE, ROUTE, AND FREQUENCY OF ADMINISTRATION	INDICATIONS FOR USE	DRUG INTERACTIONS
testosterone (short-acting injectable)	Histerone	25-50 mg IM 2-3 × per wk	Replacement therapy Postpartal breast pain	Oral anticoagulants
	T pellets	q3-6 mo 2-6 pellets SC	Palliation of metastatic breast cancer	
testosterone (transdermal)	Transderm, Androderm	1 patch q24h		
testosterone (topical)	Androgel 1%, Testin	Apply 5 mg topically daily		
testosterone (buccal)	Striant	1 buccal application q12h		
testosterone propionate	Testex	50-400 mg IM q2-4wk* 50-100 mg IM 3 ×/wk†		
testosterone (long-acting injectable)	Delatestryl, Depo-Testosterone, Depotest, Duratest	50-400 mg IM q2wk* 200-400 mg IM q2-4wk†		
fluoxymesterone	Halotestin	5-20 mg/day* po 5-10 mg × 4-5 days† po 10-40 mg/day† po buccal		
methyltestosterone	Oreton, Adroid-25, Testred, Virilon	10-50 mg/day* 80 mg/day × 3-5 days† po 50-200 mg/day‡ po		
testolactone	Teslac	250 mg po qid‡		
danazol	Danocrine	400 mg po bid	Endometriosis	lovastatin, oral anticoagulants

MAJOR SIDE EFFECTS: Females—oily skin, acne, increased hair growth, increased libido, irregular menses, deepening voice; **Males**—urinary urgency, swelling or tenderness of breasts, frequent erections, priapism; **Both genders**—change of skin color, abdominal pain, insomnia, mouth soreness, diarrhea, constipation, dizziness, headaches, confusion, depression, edema of legs.

IM, Intramuscular; *SC*, subcutaneous.
* Used as replacement therapy.
† Used for postpartum breast pain.
‡ Used to palliate metastatic breast cancer.

TABLE 29-2 *Anabolic Steroids*

GENERIC NAME	TRADE NAME	USUAL ADULT DOSE, ROUTE, AND FREQUENCY OF ADMINISTRATION	INDICATIONS FOR USE	DRUG INTERACTIONS
nandrolone	Durabolin	50-100 mg/wk IM	Breast cancer and anemias due to renal disease	anticoagulants, antidiabetics, immunosuppressants

MAJOR SIDE EFFECTS: Rash, hematuria, elevated blood pressure, amenorrhea, nausea, vomiting, decreased libido, fatigue, tremors.

IM, Intramuscular.

Patient Education for Compliance

1. Patients using Testoderm should shave the scrotum before applying the patch.
2. Sodium and water retention may occur with the use of testosterone, with resultant weight gain and edema of the extremities.
3. Signs of hepatic toxicity such as jaundice, chalky stools, and pain in the right shoulder, should be reported immediately when taking androgens.
4. Oral androgens should be taken with a snack to avoid gastrointestinal upset.
5. Buccal testosterone should be placed with the rounded surface against the gum and held in place for 30 seconds with a finger over the lip.
6. Do not chew or swallow buccal application of testosterone.

IMPORTANT FACTS ABOUT ANDROGEN PREPARATIONS

- Testosterone is the principal androgen.
- Androgens stimulate the production of red blood cells and increase muscle mass. Androgens are used therapeutically to treat anemias due to renal disease, as replacement therapy in cases of deficiencies, to treat breast engorgement in the female, and palliatively in metastatic breast cancer.
- Two transdermal forms of testosterone are available. One is applied to the scrotum; the other is applied to the extremities or back, but not to the scrotum.
- A testosterone gel and buccal tablet are also available for ease of administration.
- Testosterone taken orally is metabolized by the liver prior to absorption, so testosterone is usually given by injection or transdermally.
- Anabolic steroids have toxic effects on the liver.

Medications for Benign Prostatic Hypertrophy

Benign prostatic hypertrophy (BPH) is an increase in the glandular and connective tissue mass of the prostate, which surrounds the urethra in males. The development of BPH is considered a normal age-related change in men after the age of 40, with 73% of men by age 70 having symptoms of BPH that require medical intervention. BPH obstructs the bladder neck and compresses the urethra, resulting in urinary retention and an increased risk of urinary tract infections. The symptoms of BPH are hesitancy on urination, a decrease in the stream and force of urine, postvoiding dribbling, and the sensation of incomplete emptying of the bladder, resulting in frequency and nocturia.

The goal of treatment of BPH is to relieve bothersome symptoms. α-Adrenergic blockers such as tamsulosin (Flomax), terazosin (Hytrin), and doxazosin (Cardura) are preferred for treatment of BPH in patients with relatively small prostates. These medications relax the smooth muscles of the bladder neck and prostate for ease of voiding. They are also hypotensives and so are useful for patients with both prostate disease and hypertension. The patient should be warned to take the first medications at bedtime to reduce the first-dose phenomenon of hypotension and dizziness.

Finasteride (Proscar) is appropriate for patients with large prostate glands to promote shrinkage of the prostate. The benefits are slow in developing, taking up to 6 to 12 months to appear. The medication prevents the conversion of testosterone to dihydrotestosterone (DHT), the androgen found in the prostate gland. Finasteride shrinks the prostate by decreasing the DHT available for the growth of the prostate, which relieves the symptoms of BPH. Females of childbearing age should not handle this medication because any amount absorbed through the skin may cause birth defects. Females of childbearing age whose partners are on finasteride therapy should use contraception (Table 29-3).

Patient Education for Compliance

1. Patients taking α-adrenergic blockers should be aware of "first-dose" orthostatic hypotension and dizziness.
2. The treatment for benign prostatic hypertrophy is suppressive rather than curative, and the symptoms may return if the medication is withdrawn.
3. Finasteride may be teratogenic to a male fetus, so all women of childbearing age should not handle the drug. The sexual partner should not become pregnant while the patient is taking the drug.

IMPORTANT FACTS ABOUT DRUGS TO TREAT BENIGN PROSTATIC HYPERTROPHY

- Benign prostatic hypertrophy (BPH) occurs in 75% of men by age 70, causing sufficient symptoms to require medical intervention with drugs such as finasteride.
- α-Adrenergic blockers, which are also used as antihypertensives, relax the smooth muscles of the bladder and prostate to relieve the symptoms of BPH.
- The symptoms of BPH result from mechanical obstruction of the urethra from overgrowth of epithelial cells or of smooth muscle cells.
- Finasteride promotes regression of prostate epithelial tissue and reduces mechanical obstruction. Finasteride is more effective in men whose prostate is significantly enlarged.

TABLE 29-3 *Drugs Used to Treat Benign Prostatic Hypertrophy*

GENERIC NAME	TRADE NAME	USUAL ADULT DOSE, ROUTE, AND FREQUENCY OF ADMINISTRATION	INDICATIONS FOR USE	DRUG INTERACTIONS
ADRENERGIC ANTAGONISTS			Benign prostatic hypertrophy	
terazosin	Hytrin	1 mg po hs, up to 10 mg/day		ACE inhibitors, NSAIDs, propranolol
tamsulosin	Flomax	0.4 mg/day po		
doxazosin	Cardura	1 mg po qid		ACE inhibitors, indomethacin, verapamil, nifedipine
alfuzosin	Uroxatral	10 mg po qd		alcohol
dutasteride	Avodart	0.5 mg po qd		None

MAJOR SIDE EFFECTS OF ADRENERGIC ANTAGONISTS: Dizziness, syncope, orthostatic hypotension, nausea, decreased libido, bitter taste.

GENERIC NAME	TRADE NAME	USUAL ADULT DOSE, ROUTE, AND FREQUENCY OF ADMINISTRATION	INDICATIONS FOR USE	DRUG INTERACTIONS
OTHERS				
finasteride	Proscar	5 mg po qd		No significant interactions but should not be handled by females of childbearing age

MAJOR SIDE EFFECTS: Increased breast size, rash, stomach/back pain, diarrhea, headache, decreased libido, impotency.

ACE, Angiotension-converting enzyme; *NSAIDs*, nonsteroidal antiinflammatory drugs.

Drugs That Affect the Female Reproductive System

The medications used therapeutically to treat conditions of the female reproductive system are similar to the hormones naturally produced by females. The medications—provided as female hormones, estrogen and progesterone (or progestin, the synthetic equivalent)—are prescribed to supplement low levels of natural hormones such as during menopause, to correct the hormone imbalance that causes abnormal uterine bleeding, to reverse abnormal ovulation, to enhance fertility, and for oral contraception. In some cases women are treated with androgens palliatively for metastatic breast cancer and as therapy for postpartum breast engorgement, endometriosis, and fibrocystic breast disease. Women receiving androgen preparations may have irreversible deepening of the voice.

Estrogens

Estrogens are the dominant form of medicinal therapy for conditions of the female reproductive system because of the effects on the system, as well as bone and cardiovascular function and insulin sensitivity. Estrogens reduce the levels of low-density lipoproteins (LDLs) and increase the levels of high-density lipoproteins (HDLs). This action is thought to reduce the risk of heart at-

tacks in premenopausal women. When estrogen levels begin to fall during menopause, the incidence of heart attacks in females rises. Estrogens also increase the cholesterol content of bile, which may explain why women taking estrogens may develop gallstones.

Estrogens support the development and maintenance of reproductive organs and the secondary sex characteristics in females. These hormones also have profound influences on the physiology of reproduction, from their actions during the menstrual cycle to their actions that stimulate uterine growth and blood flow during pregnancy. In premenopausal women the ovary is the principal organ of estrogen production in the form of estradiol. Estradiol may be converted to estrone and estriol before being eliminated by a combination of hepatic metabolism and urinary excretion.

Estrogens have the positive effect of blocking bone mass resorption and promoting deposits of minerals. During puberty, estrogens promote the growth of long bones. In postmenopausal women, estrogen replacement helps to maintain bone mass.

Uses of Estrogen

The estrogens have several uses in both genders including adjuvant therapy for certain cancers— prostate cancer in the male and non–estrogen-dependent breast cancers in both genders. Hormone replacement therapy (HRT) using estrogen preparations is prescribed for women who have had their ovaries removed during the reproductive years and in older women for the prevention and treatment of osteoporosis.

- The use of estrogen without added **progestins** in postmenopausal women increases the risk of endometrial hyperplasia and of endometrial and breast cancer. The estrogens alone cause proliferation of the endometrial lining. A woman with an intact uterus who receives replacement therapy should be followed closely with physical examinations and Pap smears to ensure early detection of possible diseases.
- Estrogen use over a long period of time without progestins is associated with an increased risk of developing endometrial cancer. The addition of progestins reduces the risk of endometrial cancer by down-regulating the estrogen receptors.
- Recent studies have shown that among postmenopausal women who take conjugated estrogens for 10 years for HRT, the risk of death from any cause was decreased by 37%. The risk of death from heart disease was decreased by 53%, and the risk of death from stroke was decreased by 32%. However some scientists are of the opinion that HRT may be more harmful than helpful because of the increased risk of cancer of the reproductive tract. Some women who are given prescriptions for estrogen replacement therapy never fill the prescription out of fear of developing endometrial or breast cancer associated with HRT use.
- Women who had an early menarche and a late menopause and who take HRT appear to have a greater incidence of breast cancer. Whether the incidence is higher because of an actual increase in the disease in women taking HRT or because of earlier detection of breast cancer in women who have regular, frequent examinations is not known.
- A family or personal history of breast cancer is a contraindication to the use of HRT.
- Estrogens are available in conjugated doses from natural sources, the urine of pregnant mares, and have also been synthetically formulated. Estradiol and estrone are naturally occurring steroidal estrogens.
- Conjugated estrogens are available in mixtures of estrogenic medications that are available in oral, parenteral, transdermal, or percutaneous forms such as vaginal creams.

- Use of estradiol in women with estrogen deficiency may be transdermal to provide continuous release of estrogen.
- The lowest dose of estrogen needed to produce the desired effect should be administered over the shortest period of time to reduce the potential for serious side effects.
- Estrogens should be used with caution in patients with endometriosis, gallbladder disease, liver disease, pancreatitis, and elevated lipoprotein levels.
- Women with a history of estrogen hypersensitivity, hypercalcemia, and thrombophlebitis/thromboembolic disease should avoid estrogens unless the benefit outweighs the risk.
- Glucose tolerance is decreased with estrogen therapy, occasionally leading to symptoms of diabetes mellitus.
- Estrogens tend to cause retention of sodium and water, causing weight gain, edema, and hypertension. These symptoms may aggravate asthma, epilepsy, migraines, heart disease, and kidney disease.
- People wearing contact lenses may note intolerance for lens wear because edema changes the shape of the corneas and results in improper fit of lenses.

Forms of Estrogen Preparations

- Estrogens are available in several forms that have unique means of administration. Estrogen and progesterone products are available orally, parenterally (intramuscularly), vaginally, topically, and as implants under the skin.
- To lengthen the onset and duration of action of the medications, the hormone can be administered parenterally in an oil base—the "depot" form—for slower absorption from the muscle tissue. Using this injectable type of medication assists with patient compliance in medication administration.
- Transdermal administration bypasses hepatic metabolism. The estrogen patches are applied to the dry surface of the abdomen or buttocks for absorption through the skin. The metabolism of estradiol from transdermal absorbtion is affected very little so that the initial levels in the blood are higher than when estrogen is taken orally. The dosing with transdermal medication is one to two times a week, rather than daily.
- A new form of estrogen therapy for hot flashes of menopause has recently been introduced as an estradiol emulsion that is rubbed

on each leg daily in the morning, much like a lotion. The lower dose of estradiol is absorbed through the skin into the blood stream. The patient must be told to avoid sunscreens with this form of estrogen.

- Another unique delivery system is the vaginal ring. The drug-laden device is pressed into the vaginal canal for the continuous release of medication into local tissues.
- Vaginal inserts and creams are also formulated to release hormones into the vagina on contact.
- The new oral forms are most commonly used with the trend toward long-acting products that are taken daily for up to 3 months prior to the stoppage to allow for a menstrual period. A recent development of the FDA is to allow indefinite use of some medications for the prevention of menses, as well as for oral contraception.
- Implants containing contraceptives are surgically placed under the skin of the upper arm to prevent pregnancy. The older forms of implants contained multiple rods that were changed every 5 years. The newest implant consists of one rod with a 3-year duration. This product is expected to stop menstruation in most women.
- Estrogen may be prescribed for cyclic dosing, in which 3 weeks of estrogen are followed by a week off, or by the addition of progestin for the last 10 to 13 days.
- The new low-dose oral contraceptives rarely include more than 50 mcg of estrogen; in most cases, 20 to 30 mcg of estrogen is adequate for birth control. The lower doses with effective coverage improve the safety of the oral contraceptives (Table 29-4).

Progesterone

Progesterone, stimulated by LH and produced by the ovaries, is a naturally occurring progestin, but also may be made synthetically with similar pharmacologic effects in the body.

- Progesterone is not always therapeutically satisfactory, so a progestin is often used.
- The advantages of progestin are that a lower dose is necessary to produce the desired response, progestin has a longer duration of action than progesterone, and progestin is available in oral or sublingual forms for easier administration.
- Progestin is used for treating amenorrhea and abnormal uterine bleeding from hormone imbalances, for contraception, in combination

with estrogen for postmenopausal HRT, and as adjuvant or palliative therapy for renal or endometrial cancer. Progestin is often prescribed in combination with estrogen preparations.

- In such medications, the estrogen component of the oral contraceptives is most often stated in micrograms and the progestin component is stated in milligrams.
- A combined-continuous regimen, in which estrogen and progestin are combined in a single tablet for daily administration, is also used for HRT.
- Patients with a history of migraines, diabetes mellitus, hyperlipidemia, thrombophlebitis, and undiagnosed bleeding from the reproductive tract should be watched closely when taking progestin (see Table 29-4).

Patient Education for Compliance

1. Before starting any estrogen therapy, the female patient should undergo a full physical examination including breast and pelvic examinations, Pap smear, blood pressure, and lipid profile, followed by yearly re-examinations and monthly breast self-examinations. For women older than age 40, a mammogram may be indicated prior to beginning therapy.
2. Estrogens can cause genital abnormalities in the male fetus and vaginal cancer in the female fetus. Estrogens should be discontinued immediately if pregnancy is suspected.
3. To reduce the side effects of estrogen and progesterone, take the medication with food.
4. If persistent vaginal bleeding develops in the menopausal female, the physician should be notified.
5. Estrogen and progestin may cause a sunburn-like reaction on exposure to sunlight or ultraviolet light.
6. Blood glucose levels and urine should be checked more frequently in people with diabetes mellitus who are taking estrogens and progestins.
7. Estradiol transdermal patches should be applied to a clean, dry area of intact skin on the abdomen or trunk. After application, the patch should be pressed firmly in place with the palm of the hand for 10 seconds. If the patch falls off, the same patch is reapplied. The application site should be changed with each new patch.
8. Avoid applying estradiol transdermal patches at the waist or breasts, or in places where clothing will loosen the edges of the patch.
9. Intravaginal estrogen preparations should be positioned high in the vagina.
10. When using intravaginal estrogens, maintain a recumbent position for 30 minutes following application.

TABLE 29-4 *Select Estrogens and Progestins*

GENERIC NAME	TRADE NAME	USUAL ADULT DOSE, ROUTE, AND FREQUENCY OF ADMINISTRATION	INDICATIONS FOR USE	DRUG INTERACTIONS
ESTROGENS				
estradiol	Estrace	0.5-2 mg/day po in cycles	Menopausal symptoms, hypogonadism	bromocriptine, hepatotoxic drugs
	Estraderm, Vivelle	0.05-0.1 mg patch 2× a wk		
	Climara	0.05-0.1 mg patch 1× a wk		
	Estring	Change ring every 3 mo		
	Estrasorb	Apply package to each leg qAM (emulsion)		
estradiol valerate	Delestrogen	5-20 mg IM q2-3wk	Menopausal symptoms, hypogonadism, and prostatic cancer	tobacco
	Gynogen LA	50 mg IM q1-2wk		
estradiol, ethinyl	Estinyl	1-2 mg po tid	Prostatic cancer	
esterified estrogen	Estratab, Menest	0.3-1.25 mg po qd		
esterified estrogen with methyltestosterone	Estratest	1.25-2.5 mg po qd	Menopausal symptoms, hypogonadism, and breast cancer	None noted
conjugated estrogens	Premarin, Cenestin	0.3-2.5 mg/day po in cycles 25 mg IM q6-12h for breast cancer 2-4 g qd in vagina in cycles	Menopausal symptoms, osteoporosis prevention, prostate cancer, breast cancer, hypogonadism, and atrophic vaginitis	None noted
esterified estrogen with medroxy-progesterone	Prempro (0.625 mg/2.5 mg to 0.625 mg/5 mg)	1 tab po qd	Same as other estrogens	None noted
	Premphase (0.625 mg/2.5 mg estrogen + 15 mg progesterone)	1 tab po qd		None noted
estropipate	Ogen, Ortho-Est	0.75-3 mg/day po in cycles 0.75 mg/day po for 7 days per mo	Same as other estrogens and osteoporosis	None noted
diethylstilbestrol (DES)		1-3 mg po qd 15 mg/day po 25 mg bid × 5 days, po starting within 72 hr of intercourse	Prostate cancer Breast cancer Postcoital contraception	None noted

MAJOR SIDE EFFECTS OF ESTROGENS: Female—Stomach cramping, flatulence, anorexia, nausea, chloasma, headache, changes in libido, edema of legs, breast discomfort and enlargement. **Male**—feminization, loss of body/facial hair, atrophy of sex organs, decreased libido; additionally, estradiol is hepatotoxic.

TABLE 29-4 *Select Estrogens and Progestins—cont'd*

GENERIC NAME	TRADE NAME	USUAL ADULT DOSE, ROUTE, AND FREQUENCY OF ADMINISTRATION	INDICATIONS FOR USE	DRUG INTERACTIONS
PROGESTINS				
progesterone	Crinone,	5-10 mg/day × 6-8 days IM	Amenorrhea, abnormal uterine bleeding	None noted
	Prometrium	Vaginal gel q other day × 6 doses, 200 mg/day po × 12 days		
medroxy-progesterone	Provera, Amen	2-10 mg/day po × 5-10 days	Endometrial hyperplasia, secondary amenorrhea, abnormal uterine bleeding	None noted
	Depo-Provera	150 mg q3mo IM	Contraception	
		400-1000 mg qwk	Endometrial carcinoma	
hydroxyprogesterone	Hylutin	375 mg q4wk IM	Amenorrhea/uterine bleeding	aminoglycosides
		1-7 g/wk	Endometrial cancer	
megestrol	Megace	40 mg po qid for at least 2 mo	Breast cancer	None noted
		40-320 mg/day po in divided doses	Endometrial cancer	
		800 mg/day po	Anorexia, cachexia	
norethindrone	Micronor, Norlutin	2.5-10 mg in cycles po	Amenorrhea/abnormal uterine bleeding	None noted
		5 mg po × 14 days po, then increasing doses	Endometriosis	
		0.35 mg/day po	Contraception	
		5 mg po for 10-13 days in cycles	Prevention of endometrial hyperplasia with estrogen therapy	

MAJOR SIDE EFFECTS OF PROGESTINS: Weight gain, stomach pain/cramping, swelling of face and legs, headaches, mood variations, anxiety, weakness, nervousness, rash, acne, insomnia, hot flashes, amenorrhea.

IM, Intramuscular.

IMPORTANT FACTS ABOUT ESTROGEN/PROGESTERONE PREPARATIONS

- Estradiol is the principal endogenous estrogen.
- In addition to their role in the menstrual cycle, estrogens are required for the growth and maturation of the reproductive organs.
- Estrogens raise levels of HDL cholesterol and reduce levels of LDL cholesterol, which may explain why premenopausal women may not be susceptible to coronary heart disease.
- Nausea is the most common side effect of estrogen preparations.
- Prolonged use of estrogens alone is associated with an increased risk of endometrial carcinoma; when used with progesterone, there is little or no risk of uterine cancer.

IMPORTANT FACTS ABOUT ESTROGEN/PROGESTERONE PREPARATIONS—*Cont'd*

- Estrogens taken for less than 5 years pose less risk for breast cancer. When taken for longer than 5 years, they may or may not pose a risk.
- Progestins may cause breakthrough bleeding, spotting, and amenorrhea.
- Estrogen losses in menopause may cause hot flashes, loss of bone mass, and an increased risk for coronary heart disease.
- Hormone replacement therapy in postmenopausal women usually consists of estrogen combined with progestin.
- Estrogens and progestins are contraindicated during pregnancy and in women with estrogen-dependent carcinomas, undiagnosed abnormal vaginal bleeding, and thromboembolytic disorders.

Forms of Contraception

Contraception, commonly referred to as *birth control*, denotes prevention of fertilization of the ovum or the subsequent onset of pregnancy. Birth control may be accomplished using pharmacologic methods such as oral contraceptives, medication-laden implants, injectable hormones, and intrauterine devices (IUDs). Nonpharmacologic methods include surgical sterilization, mechanical devices, and the rhythm method.

The safety of birth control measures is a complex area. Of the contraceptive methods available, oral contraceptives have the largest spectrum of adverse effects—from nausea to menstrual abnormalities to rare thromboembolytic disorders. The lowest mortality rate is seen with barrier methods, but oral contraceptives are relatively safe in nonsmoking women with normal cardiovascular function.

Women at risk for sexually transmitted diseases should not use an intrauterine device (IUD). The chief factors to consider when choosing a method of birth control are effectiveness, safety, and personal preference. The best form of contraception will be ineffective if improperly practiced.

Oral Contraceptives

Oral contraceptives are the most effective form of easily reversible birth control presently available. First made available in the late 1950s, these medications have had a large impact on socioeconomic conditions in the United States. The use of oral contraceptives has reduced family size since their introduction. The early dosages of the contraceptives were much stronger with greater side effects than those found today. Millions of women have used these medications, and through this experience the risk factors, dosages, and effectiveness have been evaluated and modified. The newer low-dose oral contraceptives are associated with a lower risk for adverse cardiovascular effects, thromboembolytic disease and stroke, ectopic pregnancies, and endometrial, cervical, and liver cancer, but a possible earlier onset of breast cancer or coronary artery disease in women older than 35 who smoke.

- The combination oral contraceptives, which consist of some formulation of estrogen and progestin, inhibit ovulation by increasing hormone levels and increasing the viscosity of the cervical mucus, thus creating a barrier to sperm.
- The medications are nearly 100% effective for birth control.

- The two main categories of oral contraceptives are (1) those that contain estrogen and progestin, known as *combination oral contraceptives*, and (2) those that contain only progestins, or "minipills."
- The combination oral contraceptives occur in monophasic, biphasic, triphasic, and estrophasic formulations.
  - In the monophasic regimen the daily doses of estrogen and progestin remain constant throughout the menstrual cycle.
  - In the biphasic regimen the estrogen dose remains constant, but the progestin dose is increased during the second half of the cycle.
  - The triphasic regimen divides the menstrual cycle into three phases, with the amount of progestin changed in each phase of the cycle.
  - In the estrophasic regimen, the amount of progestin remains constant and the estrogen dose is gradually increased throughout the cycle.
- The estrogen components have been associated with venous and arterial thromboembolism, causing myocardial infarctions and strokes. The risk of the associated hypertension increases with the prolonged use of oral contraceptives and increasing age.
- The risk of adverse cardiovascular reactions is greatly increased in women who smoke and take oral contraceptives.
- The risk of cancer is low, especially when compared with the risk of endometrial cancer with postmenopausal estrogen therapy.
- Oral contraceptives containing progestins can elevate blood sugar levels and cause gallbladder disease.
- The efficacy of oral contraceptives can be affected by medications, and oral contraceptives in turn can affect the dosage of some medications (Box 29-1).

Effectively Taking Oral Contraceptives

Most oral contraceptives are taken in a sequence of 21 days, followed by 7 days of no pill, an inert pill, or an iron-containing pill. Some of the oral contraceptives (OC) are started on the fifth day of the menstrual cycle and are taken at the same time each day. The successive cycles begin every 28 days. Other OCs are started on the first day of the menstrual cycle and are continued daily throughout the month. These medications may contain iron supplements or placebos during the last 7 days of the cycle. During the first cycle of use, other forms of birth control should be used. If a single dose of

---

Possible Increased Doses Needed with Oral Contraceptives

rifampin (tuberculosis)

phenobarbital, phenytoin, and primidone (antiseizure)

tetracycline and ampicillin (antibiotics)

Increased Doses Needed with Oral Contraceptives

warfarin (anticoagulant)

insulin and other hypoglycemic agents (for diabetes mellitus)

Decreased Doses Needed with Oral Contraceptives

theophylline (for asthma)

imipramine (for depression)

---

oral contraceptive is missed, the chance of ovulation is small. However, the risk of pregnancy becomes greater with each consecutive pill omitted. If one dose is missed, it should be taken the next day. If two doses are missed, two tablets should be taken on the next 2 days. If three doses are missed, a new cycle of the medication should be started 7 days after the last pill was taken. Additional birth control should be used during the first 2 weeks of the new cycle. If this routine is not followed, pregnancy may occur (Table 29-5).

Patient Education for Compliance

1. Breakthrough bleeding, spotting, amenorrhea, and breast tenderness are possible with estrogen and progestin preparations.
2. The woman should take oral contraceptives at the same time each day, beginning at the appropriate time during the menstrual cycle. Monophasic medications are taken for 21 days, followed by no drug for 7 days. Other dosages may provide tablets containing iron or placebos so a tablet is taken on a daily basis throughout the month.
3. Shortness of breath, leg tenderness, chest pain, headaches, or visual disturbances while taking oral contraceptives should be reported immediately to the physician. Yearly physical examinations are necessary.
4. If two consecutive menstrual periods are missed, the possibility of pregnancy must be evaluated.
5. Menses may be irregular for several months following the discontinuation of oral contraceptives.
6. Oral contraceptives cannot be used during breastfeeding because the hormones will enter the breast milk and be passed to the nursing infant.

Patient Education for Compliance— cont'd

7. The person with diabetes mellitus taking oral contraceptives should monitor blood glucose levels closely. An increase in insulin or hypoglycemics may be necessary for the person taking oral contraceptives.
8. The incidence of multiple births is increased if conception occurs shortly after oral contraceptives are stopped. To reduce this chance, other forms of birth control should be used for 3 months following the termination of oral contraceptive use.
9. Additional forms of contraception should be used during the initial cycle of oral contraceptive use.

IMPORTANT FACTS ABOUT ORAL CONTRACEPTIVES

- Oral contraceptives are a common form of birth control.
- The two main categories of oral contraceptives are combinations of estrogen plus progestin and progestin-only medications (minipills).
- Combination oral contraceptives primarily inhibit ovulation.
- Serious adverse reactions from oral contraceptive use are rare, although side effects and some complications occur. Adjusting the estrogen and progestin content may minimize problems.
- Low-estrogen combination oral contraceptives pose only a minimal risk of thromboembolism except in women with a past history of thromboembolytic disease or in those who smoke.
- Combination oral contraceptives protect against ovarian and endometrial cancer.
- Oral contraceptives are teratogenic and may cause cancer in female offspring; thus they are contraindicated during pregnancy.
- Progestins are slightly safer than combination oral contraceptives but are less effective and cause more menstrual irregularity.
- Progestin-only oral contraceptives increase the viscosity of the mucus in the cervix, creating a barrier to sperm and suppressing growth of the endometrium to prevent implantation of the fertilized ovum.

Other Forms of Contraception

Implants and Transdermal Patches

Other medications are used as long-acting contraceptives. A subdermal system, the Norplant implant, provides the synthetic progestin levonorgestrel as a long-term, reversible method of contraception. The six tiny capsules that are surgically implanted inside the upper arm contain the synthetic progestin and are the most effective form of contraception. The

TABLE 29-5 *Select Contraceptives**

GENERIC NAME	TRADE NAME	USUAL ADULT DOSE, ROUTE, AND FREQUENCY OF ADMINISTRATION	INDICATIONS FOR USE	DRUG INTERACTIONS
MONOPHASIC COMBINATION MEDICATIONS			Prevention of pregnancy	See Box 29-1 for drug interactions with this group of drugs
ethinyl estradiol/ norethindrone (in various strengths)	Loestrin, Loestrin 24 PE, Ovcon 1-50, NEE, Brevicon, Genora, Modicon, Nelova, Norethin, Norinyl, Ortho-Novum	po in cycles (the estrogen component is in mcg; the progestin component is in mg)		
ethinyl estradiol/ drospirenone	Yasmin	1 tab daily po in cycles		
ethinyl estradiol/ norelgestromin	Ortho-Evra	apply patch qwk x 3; skip 1 wk and begin cycle again		
ethinyl-estradiol/ etonogesterol	NuvaRenz	Insert vaginally q mo		
estinyl estradiol/ levo-norgestrel	Alesse, Levlen, Nordette	po in cycles		
estinyl estradiol/ norgestrel	Lo-Ovral, Ovral	po in cycles		
estinyl estradiol/ desogestrel	Desogen, Ortho-Cept, Mircette	po in cycles		
estinyl estradiol/ norgestimate	Levora, Ortho-cyclin	po in cycles		
estinyl estradiol/ ethynodiol diacetate	Demulen	po in cycles		
mestranol/ norethindrone	Genora 1/50, Norinyl, Nelova 1/50, Norethin, Ortho-Novum	po in cycles		
estrogen/progestin	Necon 1/35, Alesse-28, Ortho-Novum 1/35	po in cycles		
BIPHASIC COMBINATION MEDICATIONS				
ethinyl estradiol/ norethindrone	Ortho-Novum 10/11, Nelova 10/11, Jenest-28	po in cycles		
TRIPHASIC COMBINATION MEDICATIONS				
ethinyl estradiol/ norethindrone	Tri/Norinyl, Ortho-Novum 7/7/7	po in cycles		
ethinyl estradiol/ levonorgestrel	Triphasil, Tri-Levlen	po in cycles		
ethinyl estradiol/ norgestimate	Ortho Tri-cyclin†	po in cycles		

TABLE 29-5 *Select Contraceptives*—cont'd

GENERIC NAME	TRADE NAME	USUAL ADULT DOSE, ROUTE, AND FREQUENCY OF ADMINISTRATION	INDICATIONS FOR USE	DRUG INTERACTIONS
ESTROPHASIC COMBINATION MEDICATIONS				
ethinyl estradiol/ norethindrone	Estrostep	po in cycles		
PROGESTIN-ONLY MEDICATIONS				
norethindrone	Micronor, Nor-QD	po in cycles		
norgestrel	Ovrette	po in cycles		

MAJOR SIDE EFFECTS OF MONOPHASIC, BIPHASIC, TRIPHASIC, AND ESTROPHASIC COMBINATIONS AND PROGESTIN-ONLY CONTRACEPTIVES: Nausea, hirsutism, acne, weight gain, edema, elevated blood glucose, diarrhea, headache, fatigue, dizziness, chloasma, rash.

LONG-ACTING CONTRACEPTIVES				
ethyl estradiol/ levonorgestrel	Seasonale, Seasonque	1 tab daily for 91-day cycle		
	Lybrel	1 tab daily indefinitely		
medroxyprogesterone with estradiol	Depo-Provera	q3mo IM		
	Lunelle	q mo IM		
levonorgestrel	Norplant,	q5yr subdermal		
	Implanon	one rod subdermal q3yr		

MAJOR SIDE EFFECTS OF LONG-ACTING CONTRACEPTIVES: Dizziness, headache, nervousness, change in appetite, vaginitis, depression, fluid retention, alopecia, pain and itching at site, weight gain; **implants/transdermal patches**: cervical erosion, rash, nausea, vomiting, dysmenorrhea, anorexia, breakthrough bleeding, amenorrhea, breast discharge, vaginitis, cervicitis, musculoskeletal pain.

INTRAUTERINE PROGESTERONE CONTRACEPTIVE SYSTEM	Progestasert	IUD annually	None noted	
	Mirena	IUD q5 years	None noted	

MAJOR SIDE EFFECTS OF IUD CONTRACEPTIVES: Abdominal cramping, increased menstrual bleeding.

IM, Intramuscular; *IUD*, intrauterine device.
*For drugs separated by a slash, the first drug listed is an estrogen component and the second drug is a progestin component.
†Federal Drug Administration approved for use with acne.

levonorgestrel diffuses slowly and continuously at the rate of about 80 mcg/day to provide contraception for up to 5 years. The implant must be surgically removed when no longer desired or effective.

A transdermal patch for contraception is a monophasic patch that holds a combination of ethinyl estradiol and norelgestromin to provide contraception much like oral preparations with the same indications and contraindications. These patches are applied to the upper arms, back, abdomen, or buttocks and are to be worn either weekly or biweekly in cycles. The patch is applied on the same day of the week, with the fourth week being patch free. With correct use, the effectiveness of this type of contraception is equal to that of oral medications and the need to remember to take the daily doses of medication is eliminated.

• This medication has proved less effective in women weighing 198 lb or more, indicating the need for other means of contraception in obese women.

- Women using this medication should not be without the patch for longer than 7 days in a row, or pregnancy is possible.
- If the patch becomes loose or falls off for less than 1 day, either the patch should be reapplied or a new patch should be applied and the regular day for change should remain the same.
- If the patch is off for more than 1 day or if the time off is unknown, a new 4-week cycle should begin immediately and a backup method of contraception should be used for the first week of the cycle.

Contraception by Injection

A single injection of medroxyprogesterone (Depo-Provera) provides contraception safely and effectively for 3 months or more.

- The injections prevent pregnancy in three ways: (1) by suppressing ovulation, (2) by thickening the cervical mucus, and (3) by altering the endometrium to discourage implantation of the fertilized ovum.
- When injections are discontinued, an average of 12 months is required for fertility to return, with some women remaining infertile for 2 or more years (see Table 29-5).

Intrauterine Devices

Intrauterine devices, another relatively long-term effective reversible form of birth control, are inserted using minor surgical procedures.

- The principal problem with IUD use is pelvic inflammatory disease with its associated risk of infertility.
- The major side effect is cramping.
- The IUD should be used by women at low risk for STDs.
- Two IUDs are available: the Copper T 380A (ParaGard) IUD and the intrauterine progesterone contraceptive system (Progestasert). ParaGard may remain in place for 8 years and is the more widely used. Progestasert must be replaced annually (see Table 29-5).

Spermicides

Spermicides come in foams, gels, creams, and suppositories. All of these preparations may be purchased without a prescription. Spermicides,

nonoxynol-9 (Delfen, Ensure) and octoxynol-9 (Ortho-Gynol, Koromex Cream), provide effective contraception when used as directed but are more effective when used with a diaphragm or condom. The active ingredient is a chemical surfactant that kills sperm by destroying their cell membranes. The adverse reactions are minimal.

- Correct use of spermicides is essential for contraception efficacy. The spermicide must be applied prior to coitus but no more than 1 hour in advance if used alone. Spermicides must be reapplied each time intercourse is anticipated.
- Foams must be thoroughly shaken before each use to ensure dispersal of the active ingredients.
- Suppositories or tablets should be inserted into the vagina a minimum of 10 to 15 minutes prior to intercourse to allow time for these forms of contraception to dissolve.
- Douching should be postponed for at least 6 hours after coitus with any spermicidal use.
- Recent data indicates that use of nonoxynol-9, the ingredient in most spermicides, can increase the risk of HIV transmission (Table 29-6).

Barrier Devices

Barrier devices are nonpharmacologic methods of birth control. These devices include male and female condoms, diaphragms, and the cervical cap. The most commonly used barrier contraceptive device is the male condom.

- Condoms are made from three materials—latex, polyurethane, and lamb intestine. Most condoms in the United States are made from latex, which is impenetrable by bacteria and viruses. So, in addition to use for contraception, the latex condom protects against STDs. Lubricants that contain mineral oil can decrease the barrier strength of latex by as much as 90% and should therefore be avoided. Allergies to latex may develop in both men and women. Polyurethane condoms are thinner, possibly stronger, and do not cause allergies, while still providing protection against STDs. Lamb intestine condoms allow the transmission of viruses and are not protection for viral STDs. Male condoms have a failure rate in preventing pregnancy of 12%.
- The female condom, Reality, is a loose-fitting tubular polyurethane pouch with flexible rings at both ends. The ring at the closed end anchors the pouch on the cervix. The pouch on the open

TABLE 29-6 *Common Spermicidals*

MEDICATION TYPE	ACTIVE INGREDIENT*	TRADE NAME
Foam	nonoxynol-9	Delfen, Koromex, Because, Emko
Jelly	nonoxynol-9	Ramses, Koromex, Gynol II
Gel	nonoxynol-9	Conceptrol, Crystal Clear, Advantage-24[†], K-Y Plus[†], Gynol II[†], Koromex[†]
	octoxynol-9	Ortho-Gynol[†]
Cream	octoxynol-9	Koromex[†]
	nonoxynol-9	Conceptrol, Ortho Crème[†]
Suppository	nonoxynol-9	Encare, Semicid, Conceptrol
Vaginal film	nonoxynol-9	VCF

MAJOR SIDE EFFECTS: Nausea, vomiting, infertility, breast tenderness, ectopic pregnancy, blood clot formation.

*Side effects minimal.
[†] To be used only in combination with a diaphragm.

end has a larger ring that is placed over the labia for an external anchor. This mechanism, as with the male condom, provides some protection against STDs. The Reality condom is prelubricated, available over the counter (OTC), and cannot be combined with a male condom. The failure rate for pregnancy is about 21%.

- The diaphragm is a soft rubber cap with a metal spring that reinforces the rim. The device must be fitted by a health care provider for proper sizing and is bought with a prescription. Before insertion, the diaphragm should be filled with spermicide to completely block the cervix. The diaphragm may be inserted up to 6 hours before intercourse but must remain in place for at least 6 hours after. The failure rate for pregnancy is about 18%.
- The cervical cap is a small, pliant, cup-shaped device that fits directly over the cervix, where it is held in place by suction. Like the diaphragm, the cap is not available OTC but must be fitted by a health care professional and spermicides must be used as a barrier. The failure rate for women who have previously given childbirth is around 40%, whereas the failure rate is about 20% for women who have not given childbirth.

Postcoital Contraception

Medications used as postcoital contraceptives may be either "morning after" pills or the "abortion" pill to prevent pregnancy following intercourse. To be effective, the morning after medication must be taken no later than 72 hours after intercourse. The pill may be taken immediately after the unprotected intercourse, but the first pill must be taken within the first 72-hour period. A second pill must be taken 12 hours after the first dose. This drug should not be considered a routine means of contraception because of potential side effects. Emergency contraception pills (ECPs) are meant to provide one-time emergency protection. They should be used to prevent unplanned and unwanted pregnancies from unprotected sexual intercourse due to sexual attack, contraception failure, and the like.

- The morning after pill has three possible modes of action: (1) inhibition of ovulation, (2) alteration of the menstrual cycle so that ovulation cannot take place, and (3) irritation of the lining of the uterus so that the body rejects the possible fertilized egg.
- The morning after pill is a high-dose oral contraceptive formulated of either progestin alone, estrogen alone, or both of these artificial steroids together. Medications with combined hormones are called combined ECPs. Preven is a specially packaged combination of high doses of estrogen and progestin with a dose of two pills. The combined ECPs are 75% effective in women who would otherwise become pregnant from unprotected sex.
- The other type of ECP contains only progestin, or progestin-only ECP, with a dose of one tablet. This type is packaged under the name Plan B and is even more effective, at an 85% rate.
- The danger signals for a few weeks following the use of morning after pills are severe pain in the legs, severe abdominal pain, chest pain, shortness of breath, blurred vision, trouble speaking, loss of vision, or jaundice. The next menstrual period may be earlier or later than usual. If the menstrual period does not begin

TABLE 29-7 *Select Medications That May Be Used as Emergency Contraceptives*

TYPE OF MEDICATION	TRADE NAME	USUAL DOSE, ROUTE, AND FREQUENCY
progestin-only ECP	Plan B*	1 pill within 72 hr and another 12 hr later
oral contraceptive	Ovrette	20 pills within 72 hr and 20 pills 12 hr later
Combined ECP	Preven	2 pills within 72 hr and 2 more pills 12 hr later
Combined oral contraceptive	Ovral	2 pills within 72 hr and 2 pills 12 hr later
	Nordette, Levlen, Levora Lo/Ovral, Low-Ogestrol	4 pills within 72 hr and 4 pills 12 hr later
	Alesse, Levlite	5 pills within 72 hr and 5 pills 12 hr later
mifepristone (RU-486)	Mifeprex	3 pills within 63 days of LMP, 2 tab misoprostol 2 days later

MAJOR SIDE EFFECTS: Excessive bleeding, cramping, nausea, vomiting, fatigue, weakness, headache, diarrhea.

LMP, Last menstrual period.
* As of February 2007, Plan B is available over the counter in some states.

for 3 weeks, a pregnancy test should be done, as well as a pelvic examination. If pregnancy occurs, an abortion should be considered because of the teratogenicity of estrogen to the fetus. (For a list of oral contraceptives that can be used as ECPs, see Table 29-7.)

IMPORTANT FACTS ABOUT METHODS OF CONTRACEPTION

- The long-lasting methods of birth control, such as Norplant implants, intramuscular medroxyprogesterone, IUDs, and sterilization, should be used when compliance may be a problem. The oral contraceptives are a close second for effectiveness of birth control.
- Norplant, which acts similarly to progestin, is effective for 5 years and is the most effective method of contraception.
- Depo-Provera works for 3 months and is highly effective.
- The morning after pill is for emergency-only postcoital contraception. It may be a combination of estrogen and progestin or a progestin-only medication.

RU-486 (Abortion Pill)

RU-486 (mifepristone) is approved by the FDA as a postcoital contraceptive agent to stop the gestation of an early pregnancy. Similar in structure to progesterone, mifepristone (Mifeprex) is the first of a new generation of birth control pills called antiprogestins. It works only in the first 9 weeks of pregnancy, or up to 63 days from the start of the last menstrual period to produce a medical-chemical abortion by stimulating uterine contractions and preventing the

fertilized egg from attaching to the uterus. After the first 7 weeks of pregnancy, the natural progesterone found in the pregnant woman is too great to allow the medication to be effective. Bleeding and cramping typically occur after administration of the pill. The bleeding is similar to or greater than a heavy menstrual period and lasts for 9 to 16 days. The efficacy is between 92% and 95%.

Women using this medication must be carefully screened, and the medicine must be administered by a specially trained health care provider who has the capability of surgical intervention if needed for an incomplete abortion or for excessive bleeding. Mifepristone should not be used with the following conditions:

- Confirmed or suspected tubal pregnancies
- IUD in place
- Chronic adrenal gland disease
- Current long-term therapy with corticosteroids
- History of allergy to mifepristone, misoprostol, or other prostaglandins
- Bleeding disorders or current anticoagulant therapy

Eligible women will need to see the health care provider three times for completion of the entire procedure:

1. Initially, to receive a three-pill dose by mouth.
2. To take misoprostol, a prostaglandin, 2 days later to complete the abortion.
3. Finally, a return visit approximately 2 weeks later to be certain the abortion was complete. If the abortion is not complete, a surgical procedure will be necessary to terminate the

pregnancy, although there is no evidence that RU-486 causes birth defects or genetic damage.

DID YOU KNOW?

The medical community has identified RU-486 as having promising effects in the treatment of some breast cancers, endometrial cancer, brain tumors, endometriosis and uterine fibroid tumors, adrenal cancer, glaucoma, and as an agent to induce labor.

New Forms of Contraception on the Horizon

Researchers are also pursuing new implants with fewer rods than Norplant and vaccines for both men and women. The male vaccine has been shown to be 99% effective in suppressing sperm production. The vaccine requires weekly injections of testosterone at present, but scientists are looking at implants or longer-acting injections for this use.

Patient Education for Compliance

1. Barrier contraceptives used by females should remain in place for the prescribed time following sexual intercourse and should be used with a spermicide as suggested by the manufacturers.
2. Lubricants containing mineral oil should not be used with latex condoms because the strength of the latex may be decreased by as much as 90%.
3. Barrier contraception devices such as diaphragms and cervical caps must be fitted professionally.
4. "Morning after" contraception must be accomplished within 72 hours of unprotected sex.
5. The "abortion pill" must be administered by a health care professional within 7 weeks of the last menstrual period. Pregnancy should be confirmed prior to using RU-486.

Drugs for Premenstrual Syndrome and Dysmenorrhea

Premenstrual syndrome (PMS) is a group of physical and psychologic symptoms that develop just before menstruation and resolve a few days after the onset of menses. See Box 29-2 for the common symptoms of PMS. For PMS to be diagnosed, the symptoms must be intense and must exhibit a relationship with the woman's menstrual cycle. For mild symptoms, lifestyle changes including dietary

---

BOX 29-2 COMMON SYMPTOMS OF PREMENSTRUAL SYNDROME

Psychologic and Behavioral Symptoms

Irritability and crying
Depression, sadness, helplessness
Alternating sadness and anger
Hypersensitivity to trivial events
Social withdrawal
Anxiety and tension
Difficulty concentrating
Reduced efficiency in work performance
Restlessness and agitation

Physical Symptoms

Acne
Breast tenderness
Abdominal bloating, ankle edema
Weight gain from water retention
Food cravings
Fatigue
Headache
Backache, joint and muscle pain
Nausea, vomiting, constipation, or diarrhea

---

supplement, exercise, eating carbohydrate-rich foods, and reducing salt intake are the first line of treatment. For more severe symptoms, drug therapy including different agents is indicated. Two types of drugs are most often those prescribed—mood-altering drugs and medications to suppress ovulation, although other medications may be used to relieve specific symptoms.

Mood-altering drugs that are often used are as follows:

- Serotonin selective reuptake inhibitors (SSRIs) such as fluoxetine (Prozac) and sertraline (Zoloft) are the first drugs of choice to relieve the psychologic symptoms of PMS (see Chapter 31).
- Alprazolam (Xanax), a member of the benzodiazepine family, is an alternative medication and is also used to reduce the irritability, anxiety, and tension of PMS.

Ovulation suppressants include two classes of drugs—oral contraceptives and gonadotropin-releasing agents (GnRH).

- Leuprolide (Lupron) can be used to reduce breast tenderness, bloating, anxiety, and nervous tension.
- Oral contraceptives are helpful with primarily physical symptoms.

Other medications for specific symptoms include the following:

- Spironolactone (Aldactone), a potassium-sparing diuretic, is used to treat bloating and urine retention.
- Calcium decreases mood swings and depression, aches, pains, food cravings, and water retention.
- Analgesics such as aspirin, acetaminophen, naproxen, and ibuprofen may relieve cramps, headaches, dysmenorrhea, and muscle and joint pain.
- Ibuprofen is considered the superior medication for the relief of primary dysmenorrhea.
- Aspirin relieves primary dysmenorrhea because it suppresses the prostaglandins that cause smooth muscle cramping.
- Naproxen (Naprosyn) also inhibits the synthesis of prostaglandins.
- Drugs known not to work are progesterone, pyridoxine, tamoxifen, lithium, and magnesium.

Medications for Infertility

Infertility is the decreased ability to reproduce; *sterility* is the absence of reproductive ability. Infertility is experienced by 15% of couples trying to conceive children and it may be the result of reproductive dysfunction in either partner or both. With medical care, approximately half of the couples are able to achieve pregnancy. In treatment, the medication must be matched to the cause of the infertility.

Fertility depends on the endocrine system secreting proper amounts of hormones for the reproductive system to work adequately and function properly. Deficiencies in the hormones responsible for the production of ova or sperm may lead to infertility. Cysts, tumors, or infections of the reproductive organs or obstruction of the tubal structures that transport ova or sperm may cause difficulty in conception. Some of these conditions can be treated with medications; others require surgical intervention.

Anovulation is a cause of infertility that frequently can be corrected by pharmaceutic means. The agents used to promote maturation of the follicle and the production of ovulation are clomiphene (Clomid), gonadorelin (Factrel, Lutrepulse), menotropin (Pergonal), urofollitropin (Metrodin), and human chorionic gonadotropin (hCG).

- Clomiphene and gonadorelin induce follicular maturation and ovulation by releasing FSH and LH from the pituitary gland.

- Menotropin and urofollitropin act on the ovary to promote follicular maturation.
- hCG may be given to induce ovulation after the use of other medications.

Treatment by Follicular Stimulation

- Clomiphene (Clomid) is used to promote follicular maturation and ovulation. This drug has antiestrogenic effects to cause ovarian stimulation, maturation of the ovarian follicles, and development of the corpus luteum.
- Menotropin (Pergonal and Humegon) is a hormonal preparation with LH and FSH activity in equal amounts. These medications are used to provide adequate ovarian stimulation when the pituitary hormones are insufficient. The cost for a single treatment can be as high as $1500, but the rate of ovulation approaches 100%. hCG is given after 4 days of menotropin to stimulate ovulation. These medications are also used to treat infertility in males.
- Urofollitropin (Metrodin), similar to menotropin, is obtained from the urine of postmenopausal women and contains FSH. hCG is administered following urofollitropin to stimulate natural ovulation.

Treatment of Amenorrhea

Bromocriptine (Parlodel) is used to correct amenorrhea and infertility associated with excessive prolactin secretion. In some persons, a common first-dose side effect is the phenomenon of dizziness or syncope on change of position. Some conditions of the female reproductive tract such as polycystic ovaries, endometriosis, and uterine fibroid tumors may be exacerbated. The medication is contraindicated in women with these conditions (Table 29-8).

Male Infertility

Infertility is due to dysfunction of the male reproductive system in 30% of infertile couples. This failure may be due to decreased density or motility of the sperm or to abnormal quality or volume of the semen. Male infertility is frequently unresponsive to medications. In men who do not produce sperm because of insufficient secretion of hormones, drug therapy may be helpful. Sperm counts may be increased with the use of hCG alone or in combination with menotropin. This combination therapy is expensive and may require prolonged treatment for 3 to 4 years. If the hormone deficiency is severe, androgens may be used for drug therapy.

TABLE 29-8 *Drugs Used to Treat Infertility*

GENERIC NAME	TRADE NAME	USUAL ADULT DOSE, ROUTE, AND FREQUENCY OF ADMINISTRATION	INDICATIONS FOR USE	DRUG INTERACTIONS
clomiphene	Clomid, Serophene	50 mg po qd × 5 days, starting on the fifth day of menstrual cycle; may be used for 3-4 cycles and then increased to 75-100 mg/day	Female infertility	None noted
menotropin	Pergonal	75 U each IM of FSH/LH	Stimulate follicles to mature by acting on FSH and LH	None noted
	Humegon	150 U each IM of FSH/LH injected daily 4 days for 9-12 cycles, followed by hCG the next day		
urofollitropin	Metrodin	75 mg/day × 1 week po or more, followed by 5000 to 10,000 U of hCG on day following last dose of urofollitropin	Stimulate follicle maturity in males and females	None noted
bromocriptine	Parlodel	2.5-7.5 mg/day po with food		None noted
human chorionic gonadotropin	hCG, A.P.L., Pregnyl, Chorex-5	5000-10,000 U IM on day 1 after last dose of tropins	Stimulate production of progesterone from the corpus luteum	None noted

MAJOR SIDE EFFECTS: menotropin: hot flashes, abdominal discomfort, spotting, weakness, photophobia; **urofollitropin:** hot flashes, abdominal discomfort, spotting, weakness, photophobia, severe stomach pain, decreased urination, weight gain, swelling of legs, breathing difficulties; **bromocriptine:** headache, dizziness, fatigue, abdominal cramping, nausea.

FSH, Follicle-stimulating hormone; *IM*, intramuscular; *LH*, luteinizing hormone.

IMPORTANT FACTS ABOUT MEDICATIONS FOR INFERTILITY
- Infertility is the decreased ability to reproduce; sterility is absence of the ability to reproduce.
- Infertility may occur in either partner or both.
- Clomiphene promotes follicular maturation and ovulation.
- Menotropin is a 50:50 mixture of LH and FSH and promotes follicular maturation and ovulation.

Medications for Miscellaneous Reproductive Conditions

Danazol (Danocrine) is used to treat endometriosis and the associated infertility. Danazol may temporarily impair the ability of the endometrium to support a pregnancy, so attempts at conception should be postponed for 3 months following completion of treatment. The medication causes atrophy of the endometrial tissue and is weakly androgenic (see Table 29-1).

Goserelin (Zoladex) is an injectable implant administered into the abdomen wall every 4 weeks for 6 months for the treatment of endometriosis. The pregnancy category is X. (Goserelin is also used as an antineoplastic agent in breast and prostate cancer.)

Two gonadotropin releasing hormone (GnRH) agents are used for endometriosis—leuprolide (Lupron) and nafarelin (Synarel). Nafarelin (Synarel) is a gonadotropin used to treat endometriosis in females and precocious puberty in both sexes. Because the route of administration is nasal, rhinitis may occur. Nafarelin is the drug of choice for treating endometriosis if future fertility is an issue. Leuprolide (Lupron) is similar to goserelin in action and side effects and is also used for uterine fibroids. Like goserelin, nafarelin may also be used to treat prostate cancer (Table 29-9).

TABLE 29-9 *Miscellaneous Medications Used for Reproductive Tract Conditions*

GENERIC NAME	TRADE NAME	USUAL ADULT DOSE, ROUTE, AND FREQUENCY OF ADMINISTRATION	INDICATIONS FOR USE	DRUG INTERACTIONS
DRUGS FOR ENDOMETRIOSIS				
danazol	Danocrine	200-800 mg po per day in 2 divided doses for 3-9 mo		
goserelin	Zoladex	3.6 mg SC q28 days for 6 mo	Endometriosis	None noted
GnRH AGONISTS				
leuprolide	Lupron	3.75 mg/dose IM for each monthly dose for 6 mo	Endometriosis and uterine fibroids	None noted
nafarelin	Synarel	400 mcg/day—200 mcg in AM and 200 mcg in PM as nasal spray in opposite nostrils for 6 mo	Endometriosis and precocious puberty	Nasal topical decongestants

MAJOR SIDE EFFECTS OF DRUGS FOR ENDOMETRIOSIS: Anxiety, headaches, CVA, hot flashes, breakthrough bleeding, breast tenderness.

GENERIC NAME	TRADE NAME	USUAL ADULT DOSE, ROUTE, AND FREQUENCY OF ADMINISTRATION	INDICATIONS FOR USE	DRUG INTERACTIONS
DRUGS FOR ERECTILE DYSFUNCTION				
sildenafil	Viagra	50 mg taken 1 hr prior to sexual activity	Erectile dysfunction in male	nitrate preparations
tadalafil	Cialis	10 mg po prior to sexual activity q24h		nitrates, some antivirals
vardenafil	Levitra	5 mg po prior to sexual activity		nitrates

MAJOR SIDE EFFECTS OF DRUGS FOR ERECTILE DYSFUNCTION: Headache, flushing, GI upset, nasal congestion, diarrhea, rash, visual disturbances.

CVA, Cardiovascular accident; *IM,* intramuscular; *SC,* subcutaneous.

Patient Education for Compliance

1. Women taking danazol for endometriosis should refrain from becoming pregnant for 3 months following treatment.
2. Danazol may cause masculinization.

Medications for Erectile Dysfunction

Sildenafil (Viagra), the first medication for the treatment of impotency, was first released for use as a cardiovascular agent to lower blood pressure; today it is used for erectile dysfunction in men. Newer drugs such as tadalafil (Cialis) and vardenafil (Levitra) have rapidly joined this medication for use with erectile dysfunction. The medications act to increase blood flow that produces penile ri-gidity associated with sexual stimulation. The drug does not cause an erection in the absence of sexual stimulation. Sildenafil and vardenafil should be taken 1 hour prior to sexual activity and not more than once a day. However, tadalafil has a more rapid onset and prolonged effects, providing effectiveness for up to 36 hours. As with the other medications in this class, tadalafil should not be taken more than once a day. Investigations are being conducted to evaluate the potential effectiveness of the drug's use in women.

- Patients taking nitrates should not take sildenafil because a synergistic decrease in blood pressure may cause severe hypotension. The hypotension may lead to myocardial ischemia and a resultant myocardial infarction.
- These medications have not been associated with **priapism,** but these drugs should be used with care in the patient who is predisposed to

the condition. An erection lasting longer than 4 hours should be reported to the physician (see Table 29-9).

CLINICAL TIP

Drugs for erectile dysfunction should not be given with nitrates because of severe hypotension and the danger of myocardial infarction.

LEARNING TIP

The generic name for medications for erectile dysfunction end in -afil.

Medications That Impair or Enhance Libido as a Side Effect

Various medications can have side effects or adverse reactions that decrease libido in both genders. Decreased levels of testosterone in either gender lowers the sex drive. Centrally acting α_2 agonists (methyldopa [Aldomet], clonidine [Catapres], guanabenz [Wytensin], and guanfacine [Tencx]) for hypertension have been associated with impotency and sexual dysfunction. Guanethidine (Ismelin) and reserpine have been reported to cause difficulty with ejaculation in the male. Anticholinergic agents used for hypertension may also cause impotence. Thiazide diuretics may induce sexual dysfunction and decrease libido, with impotency and breast changes. Spironolactone (Aldactone) seems to be the chief agent of the group to cause sexual dysfunction.

Continuous use of antihistamines will also interfere with sexual activity. Some well-known medications such as diphenhydramine (Benadryl), promethazine (Phenergan), and chlorpheniramine (Chlor-Trimeton) are used as antiemetics, sedatives, and to control allergy symptoms, but they also block the parasympathetic nerve impulses to the sex glands and organs.

Many of the centrally acting antianxiety and psychotropic medications affect sexual interest and capability. The phenothiazines decrease sexual interest in persons undergoing therapy. Phenothiazines also inhibit sexual function, causing decreased libido, inability to ejaculate, impotence, and prolonged amenorrhea. Benzodiazepine compounds such as diazepam (Valium) decrease sexual interest and may prevent orgasm.

Ethyl alcohol is a sexual depressant, although moderate amounts may enhance sexual activity by decreasing inhibitions.

The H$_2$-receptor antagonists cimetidine (Tagamet) and ranitidine (Zantac) lead to impotency when used for long periods of time. Some calcium channel blockers cause erectile dysfunction, and β-blockers, especially propranolol (Inderal), have been associated with decreased libido and erectile dysfunction.

The tricyclic antidepressant clomipramine (Anafranil) may induce a spontaneous orgasm as a side effect.

Opioids and psychotic agents such as LSD, cocaine, marijuana, and amphetamines are considered aphrodisiacs in contemporary society. More commonly, sexual behavior is decreased. The user's state of mind and the amount of medication consumed contribute to the sexual effect of the medication.

Some elderly patients taking levodopa (Dopar) have observed a sexual rejuvenation. Amyl nitrate, a vasodilator used for angina pectoris, has been alleged to enhance sexual activity and to intensify the orgasmic experience for men. Loss of erection and delayed ejaculation may also result from the use of amyl nitrate.

Many medications, both legal and illegal, may affect sexuality and sexual behavior. For the patient taking therapeutic doses of medications that interfere with sexual behavior, the allied health care professional should take an accurate history to provide awareness of the patient's needs and report this information to the physician so that alteration of treatment as needed will ensure medication compliance. Listening to patients' concerns about medications and sexual function is an important role of the allied health professional.

Patient Education for Compliance

Some drugs cause impairment of sexual function. These concerns should be discussed with the health care professional to allow changes in medications if possible.

Summary

Androgens are necessary for the normal development of male sex characteristics and for spermatogenesis. Androgens may be used therapeutically as hormonal replacement therapy in the male or for the treatment of breast cancer. A common problem with the reproductive system in the older male is benign prostatic hypertrophy. Finasteride is a drug specific for benign prostatic hypertrophy.

Anabolic steroids are synthetic androgens often used by athletes to enhance performance. Although the steroids have potential, the risks that accompany their use are substantial, making these medications Schedule III drugs because of the danger of abuse.

Estrogens and progestins are necessary for female reproduction and for the development of female sex characteristics. Estrogens and progestins are used for contraception and for noncontraceptive applications such as HRT and the treatment of breast and prostate cancer. Estrogens reduce the incidence of osteoporosis and coronary artery disease; therefore postmenopausal women should be evaluated for prophylactic use. Progestins are indicated for HRT and also for the treatment of endometriosis and carcinomas, as well as to prevent pregnancy. Estrogens, progestins, and androgens are teratogenic.

Oral contraceptives containing combinations of estrogens and progestins are an effective form of birth control. These medications are widely used because of the ease of administration. Thromboembolytic disease is one of the dangerous adverse reactions.

Medications are available for the treatment of infertility and sexual dysfunction. These medications should be used with care because of their side effects. The drugs for female infertility must be taken exactly as ordered, with coitus occurring at a specific time in relation to drug administration to encourage pregnancy.

New products are available for erectile dysfunction and for postcoital contraception. Medications for erectile dysfunction should not be used with nitrates. The morning after pill must be taken within 72 hours after unprotected intercourse. The "abortion pill" must be administered by a specially trained health care professional and requires a specific regimen requiring three office visits.

The use of hormones for any reproductive condition is a sensitive area for most patients. The allied health professional should be empathic and discreet when discussing reproductive tract conditions and their treatments with clients.

Critical Thinking Exercises

SCENARIO

Erin is taking an oral contraceptive but states that when she had the flu, she forgot to take her pills for 3 days. Also, the physician gave her a prescription for ampicillin for a bacterial infection.

1. Does the ampicillin have any bearing on the efficacy of the oral contraceptive? If so, what?
2. What should Erin do to resume her schedule of oral contraceptive use?
3. Should she use additional means of contraception at any point?
4. Erin wants to know why 21 tablets look alike and 7 look different. What is your response?

DRUG CALCULATIONS

1. Order: medroxyprogesterone acetate 0.2 g stat
   Available medication:

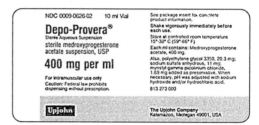

   Volume to be administered: _____

   Show the volume of medication on the syringe shown.

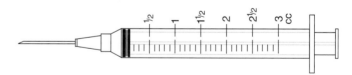

2. Order: Premarin 1.25 mg po qd
   Available medication: Premarin 0.625 mg
   Amount to be administered with each dose:

   _____

REVIEW QUESTIONS

1. What is the collective name for male sex hormones? _____

2. What hormone is primarily responsible for the development of secondary sex characteristics in the male? _____

3. What is the goal of pharmaceutic treatment for benign prostatic hypertrophy? _____

4. What are some of the risks associated with female hormone replacement therapy? _____

5. What does *conjugated estrogen* mean? _____

6. What are some of the side effects of estrogen therapy? _____

7. Why are combination oral contraceptives so effective? _____

8. What is the main component of the minipill? _____

9. Explain the differences among monophasic, biphasic, triphasic, and estrophasic oral contraceptives. _____

10. What medications reduce the effectiveness of oral contraceptives? _____

11. What medication category is most effective for dysmenorrhea? _____

12. What medications are considered dangerous for use with sildenafil? _____

CHAPTER 30

Neurologic System Disorders

OBJECTIVES

After studying this chapter, you should be capable of doing the following:

- Briefly describing how analgesics and general anesthetics work.
- Explaining the actions of local anesthetics.
- Discussing how hypnotics and sedatives affect the body.
- Describing the antiseizure medications and their actions.
- Explaining how medications can be used to relieve the symptoms of Parkinson's disease.
- Describing how medications are used for headaches and migraines.
- Discussing how drugs are used to relieve spasticity.
- Identifying central nervous system stimulants and their actions.
- Explaining the action of medications on the autonomic and peripheral nervous system.

Katherine, age 32, has a family history of migraine headaches with auras. In the past few months, Katherine has had two migraine headaches related to menstruation. She thinks these may be due to tension and fatigue from her new job.

What nondrug measures might Katherine try for relief early in the headache?

What are causes of nonmigraine headaches?

What is the group of medications specific for migraine headaches?

KEY TERMS

Absence or petit mal seizures
Acetylcholine
Adrenergic (sympathomimetic)
    agent
Analeptics
Analgesic
Anesthesia
Anorexiant
Aura
Autonomic nervous system
Blood-brain barrier
Cataplexy
Catecholamines
Central nervous system (CNS)
Cholinergic (or
    parasympathomimetic) agent

Clonic
Convulsion
Diaphoresis
Dyskinesia
Dystonia
Euphoria
Focal (partial) seizure
Generalized seizure
Grand mal seizure
Hypnotic
Narcolepsy
Neurohormones
Neuron
Parasympathetic nervous system

Parasympatholytic
    (anticholinergic or
    cholinergic blocking) agent
Peripheral nervous system
Physical dependence
Restless legs syndrome (RLS)
Sedative
Seizure
Spasticity
Sympathetic nervous system
Sympatholytic (or adrenergic
    blocking) agent
Tolerance
Tonic

Common Signs and Symptoms of Neurologic Disorders

Headaches and fever
Nausea and vomiting
Weakness and motor disturbances
Mood swings and memory impairment
Drowsiness/stupor/coma
Seizures, paralysis, convulsions, numbness
Muscle rigidity or flaccidity
Disturbances in speech, vision, hearing, taste
Tremors
Radiating pain

Common Side Effects of Medications for Neurologic Disorders

Visual disturbances
Lack of muscular coordination
Skin rashes
Drowsiness
Anorexia
Irritability
Headaches
Impotence
Dry mouth
Nightmares

Easy Working Knowledge of Drugs Used in Neurologic System Disorders

DRUG CLASS	PRESCRIPTION	OTC	PREGNANCY CATEGORY	MAJOR INDICATIONS
Analgesics	Yes	Yes	B, C, D	Relief of pain, RLS
Anesthetics	Yes	Yes		Blocking nerve endings causing pain
Sedatives/hypnotics	Yes	Yes (alcohol)		Sedation and treatment of insomnia, RLS
Antiseizure medications	Yes	No	C, D	Epilepsy and associated seizure disorders, RLS
Antiparkinsonism medications	Yes	No	B, C	Parkinson's disease and Parkinson's syndrome, RLS
Medications for headaches	Yes	Yes	B, C, X (ergot preparations and sumatriptan)	Headaches, especially migraine headaches
Medications for spasticity	Yes	Yes	C	Muscle spasticity
CNS stimulants	Yes	Yes	B, C	ADD, ADHD, anorexiants, fatigue
Cholinergics	Yes	No	C, X (isoflurophates)	Glaucoma, myasthenia gravis
Anticholinergics	Yes	No	B, C	Gastric antispasmodic and antiulcer treatment, mydriatic
Adrenergic	Yes	Yes	B, C, D	Cardiovascular and respiratory conditions
Adrenergic blockers	Yes	Yes	B, C	Hypertension, angina, glaucoma

The nervous system is composed of the brain, spinal cord, and nerves (Figure 30-1). Neurons are the basic cells of the nervous system, carrying nerve impulses from one part of the body to another. Axons carry nerve information away from the nerve cell body, and dendrites carry information to the nerve cell body (Figure 30-2). At the junction of neurons, the continuation of the messages is performed by neurotransmitters such as acetylcholine (ACh), which stimulates the nerve ending, and cholinesterase, which enzymatically breaks down ACh to inhibit its actions (Figure 30-3). Other neurotransmitters, or neurohormones, include the catecholamines, serotonin, and peptides such as the endorphins.

Incoming messages to neurons are received in the dendrites, passed through the dendrites, pro-cessed in the cell body, and transported to the axon. Messages exit by the axon terminal. They continue by either electrical or chemical transport across the synapse. The electrical impulses are generated and pumped at the junctions for moving the impulse through the nerve tract, allowing the nerve to react. Drugs can act directly on the impulses and their receptors to induce or reduce nerve transmission.

As a neurotransmitter ACh has various parasympathetic effects such as gastric peristalsis, vasodilation, and cardiac inhibition. Striated, or voluntary, muscles are contracted by the release of ACh at the neuromuscular junction, causing the muscle fibers to contract simultaneously for smooth body movement. Variations in the transmission of ACh and the inhibition of cholinesterase cause diseases related to body movement.

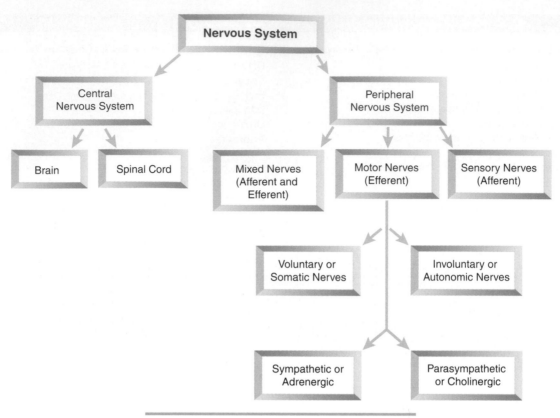

Figure 30-1 Components of the nervous system.

The catecholamines are stored in the brain and are attached to the sympathetic effector cells of the **autonomic nervous system** to depress stimulation of the brain. An increase in catecholamines and serotonin causes cerebral stimulation, so these drugs have a depressing effect on the brain.

The neuroactive peptides such as endorphins or enkephalins affect neuron activity by either increasing or decreasing the synthesis, release, or breakdown of the neurotransmitters at the synapse. Endorphins are the peptides that suppress pain and are the basis for acupuncture and transcutaneous electrical nerve stimulation (TENS) for pain relief. Enkephalins decrease the perception and emotional aspects of pain by blocking the receptors in the spinal cord.

The brain is covered by nerve cells that encircle the brain's capillary walls to form a **blood-brain barrier** that prevents the passage of many drugs and large molecules into the brain but allows small molecules (such as water, alcohol, oxygen, and carbon dioxide, as well as glucose and lipid-soluble materials) to pass for absorption. This blood-brain barrier is a type of security system against the toxic effects of some drugs on the **central nervous system** (CNS). Today's pharmaceutical

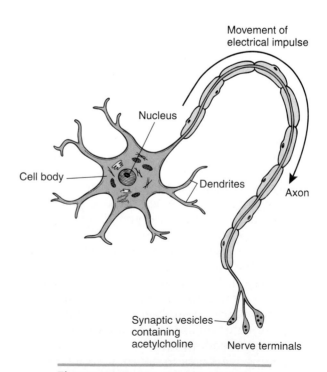

Figure 30-2 Components of a neuron.

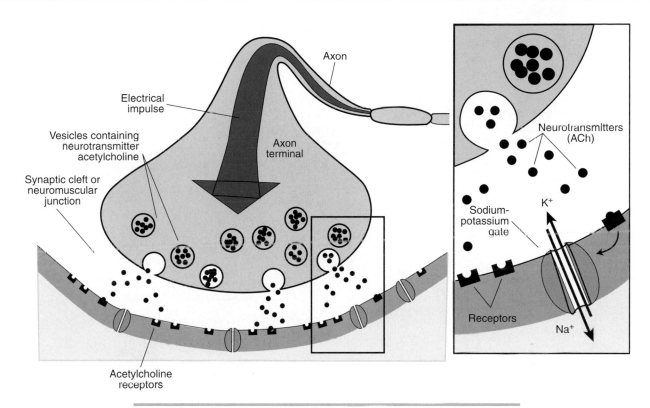

Figure 30-3 The continuation of nerve messages by neurotransmitters.

research involves ways to increase the permeability of the blood-brain barrier so that specific medications needed for treatment of diseases of the brain can be absorbed into the brain for direct treatment. Drug actions that require the use of the brain are directly related to the part of the brain affected by the medications. Figure 30-4 shows the areas of the brain and their specific function.

When neurons are too active or hyperexcited, too many messages are transmitted at a rapid, irregular rate, leading to distortion and interpretations of stimuli that are incorrect. These mixed messages lead to **seizures** of different types. If the neurons are not receiving sufficient stimulation, the neurons cannot detect the transmission and this decreases body function. Thus the medications for the nervous system are dependent on neuron stimulation, as well as the ability to cross the brain-blood barrier and the neuromuscular junctions.

The autonomic nervous system is also dependent on the actions of the neurons. The **sympathetic** nerves, also called **adrenergic,** are responsible for body safety through the "fight-or-flight" mechanism using the stimulation by two neurohormones—epinephrine or adrenalin and norepinephrine or noradrenalin. This mechanism provides the functions vital to body survival when the person must either react (fight) or run away (flight). When the

autonomic nervous system responds to stimuli, the blood and nerve stimulation bypasses body parts and organs that are not vital for survival, causing extra blood and nerve stimulation to be sent to areas of stress. The **parasympathetic,** or **cholinergic,** nervous system works to conserve energy through the neurohormone ACh and the enzyme cholinesterase. The parasympathetic system controls the "feed-or-breed" functions of the body by slowing the heart, digesting food, eliminating waste, and producing sex hormones.

Effects of Long-Term Drug Use on the Central Nervous System

When medications for the CNS are taken chronically, the effects over the long course may differ from those seen when the agent was first used because the brain adapts to the drug over time. When the adaptation is beneficial, it is considered therapeutic; when the adaptation is detrimental, it is considered a side effect. When some CNS medications are taken for a long time, the intensity of side effects may diminish while the therapeutic effect remains the same. This effect is desired in some medications (e.g., phenobarbital used in the

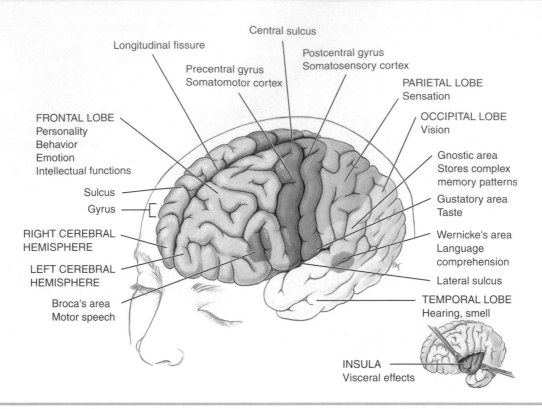

Figure 30-4   The areas of the brain and their function in homeostasis. (From Applegate EJ: *The anatomy and physiology learning system,* ed 3, St Louis, 2006, Saunders.)

treatment of epilepsy) because less sedation occurs over time. The undesired sedative effect of phenobarbital is decreased, whereas the desired anticonvulsant therapy is retained.

Certain drugs, typically the antipsychotics and antidepressants, must be taken for several weeks before the full therapeutic effects appear, although side effects may occur immediately after starting the medication. These drugs have an increased therapeutic effect that is not seen until the CNS responds and modifies its response to the prolonged drug exposure.

Tolerance and **physical dependence** are also manifestations of the CNS and its adaptive abilities. These responses are seen with medications used over prolonged periods. Tolerance is an adaptation of the brain to a medication, whereas physical dependence occurs when the drug-adapted brain requires the medication or withdrawal symptoms to occur when the medication is stopped.

Analgesics

Analgesics are used to relieve pain. Pain, a highly individualized response to a painful stimulus, is a unique and subjective symptom experienced by nearly everyone at some point in his or her life.

A feared symptom, pain is important because it warns the body that it is malfunctioning or is out of homeostasis. Only the person experiencing the pain can describe the symptoms, its intensity, and its site. The allied health professional must be aware of the types, signs, and symptoms of pain and the interventions for controlling or for preventing pain.

Analgesics are the subject of Chapter 16 but are included here in a short review because of their interactions with the nervous system and the person's perceptions of the treatment for effectiveness. The physical discomfort of pain may cause autonomic nervous system responses such as hypertension, **diaphoresis,** pallor, restlessness, anxiety, tensed muscles, and the inability to concentrate. Pain impulses are transmitted on afferent, or sensory, nerve fibers to the spinal cord and brain for interpretation. The brain releases the natural pain relievers, enkephalins and endorphins, to control pain. If these are not fully effective, analgesics are ordered for pain relief.

Classes of Analgesics: Narcotics and Nonnarcotics

Analgesics come in two main groups—narcotics and nonnarcotics (see tables in Chapter 16). Narcotic analgesics are either opioids—naturally occurring—

or opiates—synthetically produced—medications. The opioids and some nonopioids may be regulated by the Drug Enforcement Administration (DEA), others are prescription items without regulation, and some may even be bought over the counter (OTC). A great range in the potential for addiction and misuse is found with nonopioid analgesics.

Patient Education for Compliance

1. Opioids are given in specific doses that should not be adjusted or abruptly discontinued without the knowledge of the physician.
2. Increased fiber and increased fluids should be included in the diet when taking analgesics, especially with opioids, to prevent constipation. If constipation occurs, a laxative may be indicated.
3. Initial doses of opioids may cause nausea and vomiting, but this can be minimized with an antiemetic and remaining calm. The side effects usually subside with each subsequently administered dose.
4. Analgesics may cause drowsiness, decreased mental alertness, and decreased physical coordination, so hazardous activities should be stopped until the drowsiness can be evaluated to prevent accidents and falls.
5. Orthostatic hypotension may occur with analgesics, especially opioids, and the patient should take care in position changes while adjusting to the medication. Opioid medications may increase the effects of antihypertensives, especially causing orthostatic hypotension.
6. Severe or recurrent pain for more than 10 days or high continuous fever for more than 3 days should be reported to a health care provider.
7. Potential for physical and psychologic dependence and tolerance with opioids, sedatives, analgesics, and hypnotics exists. These drugs should be taken on a limited basis for short periods of time *except* by terminally ill patients.

IMPORTANT FACTS ABOUT ANALGESICS

- Analgesics are medications used to relieve pain without loss of consciousness. Some types of pain such as neuropathic pain and pain from inflammatory processes may not respond to opioid medications.
- Opioids are the most effective analgesics, with morphine being the prototype for analgesic relief.
- Respiratory depression is a serious adverse reaction to opioids. Other adverse effects are constipation, urinary retention, orthostatic hypotension, and vomiting.

IMPORTANT FACTS ABOUT ANALGESICS—Cont'd

- Prolonged opioid usage leads to physical dependence and abrupt stoppage will lead to withdrawal symptoms. Therefore opioids should be gradually withdrawn.
- Patients should avoid alcohol and other CNS depressants when taking opioid analgesics. Patients should also avoid antihistamines, tricyclic antidepressants, and atropine-like anticholinergic medications.
- Opioid dosage must be individualized. Patients with a low pain tolerance or with extremely painful conditions need higher doses. Patients with sharp, stabbing pain need higher doses that dull pain. The elderly require lower doses of opioids to be effective.
- Terminally ill patients should be given as much medication as needed to relieve pain.

Anesthetics

A short explanation of general anesthesia is included only as a general introduction to the area. In most instances the allied health professional will not see this in the outpatient setting, but the health care worker must understand the terms commonly used with general anesthesia for patient education.

The two types of **anesthesia** are general and local. Anesthesia by definition is used to produce a loss of sensation.

General Anesthetics

General anesthetics produce the desired effects throughout the body by blocking all sensory impulses to the brain, causing unconsciousness. The stages of anesthesia are the guidelines for the level or depth of anesthesia. The depths of anesthesia are controlled and passed through during induction and are reversed during recovery. The patient undergoing surgery is taken to stage 3 to allow muscular relaxation.

Stage 1: Analgesia This stage starts with the administration of anesthetic and lasts to loss of consciousness. The characteristics are euphoria, distortions of perceptions, and amnesia. Some surgery can be performed at this level.

Stage 2: Delirium This stage begins with loss of consciousness and extends to the beginning of surgical anesthesia. During this stage, the involuntary muscles are active, breathing is irregular, and hypertension and tachycardia may occur due to the excitability of muscles. Patients are taken through this stage rapidly.

Stage 3: Surgical anesthesia During this stage, muscle relaxation occurs and respiratory depression occurs. This stage lasts until spontaneous respirations cease.

Stage 4: Medullary depression This stage, usually caused by anesthesia overdose, begins with cessation of respirations and ends with circulatory collapse. Because of the circulatory and respiratory collapse, death occurs.

The most common route of administration for general anesthesia is inhalation, although some general anesthetics are given intravenously (IV). The main IV drugs are thiopental (Pentothal), ketamine (Ketalar), diazepam (Valium), and midazolam (Versed). Diazepam is used as an aid for induction of the anesthesia or as a preoperative medication.

Preanesthetic Medications

Preanesthetic medications are given to reduce anxiety, to produce preoperative amnesia, and to relieve preoperative and postoperative pain. These medications are often used prophylactically to reduce adverse reactions from anesthetics such as excessive salivation, coughing, vomiting, and increased bronchial secretions. Benzodiazepines such as diazepam and barbiturates such as secobarbital or pentobarbital are given to reduce anxiety and produce amnesia by producing mild sedation. The opioids are used to suppress coughing and relieve pain. Anticholinergic medications such as atropine decrease the risk of bradycardia during surgery and also dry secretions.

Midazolam

Intravenous midazolam (Versed) may be used for the induction of anesthesia or for conscious sedation. Conscious sedation is characterized by sedation, analgesia, amnesia, and lack of anxiety. The patient is unperturbed and passive but is capable of responding to commands needed for minor surgery or endoscopic procedures. This medication, used in outpatient settings where endoscopic examinations are performed, should not be administered unless resuscitation equipment is available because Versed causes respiratory and cardiac depression.

Patients are often fearful when anticipating surgery because of the surgery itself or the fear of feeling pain during the procedure. The allied health professional should attempt to dispel fear by assuring the patient that anesthesia provides sleep throughout the procedure with amnesia about the experience. This educational step is important because excessive fear may disrupt surgical procedures.

Local Anesthetics

Local anesthetics work by interfering with nerve conduction and pain perception from an area of the body to the CNS. The great advantage over general anesthesia is that the pain is suppressed without the loss of consciousness and depression of the entire nervous system, allowing medical and surgical procedures to be performed at less risk and pain for the patient. Pain perception is the first sensation lost, followed by cold, warmth, touch, and deep pressure, in order.

The onset of most local anesthetics is rapid; most last longer than necessary, whereas prolonged procedures may require repeated administration. Vasoconstrictors—usually epinephrine—are often added to local anesthetics to prolong the anesthesia and reduce the risk of toxicity. Systemic reactions such as palpitations, tachycardia, nervousness, and hypertension may occur with the use of vasoconstrictors.

Blood flow to the area is important in determining how long the anesthetic will last. In areas with many blood vessels, the anesthetic is quickly carried away; in areas where few blood vessels are found or the blood flow is restricted, a prolonged duration will occur. If local anesthetics are absorbed into the bloodstream, adverse reactions such as bradycardia and symptoms related to the conduction impulse of the heart may occur. If large doses are given, CNS excitability followed by depression and drowsiness may occur. Allergic reactions with local anesthetics are not common but may occur.

Local anesthetics may be administered two ways—topically as a surface anesthetic and by infiltration as an injection. Surface anesthesia may be applied to the skin or a mucous membrane. Toxicities to these medications are more likely to occur when the anesthetic is applied to a mucous membrane. The therapeutic uses for topically applied anesthetics are to relieve pain, itching, and soreness for such reasons as infections, burns, sunburns, diaper rash, wounds, bruises, abrasions, plant poisoning, and insect bites and for neuropathic-type pain. Applications to mucous membranes include those in the nose, mouth, pharynx, larynx, trachea, vagina, and urethra. Local anesthetics may also be used for hemorrhoids, anal fissures, and anal pruritus.

Infiltration anesthesia is injecting local anesthesia into an immediate area for surgery or orthopedic manipulation. The most commonly used infiltrates are procaine and lidocaine, which stop the conduction of nerve impulses and block motor neurons.

TABLE 30-1 *Topical Local Anesthetics*

GENERIC NAME	TRADE NAME	SITES OF APPLICATION	TIME TO PEAK EFFECT (MINUTES)	DURATION OF ACTION (MINUTES)
dibucaine	Nupercainal	Skin	<5	15-45
lidocaine	Xylocaine	Skin, mucous membranes	2-5	15-45
benzocaine	Many names	Skin, mucous membranes	<5	30-60
cocaine		Mucous membranes	3-8	30-60
tetracaine	Pontocaine	Skin, mucous membranes	3-8	30-60

Procaine

Procaine (Novocain) is a local anesthetic agent first made in 1905. Not effective topically, it must be administered by injection and is often given in combination with epinephrine to slow the absorption. Procaine is available in 1%, 2%, and 10% solutions for injection with epinephrine in ratios of 1:1000, 1:10,000, and 1:50,000. The allied health professional should carefully read the labels to ensure the selection of the correct medication by percentage of procaine and the correct ratio of epinephrine if it is ordered.

Lidocaine

Lidocaine (Xylocaine) was introduced in 1948 and is one of the most widely used local anesthetics today because it may be administered topically or by injection. This agent produces anesthesia more rapidly, more intensely, and has a more prolonged effect than procaine. The effects may be prolonged further by adding epinephrine, as with procaine. The injectable lidocaine comes in concentrations ranging from 0.5% to 20%. Allergic reactions are rare. Forms of lidocaine include creams, ointments, gels, aerosols, and solutions.

> **DID YOU KNOW?**
> Because lidocaine suppresses cardiac muscle excitability by blocking sodium channels, it is used to treat cardiac arrhythmias.

Cocaine

Cocaine, an excellent local topical anesthetic, is used primarily for anesthesia of the ear, nose, and throat. The anesthesia occurs rapidly and lasts for about an hour. Cocaine is a vasoconstrictor and should not be given with epinephrine because of an increased risk of cardiovascular toxicity. A Schedule II controlled substance, cocaine is available as soluble tablets, powder, and 4% solution, the usual form that is used (Tables 30-1 and 30-2).

TABLE 30-2 *Injectable Local Anesthetics*

GENERIC NAME	TRADE NAME	ONSET OF ACTION (MIN)	DURATION OF ACTION (MIN)*
procaine	Novocain	2-5	15-60
tetracaine	Pontocaine	≤15	120-180
lidocaine	Xylocaine and others	<2	30-60
mepivacaine	Carbocaine, Polocaine	3-5	45-90
bupivacaine	Marcaine, Sensorcaine	5	120-240

*Epinephrine may increase anesthesia duration by 2-3 times.

Patient Education for Compliance

Patients who have received local anesthetics should take care to avoid activities that might injure the anesthetized area while it is still numb and cannot respond to pain signals.

IMPORTANT FACTS ABOUT ANESTHETICS

- General anesthetics produce unconsciousness and insensitivity to painful stimuli. Local analgesics reduce sensitivity to pain without loss of consciousness.
- Local anesthetics may be mixed with epinephrine to cause vasoconstriction and prolong the effects of the anesthesia.

Sedatives and Hypnotics

The CNS influences the activity of the entire body. Depression of the CNS reduces physical and mental activity and is often related to the use of barbiturates and alcohol (see Chapter 31). **Sedatives** and **hypnotics** such as pentobarbital (Nembutal) and phenobarbital (Luminal) are used therapeutically to decrease CNS activity. The major difference between drugs being used as hypnotics and sedatives is the amount of depression and sedation induced. A small dose of a medication may be used for daytime sedation, whereas larger doses of the same drug may be used to produce hypnotic effects and produce induction of sleep (Tables 30-3 and 30-4).

TABLE 30-3 *Effects of Sedatives and Hypnotics on the Central Nervous System (CNS)*

INCREASED DOSAGE OF MEDICATION	EFFECTS OF DRUG	PSYCHOLOGIC/ PHYSICAL RESPONSE	CNS STIMULATION
Low dosage	No drug	Stress/ tension	CNS stimulated
	Tranquilizing	Calm	Gradual depression of CNS
	Sedative	Relaxed/ drowsy	
High dosage	Hypnotic	Sleep	Depressed CNS

TABLE 30-4 *Action Times of Barbiturates*

CLASSIFICATION	DURATION OF ACTION	TYPICAL MEDICATIONS
Ultra-short-acting	20 minutes or less	thiopental (Pentothal)
Short-acting	3-4 hr	secobarbital (Seconal) pentobarbital (Nembutal)
Intermediate-acting	6-8 hr	amobarbital (Amytal) aprobarbital (Alurate) butabarbital (Butisol)
Long-acting	10-16 hr	phenobarbital (Luminal) mephobarbital (Mebaral)

- Sedatives are used to reduce the desire for physical activity and reduce nervousness, excitability, and irritability, producing a calming effect. When various emotional or medical conditions cause anxiety or tension, the person's sleep may be interrupted and sedation may be indicated. Benzodiazepines such as diazepam (Valium) and lorazepam (Ativan) are used for their sedative effects (Table 30-5).
- Hypnotics are used to induce and maintain sleep and should be used intermittently only when needed for transient insomnia. Some drugs that are more frequently used as hypnotics are chloral hydrate (Noctec) and buspirone (BuSpar).

- Tolerance to hypnotics develops, and the effectiveness decreases after several weeks of continuous use. Therefore hypnotics use should be limited to 2 to 4 weeks.
- Benzodiazepines are frequently used over barbiturates as sedatives or hypnotics because of their safety.
- Other CNS depressants such as alcohol should not be used with antianxiety drugs and hypnotics/sedatives.
- Box 30-1 lists general rules for treatment of transient insomnia.
- Sedating medication such as diazepam and lorazepam may be therapeutically prescribed for its sedative effect in controlling stress related to hypertension.

Treatment of Sleep Disorders

Barbiturates

Barbiturates, some of the oldest drugs, produce a dose-dependent depression of the CNS for specific time periods. Most of these medications are classified as either Schedule II or III medications, although phenobarbital is a Schedule IV drug in most states (see Table 30-5).

- Barbiturates, depending on the amount given, produce depression of the CNS and mood alteration from reduced excitation to sedation followed by hypnosis and a deep coma. After 2 weeks of continuous use, these medications do not produce the desired effects at the same dosage. The tendency then is to increase the dose to produce the desired effects, leading to physical and psychologic dependence.
- After prolonged use of barbiturates, withdrawal symptoms may occur when the medication is stopped.
- These medications must be used carefully with elderly, debilitated persons, those with severe renal and liver disease, and those who have suicidal tendencies.
- The elderly consume between one third and one half of the sedatives and hypnotics prescribed because most have changes in sleep patterns that come with age. Older women report more sleep difficulties than men. The most common reasons the elderly give for being unable to sleep include respiratory problems, pain, and cramping of leg muscles.
- Of concern is that the elderly are susceptible to the many side effects that occur with sedatives and hypnotics. The elderly need to be watched

TABLE 30-5 *Select Sedatives and Hypnotics*

GENERIC NAME (SCHEDULE)	TRADE NAME	USUAL ADULT DOSE, ROUTE, AND FREQUENCY OF ADMINISTRATION	INDICATIONS FOR USE	DRUG INTERACTIONS
BARBITURATES			Hypnotic/sedative	alcohol, analgesics MAO inhibitors, other sedatives, theophylline, corticosteroids, oral contraceptives, oral anticoagulants
amobarbital (II)*	Amytal	Sedative: po 15-120 mg bid-qid; IM 30-50 mg q4-6h Hypnotic: 65-200 mg IM, IV		
aprobarbital (III)*	Alurate	Sedative: 40 mg po tid Hypnotic: 40-60 mg po tid		
butabarbital (III)*	Butisol	Sedative: 15-30 mg po tid Hypnotic: 50-100 mg po qd		
mephobarbital (IV)†	Mebaral	Sedative: 32-100 mg po tid-qid Epilepsy: 400-600 mg po tid-qid	Also used with epilepsy	
pentobarbital (II)*	Nembutal	Sedative: 30-120 mg/day po, IM, IV in 2-3 divided doses Hypnotic: 100-200 mg hs Preop: 100-200 mg IM		
secobarbital (II)‡	Seconal	Hypnotic: 100-200 mg po IM, 50-250 mg IV		
phenobarbital (IV)†	Luminal	Sedative: 30-120 mg/day po, IM in 2-3 divided doses Hypnotic: 100-320 mg		

MAJOR SIDE EFFECTS OF BARBITURATES: Ataxia, drowsiness, dizziness, hangover effects, nausea and vomiting, insomnia, constipation, headaches, night terrors, faintness.

BENZODIAZEPINES (IV)				
alprazolam*‡ (III)	Xanax	0.25-1 mg po qid	Sedative, anxiety, alcohol withdrawal	cimetidine, digoxin, macrolides, ethanol, grapefruit juice, phenytoin, carbamazepine
chlordiazepoxide† (IV)	Librium	5-25 mg po tid-qid 50-100 mg q2-4h IM, IV		ethanol, cimetidine, fluconazole, levodopa
clonazepam*‡ (IV)	Klonopin	0.5-2 mg po tid	Also used with seizures	valproic acid, disulfiram
clorazepate† (III)	Tranxene	7.5-15 mg po bid-qid	Also used with seizures	cimetidine, ethanol, rifampin, disulfiram
diazepam† (III)	Valium	2-10 mg po, IM, IV tid-qid	Also used with skeletal muscle relaxants and for seizures	See alprazolam
estazolam*‡ (IV)	Pro-Som	1-2 mg po hs	Insomnia	ethanol, cimetidine, disulfiram, macrolides, rifampin
flurazepam† (IV)	Dalmane	15-30 mg po hs	Insomnia	β-blockers, INH, cimetidine, clozapine, disulfiram. loxapine, macrolides, rifampin, omeprazole

(continued)

TABLE 30-5 *Select Sedatives and Hypnotics—cont'd*

GENERIC NAME (SCHEDULE)	TRADE NAME	USUAL ADULT DOSE, ROUTE, AND FREQUENCY OF ADMINISTRATION	INDICATIONS FOR USE	DRUG INTERACTIONS
lorazepam[†] (III)	Ativan	1-10 mg po in divided doses bid-tid	Anxiety, insomnia, alcohol withdrawal	ethanol, fluconazole, itraconazole
midazolam[‡] (II)	Versed	IM, IV varies with level of sedation	Sedation	calcium channel blockers, macrolides, lorazepam, and those with ethanol
oxazepam*[‡] (III)	Serax	10-30 mg po tid-qid	Anxiety, alcohol withdrawal	
prazepam[†] (IV)	Centrax	20-40 mg/day po	Anxiety, alcohol withdrawal	See estazolam
temazepam*[‡] (IV)	Restoril	15-30 mg po	Sedative, hypnotic	alcohol, CNS depressants
triazolam*[‡] (IV)	Halcion	0.125-0.5 mg po hs	Hypnotic, insomnia	alcohol, CNS depressants

MAJOR SIDE EFFECTS OF BENZODIAZEPINES: Drowsiness, hiccups, lassitude, dry mouth, nausea and vomiting, headaches, constipation, dizziness, blurred vision, insomnia, excitability, confusion, muscle weakness; additionally worsening of depression, decreased libido, and decreased fertility with ramelteon.

NONBENZODIAZEPINE AGENTS

zaleplon (IV)	Sonata	5-10 mg po hs; may be repeated if >4 hr of sleep remains	Insomnia	alcohol
eszopiclone (IV)	Lunesta	1-3 mg po hs	Same	alcohol
ramelteon	Rozerem	1 tab po 30 min prior to hs	Insomnia	rifampin

MAJOR SIDE EFFECTS OF NONBENZODIAZEPINES: eszopeclone: unpleasant taste, headache, dry mouth, dizziness; **ramelteon:** drowsiness, worsening of depression, decreased libido, decreased fertility.

MISCELLANEOUS HYPNOTICS/SEDATIVES

chloral hydrate (IV)	Noctec	250 mg po tid or 0.5-1 g hs	Sedative/hypnotic	alcohol, anticoagulants
zolpidem (IV)	Ambien	5-10 mg po	Hypnotic	CNS depressants, alcohol
buspirone[§]	BuSpar	5 mg po tid	Hypnotic	MAO inhibitors
hydroxyzine[§]	Atarax	10-100 mg tid-qid po, IM	Antianxiety, antiemetic,	alcohol
	Vistaril	25-100 mg q4-6h po, IM	Sedative/hypnotic	

MAJOR SIDE EFFECTS OF MISCELLANEOUS HYPNOTICS/SEDATIVES: Headache, nausea, nervousness, faintness, GI distress, dry mouth, blurred vision, inability to concentrate, depression, confusion.

ANTIHISTAMINES USED FOR INSOMNIA

			Insomnia	
diphenhydramine (OTC)	Nytol, Sominex, Sleep-Eeze	According to package instructions		alcohol
doxylamine (OTC)	Unisom	According to package instructions		

CNS, Central nervous system; *GI,* gastrointestinal; *IV,* intravenous; *IM,* intramuscular; *MAO,* monoamine oxidase; *OTC,* over the counter.
* Intermediate acting.
[†] Long acting.
[‡] Short acting.
[§] Not on Controlled Substances Act—no evidence for abuse.

for increased excitability, hostility, confusion, and hallucinations. Barbiturates should be avoided in the geriatric patient because CNS depression, confusion, and ataxia are often reported, especially with the elderly (Box 30-2).

- The short-acting benzodiazepines are safer agents than barbiturates.

BOX 30-1   GENERAL GUIDELINES FOR DRUG THERAPY FOR TRANSIENT INSOMNIA

Use short-term therapy with the lowest effective dose for the shortest period of time.
Assess patient regularly to ensure need for continued therapy.
Ensure no underlying pathology is the cause of insomnia.
Interrupt therapy to allow tolerance to decline.
Use hypnotics cautiously with those who snore heavily, are in respiratory distress, or are pregnant or suicidal.

BOX 30-2   IMPLICATIONS OF SEDATIVE/HYPNOTIC USE IN THE ELDERLY

Sleep disturbances are common with the elderly because preexisting conditions such as arthritis, dyspnea, and cardiac arrhythmias may cause interrupted sleep.
Hypnotics should be used for a short duration to treat acute insomnia and should not be given long enough to develop a tolerance/dependency.
Daytime sedation may occur when long-acting hypnotics are prescribed.
The use of relaxation techniques, the establishment of regular bedtimes, and avoidance of caffeine should be attempted prior to using hypnotic medications.
OTC sleeping aids often contain antihistamines, which cause dizziness, tinnitus, blurred vision, gastrointestinal disturbances, and dry mouth.

 LEARNING TIP

Most generic names for barbiturates end in -barbital, and the trade names end in -al.

Benzodiazepines

Benzodiazepines, or anxiolytics, are among the most widely prescribed medications because of their many advantages over the older medicines such as barbiturates, meprobamate, and alcohol.

- Diazepam (Valium) is the prototype of this class of medications.
- The indications for benzodiazepines include anxiety disorders, alcohol withdrawal, preop-

TABLE 30-6 *Safety of Benzodiazepines versus Barbiturates*

FACTORS RELATED TO SAFETY	BENZODIAZEPINES	BARBITURATES
Relative safety	High	Low
Depression of CNS function	Low	High
Respiratory depression	Low	High
Potential for suicide	Low	High
Chance of causing physical dependency	Low	High
Potential for abuse	Low	High
Tolerance potential	Low	High

erative medications, insomnia, seizures, and neuromuscular diseases such as skeletal muscle spasms or neuron dysfunction.

- Like barbiturates, the benzodiazepines have short- to long-acting duration.
- This group of drugs may be Schedule III and IV medications.
- The benzodiazepines have fewer deaths from toxicity and overdose, a lower potential for abuse and side effects, and fewer drug interactions.
- These drugs have muscle relaxant, antianxiety, anticonvulsant, and sedating/hypnotic effects.
- The newer benzodiazepines are even safer and shorter acting (see Table 30-5).

 LEARNING TIP

Many of the generic names for benzodiazepines end in -pam or -lam.

When comparing barbiturates and benzodiazepines for psychosocial uses or abuses, these medications are at opposite poles. Whereas the barbiturates are dangerous, the benzodiazepines are much safer (Table 30-6).

Other Medications Used as Sedatives/Hypnotics

A number of antianxiety drugs and sedatives/hypnotics do not fall into the categories of barbiturates or benzodiazepines. The actions are similar, causing sedation and hypnosis, making these agents such as zolpidem (Ambien) Schedule III and IV medications with a potential for misuse and abuse. As with barbiturates and benzodiazepines, these medications must be used with care in the elderly (see Table 30-5).

Other Products Available Over the Counter for Insomnia

Antihistamines, occasionally used for sedation, may cause excessive drowsiness when given with sedatives/hypnotics and may even produce a "hangover," or sedative effect, the day after they are taken. The Food and Drug Administration (FDA) has approved two antihistamines for use with insomnia—diphenhydramine (Nytol, Sominex) and doxylamine (Unisom). These medications are not as effective as benzodiazepines, and tolerance to the hypnotic effect develops quickly, often in less than 2 weeks. Daytime drowsiness often occurs (see Table 30-5).

Alternative products that do not require a prescription such as valerian root (an herbal supplement) and melatonin (a dietary supplement) have been employed to promote sleep. Valerian root can assist with falling asleep but does not help maintain sleep. Also, the supplement must be taken for a week or more to be effective. Melatonin is secreted by the pineal gland with an action that is stimulated with darkness. Some trials have indicated that melatonin supplement can promote sleep. Large doses have side effects such as headaches, hangover, nightmares, hypothermia, and transient depression.

Patient Education for Compliance

1. The potential for overdose with the elderly is always present, and signs of confusion, agitation, hallucinations, and hyperexcitability may show that this reaction is occurring.
2. Withdrawal from analgesics, hypnotics, and sedatives after long use may lead to nightmares, hallucinations, insomnia, or a combination of these.
3. With sedatives and hypnotics, daytime sedation is possible and individuals taking these drugs should avoid hazardous activities.
4. Medications for sedation and sleep should be taken in the lowest dose for the shortest period of time.
5. Alcohol and all other CNS depressants such as antihistamines should be avoided when taking sedatives.
6. The patient having difficulty sleeping should try to identify the cause. Ideally, the cause rather than the sleep disturbance should be treated.
7. Patients should not use OTC cold, cough, or allergy medications while taking sedatives/hypnotics. Some contain antihistamines that accentuate the drowsiness, whereas others contain CNS stimulants that defeat the purpose of sedatives.

IMPORTANT FACTS ABOUT SEDATIVES/HYPNOTICS

- Drugs that promote sleep are called hypnotics, with a chief side effect of causing daytime sedation and amnesia.
- Barbiturates, regulated by the DEA, have high potential for abuse and cause significant tolerance and physical dependence.
- Benzodiazepines are preferred to barbiturates and other general CNS depressants because benzodiazepines are much safer, have a low abuse potential, and cause less tolerance and dependence.
- Benzodiazepines can cause physical dependence, but the withdrawal syndrome is usually mild. To minimize withdrawal symptoms, benzodiazepine drugs should be decreased over several weeks to months.
- The principal indications for benzodiazepines are insomnia, anxiety, and seizure disorders. Benzodiazepines are the drugs of choice for transient insomnia. The dosage should be intermittent and should last only 2 to 3 weeks.
- Buspirone (BuSpar) does not cause sedation, has no abuse potential, does not intensify the CNS depressants, and the antianxiety effects take an extended time to develop. This medication may be the drug of choice for some patients because of these properties.

Antiseizure Medications

Epilepsy is a group of disorders that are characterized by hyperexcitability within the CNS. The abnormal stimuli can produce many symptoms from short periods of unconsciousness to violent **convulsions.** Approximately 2.5 million Americans have epilepsy. **Seizure** is a term for all epileptic events, whereas **convulsion** relates to abnormal motor movements such as the jerking movements of **grand mal** attacks. The seizures are of two broad types: **focal** or **partial seizures** and **generalized seizures.** Box 30-3 compares the different types of seizures.

Epilepsy cannot be cured but may be controlled. The first steps in control of epilepsy were in the mid-nineteenth century, when bromides were used to reduce seizures. In 1912 phenobarbital was found to produce depression of the motor cortex of the brain and thereby reduce the number of seizures. Phenobarbital had the unpleasant side effect of depressing sensory areas as well as the motor areas. Since the early 1900s, many drugs that bring epilepsy under control have been introduced.

Antiseizure medications allow individuals to have greater control of their lives by suppressing

I. Focal or partial seizures (limited spread)
  A. Simple seizures: Convulsion of single limb or muscle group with no loss of consciousness
  B. Complex partial seizures: Confused bizarre behavior with impaired consciousness
II. Generalized seizures (generally produce loss of consciousness)
  A. Nonconvulsive
    1. Absence or petit mal seizures: Loss of consciousness for a short time (10 to 30 seconds) with mild symmetric motor activity to no motor activity at all—may be as mild as only eye blinking
  B. Convulsive
    1. Tonic/clonic or grand mal seizures: Major convulsions with muscle rigidity and synchronous muscle jerks; marked impairment of consciousness
    2. Tonic/psychomotor seizures: Tonic muscle contractions
     a. Uncontrolled seizures: Usually children; multiple seizures per day (up to 100)
     b. Atonic or akinetic seizures: Sudden loss of muscle tone causing collapse of the body or body part without muscular contractions
     c. Myoclonic seizures: Sudden, rapid muscle contractions
     d. Febrile seizures: Tonic/clonic seizures of short duration, usually seen in children with moderate to high temperature levels (children more likely to develop epilepsy later)
    3. Status epilepticus: Uncontrolled seizures lasting 30 minutes or more; may be life threatening

the malfunction of neurons at the seizure focus. The reduction in the excitability of brain cells reduces the incidence and severity of seizures. Medications control 40% of petit mal seizures and reduce the frequency of another 35%. Tonic/clonic seizures are better controlled, with 50% being completely controlled and greatly reduced frequency in another 35%. Tonic, or psychomotor, seizures are controlled in only 35% of cases, but the frequency is reduced in another 50% of patients. Antiseizure medicines require dosage adjustments during times of stress, severe illness, or with medication taken for conditions other than seizure disorders.

• Medications for seizures include barbiturates (discussed earlier) that have anticonvulsant properties, but one—phenobarbital—is used most frequently for its antiepileptic properties. The sedative and hypnotic effects are unde-

sired in antiseizure uses. The tolerance that develops with these medications is a positive effect when used chronically to treat seizures. The sudden withdrawal of barbiturates with seizure-prone patients can produce convulsions. Therefore if withdrawal of barbiturates is desired, the dose should be gradually reduced (see Table 30-5).

• The benzodiazepines diazepam (Valium), clonazepam (Klonopin), and lorazepam (Ativan) are used as antiseizure drugs. Diazepam and lorazepam are used to stop seizures in progress. Clonazepam is used for myoclonic, akinetic/atonic, and absence seizures (see Table 30-5).

• The hydantoin class includes phenytoin (Dilantin), a potent broad-spectrum antiseizure medication for partial and tonic/clonic seizures. Phenytoin was the first medication that would suppress seizures without depressing the entire CNS and causing sedation. The hydantoins change the excitability of nerve cells by decreasing the effect of sodium in the brain. Because the hyperexcitability of the cells is decreased, a reduction in seizures occurs in most patients. Good dental hygiene and gum care are important with patients taking hydantoins (Table 30-7).

• Fosphenytoin (Cerebyx) is used parenterally for status epilepticus and when substitution for oral antiseizure medications is necessary, such as with surgical conditions (see Table 30-7).

LEARNING TIP
Most hydantoins end in -nytoin.

• Succinimides are also used exclusively for the treatment of petit mal or absence seizures. This classification of drugs decreases calcium currents in the brain that play an important role in absence seizures. The most commonly used succinimide is ethosuximide (Zarontin), with methsuximide (Celontin) and phensuximide (Milontin) being two other medications in the group (see Table 30-7).

LEARNING TIP
The generic names of the succinimides end in -mide, and the trade names end in -tin.

• Other antiseizure medications include new drugs, as well as drugs that have been around for a long time.
  • Carbamazepine (Tegretol) is similar to tricyclic antidepressants. Carbamazepine

TABLE 30-7 *Antiseizure Medications*

GENERIC NAME	TRADE NAME	USUAL ADULT DOSE, ROUTE, AND FREQUENCY OF ADMINISTRATION	INDICATIONS FOR USE	DRUG INTERACTIONS
BARBITURATES phenobarbital, mephobarbital, etc. (see Table 30-5)			Epilepsy—partial tonic/clonic seizures	See Table 30-5
BENZODIAZEPINES diazepam, clonazepam, lorazepam, clorazepate (see Table 30-5)			Myoclonic, absence, and akinetic seizures and status epilepticus	See Table 30-5
HYDANTOINS		All are highly individualized	Partial and tonic/clonic seizures	Oral contraceptives for all
phenytoin	Dilantin	50-200 mg po bid-tid		glucocorticoids, INH, diazepam, amantadine, phenobarbital, alcohol
fosphenytoin	Cerebyx	Individualized, IM, IV	For use when oral meds cannot be used	

MAJOR SIDE EFFECTS OF HYDANTOINS: Skin rashes, hirsutism, overgrowth of mouth gums, gingivitis, dizziness, visual disturbances, postural imbalance.

GENERIC NAME	TRADE NAME	USUAL ADULT DOSE, ROUTE, AND FREQUENCY OF ADMINISTRATION	INDICATIONS FOR USE	DRUG INTERACTIONS
SUCCINIMIDES			Absence seizures	None indicated
ethosuximide	Zarontin	500 mg/day po		
phensuximide	Milontin	1-3 g/day po in divided doses		
methsuximide	Celontin	300-1200 mg/day po		
zonisamide	Zonegran	500 mg po qd	Partial seizures	

MAJOR SIDE EFFECTS OF SUCCINIMIDES: GI symptoms, drowsiness, diarrhea, dizziness, blood dyscrasias.

GENERIC NAME	TRADE NAME	USUAL ADULT DOSE, ROUTE, AND FREQUENCY OF ADMINISTRATION	INDICATIONS FOR USE	DRUG INTERACTIONS
MISCELLANEOUS ANTISEIZURE AGENTS			Partial and generalized tonic/clonic seizures and mixed seizures	steroids, cimetidine, anticoagulants, lithium,
carbamazepine	Tegretol	100-400 mg po tid		acetaminophen, antidepressants, oral contraceptives, calcium channel blockers
valproic acid	Depakene	100-200 mg po bid	All generalized seizures and partial seizures	Other antiseizure drugs, medications for TB, salicylates, macrolides

TABLE 30-7 *Antiseizure Medications—cont'd*

GENERIC NAME	TRADE NAME	USUAL ADULT DOSE, ROUTE, AND FREQUENCY OF ADMINISTRATION	INDICATIONS FOR USE	DRUG INTERACTIONS
valproate	Depakote	125-250 mg po bid-qid (as sprinkle or tablet)	As with valproic acid	Same as valproic acid
primidone	Mysoline	250 mg-2 g po in divided doses	Psychomotor seizures	digoxin, alcohol, oral anticoagulants, valproic acid, carbamazepine
gabapentin	Neurontin	100-800 mg po tid-qid	Partial seizures	antacids
lamotrigine	Lamictal	50-100 mg po/day	Partial seizures	carbamazole, valproic acid, phenytoin, phenobarbital
levetiracetam	Keppra	500 mg po bid		Basically none
oxcarbazepine	Trileptal	600-2400 mg po/day	Partial seizures	Same
topiramate	Topamax	4-56 mg/day	Partial seizures	Same
tiagabine	Gabitril	25-1600 mg po qd	Partial tonic/clonic seizures, migraine headaches, alcohol treatment	Same, oral contraceptives
zonisamide	Zonegran	100 mg po daily	Partial seizures	Antifungals

MAJOR SIDE EFFECTS OF MISCELLANEOUS ANTISEIZURE AGENTS: carbamazepine: sedation, GI symptoms; **valproic acid** and **valproate:** nausea, vomiting, diarrhea, tremors; **primidone:** GI symptoms, anorexia, drowsiness; **gabapentin:** sleepiness, ataxia, fatigue, nausea, severe dizziness; **lamotrigine:** dizziness, diplopia, headache, ataxia, somnolence; **levetiracetam:** drowsiness, asthenia; **oxcarbazepine:** dizziness, nausea, headache, diarrhea, ataxia, nervousness; **topiramate:** dizziness, asthenia, somnolence, confusion, headache, tremors; **tiagabine:** somnolence, dizziness, ataxia, diplopia, nystagmus, nervousness, nausea, tremor; **zonisamide:** drowsiness, dizziness, headaches, nausea, impaired speech.

GI, Gastrointestinal; IM, intramuscular; INH, inhalation; IV, intravenous.

blocks sodium ion channels, much like phenytoin. This medication also possesses analgesic properties for neuralgia and to treat bipolar disorders.

- Oxcarbazepine (Trileptal), a derivative of carbamazepine, is better tolerated and may be used for partial seizures in adults and children.
- Valproic acid (Depakene) and valproate (Depakote) can be used for all types of seizures, as well as with migraine headache prophylaxis, by inhibiting neurotransmitters to the CNS. The reason these medications are not used more frequently is the potentially fatal liver toxicity.
- Primidone (Mysoline) is related chemically to barbiturates and is metabolized and converted in the body into phenobarbital.

- Gabapentin (Neurontin) suppresses the excitability of the neurons that initiate the epileptic seizures by acting in a manner similar to the same neurons of the brain.
- Several new drugs such as lamotrigine (Lamictal), tiagabine (Gabitril), and zonisamide (Zonegran) for control of partial seizures have been introduced. Topiramate (Topamax) has also been introduced for partial seizures and tonic/clonic seizures, as well as treatment of alcoholism and prevention of migraine headaches.
- Levetiracetam (Keppra) is used for adjunctive therapy in partial seizures in adults. The advantage of this medication is that it does not interact with other medications. For those patients who require IV medication for partial seizures, this medication has recently been approved for IV use (see Table 30-7).

Patient Education for Compliance

1. The person taking antiseizure medications should not omit, increase, or decrease medications without permission from the health care provider.
2. Antiseizure medications should not be discontinued abruptly.
3. Antiseizure medications may cause drowsiness or dizziness; therefore avoid hazardous tasks until the side effects are evaluated.
4. OTC medications should not be used with antiseizure medications without permission.
5. No alcohol should be consumed while taking antiseizure medications.
6. Use good dental hygiene following each meal, especially with hydantoins, because of the overgrowth of gum tissue.
7. Keep a record of all seizures—date, time, length, and so forth.

IMPORTANT FACTS ABOUT ANTISEIZURE MEDICATIONS

- Seizures are initiated by hyperexcitability of neurons. In partial seizures, the excitation takes place throughout certain areas of the brain. Generalized seizure excitation spreads throughout both hemispheres of the brain.
- The goal of antiseizure medication is to reduce seizures to an extent that the patient can live a normal life. Complete elimination of seizures may not be possible. Most antiseizure medications are selective for particular seizure types. Successful treatment depends on finding the most effective drug for each individual patient.
- Noncompliance is the main reason for seizure treatment failure.
- Withdrawal of antiseizure medication must be tapered and not abruptly withdrawn to prevent seizure activity.
- Most antiseizure medication causes CNS depression, and other CNS depressants such as alcohol, opioids, and antihistamines should not be used concurrently.
- Phenytoin, phenobarbital, and carbamazepine are active against partial seizures and tonic/clonic seizures but not absence seizures.
- Phenytoin causes gingival hyperplasia.

Drugs for Parkinson's Disease

Parkinson's disease is thought to be caused by a deficiency of dopamine and an excess of ACh within the CNS. The basal ganglia, a group of cell bodies within the medulla, help to regulate skeletal muscle tone and body movement by manufacturing dopamine. When regulating voluntary muscle movements, ACh is an excitatory neurotransmitter, whereas dopamine inhibits, or stops, the neurotransmitters to decrease muscle movements. Normally ACh and dopamine are balanced, providing smooth, better-controlled muscle movement. A decrease in dopamine produces excesses in ACh, causing the tremors and muscle rigidity typical of parkinsonism. Drug treatment is effective in reducing symptoms, but patients with Parkinson's disease become progressively disabled and may become immobile in later stages. Depression or dementia may occur, causing memory impairment and alterations in thinking. Appropriate medications may be used to treat the symptoms associated with parkinsonism. The medications for parkinsonism are to either increase the level of dopamine by administering levodopa—a precursor of dopamine—or the administration of medications that stimulate dopamine receptors. Reduction of ACh activity is another approach to drug therapy for parkinsonism.

- Levodopa is a medication that is converted into dopamine to lessen the symptoms of parkinsonism and to provide significant improvement in physical activity. The improvement may be such that many patients are able to resume normal activity. Levodopa can cross the blood-brain barrier (dopamine does not have this capability), and it is then metabolized by the body into dopamine.
- Carbidopa (Lodosyn) is given with levodopa to prevent the peripheral conversion of levodopa to dopamine, thus making more levodopa available to enter the brain. Carbidopa has no therapeutic effect and no side effects when given alone. Sinemet is a combination of carbidopa and levodopa and is available in three different proportions.
- Entacapone (Comtan) and tolcapone (Tasmar) are used with levodopa/carbidopa to improve the ability of patients with parkinsonism to accomplish activities of daily living by inhibiting the metabolism of levodopa (Table 30-8).
- The action of amantadine (Symmetrel) is to promote the release of dopamine. The effects of amantadine for parkinsonism were found

TABLE 30-8 *Medications Used for Parkinsonism*

GENERIC NAME	TRADE NAME	USUAL ADULT DOSE, ROUTE, AND FREQUENCY OF ADMINISTRATION	INDICATIONS FOR USE	DRUG INTERACTIONS
DRUGS TO INCREASE DOPAMINE			Parkinsonism	vitamin B$_6$, antipsychotics, carbidopa, anticholinergics, amantadine, pergolide, MAO inhibitors
levodopa	Dopar, Larodopa, L-Dopa	0.5-1 g po daily initially ↑ to 4-8 g daily in divided doses		
carbidopa/ levodopa	Sinemet 10/100 Sinemet 25/100 Sinemet 25/250	Individualized but usually 1 tab tid-qid po		
amantadine*	Symmetrel	100-200 mg po daily		alcohol
selegiline	Eldepryl Zelapar	5 mg po bid One orally dissolving tablet per day	Increases response to levodopa/ carbidopa	meperidine, tricyclic antidepressants
rasagiline	Azilect	0.5 mg-1 mg po qd	Same as above	meperidine, MAO inhibitors, antidepressants, dextromethorphan

MAJOR SIDE EFFECTS OF DRUGS TO INCREASE DOPAMINE: levodopa and **carbidopa/levodopa:** dystonia, nausea, vomiting, abdominal pain, dysphagia, dry mouth, mental changes, headache, dizziness, hand tremors, dyskinesia; **amantadine:** dry mouth, GI disturbances, CHF, visual disturbances, dizziness, confusion; **selegiline:** nausea, hallucinations, confusion, depression, loss of balance, dizziness; **rasagiline:** visual disturbances, headaches, seizures, nausea and vomiting.

DOPAMINE AGONISTS				
bromocriptine	Parlodel	1.25-100 mg/day po in divided doses		neuroleptics, erythromycin
entacapone	Comtan	200 mg with each dose of carbidopa/ levodopa		methyldopa, dobutamine, isoproterenol
pergolide	Permax	0.05-5 mg/day po in divided doses		
pramipexole	Mirapex	1.5-4.5 mg/day po in divided doses	Early or late parkinsonism and restless legs syndrome	cimetidine, dopamine antagonists, levodopa, ciprofloxin, estrogens
ropinirole	Requip	0.25 mg po tid		
tolcapone	Tasmar	100-200 mg po tid		levodopa, dopamine antagonists

MAJOR SIDE EFFECTS OF DOPAMINE AGONISTS: bromocriptine and **pergolide:** nausea, psychotic reactions, confusion, nightmares, agitation, hallucinations, paranoia; **entacapone:** nausea/vomiting, dyskinesias, orthostatic hypotension, hallucinations, sleep disturbances; **pramipexole, ropinirole, tolcapone, pramipexole:** nausea, dizziness, somnolence, hallucinations, orthostatic hypotension, agitation, confusion.

(continued)

TABLE 30-8 *Medications Used for Parkinsonism—cont'd*

GENERIC NAME	TRADE NAME	USUAL ADULT DOSE, ROUTE, AND FREQUENCY OF ADMINISTRATION	INDICATIONS FOR USE	DRUG INTERACTIONS
ANTICHOLINERGIC MEDICATIONS			Adjunctive treatment for parkinsonism	alcohol, amantadine, quinidine, procainamide
benztropine mesylate	Cogentin	1-6 mg/day po, IM, IV		
trihexyphenidyl	Artane, Trihexy	1-15 mg/day po in divided doses		
procyclidine	Kemadrin	2.5-5 mg po tid		
ANTIHISTAMINES			Reduce drug-induced extrapyramidal effects	alcohol
diphenhydramine	Benadryl	25-50 mg po, IM, IV in divided doses		

CHF, Congestive heart failure; *GI*, gastrointestinal; *IM*, intramuscular; *IV*, intravenous; *MAO*, monoamine oxidase.
* Also used with influenza to relieve aching and muscle shaking.

by accident while it was being used primarily as an antiviral. The principal indication for use with levodopa is to treat drug-induced dyskinesia. Amantadine is also associated with the release of dopamine from its storage site in the brain. Some patients experience a skin discoloration that disappears on discontinuation of the drug.

- Selegiline (Eldepryl, Cortex), a monoamine oxydase (MAO) inhibitor, reduces the "wearing out" effect of levodopa and is neuroprotective to delay the progression of the disease (see Table 30-8).
- Bromocriptine (Parlodel) is a direct-acting dopamine agonist and is often used with levodopa to decrease dyskinesias.
- Pergolide (Permax) is similar to bromocriptine in actions, uses, and adverse reactions. When given with levodopa, pergolide can prolong control of parkinsonism symptoms, reduce the fluctuations in motor response, and reduce the dyskinesia induced by levodopa.
- Two new dopamine receptor agonists have recently been approved. Pramipexole (Mirapex) and ropinirole (Requip) may be used alone in early Parkinson's or may be used with levodopa as the disease progresses and greater drug therapy is required (see Table 30-8).

Patient Education for Compliance

1. Antiparkinsonism medications may cause dizziness, drowsiness, and blurred vision. No alcohol should be consumed with these drugs.

Patient Education for Compliance—cont'd

2. Medications for parkinsonism should be taken with food to prevent the gastrointestinal disturbances that may occur.
3. Avoid vitamin B_6 with levodopa because it accelerates the breakdown of dopamine, thus decreasing the effects of levodopa.

IMPORTANT FACTS ABOUT ANTIPARKINSONISM MEDICATIONS

- Parkinson's disease is characterized by tremors, rigidity, bradykinesia, and postural instability. Parkinsonism is caused by degeneration of the neurons supplying dopamine, causing an imbalance between dopamine and acetylcholine.
- Parkinsonism is treated by activating dopamine receptors and by the use of drugs that block ACh.
- Levodopa is the most effective treatment for Parkinson's disease.
- Levodopa and MAO inhibitors taken together can cause a hypertensive crisis.
- Amantadine relieves the symptoms of early parkinsonism.

Drugs for Restless Legs Syndrome

Restless legs syndrome (RLS), affecting 2 out of 10 Americans, is characterized by an uncontrollable urge to move the legs when sitting or lying down. The person simply cannot sit still.

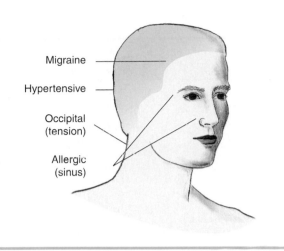

Figure 30-5 Differentiation of headaches by location of pain.

The cause is unknown, although the syndrome may be familial. Treatment includes using medications for parkinsonism, such as pramipexole (Mirapex) (see Table 30-8), opioids, muscle relaxants (see Table 30-5), and medications for epilepsy (see Table 30-7). The only drug approved by the FDA for RLS is ropinirole (Requip) (see Table 30-8).

Drugs for Migraine Headaches

Headaches are common symptoms caused by a variety of reasons including fatigue, illness, alcohol, and stress. Many headaches are relieved by OTC medications, but some patients have headaches that are debilitating, severe, recurrent, and require frequent medical attention (Figure 30-5). Severe headaches may be further subdivided into those with identifiable causes such as infections, hypertension, or tumors and those with no identifiable cause such as migraine or cluster headaches. If the cause of the headache is known, that cause is the center of treatment.

Migraine Headaches

Migraine headaches are characterized by unilateral, throbbing or nonthrobbing pain often accompanied by nausea, vomiting, and sensitivity to noise and light. Some migraines have an **aura** (formerly known as *classic migraines*), and some have no aura (formerly known as *common migraines*), the type most commonly found. Because migraine attacks are worse during menstruation and women seem to cease having migraines with menopause, hormones may be a component of the attacks. Familial tendencies are another common cause for migraine headaches. Some medical professio-

nals feel that migraine headaches are vascular in origin.

Drugs for migraines may be used in two ways: to treat a headache that is ongoing and to prevent attacks from beginning. The therapy must be carefully individualized because some headache medications can cause dependency.

Treatment of Migraines

Treatments of migraines that are ongoing are nonsteroidal antiinflammatory drugs (NSAIDs), opioid analgesics, ergot alkaloids, and sumatriptan. Aspirin, acetaminophen, ibuprofen, and other aspirin-like NSAIDs can relieve mild to moderate migraine headaches. These drugs may be combined with metoclopramide (Reglan) for the enhancement of absorption of aspirin. Fiorinal is an aspirin-containing medication with an added barbiturate sedative and caffeine. Fioricet is similar to Fiorinal but contains acetaminophen rather than aspirin. Another popular combination is Midrin (acetaminophen, a sedative, and a sympathomimetic) for pain relief. Midrin is contraindicated with glaucoma, severe renal disease, severe liver disease, and heart disease because of vasoconstriction.

- Opioid analgesics are used with severe headaches that do not respond to nonopioid analgesics. The most frequently used are meperidine (Demerol) and butorphanol nasal spray (Stadol NS). (See analgesics in Chapter 16).
- A specific medication for migraine headaches is a triptan, eletriptan (Relpax). By reducing the swelling of blood vessels surrounding the brain, it has a fairly rapid onset with relief for most people in 2 hours. Persons with vascular or coronary diseases should not use this medication.
- Sumatriptan (Imitrex), related to serotonin, relieves both headaches and the accompanying symptoms. This medication is available for oral and subcutaneous administration. Sumatriptan is teratogenic and should not be used in pregnancy.
- Other triptans include zolmitriptan (Zomig) and rizatriptan (Maxalt), which are similar to sumatriptan, with similar effects and side effects (Table 30-9).

Medications to Prevent Migraine Headaches

Nondrug measures such as biofeedback and other relaxation techniques are helpful in controlling or eliminating causative factors of migraine

TABLE 30-9 *Medications Specific for Use with Headaches*

GENERIC NAME (SCHEDULE)	TRADE NAME	USUAL ADULT DOSE, ROUTE, AND FREQUENCY OF ADMINISTRATION	INDICATIONS FOR USE	DRUG INTERACTIONS
NONOPIOID ANALGESICS				
aspirin 325 mg/caffeine 40 mg/butalbital 50 mg (III)	Fiorinal*	q3-4h po prn headache	Tension headache	Same as the ingredients included
acetaminophen 325 mg/caffeine 40 mg/butalbital 50 mg (III)	Fioricet*	q3-4n po prn headache	Tension headache	Same as Fiorinal
acetaminophen 325 mg/ dichloralphenazone 100 mg/isometheptene 65 mg	Midrin	1-2 caps po q4h, up to 8 per day	Tension/vascular headache	bromocriptine
sumatriptan	Imitrex	25-100 mg po followed by second dose in 2 hr	Severe migraine or cluster headaches	ergotamine, dihydroergotamine
zolmitriptan	Zomig	6 mg SC 2.5-5 mg po		

MAJOR SIDE EFFECTS OF NONOPOID ANALGESICS: sumatriptan, zolmitriptan: angina-like pain, pain in neck/throat, vertigo, malaise, fatigue.

GENERIC NAME (SCHEDULE)	TRADE NAME	USUAL ADULT DOSE, ROUTE, AND FREQUENCY OF ADMINISTRATION	INDICATIONS FOR USE	DRUG INTERACTIONS
TRIPTANS				
naratriptan	Amerge	2.5 mg po (5 mg max in 24 hr)	Migraine headaches	ergot preparations, other 5HT$_1$ agonists, MAO inhibitors
almotriptan	Axert	12.5 mg po (25 mg max in 24 hr)	Migraine headaches	Same as Amerge
rizatriptan	Maxalt	5-10 mg po (30 mg max in 24 hr)	Migraine headaches	Same as Amerge
eletriptan	Relpax	20-40 mg po followed by second dose in 2 hrs	Migraine headaches	ergotamine antifungals, nefazodone, macrolides, antivirals
frovatriptan	Frova	2.5 mg po q2hr up to 3 doses/day	Migraine headaches	ergotamine, oral contraceptives, propranolol

MAJOR SIDE EFFECTS OF TRIPTANS: eletriptan: dizziness, nausea, weakness, fatigue, pressure sensation in chest/throat; **frovatriptan:** hot/cold sensations, dizziness, fatigue, chest pain, skeletal pain, dry mouth, dyspepsia, flushing.

*May have codeine added in gr $\frac{1}{8}$, gr $\frac{1}{4}$, or gr $\frac{1}{2}$.

headaches. Rest in a quiet, dark atmosphere is often indicated as prophylaxis early in the headache. Some medications are given prophylactically to reduce the frequency and intensity of migraine attacks. These medications include β-blockers, amitriptyline (Elavil), calcium channel blockers, methysergide (Sansert), and valproic acid (Depakene) among others. Prophylaxis is indicated for those who have frequent or severe migraines or for those who do not respond adequately to other therapy.

- β-Adrenergic blockers (Chapter 27) are effective against migraines in approximately 70% of the patients.
- Amitriptyline (Elavil), a tricyclic antidepressant, is effective in prophylaxis against migraines (Chapter 31).

- Calcium channel blockers are also effective in reducing migraine attacks (Chapter 27).
- Phenelzine (Nardil), an MAO inhibitor-type antidepressant, is active against migraines. Nardil is potentially dangerous, so it is not used routinely (Chapter 31).
- Valproic acid (Depakene) and valproate (Depakote), used to treat epilepsy and bipolar disorder, are used as prophylaxis for migraines by reducing the number of attacks. This medication does not diminish the intensity or duration of the attacks (see Table 30-7).

IMPORTANT FACTS ABOUT MEDICATIONS FOR MIGRAINE HEADACHES

- Drugs for migraine headaches are used for either treatment of existing headaches or prophylaxis.
- The goal of treatment for migraine headaches is to eliminate the pain, nausea, and vomiting associated with the headaches.
- The goal of prophylactic therapy is to reduce the incidence of migraine attacks.
- Aspirin-like analgesics are effective for treating mild to moderate migraines.
- Opioids may be used for severe migraine headaches that have not responded to other medications.
- Propranolol, a β-blocker, is the drug of choice for prophylactic migraine therapy.

Drugs for Other Headaches

Cluster Headaches

Cluster headaches occur in a series or cluster, with each attack lasting 15 minutes to 2 hours. Severe, nonthrobbing, unilateral pain is usually located around the eye but is not preceded by an aura, does not include nausea and vomiting, is not familial in nature, and occurs mostly in males. These attacks consist of one or more every day for 4 to 12 weeks with an interval of months to years of separation in each cluster. Verapamil (Calan), a calcium channel blocker, lithium (Chapter 31), and glucocorticoids (Chapter 21) are used in cluster headaches.

Tension Headaches

Tension or muscle contraction headaches, the most common types of headaches, are characterized by moderate, nonthrobbing pain located in a distribution of the head, neck, and scalp with tightness and pressurelike pain. Precipitating factors are stress, frustrations, and eye strain. Tension headache may occur together with a migraine. An acute attack is treated with combination medications such as butalbital and muscle relaxants such as cyclobenzaprine (Flexeril) (see Table 30-9). Amitriptyline, a tricyclic antidepressant, is the drug of choice for prophylaxis.

Patient Education for Compliance

1. Patients may be able to find ways to avoid, control, or eliminate the factors that precipitate headaches.
2. Rest in a quiet, dark room for 2 to 3 hours after taking medications for headaches will ease the pain.
3. The possible causes of headaches such as eye diseases, sinusitis, or infections should be identified and treated.
4. Medications for headaches should be taken at the onset of symptoms unless prophylactic therapy is prescribed for patients with frequent migraine headaches.

Drugs for Spasticity

Spasticity is a phenomenon in which uncoordinated movements are caused by CNS overstimulation. The loss of dexterity, spasm, and increased muscle tone characterize spasticity, such as found with multiple sclerosis or muscular dystrophy. Trauma of the spinal cord or strokes may also cause the muscle spasms. Muscle relaxants are not effective in treating spasticity. Drugs and physical therapy are the treatments of choice.

- Baclofen (Lioresal) is used to reduce spasticity of multiple sclerosis, spinal cord injury, and cerebral palsy but not for strokes. The drug decreases flexor and extensor muscle spasm, reducing the discomfort of spasticity. If the medication is stopped, the withdrawal should be done slowly over 1 to 2 weeks.
- Diazepam (Valium) has similar actions but does not affect skeletal muscles directly.
- Dantrolene (Dantrium) is related to phenytoin and directly relaxes skeletal muscles by interfering with the release of calcium, decreasing skeletal muscles' ability to contract. This medicine is used with multiple sclerosis, cerebral palsy, and spinal cord injuries, and the medication may take as long as 45 days to develop effectiveness. Dantrium has a dose-related liver toxicity (Table 30-10).

TABLE 30-10 *Drugs for Spasticity*

GENERIC NAME	TRADE NAME	USUAL ADULT DOSE, ROUTE, AND FREQUENCY OF ADMINISTRATION	INDICATIONS FOR USE	DRUG INTERACTIONS
baclofen	Lioresal	10-20 mg po 3-4 × 3 per day	Muscle spasticity of CNS origin	alcohol, insulin
dantrolene	Dantrium	25-100 mg po bid-qid		calcium channel blockers, alcohol, estrogens

MAJOR SIDE EFFECTS: baclofen: drowsiness, dizziness, weakness, fatigue, nausea, constipation, urinary retention; **dantrolene:** muscle weakness, drowsiness, diarrhea, anorexia, nausea and vomiting, acne-like rashes.

Central Nervous System Stimulants

Stimulants for the CNS increase the activity of the CNS neurons. The CNS processes information to and from the peripheral nervous system and is the coordination center for control of the entire body. Many medications stimulate the CNS, but their therapeutic usefulness is limited because of the side effects throughout the body. Chronic use and misuse may occur, leading to drug tolerance, drug dependence, and drug misuse or abuse. We use stimulants such as caffeine on a daily basis when we drink coffee, eat chocolate, or drink caffeine-containing soft drinks. Caffeine is a stimulant that gives a "quick picker-upper."

CNS stimulants, also called **analeptics,** are used to fight fatigue, alleviate mild pain, and counteract the side effects of depressing medications to relieve respiratory distress. The most common analeptic is caffeine found in many foods, drinks, and drugs such as Excedrin, Anacin, and OTC decongestants. Prolonged high intake of caffeine may produce habituation and psychologic dependence. Withdrawal signs including headaches, irritation, nervousness, anxiety, and dizziness occur on abrupt discontinuation of caffeine. Caffeine should be used with care during pregnancy because it crosses the placenta to the fetus and will pass from the mother to child in breast milk.

In the past, CNS stimulants were prescribed for obesity, but today this use is considered obsolete and dangerous. CNS stimulants depress appetite, but tolerance usually occurs within 2 weeks and prior to the weight reduction goal if used for exogenous obesity. Amphetamines act by stimulating the cerebral cortex and have a high abuse potential because they produce euphoria and wakefulness. Because of the dangers of addiction and abuse, amphetamines are classified as Class II drugs by the DEA. The many side effects cause these drugs to have little use, but are a main therapeutic agent for the treatment of narcolepsy and hyperactivity found in attention deficit hyperactivity disorder (ADHD) and attention deficit disorder (ADD). The symptoms of

both of these conditions are the result of the improper functioning of the neurotransmitters. These medications should be avoided with patients with hyperthyroidism, hypertension, glaucoma, a history of drug abuse, and severe arteriosclerosis (Table 30-11).

- **Anorexiants,** stimulants for the short-term treatment of obesity, are used to suppress the appetite by a direct stimulation of the satiety center of the hypothalamus. Some of the agents work on the pathways of the sympathetic nervous system or adrenergic pathways, whereas others work with adrenergic and dopamine pathways. These agents have a high potential for abuse and are Schedule II through Schedule IV medications. Caution must be used when anorexiants are prescribed for people with hypertension, cardiac disease, and a history of seizures (see Table 30-11). (See Chapter 25 for further information on anorexiants.)
- Another use of stimulants is for narcolepsy, cataplexy, and auditory or visual hallucinations at the onset of sleep. CNS stimulants control daytime drowsiness and excessive sleep patterns. Stimulation results in an increase in motor function and mental alertness, a decrease in the sense of fatigue, and a state of euphoria.
- Psychomotor stimulants have uses similar to CNS stimulants that inhibit impulsive behaviors associated with ADD and ADHD. These medications are believed to activate the portions of the CNS that inhibit the impulsive behaviors (Chapter 31).

Patient Education for Compliance

1. Individuals taking CNS stimulants should be aware of the dangers of abuse and dependence. These medications should be taken exactly as prescribed. Abrupt withdrawal may result in depression, irritability, fatigue, agitation, and disturbed sleep.
2. CNS stimulants should be taken early in the day to prevent insomnia.

TABLE 30-11 *Central Nervous System Stimulants*

GENERIC NAME	TRADE NAME	USUAL ADULT DOSE, ROUTE, AND FREQUENCY OF ADMINISTRATION	INDICATIONS FOR USE	DRUG INTERACTIONS
caffeine	NoDoz (OTC), Vivarin (OTC), Caffedrine (OTC)	100-200 mg po	Mental alertness, respiratory depression	fluoroquinolone antibiotics, fluconazole

MAJOR SIDE EFFECTS OF CAFFEINE: Insomnia, nervousness, tremors.

AMPHETAMINES				
amphetamine sulfate	Adderall	5-60 mg/day po up to 40 mg/day 5-30 mg/day po	Narcolepsy, ADD Obesity	antacids, MAO inhibitors, guanethidine, cardiac glycosides, β-blockers
dextroamphetamine	Dexedrine	Same as amphetamine		None of significance
pemoline	Cylert	37.5 mg/day po	ADHD	
methylphenidate	Ritalin	5-20 mg po bid-tid	ADD and narcolepsy	

MAJOR SIDE EFFECTS OF AMPHETAMINES: amphetamine sulfate: Insomnia, weight loss, restlessness, euphoria, irritability, visual disturbances, excessive sweating, dry mouth, nausea/vomiting, anorexia, tachycardia, chest pain, impotence; **dextroamphetamine:** increased irritability, nervousness, insomnia, headaches, nausea and vomiting, sweating, tachycardia.

CENTRAL NERVOUS SYSTEM STIMULANTS USED AS ANOREXIANTS			Exogenous obesity	
diethylpropion	Tenuate, Tepanil	25 mg po tid		antihypertensives, alcohol, other CNS stimulants, MAO inhibitors
phentermine	Fastin, Ionamin, Adipex-P	8 mg po tid ac or 37.5 mg/day po		None
benzphetamine	Didrex	25-50 mg/day po		None
mazindol	Sanorex	1 mg/day po		MAO inhibitors
phendimetrazine	Bontril	35 mg po bid-tid ac		None
sibutramine	Meridia	10 mg/day po		MAO inhibitors

MAJOR SIDE EFFECTS OF CNS STIMULANTS: Increased irritability, euphoria, nervousness, insomnia, headache, nausea/vomiting, sweating, tachycardia.

ADD, Attention deficit disorder; *ADHD,* attention deficit hyperactivity disorder; *CNS,* central nervous system; *MAO,* monoamine oxidase.

Patient Education for Compliance— cont'd

3. Children taking CNS stimulants should be observed for tics, gastric disturbances, weight loss, nervousness, and insomnia.
4. Other stimulants such as caffeine should be avoided when taking prescribed CNS stimulants.

IMPORTANT FACTS ABOUT CENTRAL NERVOUS SYSTEM STIMULANTS

- Amphetamines produce most of their effect by releasing norepinephrine from neurons in the CNS and its periphery.
- Amphetamines can increase wakefulness and alertness, reduce fatigue, elevate mood, stimulate respirations, and suppress appetite.
- The principal indications for amphetamines are ADHD and narcolepsy.

Autonomic Nervous System Drugs

The autonomic nervous system can be thought of as the self-governing, involuntary, or automatic nervous system. The person has no control over this nervous system, which is divided into the sympathetic and parasympathetic divisions. These systems keep the internal organs of the body in homeostasis or at its highest level of function.

The system controls the function of the smooth muscle, cardiac muscle, and glandular secretions (Figure 30-6).

- The parasympathetic system and the sympathetic system simultaneously innervate many of the same organs, opposing each other to balance the innervations or negative feedback (Figure 30-7).

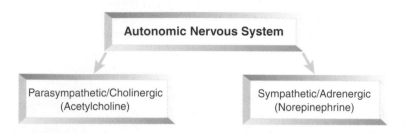

Figure 30-6 Divisions of the autonomic nervous system and the related neurotransmitters.

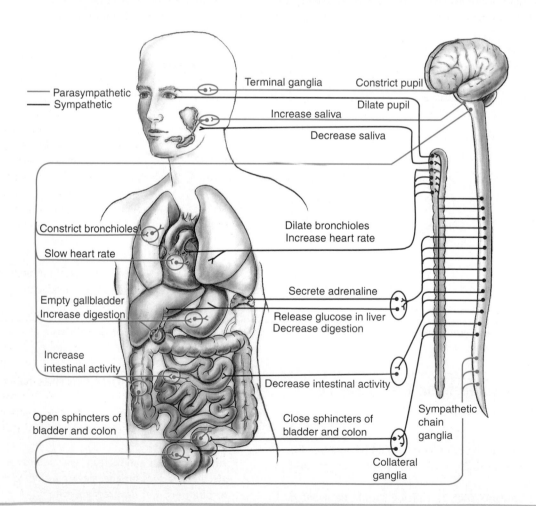

Figure 30-7 Comparison of the sympathetic and parasympathetic nervous systems. (From Applegate EJ: *The anatomy and physiology learning system*, ed 3, St Louis, 2006, Saunders.)

BOX 30-4   NOMENCLATURE FOR DRUGS ACTIVE ON THE AUTONOMIC NERVOUS SYSTEM

Division of the Autonomic Nervous System	Important Neuroactive Substances	Drugs That Promote or Reproduce Effects of This System	Drugs That Reduce or Block Effects of This System
Parasympathetic (cholinergic)	acetylcholine cholinesterase	Parasympathomimetic (cholinergic or cholinergic-acting drugs; also called cholinergic agonists)	Parasympatholytic (anticholinergic or cholinergic blocking drugs; also called cholinergic antagonists)
Sympathetic (adrenergic)	epinephrine norepinephrine dopamine	Sympathomimetic (adrenergic or adrenergic-acting drugs; also called adrenergic agonists)	Sympatholytic (antiadrenergic or adrenergic-blocking drugs; also called adrenergic antagonists)

Mime (mimetic): To reproduce, resemble closely.

Lyse (lytic): To dissolve, abate; to reduce an effect.

Agonist (agonistic): Entity that activates; in pharmacology, a drug that stimulates the activity of cell receptors normally responsive to naturally occurring chemical substances.

Antagonist (antagonistic): Entity that counteracts the action of another substance; in pharmacology, a drug that prevents stimulation of a receptor site.

- The parasympathetic system has the primary function of conserving energy and restoring the body's resources for rest and digestion, or the "feed-and-breed" system.
- The sympathetic system mobilizes the person during emergency or stress situations, or the "fight-or-flight" response. These sympathetic responses raise energy expenditures and increase body functions for response to energy requirements while decreasing digestive functions.
- The medications affecting the autonomic nervous system may mimic, intensify, or block the effects of the sympathetic or parasympathetic divisions.
  - Cholinergic medications mimic the parasympathetic system and so are called *parasympathomimetic drugs*.
  - Anticholinergic or cholinergic blocking agents, also called *parasympatholytics*, block the actions of the transmission of the parasympathetic nervous system.
  - Adrenergic drugs, or sympathomimetic agents, act to facilitate the sympathetic nervous system.
  - Adrenergic blockers, or sympatholytic drugs, block the action of the sympathetic nervous system. The terminology for substances active on the autonomic nervous system is summarized in Box 30-4.

 LEARNING TIP

Mimetic means to imitate or mimic, so *parasympathomimetic* means to mimic the parasympathetic nervous system, or acetylcholine. *Sympathomimetic* means to mimic the sympathetic nervous system transmitters such as norepinephrine and epinephrine. *Lysis* means to relieve or reduce the action of; *lytic* comes from lysis, so parasympatholytics act as cholinesterase to decrease the action of acetylcholine. Sympatholytics are used to block the sympathetic nervous system and are also called *adrenergic blockers*.

Cholinergic or Parasympathomimetic Medications

Acetylcholine is important in the transmission of nerve impulses in both phases of the autonomic nervous system. The parasympathetic nerve fibers liberate ACh as the facilitator for nerve impulses.

Cholinergic agents or parasympathomimetic drugs are obtained from plant or synthetic sources, with the synthetic medications being more stable. These are subdivided into two groups: direct-acting and indirect-acting drugs:

- The direct-acting medications such as bethanechol (Urecholine) bind to receptors to mimic ACh but have a longer action than ACh, which has a duration too short to be pharmacologically effective.

TABLE 30-12 *Cholinergic (Parasympathomimetic) Agents*

GENERIC NAME	TRADE NAME	USUAL ADULT DOSE, ROUTE, AND FREQUENCY OF ADMINISTRATION	INDICATIONS FOR USE	DRUG INTERACTIONS
DIRECT-ACTING MEDICATIONS				
acetylcholine	Miochol, Miochol-E	0.5-2 mL of 1% solution topical/ophthalmic drops	Miotic for cataract surgery	None
carbachol	Miostat	1-2 gtt bid-tid topical/ophthalmic drops	Glaucoma to lower ocular pressure	None
pilocarpine	Pilomiotin	1 gtt q4-12h topical/ophthalmic drops	Same as above	carbachol, β-blockers
	Ocusert	1 ophthalmic insert q7 days		
bethanechol	Urecholine, Duvoid	10-50 mg po bid 2.5-5 mg SC tid-qid	Urinary retention	ambenonium, neostigmine, atropine, quinidine, procainamide, epinephrine

MAJOR SIDE EFFECTS OF DIRECT-ACTING MEDICATIONS: Nausea and vomiting, diarrhea, muscle cramps, muscle weakness, slowing of heart, hypotension, respiratory depression, bronchospasm, flushing, sweating, excessive saliva, tearing.

INDIRECT-ACTING MEDICATIONS				
demecarium	Humorsol	1-2 ophthalmic gtts bid	Glaucoma	None
isoflurophate	Floropryl	¼-in strip ophthalmic ointment in conjunctival sac q8-12h	Also used with esotropia	None
physostigmine	Eserine	¼-in. strip ophthalmic ointment qd-tid 1 ophthalmic gtt qd-qid		β-blockers
ambenonium	Mytelase	5 mg po q3-4h up to 5-75 mg/dose	Myasthenia gravis	tacrine
edrophonium	Tensilon, Enlon	1-2 mg IM, IV, followed by anticholinesterase po 1 hr later	Testing for myasthenia gravis	procainamide and tacrine
neostigmine	Prostigmin	15-375 mg/day po, IM in 3-6 doses	Also used with treatment of myasthenia gravis	succinylcholine, same as bethanechol

IM, Intramuscular *IV,* intravenous; *SC,* subcutaneous.

- Indirect-acting medications such as neostigmine (Prostigmin) inhibit the enzyme acetylcholinesterase, allowing ACh to accumulate at the receptor sites.

Cholinergic medications produce actions similar to ACh and are used in conditions that require the following:

- Stimulating the intestines to increase peristalsis or the bladder to increase urination
- Lowering intraocular pressure with glaucoma because of miotic response of the eyes
- Increasing salivation and sweating

- Reversing the effects of curare-like medications used for relaxation during anesthesia

These medications are contraindicated in benign prostatic hypertrophy, gastric ulcers, intestinal obstructions, asthma, and cardiac disorders (Table 30-12).

Some physicians use cholinergic agents to increase ACh levels in the brain at the nerve synapses as a treatment of Alzheimer's disease. The memory loss, dementia, and deterioration of mental function are thought to occur because of lack of ACh in these synapses. The use of these medications in Alzheimer's disease is discussed in Chapter 31.

TABLE 30-13 *Anticholinergic (Parasympatholytic) Agents*

GENERIC NAME	TRADE NAME	USUAL ADULT DOSE, ROUTE, AND FREQUENCY OF ADMINISTRATION	INDICATIONS FOR USE	DRUG INTERACTIONS
atropine	Iso-Atropine	0.4-1 mg po q4-6h	Bradycardia, GI and GU hypermotility, Preop to ↓ secretions	amantadine, quinidine, disopyramide, levodopa, procainamide
	Ocu-tropine	1-2 ophthalmic gtt up to tid	Mydriasis	methotrimeprazine
hyoscyamine	Levsin, Cystospaz	0.125-0.25 mg tid-qid po, IM, SC, SL	Peptic ulcers, irritable bowel syndrome, vertigo, enuresis, parkinsonism, urinary tract spasms	None
scopolamine		1 patch q 3 days	Motion sickness	None
dicyclomine	Bentyl, Antispas	20-40 mg po tid-qid	Irritable bowel syndrome, infant colic, antispasmodic	amantadine, levodopa, tricyclic antidepressants, MAO inhibitors, H_1 antihistamines, phenothiazines, ketoconazole
propantheline	Pro-Banthine	15 mg qid po ac and hs		tricyclic antidepressants

MAJOR SIDE EFFECTS: atropine: flushing, blurred vision, dry mouth, constipation, urinary retention, headaches, confusion, tachycardia.

IM, Intramuscular *SC,* subcutaneous; *SL,* sublingual.

Anticholinergic or Parasympatholytic Medications

Cholinergic blocking agents such as hyoscyamine (Levsin) and scopolamine, which block cholinergic receptor sites, are referred to as *anticholinergics* or *parasympatholytic agents.*

- These medications are in competition with ACh and do not allow sufficient ACh to bind to the receptor sites to allow ACh action.
- The actions are the opposite of those found in cholinergic agents and include mydriasis (dilation) of the pupil of the eye, drying of mouth, nose, throat, and bronchi secretions, decreased secretions and motility in the gastrointestinal tract, increased heart rate, and decreased sweating.
- These medications are used as follows:
  - Antispasmodic and antisecretory agents in the gastrointestinal and genitourinary tracts
  - Neuromuscular blockers with spastic disorders

  - Antidotes for insecticide and mushroom poisoning
  - Emergency care of bradycardia and atrioventricular heart block
  - Dilation of pupils
  - Prevention and treatment of bronchospasm
- The contraindications are COPD, asthma, angle-closure glaucoma, gastrointestinal and genitourinary obstruction, cardiac arrhythmias, hypertension, hypothyroidism, and liver and renal disease (Table 30-13).

Patient Education for Compliance

1. Patients taking cholinergic medications or those exposed to insecticides such as malathion should report to a physician when such symptoms as decreased heart rate, decreased respirations, gastrointestinal distress, and excessive perspiration occur.

Patient Education for Compliance—cont'd

2. Cholinergic medications should not be combined with heart medications or antibiotics.
3. Medic-alert tags should be worn with cholinergic and antiseizure medication use.
4. Those taking cholinergic blockers should practice frequent mouth care and good dental hygiene.
5. Fluids such as water should be kept with the patient taking cholinergic blockers to combat the effects of dry mouth. Chewing gum and hard candy may also be useful.
6. Report rapid heart rate or palpitations and blurred vision when taking anticholinergics.
7. Avoid oral anticholinergics with COPD or asthma and use only prescribed inhalants. No OTC products should be used.
8. Anticholinergics may cause photophobia, so sunglasses outside and reduced light indoors may be necessary.

IMPORTANT FACTS OF ANTICHOLINERGIC MEDICATIONS

- Cholinergic medications, or parasympathomimetics, mimic the effects in the body similar to those produced by ACh and either act directly on the cholinergic receptors or indirectly by inhibiting the action of cholinesterase.
- Cholinergic medications stimulate peristalsis and urination, lower intraocular pressure with glaucoma, and treat myasthenia gravis by innervating skeletal muscles.
- Cholinergic blocking agents do not allow ACh to bind to receptor sites. As a result, these medications produce mydriasis, drying of secretions, decreased motility of the gastrointestinal tract, and increased heart rate.
- Cholinergic blocking agents, especially atropine, are used as antispasmodics and antisecretory agents, with one specific function being as an antidote for insecticide poisoning.

Adrenergic Agonists or Sympathomimetic Drugs

The sympathetic nervous system is thought of as the emergency system that can mobilize the body for quick response or action needed for response to frightening situations—the fight-or-flight response. Blood pressure, pulse, and respirations increase, the peripheral blood vessels constrict to allow flow of blood to vital organs, the pupils dilate, and the bronchioles dilate to supply more oxygen. The adrenergic agonists have a broad spectrum of clinical applications in many specialty areas from obstetrics to cardiovascular medicine.

The medications found within the *adrenergic agonists* or *sympathomimetic* classification are catecholamines and noncatecholamines.

- The catecholamines such as epinephrine (adrenalin) and dopamine (levodopa) found naturally in the body are norepinephrine, secreted at the nerve terminals, epinephrine, from the adrenal medulla, and dopamine, from sites in the brain, kidneys, and gastrointestinal tract. These same agents may be produced synthetically to produce the same effects as those naturally secreted neurotransmitters.
- The noncatecholamines including ephedrine and phenylephrine (Sudafed) have somewhat similar actions as the catecholamines but are more selective of receptor sites and are not quite as fast acting, with a longer duration.
  - Sympathomimetics are used to restore cardiac rhythm and elevate blood pressure in shock and emergency situations.
  - In the medical office, these adrenergic agonists may be used to constrict capillaries to control bleeding in relief of nosebleeds or alleviate nasal congestion.
  - The addition of these agents to local anesthetics for control of bleeding is commonly found in medical and dental practice.
  - The epinephrine-type medications are used to dilate bronchioles in asthma attacks, bronchospasm, or with anaphylactic reactions.
  - When the agents are used on lacerations found in peripheral tissues such as the nose, fingers, or toes, tissue necrosis is possible.
  - Because of the side effects, adrenergics should be used with extreme caution in patients with angina, coronary insufficiencies, hypertension, cardiac arrhythmias, angle-closure glaucoma, organic brain damage, and hyperthyroidism (Table 30-14).

Adrenergic Blocking Agents

Adrenergic blockers are also composed of two groups—α- and β-adrenergic blocking agents—depending on the receptors that are blocked. These agents plug or block the receptors, preventing other agents from stimulating the receptor sites. The α-blockers such as prazosin (Minipress) and terazosin (Hytrin) prevent norepinephrine from producing the sympathetic response. The

TABLE 30-14 *Adrenergic Agonists*

GENERIC NAME	TRADE NAME	USUAL ADULT DOSE, ROUTE, AND FREQUENCY OF ADMINISTRATION	INDICATIONS FOR USE	DRUG INTERACTIONS
α-ADRENERGIC AGONISTS				
epinephrine	Primatene[†], Bronkaid[†],	Inhalation q4h prn 0.1-0.5 mL SC, IM,	Bronchospasm, asthma, anaphylaxis, cardiac arrest,	MAO inhibitors, tricyclic, antidepressants anesthetics,
	Adrenalin	0.1-0.5 mL1% IM 0.001% as topical hemostatic with local anesthetics 1-2 gtts daily-bid ophthalmic topical 0.25%-2% solution	↑ BP, prolong local anesthesia	β-blockers, sympathomimetics
	Epi-E-Z Pen*	Inject as needed	Anaphylaxis prevention	
ephedrine	Efedron, Ectasule	25 mg po tid-qid 12.5-50 mg q3-4h IM, IV, SC 2-4 drops or small amount of gel in nostril qid for 3-4 days	Bronchodilators, nasal decongestion, ↑ BP, epistaxis, myasthenia gravis, urinary incontinence	Same as epinephrine and norepinephrine
metaraminol	Aramine	2-10 mg IM, SC; 0.5-5 mg IV	↑ BP, vasoconstriction	Same as ephedrine
methoxamine	Vasoxyl	5-20 mg IM	Same	Same
norepinephrine	Levophed	8-12 mcg/min IV	Same	Same
phenylephrine	Neo-Synephrine* Isopto-Frin*, Prefrin[†], Sinex[†], Sinarest Nasal Neo-Synephrine[†] Neo-Synephrine gel[†]	1-10 mg IV 10 mg po 1-2 gtt ophthalmic 2-3 gtt of spray or drops in nostril—0.25-0.5% solution q3-4h prn Small amounts into each nostril q3-4h prn	↑ BP, nasal decongestant, vasoconstriction, mydriasis	Same
pseudoephedrine	Sudafed, Novafed, PediaCare, etc.[†]	60 mg po q4-6h	Nasal decongestant	Other sympathomimetics, MAO inhibitors, β-blockers

MAJOR SIDE EFFECTS OF α-ADRENERGIC AGONISTS: Palpitations, tachycardia, nervousness, tremors, cardiac arrhythmias, anginal pain, hypertension, hyperglycemia, headaches, insomnia; irritation of nasal sinuses and eyes when used as decongestants.

(continued)

TABLE 30-14 *Adrenergic Agonists—cont'd*

GENERIC NAME	TRADE NAME	USUAL ADULT DOSE, ROUTE, AND FREQUENCY OF ADMINISTRATION	INDICATIONS FOR USE	DRUG INTERACTIONS
β-ADRENERGIC AGONISTS				
epinephrine	(see above)		Bronchodilator	
albuterol	Proventil Ventolin	1-2 inhalations q4-6h 2-4 mg po 3-4 × per day	Bronchodilator	epinephrine, MAO inhibitors, tricyclic antidepressants, β-blockers
isoetharine	Bronkosol, Bronkometer	Nebulizer/ inhalation various strengths and doses		
isoproterenol	Isuprel	0.02-0.06 mg IV 0.15-2 mg prn SC 10-15 mg SL q6-8h	Also used as cardiac stimulator	Same as albuterol
	Medihaler-ISO	1-2 inhalations 4-6 × per day		
metaproterenol	Alupent, Metaprel	2-3 inhalations q3-4h 20 mg po q6-8h	Bronchodilator	Same as albuterol
terbutaline	Brethine Bricanyl	2.5-5 mg po tid 0.25 mg SC at intervals, depending on use	Also used as muscle relaxant in premature labor	Same as albuterol
	Brethaire	2 inhalations separated by 1 min q4-6h		
salmeterol	Serevent	2 inhalations bid or 2 inhalations 30-60 min prior to exercise	Bronchodilator Prevent exercise-induced bronchospasm	β-blockers
dopamine	Intropin	IV based on body weight	Vasopressor for shock	Same as albuterol

BP, Blood pressure; *IM*, intramuscular; *IV*, intravenous; *SC*, subcutaneous.
* Prescription required.
† OTC medication.

major effect of α-blockade is a lowering of the blood pressure and vasodilation. The α-blockers are widely used to treat hypertension. Their antihypertensive effects are discussed in Chapter 27. These agents are also used to treat peripheral vascular conditions such as Raynaud's disease and to diagnose pheochromocytoma, a tumor of the adrenal medulla. These agents are found in the chapter tables related to the body system of use and Table 30-15.

β-Adrenergic Receptor Blockers (β-Blockers)

The β-blockers such as metoprolol (Lopressor) and nadolol (Corgard) bind to the β-adrenergic receptors, especially in the heart. The clinical use of β-blockers is to decrease the activity of the heart—heart rate, force of cardiac contractions, and impulse conduction. The reduction in heart work causes a decrease in the need for oxygen.

TABLE 30-15 *Adrenergic Blocking Agents*

GENERIC NAME	TRADE NAME	USUAL ADULT DOSE, ROUTE, AND FREQUENCY OF ADMINISTRATION	INDICATIONS FOR USE	DRUG INTERACTIONS
α-BLOCKERS				
doxazosin	Cardura	1-8 mg po 1-16 mg po	Benign prostatic hypertrophy, hypertension	ACE inhibitors, indomethacin, verapamil, nifedipine
phentolamine	Regitine	2-5 mg IM, IV	Peripheral vascular disease	Same as doxazosin
prazosin	Minipress	1-5 mg po tid	Hypertension	ACE inhibitors, NSAIDs, verapamil, β-blockers
terazosin	Hytrin	1-20 mg po daily	Hypertension	ACE inhibitors, NSAIDs, propranolol
yohimbine	Yohimex	5.4 mg po tid	Male impotence	

MAJOR SIDE EFFECTS OF α-BLOCKERS: Miosis, nasal congestion, increased GI activity, tachycardia, orthostatic hypotension, fainting.

β-BLOCKERS				
labetalol	Normodyne	100-400 mg po in divided doses	Hypertension up to 300 mg	cimetidine, NSAIDs, epinephrine
nadolol	Corgard	80-240 mg/day po in 1 dose	Also used with angina pectoris	adenosine, ampicillin, antacids, calcium channel blockers, clonidine, lidocaine, neostigmine, NSAIDs, prazosin, tacrine, verapamil
pindolol	Visken	15-60 mg/day po	Hypertension	Same and multiple others
propranolol	Inderal	120-480 mg/day po, IV in divided doses	Also used with angina pectoris, arrhythmias, migraines	NSAIDs, antidiabetic agents, barbiturates, calcium channel blockers, digoxin, epinephrine
timolol	Blocadren, Timoptic	10-60 mg bid po ophthalmic as directed	Hypertension Glaucoma	diuretics, NSAIDs
acebutolol	Sectral	400-800 mg/day po	Hypertension, ventricular arrhythmias	ampicillin, antacids, local anesthetics, digoxin, epinephrine, NSAIDs
atenolol	Tenormin	50-100 mg/day po	Hypertension, angina pectoris	neuroleptics (see literature for others)
bisoprolol	Zebeta	2.5-5 mg/day po	Hypertension	Same as acebutolol/atenolol
metoprolol	Lopressor	100 mg/day po	Hypertension, angina pectoris, myocardial infarction	Same as above

MAJOR SIDE EFFECTS OF β-BLOCKERS: Hypotension, bradycardia, fatigue, lethargy, nausea/vomiting, hypoglycemia, confusion.

ACE, Angiotensin-converting enzyme; *GI,* gastrointestinal; *NSAIDs,* nonsteroidal antiinflammatory drugs.

Because the clinical β-blockers have cardiovascular action, these agents are discussed in Chapter 27. Another use is for migraine headaches and prophylactically for neurologic conditions as found in this chapter (see Table 30-15).

 LEARNING TIP

Notice that many of the β-blockers end in *-olol*, and several of the α-blockers end in *-osin*.

Patient Education for Compliance

1. Adrenergic medications may produce anorexia. Diets high in carbohydrates and proteins and low in fats are generally well tolerated. Small meals are better tolerated than three large meals.
2. Insomnia and nervousness may accompany adrenergic medications. Caffeinated products should be avoided, especially after 5 PM. Alternative sleep aids such as relaxation techniques should be tried to reduce the insomnia.
3. Patients taking β-adrenergic blockers should be aware of the possibility of postural hypotension and use care when changing positions.
4. The pulse should be taken to assess the bradycardia that is possible with adrenergic blockers.
5. Alcohol, antihistamines, muscle relaxants, tranquilizers, and sedatives may potentiate the CNS depression and sedation found with adrenergic blockers.
6. Sexual dysfunction may be a result of β-blockers, and this symptom may mandate a dosage regulation or change to another medication.
7. β-Blockers may increase serum lipid levels, and these levels should be tested on a regular basis when prolonged therapy occurs.
8. Patients with diabetes should watch glucose levels closely when taking β-adrenergic blockers because β-blockers reduce the blood glucose levels.
9. β-blockers may cause headaches, mental confusion, and nightmares. These should be reported to the health care provider.
10. Weakness, fatigue, dizziness, and sedation are common side effects of β-blockers.

IMPORTANT FACTS ABOUT ADRENERGIC BLOCKERS

- Adrenergic agonists or sympathomimetics are classified as catecholamines or noncatecholamines. These agents mimic the fight-or-flight actions found with stimulation of the sympathetic nervous system. The naturally occurring adrenergic agonists are epinephrine, norepinephrine, and dopamine.

IMPORTANT FACTS ABOUT ADRENERGIC BLOCKERS—Cont'd

- Sympathomimetics are used to restore cardiac rhythm, elevate blood pressure, and control bleeding by vasoconstriction.
- Epinephrine is added to local anesthetics for vasoconstriction and to prolong the effects of the anesthesia.
- Sympathomimetics are used for mydriasis in ophthalmology.
- α-Adrenergic blockers are used to reduce hypertension and benign prostatic hypertrophy.
- The major adverse effects of α-blockers are orthostatic hypotension, nasal congestion, tachycardia, and sexual dysfunction.
- The first dose of α-blocker may cause fainting due to orthostatic hypotension, or the "first-dose effect."
- β-Blockers have many drug interactions that should be checked prior to adding any other medications. NSAIDs that are found OTC are products that have strong interactions with β-blockers.
- The principal indications for β-blockers are hypertension, angina pectoris, and dysrhythmias due to tachycardia, as presented in Chapter 27.
- β-Blockers must be used with caution in patients with COPD and asthma because of bronchoconstriction.
- β-Blockers reduce the conversion of glycogen to glucose in the liver or muscles to reduce blood glucose levels—a problem for people with diabetes.
- β-Blockers cause postural hypotension.
- β-Blockers are administered once or twice a day and cannot be discontinued abruptly.

Drugs Specific for Stroke Prevention

Antiplatelet medications (see Chapter 27) are indicated in the prevention of arterial thrombi and are thus used in the prevention of cerebral thrombi or strokes. Aspirin has been used for prophylaxis of thrombi, as has dipyridamole (Persantine). These drugs prevent aggregation of platelets. A combination product of two previously used agents has been released by the FDA for the prevention of recurrent strokes in people who have experienced transient ischemic attacks or who have had ischemic attacks due to thrombosis. Aggrenox is a combination of aspirin 25 mg and dipyridamole 200 mg. The combined agents reduce the risk of a stroke by a greater margin than either agent used alone. The most common side effect is a headache. The oral medication comes in capsules and is given twice a day.

Summary

The nervous system is composed of two divisions; the CNS (the brain, spinal cord, and nerves) and the peripheral nervous system. The autonomic nervous system, composed of the sympathetic and parasympathetic nervous systems, controls body functions without specific conscious innervation by the person. The CNS is controlled by nerve innervation from the peripheral nerves for interpretation and then return to the peripheral system for response. The autonomic nervous system has the fight-or-flight responses or the feed-or-breed body functions needed for the maintenance of homeostasis. Medications are used to assist with the functions of these systems.

Analgesics are used for the treatment of pain, a worldwide health symptom that disables and distresses people on a daily basis. Important is the fact that pain relief should be made available to all people at the level needed for relief. If opioids or potent analgesics are used for prolonged periods, abuse, misuse, and tolerance are possible. Short-term pain relief does not include these effects. The terminally ill person should be given long-term methods of pain relief and should be kept as pain free as possible. All people have a right to be pain free.

Anesthetics are used to interfere with conduction of nerve impulses to the CNS. General anesthesia is used in surgical procedures and may be given intravenously or by inhalation. In ambulatory care, local or regional anesthesia is achieved by topical application or through infiltration of a selected site. Local anesthesia is used to render a part of the body insensitive to pain. Additives such as epinephrine are included with local anesthetic agents to prolong their effects and to reduce bleeding by vasoconstriction, but these may also cause nervousness, palpitations, and other stimulations to body functions. These side effects are expected, but the patient should be aware this is a normal reaction.

Benzodiazepines are commonly used to treat anxiety and insomnia. These agents, because of their greater effectiveness while being safer, have replaced many of the sedatives of the barbiturate family that were used in the past. The geriatric patient is often the person needing these medications, and resultant care should be taken because of increased sensitivity to these drugs. Short-acting medications should be used in the elderly.

Before prescribing medications for insomnia, the cause should be considered and appropriate actions taken to reduce the causative factor. Medications prescribed for insomnia are habit forming when used for prolonged times; therefore a limited prescription with close monitoring of use is recommended to reduce the risk. The allied health professional should take a complete history from the patient to attempt to find the underlying cause of insomnia, possibly preventing the need for medications.

Seizures are symptoms of a discharge of disorganized electric impulses in the brain. The classification of seizures is by the causative factors and the symptoms produced. Several drug groups are used to treat seizures—barbiturates, hydantoins, succinimides, benzodiazepines, and other miscellaneous medications. These drugs produce various side effects that cause lifestyle changes in the person with epilepsy. The patient must be taught the importance of taking medications as prescribed and the necessity of reporting seizure activity that occurs while taking medications. Patient education is important with antiseizure medications.

Medications are used with diseases such as parkinsonism, RLS, and myasthenia gravis to treat the progressive symptoms that are typical. The muscle spasticity, inability to ambulate safely, and the tremors associated with these diseases are treated to allow the patient to function as independently as possible for as long as possible.

With parkinsonism, the ideal is to correct the imbalance of dopamine-acetylcholine found with the disease. The medications such as anticholinergics and antihistamines are used for central effect. Additionally, medications that increase the dopamine levels in the brain may be prescribed.

Myasthenia gravis is a debilitating disease characterized by skeletal muscle weakness and fatigue. The medications used are those that inhibit cholinesterase to provide the ACh necessary for muscle contractility. The drug therapy is for symptom control.

Medications that affect the cholinergic receptor sites are used to mimic, intensify, or inhibit the effects of the parasympathetic nervous system. Medications that affect the ACh receptors affect smooth muscle, glands, and cardiac muscles—functions that are essential with the human body. Cholinergic medications are used to stimulate the intestinal tract and the urinary bladder, lower intraocular pressure, dilate peripheral blood vessels, stimulate muscle contractility, and for the promotion of salivation and sweating. The anticholinergic medications are used to treat other illnesses that have spasticity as a symptom such as irritable bowel syndrome and urinary disorders. These medications are considered the feed-and-breed medications.

The sympathetic nervous system, or the adrenergic system, is responsible for the fight-or-flight responses of the body. The medications are used to mimic the sympathetic nervous system—sympathomimetic or adrenergic drugs. These may be direct or indirect acting or both, by affecting the α- or β-receptors.

Other medications—adrenergic blockers or sympatholytic drugs—block the receptor sites and inhibit the sympathetic response. The blocking agents have been discussed with the chapters where specific action occurs, such as hypertensives in Chapter 27. The adrenergic blockers (sympatholytics) may be α, β, or both. These medications are used for the treatment of hypertension, as well as other conditions such as benign prostatic hypertrophy and glaucoma.

Epinephrine is an important sympathomimetic drug that stimulates the α- and β-receptors. This medication is used to keep the body in homeostasis in the treatment of asthma, in emergency conditions such as anaphylaxis and cardiac emergencies, to treat local hemostasis, and in open-angle glaucoma.

Norepinephrine is used for peripheral vascular constriction to raise both systolic and diastolic blood pressure. It may also be used for vasodilation and to treat circulatory shock.

Critical Thinking Exercises

SCENARIO

Joseph, age 25, has had three tonic/clonic seizures in the past month. Until now, he has been seizure free for 2 years.

1. What questions should you ask Joseph about taking his medications?
2. Joseph tells you that he has not had the money to buy his medications for 2 weeks. Would this be important to tell the physician? Why or why not?
3. Joseph has taken Dilantin for more than 10 years. What does Joseph need to know about mouth and gum prophylactic care? Why?

DRUG CALCULATIONS

1. Order: phenobarbital 97.5 mg IM stat
   Available medication:

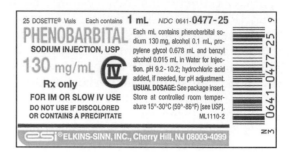

Dose to be administered: _____

Show the amount to be administered on the syringe shown.

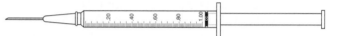

2. Order: Dilantin 60 mg po
   Available medication:

Dose to be administered: _____

REVIEW QUESTIONS

1. What is the blood-brain barrier? Why is this important in pharmacology? _____

2. What are the two groups of local anesthetics? What are typical examples of each? _____

3.   Why do we add epinephrine to local anesthetics? _____
     _____
     _____

4.   What are the actions of barbiturates? _____
     _____
     _____

5.   How do hydantoins (Dilantin) work for seizure control? _____
     _____
     _____

6.   What are the three pharmacologic categories for Parkinson's disease? _____
     _____
     _____

7.   What is the medication used prophylactically for cluster headaches? _____
     _____
     _____

8.   What diseases with spasticity can be treated with baclofen? Which cannot? _____
     _____
     _____

9.   How do cholinergic medications work? Anticholinergics? Adrenergics? Adrenergic blockers?
     _____
     _____
     _____

10. Cholinergics are used for what medical conditions? What are their side effects? _____
     _____
     _____

11. What are the side effects of anticholinergic agents? _____
     _____
     _____

12. Can anticholinergic medications be bought OTC? If so, which ones? _____
     _____
     _____

CHAPTER 31

Drugs for Mental Health and Behavioral Disorders

OBJECTIVES

After studying this chapter, you should be capable of doing the following:

- Describing mental health and deviations that are described as mental illness.
- Identifying the medications used to treat anxiety.
- Recognizing the major tranquilizers used to treat psychotic diseases.
- Identifying the principal signs of depression and the drugs used as antidepressants.
- Recognizing the agents used as antimanics and medications for bipolar disorder.
- Describing behavioral disorders found in adults and children
- Understanding the role of medications in treating Alzheimer's disease.
- Identifying drugs used for attention deficit disorder and attention deficit hyperactivity disorder.

Mrs. Jones, age 76, has become more and more disoriented and confused, and Dr. Merry has made a tentative diagnosis of Alzheimer's disease. Betty, Mrs. Jones's daughter, wants Dr. Merry to give her mother a medication to cure the disease.
  Is this possible?
  If not, why are medications given for Alzheimer's disease?
  If Aricept is prescribed, what side effects should Betty be told to look for while caring for her mother?
  What are the indications for memantine (Namenda)?

KEY TERMS

Affect	Delusion	Psychoanalysis
Affective disorders	Drug holiday	Psychologic drug dependence or
Akathisia	Dystonia	habituation
Alzheimer's disease	Extrapyramidal effects	Psychosis
Anxiolytic	Hallucination(s)	Psychotherapy
Attention deficit/hyperactivity	Neuroleptic	Schizophrenia
disorder (ADHD)	Neurosis	Tardive dyskinesia
Bipolar disorder	Obsession	Tourette's syndrome
Compulsions	Parkinson's disease	Tranquilization

EASY WORKING KNOWLEDGE OF INDICATIONS AND SIDE EFFECTS

Common Signs and Symptoms of Mental Disorders

Stress, anxiety, depression
Withdrawal from society
Disorganized thinking, hallucinations
Inappropriate or violent behavior
Crying, mood swings
Sleep disturbances, fatigue, agitation
Loss of concentration
Inability to experience pleasure
Forgetfulness
Inability to place self in environment, person, place
Paranoia

Common Side Effects of Medications for Mental Disorders

Hypotension, restlessness
Tachycardia
Dry mouth
Decreased motor and cognitive abilities
Alterations in sleep patterns
Hangover effect
Increased or decreased libido
Impotence
Dizziness, drowsiness, confusion
Extrapyramidal symptoms
Tardive dyskinesia

Easy Working Knowledge of Medications Used for Mental Disorders

DRUG CLASS	PRESCRIPTION	OTC	PREGNANCY CATEGORY	MAJOR INDICATIONS
Anxiolytics/antianxiety/minor tranquilizers	Yes	No	B, C, D	Relief of anxiety
Antipsychotics/neuroleptics/major tranquilizers	Yes	No	B, C, D	Psychotic disorders
Antidepressants				
Unipolar	Yes	No	B, C, D	Depression
Bipolar	Yes	No	D	Mania/depression
Medications for cognitive ability	Yes	No	C, X (tacrine)	Alzheimer's disease
Central nervous system stimulants	Yes	No	B, C	Attention deficit/hyperactivity disorder

The ability to cope with different types of stressors at different times of life is part of normal living or mental health. What is normal is difficult to define. The terms normal and abnormal are relative to the local environment. What is considered normal can and does vary from culture to culture, country to country, town to town, and even within towns. Daily stressors may even change normal to abnormal within short periods of time.

What Is Mental Health?

Mental health is the person's physical, cognitive, affective, behavioral, and social beings as these components interact with the environment to choose and obtain a purpose for life. The physical dimension includes physiologic aspects of the person, whereas the cognitive dimension involves the formulation of thoughts, processing information, and problem solving. The affective domain involves the person's ability to experience and express feelings and emotions. The behavioral dimension is the person's individuality, with integration of physical, cognitive, and affective domains. The social dimension is the person's ability to interact with members of the family or community effectively as a whole person. The environment is everything outside of the person. These components interact to form a continuum for a level of mental health throughout life. For example, if the transmission of nerve impulses to the brain are interrupted, the person may have disorganized thoughts—a condition that may affect social and behavioral aspects of life. Mental health is not a concrete achievable goal; rather, it is a lifelong process to form a sense of harmony and balance in the person.

What Is a Mentally Healthy Person?

Mentally healthy people are able to perceive reality accurately and control the way that emotions are experienced and expressed. They think clearly and logically and can communicate effectively while anticipating events and solving problems. The mentally healthy person can initiate and maintain meaningful relationships, develop a positive self-concept, and behave in a way that promotes personal growth and development.

Mental disorders affect almost everyone at some time during life, either personally or by association with a friend or family member. Other factors that produce mental instability include congenital deficiencies, hereditary factors, accidents, traumatic events in one's life, or drug-related toxicity. In many cases the exact cause is unknown, but mental disorders are related to the stress and pressures imposed by modern society. The pain of mental illness is real and intense, altering a person's ability to adjust to the stress found in modern society. When self-esteem is decreased, coping skills are reduced, allowing behavior to be affected. The mental disorders may be from mild to severe disruption of the person's ability to function in interpersonal relationships, in self-care, and in the ability to maintain a job in an occupational setting to be self-sufficient. When a person is able to cope and adapt to the stresses of everyday life, he or she is considered to be mentally healthy.

Role of Medication Therapy in Psychotherapy

Medications play an important role in modern psychotherapeutic care. These medications are used to reduce or alleviate symptoms of stress and allow the tense or psychotic person an opportunity to participate in other psychotherapeutic treatment.

- Drugs temporarily modify behavior, whereas **psychotherapy** may permanently change behavior, resulting in the ability to appropriately interact with the environment.
- Drugs may have additive, potentiating, or antagonistic effects on each other. Medication in psychotherapy is chosen by the diagnosis (e.g., medications that are specific for **schizophrenia,** manic depression, psychosis, or other mental illness).

- The medication selection is based on the patient's behavioral actions, pharmacologic effects, and the potential adverse reactions, as well as individual and environmental factors present.
- Elderly patients are often inappropriately prescribed psychotropic agents. In fact, about 10% of all medical visits by the elderly result in prescriptions for psychotropic agents, leading to an increased risk of an adverse or serious drug reaction and interfering with the person's cognitive and functional status.

Treatment of mental health has taken giant steps in the United States in the past 50 years with the introduction of tranquilizers. The first antipsychotic agent, chlorpromazine (Thorazine), was released in the early 1950s and remains the typical phenothiazine. Chlorpromazine was considered a tranquilizer to calm an agitated or anxious patient. Rather than being institutionalized for years, as in the past, many psychotic people are today treated at community mental health centers as outpatients. For those who are hospitalized, the course of hospitalization is usually short term—only the time necessary to stabilize the mental condition and medications and then return the person to society.

The newer medications are more selective in their action on the brain. These drugs tend to **tranquilize** or calm the patient without causing sedation or depressing the entire central nervous system (CNS). The medications are used for treating the two basic categories of mental disorders—**neurosis** and **psychosis.**

Anxiety and Daily Living

Anxiety is the major motivating factor in one's emotional life. A person usually takes a course of action to reduce stress, apprehension, tension, and uneasiness that threaten the well-being of oneself or the sense of control in a given situation. Anxiety is a lifelong emotion from infancy to older adulthood. The way in which a person confronts anxiety-causing situations, from mild anxiousness to states of panic, is an ultimate sign of mental health. Not all anxiety is harmful; mild anxiety increases alertness and increases productivity. Moderate anxiety diminishes cognitive abilities and makes learning and decision making difficult. When a person cannot adapt to anxiety or stress, homeostasis may be affected, and the person will change in an effort to maintain equilibrium. The change may be in the form of any of the defense mechanisms that protect the individual. When stress presents a crisis and the person cannot adapt and function, medications may be prescribed to decrease stress and anxiety to make adaptation more easily achieved.

When anxiety, tension, and nervousness from uncertainty or situations that are potentially threatening are prolonged, the result is behavioral and emotional changes or neurosis. Psychosomatic conditions and panic disorders are also possible with neurotic behavior. Anxiolytics, formerly called *minor tranquilizers*, are used to treat prolonged anxiety or neurosis and to calm the individual of the symptoms of severe anxiety. The anxiolytics reduce unpleasant neurotic behavior.

Neurosis versus Psychosis

Both of these basic categories display agitation, hyperactivity, and inappropriate and sometimes violent behavior. The mentally ill individual is unable to communicate with others and is unable to function in normal activities. Tranquilizers are used to treat both conditions.

Neurosis is found when a fearful individual is still in contact with reality but does not adjust favorably to his or her surroundings or life situations. Many situations in life produce fear or anxiety from either real or unknown danger. The physical and behavioral responses to fearful situations are caused by stimulation of the sympathetic nervous system, causing sleeplessness and either an increase or a decrease in appetite. With an accumulation of anxiousness and tension, emotional changes and abnormal behavior, or neurosis, may occur. Treatment involves psychotherapy to determine the cause of anxiety and drug therapy to alleviate the symptoms. The medications used are antianxiety medications, or **anxiolytics,** or minor tranquilizers. The types of anxiety-related conditions are generalized anxiety disorder, social anxiety disorder, and obsessive-compulsive disorder.

- Generalized anxiety disorder (GAD) is a chronic condition that is characterized by uncontrollable worrying for 6 months or more. In most cases GAD is accompanied by depression. Symptoms include insomnia, trembling, apprehension, and poor concentration. Physical symptoms include tachycardia, sweating, and palpitations. The drugs most commonly used are the benzodiazepines such as lorazepam (Ativan) and diazepam (Valium), buspirone (BuSpar), venlafaxine (Effexor), and the selective serotonin reuptake inhibitors (SSRIs) such as paroxetine (Paxil-SR).

- Social anxiety disorder has characteristics of intense, irrational fear in situations where the person might be scrutinized or when the person might be humiliated. The symptoms include blushing, stuttering, sweating, palpitations, muscle tension, and a dry throat. SSRIs such as paroxetine are the drugs of choice.

- Obsessive-compulsive disorder is a condition that is characterized by obsessions and compulsions that interfere with daily living. Patients may do such actions as excessive hand washing, placement of objects, or hoarding. The treatment is the use of SSRIs such as fluoxetine (Prozac) and sertraline (Zoloft) and tricyclic antidepressants (TCAs) such as clomipramine (Anafranil).

Psychosis occurs when the person is out of contact with reality and is unable to communicate satisfactorily. Psychosis involves a breakdown in personality, with thought patterns and responses to the environment unrelated to the real-life situation. The person is out of contact with reality, and communication may be impossible. Treatment may require hospitalization because this is severe mental illness.

The two major forms of psychosis are severe depression and **schizophrenia.**

- In schizophrenia, the person is usually withdrawn, with inappropriate and unpredictable behavior. **Delusions** and **hallucinations** are common.

- Delusions may be those of persecution, when the individual feels threatened and feels that others are trying to harm him or her in some way.

- Delusions of grandeur are those where the person has an exaggerated feeling of importance, knowledge, or identity.

- Treatment for both delusions and hallucinations involves psychotherapy and the use of antipsychotic medications, also called **neuroleptics** or major tranquilizers.

IMPORTANT FACTS ABOUT MENTAL HEALTH
- Mental health is difficult to define and may change from person to person, culture to culture, and time to time. Mental health is the ability to live with the stressors of daily living.
- Psychotherapeutic agents are among the most frequently prescribed medications.

Drugs for Anxiety: Anxiolytics/Minor Tranquilizers

Drugs used for the relief of anxiety may also be used as hypnotics or sedatives to promote sleep. Many of these medications have additive actions when combined with CNS depressants (see Chapter 30). The difference between using the medications as anxiolytics and hypnotics is based on dosage—a lower dose to relieve anxiety and higher doses for hypnotic effects. A single medication may be prescribed for both uses—to lower anxiety and to produce sleep. Antianxiety medications may also be used for skeletal muscle relaxants for chronic muscle pain, especially back pain and when muscle spasm is part of the pain. Occasionally minor tranquilizers are also used as antiseizure medications to reduce the numbers of convulsions and as an adjunctive medication in alcohol withdrawal. These medications are for short-term use because of the possibility of **tolerance** and **physical** and **psychologic dependence,** especially with larger doses used as sedatives at night for sleep. Sudden withdrawal of minor tranquilizers may result in seizures, agitation, psychosis, insomnia, and gastric distress. These medications may be classified as Schedule III and IV drugs. Others may be unclassified under the Controlled Substances Act, with long-term use being contraindicated (Table 31-1).

Benzodiazepines

The benzodiazepines, first introduced in the 1960s, are the drugs of choice in treating anxiety and insomnia. Today benzodiazepines are among the most widely prescribed medications in the United States, with diazepam (Valium) being the most familiar of this group. The benzodiazepines are safer than some CNS depressants because they have few actions outside the CNS, causing lower potential for abuse and producing less tolerance and physical dependence. When using benzodiazepines, the patient becomes calm without being excessively sedated. With increasing dosage, the effects increase from anxiety reduction to sedation to hypnosis to stupor.

- The oral route is the usual means of administration. Benzodiazepines are readily absorbed from the gastrointestinal tract. Diazepam (Valium), chlordiazepoxide (Librium), and lorazepam (Ativan) may also be given by injection if more rapid action is desired or required.
- The duration of action is the major difference in benzodiazepines. The long-acting agents have half-lives of more than 20 hours. Short-lived benzodiazepines have half-lives of 5 to 20 hours.
- Tremors and **extrapyramidal effects** may occur with the persistent use of benzodiazepines, especially in the elderly.
- Excessive use of benzodiazepines may lead to interference with memory and to psychotic behavior. Aggressive behavior could become a violent act with prolonged use of these drugs.
- Patients who operate machinery including driving a car should be careful of the sedating actions.
- Drug dependency with antianxiety agents seems to be more habituation than physical dependence. The patient must realize that anxiolytics only relieve symptoms and do not cure the anxiety problem. The reason for anxiety must be found and eliminated for the symptoms to be alleviated. Care should be taken that the medication does not become a crutch for relieving stress and unhappiness. Abuse of benzodiazepines is not uncommon and is more likely to occur with patients who take larger than therapeutic doses. Because of the extended action of the long-acting agents, any withdrawal symptoms remain for 1 to 2 weeks after stopping the medication. Benzodiazepines should be avoided during pregnancy and should be used with extreme caution in patients who are suicidal, who are severely depressed, or who have depressed vital signs.

LEARNING TIP
Notice that many of the benzodiazepine generic names end in *-pam.*

TABLE 31-1 *Select Medications Used as Anxiolytics/Antianxiety Medications*

GENERIC NAME (SCHEDULE)	TRADE NAME	USUAL ADULT DOSE, ROUTE, AND FREQUENCY OF ADMINISTRATION	INDICATIONS FOR USE	DRUG INTERACTIONS
SHORT-ACTING BENZODIAZEPINES			Anxiety	Other CNS depressants, alcohol, cimetidine, anticoagulants, corticosteroids, digitalis, phenytoin
alprazolam (III)	Xanax	0.25-1 mg po tid		
lorazepam (III)	Ativan	0.5-1 mg po, IM, IV tid		
quazepam (IV)	Doral	7.5-15 mg po hs		
temazepam (III)	Restoril	15-30 mg po hs		
triazolam (III)	Halcion	0.25-0.5 mg po hs	Hypnotic	+ levodopa, neuroleptics, macrolides, INH

MAJOR SIDE EFFECTS OF SHORT-ACTING BENZODIAZEPINES: Drowsiness, confusion, ataxia, nausea, constipation, dry mouth, GI disturbances, rashes, photosensitivity, menstrual irregularities, loss of libido.

GENERIC NAME (SCHEDULE)	TRADE NAME	USUAL ADULT DOSE, ROUTE, AND FREQUENCY OF ADMINISTRATION	INDICATIONS FOR USE	DRUG INTERACTIONS
LONG-ACTING BENZODIAZEPINES				Same as alprazolam
chlordiazepoxide (III)	Librium	5-10 mg po tid	Anxiolytic, alcohol withdrawal	
clonazepam (III)	Klonopin	0.5 mg po tid		Antiseizure
chlorazepate (III)	Tranxene	7.5-15 mg po tid		Antiseizure, anxiolytic, alcohol withdrawal
prazepam (III)	Centrax	10 mg po tid		Same
diazepam (III)	Valium	2-10 mg po, IM, IV tid		Same + muscle relaxant and preoperative medication
oxazepam (III)	Serax	30-120 mg po qd	Same	Same
MISCELLANEOUS ANXIOLYTICS				alcohol, CNS depressants, MAOIs
buspirone	BuSpar	5-10 mg po tid	Anxiety	
hydroxyzine	Atarax, Vistaril	25-100 mg/day po, IM	Anxiety, emesis, antipruritic, preoperative medications	
paroxetine	Paxil	10-50 mg po qd	Anxiety, depression, obsessive/compulsive disorder, panic disorder	MAOIs, cimetidine, phenytoin, risperidone
trazodone	Desyrel	100-400 mg po qd	Anxiety, depression	alcohol, CNS depressants, antihypertensives, digoxin
venlafaxine	Effexor, Effexor XR	37.5-225 mg po qd	Anxiety, depression	MAOIs

MAJOR SIDE EFFECTS OF MISCELLANEOUS ANXIOLYTICS: buspirone: dizziness, tinnitus, lightheadedness, rashes, fatigue, nausea, chest pain, nasal congestion, sore throat, CNS disturbance; **hydroxyzine, paroxetine, trazodone:** drowsiness, dry mouth, pain at injection site; additionally: diaphoresis, tremors, vomiting with paroxetine; unpleasant taste, headache with trazodone.

CNS, Central nervous system; *GI,* gastrointestinal; *INH,* inhalation; *IM,* intramuscular; *IV,* intravenous; *MAOIs,* monoamine oxidase inhibitors.

Other Anxiolytics

- An anxiolytic that produces a positive effect on depression is buspirone (BuSpar). The agent is solely an antianxiety medication with no anticonvulsant or muscle relaxing properties or sedative effect. It does not substantially impair psychomotor function. It is more effective for cognitive and interpersonal relationships such as anger and hostility, whereas the benzodiazepines are more effective for somatic symptoms. BuSpar is not a controlled substance because the potential for tolerance and drug dependency is low. This medication is well tolerated and may be increased progressively as needed (see Table 31-1).

- Hydroxyzine (Vistaril, Atarax) is a medication with many uses as an antihistamine, anxiolytic, antiemetic, or sedative. This medication may be given by mouth or by injection. When given by injection, it must be given deep intramuscularly to prevent irritation to the tissue.

- Three medications introduced as miscellaneous anxiolytics—paroxetine (Paxil), venlafaxine (Effexor), and trazodone (Desyrel)—are not Drug Enforcement Administration (DEA) scheduled drugs and are all used for anxiety and depression. Paroxetine is also used for obsessive compulsive disorder and panic disorder. Venlafaxine is also used for generalized anxiety disorder (see Table 31-1).

Patient Education for Compliance

1. Benzodiazepines should be taken with food if gastrointestinal symptoms occur.
2. Patients should take anxiolytic medications as ordered and should not increase or discontinue medications without consulting a physician. Relaxation techniques may also help reduce stress.
3. Transient insomnia usually will be relieved once the precipitating stressor has been eliminated.
4. Drowsiness occurs with benzodiazepines, so hazardous activities should be avoided until the effects of the medication can be evaluated by the patient.
5. Physical dependence is rare with most benzodiazepines, but persons using alprazolam (Xanax) have reported substantial dependence factors.
6. Benzodiazepines should not be used with pregnancy.
7. Women using oral contraceptives need to consider an alternative method of birth control when taking benzodiazepines.

IMPORTANT FACTS ABOUT ANXIOLYTICS

- Drugs used to treat anxiety are called antianxiety agents, anxiolytics, or minor tranquilizers.
- Anxiolytics may be used as hypnotics to promote sleep.
- Elderly persons generally require lower doses of psychotherapeutic agents and may experience excessive sedation when administered in the usual adult dose.
- Self-administered medications such as antihistamines and cough preparations may cause excessive sedation when combined with minor tranquilizers.
- Alcohol should not be combined with any anxiolytics.
- The potential for abuse and addiction is high when tranquilizers are used for a prolonged period of time.
- The principal indications for benzodiazepines are anxiety, insomnia, and possibly seizure disorders.
- Benzodiazepines are safer than barbiturates, have a lower abuse potential, and cause less tolerance and dependence.
- Benzodiazepines may cause severe respiratory depression when mixed with other central nervous system depressants.
- All benzodiazepines have essentially the same pharmacologic action; therefore selection is based on the differences in time of action as dictated by the patient's needs.
- Benzodiazepines are the drugs of choice for transient insomnia, with dosing being intermittent. Use should be for only 2 to 3 weeks.
- Benzodiazepines should not be used during pregnancy or by persons with sleep apnea.
- Care should be taken when using any anxiolytic or psychotherapeutic medication with persons with suicidal tendencies.
- Benzodiazepines are Schedule IV under the Controlled Substances Act, meaning there is a possibility of dependence.

Drugs for Psychosis: Neuroleptics/Major Tranquilizers

Psychosis does not have a single diagnosis, but it is clinically described as a person being out of touch with reality. The two major forms of psychosis are schizophrenia and severe depression, although other conditions are classified as psychosis (Table 31-2).

TABLE 31-2 *Select Drugs Used to Treat Psychosis*

GENERIC NAME	TRADE NAME*	USUAL ADULT DOSE, ROUTE, AND FREQUENCY OF ADMINISTRATION†	INDICATIONS FOR USE	DRUG INTERACTIONS
PHENOTHIAZINES			Psychosis	antihistamines, alcohol, analgesics, tranquilizers, narcotics, guanethidine, β-blockers, barbiturates, insulin, oral hypoglycemics, anticholinergics, levodopa, epinephrine
chlorpromazine	Thorazine (LP)	25-50 mg po, IM, IV 3-4 times/day May be up to 1000 mg/day	+ Emesis and hiccups	
fluphenazine decanoate	Prolixin (HP)	2.5-10 mg/day po in divided doses 12.5-25 mg IM q1-3wk as depot		
mesoridazine	Serentil (LP)	25-400 mg/day po		
perphenazine	Trilafon (IP)	8-24 mg/day po, 5-10 mg per dose IM, IV	+ Emesis	
prochlorperazine	Compazine (IP)	5-10 mg po tid-qid 10-20 mg per dose IM, IV 25 mg bid rectal suppository	+ Emesis	
promethazine	Phenergan (IP)	12.5-50 mg po, IM, IV, rectal supp q4-6h	+ Emesis, motion sickness	
thioridazine	Mellaril (LP)	50-800 mg/day po		
trifluoperazine	Stelazine (HP)	5-40 mg/day po, IM		
triflupromazine	Vesprin (IP)	50-150 mg po per dose		

MAJOR SIDE EFFECTS OF PHENOTHIAZINES: Postural hypotension, tachycardia, bradycardia, vertigo, dry mouth, blurred vision, fever, constipation, urinary retention, anorexia, rashes, photosensitivity, insomnia, agitation, restlessness, depression, headaches, confusion, drowsiness, weakness.

BUTYROPHENONES				
haloperidol	Haldol (HP)	0.5 mg/day po 2.5 mg q1-8h IM	Psychosis, mania	alcohol, lithium, CNS depressants, levodopa, epinephrine
THIOXANTHENES			Psychosis	Same as haloperidol
thiothixene	Navane (HP)	2 mg tid po		
DIBENZODIAZEPINES				Same as haloperidol
clozapine	Clozaril (AT)	75-450 mg po		
BENZISOXAZOLES				Same as haloperidol
risperidone	Risperdal (AT)	1-6 mg/day po		
THIENOBENZODIAZEPINES				carbamazepine, levodopa, antihypertensives
olanzapine	Zyprexa (AT)	10 mg po	Schizophrenia	

(continued)

TABLE 31-2   *Select Drugs Used to Treat Psychosis—cont'd*

GENERIC NAME	TRADE NAME*	USUAL ADULT DOSE, ROUTE, AND FREQUENCY OF ADMINISTRATION[†]	INDICATIONS FOR USE	DRUG INTERACTIONS
MISCELLANEOUS				
aripiprazole	Abilify	15-30 mg po qd	Schizophrenia	Antifungals, carbamazepine, paroxetine, fluoxetine, alcohol
ziprasidone	Geodon	40-160 mg qd, po, IM	Schizophrenia, bipolar mania	Same
quetiapine	Seroquel	25-50 mg po bid-tid	Psychosis	alcohol, opiods, lorazepam, dopamine

CNS, Central nervous system; *IM*, intramuscular; *IV*, intravenous.
*LP, Low potency; IP, intermediate potency; HP, high potency; AT, atypical agent.
[†] Given in divided doses unless otherwise noted.

- The patient with schizophrenia has the symptom of withdrawal from the social environment.
- Hallucinations and delusions are commonly found in psychotic individuals.
- Psychotic symptoms may be caused by medications used to treat these illnesses when the patient loses contact with reality.
- The patient with schizophrenia, then, has deterioration in social functioning, with disorganized thoughts, changes in **affect,** and inability to perform the tasks needed for daily living.
- Speech may be incoherent or repetitive, with wandering thoughts. Tangents, or inability to get to the point in communication, are not uncommon.
- Interpersonal relationships, work, education, and self-care are inhibited and unpurposeful.
- The patient with severe depression has a strong feeling of hopelessness.

Uses for Antipsychotics or Neuroleptics

In general, antipsychotics are effective in three major areas:

- To relieve the symptoms of psychosis or severe neurosis such as delusions, hallucinations, agitation, and combativeness.
- To be used therapeutically to relieve nausea and vomiting (see Chapter 25).
- To potentiate analgesics such as promethazine (see Chapter 16).

The dosage of these agents is regulated to modify disturbed behavior and to relieve the symptoms of severe anxiety without the profound impairment of consciousness.

- The antipsychotic medications do not cure mental disorders but are used to control the symptoms related to psychosis.
- Antipsychotic medications are also called *neuroleptics* (formerly called major tranquilizers), for use in acute and chronic psychosis.
- The most important classes of antipsychotic medications are the phenothiazines, butyrophenones, and thioxanthenes. These classes of medications are used to suppress the symptoms of schizophrenia and other psychotic conditions. The exact mechanism of action is not well understood, but it is thought that these agents act on dopamine, a neurotransmitter in the brain.
- Serotonin, another neurotransmitter, is also involved in the control of psychotic behavior. Some of the more recent drugs block serotonin to act as antipsychotic agents. These drugs are considered *atypical* antipsychotic drugs because their main action is not against dopamine.

Potency and Neuroleptics

Another way to classify antipsychotics is by **potency**—not to be confused with effectiveness of the drug. *Effectiveness* measures the therapeutic response to the individual medications. *Potency* refers to the quantity of a drug that is necessary to produce an equivalent effect as compared with a drug of the same drug classification. The antipsychotics are therefore classified by the quantity of medication needed to produce an equivalent effect when compared with drugs in the same category—low potency, intermediate potency, and high potency. An example is chlorpromazine (Thorazine). As a low-potency drug, 100 mg is considered to be the equivalent of mesoridazine (Serentil) 50 mg (an intermediate-potency drug), or haloperidol (Haldol) 2 mg (a high-potency agent).

As patients take antipsychotic medications over several months to a prolonged period of time, the medications tend to cause extrapyramidal effects by blocking dopamine receptors in the brain. **Tardive dyskinesia,** a more serious condition resulting from prolonged use of neuroleptics, includes involuntary movements of the body such as tics, movements of the lips, jaws, and tongue, and jerking movements of the extremities that cause postural imbalance. Often tardive dyskinesia appears when the medication is discontinued. At this time, either restarting the drug or increasing the dosage may suppress these symptoms, but with further prolonged use, the dyskinesia worsens and becomes unresponsive to treatment. These symptoms may then become permanent and irreversible; therefore the patient should be seen frequently to assess the progression of the dyskinesia (Figure 31-1).

Elderly patients taking neuroleptics seem more prone to *parkinsonian symptoms* such as tremors, drooling, tongue protrusion, muscular rigidity, and dysphagia. The prophylactic use of antiparkinsonism medications such as anticholinergic drugs with antipsychotic medications will not prevent the extrapyramidal symptoms, and the symptoms will only continue to worsen (see Chapter 30).

Children are more prone to dystonic reactions, which include muscle spasms of the head with twitching, facial grimacing, torticollis or wryneck, and twisting of the face, neck, and back. **Dystonia** usually appears early in treatment and subsides rapidly when the medication is discontinued. Anticholinergics are used for treating dystonia. **Akathisia,** or motor restlessness, is also more common in children. Patients manifesting signs of akathisia have continuous body movement with restlessness, pacing about, and insomnia.

Antipsychotics are contraindicated with seizure disorders, severe depression, parkinsonism, and pregnancy. These agents must be used with caution in children and elderly, patients with hepatic or renal disease, men with hypertrophy of the prostate gland, and patients with glaucoma. (Boxes 31-1 and 31-2 list implications in the elderly and children.)

- Chlorpromazine (Thorazine) was the first antipsychotic agent and remains the typical

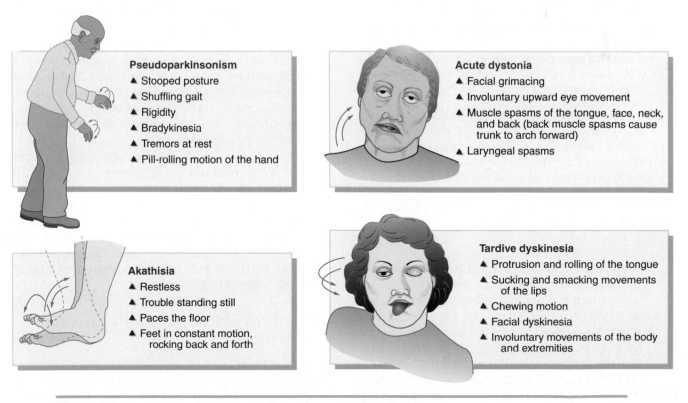

Figure 31-1 Extrapyramidal adverse effects of neuroleptic medications. (From Kee JL, Hayes ER, McCuistion LE: *Pharmacology: a nursing approach,* ed 5, St Louis, 2006, Saunders.)

BOX 31-1   PEDIATRIC IMPLICATIONS FOR USE OF PSYCHOTHERAPEUTIC AGENTS

- Children are at greater risk of developing extrapyramidal side effects, especially dystonia.
- Pediatric patients with chickenpox, central nervous system infections, measles, dehydration, gastroenteritis, or other acute illnesses are more at risk for developing severe adverse reactions and even Reye's syndrome.
- Tricyclic antidepressants are usually not recommended for depression in children younger than age 12. Some agents such as amitriptyline (Elavil), desipramine (Norpramin), and imipramine (Tofranil) may be used in children older than 6 who have major depression.
- Children are sensitive to an acute overdosage, which may be serious and even fatal.
- Increased nervousness, sleeplessness, complaints of being tired, hypertension, and stomach distress are found in children taking tricyclic antidepressants.
- Lithium may decrease bone density and bone formation when used with children.

BOX 31-2   GERIATRIC IMPLICATIONS FOR USE OF PSYCHOTHERAPEUTIC AGENTS

- Older persons tend to have higher serum levels of antipsychotic/antidepressant drugs because of changes in drug distribution from a decrease in lean body mass, less total body water, less serum albumin, and usually an increase in body fat. These patients need lower doses.
- Geriatric patients are more likely to have orthostatic hypotension, anticholinergic side effects, extrapyramidal effects, and sedation.
- Elderly patients should receive half the recommended adult dose. When clinical improvement is noted, attempts to taper or discontinue the medications should be instituted.
- Tricyclic antidepressants may cause increased anxiety in the geriatric patient. The tricyclic antidepressant increases the risk of inducing dysrhythmias, tachycardia, stroke, congestive heart failure, and myocardial infarction in the person with cardiovascular disease.
- Lithium is more toxic in the geriatric patient. The elderly are more prone to central nervous system toxicity, lithium-induced goiter, and clinical hypothyroidism.

phenothiazine. The phenothiazines possess anticholinergic, antiemetic, antihistaminic, and α-adrenergic blocking effects, as well as antipsychotic actions. Therefore these medications may also be used to treat nausea, vomiting, pruritus, and allergic reactions, although the drug is not the first choice. Phenothiazine derivatives may also be used as adjuvant therapy with tetanus and intractable hiccups, as well as for **bipolar disorder,** agitation, and delirium tremors (see Table 31-2).

 LEARNING TIP

The generic names for most phenothiazines end in *-zine*.

- Butyrophenone derivatives are chemically different from phenothiazines but have the same antipsychotic effects. Haloperidol (Haldol), the main drug found in this group, is used as an antipsychotic and antiemetic. This drug is also used for severe behavioral problems in children and for **Tourette's syndrome,** a CNS disease with rapid, involuntary, repetitive motor movements of muscles and involuntary vocal tics or noises. Low doses of haloperidol have been used to treat severe agitation, combativeness, and psychosis in demented persons. Butyrophenones cause greater movement disturbances than the phenothiazines. Lowered doses should be used with geriatric patients (see Table 31-2).
- Thioxanthenes are chemically similar to phenothiazines. Thiothixene (Navane) is the typical drug in this group. These agents also exert antipsychotic effects by blocking dopamine in the brain. They are more selective but do cause extrapyramidal effects.
- Loxapine (Loxitane), similar to the antipsychotic phenothiazines, causes a moderate degree of sedation and has a high incidence of extrapyramidal symptoms.
- *Atypical antipsychotic medications* are agents that block receptors in the brain in addition to dopamine receptors. Clozapine (Clozaril) significantly blocks serotonin receptors. Sedation, hypotension, and anticholinergic effects are prominent, but extrapyramidal effects occur only with large doses.
- Olanzapine (Zyprexa) is used for the treatment of schizophrenia by blocking serotonin and dopamine.
- The newer atypical antipsychotic agents such as aripiprazole (Abilify) and ziprasidone (Geodon) have lower incidences of side effects of sedation, extrapyramidal effects, and hypotension, making these medications more patient friendly (see Table 31-2).

Treatment of Psychosis with Parenteral Medications

For long-term maintenance therapy of schizophrenia, depot injectable antipsychotics with long-acting capabilities are used. By using these preparations, the patient who may not be compliant on a daily basis or tends to be generally noncompliant is given parenteral medication to prevent relapses and maintain the highest possible level of functioning. The depot preparations pose no increased risk of side effects than those found with oral preparations, and the risk of tardive dyskinesia is actually reduced. The most commonly used medications for depot administration are haloperidol (Haldol) and fluphenazine (Prolixin).

Treatment of Schizophrenia

Treatment for schizophrenia is chronic and prolonged and has three major objectives:

- Suppress acute episodes of psychosis
- Prevent acute exacerbations of the disease
- Maintain the highest possible level of functioning

Unless contraindicated, a high-potency traditional agent is used. The exact drug depends on the patient because some patients respond more successfully to specific medications. Sometimes the selection even comes to trial medications to obtain the drug with the fewest side effects and with the maximum comfort and promotion of compliance. Atypical agents are an alternative to traditional drugs. The atypical agents have the advantages of not causing tardive dyskinesia and are well-suited for patients who have extrapyramidal symptoms.

The patient should have an attempt at discontinuation of treatment after a year of therapy; approximately 25% will not need drugs after that time. The time for tapered attempted discontinuation should not be a time of stress. With long-term therapy, the depot method may be more effective, with fewer withdrawal symptoms, fewer side effects, and better compliance.

Patient Education for Compliance

1. The patient should be aware of the potential for psychologic and physical dependence with prolonged use of psychotropic medications. Medicines should be taken in the prescribed dosage for the time set by the physician.
2. No CNS depressants—analgesics, alcohol, muscle relaxants, antihistamines, antiemetics, cardiac medications, and antihypertensives—should be taken with psychotropics unless ordered by a physician.
3. Be careful when taking any medications with antipsychotics because of the many drug interactions. OTC medications, especially OTC antihistamines and sleeping aids, should not be taken with psychotropic medications.

Patient Education for Compliance—cont'd

4. The patient taking psychotropic medications should be educated about orthostatic hypotension and the dangers of changing positions rapidly.
5. Avoid exposure to sun when taking antipsychotics because of the danger of sunburn.
6. Report restlessness, muscle spasms, rigidity, tremors, drooling, visual disturbances, weakness, and faintness to the physician when taking antipsychotics.
7. Oral antipsychotic liquid medications should be protected from light.
8. Dilution of oral liquid antipsychotics should be achieved by fruit juice to increase palatability.
9. Oral antipsychotic liquids may cause contact dermatitis, so contact with the skin should be avoided.
10. Be sure patients have written and verbal instructions on the dosage and timing of medications. Have family members assist with medication compliance with persons taking psychiatric medications.
11. Be sure patients are aware of early signs of extrapyramidal symptoms such as spasticity in face, neck, and tongue and restlessness.
12. Inform patients that dry mouth, blurred vision, photophobia, urinary hesitancy, and constipation are possible but should be reported. If symptoms are severe the medication may have to be stopped or a reduced dosage attempted. Dryness of the mouth may be relieved by chewing gum or sucking on hard candy.
13. Sexual dysfunction is possible with antipsychotics and should be reported for dosage reduction or possible changing of medications.
14. Encourage patients to attend all psychotherapeutic sessions when taking medications for psychotic conditions.
15. Antipsychotics cause drowsiness. The patient should not perform tasks that require mental alertness until the effects of the medications are known.
16. The patient should eat high-fiber diets and may need a stool softener when taking antipsychotics.

IMPORTANT FACTS ABOUT ANTIPSYCHOTICS

- Antipsychotics are effective in three major areas:
  - To relieve psychosis or severe neurosis
  - To relieve nausea and vomiting
  - To potentiate analgesics
- Antipsychotic medications fall into two groups, traditional and atypical. Traditional drugs are thought to relieve symptoms by blocking neurotransmitter receptors such as dopamine. Atypical medications block other neurotransmitters such as serotonin.

- The major indication for antipsychotics is schizophrenia. Schizophrenia is a chronic illness marked by hallucinations, delusions, and agitation along with disorganized thoughts and loss of reality. Social withdrawal is often seen.
- Low-potency to high-potency traditional drugs have equal therapeutic effect.
- Low-potency agents produce more sedation, orthostatic hypotension, and anticholinergic effects than high-potency agents.
- The therapeutic effects of antipsychotic medications develop slowly, often taking several weeks to be effective.
- Traditional antipsychotic medications may cause three types of extrapyramidal effects to occur: tardive dyskinesia, acute dystonia, and akathisia.
- Atypical antipsychotics cause few or no extrapyramidal effects.
- Antipsychotic agents with depot parenteral preparations are used for long-term maintenance therapy of schizophrenia and for those who tend to be noncompliant.
- Chlorpromazine (Thorazine) was the first low-potency agent and is the prototype for antipsychotic medications. Haloperidol (Haldol) is the prototype for high-potency agents.

Depression and Its Treatment

Depression, one of the most common psychiatric disorders, is characterized by feelings of intense sadness, helplessness and worthlessness, and impaired functioning. Appetite disturbances such as anorexia or overeating, sleep disturbances, and loss of interest in previously enjoyed activities including family and work are the physical and psychologic symptoms of depression. Generally the diagnosis of depression includes mood changes with despondency, anxiety, self-pity, and so on, psychologic symptoms of low self-esteem, poor concentration, hopelessness and helplessness, physiologic manifestations of either insomnia or hypersomnia, headaches, loss of energy, and complaints of fatigue, and thought alterations including decreased concentration, poor memory, confusion, and delusions. The mood swings are often diurnal or related to specific times of day and are often worse in the mornings.

Mood disorders are also called **affective disorders** and include depression, as well as mania or elation. Major depression is presently referred to as *unipolar affective disorder*. Those disorders that include mixed-type reactions or mood changes from elation to depression are called *bipolar disorder* (previously known as *manic-depressive disorder*). Dysthymia is a milder form of depression in which the patient is sad or "down in the dumps." The person is chronically depressed and finding little joy or excitement in life, having more days of depression than not for at least 2 years. Dysthymia is a common condition—approximately 6% of the entire population experiences dysthymia at some point in their life with about 3% affected at any given time. These processes have no single cause, but psychiatrists believe that stressful events or mental conflicts precede depression. Many factors including genetics, psychosocial events, physiologic stress, and personality traits are precipitating factors with affective disorders.

Classification of Depression

Through the years, many classifications of depression have been used to describe the affective disorders. Some professionals have used the time in life when depression occurred, such as childhood, adolescent, adult, and senile, to characterize depression. Others prefer using the reason for depression, such as exogenous, or reactive, depression and endogenous depression such as chemical imbalances or maladjustments (Box 31-3).

Exogenous depression is often a response to a loss or disappointment such as the death of a loved one, loss of a job, or the presence of a debilitating illness. This type of depression is often called "the blues." After a period of adjustment, the depression resolves and life goes on. Reactive or exogenous depression is usually self-limiting, and the support system of family and friends is sufficient to get through the crisis without the need for antidepressant medications and psychotherapy to make the readjustment.

Endogenous depression or unipolar disorder is characterized by depression that has no external

BOX 31-3   RECOGNIZING DEPRESSION

Signs of depression include the following:
- Minor fluctuations in mood, becoming an overall "down" feeling
- Feeling overwhelmed by responsibilities
- Future seems dismal
- Negative opinion of self
- Criticizing and blaming self repeatedly
- Smallest incidents of life are bothersome

cause and may be the result of genetic factors or biochemical changes in the brain. This type of depression originates within the person, and causes are difficult to recognize. Psychotherapy and antidepressant medications are usually necessary for treatment of these episodes of depression that occur throughout a lifetime.

Antidepressant Medications

The major antidepressant drug classes include monoamine oxidase inhibitors (MAOIs), tricyclic antidepressants (TCAs), selective serotonin reuptake inhibitors (SSRIs), and selective norepinephrine uptake inhibitors (SNRIs). Some herbal supplements, called natural reuptake inhibitors (NRIs), have been indicated as effective as antidepressants. The therapeutic response rate with all antidepressants is similar, so the selection of the proper agent is dependent on the side effects that the patient experiences from the drugs. Selection of the antidepressant to be used takes into account the side effect potential compared with the medical problems of the individual. Some patients will need sedation for their agitation, so a sedating antidepressant is ordered. The Depression Guideline Panel in 1993 established the manner of selection of the medications (Box 31-4).

Tricyclic Antidepressants

Tricyclic antidepressants (TCAs), so named because of their triple-ring structure, are the drugs used with major depression because they are inexpensive, effective, easy to administer, and relatively safe. TCAs block the uptake of serotonin and norepinephrine to result in stimulation of the CNS. The first tricyclic agent, imipramine (Tofranil), was introduced in the 1950s, leading to a group of medications that have the ability to relieve depressive symptoms by blocking the reuptake of the endogenous neurohormones. TCAs may also benefit patients for pain control, chronic insomnia, and attention deficit/hyperactivity disorder (ADHD). These medications are also used for obsessive-compulsive disorders and for enuresis in children.

Nine tricyclic antidepressants are available in the United States; all are equally effective. Geriatric patients are usually started on one third to one half of the usual adult dose followed by evaluation of the therapeutic response, the presence or absence of undesirable side effects being the criterion for dosage adjustment (Table 31-3).

BOX 31-4	SELECTION OF ANTIDEPRESSANT MEDICATIONS FOR DEPRESSED PATIENTS

A. First-and second-line choices
   1. Secondary amine tricyclic antidepressants
   2. bupropion (Wellbutrin, Zyban)—second-generation TCA
   3. fluoxetine (Prozac)—SSRI
   4. paroxetine (Paxil)—SSRI
   5. sertraline (Zoloft)—SSRI
   6. trazodone (Desyrel)—second-generation TCA
B. Alternative agents for patients with special medical considerations
   1. Tertiary amine TCAs for the following:
      a. Absence of serious medical illness including cardiac disease
      b. Need for rapid sedation
   2. MAOIs
      a. Unresponsiveness or intolerance to at least one TCA
      b. Family or personal history of response to MAOI
      c. Atypical depression symptoms
   3. Select anxiolytic medications
      a. Medical contraindications to FDA-approved antidepressant medications
      b. No adverse cardiovascular effects
      c. Low side-effect profile
      d. No history of substance abuse
      e. Need for quick action
      f. Short, limited exposure time needed for medication

Atypical Antidepressants

Atypical antidepressants are second-generation antidepressants that became available in the 1980s for use with major depression, reactive depression, and anxiety. These medications affect one or two of the neurotransmitters—serotonin, norepinephrine, and dopamine—and should not be taken with MAOIs.

- Bupropion (Wellbutrin, Zyban) weakly blocks the reuptake of neurotransmitters and is used for people who are unresponsive to other antidepressants. It is one of the drugs of choice for smoking cessation therapy.
- Mirtazapine (Remeron) is the first drug in a new, well-tolerated class of medications that increase the release of serotonin and norepinephrine to relieve depression, anxiety, and insomnia. A related drug that is indicated only for depression is nefazodone (Serzone).
- Trazodone (Desyrel) is a second-line agent for depression and can be helpful for patients with antidepressant-induced insomnia. A major side effect is priapism.

TABLE 31-3 *Drugs Used to Treat Depression*

GENERIC NAME	TRADE NAME	USUAL ADULT DOSE, ROUTE, AND FREQUENCY OF ADMINISTRATION	INDICATIONS FOR USE	DRUG INTERACTIONS
TRICYCLIC ANTIDEPRESSANTS				alcohol, amphetamines, anticholinergics, antihistamines, antiseizure medications, barbiturates, MAOIs, phenothiazines, antidysrhythmics
clomipramine	Anafranil	25-250 mg/day	Obsessive-compulsive disorder, depression	
desipramine	Norpramin	100-300 mg/day	Depression	
nortriptyline	Aventyl, Pamelor	25 mg tid to 150 mg/day		
maprotiline	Ludiomil	100-150 mg po per day		
protriptyline	Vivactil	15-40 mg po per day		
trimipramine	Surmontil	100-200 mg po per day		
amitriptyline	Elavil, Endep	Up to 300 mg/day po, IM		
doxepin	Sinequan, Adapin	10-300 mg/day po		
imipramine	Tofranil	50-150 mg/day po, IM		

MAJOR SIDE EFFECTS OF TRICYCLIC ANTIDEPRESSANTS: Dry mouth, constipation, urinary retention, tachycardia, orthostatic hypotension, blurred vision, drowsiness, restlessness, tremors, mania, sexual dysfunction.

GENERIC NAME	TRADE NAME	USUAL ADULT DOSE, ROUTE, AND FREQUENCY OF ADMINISTRATION	INDICATIONS FOR USE	DRUG INTERACTIONS
ATYPICAL ANTIDEPRESSANTS			Depression	anticholinergics, guanethidine, phenothiazines
bupropion	Wellbutrin, Zyban	100-450 mg/day po		
mirtazapine	Remeron	15-30 mg/day po		
nefazodone	Serzone	50-100 mg bid po		
trazodone	Desyrel	100-400 mg/day po		+ terfenadine, astemizole
venlafaxine	Effexor	75-375 mg/day po		Same as amoxapine
amoxapine	Asendin	50-100 mg po per day		

MAJOR SIDE EFFECTS OF ATYPICAL ANTIDEPRESSANTS: bupropion: same as tricyclic antidepressants plus agitation, insomnia; **mirtazapine:** somnolence with unusual dreams, increased appetite, weight gain, elevated cholesterol, flulike symptoms; **nefazodone:** somnolence, sexual dysfunction; **trazodone:** sedation, nausea, vomiting; **venlafaxine:** diastolic hypertension; **amoxapine:** EPS, tardive dyskinesia.

GENERIC NAME	TRADE NAME	USUAL ADULT DOSE, ROUTE, AND FREQUENCY OF ADMINISTRATION	INDICATIONS FOR USE	DRUG INTERACTIONS
MAOIs			Neurosis or atypical depression	See Table 31-5
phenelzine	Nardil	15-75 mg po		
tranylcypromine	Parnate	10-40 mg po qd		

MAJOR SIDE EFFECTS OF MAOIs: Postural hypotension, dry mouth, constipation, urinary retention, blurred vision, impotence, insomnia, tremors, convulsions.

GENERIC NAME	TRADE NAME	USUAL ADULT DOSE, ROUTE, AND FREQUENCY OF ADMINISTRATION	INDICATIONS FOR USE	DRUG INTERACTIONS
SELECTIVE SEROTONIN REUPTAKE INHIBITORS			Depression, obsessive compulsive disorder	alcohol, digitalis, anticholinergics, MAOIs, phenytoin, tryptophan
escitalopram	Lexapro	20-60 mg po qd		
fluoxetine	Prozac, Sarafem	20-80 mg/day po in divided doses		
citalopram	Celexa	20-40 mg/day po		+ cimetidine
fluvoxamine	Luvox	100-200 mg po		

TABLE 31-3 *Drugs Used to Treat Depression—cont'd*

GENERIC NAME	TRADE NAME	USUAL ADULT DOSE, ROUTE, AND FREQUENCY OF ADMINISTRATION	INDICATIONS FOR USE	DRUG INTERACTIONS
paroxetine	Paxil	20-40 mg/day po		
sertraline	Zoloft	50-100 mg/day po		
duloxetine	Cymbalta	60 mg po qd		+ thioridazine

MAJOR SIDE EFFECTS OF SELECTIVE SEROTONIN REUPTAKE INHIBITORS: All except duloxetine: sexual dysfunction, nausea, headache, nervousness, insomnia, anxiety, dizziness, fatigue, diarrhea, anorexia, diaphoresis; **duloxetine:** nausea, dry mouth constipation, decreased appetite, sleepiness.

GENERIC NAME	TRADE NAME	USUAL ADULT DOSE, ROUTE, AND FREQUENCY OF ADMINISTRATION	INDICATIONS FOR USE	DRUG INTERACTIONS
RESELECTIVE NOREPINEPHRINE REUPTAKE INHIBITORS				
reboxetine	Vesta	4 mg po bid		MAOIs

MAJOR SIDE EFFECTS OF SELECTIVE NOREPINEPHRINE UPTAKE INHIBITORS: Dry mouth, tremors, hypotension, constipation, decreased libido, urinary retention, dizziness, headache, insomnia, diaphoresis.

GENERIC NAME	TRADE NAME	USUAL ADULT DOSE, ROUTE, AND FREQUENCY OF ADMINISTRATION	INDICATIONS FOR USE	DRUG INTERACTIONS
MEDICATIONS FOR BIPOLAR DISORDER				
lithium carbonate	Eskalith, Lithobid	600 mg bid po or 300 mg tid-qid po	Mania	Diuretics, fluoxetine, antithyroid, haloperidol, anticholinergics, phenytoin, NSAIDs
lithium citrate	Cibalith-S (syrup)	Varies with individual		
carbamazepine	Tegretol	200-400 mg po initially, up to 1200 mg/day po		Multiple
valproic acid	Depakene	500-1000 mg/day po		alcohol, aspirin, warfarin, cimetidine, clonazepam
valproate	Depakote	500-1000 mg/day po		
aripiprazol	Abilify	15-30 mg po qd	See Table 31-2	

MAJOR SIDE EFFECTS OF BIPOLAR DISORDER MEDICATIONS: lithium carbonate: nausea, tremors, vomiting, diarrhea, drowsiness, loss of equilibrium, tinnitus, frequency of urination; **carbamazepine:** sedation, GI disturbances, tremors, leukopenia; **valproic acid:** sedation, nausea, tremors, hair loss.

GI, Gastrointestinal; *MAOIs,* monoamine oxidase inhibitors; *NSAIDs,* nonsteroidal anti-inflammatory drugs.

- Venlafaxine (Effexor) is used for anxiety and depression by blocking norepinephrine and serotonin and more weakly blocks dopamine. The drug has the potential to produce a complete remission.
- An agent that has both an antidepressant and antipsychotic properties is amoxapine (Asendin). Because of the side effects, this medication should be used only for psychotic depression (see Table 31-3).

Monoamine Oxidase Inhibitors

Monoamine oxidase inhibitors (MAOIs), such as phenelzine (Nardil), are antidepressants that are used only for atypical depression when other medications have not been effective. These medications have numerous interactions with prescription and OTC medications and caffeine- and tyramine-containing foods and beverages (Tables 31-4 and 31-5). These food products cause sudden and severe hypertension that may progress to vascular collapse if untreated.

MAOIs inhibit the breakdown of norepinephrine and serotonin to permit the increase of these neurotransmitters in the brain, allowing stimulation of the CNS with clinical improvement of depression. Initially these drugs cause a decrease in appetite and insomnia that improves after 2 weeks of therapy, and the same effects continue for approximately 2 weeks after therapy is discontinued. MAOIs are indicated primarily for resistant depression and anxious hostile depression, especially with panic attacks or when phobic symptoms are involved. In general MAOIs are most effective in reversing dysphoric states, but they may be used

TABLE 31-4 *Foods That Are Safe and Unsafe to Consume When Taking MAO Inhibitors*

CATEGORY	UNSAFE	SAFE
Cheeses/milk products	Practically all cheeses, sour cream, yogurt	Milk, cottage cheese, cream cheese
Meats, fresh sausage	Beef and chicken liver; fermented, smoked, aged meats; bologna, pepperoni, salami; dried or cured fish	Fresh meats, fresh fish
Fruits and vegetables	Avocado, fava beans, figs, raisins, bananas, sauerkraut	Most fruits and vegetables
Foods with yeast	Yeast extract	Baked goods with yeast
Beer, wine	Imported beer, Chianti wine, ale	Domestic beers and wines
Other foods	Protein dietary supplements, soups, shrimp paste, soy sauce	Most other foods
Caffeinated beverages	Colas, tea, coffee, chocolate drinks	Noncaffeinated beverages
Chocolate	Any chocolate product	Nonchocolate products
Ginseng	Herbal products containing ginseng	Nonginseng herbals

TABLE 31-5 *Drug Interactions with Monoamine Oxidase Inhibitors*

DRUG	POSSIBLE EFFECTS
alcohol, CNS depressants	Enhanced CNS depression
local anesthetic	Severe hypertensive reaction
antidepressants	Elevated temperatures, hypertensive crisis, seizures, death
hypoglycemic agents	Enhancement of hypoglycemics
bupropion	Increased risk of toxicity
buspirone	Hypertension
caffeine	Cardiac dysrhythmias, hypertension
dextromethorphan	Increased excitability, increased fever, hypertension
fluoxetine	Agitation, restlessness, gastrointestinal distress, seizures, hypertensive crisis
guanadrel, guanethidine, rauwolfia alkaloids	Severe hypertension
levodopa	Severe, sudden hypertensive crisis
meperidine and other opioids	Severe hypertension, increased excitability, sweating, and rigidity
methyldopa	Severe headaches, hypertension, hallucinations
methylphenidate	Hypertensive crisis
systemic sympathomimetics	Severe hypertensive crisis, increased temperature, cardiac arrhythmias, headache, vomiting
tryptophan and tranylcypromine	Hyperventilation, increased temperature, disorientation, mania
tyramine or foods containing large amounts of pressors (see Table 31-4)	Sudden, severe hypertensive crisis

CNS, Central nervous system.

to treat bulimia and obsessive-compulsive disorders (see Table 31-3).

Selective Serotonin Reuptake Inhibitors

Selective serotonin reuptake inhibitors (SSRIs) are newer antidepressant drugs that block the reuptake and inactivation of serotonin in the brain, causing a stimulant to reverse depression. But unlike the TCAs, the SSRIs have little action to block cholinergic, adrenergic, or histamine receptors. Therefore SSRIs produce fewer side effects and are the most widely used antidepressant drugs. They should be administered in the morning because of the chance of nervousness and insomnia.

Used primarily to treat major depression, the SSRIs are effective orally and are approved for obsessive-compulsive disorders. The patient should take care in participation in hazardous activities until symptoms of dizziness can be evaluated.

- Fluoxetine (Prozac) was the first drug and is often prescribed for this class. This medication is a widely prescribed antidepressant in the United States because it is as effective as the TCAs with fewer side effects and is less dangerous when taken in overdose. Although not approved for these uses by the FDA, Prozac is the preferred agent for panic disorders and for premenstrual syndrome. Investigational uses include bulimia, alcoholism, attention deficit/hyperactivity disorder (ADHD), bipolar disorder, migraine headaches, and obesity. Prozac should be used with care in patients with diabetes mellitus and those with suicidal tendencies.

- Sertraline (Zoloft) is also frequently used for posttraumatic stress syndrome as well as for depression.
- Citalopram hydrobromide (Celexa) and escitalopram (Lexapro) are two of the newer SSRI-type medications for use only with depression. Having fewer side effects, these agents do not produce a sympathomimetic response or anticholinergic activity. This medication cannot be used with MAOIs and should not be given until 2 weeks after stopping any MAOIs (see Table 31-3).

Selective Norepinephrine Reuptake Inhibitors

SNRIs are not related to TCAs, MAOIs, or SSRIs; rather, the two medications in this category, reboxetine (Vestra) and atomoxetine (Strattera) enhance the transmission of norepinephrine. These medications induce remission when used for short-term therapy and prevent relapses in long-term use. The chief indication for use is for patients with severe depression and for those who have difficulty with social functioning (see Table 31-3).

Natural Reuptake Inhibitors

In recent years an increased interest in using herbal supplements that act as natural reuptake inhibitors (NRIs) for treatment of depression has occurred. These products stabilize serotonin and norepinephrine. Studies have shown that St. John's Wort is helpful for mild to moderate depression but not for severe depression. However, the herbal does interact adversely with many drugs. Other natural products including SAM-e and 5-HTP that increase the production of serotonin to regulate mood and emotion are being used. Ginseng and gingko have also been tried with depression.

Antimanic Medications

Antimanic medications are used for the patient with bipolar disorder, formerly called *manic-depressive disorder*. Typically the patient experiences alternating episodes of mania and depression. In the manic state the patient has a heightened mood, with hyperactivity, excessive enthusiasm, overactivity at work or play, and a reduced need

for sleep. Extreme self-confidence, excessive sociability, and extreme talkativeness are characteristic signs. Thoughts and ideations are unrealistic in the manic phase. Ideally, bipolar disorder is treated with a combination of medications and psychotherapy because drug therapy alone is not optimal. Poor patient compliance is often found during manic episodes because the patient sees nothing wrong with their thinking or behavior. Furthermore, the manic episode may not be an unpleasant experience. The family is an important factor in ensuring patient compliance with medication administration during mania and depression.

- Lithium, the most commonly used medication for mania, is a mood stabilizer. Used to prophylactically reduce the frequency and severity of mania in the person with bipolar disorder, lithium appears to reduce hyperactivity and excitement while allowing organization of thought patterns. It is indicated for the treatment of individuals who experience large shifts in mood, mania, or alternating cycles of depression and mania. Lithium can control symptoms in both the manic and depressive phases of the disorder. In the acute manic state, lithium reduces hyperactivity without sedation and it may be combined with a benzodiazepine or an antipsychotic agent that suppresses symptoms until the lithium can be effective. In the depressive state, tricyclic antidepressants or bupropion (Wellbutrin) may be given. If depression occurs, an antidepressant must be given because lithium does not prevent episodes of depression, although it may control early symptoms (see Table 31-3).
- Carbamazepine (Tegretol), valproic acid (Depakene), and valproate (Depakote) were originally marketed for seizure disorders. Recently these medications have been used to treat bipolar disorder.
  - Carbamazepine reduces symptoms during manic and depressive attacks and is prophylactically used for repeated attacks.
  - Valproic acid and valproate are promising alternatives for lithium in the patient who has not responded to lithium or cannot tolerate the side effects. Both of these medications control acute manic episodes and may prevent recurrent episodes of mania and depression. These agents seem to be especially useful with rapidly cycling bipolar disorder. For more information about carbamazepine, valproic acid, and valproate, see Chapter 30.

Patient Education for Compliance

1. Patients taking MAOIs should keep a list of foods and OTC medications that contain tyramine so that these can be avoided.
2. MAOIs cause dizziness, low blood pressure, dry mouth, constipation, blurred vision, and impotence in males.
3. Patients should report feelings of faintness, difficulty with urination, agitation, or jaundice when taking MAOIs.
4. Patients should monitor blood pressure and pulse when taking tricyclic antidepressants.
5. Anyone taking tricyclic antidepressants should not take any medications, especially OTC medications, without permission from the physician.
6. Insomnia, nausea, loss of appetite, headaches, and nervousness are common side effects of SSRIs.
7. Noncompliance is common with any psychotropic or antidepressant medications. Patients should be encouraged to take medications as prescribed.
8. The therapeutic effects of psychotropic medications may not occur for several weeks.
9. Inform all health care professionals of current antidepressant therapy.
10. Antidepressants should be taken on a daily basis, not as needed.
11. All SSRIs should be administered with food.
12. Patients taking lithium should be monitored for hyperglycemia.
13. Patients must maintain adequate sodium intake when taking lithium; a reduced sodium level causes an increased lithium level.
14. Patients taking lithium should drink at least 10 glasses of fluid a day.

IMPORTANT FACTS ABOUT ANTIDEPRESSANTS AND ANTIMANICS

- Symptoms of major depression are depressed mood and loss of pleasure or interest in one's usual activities and pastimes.
- Antidepressants are slow to provide therapeutic responses. The initial responses develop in 1 to 3 weeks, but the maximum response develops in 1 to 2 months.
- Antidepressant therapy should continue for 6 to 12 months following the relief of symptoms.
- Tricyclic antidepressants (TCAs) cause sedation, orthostatic hypotension, dry mouth, and constipation.
- TCAs and MAOIs cannot be combined because of the danger of hypertensive crisis.
- SSRIs have fewer side effects and are safer in overdose than TCAs.

IMPORTANT FACTS ABOUT ANTIDEPRESSANTS AND ANTIMANICS—Cont'd

- SSRIs may cause insomnia and nervousness. TCAs may cause sedation.
- Sexual dysfunction is more common with SSRIs than with other antidepressants.
- TCAs and MAOIs may cause orthostatic hypotension, whereas SSRIs do not.
- Suicidal tendencies should be evaluated in all depressed patients.
- Lithium is used for bipolar disorder and is teratogenic.

Drugs for Alzheimer's Disease

Alzheimer's disease is a devastating illness characterized by progressive memory failure, impaired thinking, confusion, disorientation, personality changes, restlessness, speech disturbances, and inability to perform routine tasks. Tragically, the disease is incurable and affects about 250,000 new individuals per year. Clinically, the progressive decline of intellectual functions and reduction or deterioration of the nerve pathways have recently been shown to respond to therapy with cholinesterase inhibitors and memantine (Namenda). Most pharmacotherapy is focused on improving cognitive functioning or limiting the disease progression, and symptom control. In Alzheimer's disease, acetylcholine (ACh) is decreased (ACh is necessary for neurotransmission and for forming memories) and thus cholinesterase inhibitors are used. With the loss of memory comes confusion, wandering, agitation, and pacing, which seem to intensify in the early evening, or "sundowning." No specific test for Alzheimer's disease exists; therefore a definitive diagnosis is possible only on autopsy and possibly changes in brain tissue as seen on computed tomography scans. When all other causes of dementia have been ruled out, Alzheimer's is the probable diagnosis.

- Tacrine (Cognex) enhances the transmission of cholinergic neurons that have not been destroyed. Tacrine does not slow the actual disease process but has been approved for patients with mild to moderate Alzheimer's disease to improve transmission of thought processes. The improvements from tacrine are not universal, dramatic, and long-lasting; rather, they are modest and short lived. A significant risk of liver damage exists, but the benefits are worth the risk of devastation from the disease.

- Donepezil (Aricept) is similar in mechanism of action to tacrine and has the same effectiveness. Approved by the FDA for Alzheimer's disease, donepezil does not affect the underlying disease process. Unlike tacrine, donepezil does not damage the liver.
- Galantamine (Reminyl), an antidementia medication, elevates ACh concentrations in the brain by slowing degeneration. The decrease of ACh is thought to be one of the causes of Alzheimer's disease.
- Memantine (Namenda) is the most recent medication approved as an anti-Alzheimer agent. It is used to reduce the deterioration of cholinergic nerve pathways with moderate to severe Alzheimer's disease (Table 31-6).

Investigation is being done into the use of NSAIDs and vitamin E to decrease the risk of and prevent and treat early symptoms of Alzheimer's disease. Evidence indicates that a link exists between Alzheimer's and inflammation. Estrogens appear to reduce the risk of the disease in postmenopausal women because estrogens seem to improve memory.

If needed, medications for delusions, agitation, depression, or anxiety may be used for Alzheimer's disease. Tricyclic antidepressants must be used with care because of their significant anticholinergic actions.

> **DID YOU KNOW?**
> Reminyl, a medication for the slowing of Alzheimer's disease, is derived from daffodil bulbs.

> **IMPORTANT FACTS ABOUT MEDICATIONS FOR ALZHEIMER'S DISEASE**
> - Alzheimer's disease is a relentless illness characterized by progressive memory loss, impaired thinking, personality changes, and the progressive inability to perform routine tasks.
> - The major risk factor for Alzheimer's disease is age.
> - Tacrine causes modest improvement in 30% of Alzheimer's disease patients; the other 70% do not respond.
> - Several medication categories are being investigated for use in Alzheimer's patients.

Drugs Used for Attention Deficit/Hyperactivity Disorder

ADHD is a common behavioral disorder in children, with an average of one ADHD child in each classroom. The symptoms of inattention, hyperactivity, and impulsivity begin between ages 3 and 7 and persist into the teenage years. Boys are four to eight times more likely to have ADHD than girls.

Children with ADHD are fidgety and unable to complete tasks, jumping from one activity to another. They have an inability to concentrate on schoolwork and tend to be impatient in class, never waiting their turn. The diagnosis is made when symptoms occur before 7 years of age and last for 6 months. The exact underlying pathology is unknown, but the symptoms do respond to stimulant medications (see Chapter 30).

Central nervous system stimulants should not be given for more than a year without interruption

TABLE 31-6 *Drugs Used with Alzheimer's Disease*

GENERIC NAME	TRADE NAME	USUAL ADULT DOSE, ROUTE, AND FREQUENCY OF ADMINISTRATION	INDICATIONS FOR USE	DRUG INTERACTIONS
tacrine	Cognex	10-40 mg po qid	Alzheimer's disease	NSAIDs, anticholinergic, cimetidine, fluvoxamine, theophylline
donepezil	Aricept	5-10 mg/day po	Same	anticholinergics
ergoloid mesylates	Hydergine	3 mg po tid	Same	None
rivastigmine	Exelon	1.5-3 mg po bid	Same	None
memantine	Namenda	5-20 mg po qd	Same	Carbonic anhydrase inhibitors
galantamine	Reminyl	4 mg po bid	Same	cimetidine, ketoconazole, paroxetine, erythromycin

MAJOR SIDE EFFECTS: tacrine: nausea, vomiting, diarrhea, dyspepsia, myalgia, headache, ataxia; **donepezil:** nausea, diarrhea; **memantine:** dizziness, headache, confusion, constipation, hypertension, cough.

NSAIDs, Nonsteroidal antiinflammatory drugs.

because of the suppression of growth. More important, the need for continued treatment should be assessed yearly. The summer break is a good period for long-term interruption, and weekends and holidays are good times for short-term interruption of medications.

The mainstay drugs for ADHD are methylphenidate (Ritalin, Concerta), dextroamphetamine (Dexedrine), amphetamine sulfate (Adderall), atomoxetine (Strattera), and lisdexamfetamine (Vyvanse). These drugs will have increased warnings because of the heart disease and psychiatric effects that have been found to happen in later life for children who take these medications.

- Methylphenidate (Ritalin), a Schedule II medication, is the most commonly prescribed drug; children respond dramatically to this drug. The child has an increased attention span and well-focused behavior, with decreased distractibility, hyperactivity, restlessness, and impulsiveness. Cognitive functions of memory, reading, and arithmetic improve significantly. The use of a stimulant would seem to be the opposite of the expected; methylphenidate does not suppress rowdy behavior but improves attention and focus. Because the child can concentrate on the task at hand, the impulsiveness and hyperactivity decline.
  - Methylphenidate comes in standard and sustained-release tablets. Standard tablets are given two to three times a day, whereas sustained-release tablets are given once a day.
  - The standard tablet is given in the morning and at noon, but it may be given at 4 PM if the behavior is impulsive at home after school. Dosage is individualized according to improvement in symptoms and the appearance of side effects.
  - If possible, the medication is not given on weekends and during the summer, to allow growth to catch up. The break between administration of medication is known as a **drug holiday.**
- Dextroamphetamine (Dexedrine and others), also a Schedule II drug, is as effective as methylphenidate; in fact, some children who do not respond to Ritalin will respond to dextroamphetamine. Dexedrine has a rapid time of action, with dosing being at 8 AM and 4 PM.
- Another amphetamine-based CNS stimulant is lisdexamfetamine (Vyvanse) that provides consistent 12-hour control of ADHD. Only one dose per day is needed for therapeutic effects.
- Tricyclic antidepressants may be used to decrease hyperactivity but have little effect on

impulsivity and inattention. Tolerance frequently develops within a few months, and the medication cannot be discontinued on weekends. These medications are less effective and more dangerous than the central nervous system stimulants, so they should be given as medications of second choice.
- Clonidine, a medication for hypertension, reduces hyperactivity and impulsiveness. The sedation and hypotension found with this medication make clonidine an alternate medication to be used only if needed.
- The newest medication used for ADHD is atomoxetine (Strattera), which is not a scheduled medication. It selectively inhibits the uptake of norepinephrine, causing a calming effect. This drug also is being used as an antidepressant (Table 31-7).

Patient Education for Compliance

Children taking medications for ADHD who require more than one dose per day should take the morning dose after breakfast and the last dose by 4 PM.

IMPORTANT FACTS ABOUT MEDICATIONS FOR ADHD

- Most medications for ADHD are classified as Schedule II medications under the Controlled Substances Act and should be treated with the proper precautions.
- The goals of ADHD medications are to reduce the symptoms of hyperactivity and reduce sleep attacks in patients with narcolepsy.
- The common side effects of amphetamines are insomnia and weight loss.

Summary

The ability to cope with life's stressors at different stages of life is the basis for mental health. "Normal" can be difficult to define; it varies from time to time, culture to culture, and person to person. Mental illness affects almost everyone at some point during life, either themselves or their family members. The causes of mental illness may be congenital deficiencies, hereditary factors, or traumatic events. The treatment of mental illness has made giant steps in the past 50 years. With the introduction of new psychiatric medications, many mentally ill persons are today treated as outpatients rather than institutionalized as previously.

TABLE 31-7   *Drugs Used for Attention Deficit/Hyperactivity Disorder*

GENERIC NAME (SCHEDULE)	TRADE NAME	USUAL DOSE, ROUTE, AND FREQUENCY OF ADMINISTRATION	INDICATIONS FOR USE	DRUG INTERACTIONS
methylphenidate (II)	Ritalin	5-30 mg/day po	ADHD	Other CNS
	Ritalin SR	20 mg po once a day		stimulants
	Concerta	18-36 po once a day		and MAOIs
dextroamphetamine (II)	Dexedrine	5-15 mg/day po		
lisdexamfetamine (II)	Vyvanse	30 mg-70 mg po qd		
pemoline (IV)	Cylert	37.5 mg po at 8 AM; may be increased by 18.75 mg/week po to a maximum of 112.5 mg/day po		
amphetamine sulfate (II)	Adderall	5-30 mg po daily		
atomoxetine	Strattera	40 mg po qd		

MAJOR SIDE EFFECTS: methylphenidate: insomnia, growth suppression, headache, abdominal pain, lethargy, listlessness, weight loss, dry mouth, irritability; **tomoxetine:** headache, dyspepsia, nausea and vomiting, fatigue, decreased appetite, dizziness, altered mood.

ADHD, Attention deficit hyperactivity disorder; CNS, central nervous system; MAOIs, monoamine oxidase inhibitors.

The two main categories of mental illness are neurosis and psychosis, both of which produce such symptoms as agitation, hyperactivity, and inappropriate behavior. Neurosis produces fear or anxiety from either real or unknown dangers. The response may cause many symptoms, and drug therapy with anxiolytics, or minor tranquilizers, is used to alleviate the symptoms. Psychosis occurs when the person is out of control, out of touch with reality, and unable to communicate. The treatment for psychosis includes psychotherapy and antipsychotic medications, also called *neuroleptics* or *major tranquilizers.*

Anxiolytics may be used to treat prolonged anxiety, but these medications may be used as hypnotics/sedatives, as muscle relaxants, as adjuvant medications for convulsions, and with treatment for withdrawal from alcohol abuse. Antianxiety medications cannot be used for prolonged periods of time because tolerance, habituation, and physical and psychologic dependence may occur. Benzodiazepines were introduced in the 1960s and continue to be some of the most widely prescribed anxiolytic medications.

The first antipsychotic agent was introduced in the 1950s, and these medications have changed the world of mental health treatment. These agents are used to suppress the symptoms of schizophrenia and other psychotic conditions. All of these medications act on dopamine in the brain. The major side effects with these drugs are extrapyramidal symptoms, tardive dyskinesia, parkinsonism-

like symptoms, akathisia, and dystonic reactions. Dystonic reactions are more likely to occur in children. In general the antipsychotics are used to relieve the symptoms of psychosis or severe neurosis, to relieve nausea and vomiting, and for the potentiation of analgesics. Children and geriatric patients require special care when using neuroleptics.

Depot antipsychotics are used for long-term maintenance therapy. By giving these injectable medications, patient compliance is enhanced and the patient is maintained at the highest possible level of functioning.

Antidepressants are used for both endogenous and exogenous depression. In many depressed people the neurotransmitters in the brain, serotonin and norepinephrine, are in short supply, keeping nerve cells from functioning. Drugs are used to increase the levels of these monoamines in the brain to elevate moods. Groups of medications used for depression include TCAs, MAOIs, SSRIs, and SNRIs. The TCAs are the usual first line of medication for use, followed by SSRIs or SNRIs. MAOIs have many side effects, have drug interactions, and require severe dietary restrictions; therefore they are used only when other antidepressants do not provide relief. In recent years herbal supplements have been studied and used as agents to relieve mild to moderate depression.

Lithium is the medication of choice for bipolar disorder or manic-depressive disorder. It is the most effective drug for use in acute manic attacks, but benzodiazepines or other antipsychotic agents may be used until lithium becomes effective. This drug is also used prophylactically to prevent manic attacks.

Alzheimer's disease is a progressive illness that causes a decline in intellectual functions. Five medications have been specifically approved for use with this condition. These drugs may slow the advance of the disease, but they are not cures for the progressive devastation caused by the brain changes. Investigation is being done to study the use of NSAIDs, vitamin E, and estrogens with Alzheimer's disease.

Methylphenidate (Ritalin) is the drug of choice for ADHD, but amphetamine sulfate (Adderall), dextroamphetamine, or lisdexamfetamine (Vyvanse) may be used. These drugs increase a child's attention span and enable goal-oriented behavior. Children taking these drugs should have drug holidays, or nonadministration, on weekends and during the summer to overcome the growth suppression that is a major side effect of the medication. One of the newest drugs for this condition, atomoxetine (Strattera) does not have an amphetamine base and causes calming by inhibiting the uptake of norepinephrine.

Within the past half century, medications for mental health have increased rapidly since the introduction of anxiolytic and antipsychotics. These drugs have changed the world of health care in many ways, but perhaps the greatest is that now most mentally imbalanced persons are able to live and work in their home communities and may be contributing members of society.

Critical Thinking Exercises

SCENARIO

Lakeesha is a 10-year-old who has been diagnosed with ADHD and is treated with methylphenidate three times a day. Her mother calls to tell you that she is giving the medicine in the morning, at school, and at supper, and Lakeesha is unable to sleep.

1. At what times do you think Dr. Merry intended Lakeesha to take the medication?
2. Her mother also wants to know why Lakeesha cannot take the medications on weekends and during the summer to help with her hyperactivity. What reasons do you think Dr. Merry would give Lakeesha's mother?
3. What side effects can Lakeesha and her mother expect?
4. What class of controlled substances is methylphenidate?
5. What does that mean to her family when prescriptions for Lakeesha are necessary?
6. How is the drug effective against ADHD?

DRUG CALCULATIONS

1. Order: Ativan 1 mg stat then bid
   Available medication:

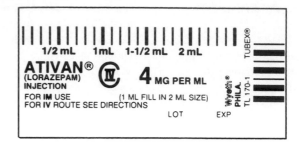

Dose to be given: _____

_____

2. Mellaril 15 mL
   Available medication:

Dose to be given: _____

_____

How should this medication be diluted prior to administration?_____

_____

_____

Show the amount of medication for dilution and the amount of diluent on the utensil provided.

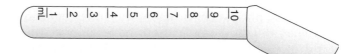

REVIEW QUESTIONS

1. What drugs are used to treat neurosis? Psychosis? _____
_____
_____

2. What are other names used for anxiolytics? _____
_____
_____

3. What are three uses for anxiolytics other than reduction of anxiety? _____
_____
_____

4. What three drug classes are used to treat psychosis? _____
_____
_____

5. What are the uses of neuroleptics? How are they effective in the treatment of schizophrenia? ____
_____
_____

6. What is meant by a low-potency antipsychotic? Intermediate-potency? High-potency?_____
_____
_____

7. What is an atypical antipsychotic medication? How are these effective?_____
_____
_____

8. What is a depot antipsychotic agent? What is an indication for the use of a depot antipsychotic? __
_____
_____

9. What are the three classes of major antidepressants? _____
_____
_____

10. What is the use of lithium, and what condition does it treat? _____
_____
_____

11. Why are medications effective only in slowing the signs and symptoms of Alzheimer's disease?
_____
_____
_____

CHAPTER 32

Drugs of Abuse and Misuse

OBJECTIVES

After studying this chapter, you should be capable of doing the following:

- Discussing the dangers of drug abuse by health care workers.
- Recognizing the medications used for treatment of alcohol abuse.
- Discussing illegal drugs that are abused.
- Identifying the prescription medications that may be misused or abused.
- Describing ways that lead to misuse or abuse of prescription/nonprescription medications and identifying possible abuse/misuse situations.

Mr. Goddio, age 45, has lower back pain and early emphysema. You find Mr. Goddio's blood pressure to be elevated, and laboratory tests show an elevated lipid profile. He is known to smoke one to two packs of cigarettes per day.

How does this habit increase Mr. Goddio's chance of cardiovascular disease?

What would you tell Mr. Goddio if he asks why it is important for him to stop smoking?

What types of products are available for the physician to prescribe to help Mr. Goddio stop smoking? What are their side effects?

How would you answer Mr. Goddio if he wants to know why the dosage of medication is gradually decreased throughout the program?

Will this medication be effective if he does not want to stop smoking? Why or why not?

KEY TERMS

Cirrhosis	Dysphoria	Inebriation
Delirium tremens	Euphoria	

EASY WORKING KNOWLEDGE OF INDICATIONS AND SIDE EFFECTS

Common Signs and Symptoms of Drug Abuse and Misuse	Common Side Effects of Abused and Misused Drugs
Changes in weight and sleep habits	Drowsiness, constipation
Impaired memory	Hallucinations
Illogical thinking	Lightheadedness, dizziness, headache
Mood swings, irritability, depression, anger	Impotence
Defensiveness	Cardiac arrhythmias
Anxiety and overreaction to difficult situations	Nausea, sore mouth and throat, diarrhea
Changes in vital signs	Respiratory distress
Runny nose, nasal stuffiness, bloodshot eyes, sweating	Erythema, pruritus, local edema, rash
Changes in friends and appearance	Mental confusion

Easy Working Knowledge of Medications Used to Treat Substance Abuse

DRUG CLASS	PRESCRIPTION	OTC	PREGNANCY CATEGORY	MAJOR INDICATIONS
Substance abuse deterrents	Yes	Yes	X	Cessation of alcohol and nicotine use
Narcotic antagonists	Yes	No	B, C	Detoxification in narcotic abstinence

All drugs, prescribed or over-the-counter (OTC), including those that are used for self-medication, have the potential for abuse and misuse. The patient's actual needs for medications should be evaluated, and only medications determined to be appropriate for the patient should be prescribed. The physician who indiscriminately prescribes medications without looking into the complaints and medical conditions of the patient is misusing medications. The prolonged and unsupervised taking of medications is also drug misuse. Drug abuse is self-medication on a chronic basis in quantities that cause physical or psychologic dependence and the inability to function within socially acceptable norms. Taking antihistamines or analgesics either too frequently or in doses that are not recognized as acceptable dosages are examples of drug abuse. Some patients just enjoy feeling high and will take medications to achieve this feeling.

Drug abuse and misuse are not new phenomena; they have occurred throughout history as a way to relieve personal, physical, psychologic, social, and economic problems. Since the dawn of civilization, mind-altering drugs have held a fascination as a means to elevate mood, induce **hallucinations,** and modify thinking. Abuse is not related to any certain socioeconomic, cultural, or ethnic group, but is found in all levels of society.

BOX 32-1   DEFINITIONS OF TERMS USED IN DRUG ABUSE/MISUSE

- Drug misuse—Nonspecific or indiscriminate use of drugs
- Drug abuse—Use of a drug not prescribed by a physician or improper/excessive use of a drug
- Drug habit—Frequent and indiscriminate use of a drug, causing a problem when attempting to stop the use
- Drug dependency—Physical or psychologic need to use a drug to achieve a sense of well-being or to avoid withdrawal symptoms; not the same as addiction
- Drug habituation—Use of a drug so frequently that the drug is part of the daily activities
- Drug addiction—Compulsive, excessive, or constant use of drugs to achieve a desired state, with the results being harmful to the person, to society, or both
- Drug tolerance—Increased amount of a drug is necessary to produce the original effect because the medications produce less effect than when previously taken
- Withdrawal—Effect experienced when the drug of physical or psychologic dependence has been discontinued

---

DID YOU KNOW?

Drug or substance abuse is a multibillion-dollar-a-year problem that has a significant impact on all aspects of society and in all cultural and economic backgrounds. Substance abuse affects every person in the United States, either directly or indirectly, in social, economic, medical, or interpersonal ways. Assaults, rape, and child abuse are often related to substance abuse, whereas traffic accidents and fatalities often involve alcohol impairment.

DID YOU KNOW?

Mind-altering medications are still used in some cultures today during religious ceremonies. These may come from sources considered socially acceptable such as herbals.

What Is Drug Abuse?

Drug abuse may be described as using a drug in a way that is inconsistent with the medical, social, and cultural norms of a certain population. Each instance of drug use must be evaluated for the potential for drug abuse and misuse. Large dosages of psychotherapeutic medications may be necessary in certain populations, whereas these dosages could very well be abused in other populations. An instance of acceptable medicinal use versus abuse would be the use of opioids for the relief of acute or chronic pain found with cancer and other painful conditions, which is an acceptable use, but the healthy person who takes the drug to get high would be considered to be abusing the drug. Drug abuse also has degrees of severity from occasional use to habitual, compulsive, and routine use. Box 32-1 shows the terminology of substance abuse.

Factors That Contribute to Drug Misuse and Abuse

Several factors contribute to drug abuse or the progressive involvement with drugs. Curiosity concerning the effects of a medication often leads to psychoactive drug use. Drug abuse may begin with occasional misuse to feel good and then progress to a compulsive need for the drugs—or the progression from experimentation with drugs to compulsive need and use of the substances.

- People might first try a drug out of *curiosity* or *peer pressure,* but "feeling good" leads to continued use. If the drug caused negative feelings, drug use would stop.
- *Dependence*
  - Physical dependence is based on the size of the dose and the length of time used. The more physically dependent, the more likely

withdrawal symptoms will occur. Physical dependence plays an important role when the person's need is to alleviate symptoms, although other reasons may lead to dependencies. When withdrawal symptoms begin, the person again takes the drug for the relief of symptoms, causing a desire for the drug that results in further drug abuse.

- Psychologic dependence, a craving for the drug with a strong need for a feeling of well-being, leads to addiction.

- *Social status* and *social approval*, caused by peer pressure to become a part of a desired culture, may cause continued use of medications even when the drug causes an unpleasant result. This pressure is often the reason for continued experimentation with substances of abuse.

- *Drug availability* is a factor in the development of drug abuse and the continued use of these agents.

- *Vulnerability* to drugs leads some people to be more likely to become drug abusers or misusers than others. Individual differences lead some people to experiment with a drug once and never try it again; others will try a drug one time and immediately develop a compulsive desire for the agent.

- *Psychosocial disorders* such as depression and anxiety tend to cause persons who are impulsive with little tolerance for frustration to become rebellious toward social expectations and that can lead to abuse. Once an abuser of one drug, the more likely a person will abuse other drugs.

- *Genetics*, especially with the use of alcohol, have also been proven to play a role in drug abuse and **drug misuse.** (Alcoholism and drug abuse are seen as familial tendencies and diseases.)

- *Tolerance to otherwise intolerable situations* allows the ability to alter the state of consciousness in the person, causing the individual to develop a rapid onset of desired effects and withdrawal symptoms if discontinued abruptly. The feelings of shame and inadequacy, the personal conflicts, and the predisposition to depression are avoided with drug abuse, and the person believes he or she can function acceptably in society.

DID YOU KNOW?

Different abused drugs can be detected in the urine over different lengths of time. Table 32-1 gives a sampling of these times. For certain drugs, prolonged use can extend these times.

TABLE 32-1 *Length of Time That a Drug Can Be Detected in the Urine*

DRUG	DURATION
alcohol	<1 day
amphetamines	Up to 1 day
barbiturates	Up to 1 day
benzodiazepines	Up to 2 days
cocaine	Up to 2 days
marijuana—single use	Up to 6 days
marijuana—multiple uses	Up to 1 mo
opioids (short-acting)	Up to 1 day
phenobarbital	Up to 6 days
PCP	Up to 6 days

Behaviors of Drug Abuse

Drug misuse or abuse is often unplanned, with the user beginning with experimentation and steadily increasing from there. The person who starts with weekend use next relies on the drug to assist with "difficult situations" during the week. The weekend use becomes insufficient and increases to several times a week or daily, until the drug becomes a crutch in any uncomfortable or tension-producing situation. Often the family becomes aware of the problem only when daily drug use becomes the user's mode of "surviving" or the norm.

Signs of drug abuse include the following:

- Physical signs
  - Changes in sleeping habits and in weight
  - Lack of muscle coordination, with slurring of words
  - Lethargy and illnesses on a more frequent basis
- Psychologic signs
  - Depression and apathy
  - Anxiety and overreaction
  - Concentration impairment and shortened memory
  - Inability to organize and inflexibility to changes in planned schedules
  - Illogical thinking and confusion
- Social signs
  - Mood swings, irritability, anger
  - Defensiveness and overreaction to social situations
  - Decreased school or work performance and absenteeism
  - Feelings of inadequacy
  - Disrespect for authority and discipline
  - Old friends are often cast aside

Drug withdrawal symptoms include the following:

- Nervousness, runny nose and stuffiness, sweating, bloodshot or puffy eyes, and the inability to stay still
- Changes in vital signs including variations in blood pressure and pulse with rapid respirations
- Death from rapid withdrawal is possible; this causes the abuser to become desperate for the next dose and willing to engage in any activity that will provide the needed drug

IMPORTANT FACTS ABOUT DRUG ABUSE

- Drug abuse is using a drug in a way that is inconsistent with medical, cultural, and social norms within a given population.
- Drug abuse is not a new phenomenon, but has occurred throughout history, involving prescribed or OTC medications as well as street drugs.
- Drugs used for self-medication are often those most abused or misused because of chronic use and excessive dosages.
- Curiosity is one of the leading reasons for beginning the drug's use. A desirable feeling following the use of a drug is usually the reason for continued drug abuse or misuse.
- Physical dependence has built-in conditions such as tolerance levels and withdrawal symptoms when stopping the drug.
- Psychologic dependence leads to addiction because of craving for the medication/agent.
- Drug availability, social status, and social acceptance are reasons for continued use of drugs of abuse.

Drugs That Are Abused and Misused

Drugs and alcohol are major problems in our society. One can pick up any newspaper and find articles concerning drugs that are abused, from stimulants to depressants, from those agents that cause a high to those that bring the abuser down. Drug abuse is defined as the use of a drug for purposes other than therapeutic. Drug misuse is the indiscriminate use of a drug.

The most frequently abused chemical substances are xanthines and caffeine, found in coffee, tea, caffeine-containing soft drinks, and chocolate. These drugs produce mild stimulation and euphoric effects and a physical dependence necessary to be able to perform daily tasks without having signs such as headaches, sleepiness, and lethargy.

Nicotine

The chief source of nicotine, a liquid alkaloid, is tobacco. As a drug, it has only one therapeutic use, that being to provide products for assistance with smoking cessation. But nicotine has great pharmacologic and toxicologic interest. Readily absorbed into the body through the gastrointestinal tract, the respiratory tract, and the skin, the components of tobacco smoke include materials that are potentially dangerous to the body such as carbon monoxide, hydrogen cyanide, ammonia, and coal tar, which are known carcinogens.

Smoking, using cigarettes, pipe tobacco, or cigars, is the greatest single cause of preventable illnesses and premature death and produces complex and unpredictable pharmacologic effects on the body. Secondhand smoking—inhalation of cigarette smoke by nonsmokers—has been shown by the Food and Drug Administration to lead to as many health risks and harmful effects as (or more than) the effects on the smoker. Nicotine may cause acute toxicity in children who ingest or inhale tobacco products, or chronic toxicity may occur from long-term use of or association with the products. Use of chewing tobacco and snuff lead to leukoplakia and cancer of the mucous membranes of the oral cavity. See Table 32-2 for effects of nicotine on the body systems.

Nicotine interacts with other drugs. Smoking increases the drug metabolism of acetaminophen (Tylenol), caffeine, oxazepam (Serax), pentazocine (Talwin), propranolol (Inderal), propoxyphene (Darvon), and theophylline, requiring higher or more frequent doses of these drugs. Cessation of smoking may result in an increased insulin effect, and the dosage of insulin may have to be decreased to prevent hypoglycemia.

Smoking Cessation Products

Nicotine products for smoking cessation come as tablets, gums, lozenges, nasal sprays, and transdermal systems for the patient who is experiencing acute nicotine withdrawal. Products are available as prescription items and those found over the counter. Instead of smoking, the person chews the nicotine gum, reducing the number of pieces per day over a period of 2 to 3 months. Nicotine taken this way is more slowly absorbed through the buccal mucosa than if inhaled. The transdermal patches are worn for 16 to 24 hours per day. Those worn for 16 hours mimic the daily use of cigarettes, with a lowering of serum nicotine at night when the person is usually sleeping. The nicotine nasal spray,

TABLE 32-2 *Effects of Nicotine on the Body*

BODY SYSTEM	EFFECTS
Cardiovascular system	Initially slows the heart rate but later causes acceleration
	Peripheral blood vessels constrict but later dilate, causing a drop in blood pressure
	Causes coronary heart disease, myocardial infarctions, arteriosclerosis
Nervous system	Affects the vital organ function regulated by the central nervous system
	Causes tolerance and physical dependence
	Increased levels of cortisol and **catecholamines**
Urinary system	Acts as an antidiuretic
Gastrointestinal system	Increases gastric acids
	Increases gastric muscle tone and motility
	Causes gastric ulcers and chronic dyspepsia
	Loss of appetite
Immune system	Decreases immunity
	Causes mutation of cells leading to precancerous cells
Respiratory system	Decreases lung volume
	Decreases air flow
	Causes pulmonary emphysema, acute and chronic bronchitis
	Increased risk of sudden infant death syndrome (SIDS)
Reproductive system	Low birth weights of infants born to smokers
	Increased chance of congenital abnormalities
	Increased risk of prematurity

which more closely simulates smoking, works faster than the gum or patches and has the same efficacy. The patient should not smoke while using the spray, nor should the spray be used with other nicotine products. Tablets, one of the newest forms of these products, are taken over several months to assist with abstinence. All of these agents should be used for at least 3 months but no longer than 6 months, with the dosage reduced as the body adjusts to the nonsmoking regimen. The latest smoking deterrent is a vaccine (NicVax) that is used to reduce the pleasurable effects of smoking.

Prescription medications for cessation of nicotine use include bupropion (Zyban) and the newest medication in this group, varenicline (Chantix).

- Bupropion (Zyban) has the same active ingredient as found with the antidepressant, Wellbutrin. This medication reduces the craving for nicotine and reduces nicotine withdrawal symptoms. The treatment takes about a week, while the person is still smoking, to be effective, so the person should not attempt to stop smoking until the second week of treatment. This medication should be taken for 7 to 12 weeks, although if the person has not stopped smoking by the seventh week, it is unlikely that the medication will be effective.
- Varenicline (Chantix) partially activates the nicotine receptors in the brain to reduce the craving for and the withdrawal symptoms of nicotine use. The medication reduces the urge to smoke and then blocks the effects of nicotine if smoking resumes. The treatment is 12 weeks in length and may be repeated for a second 12-week period. This medication should also be taken for 7 days prior to attempting to stop smoking (Table 32-3).

Early signs of an overdose of nicotine are nausea and vomiting, severe abdominal pain, diarrhea, cold sweat, and severe headaches. Disturbed hearing and vision, confusion with hypotension, and fast, weak, or irregular pulse are found with advanced overdosage. These smoking cessation agents should not be used by patients who have angina pectoris, cardiac dysrhythmias, insulin-dependent diabetes mellitus, hypertension, peripheral vascular disease, peptic ulcer, or a history of myocardial infarction (see Table 32-3).

Patient Education for Compliance

Smoking is carcinogenic. Only when the person desires to cease nicotine use will medications for smoking cessation assist the patient in breaking the habit.

IMPORTANT FACTS ABOUT MEDICATIONS FOR NICOTINE ABUSE

- Nicotine from cigarette smoking is absorbed in the lungs, whereas nicotine from cigars and smokeless tobacco is absorbed in the mouth.
- Nicotine increases alertness, facilitates memory, improves cognitive function, and suppresses the appetite.
- Nicotine causes tolerance and physical dependence, with craving, nervousness, restlessness, irritability, impatience, hostility, insomnia, increased appetite, weight gain, and impaired concentration occurring on its withdrawal.

TABLE 32-3 *Deterrents to Drug Abuse and Misuse*

GENERIC NAME	TRADE NAME	USUAL ADULT DOSE, ROUTE, AND FREQUENCY OF ADMINISTRATION	INDICATIONS FOR USE	DRUG INTERACTIONS
MEDICATIONS USED AS NICOTINE DETERRENTS			Use of nicotine products	
nicotine	Nicotrol	1 mg = 2 sprays/nostril (1-2 doses/hr up to 40 doses per day)		None indicated
	Nicorette (OTC)	9-12 pieces of gum at 1-2 hr intervals (up to 30 pieces/day) Dissolve lozenges in mouth as above		
	Nicotrol	1 transdermal patch per day; wear for 16 hr		
	ProStep, Nicoderm CQ	1 transdermal patch per day; wear for 24 hr		
	NicVAX (to be released in 2008)	Injectable		
varenidine	Chantix	0.5 mg-1 mg tab po qd in 12-wk cycle		
bupropion	Zyban, Wellbutrin	150 mg po qd × 3 days, then 150 mg po bid		alcohol, TCA, lithium, ritonavir, trazodone

MAJOR SIDE EFFECTS OF NICOTINE DETERRENTS: All: Nausea, tachycardia, Headaches/dizziness, increased appetite, indigestion, insomnia; additionally, damage to mouth, teeth, and dental work with gums and lozenges; local rash or pruritus with transdermal patches.

GENERIC NAME	TRADE NAME	USUAL ADULT DOSE, ROUTE, AND FREQUENCY OF ADMINISTRATION	INDICATIONS FOR USE	DRUG INTERACTIONS
MEDICATIONS USED AS ALCOHOL/OPIOID DETERRENTS				
naltrexone	Revia	50 mg po as maintenance dose, or 100-150 mg po 3x/wk	Alcoholism, opioid misuse	Analgesics, cough preparations, any preparation with alcohol base
disulfiram	Antabuse	125-500 mg po daily in AM	Alcoholism	alcohol, paraldehyde, isoniazid, warfarin
acamprosate	Campral	180 mg po tid	Alcoholism	
methadone	Dolophine	15-40 mg/day po, SC, IM, usually maintained at 20-120 mg/day	Opioid abuse	In addition, cimetidine, selegiline, furazolidone

MAJOR SIDE EFFECTS OF ALCOHOL/OPIOID DETERRENTS: disulfiram: Drowsiness; (side effects such as nausea and vomiting are desired); **acamprosate:** diarrhea, gas, loss of appetite, dizziness, weakness, itching.

IM, Intramuscular; *SC,* subcutaneous; *TCA,* tricyclic antidepressants.

IMPORTANT FACTS ABOUT MEDICATIONS FOR NICOTINE ABUSE—*Cont'd*
- Few people achieve long-term success when attempting to quit smoking, even with nicotine replacement therapy.
- Nicotine replacement therapy is available in six forms: tablets, transdermal patches, chewing gum, lozenges, and nasal sprays that are available by prescription and OTC, and, beginning in 2008, a vaccine.

IMPORTANT FACTS ABOUT MEDICATIONS FOR NICOTINE ABUSE—*Cont'd*
- Smoking cessation agents cause belching, tachycardia, headaches, increased appetite, soreness of the mouth and throat, dizziness, and insomnia.
- The fastest-working nicotine substitute is the nasal spray. It has the same efficacy as the patches.
- Transdermal patches may cause local irritation.

Ethyl Alcohol or Ethanol

Alcohol is one of the oldest and most abused drugs used in the United States. A central nervous system depressant, alcohol does have some medicinal uses such as a vehicle for cough suppressants and as a germicidal in mouthwashes. Alcohol is often abused or misused through the use of OTC medications such as nighttime cough and cold preparations containing antihistamines that may have as much as 25% alcohol (or 50 proof). The elderly may use these ethyl alcohol–based medications as appetite stimulants during periods of disability or convalescence or may use alcohol preparations for rest when other hypnotics cannot be tolerated.

The effects are dose dependent, with high doses causing depression of the medulla and the basic functions of life. The most common concern is the nonmedical chronic use of alcohol by heavy drinkers, which causes atrophy of the cerebrum and a loss of intellectual functions. In extreme doses, alcohol may produce anesthesia that could be lethal.

DID YOU KNOW?
- According to the U.S. Department of Health, alcoholism is the third most serious public health problem, following heart disease and cancer.
- The mouthwash Cepacol contains 14.5% alcohol (29 proof), whereas Listerine is approximately 27% alcohol or 54 proof. Vicks 44 and Vicks Nyquil are 10% (20 proof) alcohol. The liquid appetite stimulants such as Allertonic, Eldertonic, and Hadacol are actually multivitamins in alcohol bases.

When used in moderation, some research has shown that alcohol can prolong life and improve coronary health, but used in excess, alcohol diminishes the quality and length of life. The U.S. Department of Health suggests that moderate consumption of alcohol (≤two drinks per day for men, ≤one drink per day for women) dilates the blood vessels at the skin level, leading to less coronary heart disease. Alcohol may also protect the heart by raising the "good cholesterol"—high-density lipoprotein (HDL). Another protective mechanism is its ability to activate the body system to dissolve blood clots. Abuse of alcohol has the opposite effect by damaging heart muscle and increasing the risk of heart failure. Those persons who are advised to use alcohol as a medicinal agent need to be carefully screened for no addictive history.

The National Institute of Alcohol Abuse and Alcoholism has identified the following as those who should avoid alcohol:

- Women who are pregnant or trying to conceive
- People who plan to drive or perform other activities that require unimpaired attention or muscular coordination
- People taking antihistamines, sedatives, or other drugs that can intensify alcohol's effects
- Recovering alcoholics
- People younger than the age of 21

Caution is also indicated for people with strong family histories of alcoholism and for those with diabetes and peptic ulcer disease.

Physical dependence causing the use of larger and larger amounts of alcohol with denial and tolerance of the drug is common with chronic use. Those who have physical dependence to alcohol tend to have cross-dependence on other central nervous system depressants such as barbiturates and benzodiazepines. When the alcohol is discontinued following physical dependence, the body may respond with **delirium tremens.**

With the chronic use of alcohol, detrimental effects to body systems that will shorten the life of the chronic drinker are common (Table 32-4).

Drug Interactions with Alcohol

Drug interactions with alcohol and other medications may be additive or may just change the effectiveness of the medications. The alcohol plus the other medication may cause many detrimental symptoms, even life-threatening ones (Table 32-5). A general rule to be followed with medications is that alcohol should be avoided when taking prescription or OTC medications unless prescribed by a physician who is aware of the patient's alcohol consumption.

Drugs Used with Alcoholism

For those who have chronic alcohol intake with dependence or alcoholism, certain medications may assist with the withdrawal symptoms. Benzodiazepines (tranquilizers; Chapter 31), atenolol (Tenormin; Chapter 27), and naltrexone (Revia) are used to suppress symptoms caused by abstinence. Research has shown decreased craving for alcohol, fewer drinks consumed, and less relapse with use of naltrexone. Once abstinence has been accomplished, continued abstinence may be maintained by the use of disulfiram (Antabuse) or the relatively new medication, acamprosate (Campral).

TABLE 32-4 *Effects of Alcohol on the Body*

BODY SYSTEM	EFFECTS
Gastrointestinal system	Liver damage by accumulating fats and proteins
	Leads to **cirrhosis** and hepatitis
	Erosion of the gastric mucosa with gastric bleeding
	Esophageal varices
	Pancreatitis
Nervous system	Hepatic encephalopathy
Urinary system	Acts as diuretic by suppressing antidiuretic hormone
Respiratory system	Depresses respirations
Nervous system	Produces tolerance
	Central nervous system depressant

TABLE 32-5 *Interactions Between Medications and Alcohol*

ALCOHOL COMBINED WITH	MAY CAUSE
Medication for sleep/ tranquilizers	Increased physical and psychological dependence
Antidepressants	Rapid intoxication
Motion sickness medications	Excessive drowsiness
Pain relievers, muscle relaxants, antiallergics, antihistamines	Mental confusion
Medications for angina pectoris	Dizziness, fainting
Antihypertensives	Lack of skeletal muscle coordination
aspirin, NSAIDS, anticoagulants, potassium supplements	Increased gastric irritation and bleeding
Some antibiotics, metronidazole	Nausea, vomiting, and flushing
Oral hypoglycemics	Tachycardia, dyspnea
Anticoagulants, seizure medications, hypoglycemics	Changes in the effectiveness of the medications in controlling the specific illness

- The only use of disulfiram is its known interactions with alcohol, discouraging the person from drinking by causing severe side effects when mixed with alcohol ingestion. The desired side effects include nausea, copious vomiting, flushing, palpitations, headache, thirst, sweating, chest pain, blurred vision, weakness, and hypotension. Because these symptoms may be severe and may last from 30 minutes to several hours with even the smallest absorption of alcohol (as little as 7 mL), this medication is not used as frequently as in the past. The person who does not have the determination to stop the use of alcohol should not be treated with disulfiram because of the severe adverse effects when combined with alcohol (see Table 32-3).

- Patient education with disulfiram is extremely important: The patient must be thoroughly informed of the potential hazards of the drug's use. Any consumption of alcohol may produce a severe and potentially fatal reaction; therefore any form of alcohol (e.g., in sauces, cough syrups, cooking, mouthwashes, and applications to skin such as liniments, aftershave lotions, perfumes, and any product containing alcohol) may cause problems.

- Acamprosate is used along with counseling and social support to help persons avoid the craving for and drinking of large amounts of alcohol. It is a delayed-release tablet that must be administered three times a day. Acamprosate does not cause alcohol aversion as found with disulfiram and does not cause a reaction when alcohol is ingested. However, the medication does increase suicidal tendencies.

Other Alcohol Preparations

Toxic alcohols include isopropyl alcohol and methyl or wood alcohol. When unable to purchase ethyl alcohol or ethanol, some alcoholics will substitute isopropyl (rubbing) alcohol or methyl alcohol (antifreeze) for consumption. Either of these will prevent alcohol withdrawal symptoms but may also cause poisoning or death.

Patient Education for Compliance

1. Disulfiram should not be administered until at least 12 hours have passed since the last ingestion of alcohol. Patients should avoid all alcohol products, no matter what the form, while taking Antabuse.
2. Many home remedies containing alcohol cause sedation and hypnosis without the person taking the medication being aware of their content.
3. People may become less self-conscious when drinking alcohol and may not realize the dangers from excessive drinking.
4. Some states require a witness for administration of disulfiram in patients with a history of driving under the influence.

IMPORTANT FACTS ABOUT MEDICATIONS FOR ALCOHOLISM

- Alcohol, opioids, and opiates are depressant drugs.
- Alcohol produces an increase in blood pressure correlated to the amount of alcohol consumed. Alcohol depresses respirations and may cause hepatitis, cirrhosis of the liver, and erosive gastritis. Alcohol is cardioprotective when used in moderation and low volumes.
- The chronic use of alcohol produces a tolerance to many effects and to central nervous system depressants except opioids.
- Alcohol is an additive to central nervous system depressants.
- Acamprosate may be used to assist with avoiding alcohol consumption.
- Disulfiram is given to alcoholics to assist in refraining from alcohol consumption.
- Patient education concerning alcohol is very important when prescribing disulfiram. Only patients desiring to withdraw from the chronic use of alcohol should be prescribed disulfiram because of the dangers of side effects.
- Research has shown that alcoholism tends to be familial.
- Alcoholics, to obtain alcohol, may use OTC medications and agents containing alcohol as drugs of abuse.

Opiates and Opioids

Drugs that are abused and misused frequently are the opioids and opiates, including those from natural sources (opiates) such as opium alkaloids of heroin and morphine; the semisynthetic drugs (hydromorphone, oxymorphone); and the synthetic agents (hydrocodone, methadone, oxycodone) (see Chapter 16 for more information). The most frequently abused pain relievers are meperidine (Demerol), propoxyphene (Darvon), oxycodone drugs (OxyContin, Percodan, and Percocet), and morphine. The most frequently abused street drugs are marijuana, heroin, cocaine, and oxycodone, with oxycodone and meperidine being the legal drugs most frequently abused by health care professionals. These medications may be taken by mouth, by percutaneous means for absorption through mucous membranes, by injection, by direct administration into veins (or mainlining), or by sniffing and snorting.

DID YOU KNOW?

In 1898 the Bayer Company advertised a new drug to be used as a cure for morphine withdrawal. Morphine was a widely abused drug at that time. The new agent was thought to be nonaddictive. The new "safe" drug was heroin—a drug that we now know is not the expected nonaddicting cure but a powerful addicting central nervous system depressant classified as a narcotic.

The beginning of opioid use occurs either socially or for pain management in a medical setting, whereas most abuse starts with the illegal use of a street drug or unneeded use of prescription pain medications. Opioids relieve pain, elevate the mood, relieve tension, fear, and anxiety, and produce tranquility and peace, with **euphoria.** Other effects include suppression of cough and appetite. These feelings lead to psychologic and physical dependence. With opiates, the expected results include warm, flushing sensations that are described as similar to a sexual orgasm. The long-term continued use is based on the feelings of "all is well" rather than the rush that occurs with earlier administration. The user/abuser has the perception that the world is rosy and bright and that no problems exist. Researchers feel that the psychologic dependence for opioids continues throughout life, although the desire may be controlled with strong willpower and the desire to remain drug free.

Toxicity levels, often found with abuse of these medications, cause signs such as slow, shallow breathing with hypoxia; cold, clammy, skin; pinpoint pupils; depressed blood pressure; and depressed sensory perception. Because these agents also tend to decrease gastric motility and reduce peristalsis, more of the medication may be absorbed.

Signs and Symptoms of Opioid/Opiate Withdrawal

Withdrawal from opioids or alcohol for the person with physical dependence will produce symptoms that start approximately 2 to 48 hours after the last dose of the drug, depending on which drug has been abused. The person will experience restlessness, chills and hot flashes, restless sleep, piloerection (or goose bumps), rhinorrhea (runny nose), tearing, and dilation of the pupils of the eye during the first 24 hours. Sneezing, yawning, cramping of legs, vomiting, diarrhea, loss of appetite, sweating, muscle twitches, insomnia, elevated vital signs, and a craving for the drug follow as these early symptoms subside. Withdrawal symptoms may progress to cardiovascular collapse.

Withdrawal programs provide a therapeutic means of handling the symptoms that abrupt withdrawal, or cold turkey, might produce by tapering the drug dosage over a period of days, using a substitution of methadone for the opioid/opiate. Methadone, a synthetic opioid analgesic that permits substitution by cross-tolerance, stalls the euphoric effects of heroin and other opioids and reduces the craving for the drug without the physical and mental effects. Methadone treatment programs cause dependence on methadone, but the withdrawal symptoms are less severe and the person is given supplemental programs such as vocational rehabilitation and social skills to then stop the methadone (see Table 32-3).

IMPORTANT FACTS ABOUT OPIOID/OPIATE ABUSE

- One of the most abused/misused groups of drugs is the opioids/opiates, which are used as pain relievers. Morphine, OxyContin, meperidine, and hydromorphone are the prescription items used most frequently.
- Opiates produce mental depression and analgesia, as well as depression of cough and appetite. The abuser likes the feelings of well-being and euphoria rather than the rush that occurs immediately after administration.
- Withdrawal symptoms such as restlessness, cramping of the legs, vomiting, diarrhea, insomnia, and craving for the drug occur with prolonged use of opioids.
- Methadone, a substitution for opioids, is used in withdrawal programs for opioid abuse.

Abused Central Nervous System Stimulants

Amphetamines

Amphetamines, called "uppers" or "speed," have both legal and illegal uses. Legally prescribed, amphetamines are classified as Schedule II drugs and are used to treat chronic fatigue syndrome, obesity, narcolepsy, attention deficit disorder, and mental depression and to combat the side effects of narcotics in the terminally ill patient (see Chapter 30). When used illegally, they increase physical performance and provide psychologic stimulus. The most frequently abused amphetamines are methamphetamine ("ice" or "crystal meth"), which may be smoked and may be taken orally or by intravenous use. The rapid rise of the use of methamphetamine and the use of OTC medications such as cold and allergy products containing pseudoephedrine that are used for its manufacture have caused many states to place limits on these OTC sales. To be able to partially control the sale of these medications, many stores have moved them into the pharmacy or behind the checkout area for safekeeping. Amphetamines cause more confidence, alertness, and talkativeness. The person is generally hyperactive, with a feeling of euphoria and a sense of arousal. The amphetamines are also anorexics, so the person feels no need for food and therefore weight loss occurs. Other symptoms of possible illicit use include irritability, confusion, social withdrawal, chewing or tooth grinding, photophobia, and paranoia. Compulsive behaviors drive the user to repeat the drug use again and again to maintain the euphoria. Physical dependence is moderate, but psychologic dependence may be intense.

Signs of toxicity are flushing or pallor of the skin, palpitations, tremors, extreme fluctuations of pulse and blood pressure, chest pain, sweating, dilated pupils, and mental disturbances. Treatment is symptomatic as no antidote is available for amphetamines. Abrupt withdrawal will produce a disagreeable and depressed mood—an experience known as a "crash." These manifestations, especially the depression, may persist for months and are often the reason for resuming the use of amphetamines.

Cocaine

Cocaine has been used for years by native Indians of South America to ward off fatigue and hunger. In the nineteenth century in the United States cocaine was a "wonder drug" for numerous medical conditions, including to ward off fatigue and hunger. In 1914 legislation restricted its use; however, its use dramatically increased as a recreational drug beginning in the 1970s. This return has dramatically caused numerous social and medical problems. The only approved medicinal use of cocaine is as a local anesthetic applied topically, usually for nasal procedures because of the anesthetic and vasoconstrictive properties.

DID YOU KNOW?
Coca-Cola originally contained cocaine from the coca plant—hence the name and nickname *coke*.

The effects of cocaine are similar to those of amphetamine. The intensity and duration of the drug effects are dependent on the purity of the preparation and the method of administration.

Cocaine, because of its derivation from coca leaves, can be converted to a water-soluble hydrochloride salt in a powder form that can be administered orally, intranasally, and intravenously. When it is used as a drug of abuse, the usual route is intranasal, or "snorted," for rapid absorption through the nasal mucous membranes.

Cocaine base, which is in a crystalline rock form, gets the name "crack" from the cracking sound it makes as it burns. The powdered, pure cocaine is cut by adding such substances as cornstarch or baking soda to raise the volume of the drug, thus increasing the street value. Unfortunately, the purity or amount of the cocaine for each use is not predictable and potency will vary greatly from one dose to the next. When cocaine base ("crack") is smoked (or free-based), a rapid absorption occurs through the lungs. The euphoria (highs) received from the smoked crack cocaine is rapidly replaced by **dysphoria,** a down, and the cocaine user repeats doses to maintain the high.

The half-life of cocaine is short, leading to acute intoxication, which occurs in the first few hours, so the symptoms subside in 1 to 2 hours. As a person uses cocaine, tolerance occurs, causing an increase in need for or in the amount of cocaine used to obtain the same feelings of euphoria. For this reason and others, cocaine addiction is difficult to treat and no antidote is available for toxicity (Table 32-6).

IMPORTANT FACTS ABOUT MEDICATIONS USED AS STIMULANTS

- Amphetamines, nicotine, and cocaine are central nervous system stimulants that are often abused.
- Amphetamines are called "uppers" or "speed" and have both medicinal and illicit implications.
- Amphetamines produce compulsive behaviors, causing the user to repeat drug use again and again.
- No antidote for amphetamine or cocaine toxicity is known, and treatment must be symptomatic.

Abused Central Nervous System Depressants

Barbiturates and benzodiazepines (as well as alcohol, discussed earlier) are central nervous system depressants that are often abused. These medications have many therapeutic uses and are safe when used as designed by the manufacturer and as prescribed by the physician. However, because of the potential for abuse, tolerance, and physical dependence, these medications are regulated under the Controlled Substances Act.

TABLE 32-6 *Effects of Cocaine on the Body*

BODY SYSTEM	EFFECTS
Cardiovascular system	Tachycardia
	Hypertension
	Myocardial infarction and thrombi
Respiratory system	Lung infections and abscesses
	Pulmonary edema
	Pneumonitis
	Atrophy of the nasal mucosa with snorted cocaine with a loss of smell
	Necrosis and perforation of the nasal passages with intranasal use
	Severe respiratory system damage occurs when other substances of abuse are used in conjunction with cocaine
Urinary system	Acute renal failure
Nervous system	Seizures
	Strokes and increased intracranial pressure
Reproductive system	Leads to stillbirths and preterm labor
	Congenital deformities
	Acute withdrawal symptoms in the infant with behavioral delays throughout life
Psychologic health	Paranoia and depression
	Psychosis
	Suicide
	Dependence with severe anxiety and auditory, visual, and tactile hallucinations

Barbiturates

Barbiturates (see Chapter 30) typify the central nervous system depressants that are used for illicit purposes. The depressant effects are dose dependent and range from mild sedation to sleep or coma such as the use of phenobarbital for seizures and seconal (Nembutal) for sleep.

Used indiscriminately, barbiturates are called "downers." The route of administration is oral or injected intravenously in a liquid form producing symptoms that include drowsiness, confusion, impaired judgment, slurred speech, and lack of facial expression. Acute toxicity produces three expected signs: respiratory depression, coma, and pupils constricted to pinpoints. Other signs are nausea and loss of appetite. Rebound rapid eye movement sleep and nightmares occur on withdrawal of the medications. No specific antidote is available for barbiturate intoxication.

Benzodiazepines

Benzodiazepines are commonly prescribed for anxiety and insomnia (Chapter 31). These medications are safer than the barbiturates and are rarely lethal when taken alone. The danger comes when the drugs are combined with other central nervous system depressants such as alcohol. Benzodiazepines are generally not considered street drugs, but misuse, abuse, and dependencies have been reported, especially with diazepam (Valium), alprazolam (Xanax), and lorazepam (Ativan). As a rule, tolerance and physical dependence are only minimal when taken for legitimate indications, but the problem can be substantial with misuse or abuse.

For the patient who has built a tolerance and abuse level of these agents, gradual withdrawal and changing to a long-acting benzodiazepine are recommended. Symptoms of withdrawal include increased anxiety and irritability, twitching, aching, muscle weakness, tremors, headaches, nausea, anorexia, depression, lethargy, hypersensitivity to stimuli, blurred vision, and sleep disturbances. The health care professional should be aware of the danger of prolonged use of benzodiazepines even for therapeutic reasons, especially important with the elderly who use these medications for insomnia and daily anxieties. Flumazenil (Romazicon) is specific as an antagonist for benzodiazepine toxicity and sedation reversal.

IMPORTANT FACTS ABOUT ABUSED CENTRAL NERVOUS SYSTEM DEPRESSANTS

- Barbiturates and benzodiazepines are commonly abused prescription medications because of their use for anxiety relief.
- Tolerance is a common effect of barbiturate and benzodiazepine usage, leading to physical dependence on the drug. Therefore these medications should be used for short-term therapy.
- Barbiturates are used as downers.
- Withdrawal from barbiturates and benzodiazepines should be gradual when these agents have been used for prolonged lengths of time.

Marijuana and Hashish

Marijuana and hashish, classified as central nervous system depressants, cause euphoria, sedation, and hallucinations and are derived from the hemp plant, *Cannabis sativa*. The potency of the drug, tetrahydrocannabinol (THC), varies with the conditions under which the plants were grown. The resin from the female plants is known as hashish, and the dried plant (seed, flower, twigs, and leaves) is the basis for marijuana. These drugs, known as cannabinoids, have street names such as grass, weed, hemp, Mary Jane, pot, and dope, whereas the cigarettes of marijuana are known as bowls, stogies, joints, or reefers.

When smoked, marijuana has its effect in 5 to 15 minutes, peaking at 30 to 90 minutes, with duration of 3 to 4 hours. Because of fat solubility, THC is taken up in the fatty tissues of the body and thus metabolizes slowly with 30% to 50% of the drug remaining in the body a week later. When smoked, hashish is absorbed rapidly through the lungs. The major side effect of marijuana is damage to the lungs with a greater risk of cancers. Marijuana produces a greater amount of tar than its equivalent weight in tobacco and contains more carcinogens than tobacco smoke.

When taken orally, practically all of the THC is absorbed but is inactivated by the first pass through the liver, requiring 3 to 10 times as much marijuana or hashish to obtain the same effect as found with smoking. When ingested, marijuana may have some effectiveness for up to 12 hours.

Effects of Marijuana

Marijuana produces three subjective effects: sedation, euphoria, and sometimes hallucinations. No other drug produces all three responses, placing marijuana in a class by itself (Table 32-7).

Tolerance occurs with marijuana and is rapidly reversed after cessation of its use. Abrupt cessation after prolonged use has been indicated in some psychologic rather than physical dependence. The symptoms include dysphoria, anxiety, tremors, eating and sleeping disturbances, and increased sweating. Psychotic reactions and acute panic-anxiety reactions may occur with inexperienced users who are unfamiliar with the effects of marijuana or with those who have taken high doses or have experienced prolonged use of marijuana.

IMPORTANT FACTS ABOUT MARIJUANA USE

- Marijuana is considered to be a central nervous system depressant, although it causes euphoria prior to sedation and hallucinations.
- Marijuana is fat soluble, leading to absorption in the fatty body tissues, thus providing prolonged effects of the drug.

- Marijuana produces three effects— euphoria with gaiety and heightened sense of humor, sedation with lethargy and memory loss, and sometimes hallucinations caused by perceptual inadequacies and increased sensory stimuli.
- Tolerance occurs with marijuana and is rapidly reversed with cessation of use.

TABLE 32-7 *Effects of Marijuana on the Body*

BODY SYSTEM	EFFECTS
Cardiovascular system	Tachycardia
Gastrointestinal system	Increased appetite
Respiratory system	Bronchodilation
	Lung irritations and cough
Sensory System	Conjunctival redness
	Increased sense of taste, touch, and smell
	Distortion of time perception
	Perceptual inaccuracies
Nervous system	Short term memory loss
	Impaired learning with decreased intellectual performances
	Impaired reflex reaction with inability to multitask
Reproductive system	Decreased sperm counts and reduced testosterone levels
	Irregular menses and sporadic ovulation
	Reduced estrogen levels
	Teratogenic to fetus and lowered birth weights
Psychologic health	Euphoria and relaxation with gaiety and heightened sense of humor
	Apathy, dullness, lethargy, poor grooming
	Reduced interest in achievement (amotivational syndrome)
	Paranoia and depression
	Psychosis
	Suicide
	Dependence with severe anxiety and auditory, visual, and tactile hallucinations

Hallucinogens, Psychedelics, and Psychomimetics

Hallucinogens and psychedelics (mind-altering drugs) are agents that produce auditory and visual hallucinations, or a "psychedelic" state. The psychoactive effects of these medications occur in 1 to 2 hours after administration and may be in the form of euphoria to panic and severe depression. The person, who often does not realize the difference in self and nonself, has an increased awareness of sensory stimuli and often believes that the world around him or her is harmonious and beautiful. The psychedelics are different from other drugs because the agents have the ability to bring about the types of alterations in thought, perception, and feeling that otherwise occur in dreams; or the psychedelics can cause dreaming without loss of consciousness. Lysergic acid diethylamide (LSD), dimethyltryptamine (DMT), phencyclidine (PCP), mescaline, psilocybin, and MDMA (ecstasy) are examples of these agents, with LSD considered the prototype.

Lysergic Acid Diethylamide

LSD is a potent hallucinogenic street drug used with no idea of its real strength with tolerance to the drug developing rapidly. As with most street drugs, strengths vary, causing many problems for the user. The unpredictable effects that take place in 20 minutes include hypertension, dilated pupils, hyperthermia, tachycardia, and enhanced awareness of activities after use. The unpleasant experiences are frequent: the altered states of consciousness may cause psychosis to develop, or the drug may trigger latent psychosis to become observable. Homicidal thoughts may be the result of the acute panic or paranoia that accompanies the drug. After alternating and altering levels of consciousness, the user generally feels a complete state of exhaustion as the drug's effects wear off—a time when suicide is a risk.

The significant unfavorable reactions induced by LSD may be prolonged, delayed, and recurrent flashbacks ("bad trip") including paranoia, depression, and schizophrenic psychotic reactions.

Mescaline

Mescaline, from the flower heads of the peyote cactus, produces effects similar to those of LSD. The flower may be dried and smoked, or a soluble crystalline powder may be used for ingestion, either as a tea or capsule. The effects of mescaline include abdominal pain, nausea, vomiting, and diarrhea, followed by vivid, colorful hallucinations. Anxiety, stimulation of reflexes, tremors, and psychic disturbances are encountered with the use of this drug.

Psilocybin

Psilocybin comes from Mexican mushrooms, producing hallucinogenic dysphoria similar to mescaline but of a shorter duration. The mood may be pleasant for some people, whereas the drug produces apprehension in others. The capacity to make critical judgments is poor, and performance abilities are impaired, with compulsive hyperkinetic movements, laughter, dilation of pupils, vertigo, ataxia, paresthesia, muscle weakness, drowsiness, and sleep.

MDMA (Ecstasy)

MDMA (3,4-methylenedioxymethamphetamine), or "ecstasy," became a drug of prominence in the mid-1980s. At first it was not a regulated drug, but it soon became classified as a Schedule I Controlled Substance. Ecstasy acts as both a psychedelic and psychostimulant agent. Taken orally, this amphetamine derivative produces central nervous system stimulation, euphoria, and visual disturbances. Those who use MDMA report a sense of closeness with people, a lowering of defenses, reduced anxiety, enhanced communication skills, and increased sociability. When taken in large doses, the results are panic, anxiety, paranoia, and signs of sympathetic nervous system stimulation such as increased heart rate, irregular pulse and respirations, dilated pupils, and vasoconstriction of the blood vessels in the skin, causing a decreased body temperature.

Phencyclidine (PCP)

Phencyclidine (PCP), or "angel dust," "acid," or "purple haze," was first studied for use as a general anesthetic for humans. Therapeutic human use was subsequently dropped because of the high incidence of delirium, although it is still used in veterinary practices. The use and cheapness of production of the agent by amateurs have led to this being widely abused. The effects of PCP make it one of the most dangerous and most unpredictable of the abused street substances. PCP may be administered orally, intranasally, intravenously, and by smoking. Because of its high solubility, PCP is rapidly absorbed from all sites. Absorption begins in the stomach, followed by

recirculation of the blood back to the acid environment of the stomach, where the drug reenters the intestine for reabsorption to the blood. This constant recycling through the body leads to prolonged drug action.

Low PCP doses cause central nervous system stimulation, euphoria, and sympathetic nervous system stimulation, similar to the effects of amphetamines or alcohol. With increased doses, thought processes become disorientated and motor incoordination and slurred speech occur. The euphoria leads to release of rapidly changing inhibitions and emotional swings. Bizarre behavior may occur with high doses, progressing to dysphoria, catatonia, muscle rigidity, hypertensive crisis, coma, and death.

Treatment for PCP use includes protection by removing the person from external stimuli because antipsychotics and psychotherapy are rarely effective. Symptoms of withdrawal must be treated in ways to provide life support.

IMPORTANT FACTS ABOUT HALLUCINOGENS, PSYCHEDELICS, AND PSYCHOMIMETICS

- Hallucinogens and psychedelics produce auditory and visual hallucinations because of increased awareness of sensory stimuli.
- LSD is a potent hallucinogen that causes unpredictable responses, some pleasant and some unpleasant.
- LSD may produce prolonged, delayed, and recurrent reactions of depression and schizophrenic and psychotic reactions, with the rapid development of tolerance.
- Mescaline is similar to LSD, with vivid, colorful hallucinations.
- Psilocybin produces hallucinogenic effects that are less prolonged than LSD or mescaline.
- MDMA, or ecstasy, acts as a psychedelic and a psychostimulant. It is a derivative of amphetamine.
- PCP produces stimulation and euphoria, similar to alcohol or amphetamines. The euphoria leads to release of inhibitions and produces emotional changes on a rapid basis.

Inhalants

Benzine (used in dyes and drugs), acetone (nail polish and paint removers), carbon tetrachloride (dry cleaning fluid), gasoline, trichloroethylene (anesthetic), and toluene are volatile hydrocarbons used for sniffing. Many of these chemicals are found in common household products that use hydrocarbons as propellants. These products are relatively inexpensive and easily bought legally including gasoline, kerosene, ink correction fluids, the gas found in aerosol containers, and even helium found in balloons. Therefore these agents have become more popular with young people and those who cannot afford the illegal substances. Although children including teens are the most likely to use hydrocarbons for sniffing, some adults are also abusers.

Bagging, huffing, and sniffing processes are used for inhalation. Bagging is performed by pouring solvents in a plastic bag and inhaling the vapors. Huffing is pouring the solvent on a rag and inhaling the vapor. Sniffing is inhaling the solvent from its original container. All three means of inhalation produce rapid general central nervous system depression with marked **inebriation,** dizziness, lightheadedness, and intense feelings of well-being similar to alcohol intoxication. Euphoria and hallucinations that usually last for 15 to 45 minutes are the desired and expected results. Some users experience feelings of reckless abandonment and increased power, with resultant aggressiveness, headaches, vertigo, and ataxia. High doses lead to confusion, brain damage, and coma causing permanent disability or death. Sudden death is possible, caused by anoxia, respiratory depression, increased heart rates, and dysrhythmias. For the person in poverty or economic deprivation, glue sniffing may be the drug of choice. Tolerance of inhalants commonly occurs. The person starting with a single tube of glue per day may progress to three, four, or more tubes to maintain the same effect.

IMPORTANT FACTS ABOUT INHALANTS
- Commonly found inhalants such as cleansing products, glue, hairsprays, lacquers, and paints are abused, especially by young people and the economically depressed.
- Inhalants provide euphoria and hallucinations.

Anabolic Steroids

A growing problem with drugs of misuse/abuse includes many athletes taking anabolic (adrenergic) steroids to enhance athletic performance and increase their chances of winning in sports events. People also take these hormones to increase body weight and strength and to "look good."

Many anabolic-adrenergic steroidal preparations are available for oral or parenteral use, and these preparations from the male hormone testosterone have been prescribed, especially for the under-

weight and those wanting the athletic edge. Many organizations, like the National Collegiate Athletic Associations, the International Olympics Committee, and major league sports, have banned the use of these substances. The U.S. Congress has even had hearings because of the increased use of these products. The misuse led to addition of anabolic steroids to the Drug Enforcement Administration (DEA) controlled substances in 1982. "Stacking" of steroids, or taking multiple metabolic steroids at one time, is still a practice used illegally and unethically by some athletes. At the same time as the steroid use, a program of strenuous exercise and a high-protein diet are used to increase muscle mass and stamina. Short-term effects include increased aggressive behavior and masculinization in females. Because of the misuses/abuses, steroids are Schedule III drugs in all states, with some states making these drugs Schedule II agents with a high potential for abuse/misuse (see Table 29-2).

IMPORTANT FACTS ABOUT ANABOLIC STEROIDS
- Anabolic steroids are used by athletes to increase body weight and strength.
- Anabolic steroids are prepared from the male hormone testosterone, thus tending to masculinize users.

Care of Drug Abuse and Misuse Patients

The health care professional needs a knowledge of the psychotropic drugs, their actions, and side effects. When giving care to persons with drug abuse/misuse problems, the professional should be nonjudgmental but willing to work with the patient, family, and members of the community for education to provide the needed support for treatment.

Through education and recognition of the signs and symptoms of drug abuse, proper referrals for care may be made. Some of the more common signs of drug abuse/misuse include the following:

- Abrupt changes in work or school attendance, the quality of work, work output, grades, and discipline
- Unusual flare-ups or outbreaks of rage or temper
- Withdrawal from responsibility
- General changes in overall attitude
- Deterioration in physical appearance and grooming
- Wearing sunglasses at inappropriate times
- Continual wearing of long-sleeved garments, particularly in hot weather, or the reluctance to wear a short-sleeved garment

TABLE 32-8 *Symptoms Specific to Abused Drugs*

SUBSTANCE	SYMPTOMS
inhalants	Nausea, dizziness, headaches, lack of coordination, odor of substance on breath
heroin and narcotics	Euphoria, drowsiness, nausea, vomiting, pinpoint pupils, needle tracks on arms
cocaine and amphetamines	Talkativeness, hyperalert state, increased blood pressure, history of weight loss, hyperactivity, ulcers in nose and throat, hallucinations and paranoia
barbiturates, heroin, and benzodiazepines	Slow pulse and respiratory rates, doctor-hopping with vague complaints, slurred speech
hallucinogens (PCP, LSD)	Mood/mind alteration, panic, extreme focus on details, symptoms of fear and paranoia, unpredictable violent behavior
Marijuana	Red eyes, dry mouth, altered perceptions of surroundings, euphoria, inappropriate laughing and manner, smell of burnt rope, panic reactions, impaired memory

- Association with known drug abusers
- Secretive behavior about actions and behaviors; poorly concealed attempts to avoid attention and suspicion such as frequent trips to restrooms, basements, and like areas
- Stealing of items from home, work, or school
- Glazed appearance in the eyes
- Odor on breath
- Changes in health habits
- Asking for particular medications for pain and accepting only those medications

The knowledge of symptoms of drug use will enable the health care professional to assess drug usage (Table 32-8). Through asking questions that will assist with interventions in the drug abuse cycle, the uncomfortable withdrawal symptoms may be eased and the possibility of severe or life-threatening effects may be avoided. Remember that substance abuse is not limited to street drugs but may be found with use of prescription medications.

Low self-esteem, a feeling of not belonging in society, a high risk for social approval, and inadequate communication skills are risk factors that increase drug abuse and misuse. The inability to feel gratification and nonbonding with families and friends predispose an individual to substance abuse. The person with a family history of alcoholism or drug abuse is also more likely to become an abuser as a way of facing personal confrontation. The health care worker should assist the patient and family.

Patient Education for Compliance

The best patient education is teaching prevention of the abuse and misuse of medications including therapeutic medicines such as antibiotics and steroids.

Summary

Drug abuse is the self-medication of drugs on a chronic basis, using excessive quantities that may cause physical and/or psychological dependence. The allied health professional should be aware of the dangers of drug abuse/misuse. Drugs, from therapeutically prescribed medications to street drugs, may be abused or misused. Prior to prescribing medications, the physician will establish a definite need by the patient that the drug is necessary.

Drug abuse, not a new phenomenon, is using a drug in a way that is inconsistent with medical, social, and cultural norms of a certain population. Important is the fact that the definition of drug abuse is related to social and cultural norms and to specific situations where medications are prescribed. No socioeconomic, ethnic, and cultural classes are exempt from drug and substance abuse.

Physical and psychologic dependence occur with the misuse or abuse of drugs. Dependence and tolerance lead to greater doses of drugs. The availability of the drugs is another factor leading to dependency and the continued use of drugs. Abuse can only occur if the drugs can be obtained. Vulnerability to abuse can be a familial tendency, as well as the dependence as a crutch to cope with everyday tensions.

Physical signs of drug abuse include weight loss, changes in sleeping habits that cause lethargy, and frequent illnesses. Psychologic signs include inability to concentrate, lack of memory, apathy, and inability to function due to illogical thought processes. Socially the person has mood swings, irritability, anger, and becomes isolated from the environment including a change of surroundings and friends. The drug abuser may become anxious in social situations and may over-react including defensiveness and unexplained anger in social settings.

Two of the most abused drugs are readily available and are legally purchased by adults—nicotine and alcohol. The dangers from addiction to these drugs far outweigh any positive effects. Tolerance levels occur with both drugs. Alcohol has interactions with many other drugs, causing severe physiologic effects. Disulfiram and acamprosate are the medications used in the specific therapeutic treatment of alcohol abuse. Patient education in many areas is absolutely necessary when these medications are prescribed.

The use of illicit drugs is a major problem—societal and personal—in the United States today. Some of the abused substances are easily obtained such as glue, household chemicals, or acetaminophen, whereas others are more difficult such as narcotics, making the agents expensive at the street level. Some problems of misuse are from the administration of medications by the patient or even from unintentional misuse of prescribed medicines.

One of the main dangers of illicit drugs consists of changes in the strengths of drugs caused by manufacture on the street level—cutting drugs for increased profits. Because each dose is different and there is no control of these illegal medicines, the user is at risk for overdose. The health care professional must be aware of and recognize the many schemes used to obtain these prescription medications such as opiates and opioids for illicit use. A physical disease may be replaced by a physical and psychologic dependence with tolerance of the medication, requiring the person to use more and more of the drug to achieve the same results.

Of great importance for the health care professional to remember is that all medicinal agents have the potential for misuse and abuse. Innocently using medications when there are insufficient symptoms is abusing drugs—that is, using drugs too frequently or using excessive dosages. These abuse/misuse problems are frequently seen in health care facilities today.

Critical Thinking Scenario

Mrs. Svensdottir comes to the physician's office for a migraine headache. Dr. Merry prescribes a narcotic medication for pain. Mrs. Svensdottir mentions that she has been drinking wine nightly with her dinner and has another glass of wine before bedtime when she feels she will not sleep well.

1. Does Dr. Merry need this information? Why or why not?
2. Could the use of wine at night be a kind of drug misuse? Why or why not?
3. Mrs. Svensdottir denies that she has an alcohol abuse problem and states that she has "everything under control." How is this a typical response from someone who is alcohol dependent?

REVIEW QUESTIONS

1. What is drug abuse? Drug misuse? Why are these so prevalent? _____
   _____
   _____

2. How can a drug be used therapeutically and abused by the same person? _____
   _____
   _____
   _____

3. How does drug availability affect drug abuse? _____
   _____
   _____

4. What are the psychologic symptoms of drug abuse? Physical signs? Social effects? _____
   _____
   _____

5.   What is the effect of alcohol on the body? What groups should avoid the use of alcohol? _____
     _____
     _____

6.   What distinct patient education must occur with disulfiram? _____
     _____
     _____

7.   Explain what tolerance of medications means and how this increases the dangers of drug abuse.
     _____
     _____

8.   What is a hallucinogen/psychedelic? Why are these agents dangerous? _____
     _____
     _____

9.   Have anabolic steroids been placed on the DEA's list of scheduled drugs? If so, what schedule?
     _____
     _____

10. What are the implications for the medical assistant when confronted by a drug abuser/misuser?
     _____
     _____

Basic Intravenous Therapy Medications

This appendix provides a basic overview of medications that are administered intravenously. Each medication is not listed, but the drug categories are provided to allow a better understanding of the intravenous (IV) medication process.

Intravenous Antiinfective Agents

Antiinfective agents—antibiotics, antifungals, and antiviral medications—are the most frequently used of the IV medications, especially antibiotics. The professional administering IV antiinfectives should know normal dosage for the drug, the side effects, and incompatibilities, just as with administration of medications by other routes. Important also is knowing the time limit for the stability of the medication after reconstitution if this is a factor in timing the reconstitution and administration. Being familiar with side effects and adverse reactions is important, and with antibiotics the professional should always be alert for drug sensitivity and possible anaphylaxis.

Antibiotics

Penicillins

Penicillins are both natural and semisynthetic antibiotics that are derived from the fungus *Penicillium*. With the low cost, low toxicity, and good clinical efficacy, the penicillins, both natural and semisynthetic, are often ordered when the microorganism is susceptible and the person is not allergic to the medication. The disadvantages to these medications are the possibility of phlebitis and drug interactions with other antibiotics. Aminoglycosides cannot be delivered in the same container or tubing as penicillins. Importantly, procaine penicillin should never be given intravenously.

Penicillin G potassium (Pfizerpen), a natural penicillin, may be given either as continuous or intermittent IV therapy for bactericidal action. Penicillin G is relatively nontoxic, although it does have hypersensitivity issues, as do other penicillins. Treatment of severe infections is one of the main indications for use. Hypersensitivity manifestations are similar to those found with all penicillins (see Chapter 18).

Penicillinase-resistant penicillins such as methicillin sodium (Staphcillin) are used intravenously to treat *Staphylococcus aureus* or *Staphylococcus epidermidis* infections. These medications tend to cause phlebitis and kidney reactions. Nafcillin sodium (Nafcil) is more likely to cause phlebitis, although it does not cause as many kidney reactions.

Aminopenicillins such as ampicillin sodium (Totacillin-N) may be injected intravenously directly or by the more common means of an intermittent infusion. The stability of ampicillin after reconstitution is about 4 hours when added to a solution containing dextrose. However, if the medication is added to normal saline (NS) without dextrose, the time is extended to 8 hours. Finally, when placed in a minibag, the stability may last for 48 hours.

Some penicillins have extended or wider spectrums against microorganisms that have been identified by laboratory testing. Mezlocillin (Mezlin) and piperacillin (Pipracil) are typical of this group of antibiotics. Administration may be direct injection, intermittent infusion, or continuous infusion. Following the recommended rate of infusion and not exceeding the flow rate are important because rapid infusion of some of these medications may result in seizures. These drugs have similar dermatologic and hematologic reactions as the other penicillins, and the systemic reactions are found in Chapter 18.

Cephalosporins

Cephalosporins are similar to the penicillins, having similar indications as bactericides, side effects, and contraindications as found in Chapter 18. Cephalosporins are known to present a high risk for phlebitis, so the infusion site should be rotated frequently.

First-generation IV agents such as cefazolin (Ancef and Kefzol) and cephradine (Anspor and Velosef) are used with such bacteria as *Staphylococcus* microorganisms. Second-generation cephalosporin agents used intravenously include cefoxitin sodium (Mefoxin), cefamandole nafate (Mandol), and cefotetan disodium (Cefotan) with anaerobic microorganisms. With the ability to cross the blood-brain barrier, third-generation cephalosporins are often used by IV means with neurologic infections. Medications typical of this category are cefotaxime sodium (Claforan), ceftazidime (Fortaz and Tazidime), and ceftriaxone sodium (Rocephin). These are usually used in home care IV therapy because the medication is given as a once-daily dose. Fourth-generation cephalosporins such as cefepime (Maxipime) are relatively new but are being accepted by the Food and Drug Administration for use with severe infections, especially of the urinary tract and in dermatology.

Aminoglycosides

The aminoglycosides that are used intravenously as bactericidal agents will cause balance and hearing loss by damaging the eighth cranial nerve just as with the oral medications. Therefore the patient receiving aminoglycosides over a period of time should be assessed for this adverse reaction. Chapter 18 contains the information on further side effects. Remember that with these medications the margin between therapeutic and toxic is small, but an advantage is the length of time the medication remains in the body for further therapeutic effect. Aminoglycosides such as gentamicin, amikacin sulfate, and tobramycin sulfate may be given as a single larger dose instead of in multiple daily doses. The single large dose administered over 60 minutes seems to reduce the toxicity.

Tetracyclines

Tetracyclines such as minocycline (Minocin) are considered both bactericidal and bacteriostatic. These drugs may be used when penicillin therapy is contraindicated. The infusion site should be rotated more frequently than every 48 hours because this classification of medications tends to cause venous irritation and thrombophlebitis. An intermittent infusion over a period of 1 to 4 hours is the most commonly used means of administration for tetracyclines.

Macrolides

Closely related to tetracyclines, **macrolides** are considered to be bacteriostatic and may have some bactericidal activity when administered in high dosages. Macrolides that can be administered intravenously include erythromycin (erythromycin lactobionate [Erythrocin] or erythromycin gluceptate [Ilotycin]), azithromycin (Zithromax), and troleandomycin (TAO). These medications tend to cause phlebitis and must be diluted in at least 100 mL of solvent such as NS or 5% dextrose solutions and must be given over a longer period of time than other antibiotics. Dilution and rotating the infusion site make these medications less irritating for the patient. These medications are considered to be relatively free of serious side effects and are therefore considered among the safest.

Chloramphenicol

Chloramphenicol (Chloromycetin) is found in IV forms for use with serious infections. This medication should be administered by intermittent infusion and may be administered concurrently with penicillin G for serious anaerobic infections. Because of the potential for serious and possibly fatal reactions, chloramphenicol should not be used unless no other medication is effective. The patient must be closely monitored during the time this medication is administered.

Fluoroquinolones

Fluoroquinolones are such drugs as ciprofloxacin (Cipro), levofloxacin (Levaquin), gatifloxacin (Tequin), and ofloxacin (Floxin) and may be used as bactericidal agents in gram-positive and gram-negative organisms and, with large doses, are effective with anaerobic microorganisms. Because most of the medications require only once-daily dosing intravenously, these drugs are often given intermittently with home infusion and in hospital settings to reduce the damage to veins.

Other Antibiotics

Other antibiotics such as vancomycin (Vancocin), clindamycin (Cleocin), and lincomycin (Lincocin) are introduced on a regular basis to reduce the chance of bacteria resistance. Before administering any of these medications, as should be done with all medications, be sure to read the literature for the proper time of administration, as well as the side effects and adverse reactions. Remember that patient safety is of utmost consideration and importance.

Antifungals

Two antifungals most frequently administered intravenously are amphotericin B (Fungazone) and fluconazole (Diflucan). Because most antifungals are suspensions, these medications should be administered using an in-line filter as directed by the manufacturer. These drugs should not be added to saline solution because a precipitate will form. The infusion should run over 2 to 6 hours, using the most distal vein available to prevent irritation of the veins proximal to the body. Thrombophlebitis is an expected adverse reaction when these medications are administered, but this can be decreased by adding heparin to the fluids. Rapid infusion may cause circulatory collapse, a danger with these medications. Amphotericin B is light sensitive and should not be mixed with any other drugs because of the numerous incompatibilities. Fluconazole must be administered in a glass container and should not have other medications added to the container. Careful monitoring of the patient is essential with these medications.

Antivirals

Used to treat viral diseases, antivirals such as acyclovir (Zovirax), ganciclovir (Cytovene), and cidofovir (Vistide) must be used after a patient has been prehydrated to prevent renal toxicity. These medications prevent the replication of viruses. These antivirals are given as intermittent infusions two to three times a day. Headaches and thrombophlebitis are common adverse reactions even if the medication is infused over a period of at least an hour.

Antiretrovirals

Antiretrovirals are administered intravenously only until oral therapy can be administered. These medications must run over a period of at least an hour at a constant rate and should be diluted in D-5-W or NS. Medications that include zidovudine (Retrovir) have many drug incompatibilities that should be checked before adding to fluids containing other medications.

Sulfonamides

Sulfonamides such as trimethoprim-sulfamethoxazole (Bactrim, Septra) have been used for more than 50 years to treat infections, especially those of the urinary tract. These medications inhibit growth and reproduction of the microorganism and are administered as intermittent infusions of up to 3 to 4 doses daily.

Intravenous Medications for Central Nervous System

Drugs that are most frequently administered intravenously for the central nervous system are analgesics (see Chapter 16). Other types of medications may include sedatives, hypnotics, and some that are specific such as anticonvulsants (see Chapter 30).

Analgesics

Prior to infusing any analgesic the patient should be assessed for the location of the pain, its intensity, quality, frequency, onset, duration, and any aggravating or alleviating factors because the physician may order different dosages of analgesics for different levels of patient pain. Parenteral dosing may be by continuous infusion or by intermittent routes. Continuous infusion provides continuous levels of pain control without the peaks of side effects or breakthrough pain. Intermittent dosing can be accomplished by patient-controlled analgesia or through direct injection of the medication into the IV line at the time analgesia is necessary.

The most commonly used controlled analgesic for continuous IV use is morphine. Other controlled analgesics are meperidine (Demerol) and hydromorphone (Dilaudid). The main indications for these types of medications, especially morphine, are the pain of coronary occlusion, chronic pain of malignancies, and acute pain following surgery.

Morphine

Morphine may be administered by slow, direct injection or by continuous infusion and should never be given full strength but should be diluted prior to administration. The major side effect is respiratory depression, and patients with respiratory disease must be carefully monitored. Most analgesics are potentiated by other central nervous system depressants, neuromuscular blockers, adrenergic blockers, phenothiazines, and monoamine oxidase inhibitors. Care with obtaining a full patient history is important to prevent adverse reactions due to drug interactions.

Hydromorphone and Meperidine

Hydromorphone (Dilaudid) is 5 to 10 times more potent than morphine, whereas meperidine (Demerol) has about 20% of the analgesic potency and a shorter duration of action. These two medications also require the same safety measures as found with morphine. These two medications should also be diluted prior to infusing, and patients should be evaluated prior to administration, during the administration, and following the infusion in the same manner as with morphine.

Opiate Agonists and Antagonists

Opiate agonists include pentazocine (Talwin), nalbuphine (Nubain), and butorphanol (Stadol). These medications may be administered undiluted as IV injections (IV push) and have lower addictive levels than found with the opiate and opioid medications (narcotics). When these medications are given to a patient who has not previously received a narcotic analgesic, the medication behaves as an agonist, acting much like a narcotic analgesic. However, when administered to a patient receiving a narcotic analgesic, these medications have an antagonist effect and inhibit the response of the narcotic. As with narcotics, these medications potentiate central nervous system (CNS) depressants such as tranquilizers and sedatives.

Sedatives, Hypnotics, and Anxiolytics

CNS depressants are used to cause drowsiness (sedatives), induce sleep (hypnotics), and relieve anxiety (anxiolytics). These may provide levels of sedation from mild sedation to anesthesia.

Barbiturates, drugs that produce sedation, include phenobarbital (Luminal), amobarbital (Amytal), secobarbital (Seconal), and thiopental (Pentothal) with the main difference among these being the time of onset and duration. Depending on the indication for the use of the medication, barbiturates may be administered either as intermittent doses or a one-time dose for sedation or as continuous administration for such conditions as status epilepticus. Adverse reactions include pain at the infusion site and, more importantly, the tendency to thrombophlebitis.

Benzodiazepines are different from barbiturates but are often used for the same indications. These medications reduce anxiety, produce sedation, relax muscle spasticity, and act as anticonvulsants. The common drugs in this classification are diazepam (Valium), lorazepam (Ativan), and midazolam hydrochloride (Versed). Midazolam, short-acting, has been used for conscious sedation for such minor surgical procedures as endoscopy or as a preoperative sedative. Lorazepam should be diluted with either D-5-W or NS for immediate administration directly into the vein or as close to the terminal end of the tubing as possible. Adding these drugs to other fluids is not indicated. These medications potentiate other depressants.

The preferred method of administration of diazepam is directly into the vein because of possible precipitation on administration within the plastic tubing. If given into tubing, the medication should be given as close to a vein as possible and flushed with NS prior to and after the administration.

Promethazine (Phenergan) may be given to potentiate sedative properties and to assist with the prevention of nausea and vomiting. With terminal patients it may also be given to assist with pain control. This medication is irritating to the veins and will cause phlebitis; therefore the peripheral venous access should be rotated often.

Anticonvulsants

Many of the drugs for the CNS already discussed are used as anticonvulsants, although there are specific drugs for this condition. Phenytoin (Dilantin), one of the specific anticonvulsants used, precipitates if the pH is changed; therefore the tubing must be flushed with NS prior to and after administration. NS in the amounts of 25 to 50 mL may be used for each 100 mg of phenytoin; however, the greatest dilution should be 100 mg per 100 mL of solvent. The IV solution should be prepared just prior to administration, and the infusion should be added using a filter with the infusion time to be within an hour of preparation.

Magnesium sulfate, another medication used as an anticonvulsant, is given intravenously with preeclampsia and eclampsia. This medication may be administered by IV injection or by intermittent infusion over 4 hours. The onset of action when administered intravenously is almost immediate and lasts for about 30 minutes.

Intravenous Medications for the Cardiovascular System

Drugs given for use with the cardiovascular system include those that affect cardiac strength and cardiac rhythm, reverse hypotension, control hypertension, and improve blood flow as discussed in Chapter 27. The following is only a summary of the medications because the use in this area is specialized and is most frequently administered in the hospital setting.

α- and β-Adrenergic Agonists

α- and β-Adrenergic agonists such as epinephrine (Adrenalin) imitate the responses of the sympathetic nervous system by elevating systolic blood pressure and lowering diastolic blood pressure and also by increasing the strength of the cardiac contraction and the contraction rate, thus increasing cardiac output. α- and β-Adrenergic agonists interact with many drugs including the potentiation of anesthetics and antihistamines. These medications, especially epinephrine, may be given as a bolus in emergency situations, as an IV injection or as an infusion. When given as an overdose or too rapidly, the patient may have symptoms that occur with the stimulation of the sympathetic nervous system. If the medication extravasates, severe tissue damage may occur because of its vasoconstriction properties.

α-Adrenergic Agents

This classification of medications is used for vasoconstriction and cardiac stimulation, especially with hypotension. The most commonly used medication is metaraminol bitartrate (Aramine), a drug that strengthens cardiac contractility and increases blood flow to essential body organs such as brain, kidneys, and heart and mimics naturally occurring norepinephrine. If the infusion with these medications extravasates, the tissue will be damaged, necrose, and slough.

β-Adrenergic Agonists

β-Adrenergic agonists such as dopamine (Intropin) or isoproterenol (Isuprel) are used to treat shock by acting to stimulate the heart and dilate the bronchi. These medications stimulate the contractility of the heart and increase cardiac output, blood pressure and urinary output. Dopamine may be administered as a continuous infusion with blood pressure monitored frequently.

β-Adrenergic Blockers

Propranolol hydrochloride (Inderal) is a typical β-adrenergic blocker that blocks the action of norepinephrine and epinephrine. These medications, given by slow IV injection, have an antiarrhythmic effect and are used to treat arrhythmias such as paroxysmal atrial tachycardia, atrial flutter, and atrial fibrillation.

Cardiac Glycosides

Cardiac glycosides such as digoxin (Lanoxin) are used to increase cardiac contractility and to alter the generation and conduction of electrical impulse to increase cardiac output and to slow the rate of contractions. These drugs are given either diluted with sterile water, D-5-W, or NS or undiluted by IV injection and may be repeated intermittently until the digitalizing dose is obtained. Because so many drugs interact with digoxin, all medication that the patient is taking should be evaluated before the initiation of IV therapy.

Antidysrhythmics

No drug is typical of this category of medications. Some antiarrhythmics such as quinidine gluconate and procainamide hydrochloride (Pronestyl) are used to decrease the amount of sodium that is transported through the heart tissue, thus slowing the conduction of the electrical impulse through the AV node. Another group of antidysrhythmics promote uniform conduction rates by decreasing the refractory period of the Purkinje fibers and the ventricular myocardium. This group includes lidocaine, which is given either as a bolus in the amount of 50 to 100 mg at a rate not exceeding 25 mg/minute. The bolus dose may be repeated, but then the medication would be given as a continuous infusion at the rate of 1 to 4 mg/minute. Phenytoin sodium (Dilantin) is often used when the arrhythmia is digitalis induced. Another group such as propranolol hydrochloride (Inderal), which is also used in β-blockers, may be used for arrhythmias.

The antidysrhythmics used to slow the electrical impulse by blocking the calcium influx into the cardiac cells include verapamil hydrochloride (Isoptin) and diltiazem (Cardizem). If given with digoxin, the patient must be monitored closely because these medications have potentiating interactions. Calcium blockers also have other interactions that must be closely monitored (see Chapter 27).

Intravenous Hematology Agents

Anticoagulants and thrombolytics are used to keep the body in homeostasis by keeping the coagulation factors within normal limits, as discussed in Chapter 27. If the blood tends to clot or has a treatment that could initiate a clot, an anticoagulant may be used. However, if the patient is bleeding and the clotting time needs to be shortened, a thrombolytic may be prescribed.

Anticoagulants

Anticoagulants interfere with the clotting of blood and may be used to reduce the risk of clot formation. A commonly used anticoagulant is heparin sodium, which, in small doses, inhibits the conversion of prothrombin to thrombin. Heparin is often used in the prevention of venous thrombi and pulmonary emboli, used with renal dialysis, prevention of clotting during cardiac and arterial surgery, and treatment of myocardial infarctions. To provide a constant degree of anticoagulation, heparin is often given as a continuous infusion, although it may be given as an intermittent injection. A coagulation time is necessary prior to the therapy and throughout therapy at regular intervals. Heparin is also used as a flush to retain patency of IV lines during intermittent infusions.

Thrombolytic Agents

The opposite of anticoagulants are thrombolytic agents such as streptokinase (Streptase), used to enhance formation of clots or thrombi. By degrading fibrinogen and fibrin clots, streptokinase causes lysis of coronary artery thrombi, pulmonary emboli, and deep vessel thrombi.

Intravenous Drugs for Electrolyte Balance

The medications needed for fluid and electrolyte balance and the maintenance of homeostasis were discussed in Chapter 20. Medications may be required to correct acid-base balances, excrete extra fluids from the body, or replace or maintain electrolyte or fluid levels. The replacement of electrolytes and fluids may be a reason for IV therapy on an ambulatory care basis, whereas continuous fluid infusion for replacement therapy may be prescribed in the inpatient setting.

When metabolic alkalosis occurs, acidifying agents such as ammonium chloride may be used to reverse the alkaline state. Acidifying agents will react with the bicarbonate ions to form water that is excreted by the body. The patient must be watched for respiratory distress, irregular heartbeats, headache, and disorientation.

If the body becomes acidic, alkalinizing agents such as sodium bicarbonate will be administered to reduce the acidity of the body. Sodium bicarbonate reacts with many medications, so the drugs being taken must be carefully assessed prior to starting this medication and the IV tubing must be flushed both before and after any infusion of this medication. If the medication extravasates into the tissue, severe tissue damage with necrosis and ulceration may occur. The rate of flow must not be rapid because complications such as cerebral hemorrhage may occur.

Medications for Fluid and Electrolyte Replacement

Fluid and electrolyte replacement are necessary with medical conditions such as severe vomiting and diarrhea. When the patient is dehydrated because of fluid loss, giving fluids for hydration and electrolyte replacements will be necessary. The fluids without added medications are discussed in Chapter 11, whereas electrolytes are discussed in Chapter 20. Conversely, if the patient has edema and water retention, diuresis is necessary and medications to promote fluid loss will be administered. Diuretics, discussed in Chapters 27 and 28, are used for this purpose.

Intravenous Drugs for Electrolyte Replacement

Electrolytes are replaced using IV fluids when the specific deficiency is known. The most common electrolytes that need replacement are calcium and potassium.

Calcium is most commonly replaced using calcium gluconate administered as a continuous infusion. This medication may also be given as a direct injection at a rate of 0.5 mL over a minute.

When replacing potassium, either potassium chloride or potassium phosphate is used. Loss of potassium most frequently occurs following diuretic therapy, vomiting, diarrhea, and acidosis. This medication does cause vein irritation, so the amount of medication per liter should not exceed 80 mEq. Under no circumstance should potassium be infused undiluted because this may lead to cardiac arrest.

Diuretics

Loop and thiazide diuretics may be administered intravenously. Diuretics increase the amount of water eliminated through the kidneys and are used to treat severe edema including that from cardiac and nephrotic conditions.

Loop diuretics such as furosemide (Lasix) inhibit the reabsorption of fluids in the loop of Henle to remove excess fluid from the body. Large doses of furosemide should be infused at a slow rate, whereas doses of 20 to 40 mg may be infused as a direct injection over 1 to 2 minutes.

Thiazide diuretics such as chlorothiazide sodium (Diuril) interfere with the reabsorption of sodium in the distal convoluted tubules. This medication is not as effective as the loop diuretics but is used with toxemias and diabetes insipidus. Because of the potency of chlorothiazide, oral administration is preferable.

Intravenous Hormones

Several hormones are given intravenously such as corticosteroids (See Chapter 17) for use with immunosuppressant or malignant diseases. The adverse effects are not readily seen but result in long-term therapy.

Estrogens

Estrogens, discussed in Chapters 21 and 29, are given intravenously to treat breast cancer and for prostatic enlargement. These medications such as diethylstilbestrol (Stilphostrol) are given intermittently over a period of days with the rate of each infusion increased after the first 15 minutes. This medication should always be diluted in at least 300 mL of fluids prior to administration.

Insulin

Insulin, discussed in Chapter 21, is used to treat diabetes mellitus and acts as a catalyst for carbohydrate metabolism by allowing the transport of glucose and allowing its utilization in peripheral tissues. Regular insulin may be given intravenously and may be used for emergency treatment of hyperglycemic reactions. The potency of the insulin that is given to the patient may be affected by the absorption of the medication in the tubing and IV solution containers. Insulin may be administered as a direct injection or a continuous infusion.

Incompatibilities of Fluids and Medications

In some instances the IV fluids have incompatibilities with medications. Factors that affect drug incompatibilities include solubility, drug concentration, type of administration set, pH of the fluids and medications, and duration of drug-drug or drug-solution contact. Fluids containing dextrose are slightly acidic and should be used with slightly acidic medications, whereas saline solutions are slightly alkaline and should be used with alkaline medications. Several antibiotics on the market require an acidic fluid for dilution because the medication is not stable when it is not in an acidic environment.

Drugs may be compatible with some solutions but incompatible with other solutions. The incompatibility may be when two or more medications are mixed or when specific medications are mixed in incompatible fluids. Finally, incompatibilities may occur due to the tubing and drugs that are absorbed or changed by specific tubing materials. These incompatibilities should be detected by pharmacists in inpatient settings but may become the responsibility of the person initiating the IV therapy in other environments. When in doubt of incompatibilities, check the medication reference materials and, for safety, flush the IV administration set with NS before and after medications are infused.

Some medications interact with the plastic flexible IV bags because of the PVC (polyvinyl chloride) found therein. These drugs include vitamin A acetate, insulin, warfarin, and phenothiazine tranquilizers.

Incompatibility may also occur when mixing medications due to physical properties of the drugs. Insolubility, created when a drug is added to an inappropriate fluid, is the incomplete solution or the forming of a precipitate. This is more common with multiple additives but may occur when products interact. Usually a visible precipitate occurs. The presence of calcium in a medication often indicates that a precipitate will develop when mixing two or more medications in IV fluids. Because Ringer's solutions contain calcium, always check for incompatibilities when using this solution.

Check Your Understanding Answers

Chapter 6

6-1

1. $4/4 = E$
3. $6/5 = I$
5. $3/3 = E$
7. $3/4 = P$
9. $1/1 = E$
11. $30/90 = 1/3, 2/6, 3/9, 5/15, 6/18, 10/30, 15/45$
13. $15/60 = 1/4, 3/12, 5/20$
15. $10/40 = 1/4, 2/8, 5/20$

6-2

1. $14/3 = 4\ 2/3$
3. $31/5 = 6\ 1/5$
5. $55/7 = 7\ 6/7$
7. $25/6 = 4\ 1/6$
9. $19/3 = 6\ 1/3$
11. $1\ 2/5 = 7/5$
12. $13\ 3/4 = 55/4$
13. $6\ 1/2 = 13/2$
15. $4\ 5/6 = 29/6$
17. $17\ 1/4 = 69/4$
19. $5\ 7/10 = 57/10$
21. $70/8 = 8\ 3/4$
23. $26/6 = 4\ 1/3$
25. $35/10 = 3\ 1/2$
27. $30/20 = 1\ 1/2$
29. $70/16 = 4\ 3/8$

6-3

1. $2/5, 3/8 = 40$
3. $3/4, 1/6 = 12$
5. $5/6, 4/7 = 42$
7. $2/3, 1/6 = 6$
9. $2/5, 5/7 = 35$
11. $1/2 + 3/4 = 1\ 1/4$
13. $1/8 + 1/4 = 3/8$
15. $1/7 + 1/5 = 12/35$
17. $1/4 + 2/7 = 15/28$
19. $1/3 + 4/7 = 19/21$

6-4

1. $4/7 - 1/4 = 9/28$
3. $7/8 - 1/4 = 5/8$
5. $5/9 - 2/7 = 17/63$
7. $5/8 - 3/16 = 7/16$
9. $2/3 - 1/6 = 1/2$
11. $16\ 1/2 - 4\ 1/3 = 12\ 1/6$
13. $12\ 1/4 - 6\ 5/7 = 5\ 15/28$
15. $9\ 1/8 - 7\ 2/3 = 1\ 11/24$
17. $4\ 1/4 - 2\ 1/2 = 1\ 3/4$
19. $6\ 1/6 - 5\ 4/5 = 11/30$

6-5

1. $2/3 \times 3/4 = 1/2$
3. $1/5 \times 5/8 = 1/8$
5. $1/4 \times 2/7 = 1/14$
7. $6 = 6/1$
9. $12 = 12/1$
11. $1/3 \times 2 \times 5/8 = 5/12$
13. $4 \times 1\ 3/4 \times 1/9 = 7/9$
15. $2/5 \times 3\ 3/4 \times 8 = 12$
17. $1/4 \times 2/3 \times 1/2 = 1/12$
19. $2\ 1/5 \times 2\ 1/4 \times 2\ 2/3 = 13\ 1/2$

6-6

1. $3\ 4/5 = 19/5$
3. $1\ 1/4 = 5/4$
5. $10\ 1/5 = 51/5$
7. $3\ 2/3 \div 1/3 = 11$
9. $5\ 4/9 \div 2\ 1/3 = 2\ 1/3$
11. $4 \div 5/6 = 4\ 4/5$
13. $8\ 5/9 \div 6\ 1/3 = 1\ 20/57$
15. $10\ 1/5 \div 1\ 1/4 = 8\ 4/25$

6-7

1. 3 1/2 = 7/2
3. 1 = 1/1
5. 2 1/3 = 7/3
7. 6/12 = 3/6, 1/2, 2/4
9. 8/24 = 2/6, 4/12, 1/3
11. 11/8 = 1 3/8
13. 9/5 = 1 4/5
15. 7/4 = 1 3/4
17. 20/6 = 3 1/3
19. 18/12 = 1 1/2
21. 2 1/2 + 1/4 = 2 3/4
23. 1/3 + 1 1/2 = 1 5/6
25. 6 + 1 3/8 = 7 3/8
27. 2 1/2 − 1/8 = 2 3/8
29. 2 5/8 − 3/4 = 1 7/8
31. 2 × 1/8 × 3/4 = 3/16
33. 2 5/8 × 4 × 1/3 = 3 1/2
35. 2/3 × 1/2 × 3/8 = 1/8
37. 6 2/5 ÷ 4 1/2 = 1 19/45
39. 5 ÷ 1/2 = 2 1/2

6-8

1. 0.8 = 1
3. 0.95 = 1
5. 67.6 = 68
7. 56.78 = 56.8
9. 121.334 = 121.3
11. 233.332 = 233.33
13. 88.8883 = 88.89
15. 100.0593 = 100.06
17. 234.5574 = 234.557
19. 357.9753 = 357.975

6-9

1. 5/8 = 0.625
3. 1/6 = 0.167
5. 3/8 = 0.375
7. 17/9 = 1.9
9. 8/3 = 2.7
11. 3 1/2 = 3.5
13. 4 3/4 = 4.75
15. 2 7/11 = 2.64

6-10

1. 71.4 + 16.32 + 38 = 125.72
3. 33.33 + 66.7 + 1245.121 = 1345.151
5. 0.001 + 1.34 + 654.2 = 655.541
7. 123.5 + 688.8 + 99.99 = 912.29
9. 9.1 + 8.23 + 765.124 = 782.454
11. 38.672 − 32.43 = 6.242

13. 77.4 − 37.46 = 39.94
15. 5.04 − 1.67 = 3.37
17. 98.7 − 8.662 = 90.038
19. 1.06 − 0.92 = 0.14

6-11

1. 6.34 × 42.44 = 269.07
3. 43.011 × 17.92 = 770.76
5. 31.97 × 16.3 = 521.11
7. 1.01 × 0.011 = 0.01
9. 89.98 × 76.4 = 6874.47

6-12

1. 72.6 ÷ 31.5 = 2.3
3. 41.37 ÷ 6.777 = 6.1
5. 2.3 ÷ 0.76 = 3
7. 39.7 ÷ 18.4 = 2.2
9. 99.8 ÷ 16.22 = 6.2

6-13

1. 98.6 = 98 6/10
3. 432.67 = 432 67/100
5. 27.3 = 27 3/10
7. 674.75 = 675
9. 18.99 = 19
11. 99.109 = 99.1
13. 123.456 = 123.5
15. 3.717 = 3.7
17. 0.3826 = 0.38
19. 2.653 = 2.65
21. 68.2467 = 68.247
23. 4.2468 = 4.247
25. 1047.3218 = 1047.322
27. 3 1/2 = 3.5
29. 11/8 = 1.375
31. 46.38 + 27.4 + 0.44 + 17 = 91.22
33. 16.334 + 31.6 + 34.567 + 17.889 = 100.39
35. 91.25 + 44.337 + 16.4 + 88 + 391.24 = 631.23
37. 598.7 − 394.621 = 204.1
39. 274.651 − 35.7 = 239
41. 91.47 × 16.3 = 1491
43. 31.456 × 18 = 566
45. 3 × 17.2 × 0.47 = 24
47. 77.99 ÷ 7.99 = 9.761
49. 44.333 ÷ 16.333 = 2.714

6-14

1. 2/3% = 0.67
3. 4 1/2% = 0.045
5. 31% = 0.31

7. $7\ 7/8\% = 0.08$
9. $17\ 7/10\% = 0.18$

6-15

1. $3.59 = 359\%$
3. $0.06 = 6\%$
5. $0.047 = 4.7\%$
7. $1.17 = 117\%$
9. $0.055 = 5.5\%$

6-16

1. Find 14% of $28 = 3.92$
3. Find 6 2/3% of $80 = 5.33$
5. Find 19% of $75 = 14.25$
7. Find 48% of $100 = 48$
9. Find 82% of $19 = 15.58$

6-17

1. 70 is what percent of 84? 83.3%
3. 14 is what percent of 77? 18.2%
5. 3 is what percent of 7? 42.9%
7. 2 is what percent of 13? 15.4%
9. 7 is what percent of 77? 9.1%

6-18

1. What number is 25% of 40? 10
3. 15 is 60% of what number? 25
5. 5 is 10% of what number? 50
7. What number is 25% of 500? 125
9. 12 is 40% of what number? 30

6-19

1. $1/2\% = 0.005$
3. $1.44\% = 0.0144$
5. $33\ 1/3\%\ 0.3333$
7. $72.34 = 7234$
9. $0.05 = 5$
11. 27% of $2 = 0.5$
13. 66.67% of $49 = 32.7$
15. 33 1/2% of $50 = 16.8$
17. 67 is what percent of 200? 33 1/2%
19. 30 is what percent of 45? 66.7%
21. 6 is 10% of what number? 60
23. 25 is 50% of what number? 50
25. 2 is 60% of what number? 3
27. What number is 40% of 80? 32
29. What number is 80% of 60? 50

6-20

1. $5 : x :: 4 : 20$ $x = 25$
3. $11 : 22 :: x : 44$ $x = 22$
5. $50 : x :: 3 : 9$ $x = 150$
7. $x : 14 :: 12 : 24$ $x = 7$
9. $8 : 2 :: x : 4$ $x = 16$
11. $x : 5 :: 12 : 10$ $x = 6$
13. $1 : 9 : x : 81$ $x = 9$
15. $6 : x :: 3 : 1$ $x = 2$
17. $2 : x :: 4 : 250$ $x = 125$
19. $3 : 600 :: 2 : x$ $x = 400$

6-21

1. What number is 12% of 500?   60
3. What number is 81% of 11?   9
5. What number is 34% of 60?   20
7. What number is 47% of 400?   188
9. What number is 38% of 70?   27
11. 16 is 25% of what number?   64
13. 50 is 40% of what number?   125
15. 14 is 75% of what number?   19
17. 7 is 15% of what number?   47
19. 72 is 90% of what number?   80

6-22

1. $1 : x :: 3 : 12$ $x = 4$
3. $4 : 5 :: 16 : x$ $x = 20$
5. $0.2 : 0.8 :: x : 0.16$ $x = 0.04$
7. 56 tablets
9. 1 1/2 tablet
11. 0.2 mL
13. 95 kg
15. 2 tab
17. 3/4
19. 900 mg

Chapter 7

7-1

1. centi: less than
3. deka: greater than
5. kilo: greater than
7. milli: less than
9. basic unit of weight: gram
11. 1.00100: 1.001
13. 0.00110: 0.0011
15. .101010: 0.10101

16. liquid (volume), 0.4 mL
18. solid (weight), 624 mg
20. liquid (volume), 2.3 L
22. solid (weight), 10 g
24. liquid (volume), 1.5 L

7-2

1. 4.5 m = 4500 mm
3. 6.5 m = 650 cm
5. 9.2 m = 920 cm
7. 120 cm = 1.2 m
9. 1450 cm = 145 m
11. 6900 mm = 6.9 m (D)
13. 4.3 cm = 0.043 m (D)
15. 90 mm = 9 cm (D)
17. 8.8 cm = 88 mm (M)
19. 1200 mm = 120 cm (D)
21. 425 mm
23. 50 cm
25. 100 cm

7-3

1. 1.4 L = 1400 mL
3. 5 L = 5000 mL
5. 6.6 L = 6600 mL
7. 200 mL = 0.2 L
9. 1000 mL = 1 L
11. 1 mL = 0.001 L (D)
13. 6.4 L = 6400 mL (M)
15. 500 mL = 0.5 L (D)
17. 1450 mL = 1.45 L (D)
19. 100 mL = 0.1 L (D)
21. 2000 mL
23. 1 L
25. 3 L

7-4

1. 4 kg = 4000 g
3. 9 mg = 9000 mcg
5. 0.003 g = 3 mg
7. 25 mg = 0.025 g
9. 330 g = 0.33 kg
11. 1500 mcg = 1.5 mg (D)
13. 6.5 g = 6500 mg (M)
15. 0.34 kg = 340 g (M)
17. 0.09 g = 90 mg (M)
19. 0.03 kg = 30 g (M)
21. 2200 g
23. 0.5 mg
25. 1 tab = 0.088 mg

7-5

1. tablespoon
3. cup
5. tablespoon
7. greater than
9. less than
11. Dissolve 2 teaspoons of magnesium sulfate in 1 cup of water and take by mouth.
13. Take 1 teaspoon of Benadryl elixir every 4 hours. Do not exceed 6 doses daily.
15. Place 2 drops of Liquifilm tears in each eye as needed.

Chapter 8

8-1

1. 4:40 AM = 0440
3. 11:02 AM = 1102
5. 10:45 PM = 2245
7. 12:33 AM = 0033
9. 3:33 PM = 1533
11. 2121 = 9:21 PM
13. 0045 = 12:45 AM
15. 2400 = midnight
17. 0210 = 2:10 AM
19. 1515 = 3:15 PM

8-2

A. 96.4° F
C. 100.4° F
E. 105.4° F

8-3

1. 37.6° C = 99.6° F
3. 39.4° C = 103° F
5. 26.7° C = 80° F
7. 100° C = 212° F
9. −17.7° C = 0° F
11. 57.2° F = 14° C
13. 41° F = 5° C
15. 204.8° F = 96° C
17. 108.1° F = 42.3° C
19. 51.8° F = 11° C

8-4

1. 1:5 = 1/5
3. 2:5 = 2/5
5. 9:10 = 9/10

7. 1/2 = 1:2
9. 1/100 = 1:100
11. 8 mL
13. 14 tabs
15. 2 tabs

8-5

1. 45 mL = 3 tbsp
3. 1 mL = 15 (16)* gtt
5. 3 fluid oz = 90 mL
7. 250 mL = 1 c
9. 1 pt = 480 (500)* mL
11. 2 T
13. 2 qts or 4 pts
15. 1 oz

8-6

1. gr 3/4 = 45 mg
3. gr 15 = 900 mg
5. gr v = 0.33 g
7. 360 mg = 0.36 g
9. gr vi = 360 mg
11. 3 lb
13. 4250 mg
15. 75 g

8-7

1. 8 in = 20 cm
3. 3 m = 10 ft
5. 60 cm = 2 ft
7. 75 in = 2 m
9. 3 1/2 ft = 1 m
11. 25 mm (2.5 cm), yes
13. 45 cm
15. 0.6 inches

Chapter 9

9-1

1. 3 tsp
3. 6 mL
5. 5 mL

9-2

1. 2:3 = 2/3
3. 1:150 = 1/150
5. 2:7 = 2/7

7. 1/250 = 1:250
9. 1/1000 = 1:1000
11. 1 1/2 tabs
13. 2 tabs
15. 4 tabs

9-3

1.
a. What the doctor ordered: 500 mg
b. What strength is on the shelf: 1000 mg
c. What is the unit of measure: mL
d. How much of the drug will be administered: 1.5 mL
3.
a. What the doctor ordered: 160 mg
b. What strength is on the shelf: 320 mg
c. What is the unit of measure: tablets
d. How much of the drug will be administered: 1/2 tablet
5.
a. What the doctor ordered: 400 mg
b. What strength is on the shelf: 200 mg
c. What is the unit of measure: mL
d. How much of the drug will be administered: 10 mL
7. 1 1/2 tab
9. 20 mL; 4 tsp

9-4

1. 500 mg/1
3. 1 tab/500 mg
5. 15 gtt/1 mL
7. 1 1/2 tab
9. 20 mL; 4 tsp

9-5

1. Dose to be given: two tabs by mouth twice a day
3. Dose to be given: two tabs by mouth 4 times a day
5. Dose to be given: four tabs by mouth daily
7. Dose to be given: 1/2 tab by mouth daily
9. Dose to be given: 1 tab by mouth twice a day

9-6

1. 1200 mg
3. 30 mL
5. Yes, 1 teaspoon = 5 mL; use dose syringe for accuracy

7. 200 mg
9. 6 days
11. 87 mL
13. First, loosen the powder by tapping on the bottle. Add about half the water and shake. Add the final amount of water and shake well.
15. No, the bottle sizes are 60 mL and 100 mL. Add more water to the bottle for a final volume of 100 mL.

9-7

1. 0.35 BSA
3. 1.0 BSA
5. 1.2 BSA

9-8

1. 0.92 m^2; 135 mg; 2.7 mL or 1/2 tsp
3. 1.36 m^2; 4 mg or 4 mL
5. 1.08 m^2; 318 mg; 6.4 mL
7. 0.26 m^2; 76.5 mg or 8 mg; 3 mL (should be measured in dose syringe for this amount)

9-9

1. 250 mg; 5 mL
3. 380 mg/day; 127 mg/dose or 125 mg/dose; 5 mL/dose; 1 tsp
5. 500 mg/dose; 10 mL/dose; 2 tsps

Chapter 10

10-1

1. 2.3 mL
3. 0.7 mL
5. 2.8 mL
7. Draw a line at 0.9 mL
9. Draw a line at 1.1 mL
11. Draw a line at 0.3 mL
13. Draw a line at 1.9 mL
15. Draw a line at 2.9 mL

10-2

1. 2.5 mL
3. 0.5 mL
5. 3 mL

10-3

1. 52 units
3. 14 units
5. 26 units
7. 46 units
9. 0.5 mL

10-4

1. Desired dose: 35 units
3. Desired dose: 84 units
5. Desired dose: 15 units
7. Desired dose: 1 mL (100,000 U/dose)
9. 1.8 mL

10-5

1. 0.5 mL
3. 2 mL
5. 0.2 mL; tuberculin syringe

Chapter 11

11-1

1. 56 gtt/min
3. 56 gtt/min
5. 25 gtt/min

11-2

1. 333 min; 5.6 hr
3. 10 min
5. 13 hr 54 min

11-3

1. 5 mL; 4 mL
3. 2.5 mL; 100 mg
5. 5 mL; 250 mg; 312.5 mg

Drug-Food and Drug-Drug Interactions

Drug-Food Interactions

calcium carbonate (Tums): dairy products, bran and other whole grains

Erythromycin, penicillins: acidic juices, citrus fruits, soft drinks

All statins (Mevacor): grapefruit juice

Tetracyclines: calcium-containing foods such as ice cream, cheese, and milk

warfarin sodium: beef liver, spinach, cabbage, Brussel sprouts, broccoli

Monoamine oxidase inhibitors: foods high in tyramine such as cheese, sour cream, yogurt, meat tenderizers, beer and wine, aged meats

Clinically Significant Drug-Drug Interactions

carbamazepine (Tegretol): charcoal, erythromycin, clozapine

chlorpropamide (Diabinese): ethyl alcohol

clonidine (Catapres): propranolol (Inderal)

clozapine (Clozaril): carbamazepine (Tegretol)

digitoxin: rifampin (Rifadin)

digoxin (Lanoxin): amiodarone (Cordarone), erythromycin base, quinidine, tetracycline, verapamil (Calan)

diltiazem (Cardizem): cyclosporine (Neoral)

erythromycin: cyclosporine (Neoral)

ether: neomycin

ethyl alcohol: disulfiram (Antabuse)

gentamicin (Garamycin): carbenicillin (Geocillin), cephalothin (Keflin)

heparin: aspirin

insulin: propranolol (Inderal)

ketoconazole (Nizoral): cyclosporine (Neoral)

lidocaine (Xylocaine): cimetidine (Tagamet)

lincomycin (Lincocin): kaolin

lithium carbonate (Lithobid): acetazolamide (Diamox), chlorothiazide (Diuril)

meperidine (Demerol): phenelzine (Nardil)

methotrexate (Folex): aspirin, probenecid (Bencmid), sulfamethoxazole-trimethoprim (Septra, Bactrim)

phenelzine (Nardil): levodopa (L-Dopa)

phenytoin (Dilantin): cimetidine (Tagamet), disulfiram (Antabuse), dopamine (Dopastat, Entropion), fluconazole (Diflucan)

propranolol (Inderal): cimetidine (Tagamet), epinephrine

pyridoxine (vitamin B_6): levodopa (L-Dopa)

quinidine: amiodarone (Cordarone), verapamil (Calan)

rifampin (Rifadin): cyclosporine (Neoral), oral contraceptive agents

spironolactone (Aldactone): potassium chloride (K-Tabs)

tetracycline: aluminum hydroxide (Amphojel), ferrous sulfate

theophylline (Elixophyllin, Theo-Dur): charcoal, cimetidine (Tagamet), erythromycin, tobacco

triazolam (Halcion): ketoconazole (Nizoral)

warfarin (Coumadin): amiodarone (Cordarone), aspirin, cimetidine (Tagamet), clofibrate (Atromid-S), disulfiram (Antabuse), erythromycin, glucagon, methyltestosterone, nalidixic acid (NegGram), phenobarbital, phenylbutazone (Alka Butazolidin), phytonadione (vitamin K), rifampin (Rifadin), sulfamethoxazole (Gantanol), sulfinpyrazone (Anturane), thyroid (Synthroid)

Source for drug-drug interactions: *Pocket guide to evaluations of drug interactions,* ed 4, Washington, DC, 2002, American Pharmaceutical Association.

Absence or petit mal seizures Loss of consciousness for a short period of time due to seizure activity

Absorption Uptake of medications for distribution in the body through or across tissues

Accommodation Change in shape of the lens of the eye to adjust to viewing objects at different distances

Acetylcholine Chemical neurotransmitter in the parasympathetic nervous system

Acid Any substance with a hydrogen ion that is released in a solution and reacts with metals to form salts; pH below 7

Acid rebound Increase in gastric acid secretions that neutralize antacids that have been taken for a prolonged period of time

Acne Inflammation of the hair follicles and sebaceous glands characterized by comedones, pustules, and papules (raised areas)

Acquired immunity Immunity that is the result of exposure to a disease antigen or the injection of immune globulins or through immunizations

Actinic keratosis Horny, premalignant lesions of the skin caused by excessive exposure to sunlight

Active immunity Immunity resulting from the development of antibodies within a person's body that renders the person immune; may occur from exposure through a disease process or from immunizations

Active ingredient Medicinal ingredient in a pure, undiluted form of the chemical that has effects on body functions

Adjuvant medication Medication used to increase or hasten the action of the principal medications

Adjuvant treatment Form of treatment used in addition to primary treatment

Administer To give or apply medication to a person

Adrenergic (sympathomimetic) agent or agonist Agent that stimulates the action of the sympathetic nervous system or mimics the sympathetic nervous system

Adsorbent Liquid or gas substance that readily adheres the surface of a solid material to the surface of another substance

Adverse reaction Unintended, undesirable, and often unpredictable effect of a medication that causes pain, discomfort, or unwanted symptoms; more severe than a side effect

Aerobic bacteria Bacteria that live in an environment containing oxygen

Aerosol Liquid in a pressurized container that dispenses medication to sites of absorption

Aerosol foam Water-in-oil emulsion that dispenses into a foam when mixed with air

Affect Emotion or emotional response

Affective disorders Group of disorders characterized by disturbances in mood, from partial to full mania or depression

Agonist Medication that binds to the receptor site and stimulates the function of that site; drug that mimics a function of the body

Akathisia Restlessness, inability to sit still, urgent need to move

Alkaloid Organic compound that is alkaline in nature and is combined with acids to make salts

Alkylating agent Substance that interferes with cell metabolism and growth by introducing an alkyl agent or compound; agent used to treat malignancies

Allergic reaction Hypersensitivity to a drug that may occur after only one dose is taken (see **Hypersensitivity reaction**)

Alopecia Loss of hair

Alternative medicine Practice of using products for which scientific evidence of safety and efficacy is lacking (e.g., most herbal preparations, copper bracelets for arthritis)

Alzheimer's disease Progressive disease that is characterized by memory loss and inability to carry through on thought processes

Ampule Small glass container that is sealed and holds a single dose of medication, usually for injection

Anabolic steroids Synthetically produced androgens

Anabolism Constructive metabolic process by which substances are converted by an organism into other components of the organism's chemical structure; in the example of anabolic steroids such as testosterone, the result is greater muscle mass

Anaerobic bacteria Bacteria that live in an environment free of oxygen

Analeptics Drugs that stimulate the central nervous system

Analgesic Medication with pain-relieving property

Anaphylaxis Severe allergic reaction, possibly fatal, to a drug that occurs a short time after a drug has been administered to a person who is hypersensitive to it

Androgen Any male sex hormone

Anesthesia Loss of sensation, either of the entire body or of certain body areas

Angina pectoris Insufficient blood flow to the heart, with resultant spasm of the cardiac muscle causing chest pain

Anion Negatively charged ion

Ankylosing spondylitis Change in spine, similar to rheumatoid arthritis, which causes stiffening of the back

Ankylosis Immobility of joints, caused by congenital conditions, surgery, trauma, or diseases

Anomaly Any deviation from normal

Anorectal Pertaining to the anus and rectum

Anorexia Loss of appetite

Anorexiant Medication used to suppress appetite

Antagonism Cancellation or reduction of one drug's effect by another drug

Antagonist Medication that binds at receptor sites to prevent other medications from binding to those same sites

Anthelmintics Agents used for treatment of intestinal worms

Antibacterial drugs Drugs with the ability for destruction or inhibition of growth of bacteria

Antibiotic Natural or synthetic substance, originally derived from plant or animal sources, that kills or inhibits the growth of microorganisms

Antibody Protein that develops in response to the presence of an antigen in the body and reacts with the antigen on the next exposure. Antibodies may be formed from infections, immunizations, transfer from the mother to a child, or from no known antigen stimulation.

Antibody titer Quantity of viable antibodies required to respond to a given quantity of antigen as determined by a laboratory (serologic) test

Anticholinergic agents or anticholinergics Agents that block the parasympathetic nerve impulse (e.g., causing dilation of the pupil)

Antidiarrheal Agent or substance that prevents or treats diarrhea

Antidote Drug or substance given to stop a toxic effect

Antiemetic Agent that prevents or relieves nausea or vomiting

Antiflatulent Agent that decreases excessive gas in the stomach or intestines

Antigen Substance that is either introduced into the body or formed by the body to induce the formation of antibodies specific to that antigen

Antigen-antibody response Neutralization or destruction of antigen by antibodies

Antihistamine Agent that decreases histamine release

Antiinflammatory Medication with inflammation-reducing property

Antimetabolite Agent that disrupts essential cell metabolic processes and is used to treat malignancies by opposing the actions of or replacing a metabolite necessary for cell growth by interfering with DNA metabolism

Antimicrobial Pertaining to destruction or inhibition of growth of microorganisms; when said of drugs, includes both those of organic origin (*antibiotics*) and nonorganic origin (e.g., silver, sulfur, and mercury)

Antipyretic Medication with fever-reducing property

Antisecretory agent Agent that inhibits secretions of a gland or organ

Antiseptic Agent that reduces, prevents, or inhibits the growth of microbial flora of the skin and mucous membranes without necessarily killing them

Antiserum Serum containing antibodies to a specific antigen; usually of human or animal origin

Antispasmodics Agents that prevent or decrease intestinal spasms

Antitoxin Agent that provides antibodies produced in response to a specific toxin that has the ability to neutralize that same toxin in another person (e.g., tetanus antitoxin)

Antitussive Agent that relieves or suppresses coughing

Antiviral Agent that opposes the action of a virus; medication specifically for treating viral conditions

Anxiolytic Medication to relieve anxiety; minor tranquilizer

Apothecary Pharmacist or druggist

Apothecary system One of the oldest measurement systems based on grains and drams used to calculate drug orders

Aqueous solution Water soluble solution; when referring to injections, the aqueous solution is considered as thin or watery

Arrhythmia Irregular rhythm (i.e., irregular heartbeat)

Arteriosclerosis Thickening of walls of arterioles causing loss of elasticity and loss of ability to contract

Arthritis Inflammation of joint, accompanied by pain, swelling, and bony changes in the joint

Articulate To join bones in joints

Artificially acquired active immunity Long-term immunity provided by immunization with a specific agent to develop antibodies to a specific disease process

Artificially acquired passive immunity Short-term immunity provided from other persons or animals that have the antibodies for a specific disease (e.g., immune globulins, antitoxins)

Astringent Agent that causes shrinking or constricting action, usually applied topically or locally

Ataxia Difficulty with balance

Atherosclerosis Form of arteriosclerosis characterized by buildup of fatty plaques on the walls of arteries and arterioles

Attention deficit/hyperactivity disorder (ADHD) Disease found most frequently in children that is characterized by inattention, hyperactivity, and impulsiveness

Attenuated Lessened, abbreviated; in reference to immunity, lessened virulence of a pathogen

Auditory ossicles Bones of the middle ear that vibrate to amplify received sound waves and transmit the waves to the inner ear

Aura Neurological visual phenomenon (e.g., light flashes, blank areas in the field of vision) that may precede epileptic seizures and migraine headaches

Auralgia Ear pain; also called *otalgia* or *otodynia*

Automaticity Automatic spontaneous initiation of a heart impulse

Autonomic nervous system Self-governing, involuntary nervous system

Avitaminosis Any disease caused by lack of vitamin production or intake

Bacteria One-celled organisms that can synthesize DNA, RNA, or other essential products and can reproduce, but live on food supplied by a host or by a supportive environment (singular: bacterium)

Bactericidal Pertaining to destruction of bacteria; drugs or chemicals with this ability

Bacteriostatic Inhibiting or retarding the growth of bacteria; drugs or chemicals with this ability

Base Any substance that combines with hydrogen to form a salt; pH above 7 or alkaline in nature

Bath Method of cleansing the body or its parts or treating the body therapeutically with a cleansing agent

Benign Nonmalignant

Bevel   Slanted surface on end of a hypodermic needle, including the point and the lumen

Bioequivalency   State or property of having the same strength and availability for absorption in the body as the same dosage of another available source of that drug

Bipolar disorder   Psychiatric condition characterized by alternating periods of mania and depressive states; previously called *manic-depressive disorder*

Bleb   Irregularly raised elevation of the epidermis

Blepharitis   Inflammation of the eyelids from bacterial infections or allergies

Blood-brain barrier   Capillary walls of the brain, which can act to prevent potentially harmful substances from moving out of the bloodstream and entering the meninges in the brain or cerebral spinal fluid

Body surface area (BSA) calculation   Process of calculating dosages based on weight and height using a nomogram

Bolus   Concentrated amount of medication given rapidly intravenously

Brand-name drug   Proprietary ("brand-name") drug with a trademark (such drugs are marked with ®)

Broad-spectrum antibiotic   Antibiotic effective against a variety of gram-positive and gram-negative microorganisms

Buccal tablet   Tablet placed in the mouth between cheek and gum (buccal area) for absorption

Buffered tablet   Medication combined with an antacid to reduce irritation to the stomach when ingested

Cancer   Malignant neoplasm; uncontrolled growth and spread of abnormal cells

Caplet   Long, oblong tablet with a smooth film-coated covering for ease of swallowing

Capsule   Small gelatin container filled with medication in powder or granule form

Carbuncle   Lesion of the skin with inflammation of the skin and deeper tissues that produces suppuration and sloughing of the tissue; similar to a boil or furuncle

Carcinogenic agent   Substance or agent that has potential to produce cancer or increase the risk of cancer

Caries   Cavities in teeth

Carminative   Agent that helps prevent formation of gas in the gastrointestinal tract

Cataract   Opacity (loss of transparency) on or in the lens or capsule of the eye

Catecholamines   Epinephrine, norepinephrine, and dopamine, derived from tyrosamine

Cathartics   Active agents that cause a bowel movement

Cation   Positively charged ion

Ceiling effect   Dose beyond which no further response occurs (e.g., an analgesic ceiling effect)

Cell cycle phase   Steps that occur in the growth and development of a cell

Central nervous system   Brain and spinal cord

Cerumen   Ear wax

Chalazion   Hard eyelid cyst resulting from chronic inflammation of a meibomian gland

Chelator   Agent used to treat metal poisonings

Chemical biotransformation   Alteration of medications within the body to prepare for excretion from the body; metabolism

Chemotherapy   Treatment of disease using chemical agents

Chewable tablet   Tablet with a sugar or flavored base, designed to be chewed

Chloasma   Darkening of the skin around the eyes

Cholelithiasis   Formation or presence of calculi or bile stones in the gallbladder

Cholinergic (or parasympathomimetic) agent   Drug that mimics the parasympathetic nervous system; agent that acts to transmit nerve stimulations in the parasympathetic nervous system (e.g., causing constriction of the pupil in the eye)

Chronotropic effect   Increase or decrease in the heart rate

Cirrhosis   Chronic liver disease frequently found in persons with long-term alcohol abuse

Clinical pharmacology   Study of drug effects in humans

Clonic   Pertaining to alternating contracting and relaxing of muscles

Co-analgesia   Administration of two or more medications (analgesics) together for synergistic effect

Colloid suspension/solution   Suspension with alcohol, water, or ether as a solvent; a thin layer of medication is left on the skin when the solvent evaporates

Comedo/comedones   Skin lesion found with acne vulgaris; commonly called *whitehead* or *blackhead*

Compatible   Suitable for mixing without unfavorable actions; in pharmacology, refers to mixing two or more medications

Complementary medicine   Alternative medical techniques that have been proved effective by scientific research as a basis for use and that are accepted as part of good medical practice (e.g., acupuncture, massage therapy)

Compounding   Mixing a prescription according to the physician's order

Conjunctivitis   Acute inflammation of the conjunctiva from bacterial or viral infection, usually self-limiting; also called "pink-eye"

Contraception   Prevention of fertilization of the ovum and the subsequent onset of pregnancy

Contraindication   Condition in which use of given medication should be avoided

Controlled substance   Medication that is controlled by the Drug Enforcement Administration because of its potential for abuse and misuse

Conversion factor   Known equivalency of two values in different measurement systems; may be written as a fraction or a ratio

Convert   Change from one form to another

Convulsion   Abnormal motor movements such as the jerking movement of a grand mal seizure

Coryza   Inflammation of the mucous membranes of the nose with a profuse nasal discharge; commonly called a "head cold"

Cream   Semisolid preparation in a base that is absorbed into the tissue for slow, sustained release

Crepitus   Crackling sounds in joints due to arthritis

Cumulation   Increasing storage of a medication in the body caused by the body's inability to metabolize or excrete the medication before another dose is taken

Curative (healing) medication   Medication prescribed to kill or remove the causative agent of a disease

Cycloplegia   Paralysis of the ciliary muscle

Cytotoxic agent   Compound that causes cell destruction

Dangerous drug   Drug that can cause addiction or that is detrimental to the body

Decongestant   Agent that reduces swelling and congestion in the respiratory tract

Defecation Passage of feces from the body; bowel movement

Delayed-action capsule Capsule prepared to release drug at a particular site or to provide a steady release of medication over a period of time

Delirium tremens Restlessness, confusion, insomnia, irritability, with visual, tactile, and auditory hallucinations caused by abstinence of alcohol consumption in an alcohol abuser

Delusion False belief that cannot be changed with reason

Demulcent Drug used to soothe a body part or to relieve symptoms of irritation

Dentifrice Substance for cleaning teeth

Depot injectable Medication given parenterally that is stored in the fatty tissue for slow release in the body

Depressant Drug that acts to lower or lessen the activity of a body part

Desired effect Intended response to a medication

Destructive agent Substance that destroys cells and tissues; from bactericidals to chemotherapy

Diagnostic agent Medication used to assist in diagnosing diseases

Diaphoresis Excessive perspiration

Digitalization Rapid dosing of digitalis to reach a therapeutic level

Diluent Agent that dilutes a substance; in pharmacology, the liquid added to a powder to change the powder to a liquid form for parenteral administration or for unstable oral preparations

Disease-modifying antirheumatic drug (DMARD) Drug that modifies rheumatic diseases

Disinfectant/germicidal agent Agent that decreases the number of microorganisms on inanimate objects and prevents infection by killing bacteria on inanimate surfaces

Dispense To give medications to a patient to be taken at a later time

Dispersion Scattering of medication particles throughout the body or throughout a liquid

Distribution Dispersion of medication to sites in the body

Diuresis Loss of water in the body

Documentation Written notation in a medical record of information obtained from a patient and procedures that have been performed in the medical setting

Dosage Regimen of administering individual doses of medication, expressed in quantity per unit of time

Dose Exact amount of a medication to be given or taken at one time

Dram Unit of measure for liquid volume in the apothecary system

Dromotropic effect Increase or decrease in the conduction of cardiac electrical impulses

Drug Any chemical that has an effect on living processes

Drug abuse Misuse or overuse of drugs in a manner that deviates from the prescribed manner, which might lead to physical or psychologic dependence, usually by self-medication

Drug addiction Compulsive use of drugs or substances that results in physical, psychologic, or social harm

Drug blood level Amount of a drug circulating in the bloodstream; also known as the *reference value in laboratory reports*

Drug dependence Compulsion to take a drug, either continuously or periodically, to relieve a real or imagined physical or psychologic need

Drug efficacy Ability of a drug to produce the desired chemical change in the body

Drug Enforcement Administration (DEA) Agency in the Department of Justice with the legal responsibility to enforce the statutes of the Comprehensive Drug Abuse and Prevention Act of 1970

Drug Facts and Comparisons Publication updated monthly by Facts and Comparisons giving in-depth information concerning medications, usually used by pharmacists

Drug habituation Taking of medication as a matter of course, not out of need

Drug half-life Time in which half of the available drug is metabolized by the body for excretion

Drug holiday Period during which drug dosages are withheld to allow reversal of side effects or adverse reactions

Drug interaction Effects of medications taken together

Drug misuse Nonspecific or indiscriminate use of drugs; the use of drugs for purposes other than therapeutic intentions

Drug nomenclature Process of naming drugs (i.e., chemical, generic, and brand names)

Drug purity Quality or state of having the type and concentration of substances set forth by FDA standards for production of a drug

Drug quality State or condition of ensuring that each time a medication is taken as ordered or in compliance with the manufacturer's directions, it meets the same drug standards

Drug sample Medication left by a manufacturer's representative in a physician's office to be given, not sold, to a patient with the main purpose of ensuring the patient can effectively take the medication

Drug standards Rules and regulations to ensure consumers that they are receiving medications with therapeutic consistency

Drug strength or potency Concentration of active ingredient(s) in a medicinal preparation

Drug tolerance Accustomization to a medication resulting in a decreased response to the usual dose

Dry powder inhaler (DPI) Drug delivery system that dispenses a given amount of medication as a dry powder directly to the mucous membranes of the respiratory tract

Dyskinesia Excessive involuntary body movements

Dyspareunia Painful sexual intercourse

Dysphonia Difficulty speaking or hoarseness

Dysphoria Exaggerated feeling of depression or unrest

Dystonia Weak, slow body movements caused by lack of muscle coordination or impaired muscle tone

Dysuria Painful urination

Eczema Acute or chronic skin irritation that has erythema, papules, vesicles, pustules, scales, crusts, or scabs, either alone or in combination

Edema Excessive amount of tissue fluid; swelling

Effervescence Formation of gas bubbles on the surface of a liquid

Effervescent powder Coarsely ground medicinal agent that has been mixed with an effervescent salt to release carbon dioxide when a liquid is added

Electrolyte Substance that uncouples into ions in solution and can then conduct an electrical charge; in human physiology, an ionized salt such as sodium and chloride found in blood, tissue fluids, and cells

Elixir Clear, sweetened, flavored medication containing alcohol and water

Embolus Obstruction of a blood vessel by a foreign substance or a blood clot

Emesis Act of vomiting

Emetic Agent that initiates vomiting

Emollient   Agent that softens and soothes the surface to which it is applied, usually the skin

Emulsion   Water-and-oil mixture containing medication in pharmacology

Endemic   Pertaining to continuous or cyclical presence of disease in a given geographic area

Endogenous   Arising from within a cell, organ, or organism itself

Endorphin   Naturally occurring opioid-like substance, produced by the body, that blocks pain stimuli

Enema   Instillation of a liquid into the rectum

Enkephalin   Neurotransmitter that acts as an opiate to produce analgesia by blocking pain receptor sites

Enteral route   Gastrointestinal tract route of medication administration (i.e., oral or rectal). The medication is absorbed from the gastrointestinal tract.

Enteric-coated tablet   Tablet coated with a film, formulated to pass through the stomach into the small intestines for absorption; prevents irritation of the gastric mucosa

Enuresis   Involuntary discharge of urine after an age when bladder control should be achieved; usually called bedwetting because the person does not wake up at night

Epistaxis   Nosebleed

Eschar   Sloughing of skin following a burn

Estrogen   Female sex hormone

Euphoria   Exaggerated feeling of well-being

Exacerbate   To aggravate symptoms or cause increased symptomatology of a disease

Excoriation   Abrasion of the skin

Excretion   Elimination of medication from the body through respiration, perspiration, urination, or defecation

Exogenous   Originating outside an organ or organism itself

Expectorant   Agent that assists with the removal of mucous secretions from the lower respiratory tract

Expectorate   Act or process of spitting out saliva or coughing materials from the air passages

Extract and fluid extract   Highly concentrated preparation of liquid medication achieved through evaporation of a solution

Extrapyramidal effects   Tremors, dystonia, or slow irregular, involuntary movements of the upper extremities, especially hands and fingers; symptoms of motor imbalance and lack of muscle tone

Extravasation   Escape of fluid from vessels into surrounding tissues; in pharmacology, refers to drugs that escape from blood vessels into tissues

Facultative   Pertaining to ability to thrive in dissimilar environments; when said of microbes, denotes those able to live in either aerobic or anaerobic conditions

Fibromyalgia   Debilitating disease with chronic pain of muscles and soft tissues surrounding the joints

Filter needle   Hypodermic needle that contains a small filter system to prevent aspiration of small glass particles from ampules into the syringe; should be removed from the syringe and replaced with a hypodermic needle prior to injection

First-pass effect   Rapid inactivation of some oral medications as they pass through the liver for the first time before entering the systemic circulation

Focal (partial) seizure   Seizure with limited spread in the brain, usually affecting a single muscle group

Folk medicine   Remedies for illnesses passed down from generation to generation in families or in a culture for the treatment of specific symptoms (e.g., cobwebs to stop bleeding, meat tenderizer to relieve the itching of insect bites)

Food and Drug Administration (FDA)   Agency responsible for the safety, efficacy, and purity of drugs marketed in the United States

Formula method   Substitution of information into a formula

Free or unbound drug   Drug that has reached the bloodstream and is ready for use in the body

Fungus   Spore-forming, plantlike, single-celled microorganism that thrives on dead organic matter; usually part of normal body flora (plural: fungi)

Furuncle   Acute, deep-seated inflammation of the skin that begins in a hair follicle or sweat gland and produces suppuration and necrosis; boil

Fusion   Joining together of two lines, such as bone fusion where two sections of bone are permanently joined together

Galactorrhea   Excessive secretion of milk

Gastroesophageal reflux disease (GERD)   Condition in which acidic contents of the stomach flow backward into the esophagus

Gauge   Standard of measurement indicating the diameter of the lumen of a hypodermic needle

Gel/jelly   Semisolid in a water base with a thickening agent for absorption through the skin

Gelcap   Soft gelatin shell filled with liquid medication

Generalized seizure   Seizure with loss of consciousness

Generic drug   Drug not protected by a trademark but regulated by the FDA

Genetic immunity (inborn) or natural immunity   More or less permanent immunity present from birth as a result of genetic factors

GenRx   Compilation of comprehensive drug information published by Mosby; also includes such information as costs and drug comparisons not found in the PDR

Germicide   Agent with the ability to destroy germs or microorganisms

Germistatic agent   Agent that prevents growth of microorganisms

Gingivitis   Inflammation of the gums

Glaucoma   Disease of the eye characterized by increased intraocular pressure

Glucocorticoid   Hormone secreted by the adrenal cortex that protects against stress and is used in protein and carbohydrate metabolism

Glycoside   Active plant substance that yields a sugar (glyco-) plus an active ingredient

Goiter   Enlargement of the thyroid gland

Grain   Basic unit of measure for solid weight in the apothecary system; compared with one grain of wheat or rice

Gram   Basic unit of measure for solid weight in the metric system

Grand mal seizure   Generalized tonic/clonic seizure

Growth hormone   Hormone secreted by the anterior pituitary that regulates cell division and protein synthesis needed for growth

Gum   Thick solution that can hold water and swell

Halitosis   Bad breath

Hallucination(s)   Perception(s) that have no basis in reality; may be visual, auditory, tactile, or olfactory

Hematuria   Blood in urine

Hemoptysis   Cough that contains blood expectorated from either the oral cavity or from another part of the respiratory tract

Hemostasis   Arrest of bleeding

High-density lipoprotein (HDL)   Simple protein that is combined with the lipids—cholesterol, phospholipids, and triglycerides; a high level of HDL lipoproteins is desirable

Hives   Vascular skin condition characterized by papules and wheals, producing intense itching

Homeostasis   Equilibrium of the body that is maintained by ever-changing feedback and regulation processes in response to external or internal changes; state of equilibrium in the internal environment of the body

Home remedy   Treatment devised and applied at home without professional medical advice; may or may not have therapeutic value (e.g., preparations from plants grown in herb gardens to treat toothache, itching from poison ivy, nausea, and the like)

Hordeolum   Localized, purulent, inflammatory bacterial infection of sebaceous glands of the eyelids, usually with small abscesses; also called a *stye*

Hormone   Substance originating in an organ, gland, or body part that is secreted directly into the bloodstream and carried to another part of the body to begin a chemical action to increase the activity of that part or to increase another secretion

Host   Organism that provides nourishment for a parasite

Household system   System of measurement that uses common kitchen measuring devices

Hyperglycemia   Elevated blood glucose level

Hypersensitivity reaction   Heightened immune reaction or allergic reaction to a medication

Hypertension   Elevation of blood pressure above normal limits

Hyperuricemia   Excessive amounts of uric acid in blood

Hypervitaminosis   Condition resulting from the excess intake of vitamins, usually vitamin compounds; usually found with lipid-soluble vitamins

Hypnotic   Medication used to induce or maintain sleep

Hypoglycemia   Decreased blood glucose level

Hypothalamus   Portion of the brain that lies directly under the thalamus; it has many functions including secretion of releasing and inhibiting hormones

Ideal drug   Drug that is both effective and safe, producing no side effects or adverse reactions; only a theoretical construct

Idiosyncratic drug reaction   Unexpected, unusual response to a drug

Immune serum   Serum from an animal immune against a specific pathogen for injection into a patient with the disease from the same organism; a blood component

Immunity   Antibody protection against a disease, especially infectious diseases

Immunodeficiency   Decreased or compromised ability of the body to respond to an antigen with an appropriate immune response

Immunoglobulins or immune globulins   Blood products that contain disease-specific antibodies for passive immunity

Immunostimulant   Agent that stimulates the activity of the immune system

Immunosuppressant   Agent that interferes with the normal reactions of the immune system to an antigen; used in arthritis treatment and organ transplantation to prevent the production of antibodies to foreign antigens

Impetigo   Inflammatory skin disease with isolated pustules that become crusted and break down; usually caused by streptococci or staphylococci

Implant   Form of medication placed under the skin for long-term, controlled release; also called a *pellet*

Incontinence   Inability to hold or retain urine

Indication   Reason to use a particular drug for a particular disorder

Inebriation   State of intoxication or drunkenness

Inert ingredient   Ingredient that has little or no effect on body functions; used to provide substance to active ingredient

Inotropic effect   Increase or decrease in the force of myocardial contraction

Inscription   Part of the prescription that indicates the name of a drug and dosage prescribed

Intermittent claudication   Severe pain in the calf muscles that occurs during exercise because of inadequate blood supply to the lower extremities

Intradermal   Into or within the dermis of the skin

Intramuscular   Into or within a muscle

Intravenous   Into or within a vein

Ion   Atom or molecule bearing a positive (cation) or negative (anion) electric charge; in aqueous solutions and in the body fluids, ions are charged electrolytes

Irritant   Drug applied to produce inflammation at the site of administration

Islets of Langerhans   Cluster of cells in the pancreas that produce insulin

Isotonic   Referring to solutions with the same tonicity; in physiology, solutions that are compatible with normal body tissue on the basis of having the same concentration of solutes as is found in that body tissue (e.g., physiologic salt solution and normal saline)

Keratin   Tough protein substance in the hair, nails, and stratum corneum

Keratitis   Inflammation of the cornea

Keratolytic agent   Agent that causes or promotes the shedding of skin

Kernicterus   Jaundice occurring in infants during the second to eighth day of life

Killed vaccines   Vaccines made from whole killed microbes and their components

Laxative   Substance that acts to promote and facilitate the evacuation of bowel contents, thus alleviating constipation

Legend drug   Drug that requires an order from a licensed health care provider for dispensing (synonym: prescription drug)

Lethargy   Feeling of sluggishness

Liniment   Medication that combines oil, soap, water, or alcohol and is placed on the skin to produce heat

Liter   Basic measurement unit of volume (liquid/gas) in the metric system

Live vaccines   Vaccines composed of live microbes that have been rendered avirulent

Local action   Drug action of a medication at the site of administration or in the surrounding tissues

Lotion   Free-flowing liquid or formulation with ingredients suspended in water, for application to the skin

Low-density lipoprotein (LDL)   Simple proteins that are combined with lipids—cholesterol, phospholipids, and triglycerides; a high level of LDL lipoproteins is undesirable

Lozenge   Hard, dry medication held in the mouth to dissolve

Magma   Suspension of fine particles in small amount of water

Maintenance medication   Medication prescribed to maintain a condition of health; usually used with a chronic disease process

Malaise   Discomfort or a nonspecific feeling of uneasiness, often a sign of illness

Malignant   Cancerous

Managed health care   Methods for financing and organizing the delivery of health care in which costs are contained by controlling the services provided

Medication administration   Introduction of a medication into the body or its application to the body; the giving of a dose of medicine

Medication error   Mistake made in prescribing, administering, or dispensing a medication. This may include administering the wrong medicine or the incorrect dose, using the incorrect route, failing to administer a medicine that has been ordered, giving the medicine at the incorrect time, or giving the medicine to the wrong patient.

Medication order   Written or verbal (oral) order for administration of a medication in a health care setting

Meniscus   Concave curvature made by a solution when poured into a container; in pharmacology, the liquid is poured into a calibrated measuring cup

Metabolism   Physical or chemical processes in the body that inactivate a drug for excretion from the body; biotransformation

Metastasis   Change in the location of a disease or its manifestations from one body organ or area to another; a secondary growth of malignant cells in a new location

Meter   Basic measurement unit of length in the metric system

Metered dose inhaler   Breath-activated device that delivers a given amount of a fine mist of medication directly to the mucous membranes of the respiratory tract

Metric system   Measurement system based on powers of 10 considered to be the international standard for scientific and industrial measurements using grams, liters, and meters

Microbe   Unicellular or small multicellular organism

Microbiology   Study of microscopic organisms

Milliequivalent   Weight of a drug (usually milligrams) in a volume (usually liters) of solution

Mineral   Inorganic (neither plant nor animal) solid substance, usually a component of the earth's crust

Mineralocorticoid   Hormone secreted by the adrenal cortex that is primarily involved in the regulation of fluid and electrolytes through actions on ion transport and the renal tubules

Minim   Smallest unit of volume (liquid) in the apothecary system; approximately a drop in household measure

Miosis   Constriction of the pupil

Miotic   Agent that causes the pupil to constrict (contract)

Mitotic alkaloids   Group of alkaline materials obtained from plants that interfere with cell division

Morbidity   Illness or disease state

Mortality   Death

Mucokinetic agent   Medication that removes excessive or abnormal secretions from the respiratory tract

Mucolytic   Agent that decreases the viscosity or thickness of sputum or other secretions of the respiratory tract

Mucus   Viscid fluid secreted by mucous membranes and glands containing mucin, white cells, epithelial cells, and water and salts such as the fluids from the mucous glands of the mouth

Muscle spasm   Sudden involuntary muscular contraction

Muscle spasticity   Increased tone or contractions of muscle, causing stiff and awkward movements

Mutagenic   Causing a change in genetic structure

Myasthenia gravis   Disease with symptoms of great muscular weakness (without muscle atrophy) and progressive fatigue on exertion

Mydriasis   Dilation of the pupil

Myocardial infarction (MI)   Deprivation of the myocardium of blood supply to the heart owing to blockage of the coronary arteries with resultant necrosis of the myocardium; heart attack

Myopia   Visual refractive error; nearsightedness

Narcotic   Older term for a controlled drug that depresses the central nervous system to relieve pain and has the potential to cause habituation or addiction

Narrow-spectrum antibiotic   Antibiotic effective against only a few or specific microorganisms

National Drug Code (NDC)   Number on drug label that identifies the manufacturer, product substances, and size of container

National Formulary (NF)   List of officially recognized names of drugs that have an established usefulness

Natural immunity   Immunity that is genetically determined by species, families, or populations

Naturally acquired active immunity   Immunity that is more or less permanent by species or from disease processes forming antibodies

Naturally acquired passive immunity   Immunity passed from mother to child, either in utero or in breast milk; immunity from natural inherent factors

Nebulizer   Breath-activated device that delivers a fine spray of micronized powder into the mucous membranes of the respiratory tract

Necrosis   Death of tissue or bone in areas that are surrounded by healthy tissue

Negative feedback   Control mechanism in which a stimulus produces a response that reverses or reduces a previous stimulation, thereby stopping the initial response

Neoplasm   New and abnormal formation of tissue

Neurohormones   Hormones found in portions of the nervous system such as the catecholamines

Neuroleptic   Another name for medication used to treat psychosis

Neuron   Nerve cell

Neurosis   Abnormal behavior from increased anxiety, tension, or emotional imbalance

Nits   Eggs of lice

Nocturia   Excessive urination at night

Nomogram   Measuring device used to show relationships among numerical values; set up as a graph, it is the most accurate means of calculating the dose of medication based on weight and height, usually used with pediatric and geriatric patients

Nonopioid analgesic   Analgesic that contains no opium, its derivatives, or synthetic opioid medications

Nonparenteral medications   Medications taken by mouth or through mucous membranes or skin such as ears, eyes, nose, or rectum

Nonproductive cough   Cough in which no exudate is expelled

Nonsalicylate   Antiinflammatory agent that does not contain salicylic acid (e.g., Tylenol, naproxen)

Nonsteroidal antiinflammatory drug (NSAID)   Antiinflammatory medication that does not contain a steroid preparation

Normal flora   Bacteria and microorganisms normally found on or within the body; may be potentially pathogenic when the body is not in homeostasis

Novolin pen   Prefilled, multiuse cartridge of insulin that allows a dosage to be dialed for administration of correct dose

Nutrient   Food or substance that supplies the body with the necessary elements for metabolism and body nourishment

Nystagmus   Constant involuntary movement of the eye in any direction

Occlusive dressing   Dressing that does not allow air to enter under the dressing (e.g., plastic wrap)

Ocular insert   Medication enclosed in small transparent membranes for placement in the eye

Oil   Thick, greasy liquid that is either volatile (to impact an aroma) or fixed

Ointment   Semisolid in greasy base that is not absorbed into the skin, but the medication is absorbed from the greasy base

Ophthalmic preparations   Medications used in the eye

Opiate   Drug containing or derived from opium; a narcotic

Opioid analgesic   Drug that is a synthetic pain medication with the strength of a morphine-like substance but is not derived from opium

Opportunistic infection   Infection that is present because the immune system cannot fight the normal flora found on the body or in the environment; resident flora proliferate and infect the body

Orthostatic hypotension   Drop in blood pressure that a person experiences when changing from a supine to an upright position

Ossification   Formation of bone

Osteoarthritis   Chronic noninflammatory autoimmune disease of the joints, especially weightbearing joints, that causes destruction of the joints

Osteomalacia   Disease in which softening of the bones causes flexibility and brittleness, leading to deformities; the adult form of rickets in children

Osteoporosis   Disease with reduction of bone mass that tends to occur in the elderly; bones become porous

Otic preparations   Medications used in the ear

Otitis media   Infection of the middle ear; also called tympanitis

Ototoxicity   Detrimental effect from medications on the eighth cranial nerve or the organ of hearing

Over-the-counter (OTC) drug   Drug that does not require a prescription; nonlegend drug

Package insert   Comprehensive, concise description of a medication developed by the manufacturer that accompanies any legend drug; required by the Food and Drug Administration for all pharmaceutics

Pain perception   Point at which a person becomes aware of a painful stimulus

Pain threshold   Point at which a person acknowledges that the stimulus is painful

Pain tolerance   Person's ability to tolerate pain

Palliative   Alleviating a symptom without curing the condition causing the symptom

Palliative medication   Medication prescribed to reduce the severity of condition or disease or its symptoms but not to provide a cure

Pannus   Inflamed synovial granulation tissue of joints found in rheumatoid arthritis

Papule   Small, red, elevated area on skin that precedes pustules; pimple

Parasite   Organism that lives within, upon, or at the expense of another without contributing to survival

Parasympathetic nervous system   Portion of the autonomic nervous system that conserves energy and restores body resources in rest and digestion ("feed-or-breed" action)

Parasympatholytic (anticholinergic or cholinergic blocking agent)   Agent that blocks the action of the parasympathetic nervous system

Parenteral route   Route by which medications are given through the skin by injection such as intramuscular, intradermal, subcutaneous, intravenous

Paresthesia   Sensation of numbness, prickling, or tingling

Parkinson's disease   Chronic nervous system disease characterized by fine, slowly spreading tremors and muscular weakness and rigidity, accompanied by a characteristic shuffling gait

Passive immunity   Immunity acquired from the injection or passage of antibodies from an immune person or animal to another or short-term immunity or immunity passed from mother to child

Paste   Stiff, thick, semisolid medicated preparation that adheres to the skin

Patent   State where an object is open, as in an open airway

Pathogen   Organism capable of causing disease; usually a microorganism

Pathology   Study of the causes of diseases, involving structure or function; condition produced by disease

Pediculicide   Agent that kills lice

Pellet   See *implant*

Percutaneous   Route through the skin; in pharmacology, refers to medications absorbed through the skin or mucous membranes such as topical, buccal, transdermal

Percutaneous route   Route by which medications are applied to the skin or mucous membranes such as topical, buccal, transdermal

Peripheral nervous system   Portions of the nervous system outside the brain and spinal cord

Peripheral vascular resistance   Resistance of blood flow through the arterial vascular system, especially arterioles and capillaries

Peristalsis   Progressive wavelike involuntary movement that occurs in a hollow tubular body organ; for moving food and waste materials through the gastrointestinal tract

Pharmacodynamic agent   Substance that alters normal body function in some way

Pharmacodynamics   Interactions of drugs and living tissues

Pharmacognosy   Branch of pharmacology dealing with the origins of drugs (natural or manufactured sources)

Pharmacokinetics   Processing of drugs by the body

Pharmacology   Study of drugs, their uses, and their interactions with living systems

Pharmacotherapeutics   Effects of drugs in the treatment of disease

Photophobia   Abnormal intolerance of light

Physical dependence   Craving for drugs because of extended use, so the drugs have taken over the individual's life and have affected normal body functioning; discontinuation of use of the drug typically results in withdrawal symptoms

***Physicians' Desk Reference* (PDR)**   Book, published yearly, that is a compilation of drug package inserts

Placebo   Medication with no pharmacologic or therapeutic effect that is used to satisfy a patient's psychologic need for medication

Plant alkaloids   Group of organic alkaline substances obtained from plants for medicinal purposes

Plaster   Solid or semisolid, medicated or nonmedicated preparation that adheres to the skin

Point of maximum impulse (PMI)   Landmark in the fifth intercostal space, 2 inches to the left of midline, where the pulse of the heart can be felt most strongly

Polypharmacy   Indiscriminate use, whether intentional or unintentional, of multiple drugs at the same time (commonly found with the elderly)

Potency   Strength of a medication

Potentiation   Prolongation or increase in the effect of a drug by another drug

Powder   Medication in fine particle form; may be reconstituted into other forms of medications or used as a powder

Precaution   Specific warning to consider when prescribing or administering medications

Precipitate   Insoluble granules or solid particles that separate from a solution

Premeasured cartridge   Premeasured, one-dose amount of medication in a disposable cartridge

Presbyopia   Inability of the lens to accommodate to near objects because of the rigidity of the lens caused by aging

Prescribe   To indicate, either in writing or orally, a medication to be given

Prescription   Written order for dispensing or administering medications, usually by a physician, dentist, or other licensed health care provider as allowed by law

Preventive (prophylactic) medication   Medication prescribed to prevent a disease or illness, or to lessen its severity

Priapism   Frequent or continuous erections in the male

Productive cough   Cough in which mucus or an exudate is expelled

Progestin   Female sex hormone secreted by the corpus luteum

Prokinetic agent   Agent used to stimulate gastrointestinal motility by reducing esophageal sphincter pressure and accelerating gastric and intestinal emptying

Proliferation   Rapid and repeated reproduction by cell division

Prophylactic agent   Drug used to prevent pregnancy or illness

Proportional method   Process of setting up dosage problems by comparing the relationships between two ratios that are considered equivalent

Proteolytic enzyme   Enzyme that helps break down proteins into usable peptides

Protozoa   Single-celled parasitic organisms (singular: protozoon)

PSD   Packaging, storage, and distribution

Psoriasis   Chronic disease of the skin with silvery, yellow-white lesions that form plaques with distinct borders

Psychoanalysis   Method of obtaining mental and emotional history of past experiences that are currently affecting mental disorders

Psychologic drug dependence or habituation   Accustomization to a drug through frequent use or exposure or repeated administration of medications for the patient's mental sense of well-being; the craving for a drug because of frequent use

Psychosis   Mental illness accompanied by bizarre behavior and altered personality with failure to perceive reality

Psychotherapy   Treatment of mental illness through mental means rather than physical or chemical therapy

Pustule   Small elevation of the skin filled with lymph or pus

Pyuria   Pus in the urine

Radioisotope   Radioactive form of an element; used to diagnose or treat neoplasms

Ratio   Expression that compares two quantities; a colon usually separates the two quantities

Rebound congestion   Reflex response of nasal congestion that occurs following the prolonged daily use of decongestants; nasal congestion caused by the body's response to prolonged depression of the mucous membranes' secretions by medication

Receptor site   Cell component that combines with a drug to alter cell function; in pharmacology, the part of a cell that interacts with drugs

Recombinant DNA technology   Genetic engineering technology used to create new drugs

Reconstitution   Process of adding a fluid such as water or saline to a powdered form of a drug, making a specific dosage strength

Refill   Additional medication or treatment to be dispensed if prescribed

Regurgitation   Backward flow; the return of stomach contents to the mouth, as in vomitus

Replacement medication   Medication used to replace missing chemicals in the body

Replacement therapy   Therapeutic replacement of lost body substances including hormones, electrolytes, and fluids

Respondeat superior   Legal premise in which the employer is held responsible/liable for the wrongful actions of an employee that may cause injury or damage as long as the employee works within the scope of practice; literally, "Let the master answer"

Rhinitis   Inflammation of the nasal mucous membranes

Rhinorrhea   Runny nose

Safe drug   Drug that causes no harmful effects when taken in high doses over a long period of time

Salicylate   Antiinflammatory drug compound containing salicylic acid (e.g., aspirin)

Salt   Chemical compound resulting from the interaction of an acid and a base

Sanitization   Process of cleaning and removing dirt from objects

Scabicide   Agent that kills scabies

Schizophrenia   Group of mental disorders of unknown etiology that affect thinking, affect, and behavior

Seborrheic dermatitis   Inflammatory skin disease of unknown etiology that exhibits yellow or brown-gray greasy scales

Sebum   Fatty secretion from the sebaceous glands of the skin

Sedative   Medication used to reduce the desire for physical activity and produce a calming effect

Seizure   Epileptic event

Side effect   Mild or annoying but expected and fairly common undesirable response to a medication

Signature (Sig or Signa)   Part of prescription that indicates the proper dosage of medication to be taken

Skin cleanser   Agent used as soap to remove debris, bacteria, and waste products from the skin

Solubility   Ability of particles to be dissolved

Solute   Substance dissolved in a solution or body fluids

Solution   Medication dissolved in a liquid vehicle

Solvent   Liquid in which substances are dissolved (e.g., water in the body)

Spacer   Aerochamber used with metered dose inhalers

Spasticity   Phenomenon in which uncoordinated movements are caused by CNS overstimulation

Spirits   Alcoholic or hydroalcoholic solutions containing volatile aromatic ingredients

Sputum   Substance obtained and expelled from coughing or clearing of the throat containing a variety of materials from the respiratory tract

Standardization   See *drug standards*

Standard protocol Written description of one or more steps to be taken in treating specific medical problems; this should be signed by the appropriate health care provider

Standing order Request for a procedure that is a routine for certain medical treatments under certain conditions

Sterilization Process of destroying all microorganisms and spores

Steroid Hormone produced by the adrenal cortex

Stimulant Drug that acts to increase the function or activity of a body part

Stomatitis Inflammation of the mouth

Subcutaneous Beneath the skin; injected into the subcutaneous tissue

Sublingual tablet Tablet designed to dissolve under the tongue

Subscription Part of the prescription containing the directions for the pharmacist with the information for compounding ingredients if necessary

Summation Combining of drugs to achieve the expected effect of each drug

Superinfection New infection that appears during the course of treatment for a primary infection

Superscription Portion of a prescription designated with the symbol R_x

Supplemental medication Medication used to avoid deficiencies or to achieve necessary levels of existing body chemicals

Supportive medication Medication prescribed to assist with maintenance of homeostasis until a disease process can be resolved

Suppository Medication carried in cocoa butter, hydrogenated vegetable oil, or glycerinated gelatin to form a solid dose for insertion into a body orifice such as the vagina, urethra, or rectum

Suspension Medication in the form of undissolved particles dispersed in a liquid vehicle

Sustained-release tablet Tablet form of medication in which the medication is released over a period of time; also called *controlled-release tablet*

Sustained-released/timed-release capsule Capsule form of medication in which the medication is released over a desired period of time of known duration

Sympathetic nervous system Portion of autonomic nervous system that mobilizes a person in an emergency situation ("fight-or-flight" reaction)

Sympatholytic (or adrenergic blocking) agent Agent that blocks the action of the sympathetic nervous system

Sympathomimetic agent Agent that acts to simulate or mimic the sympathetic nervous system

Synergism Working together of two or more drugs to produce a stronger effect than could be achieved with each drug taken alone

Synthetic or manufactured drug Drug that has been created chemically in the laboratory without the use of plant or animal products

Syrup Aqueous solution sweetened with sugar or a sugar substitute to disguise taste

Systemic action Drug action found at more than the site of administration, usually tissues throughout the body

Tablet Dried powder form of medication that has been compressed into a small disk

Tardive dyskinesia Slow, rhythmical, involuntary movement as a result of the use of psychotropic drugs

Target organ Site to which the effects of a drug, hormone, or therapeutic agent are primarily directed

Tenacious Thick, viscous

Tenacious cough Stubborn, retentive, or persistent cough with thick, viscous exudate

Teratogen Agent that adversely affects the development of an embryo or fetus

Teratogenic Capable of causing abnormal cellular development of an embryo or fetus

Tetany Hyperexcitability of nerves and muscles characterized by spasms, cramps, and twitching

Therapeutic medication/agent Medication used in the treatment of a condition or disease to relieve symptoms or effect a cure

Thromboembolism Embolism; the blocking of a blood vessel by a detached embolus

Thrombus Blood clot that obstructs the lumen of a blood vessel

Tincture Alcohol-based liquid used as a skin disinfectant

Tinnitus Ringing in the ears

Tolerance Decreased response to a medication following prolonged use of a drug

Tonic Pertaining to muscular tension or contraction

Tonometry Measurement of intraocular pressure; used to diagnose glaucoma

Topical Adjective denoting surface; in pharmacology, refers to medications applied to a surface area or locally to the skin or mucous membrane

Tourette's syndrome Rare disease of unknown etiology characterized by lack of muscle control, tics, purposeless movements, and incoherent grunts and barks

Toxic Poisonous

Toxicology Study of poisonous effects of drugs

Toxoid Bacteria toxins that have been changed to a nontoxic state for immunization

Trade name Brand name given to a drug by its manufacturer

Tranquilization State of reduced mental tension characterized by calmness, but without significant sedation or mental confusion

Transdermal Through the skin; in pharmacology, refers to medications that are applied to the skin for local or systemic effect

Transdermal patch/disk Drug-containing patch or disk that is applied to the skin, through which the drug is absorbed

Troche Hard disk of medication designed to dissolve in the mouth for local effect; similar to lozenge

Tropic hormone Hormone secreted by the pituitary gland that stimulates the production of another hormone; also known as a *stimulating hormone* (e.g., thyroid-stimulating hormone)

Tumor Swelling or enlargement; new growth formation

Tympanic membrane Eardrum

Ulcer Open sore including sores of mucous membranes, as in the stomach and duodenum

Ulceration Lesion of the skin or mucous membrane accompanied by sloughing of the inflamed necrotic tissue

Unit Basic quantity used when calculating desired dosages to indicate the strength of a particular medication; the unit is unique for each drug, based on the drug's strength in a basic measurement system (e.g., grain, gram, milligram)

United States Pharmacopoeia (USP) Official guide prepared by a national group of pharmaceutical professionals and issued every 5 years (with periodic supplements) by the U.S. government giving the approved formulas and information on the preparation and dispensing of medications found in the United States

United States Pharmacopoeia/Dispensing Information (USP/DI) Compendium of practical information about medications approved by USP

United States Pharmacopoeia/National Formulary (USP/NF) Official drug reference book for medications approved in the United States; combination of USP and NF

Urgency Sudden, uncontrollable need to urinate

Usage Application/administration of a medication for a given purpose

Uveitis Inflammation of the uveal tract (iris, choroid, and ciliary body)

Vaccination Process of immunization for prevention of diseases

Vaccine Preparation containing a suspension of whole or fractionated microorganisms that on administration causes the recipient to form antibodies to a disease

Vasocongestion Congestion of the blood vessels

Vector Carrier, usually an insect, which transmits pathogens (disease-causing organisms) from infected to noninfected individuals without the carrier itself acquiring the disease

Vehicle Inactive agent that carries an active medicinal ingredient

Verbal order Request for medications or procedures that is given orally rather than in writing

Vertigo Sense that the environment or oneself is revolving

Very-low-density lipoprotein (VLDL) Simple protein that is combined with lipid-cholesterol, phospholipids, and triglycerides; a high level of these proteins is undesirable

Vial Glass or plastic container with a metal-enclosed rubber seal for injectable medications; may hold single or multiple doses

Virulence Disease-producing strength of a microorganism

Virus Bundle of genetic material in a protein coat that requires a host for nutrition and reproduction; sometimes considered to be a one-celled microorganism

Viscosity Thickness of a substance

Viscous solution Thick, often oil-based solution; when referring to injections, a solution with a viscous base is much thicker than an aqueous solution and is, therefore, given intramuscularly

Viscous suspension Thick gummy or gelatinous compound made up of solid particles mixed, but not dissolved, in a fluid

Vitamin General term for a number of organic substances necessary in trace amounts for normal growth, development, metabolism, and release of energy from food; exclusive of proteins, carbohydrates, fats, and organic salts

Wheal Round or elongated elevation of the skin, which can be produced by intradermal injections

Index

A

Abacavir (Ziagen), 357t
Abatacept (Orencia), 486
Abbokinase (urokinase), 576
Abbreviations used in medication
    orders, 85-86
Abilify (aripiprazole), 666
Abreva (docosanol), 497
Absinthe, 399t
Absorbable gelatin foam, 578
Absorbine (tolnaftate), 248
Absorption, drug, 33-34, 34t, 35t, 67
    dermatologic, 457-58
Abuse, drug, 14, 15
    alcohol, 617, 685t, 686-88
    anabolic steroids, 694
    behaviors of, 682-83
    central nervous system
        stimulants, 689-90
    defined, 681
    factors that contribute to, 681-82
    hallucinogens, psychedelics,
        and psychomimetics, 692-93
    inhalants, 693-94
    nicotine, 683-85
    opiates and opioids, 688-89
    over-the-counter, 303
    patient care, 694-95
    preventing, 24-25
    signs of, 695-96
Acamprosate (Campral), 686, 687
Accolate (zafirlukast), 541
Accommodation, lens, 437
Accumulation, 43
Accutane (isotretinoin), 388t, 463
ACE inhibitors, 568, 571t, 580
Acetaminophen, 296, 297t
    and caffeine, 299
    codeine, and butalbital, 299t
    combinations, 298, 299t

Acetaminophen (Continued)
    for migraine headaches, 639
    and oxycodone, 299t
Acetasol Solution (hydrocortisone-
        acetic acid), 451t
Acetic acid solutions (Vo-Sol), 451t
Acetylcholine (ACh), 621, 636, 645,
        674
Acetylcysteine (Mucomyst), 536
Achromycin (tetracycline), 344t
Acid-base balance, 390, 392t, 393t
Acid rebound, 500
AcipHex (rabeprazole), 503
Acne preparations, 463, 466-68
Acquired antibiotic resistance,
        336
Acquired immunity
    active, 306, 307f, 308-11
    passive, 306, 307f, 322, 324, 326t
ACTH, 408-9
Actigall (ursodiol), 506
Actinic keratosis, 473
Actinomycin D (dactinomycin),
        376t
Action, drug. See
        Pharmacodynamics
Actiq buccal lozenges (fentanyl),
        293t
Activase (alteplase), 576
Active immunity, 307t
    artificially acquired, 306, 307f,
        315-22
    patient safety and, 321-22
Active ingredients, 30
Actonel (risedronate), 477-78
Acute pain, 290-91
Acyclovir (Zovirax), 357t, 497
Adacel, 319t
Adalat (nifedipine), 555
Adalimumab (Humira), 486
Adapalene (Differin), 466
Adderall (amphetamine sulfate),
        676

Addiction, drug, 14, 15, 24-25
Addition
    decimals, 113-14
    fractions, 103-5
Adjuvant medications, 292, 298,
        299-300t
Administration, medication
    anesthetics, 626-27
    "befores" of, 231-32, 237
    buccal and sublingual, 252
    inhaled, 59t, 257-59
    injectable, 274
    nasal, 254-56
    ophthalmic, 252-53
    oral, 238, 239-41p, 242b
    OSHA standards, 228-29, 237-38
    otic, 59t, 253-54, 255p
    parenteral, 274-81, 282-83p, 284t
    rectal, 241-45
    "rights," 232-33, 237
    routes of, 34t, 35t, 67, 234-35
        injection, 274-81, 282-83p
    3 + 7 rules, 231-33, 237
    safe, 227, 228b, 230-31
    steroids, 415, 418
    time of, 67
    topical, 34, 58, 247, 248-52
    transdermal, 58, 59t, 61f, 234,
        247-52
    vaginal, 59t, 256-57
A & D ointment, 388t
Adolescents, 312
Adrenal cortex hormones, 414-15
Adrenal steroid inhibitors, 418
Adrenergic agonists, 442, 600, 601t,
        645, 648, 649t
Adrenergic-inhibiting agents, 568,
        569-70t, 648-50
Adrenocorticotropic hormone
        (ACTH), 408-9
Adriamycin (doxorubicin), 376t
Adrucil (fluorouracil), 375t
Adsorbents, 516

Page numbers followed by b indicate
boxes; f, figures; p, procedures; t, tables.

Advair Diskus, 59t
Adverse reactions, 40, 41, 41b
　to immunizations, 314
　to insulin, 428
Advil (ibuprofen), 297t
Aerobic bacteria, 334
Aerosols, 59t, 251
　foams, 59t
Affective disorders, 668
Aftate (tolnaftate), 248
Age and drug dosing, 65, 70
Agenerase (amprenavir), 358t
Aggregation of platelets, 576
Aggrenox, 652
Airborne, 532, 533
Akathisia, 665
Albuterol MDI, 59t
Albuterol (Ventolin), 59t, 537
Alcohol
　abuse, 617, 685t, 686-88
　preparations, 360
Aldactone (spironolactone), 567,
　617
Aldomet (methyldopa), 617
Aldosterone receptor antagonists,
　568, 569t
Alefacept (Amevive), 473
Alendronate (Fosamax), 477-78
Aleve (naproxen), 297t
Alfalfa, 398t
Alkaloids, 31, 639
Alka Seltzer, 57, 296, 297t, 299t, 502t
Alkeran (melphalan), 374t
Alkylating agents, 372, 374t
Alkylating-like agents, 372
Allergic reactions, 40
　allergic rhinitis, 427, 534t
　herbal supplements for, 399b
Allied health professionals, 3, 3f
　awareness of cultural differences,
　　76-77
　drug cards for, 53-54
　duties in the medication pathway,
　　6-8
　ethics, 25-27
　legal implications for, 9
　patient confidentiality and, 89
　role in medication administration,
　　24-27
Allopurinol (Zyloprim), 487
Aloe, 397t
Alopecia, 370
Aloprim (allopurinol), 487
Aloxi (palonosetron HCL), 370t
Alpha-adrenergic blockers, 600,
　601t, 651t
Alpha/beta-blockers, 568, 569t
Alpha-glucosidase inhibitors, 429
Alpha-interferon (Roferon-A), 328,
　328t

Alpha-Keri, 458
Alpha-tocopherol, 384t, 387
Alprazolam (Xanax), 613
Alteplase (Activase), 576
Alternate-day therapy (ADT), 415
Alternative medications, 394-400
Aluminum, 500, 501
Alzheimer's disease, 646, 674-75,
　678
Amantadine (Symmetrel), 357t, 636
Ambien (zolpidem), 631
Amendment to Applications for
　FDA Approval to Market New
　Drugs, 15, 18b
Amenorrhea, 614
American Dental Association, 496
Amethopterin (methotrexate), 375t
Amevive (alefacept), 473
Amikacin (Amikin), 345t
Amikin (amikacin), 345t
Amino acids, 406
Aminoglycosides, 344, 345t
Amiodarone (Cordarone), 561
Amitriptyline (Elavil), 300t, 640
Amlodipine (Norvasc), 555
Amoxicillin (Amoxil, Trimox,
　Polymox), 339t, 504
Amoxicillin-clavulanate
　(Augmentin), 339t
Amoxil (amoxicillin), 339t
Amphetamine abuse, 689
Amphetamine sulfate (Adderall),
　676
Amphotericin B (Fungizone), 353t
Ampicillin (Principen, Omnipen,
　Polycillin), 339t
Amprenavir (Agenerase), 358t
Ampules, 58, 263, 267, 268p, 283
　mixing medications in, 273
Amyl nitrate, 551t, 617
Anabolic steroids, 598-600, 599t,
　618, 694
Anabolic Steroids Control Act of
　1990, 15
Anacin, 295, 299t
Anaerobic bacteria, 334
Anafranil (clomipramine), 617, 659
Anakinra (Kineret), 486
Analeptics, 642
Analgesics
　acetaminophen, 296
　adjuvant, 298, 299-300t
　advantages and disadvantages of,
　　301t
　for arthritis, 481-85
　in children, 300, 302
　combined, 298
　defined, 291
　in the elderly, 302
　for migraine headaches, 639, 640t

Analgesics (Continued)
　neurologic effects, 624-25, 653
　nonopioid, 291, 292, 295-98
　nonsteroidal antiinflammatory,
　　296
　opioid and opiate, 292-95
　oral versus rectal, 301t
　otic, 450, 452t
　over-the-counter, 301t, 302t
　salicylate, 295-96, 297t
　types of, 291-92
　urinary tract, 589t, 590
Anaphylaxis, 40, 336
　immunizations and, 314
Anastrozole (Arimidex), 376t, 377t
Anatomy and physiology in
　pharmacology, 3
Ancef (cefadroxil), 342t
Androgel, 598
Androgens, 596, 598, 599t, 617
Androgen (Teslac), 376t
Anemia, 392t, 579
Anesthetics
　general, 625-26, 653
　local, 626-27, 653
　mouth, 496-500
　ocular, 442
　route of administration, 626
　topical, 59t, 468, 496-500, 627
Angina pectoris, 550-56
Angiotensin converting enzyme
　inhibitors. See ACE inhibitors
Angiotensin II receptor antagonists,
　570t
Anistreplase (Eminase), 576
Ankylosis, 480
Anorectal preparations, 517-18
Anorexia, 587
Anorexiant drugs, 518-20, 521, 642
Anspor (cephradine), 342t
Antabuse (disulfiram), 57b, 686, 687
Antacids, 295, 392t, 500
Antagonism, 42
Anterior pituitary gland, 408-9
Anthelmintic drugs, 511, 518, 521
Antiallergic agents, 447
Antiandrogens, 376t
Antibacterial drugs
　aminoglycosides, 344
　cephalosporins, 340-41, 342t
　macrolides, 341, 343t
　penicillins, 332, 333, 338-40
　quinolone, 344-45
　sulfonamides, 332, 348, 349t
　tetracyclines, 69, 72, 342-44
　See also Antibiotics
Antibiotics
　acne vulgaris and, 463, 466
　antitumor, 373, 376-77t
　broad-spectrum, 333

Antibiotics *(Continued)*
  compared to antimicrobials, 334
  defined, 332-33
  factors in choice of, 335-36
  miscellaneous, 345-46, 347t
  misuse of, 337, 362
  narrow-spectrum, 333
  ointments, 59t
  otic, 451t
  over-the-counter, 346-48
  patient factors in choice of, 335-36
  peptic ulcers and, 504-5
  prophylactic use of, 336-37
  resistance, acquired, 336
  sensitivity, 335
  superinfections and, 336
  topical, 459
  See also Antibacterial drugs
Antibodies, 308, 311
  titer, 313
Anticholinergic agents, 442, 504, 507, 539t, 540, 645, 647-48
Anticoagulants, 295-96, 576, 578t
Anticonvulsants, 300t, 392t
Antidepressants
  antimanic medications, 673-74
  atypical, 669-71
  monoamine oxidase inhibitors, 671-72
  natural reuptake inhibitors (NRIs), 673
  selective norepinephrine reuptake inhibitors (SNRIs), 673
  selective serotonin reuptake inhibitors, 670-71t, 672-73
  tricyclic, 300t, 659, 669, 670t
Antidiabetic agents, 428-30
Antidiarrheal agents, 515-17, 521
Antidiuretic hormone, 409
Antidysrhythmic drugs, 558-61, 580
Antiemetics, 506-10, 521
Antiestrogens, 376t
Antiflatulents, 500, 510
Antifungals, 59t, 352-55, 362
  oral, 497
  topical, 453, 464-65t
Antigen-antibody response, 308
Antihistamines, 300t, 527-29, 543, 617
  side effects, 632
Antihypertensive therapy. *See* Hypertension
Antiinfective agents
  ophthalmic, 438-39, 440t
  otic, 450
  topical, 459, 461-63
Antiinflammatory agents
  for arthritis, 481-85
  for the gastrointestinal tract, 517

Antiinflammatory agents *(Continued)*
  ophthalmic, 438-39, 440t
  topical, 459, 461-63
Antimalarials, 356, 358t
Antimanic medications, 673-74
Antimetabolites, 369, 372, 375-76t
Antimicrobials, 313
  antibiotic resistant, 336, 345
  bactericidal versus bacteriostatic, 334-35
  compared to antibiotics, 334
  quinolone, 344-45, 346t
  safety, 362
Antiminth (pyrantel), 518
Antineoplastic agents, 366
  classes of, 372-73, 374-78t
  drug delivery systems, 373
  function, 368-69
  handling and administering, 379-80
  side effects of, 369-71
  specific, 374-78t
  See also Chemotherapy
Antiplatelet medications, 576, 652
Antipruritics, 468
Antipsychotic drugs, 662-68, 677-78
Antiretroviral drugs, 355-56
Antisecretory agents, 500, 502
Antiseizure medications, 632-36
Antiseptics, 59t, 350, 356, 358-61
  versus disinfectants, 359
  ophthalmic, 440t
  oral, 496-500
  soaps, 458
  urinary tract, 588-90
Antispasmodics, 500, 504
  urinary tract, 589t, 590
Antistaphylococcal penicillins, 338, 339t
Antithyroid medications, 412
Antitoxins, 311, 312, 326t
Antitubercular drugs, 350-52
Antitumor antibiotics, 373, 376-77t
Antitussives, 533
Antiulcer medications, 500-505, 520
Antiviral drugs, 355-56, 357t
  oral, 497
  topical, 459, 461
Antragen (tretinoin), 377t
Anturane (sulfinpyrazone), 487
Anxiety
  and daily living, 658-59
  drugs for, 660-62
  generalized, 659, 662
Anxiolytics, 659, 660-62, 677
Apidra (glulisine), 421
Apothecary system, 139
  length measurements, 159-61
  volume measurements, 152-54
  weight measurements, 154-59

Appetite suppressants, 518-20
Aquasol A, 388t
Aquasol E, 388t
Aqueous humor, 437
Aralen (chloroquine), 358t
Aricept (donepezil), 675
Arimidex (anastrozole), 376t, 377t
Aripiprazole (Abilify), 666
Aristocort (triamcinolone), 485
Aromasin (exemestane), 378t
Arteriosclerosis, 550
Arthritis. *See* Osteoarthritis
Artificially acquired active immunity, 306, 307f, 315-22
Artificially acquired passive immunity, 306, 307f, 322, 324, 326t
Ascorbic acid, 389-90, 389t
Asian medicine, 396
Asparaginase (Elspar), 377t
Aspirin, 295-96, 297t
  caffeine and, 295, 299t
  with codeine, 299t
  combinations, 298, 299t
  for migraine headaches, 639
  propoxyphene, and caffeine (Darvon compound), 299t
  therapy, 317
Asthma
  treatments for, 537-42, 543
  weed, 399t
Astragalus, 397t
Atarax (hydroxyzine), 300t, 662
Ataxia, 449
Atenolol (Tenormin), 686
Atherosclerosis, 550, 573
Ativan (lorazepam), 370t, 507, 633, 659, 660
Atomoxetine (Strattera), 676
Atorvastatin (Lipitor), 575
Atrioventricular (AV) nodes, 561
Atromid-S (clofibrate), 575
Atrophy, skin, 460f
Atrovent (ipratropium), 540
Attention deficit/hyperactivity disorder, 675-76, 678
Attenuvax, 319t
Atypical antidepressants, 669-71
Auditory ossicles, 449
Augmentin (amoxicillin-clavulanate), 339t
Auralgia, 449
Aureomycin (chlortetracycline), 344t
Automaticity of the heart, 558
Autonomic nervous system, 622
  adrenergic agonists, 648, 649t
  adrenergic blocking agents, 648-50

Autonomic nervous system
   (Continued)
   anticholinergic or
      parasympatholytic
      medications, 647-48
   beta-adrenergic receptor
      blockers, 650-52
   cholinergic or
      parasympathomimetic
      medications, 645-46
   functions, 644-45
Auxiliary labeling, 84
Avandia (rosiglitazone), 429
Aveeno, 59t, 458, 468
Avelox (moxifloxacin), 346t
Avirulent microbes, 311
Avitaminosis, 384
Azathioprine (Imuran), 327, 328t,
   486
Azelaic acid (Azelex), 466
Azelex (azelaic acid), 466
Azithromycin, 175, 176f, 177t, 341,
   343t
Azlin (azlocillin), 339t
Azlocillin (Azlin), 339t
Azole antifungals, 353t
Azulfidine (sulfasalazine), 349t, 486,
   517

B

Bacampicillin (Spectrobid), 339t
Bacille Calmette-Guérin vaccine
   (TheraCys), 317, 320t, 377t
Bacitracin, 346
Baclofen (Lioresal), 489, 641
Bacteria
   aerobic, 334
   anaerobic, 334
   classification of, 333, 359
   facultative, 334
Bactericidal versus bacteriostatic
   agents, 334-35
Bactosill (oxacillin), 339t
Bactrim (trimethoprim
   sulfamethoxazole), 349t, 588
Bactroban cream, 59t
Balsalazide (Colazal), 517
Barbiturates, 628, 629t, 631, 633,
   634t, 690
Barrier contraceptive devices,
   610-11
Base balance, acid-, 390, 392t
Baths, 458
Bayer (aspirin), 297t
B-cells, 308, 328
BCG vaccine (TheraCys), 317, 320t,
   377t
B-C Powders, 57
Beconase (fluticasone), 59t
Behaviors of drug abuse, 682-83

Belladonna (Bellafoline), 399t
Benadryl (diphenhydramine), 37,
   468, 535, 617
Benazepril (Lotensin), 568
Benemid (probenecid), 487
Ben-Gay, 59t
Benign cancer, 366, 367f, 367t
Benign prostatic hypertrophy, 600,
   601t
Benzalkonium chloride (Zephiran),
   359
Benzisoxazoles, 663t
Benzodiazepines
   abuse, 691
   for alcoholism, 686
   anxiety and, 660, 661t, 678
   gastrointestinal system disorders
      and, 507
   neurologic disorders and, 629-30t,
      631, 634t, 653
   reproductive disorders and, 617
Benzonatate (Tessalon), 535
Benzoyl peroxide (Pan-Oxyl,
   Desquam, Benzox, Persa-Gel,
   Benzagel), 466
Benzphetamine (Didrex), 520
Bepridil (vasocon), 555
Beriberi, 384
Beta-adrenergic blockers
   autonomic nervous system and,
      650-52
   for cardiovascular disorders,
      537-39, 552-55, 554t, 558,
      561, 568, 569
   for migraine headaches, 640
Beta-adrenergic receptor blockers,
   439, 443t, 650-52
Betadine, 248
Betamethasone (Celestone), 485
Betapace (sotalol), 561
Bethanechol (Urecholine), 645
Bevel, needle, 266
Biaxin (clarithromycin), 341, 343t,
   504
Bicalutamide (Casodex), 376t
BiCNU (carmustine), 374t
Biguanides, 429
Bilberry, 398t
Bile acid sequestrants, 574t, 575
Biltricide (praziquantel), 518
Bioequivalency, 16
Biofeedback, 639
Biological response modifiers,
   377t
Bipolar disorder, 666
Biotin, 389
Biotransformation, 36
Bipolar disorder, 671t, 673-74
Bisacodyl (Dulcolax), 512
Bismuth salts (Pepto-Bismol), 504

Bisphosphates, 477-78
Bladder, 588, 590
Blenoxane (bleomycin), 376t
Bleomycin (Blenoxane), 376t
Blepharitis, 438
Blinx (boric acid), 360
Blood
   -brain barrier, 36, 622
   coagulation, 295-96, 575-79
   level, drug, 35
   platelets, 576
   pressure and hypertension,
      562
   vessel diseases, 572, 573t
   vitamin E and, 384t, 387
Body fluids
   balance, 207, 392t, 584-87
   and intravenous therapy,
      206-7
Body surface area, 65-66, 178-82
Bones. See Musculoskeletal
   system
Boniva (ibandronate), 477-78
Boric acid (Blinx, Collyrium), 360
Botulism antitoxin, 326t
Bowel evacuants, 515, 521
Bowel function, 294, 392t, 510-15,
   521
Brain, 36, 622
Brand-name drugs, 16, 50, 81
Breast cancer, 602
Broad-spectrum antibiotics, 333
Broad-spectrum penicillins, 338
Bromocriptine (Parlodel), 614,
   638
Bronchodilators, 538-39t, 543
Buccal medications, 252
Buckeye, 399t
Bufferin (aspirin), for pain, 295, 296,
   297t
Bulk-forming laxatives, 512
Bullas, skin, 460f
Bupropion (Wellbutrin, Zyban), 669,
   673, 684
Bureau of Narcotics and Dangerous
   Drugs (BNDD), 15
Burns, 399b
   topical treatment of, 468-70
Bursitis, 480
BuSpar (buspirone), 628, 659,
   662
Buspirone (BuSpar), 628, 659,
   662
Busulfan (Myleran), 374t
Butenafine gentian violet (Mentax),
   354t
Butorphanol nasal spray (Stadol),
   639
Butterfly needles, 213
Butyrophenones, 663t

C

CAD. *See* Coronary artery disease (CAD)
Caffeine
  in decongestants, 532
  salicylates and, 295, 299t
Calamine lotion and cream, 59t, 249, 468
Calan (verapamil), 555, 561, 641
Calciferol, 384t, 386-87, 388t
Calcitonin, 414
Calcitonin salmon (Calcimar, Miacalcin), 478
Calcitriol, 388t
Calcium, 386, 391, 392t
  channel blockers, 554t, 555, 561, 571-72, 640, 641
  loss, 586-87
  magnesium and, 393
  osteoporosis and, 476-77
Caldcrol, 388t
Calusterone (Methosarb), 376t
Camphorated opium tincture (Paregoric), 293t, 516
Campral (acamprosate), 686, 687
Camptosar (irinotecan), 378t
Cancer
  benign versus malignant, 366, 367f, 367t
  breast, 602
  defined, 366
  metastasis, 366-68
  morbidity and mortality, 366
  tumor classification, 368
  See also Chemotherapy
Cannulas, 206
Cantharidin (Cantharone), 468
Cantharone (cantharidin), 468
Capecitabine (Xeloda), 375t
Capsules, 55, 56b, 56t
Carafate (sucralfate), 501
Carbamazepine (Tegretol), 300t, 633, 635, 673
Carbenicillin (Geocillin), 339t
Carbidopa (Lodosyn), 636
Carbonic anhydrase inhibitors, 439
Carboplatin (Paraplatin), 374t
Carcinogenic substances, 379
Cardene (nicardipine), 555
Cardiac dysrhythmias, 558-61
Cardiac glycosides, 31, 556-57, 580
Cardiovascular system, the
  angina pectoris and, 550-56
  blood vessels diseases, 572, 573t
  cardiac dysrhythmias and, 558-61
  chemotherapy effects on, 370
  coagulation and, 295-96, 575-79
  congestive heart failure and, 556-58

Cardiovascular system, the (*Continued*)
  death and diseases of, 550, 579
  drug effects on, 549-61
    ACE inhibitors, 568, 571t
    adrenergic-inhibiting agents, 568, 569-70t
    anticoagulants, 575-78
    antidysrhythmic, 558-61
    antiplatelets, 575-78
    beta-adrenergic blockers, 552-55, 554t, 558, 561
    calcium channel blockers, 554t, 555, 561, 571-72
    diuretics, 565-68
    hematopoietic/erythropoietic stimulants, 579
    nitrates, 551-52, 553t
    vasodilators, 550, 556, 561, 568, 571t
  functions of, 547-48
  hyperlipidemia and, 572-75
  hypertension and, 561-72
Cardizem (diltiazem), 555, 561
Cardura (doxazosin), 568, 600
Carisoprodol (Soma), 488
Carminatives, 510
Carmustine (BiCNU), 374t
Cascara sagrada (Ex-Lax), 512
Casodex (bicalutamide), 376t
Castor oil, 512
Catapres (clonidine), 568, 617
Cataracts, 437
Catecholamines, 622
Cathartics, 515
Catheters, over-the-needle, 214f, 214
Cayenne, 397t
CCNU (lomustine), 374t
Ceclor (cefaclor), 342t
Cecon, 389t
Cedex (ceftibuten), 342t
Cefaclor (Ceclor), 342t
Cefadroxil (Ancef), 342t
Cefadyl (cephapirin), 342t
Cefamandole (Mandol), 342t
Cefazolin (Duricef), 342t
Cefdinir (Omnicef), 342t
Cefepime (Maxipime), 340, 342t
Cefixime (Suprax), 342t
Ceforanide (Precef), 342t
Cefotan (cefotetan), 342t
Cefotaxime (Claforan), 342t
Cefotetan (Cefotan), 342t
Cefoxitin (Mefoxin), 342t
Cefpodoxime (Vantin), 342t
Cefprozil (Cefzil), 342t
Ceftazidime (Fortaz, Tazidime), 342t
Ceftibuten (Cedex), 342t

Ceftin (cefuroxime), 342t
Ceftriaxone (Rocephin), 342t
Cefuroxime (Ceftin), 342t
Cefzil (cefprozil), 342t
Ceiling effect, 293
Celestone (betamethasone), 485
CellCept (mycophenolate mofetil), 327, 328t
Cells
  cancer, 366-68
  replication cycle, 369
Centers for Disease Control and Prevention (CDC)
  recommendations on immunizations, 313, 314-15
Centrally acting adrenergic inhibitors, 568, 570t
Central nervous system, the, 622-24, 653
  barbiturates and, 628, 629t, 631
  sedatives/hypnotics and, 627-32
    abuse, 690-92
  spasticity and, 488, 490, 491, 641, 642t
  stimulants, 642-43
    abuse, 689-90
Cephradine (Anspor, Velosef), 342t
Cephalexin (Keflex, Keftab), 342t
Cephalosporins, 340-41, 342t
  for urinary tract infections, 588
Cephulac (lactulose), 511
Cerebyx (fosphenytoin), 633
Cerubidine (daunorubicin), 377t
Cerumen, 450
Ceruminolytics, 450
Cervical caps, 611
Cevimeline (Evoxac), 497
Chalazion, 438
Chantix (varenicline), 684
Chemotherapy, 206, 366, 368
  hematopoietics and, 579
  selecting patients for, 371-72
  side effects, 369-71, 507b
  See also Antineoplastic agents
Chenix (chenodiol), 506
Chenodiol (Chenix), 506
Chickenpox vaccine, 316-17, 320t, 321t, 323t
Children
  analgesics for, 300, 302
  antibiotics for, 336
  aspirin use in, 296
  with attention deficit/hyperactivity disorder, 675-76
  bowel function in, 510
  diarrhea in, 515
  ear drops for, 452
  fluoride for, 496-97
  herbal supplements for, 397t, 400

Children *(Continued)*
immunizations for, 312, 318, 324-25
neuroleptics and, 665, 666b
precautions and contraindications in, 70-72
Clonazepam (Klonopin), 629t
Chloral hydrate (Noctec), 628
Chlorambucil (Leukeran), 374t
Chloramphenicol (Chloromycetin), 345, 347t
Chlordiazepoxide (Librium), 660
Chlorine, 393t, 394
Chloromycetin (chloramphenicol), 345, 347t
Chloroquine (Aralen), 358t
Chlorpheniramine (Chlor-Trimeton), 617
Chlorpromazine (Thorazine), 664, 665-66
Chloraseptic, 496
Chlortetracycline (Aureomycin), 344t
Chlorthalidone (Hygroton), 567
Chlor-Trimeton (chlorpheniramine), 617
Cholelithiasis, 506
Cholera, 327t
Cholesterol, 399b, 572-75
Cholestyramine (Questran), 575
Cholinergic agents, 439, 645-46
Cholinesterase inhibitors, 439
Chronic obstructive pulmonary disease (COPD), 526, 529, 537-40, 543
Chronic pain, 290-91
Chronotropic medications, 550
Cialis (tadalafil), 616
Ciclopirox olamine (Loprox), 354t
Cidofovir (Vistide), 357t
Cilostazol (Pletal), 572
Ciloxan (ciprofloxacin), 337
Cimetidine (Tagamet), 502, 617
Cinobac (cinoxacin), 350t, 588
Cinoxacin (Cinobac), 350, 350t, 588
Cipro (ciprofloxacin), 346t
Ciprofloxacin (Ciloxan), 337
Ciprofloxacin (Cipro), 346t
Circulatory system, the
angina pectoris and, 550-56
blood vessel diseases, 572, 573t
cardiac dysrhythmias and, 558-61
coagulation and, 295-96, 575-79
congestive heart failure and, 556-58
death and diseases of, 550, 579

Circulatory system, the *(Continued)*
drug effects on, 549-61
adrenergic-inhibiting agents, 568, 569-70t
anticoagulants, 575-78
antidysrhythmic, 558-61
antiplatelets, 575-78
beta-adrenergic blockers, 552-55, 554t
calcium channel blockers, 554t, 555, 571-72
diuretics, 565-68
hematopoietic/erythropoietic stimulants, 579
nitrates, 551-52, 553t
vasodilators, 550, 556, 561, 568, 571t
functions of, 547-48
hyperlipidemia and, 572-75
hypertension and, 561-72
Cisplatin (Platinol), 374t
Citracal, 392t
Citroma (magnesium citrate), 392t
Citro-Nesia, 392t
Citrucel (methylcellulose), 512
Cladribine (Leustatin), 378t
Claforan (cefotaxime), 342t
Clarithromycin (Biaxin), 341, 343t, 504
Classifications
drug, 49
tumor, 368
Clinical pharmacology, 4b
Clioquinol (Vioform), 354t
Clofibrate (Atromid-S), 575
Clomid (clomiphene), 614
Clomiphene (Clomid), 614
Clomipramine (Anafranil), 617, 659
Clonazepam (Klonopin), 633
Clonidine (Catapres), 568, 617, 676
Clopidogrel (Plavix), 576
Clotrimazole (Lotrimin, Mycelex, Gyne-Lotrimin), 354t
Cloxacillin (Cloxapen, Tegopen), 339t
Cloxapen (cloxacillin), 339t
Clozapine (Clozaril), 666
Clozaril (clozapine), 666
Cluster headaches, 641
Coagulation, 575-79
Coal tar, 473
Coanalgesia, 292
Cocaine, 627, 688, 689-90
Codeine, 293t, 533-35
aspirin with, 299t
Coenzyme A, 389
Cognex (tacrine), 674
Colace (docusate sodium), 515
Colazal (balsalazide), 517
Colchicines, 487-88

Cold-Eeze, 532, 533
Colds, common, 533, 534t
Colgate Tooth Whitener, 497
Colloids, 59t
Collyrium (boric acid), 360
Combination diuretics, 567
Combination nonopioid medications, 296
Comedo/comedones, 463
Common cold, 533, 534t
Compazine (prochlorperazine), 370t
Complementary medicine, 395, 400
Compliance, medication
adrenergic, 652
alcoholism treatment, 687-88
antacids, 501
anthelmintic therapy, 518
antianginal agents, 555
antibiotic, 337
antidepressants, 674
antidiarrheals, 517
antidysrhythmic drugs, 561
antiemetics, 507
antifungals, 355
antihistamines, 529
antihypertensives, 571
antipsychotics, 667
antiulcers, 504
antivirals, 356
anxiolytics, 662
arthritis treatment, 482
asthma treatment, 542
burn treatment, 469
cephalosporins, 341
chemotherapy, 371
cholinergic/anticholinergic, 647
contraception, 613
cough medicine, 535
cultural differences and, 77
digoxin, 557
diuretics, 567
by the elderly, 74
estrogen therapy, 603
headache treatment, 641
herbal medicines, 400
hormone therapy, 409
hypolipidemics, 575
immunosuppressants, 329
insulin injections, 430-31
laxatives, 515
nasal preparations, 533
nonopioids, 297-98
ophthalmic medications, 447
opioids and opiates, 294-95, 625
oral anesthetics, 497
oral contraception, 607
osteoporosis treatment, 478-79
otic, 452
pain and, 291
parkinsonism, 638

Compliance, medication
    (Continued)
    penicillin, 340
    radioactive iodine, 412
    sedatives/hypnotics, 632
    for special populations, 74
    steroid/corticosteroids, 418
    sulfonamides, 332
    testosterone replacement, 600
    tetracyclines, 343
    thyroid replacement therapy, 412
    topical medications, 453, 459, 466,
        468, 472, 473
    tuberculosis drugs, 352
    urinary tract treatment, 588, 590
    vitamins and nutritional
        supplements, 390, 394
    See also Education, patient
Complications
    analgesic, 300, 302
    antibiotic misuse, 337
    intravenous therapy, 220
    opioid and opiates, 294
Compounding, drug, 87
Compound W (salicylic acid), 59t
Comprehensive Drug Abuse
    Prevention and Control Act
    1970, 15, 17b, 18-19
Compresses, 248
Comtan (entacapone), 636
Concentration, drug, 34
Concerta (methylphenidate), 676
Condoms, 610-11
Confidentiality, patient, 89
Congestion, nasal, 527-33
Congestive heart failure, 556-58
Conjunctivitis, 438
Conscious sedation, 626
Constipation, 294, 392t, 510-15, 521
Containers
    injectable medication, 263,
        267-69, 270-71p
    IV, 211-12
Contamination and intravenous
    therapy, 208
Contemporary medication
    indications, 38-39
Contraception
    barrier devices, 610-11
    forms of, 606, 608t
    implanted and transdermal, 607,
        609-10
    injection, 609t, 610
    intrauterine devices, 609t, 610
    oral, 59t, 466, 606-7, 608-9t, 618
    postcoital, 611-12
    RU-486, 612-13
    spermicidal, 610, 611t
Contraindications to
    immunizations, 313-14

Controlled substances
    Act of 1970, 20, 21t
    classification of, 20, 21t
    defined, 15
    inventory forms, 22f
    labels, 84
    in the medical office, 20
    ordering and securing, 20, 22-23
    record keeping and inventory
        control, 22f, 23
    regulation of, 18-19
Conversions
    decimals, 111-12, 116-17
    fractions, 112-13
    length, 159-61
    percents, 116-17
    system, 151-61
    temperature, 147-50
    time, 146-47
    volume, 152-54
    weight, 154-59
Convulsions, 632
COPD. *See* Chronic obstructive
    pulmonary disease (COPD)
Cordarone (amiodarone), 561
Corgard (nadolol), 568, 650
Cornea, 436
Coronary artery disease (CAD), 550,
    579
Cortex (selegiline), 638
Corticosteroids, 300t, 407, 432
    administration of, 415, 418
    adrenal gland secretion, 414
    creams, 59t
    drugs used as, 416-17t
    immunosuppression, 327
    otic, 450
    topical, 461-63
Cortisporin, 59t
Cosmegen (dactinomycin), 376t
Cotazym (pancrelipase), 506
Cotrim (trimethoprim
        sulfamethoxazole), 349t, 588
Cough
    medications, 533-35, 536-37, 543
    reflex, 294
Coumadin (warfarin), 576
Cox inhibitors, 485
Creams, 59t, 241-42, 248-49
Crepitus, 480
Cromolyn sodium, 511, 531, 543
Crotamiton (Eurax), 472
Crust, skin, 460f
Cryptorchidism, 598
Crysti-12, 389t
Cultural beliefs
    about hypertension, 563-64
    about pain, 303
    about sexual issues, 594
    alternative medicine and, 395-96

Cultural beliefs *(Continued)*
    concerning health and illness,
        75-77
    regarding intravenous therapy,
        221-22
Cumulation, 43
Cunica flowers, 399t
Cuprimine (penicillamine), 486
Curative/healing drugs, 38t
Cyanocobalamin, 389, 389t
Cyanoject, 389t
Cyclophosphamide (Cytoxan,
        Neosar), 374t
Cycloplegia, 437, 442
Cycloserine (Seromycin), 351t
Cyclosporine (Restasis, Neoral),
        442, 486
Cyclosporine (Sandimmune), 327,
        328t, 329
Cytarabine (Cytosar), 375t
Cytosar (cytarabine), 375t
Cytotec (misoprostol), 501
Cytotoxic medications, 369
Cytovene (ganciclovir), 357t
Cytoxan (cyclophosphamide), 374t

D

Dacarbazine (DTIC-Dome), 378t
Dactinomycin (Actinomycin D,
        Cosmegen), 376t
Daily living and anxiety, 658-59
Danazol (Danocrine), 615
Dandruff, 468
Dangers
    immunosuppressive agents, 327
    intravenous therapy, 208, 220
Danocrine (danazol), 615
Dantrium (dantrolene), 641
Dantrolene (Dantrium), 641
Daraprim (pyrimethamine), 358t
Darvocet N (acetaminophen and
        propoxyphene), 299t, 302
Darvon compound (aspirin,
        propoxyphene, and caffeine),
        299t
Darvon (propoxyphene), 294, 688
Datril (acetaminophen), 297t
Daunorubicin (Cerubidine), 377t
DDAVP (desmopressin), 591
Deadly nightshade, 399t
Decadron (dexamethasone), 300t,
        485
Decimals
    adding and subtracting,
        113-14
    changing percents to, 116-17
    conversion to percents, 117
    converting fractions to, 111-12
    dividing, 114-15
    multiplying, 113-14

Decimals *(Continued)*
  percents conversion to, 116-17
  rounding, 111-12
Decongestants, 59t, 447, 529-30
Delavirdine (Rescriptor), 357t
Delfen (nonoxynol-9), 610
Delirium tremens, 686
Delivery systems, drug
  antineoplastic, 373
  buccal and sublingual, 252
  enteral, 35t, 234-45
  inhaled, 59t, 257-59
  insulin, 423, 427-28
  labeling, 81
  nasal, 254-56
  ophthalmic, 59t, 252-53, 253p,
    254p
  oral, 55-57, 58t, 238, 239-41p
  otic, 59t, 253-54, 255p
  parenteral, 58, 60
  percutaneous, 35t, 58, 59t, 60b
  quality assurance, 229-30
  rectal, 241-45
  routes of administration and, 34t,
    35t, 67, 234-35, 247-48
  topical, 34, 58, 247, 248-52
  transdermal, 58, 59t, 61f, 234,
    247-52
  vaginal, 59t, 256-57
Deltasone (prednisone), 300t
Deltoid site for intramuscular
    injections, 279-80
Delusions, 659, 664
Demerol (meperidine HCL), 50,
    293t, 294, 639, 688
Demulcent drugs, 37t
Denavir (famciclovir-penciclovir),
    357t
Dendrid (idoxuridine), 357t
Denominators, 103-5
Dental caries, 393t, 394
Dentifrices, 497
Dentition, 73
Depakene (valproic acid), 635, 640,
    641
Depakote (valproate), 635, 673
Depo-Medrol (methylprednisolone
    acetate), 485
Depo-Provera
    (medroxyprogesterone), 610
Depressant drugs, 37t
  abuse, 690-92
  See also Sedatives
Depression, 399b
  classification of, 668-69
  medications, 300t, 659, 669-74
Dermatologic medications. *See*
    Topical medications
Desenex (undecylenic acid), 354t
Desired effects, 37, 39

Desmopressin (DDAVP), 591
Desyrel (trazodone), 662, 669
Detemir (Levemir), 421-22
Detrol-LA (tolterodine), 590
Dexamethasone (Decadron,
    Decaspray), 300t, 485
Dexedrine (dextroamphetamine),
    676
Dextroamphetamine (Dexedrine),
    676
Dextromethorphan, 535
Diabetes mellitus
  administration of insulin in type 1,
    420-23
  obesity and, 518
  treatment of, 419-20
  types, 418-19, 432
Diagnostic agents, 4b, 38t, 449t
Diaphragms, 611
Diarrhea, 399b, 510, 515-17
Diazepam (Valium), 50, 489, 507
  for anxiety, 659
  libido and, 617
  for seizures, 633
  for spasticity, 641
Dibenzodiazepines, 663t
Dicloxacillin (Dynapen, Dycill),
    339t
Didanosine (Videx, ddl), 357t
Didrex (benzphetamine), 520
Diet and drug dosing, 66
Dietary Supplement Health and
    Education Act, 396
Diethylpropion (Tenuate), 520
Diethylstilbestrol (Stilphostrol),
    376t
Differin (adapalene), 466
Diflucan (fluconazole), 353t
Digitalis, 556
Digitalization, 556-57
Digoxin, 556
Dihydrotestosterone, 600
Dilantin (phenytoin Na), 300t, 558,
    633
Diltiazem (Cardizem), 555, 561
Dimensional analysis method, 157,
    173-74, 194, 198
Dipentum (olsalazine), 517
Diphenhydramine (Benadryl), 37,
    468, 535, 617
Diphenhydramine (Nytol,
    Sominex), 632
Diphenoxylate/atropine (Lomotil),
    516
Diphtheria, tetanus, and pertussis
    vaccine, 315, 319t, 321t, 323t,
    324, 326t
Diphtheria-tetanus toxoid, 313
Dipyridamole (Persantine), 576, 652
Dirithromycin (Dynabac), 343t

Disabled persons and
    immunizations, 312
Disease-modifying antirheumatic
    drugs, 481
Diseases and drug dosing, 67
Disinfectants/germicides, 356,
    358-61, 458
  versus antiseptics, 359
Disks, transdermal, 249-51
Disopyramide (Norpace), 558
Dispersions, 57, 58b, 58t
Disposable injection units, 269,
    270-71p
Disposal, needle, 228-29
Distal tubule/potassium-sparing
    diuretics, 566t, 567
Distribution, pharmacokinetic,
    34-36
Disulfiram (Antabuse), 57b, 686,
    687
Ditropan (oxybutynin), 590
Diuresis, 221
Diuretics
  combination, 567
  for congestive heart failure, 556
  high-ceiling, 565, 566t
  for hypertension, 564-68
  kidney function and, 584
  osmotic, 442
  potassium-sparing, 566t, 567
  thiazide, 565, 567, 617
Division
  decimals, 114-15
  fractions, 108-10
  percents, 118-19
DMARDs, 486
DNA technology, recombinant, 32
Docetaxel (Taxotere), 378t
Docosanol (Abreva), 497
Documentation, vaccine, 314-15
Docusate sodium (Colace), 515
Donepezil (Aricept), 675
Dong quai, 398t
Dopamine antagonists, 507,
    636-38
Dopar (levodopa), 617, 636
Dorsogluteal site for intramuscular
    injections, 280, 281f
Dosage calculation
  age and, 65, 70
  choosing a method for, 174-75
  diet and, 66
  diseases and, 67
  gender and, 66
  genetics and, 66
  herbal supplements, 400
  history of previous medications
    and, 67
  mental state and, 67
  method introduction, 165-67

Dosage calculation *(Continued)*
  nonparenteral medications
    dimensional analysis, 173-74
    forms, 167
    formula method, 169-72
  parenteral medications
    metric system and, 194-95
    in units, 196-98
  patient compliance and, 67-68
  powder reconstitution and, 175, 177t
  time of administration and, 67
  using body surface area, 178-82
  using Mg/Kg, 182
  weight and, 65-66, 178-82
Dots, transdermal, 249-51
Douches, 61
Doxazosin (Cardura), 568, 600
Doxepin (Sinequan), 300t
Doxil (doxorubicin), 377t
Doxorubicin (Adriamycin), 376t, 377t
Doxycycline (Vibramycin, Oracea), 344t, 358t, 467t
Doxylamine (Unisom), 632
DPP-4 inhibitors, 430
Dressings, 248
Drip chambers, 212-13
Drisdol, 388t
Dromotropic drugs, 550
Drop orifices, 212
Drug administration, role of allied health professionals in, 24-27
Drug blood level, 35
Drug-drug interactions, 42-43, 44t
Drug Enforcement Agency (DEA), 6, 15, 694
  controlled substances in the medical office and, 20, 21t
  and disposing of scheduled and nonscheduled drugs, 23-24
  prescription numbers, 89
  record keeping and inventory control requirements, 22f, 23
  regulation of controlled substances, 18-19
Drug Facts and Comparisons, 53
Drug Listing Act of 1972, 15
Drug Price Competition and Patent Term Restoration Act, 15, 17b
Drug Regulation and Reform Act of 1978, 15, 17b
Drug(s)
  active ingredients, 30
  addiction, 14, 15, 24-25
  brand-name, 16, 50
  classifications, 49
  compounding, 87
  definition of, 3, 4b, 30

Drug(s) *(Continued)*
  disposing of scheduled and nonscheduled, 23-24
  errors, 9
  forms and delivery systems, 54-61
  generic, 16, 50
  half-life, 36
  ideal, 30
  indications and uses of, 38
  inert ingredients, 30
  information sources, 51-54
  interactions, 42-45, 423, 427b
  labels, 81-85
  legislation related to, 14-16, 17b, 314
  nomenclature, 50-51
  off-label uses, 49-50
  receptor sites, 41-42
  record keeping and inventory control, 22f, 23
  regulation of, 13-16
  safe, 30
  safety education, 8-10
  samples, 26
  sensitivity, 335
  solubility, 33
  sources, 31-32
  standardization of, 13
  standards and patient safety, 16-24
  strength of, 13, 14, 18, 50-51, 81
  surveillance, 18, 20t
  toxicology, 39-41
  unbound, 34
  vehicle, 30
Drying agents, otic, 450
Dry powder inhalers, 537
DTap. *See* Diphtheria, tetanus, and pertussis vaccine
DTIC-Dome (dacarbazine), 378t
Dulcolax (bisacodyl), 512
Duragesic (fentanyl), 293t, 294
Durham-Humphrey Amendment, 14, 17b
Duricef (cefazolin), 342t
Dycill (dicloxacillin), 339t
Dynabac (dirithromycin), 343t
DynaCirc, 555
Dynapen (dicloxacillin), 339t
Dysmenorrhea, 613-14
Dysphonia, 427
Dysrhythmias, cardiac, 558-61
Dystonia, 665

E

E. coli, 587, 590
Ear
  anatomy, 449, 450f
  conditions, typical, 449

Ear *(Continued)*
  medications, 59t, 253-54, 255p, 449-53
  signs of ototoxicity and, 450, 452b
Echinacea, 396, 397t, 399t
Ecotrin (aspirin), 295
Ecstasy (MDMA), 693
Ectopic beats, 558
Eczema, 461
Education, patient
  antimicrobials, 362
  for safety, 8-10
  on vaccination, 324-25
  See also Compliance, medication
Effervescent powders, 57
Effexor (venlafaxine), 659, 662
Efficacy, drug, 16
Efudex (fluorouracil), 375t, 473
Elavil (amitriptyline), 300t, 640
Eldepryl (selegiline), 638
Elderly, the. *See* Geriatric patients
Electrical conduction system, 548-50
Electrolytes, 206, 390-91, 393
  replacement therapy, 585-87
Eletriptan (Relpax), 639
Elimination, drug, 36
Elimite (permethrin), 472
Elixophyllin (theophylline/aminophylline), 540
Elspar (asparaginase), 377t
Emboli, 208, 220, 576, 577f
Emcyt (estramustine), 376t
Emergency contraception pills (ECPs), 611-12
Emesis, 370, 506-10
Emetic weed, 399t
Emetrol, 507
Eminase (anistreplase), 576
Emollients, 458
Emotional responses and pain, 290
Empirin with codeine (aspirin with codeine), 299t
Enalapril (Vasotec), 568
Encephalitis, 314
Endocrine system, the
  activities of, 405, 432
  corticosteroids/steroids, 415-18
  glands, 406f
  hormones, 405-7
  hyperglycemics, 424-26t, 431-32
  hypoglycemics, 423, 424-26t, 427b, 428-30, 430-31
  parathyroid hormones, 414
  pituitary gland hormones, 408-9
  thyroid gland hormones, 37, 409, 411-14
Endometriosis, 615-16
Endorphins, 290, 622

Enemas, medicated, 61, 242, 244p, 245f
Engerix B, 320t
Enoxacin (Penetrex), 346t
Ensure (nonoxynol-9), 610
Entacapone (Comtan), 636
Enteral routes of administration, 35t, 234
  oral, 238, 239-41p
  rectal, 241-45
Enteric-coated medications, 482
Enterobacter, 590
Entertainer's Secret, 497
Enuresis, 589t, 590-91
Environment and drug dosing, 67
Enzymes, pancreatic, 506, 520
Ephedra, 396, 398t, 399t, 537-39
Epinephrine, 537-39, 627, 654
Epistaxis, 427
Epivir (lamivudine), 357t
Eplerenone (Inspra), 568
Epsom salts (magnesium sulfate), 392t
Equipment, intravenous therapy, 208
Equivalent fractions, 101
Erectile dysfunction, 615-17, 618
Ergamisol (Levamisole), 328t, 377t
Ergocalciferol, 388t
Ergot alkaloids, 639
Erlotinib (Tarceva), 378t
Errors, medication, 9
  in elderly patients, 73-74
  intravenous therapy, 208
  reduction using 3 + 7, 231-33
  sources of, 234
Ertaczo (sertaconazole), 354t
Ery-Ped (erythromycin succinate), 343t
Erythrocin (erythromycin), 343t
Erythromycins, 341, 343t
  for acne, 463
  -sulfisoxazole, 349t
Erythropoietics, 579
Eschar, 468
Esomeprazole (Nexium), 503
Essential hypertension, 562
Estradiol, 602, 609
Estramustine (Emcyt), 376t
Estrogens, 59t, 376t, 601-3, 604t, 618
Ethambutol (Myambutol), 351, 351t
Ethics
  health care professionals, 25-27
  intravenous therapy, 222
Ethyl alcohol, 617
  abuse, 685t, 686-88
Eulexin (flutamide), 376t
Eurax (crotamiton), 472
Evista (raloxifene), 376t, 478
Evoxac (cevimeline), 497

Excedrin, 295, 299t
Excretion, drug, 36
Exemestane (Aromasin), 378t
Ex-Lax (cascara sagrada), 512
Expectoration, 536-37
Expiration dates, 84
Extended-spectrum penicillins, 339t, 340
Extracellular fluids, 207, 584-85
Extrapyramidal effects, 660
Extravasation, 372
Exubera (insulin), 427
Eye
  anatomy, 436-38
  antiinfective and antiinflammatory agents, 438-39
  artificial tears and lubrication, 442
  glaucoma, 439, 442
  See also Ophthalmic medications
Eyelashes, 437

F

Factive (gemifloxacin), 346t
Factrel (gonadorelin), 614
Facultative bacteria, 334
Famciclovir-penciclovir (Denavir), 357t
Fansidar (pyrimethamine with sulfadoxine), 358t
Fat solubility, 34, 35
Fat-soluble vitamins, 384t, 385-87, 400
Federal Narcotic Drug Act, 14, 17b
Federal Trade Commission, 84
Federal Triplicate Order, 20
Feedback, negative, 405, 407f
Felodipine (Plendil), 555
Female reproductive system, the, 59t, 376t, 595, 597f
  endometriosis and, 615-16
  hormones and, 601-5
  infertility and, 614-15
  premenstrual syndrome and, 613-14
  See also Contraception
Fentanyl patches, 59t, 293t, 294
Feosol, 392t
Feostat, 392t
Fergon, 392t
Feverfew, 396, 398t
Fevers
  immunization and, 313
  Reye's syndrome and, 296, 300
Fiber-Con (polycarbophil), 512
Fiber-Trim, 520
Fibric acid derivatives, 575
Fibromyalgia, 490-91
Finasteride (Propecia, Proscar), 473, 600

Fioricet with codeine (acetaminophen, codeine and butalbital), 299t
Fiorinal with codeine (aspirin, butalbital, and codeine), 299t
First-pass effect, 36
Fissures, skin, 460f
Flagyl (metronidazole), 345-46, 347t, 504
Flavoxate (Urispas), 590
Fleming, Alexander, 332
Flexible collodion, 59t
Flomax (tamsulosin), 600
Flonase (fluticasone), 59t
Flora, normal, 333
Flow rates, intravenous fluid, 213, 215-17
Floxin (ofloxacin), 346t
Fluconazole (Diflucan), 353t
Fluids
  body, 206-7, 584-85
  calculating amount of medication infused in amount of, 219
  electrolyte balance, 392t, 584-87
  intravenous therapy, 209
  replacement therapy, 585-87
  tonicity of, 210
Flumadine (rimantadine), 357t, 542
FluMist, 320t
Fluogen, 320t
Fluoride, 393t, 394, 496
  for children, 496-97
Fluoroquinolones, 344-45, 346t
  for urinary tract infections, 588
Fluorotab, 393t
Fluorouracil (5-FU, Efudex, Adrucil), 375t, 473
Fluoxetine (Prozac), 613, 659, 672-73
Fluoxymesterone (Halotestin), 376t
Flutamide (Eulexin), 376t
Fluticasone (Flonase, Beconase), 59t
Fluzone, 320t
Focal seizures, 632
Folic acid, 388t, 389
Folk remedies, 395-96
Follicle-stimulating hormone (FSH), 409, 595, 597
Folvite, 388t
Food
  -drug interactions, 43-45, 671, 672t
  in the stomach and drug absorption, 34
Food, Drug, and Cosmetic Act of 1938, 14, 17b
Food and Drug Administration (FDA), 14
  on adverse vaccine reactions, 314
  antihistamines regulation, 632
  on consumer information, 64-65

Food and Drug Administration (FDA) *(Continued)*
herbal supplements regulation, 396
introduction of new drugs and, 18
Modernization Act, 16, 18b
off-label uses for drugs and, 49-50
regulation of sun products, 470
Form, drug. *See* Delivery systems, drug
Formula methods for calculating doses, 169-72, 194
Fortaz (ceftazidime), 342t
Forteo (teriparatide), 478
Fosamax (alendronate), 477-78
Foscarnet (Foscavir), 357t
Foscavir (foscarnet), 357t
Fosphenytoin (Cerebyx), 633
Fraction(s)
adding, 103-5
conversion to decimals, 111-12
dividing, 108-10
equivalent, 101
improper, 101, 103
mixed numbers and, 103-5, 106-8
multiplying, 106-8
proper, 101
simplifying, 102
subtracting, 105-6
used to figure percentages, 118-21
5-FU (fluorouracil), 375t
Fulvicin (griseofulvin), 353t
Functions of body fluids, 206-7
Fungi
antifungal drugs and, 59t, 352-55, 362
classification of, 333
Fungizone (amphotericin B), 353t
Fungoid (triacetin), 354t
Furadantin (nitrofurantoin), 350t, 590
Furosemide (Lasix), 565

G

Gabapentin (Neurontin), 300t, 635
Gabitril (tiagabine), 635
Galantamine (Reminyl), 675
Gallbladder disease, 506
Gallstones, 506
Galzin, 393t
Ganciclovir (Cytovene), 357t
Gantanol (sulfamethoxazole), 349t
Gantrisin (sulfisoxazole), 349t, 588
Garamycin (gentamicin), 345t
Gardasil, 320t
Garlic, 397t, 399t
Gastroesophageal reflux disease (GERD), 500, 520
Gastrointestinal system disorders
anatomy of, 495
anorectal preparations, 517-18

Gastrointestinal system disorders *(Continued)*
antiinflammatories, 517
appetite suppressants and, 518-20
constipation, 510-15, 521
diarrhea, 510, 515-17
emesis, 506-10
functions, 495
gallbladder disease, 506
mouth, 496-500, 520
pancreatic enzyme replacements, 506
peptic ulcers, 500-505, 520
urinary tract infections and, 587
Gas-X, 510
Gatifloxacin (Tequin), 346t
Gauges, needle, 265
Gelcaps, 55
Gelfilm, 578
Gelfoam, 578
Gelfoam powder, 578
Gels, 59t, 248-49
dermatologic, 458
Gelusil, 500
Gemcitabine (Gemzar), 378t
Gemfibrozil (Lopid), 575
Gemifloxacin (Factive), 346t
Gemzar (gemcitabine), 378t
Gender and drug dosing, 66
General anesthetics, 625-26, 653
Generalized anxiety disorder (GAD), 659, 662
Generalized seizures, 632
Generic drugs, 16, 50
names, 81
Genetics and drug dosing, 66
Genotropin (somatropin), 409
GenRx, 53
Gentamicin (Garamycin), 345t
Geocillin (carbenicillin), 339t
Geodon (ziprasidone), 666
GERD (gastroesophageal reflux disease), 500, 520
Geriatric patients
analgesics for, 302
antibiotics for, 336
bowel function in, 510
calcium channel blockers and, 572b
herbal supplements for, 400
medication compliance assistance for, 74
neuroleptics and, 665, 666b
polypharmacy and, 73-74
precautions and contraindications in, 72-74
topical medications for, 251
vitamins and supplements for, 390
Germicides/disinfectants, 356, 358-61

Ginger, 398t
Gingko, 396, 397t, 399t
Ginseng, 396, 397t
Glargine (lantus insulin), 421-22, 423
Glaucoma, 439, 442, 443-44t
Globulins, immune, 312
Glucocorticoids, 414-15, 432, 531, 532t
for asthma, 540-41
Glucocorticosteroids, 485
Glucophage (metformin), 429
Glucosamine chondroitin, 394-95, 486-87
Glucose absorption inhibitors, 429
Glulisine (Apidra), 421
Glycerin, 515
suppositories, 59t
Glycosides, cardiac, 31, 556-57, 580
Goiter, 411
Golden seal, 397t, 399t
Gold salts, 486
Gonadorelin (Factrel, Lutrepulse), 614
Gonadotropin-releasing hormone (Lupron), 376t, 613, 615
Goody's powders, 296, 299t
Goserelin (Zoladex), 376t, 615
Gouty arthritis, 487-88, 491
Gram stains, 334, 359
Granisetron (Kytril), 507
Granules, 57
Grisactin (griseofulvin), 353t
Griseofulvin (Grisactin, Fulvicin), 353t
Growth hormones, 406, 408-9
inhibitors, 409
Guaifenesin, 536
Guanabenz (Wytensin), 617
Guanethidine (Ismelin), 617
Guanfacine (Tenex), 617
Guillain-Barré syndrome, 314
Gums, 31
Gyne-Lotrimin (clotrimazole), 354t

H

H, 486
H. pylori, 501, 504
Haemophilus influenzae vaccine, 316, 319t, 323t
Hair loss and growth, 472-73
Haldol (haloperidol), 665, 666
Half-life, drug, 36
Halitosis, 496
Hallucinations, 659, 664
Hallucinogens, 692-93
Haloperidol (Haldol), 665, 666
Halotestin (fluoxymesterone), 376t
Handbooks, drug, 53-54
Harrison Narcotic Act, 14, 17b

Hashish, 691
Havrix, 320t
HDL cholesterol, 573, 687
Headaches, 399b
  cluster, 641
  migraine, 639-41
  tension, 641
Health care professionals
  allied, 3, 3f, 6, 76-77
  cultural awareness of, 76-77
  ethics, 25-27
  immunizations for, 312
  pharmacology use by, 6-8
Heart, the
  anatomy of, 547-48, 549f
  angina pectoris and, 550-56
  congestive failure of, 556-58
  electrical conduction system,
    548-50
  pacemaker cells, 561
  and vessel diseases, 550
  See also Cardiovascular system,
    the
Hematomas, 221
Hematopoietics, 579
Hemlock, 399t
Hemorrheologic agents, 572
Hemostasis, 575
Hemostatics, topical, 576, 578
Heparin dosage calculations, 198
Hepatitis vaccines, 316, 320t, 323t
Herbal medicine, 394-400
  for colds, 533
  for insomnia, 632
Heroin, 688
Herplex (idoxuridine), 357t
Hexachlorophene, 359, 360
Hexavac, 318
HibTITER, 319t
Hib-vaccine. See Meningitis
High-ceiling diuretics, 565, 566t, 567
Hiprex (methenamine), 350t, 590
Histamine receptors, 300t, 502,
    527-29
History of pharmacology, 4-6
HIV
  antivirals, 355-56, 357-58t
  transmission, 610
Hivid (zalcitabine), 357t
HMG CoA reductase inhibitors. See
  Statins
Holistic beliefs on health and
    illness, 76-77
Homeostasis, 3, 405, 407f
Home remedies, 395-96
Hordeolum, 438
Hormones
  ACTH, 408-9
  adrenal cortex, 414-15
  androgens, 596, 598, 617

Hormones (Continued)
  antidiuretic, 409
  calcitonin, 414
  endocrine system, 405-7
  estrogen, 59t, 376t, 601-3, 604t, 618
  follicle-stimulating, 409, 595, 597
  functions, 407
  growth, 406, 408-9
  and hormone antagonists, 372-73,
    376t
  luteinizing, 409, 596
  nonsteroid, 406
  parathyroid, 414
  pituitary gland, 408-9
  progesterone, 603-5
  progestins, 376t, 602, 605t, 618
  prolactin, 409
  -receptor action, 406f
  replacement therapy, 598, 601-2
  reproductive, 59t, 594-96, 598
  steroid, 406, 414
  thyroid, 37, 409, 411-14
  tropic, 408
Horse chestnut, 399t
Household measurement system,
    139-40
  length measurements, 159-61
  volume measurements, 152-54
  weight measurements, 154-59
Humalog (lispro), 421, 423
Human chorionic gonadotropin
    (hCG), 614
Human papillomavirus vaccines,
    318, 320t, 324
Humatrope (somatropin), 409
Humira (adalimumab), 486
Humulin (insulin), 421, 428f
Hydantoins, 634t
Hydration, 392t
Hydrea (hydroxyurea), 378t
Hydrobexan (hydroxocobalamin),
    389t
Hydrochlorothiazide
    (HydroDIURIL), 565
Hydrocodone
  and aspirin (Lortab with ASA),
    299t
  in cough suppressants, 533-35
HydroDIURIL
    (hydrochlorothiazide), 565
Hydrogen peroxide, 360, 496
Hydromox (quinethazone), 567
Hydroxocobalamin (Hydrobexan),
    389t
Hydroxychloroquine (Plaquenil),
    358t, 486
Hydroxyurea (Hydrea), 378t
Hydroxyzine (Atarax, Vistaril),
    300t, 662
Hygroton (chlorthalidone), 567

Hyoscyamine (Levsin), 647
Hyperglycemia, 420, 421t
Hyperglycemics, 424-26t, 431-32
Hyperlipidemia, 572-75
Hypersensitivity reactions, 40
Hypertension
  adding medications for treatment
    of, 563-64
  adrenergic-inhibiting agents for,
    568, 569-70t
  cultural beliefs about, 563-64
  diuretics for, 564-68
  etiology, 561-62
  lifestyle and, 562-63
  risk factors, 562
  types of antihypertensive
    medications for, 562
  vasodilators for, 568, 571t
Hypertonic solutions, 207, 211, 536
Hyperuricemia, 487
Hypervitaminosis, 387
Hypnotics, 627-32
  abuse, 690-92
Hypoglycemia, 420, 421t
Hypoglycemics, 423, 424-26t, 427b,
    428-30
  See also Diabetes mellitus
Hypogonadism, 598
Hypolipidemics, 573-75
Hyposecretion, 411
Hypotension, orthostatic, 555
Hypothalamus, 405, 408
Hypotonic solutions, 207, 211
Hytrin (terazosin), 600

I

Ibandronate (Boniva), 477-78
Ibuprofen, 297t
  combinations, 299t
  and hydrocodone, 299t
Ideal drugs, 30
Identification of undesirable effects
    of drugs, 41
Idoxuridine (Herplex), 357t
Ifex (uracil mustard ifosfamide),
    374t
Iletin (insulin), 421
Ilosone (erythromycin estolate),
    343t
Imferon, 392t
Imipramine (Tofranil), 300t, 591
Imitrex (sumatriptan), 639
Immunity
  active and passive, 306, 307t,
    309-11
  agents
    artificially acquired active,
      315-22
    artificially acquired passive,
      322, 324

Immunity (Continued)
  artificially acquired, 306, 307f, 315-24, 326t
  immunostimulants and, 327-29
  immunosuppressants and, 325, 327
  inborn, 306, 307f, 308-11
  lymphocytes in, 307-8
  natural, 306, 307f
  types, 306, 307f, 308-11
  vaccines and, 306, 307f, 309, 311-12
Immunizations
  adverse reactions to, 314
  agents for artificially acquired active immunity, 315-22
  antitoxin, 311, 312
  BCG, 317, 377t
  chickenpox, 316-17, 320t, 321t, 323t
  for children, 312, 318, 324-25
  contraindications to, 313-14
  diphtheria, tetanus, and pertussis, 315, 319t, 321t, 323t
  documentation of, 314-15
  Haemophilus influenzae, 316, 319t, 323t
  hepatitis, 316, 320t, 323t
  human papillomavirus, 318, 320t, 324
  immunoglobulin, 312
  indications for, 313
  influenza vaccine, 317, 320t, 323t
  lyme, 320t, 321
  measles-mumps-rubella vaccine, 69, 311-12, 315-16, 321t, 323t
  meningococcal, 318, 320t, 321t, 323t
  patient education, 324-25
  patient safety with, 321-22
  pneumococcal, 317, 323t, 324
  poliomyelitis, 316, 319t, 323t
  rabies, 321, 326t, 327t
  rotavirus, 318
  routes of administration, 324
  schedule, 323t
  for specific populations, 312-13
  storage, 324
  supershots, 318, 321t
  tetanus, 315
  toxoid, 312, 315
  for travel, 325
  vaccine, 306, 307f, 309, 311-12
  zoster, 318
Immunodeficiency, 327-29
Immunoglobulins
  preparation of, 312
  rho(D), 324
Immunomodulators, 442
Immunostimulants, 327-29

Immunosuppressants, 325, 327, 328t
  arthritis and, 485-86
  cancer cells and, 373, 377t
Imodium (loperamide), 516
Imovax Rabies vaccine, 327t
Implantable contraceptives, 607, 609-10
Implantable insulin pumps, 423, 427
Implants, 61
Improper fractions, 101, 103
Imuran (azathioprine), 327, 328t, 486
Inborn versus acquired immunity, 306, 307f, 308-11
Incretin mimetics, 430
Indapamide (Lozol), 567
Inderal (propranolol), 552, 555, 558, 561, 568, 617
Indian tobacco, 399t
Indications, medication
  antibiotic, 335-36
  contemporary, 38-39
  immunization, 313
  injections, 274-81, 282-83p
  nutritional supplements, 400
  and uses of drugs, 38
Indinavir (Crixivan), 357t
Inert ingredients, 30
Infections
  ocular, 438-39
  opportunistic, 352
  or inflammation at injection sites, 208, 220
  urinary tract, 350, 399b, 587-90
  viral, 355-56
INFeD, 392t
Infertility, 614-15
Infliximab (Remicade), 486
Influenza, 534t
  vaccines, 317, 320t, 323t
  virus, 542-43
Information, drug, 51-54
Infusion pumps, 214-15
Infusion therapy
  equipment, 211-14
  screening, 220-21
Inhalant abuse, 693-94
Inhalation factors and drug absorption, 34
Inhaled medications
  administration, 257-59
  for chronic pulmonary diseases, 537-42
  metered dose inhalers, 59t, 257-59
INH (isoniazid), 351, 351t
Injectable parenteral suspensions, 60, 61f
Injection(s)
  administering, 274
  advantages and disadvantages of, 262

Injection(s) (Continued)
  ampules for, 58, 263, 267, 268p
  anesthetic, 626-27
  calculating doses for, 194-98
  contraceptive, 609t, 610
  disposable units, 269
  insulin, 423, 424-25t, 427-28, 430-31
  intradermal, 274-75, 276-77p
  intramuscular, 277, 279-81, 282-83p
  ports, 213
  preparation of medications for, 271-73, 274p
  site infection or inflammation, 208, 220
  subcutaneous, 275, 276-77p, 278-79p, 279f
  vials for, 267, 269-70p
Inserts, package, 51, 52f, 53t
Insomnia, 399b, 627-32, 653
Inspra (eplerenone), 568
Insulin
  action onset, peak and duration, 421, 423f
  administration in type 1 diabetes mellitus, 420-23
  adverse reactions to, 428
  automatic delivery systems, 62
  delivery systems, 423, 427-28
  dosage calculations, 198
  injectable, 424-25t
  interactions with other drugs, 423, 427b
  labels, 422f
  mixing, 273, 423
  patches, 428
  pens, 423, 428f
  pumps, 423, 427, 428f
  regular, 421
  resistance, 419
  syringes, 263
  See also Diabetes mellitus
Intal (cromolyn), 541
Interactions, drug
  alcohol, 687, 687t
  digoxin, 557b
  drug-drug, 42-43, 44t
  food-drug, 43, 45
  insulin, 423, 427b
  monoamine oxidase inhibitors, 671, 672t
  nicotine, 683
  oral contraceptives, 607b
Interferon alfa-2a (Roferon), 377t
Interleukin-2 (Proleukin), 328
Intermittent claudication, 572
Internet pharmacy, 5
Interstitial cell-stimulating hormone (ICSH), 595, 597

Intestinal conditions, 510-15
    parasites, 333, 518
Intracellular fluids, 584-85
Intracellular fluid, 206
Intradermal injections, 274-75,
    276-77p
Intramuscular injections, 277,
    279-81, 282-83p
Intrauterine devices, 609t, 610
Intravenous piggyback (IVPB), 210
Intravenous therapy
    administration equipment, 212-14
    containers, 211-12
    contamination and, 208
    cultural beliefs regarding, 221-22
    dangers of, 208, 220
    equipment, 208, 211-14
    flow rates, 213, 215-17
    fluid labels, 212
    history of, 206
    infection or inflammation at
        injection site, 208
    infusion times, 217-18
    intravenous screening before,
        220-21
    legal and ethical issues, 222
    medication errors, 208
    overload, 208
    physiology and, 206-7
    reasons for, 207-8, 208-9
    types of, 207-8, 208-9
    wrong solutions in, 208
Intron (interferon alfa-2b), 377t
Inventory control, 22f, 23
Invirase (saquinavir), 357t
Iodine
    preparations, 359-60
    radioactive, 412
    tincture, 59t, 359-60
Ions, 391, 585
Ipratropium (Atrovent), 540
IPV. See Poliomyelitis vaccines
Irinotecan (Camptosar), 378t
Iris, 437
Iron, 391, 392t
Irritant drugs, 37t
Islet of Langerhans, 418
Ismelin (guanethidine), 617
Isoniazid (INH, Laniazid), 351t
Isophane, 421, 423
Isoptin (verapamil), 561
Isopto Homatropine (homatropine),
    507
Isosorbide dinitrate, 551t
Isotonic solutions, 208, 211, 391
Isotretinoin (Accutane), 388t,
    463
Isoxsuprine (Vasodilan), 572
Isradipine (DynaCirc), 555
Itraconazole (Sporanox), 353t

J
Januvia (sitagliptin), 430
Jet injectors, 423
Joints, 476
    arthritis, 480
    bursitis, 480
    medications for, 481-87

K
Kanamycin (Kantrex), 345t, 351t
Kantrex (kanamycin), 345t
KAON, 393t
Kava kava, 398t
K-Dur, 393t
Kefauver-Harris Amendment of
    1961, 15, 17b, 69
Keflex (cefalexin), 342t
Keftab (cefalexin), 342t
Kelp, 398t
Keppra (levetiracetam), 635
Keratin, 457
Keratitis, 438
Keratolytic agents, 466, 468
Ketek (telithromycin), 343t
Ketoconazole (Nizoral), 353t, 497
Ketolides, 343t
Kidneys
    chemotherapy and, 370
    diuretics and, 584
    impairment, 294
Killed vaccines, 311
Kineret (anakinra), 486
Klonopin (clonazepam), 633
K-Lor, 393t
Klor-Con, 393t
K-Lyte, 393t
Koromex Cream (octoxynol-9), 610
K-Phosphate, 392t
Kwell (lindane), 472
K-Y Jelly, 249
Kytril (granisetron), 507

L
Labels
    drug
        OTC, 84-85
        parts, 81-84
    insulin, 422f
    intravenous fluid, 212
    quality assurance and, 231
Labetalol (Normodyne), 568
Lactated Ringer's solutions, 209
Lamictal (lamotrigine), 635
Lamisil (terbinafine), 353t
Lamivudine (Epivir), 357t
Lamotrigine (Lamictal), 635
Laniazid (INH), 351t
Lanolin, 458
Lansoprazole (Prevacid), 503

Lantus insulin (glargine), 421-22,
    423
Lariam (mefloquine), 358t
Lasix (furosemide), 565
Latin Americans, 395-96
Lavoris, 496
Laxatives, 392t, 510-15, 521
LDL cholesterol, 573
Legal issues regarding intravenous
    therapy, 222
Legend drugs, 6, 50-51, 301t
Legislation related to drugs, 14-16,
    17b, 314
    herbal supplements, 396
Length measurement and
    conversion in metric system,
    134, 159-61
Lente insulin, 422, 423
Lesions, skin, 460f, 473
Lethargy, 221
Leucovorin (Wellcovorin), 375t
Leukeran (chlorambucil), 374t
Leukotrienes, 541
Leuprolide (Lupron), 376t, 613, 615
Leustatin (cladribine), 378t
Levalbuterol (Xopenex), 59t
Levamisole (Ergamisol), 328t,
    377t
Levaquin (levofloxacin), 346t
Levemir (detemir), 421-22
Levetiracetam (Keppra), 635
Levitra (vardenafil), 616
Levocabastine (Livostin), 447
Levodopa (Dopar), 617, 636
Levofloxacin (Levaquin), 346t
Levsin (hyoscyamine), 647
Librium (chlordiazepoxide), 660
Lidocaine, 558
Lifestyle factors
    in gastrointestinal conditions,
        503b
    hypertension and, 562-63
    vitamin supplements and, 390,
        390t
Lincocin (lincomycin), 347t
Lincomycin (Lincocin), 345, 347t
Lindane (Kwell), 472
Liniments, 59t, 459
Lioresal (baclofen), 489, 641
Lipid solubility, 34, 35, 66
Lipitor (atorvastatin), 575
Lipoproteins, 573
Liposome products, 377t
Liquid oral preparations, 55-57, 57t,
    58b, 58t
Lisdexamfetamine (Vyvanse), 676
Lispro (Humalog), 421, 423
Listerine, 496
Lithium, 673, 677-78
Live attenuated vaccines, 311

Liver impairment, 294, 296
  anabolic steroids and, 598
  chemotherapy and, 370
  vitamin K and, 384t, 387
Live vaccines, 311
Livostin (levocabastine), 447
Lobelia, 399t
Local action, 37
Local anesthetics, 626-27, 653
Lodosyn (carbidopa), 636
Lomefloxacin (Maxaquin), 346t
Lomotil (diphenoxylate/atropine), 516
Lomustine (CCNU), 374t
Loniten (minoxidil), 568
Loop diuretics, 565, 566t, 567
Loperamide (Imodium), 516
Lopid (gemfibrozil), 575
Lopressor (metoprolol), 650
Loprox (ciclopirox olamine), 354t
Lorabid (loracarbef), 342t
Loracarbef (Lorabid), 342t
Lorazepam (Ativan), 300t, 370t, 507, 633, 659, 660
Lortab with ASA (aspirin and hydrocodone), 299t
Lotensin (benazepril), 568
Lotions, 59t, 248-49, 458-59
Lotrimin (clotrimazole), 354t
Lower respiratory tract
  acute conditions, 536-37
  chronic conditions, 526, 529, 537-42
  disorders, 535-36
Loxapine (Loxitane), 666
Loxitane (loxapine), 666
Lozenges, 55, 496, 533
Lozol (indapamide), 567
LSD (lysergic acid diethylamide), 692
Lubricant laxatives, 512, 515
Luminal (phenobarbital), 627
Lupron (gonadotropin-releasing hormone), 376t, 613, 615
Lupron (leuprolide), 613
Luride (fluoride), 393t
Luteinizing hormone (LH), 409, 596
Lutrepulse (gonadorelin), 614
Lyme vaccine, 320t, 321
Lymphocytes in immunity, 307-8
Lyrica (pregabalin), 296t
Lysodren (mitotane), 378t

M

Maalox-Plus, 500
Macrobid (nitrofurantoin), 350t, 590
Macrodantin (nitrofurantoin), 350t, 590
Macrodrip administration sets, 213, 213f
Macrolides, 341, 343t

Macrophages, 308
Macules, 460f
Madwort, 399t
Mafenide (Sulfamylon), 469
Magicoreligious beliefs on health and illness, 76-77
Magnesium, 392t, 393, 500
  loss, 587
Magnesium hydroxide (Milk of Magnesia), 511
Magnesium sulfate (Epsom salts), 392t
Mag sulfate, 392t
Ma-huang, 396
Maintenance drugs, 38t
Maintenance therapy, 207
Malaise and lethargy, 586-87
Malaria, 356, 358t
Malathion (Ovide), 472
Male reproductive system, the, 595-600, 601t, 617
  erectile dysfunction, 615-17, 618
  infertility and, 614
  See also Contraception
Malignant cancer, 366, 367f, 367t
Managed health care, 8
Mandelamine (methenamine), 350t, 590
Mandol (cefamandole), 342t
Manufactured drugs, 32
Manufacturers, drug, labeling by, 84
Marijuana, 688, 691-92
Mastication, 495
Math review
  addition
    decimals, 113-14
    fractions, 103-5
  division
    decimals, 114-15
    fractions, 108-10
    percents, 118-19
  fractions
    adding, 103-5
    conversion to decimals, 111-12
    dividing, 108-10
    equivalent, 101
    improper, 101, 103
    mixed numbers and, 103-5, 106-8
    multiplying, 106-8
    proper, 101
    simplifying, 102
    subtracting, 105-6
    used to figure percentages, 118-21
  mixed numbers
    adding, 103-5, 106
    dividing, 108-10
    multiplying, 106-8
    subtracting, 106

Math review (*Continued*)
  multiplication
    decimals, 113-14
    fractions, 106-8
    percents, 117-18
  percents
    conversion to decimals, 116-17
    decimals conversion to, 117
    dividing, 118-19
    multiplying, 117-18
    using equations to figure, 121
    using fractions to figure, 118-21
  ratios and proportions
    figuring percents using, 122-244
    practical applications, 124-25
    solving for x, 121-22
  subtraction
    decimals, 113-14
    fractions, 105-6
Matulane (procarbazine), 378t
Maxalt (rizatriptan), 639
Maxaquin (lomefloxacin), 346t
Maxipime (cefepime), 340, 342t
MDMA (Ecstasy), 693
Measles-mumps-rubella vaccine, 69, 311-12, 315-16, 319t, 321t, 323t
Measurement systems
  apothecary, 139
  conversions
    length, 159-61
    system, 151-61
    temperature, 147-50
    time, 146-47
    using ratio and proportion, 150-51
    volume, 152-54
    weight, 154-59
  current trends for symbols and abbreviations, 141, 142t
  household, 139-40
  metric, 130-39
  temperature, 147-49
  units, 140-41
Mebendazole (Vermox), 518
Mechanisms of drug interactions, 42-45
Medicated enemas, 61
Medication(s). *See* Drug(s)
Mediplast (salicylic acid), 59t
Medroxyprogesterone (Depo-Provera), 610
Mefloquine (Lariam), 358t
Mefoxin (cefoxitin), 342t
Megace (megestrol), 376t
Megestrol (Megace), 376t
Meglitinides, 429-30
Melatonin, 398t
Melphalan (Alkeran), 374t
Memantine (Namenda), 674, 675

Memory enhancement, 399b
Menactra, 321t
Meningitis, 316, 318
Meningococcal vaccine, 318, 320t, 321t, 323t
Menopause, 399b, 596, 601-2
Menotropin (Pergonal), 614
Mental health
    Alzheimer's disease and, 646, 674-75, 678
    antipsychotic drugs and, 662-68, 677
    anxiety and, 658-59, 677
    attention deficit/hyperactivity disorder, 675-76, 678
    characteristics of, 658
    defined, 657
    depression and, 399b, 668-74, 677
    neuroses and, 659-60
    psychoses and, 659-60, 662-68
    role of medication in psychotherapy and, 658, 676-78
Mental state and drug dosing, 67
Mentax (butenafine gentian violet), 354t
Meperidine HCL (Demerol), 50, 293t, 294, 639, 688
    and promethazine, 299t
Mephyton, 388t
Meprozine (meperidine and promethazine), 299t
Mercaptopurine (Purinethol), 375t
Mercury preparations, 360
Mesalamine (Rowasa), 517
Mescaline, 692-93
Mesoridazine (Serentil), 664
Mestinon (pyridostigmine), 490
Metabolism, drug, 36
Metamucil (psyllium hydrophilic), 520
Metastasis of cancer, 366-68
Metered dose inhalers, 59t, 257-59, 537
Metformin (Glucophage), 429
Methadone, 689
Methenamine (Mandelamine, Hiprex), 350, 350t, 590
Methicillin (Staphcillin), 339t
Methocarbamol (Robaxin), 488
Methosarb (testolactone calusterone), 376t
Methotrexate (Amethopterin, Mexate, Rheumatrex, MTX), 375t, 486
Methotrexate (Trexall), 377t
Methylcellulose (Citrucel), 512, 520
Methyldopa (Aldomet), 617
Methylphenidate (Ritalin, Concerta), 676

Methylprednisolone (Medrol), 485
Methylxanthines, 538-39t
Methysergide (Sansert), 640
Metoclopramide (Reglan), 370t, 505, 639
Metolazone (Zaroxolyn), 567
Metoprolol (Lopressor), 650
Metric system, the, 130-31
    length measurement and conversion in, 133-35
    mnemonics and conversion within, 131-33
    parenteral medications calculations using, 194-95
    temperature, 147-50
    volume measurement and conversion in, 135-36, 152-54
    weight measurement and conversion in, 136-38, 154-59
Metrodin (urofollitropin), 614
Metronidazole (Flagyl), 345-46, 347t, 504-5
Mexate (methotrexate), 375t
Mexiletine (Mexitil), 558
Mexitil (mexiletine), 558
Mezlin (mezlocillin), 339t
Mezlocillin (Mezlin), 339t
Miacalcin (calcitonin salmon), 478
Micafungin sodium (Mycamine), 353t
Microdrip administration sets, 213
Micro-K, 393t
Microorganisms
    classification of, 333
    gram stains, 334
    identification of, 333-35
    shape, 333
Microsulfon (sulfadiazine), 588
Midazolam (Versed), 626
Midrin, 639
Mifepristone (RU-486), 612-13
Migraine headaches, 639-41
Migrant workers, 312, 325
Milk of Magnesia, 511
Milliequivalents, 140-41
Mineralocorticoids, 414, 415, 418, 432
Minerals, 390-94
    calcium, 386, 391, 392t
    chlorine, 393t, 394
    iron, 391, 392t
    magnesium, 392t, 393
    phosphorus, 391, 393
    potassium, 393-94, 393t
    sodium, 392t, 393
    supplements, 394
Minocin (minocycline), 344t
Minocycline (Minocin, Solodyn), 344t
Minoxidil (Loniten), 568

Minoxidil (Rogaine), 50, 472-73
Mintezol (thiabendazole), 518
Miosis, 437
Miotics, 439
Mirapex (pramipexole), 638, 639
Mirtazapine (Remeron), 669
Misoprostol (Cytotec), 501
Misuse of antibiotics, 337, 362
Mithracin (mithramycin/ plicamycin), 377t
Mithramycin/plicamycin (Mithracin), 377t
Mitomycin (Mutamycin), 377t
Mitotane (Lysodren), 378t
Mitotic inhibitors, 372, 375-76t
Mixed numbers
    adding, 103-5
    dividing, 108-10
    multiplying, 106-8
    subtracting, 106
Mixing two medications, 271, 273-74p, 284
MMR. See Measles-mumps-rubella vaccine
Mnemonics and metric conversions, 131-33
MOM, 392t
Monoamine oxidase inhibitors (MAOIs), 671-72
Montelukast (Singulair), 541
Morphine sulfate (MSIR), 293t, 294
Motrin (ibuprofen), 297t
Mountain tobacco, 399t
Mouth, 496-500, 520
    See also Oral medications
Mouthwashes, 496-500
Moxifloxacin (Avelox), 346t
MSIR (morphine sulfate), 293t, 294
MTX (methotrexate), 375t
Mucokinetic agents, 536
Mucolytics, 536
Mucomyst (acetylcysteine), 536
Mucosal protectants, 501
Mucus, 536
Mugwort, 399t
Multiple-copy prescription program (MCPP), 87
Multiplication
    decimals, 114
    fractions, 106-8
    percents, 117-18
Mupirocin (Bactroban), 59t
Musculoskeletal system
    anatomy, 476, 477f, 478f, 491
    fibromyalgia, 490-91
    gouty arthritis, 487-88
    joint diseases, 480-87
    muscle diseases, 488-91, 641, 642t
    osteoporosis, 384t, 386, 412, 476-79
    spasticity, 488, 490, 491, 641, 642t

Mustargen (nitrogen mustard), 374t
Mutagenic substances, 379
Mutamycin (mitomycin), 377t
Myambutol (ethambutol), 351t
Myasthenia gravis, 490, 491, 653
Mycamine (micafungin sodium), 353t
Mycelex (clotrimazole), 354t, 497
Mycophenolate mofetil (CellCept), 327, 328t
Mycostatin (nystatin), 353t
Mydriasis, 437, 442
Mydriatics, 442
Mylanta, 500, 510
Myleran (busulfan), 374t
Myocardial infarction (MI), 550
Myocardium, 548
Myopia, 439
Mysoline (primidone), 635

N

Nadolol (Corgard), 568, 650
Nafarelin (Synarel), 615
Nafcillin (Nafcil, Unipen), 339t
Nafcil (Nafcillin), 339t
Naftifine (Naftin), 354t
Naftin (naftifine), 354t
Nalfinavir (Viracept), 357t
Naloxone (Narcan), 294
Naltrexone (Revia), 686
Namenda (memantine), 674, 675
Naproxen, 297t
Narcan (naloxone), 294
Narcotics and nonnarcotics combinations, 298, 299-300t, 624-25
Nardil (phenelzine), 641, 671
Narrow-spectrum antibiotics, 333
Narrow-spectrum antistaphylococcal penicillins, 338
Narrow-spectrum penicillins, 338, 339t
Nasal congestion, 527-33
Nasalcrom (cromolyn), 541
Nasal medications, 254-56, 531, 543
Nasal passages, 524-25
Nascobal, 389t
Nateglinide (Starlix), 429
National Childhood Vaccine Injury Act of 1986, 314
National Council on Patient Information and Education, 65
National Drug Code, 83
National Formulary (NF), 14
Native Americans, 395
Natural immunity, 306, 307f, 309-11
Natural reuptake inhibitors (NRIs), 673
Nausea, 370, 399b, 506-10

Navane (thiothixene), 666
Navelbine (vinorelbine), 375t
Nebcin (tobramycin), 345t
Nebulizers, 59t, 537
Nedocromil (Tilade), 541
Needles
  bevels, 266
  gauges, 265
  selection of, 266-67
  See also Syringes
Nefazodone (Serzone), 669
Negative feedback, 405, 407f, 596
Nembutal (pentobarbital), 627
Neobiotic (neomycin), 345t, 347
Neo-Calglucon, 392t
Neomycin (Neobiotic), 345t, 347
Neoplasms. *See* Cancer
Neoral (cyclosporine), 486
Neosar (cyclophosphamide), 374t
Neosporin, 248, 346, 347t
Neostigmine (Prostigmin), 490, 646
Neuroleptics, 659, 662-68
Neurologic system, the
  analgesics effects on, 624-25
  anesthetics and, 625-27
  autonomic nervous system, 622
    functions, 644-45
  central nervous system, 622-24
    stimulants, 642-43
  chemotherapy and, 370
  components and activities of, 621-23
  headaches and, 399b, 639-41
  parasympathetic nervous system and, 623
  Parkinson's disease and, 636-38
  restless legs syndrome and, 638-39
  sedatives/hypnotics and, 627-32
  seizures and, 623, 632-36
  stroke prevention and, 576, 652 sympathetic nervous system and, 623
Neurons, 621, 623
Neurontin (gabapentin), 300t, 635
Neuroses, 659-60
Neurotransmitters, 621
Neutra-Phos, 392t
Neutropenia, 337
Nevirapine (Viramune), 357t
Nexium (esomeprazole), 503
Niacin, 384t, 387
Niaspan, 388t
Nicardipine (Cardene), 555
Nicobid (nicotinic acid), 384t, 387, 388t, 575
Nicotine, 683-85
  patches, 59t
Nicotinic acid (Nicobid), 384t, 387, 388t, 575

NicVax, 684
Nifedipine (Adalat), 555
Nilstat (nystatin), 353t
Nitrates, 551-52, 553t, 616
Nitrofurantoin (Furadantin, Macrodantin, Macrobid), 350, 350t, 590
Nitrogen mustard (Mustargen), 374t
Nitroglycerin, 59t, 551-52
  ointment, 248, 250p, 552
  spray, 552
  sublingual, 552
  transdermal, 552
Nitrolingual, 552
Nitrosoureas, 374t
Nitrostat, 552
Nix (permethrin), 472
Nizoral (ketoconazole), 353t, 497
Noctec (chloral hydrate), 628
Nodules, skin, 460f
Nolvadex (tamoxifen), 376t
Nomenclature, drug, 50-51
Non-English speaking patients, 77
Non-HIV antivirals, 356
Nonopioids
  acetaminophen, 296
  in coanalgesia, 292
  combination, 296
  as controlled substances, 291
  cough suppressants, 534t, 535
  defined, 291
  for migraine headaches, 639, 640t
  nonsteroidal antiinflammatory, 296
  over-the-counter, 297t
  saliyclate, 295-96
  uses, 295
Nonoxynol-9 (Delfen, Ensure), 610
Nonparenteral medications
  dosage calculation methods
    choosing among, 174-75
    dimensional analysis, 173-74
    formula, 169-72
    ratio and proportion, 168-69
  dosage forms, 167
  powder reconstitution, 175, 177t
Nonproprietary drugs. *See* Generic drugs
Nonsalicylate NSAIDS, 482
Nonsteroidal antiinflammatory drugs, 296, 301t
  headaches and, 639, 640t
  for musculoskeletal disorders, 481-85, 491
Nonsteroid hormones, 406
Norelgestromin, 609
Norepinephrine, 671
Norfloxacin (Noroxin), 346t
Normal flora, 333
Normodyne (labetalol), 568

Norpace (disopyramide), 558
Norplant, 607, 613
Nortriptyline (Pamelor), 300t
Norvasc (amlodipine), 555
Norvir (ritonavir), 357t
Novocain (procaine), 627
Novolin (insulin), 421
Novolin Pen, 62
Noxafil (posaconazole), 353t
NSAIDs. *See* Nonsteroidal
    antiinflammatory drugs
Nu-Phosphate, 392t
Nuprin (ibuprofen), 297t
Nutritional supplements
    for the elderly, 390
    herbal, 394-400
    indications for, 400
    lifestyle choices and, 390, 390t
    minerals, 390-94
    over-the-counter market, 383
    vitamins
        deficiencies, 384-85
        fat-soluble, 384t, 385-87, 388t,
            400
        functions, 383-84
        sources of, 385, 386t
        water-soluble, 384t, 387-90,
            388t, 400
Nystatin (Mycostatin, Nilstat), 353t
Nytol (diphenhydramine), 632

O

Obesity, 518-20
Obsessive-compulsive disorder,
    659, 662, 672
Ocean Mist, 392t
Octoxynol-9 (Ortho-Gynol,
    Koromex Cream), 610
Octreotide (Sandostatin), 409
Ocular inserts, 59t
Ocusert (pilocarpine), 59t
Ocu-Sol, 59t
Off-label uses for medications, 49-50
Ofloxacin (Floxin), 346t
Oil-based parenteral medications,
    60
Oils, 31
Ointments, 59t, 241-42, 248-49
    nitroglycerin, 248, 250p
    ophthalmic, 440-41t, 443-46t
Olanzapine (Zyprexa), 666
Oleated oatmeal. *See* Aveeno
Olsalazine (Dipentum), 517
Omeprazole (Prilosec), 502
Omnibus Budget Reconciliation Act
    of 1990, 15, 18b
Omnicef (cefdinir), 342t
Omnipen (ampicillin), 339t
Oncovin (vincristine), 375t
Ondansetron (Zofran), 370t, 507

Ony-Clear Nails (triacetin), 354t
Ophthalmic medications, 438
    anesthetic, 442
    antiallergic and decongestant, 447
    diagnostic aids, 447, 449t
    glaucoma, 439, 442, 443-44t
    immunomodulator, 442
    instillation, 253p, 254p
    mydriatic and cycloplegic, 442
    ointments and drops, 252-53,
        440-41t
    silver nitrate, 360, 439
    solutions and suspensions, 59t
    staining agents, 447, 449t
    storage, 453
    See also Eye
Opioids/opiates
    abuse, 688-89
    antidiarrheal, 516-17
    ceiling effect, 293
    as controlled substances, 291
    cough suppressants, 533-35
    defined, 291
    libido and, 617
    neurologic effects of, 625
    oral, 301t
    patient education for compliance
        with, 294-95
    potency and classification of, 292
    precautions, 294
    rectal, 301t
    transdermal, 301t
    uses of, 292-94
Opportunistic infections, 352
OPV. *See* Poliomyelitis vaccines
Oral contraception, 59t, 466, 606-7,
    608-9t, 618
Oralgen, 427
Oral medications
    absorption rates, 34t
    analgesic, 301t
    antacid, 500-501
    antidiabetic, 428-30
    antifungal, 497
    antiseptic, 496-500
    antiulcer, 500-505
    antiviral, 497
    nasal congestion, 527-30
    route of administration, 238,
        239-41p, 242b
    saliva substitutes, 497, 520
    types, 55-57, 58t
Orders, medication
    abbreviations used in, 85-86
    components of, 86, 87b
    prescription, 87-91
    standard protocol, 86
    standing, 86
    verbal, 86
Orencia (abatacept), 486

Origins of drugs, 31-32
Orimune, 319t
Orphan Drug Act, 15, 17b
Ortho-Gynol (octoxynol-9), 610
Orthostatic hypotension, 555
Os-Cal, 392t
Oseltamivir (Tamiflu), 542-43
OSHA standards
    in medication administration,
        228-29, 237-38
    for needle handling, 263
    safety precautions for
        antineoplastic agents, 379
Osmotic diuretics, 442
Osmotic saline, 511
Osteoarthritis, 296, 480
    alternative medications for,
        394-95
    nonsteroidal antiinflammatories
        for, 481-85
Osteoporosis, 384t, 386, 412, 476-79
Otic medications, 59t, 253-54, 255p,
    449-53
    storage, 453
Otitis media, 449
Ototoxicity, 450, 452b
Over-the-counter (OTC) drugs, 6, 13
    abuse of, 303
    analgesic, 301t, 302t
    antibiotic, 346-48
    antidiarrheals, 521
    antiemetics, 507
    antiflatulents, 510
    antihistamines, 527, 529
    calcium replacement, 477
    contraceptives, 610-12
    cough medicines, 535b
    labeling, 84-85
    laxatives, 511-15
    mouthwashes and local
        anesthetics, 496
    nonopioid, 297t
    nutritional supplements, 383
    patient teaching, 226-27
    percutaneous, 247
    safety and standards, 16
    steroid, 418t
    strength of, 18, 50-51
    for upper respiratory conditions,
        531-33
Over-the-needle catheters, 214f, 214
Ovide (malathion), 472
Ovulation, 595, 596, 610
    infertility and, 614
    suppressants, 613
Oxacillin (Bactocill, Prostaphlin),
    339t
Oxcarbazepine (Trileptal), 635
Oxiconazole (Oxistat), 354t
Oxidized cellulose, 578

Oxistat (oxiconazole), 354t
Oxybutynin (Ditropan), 590
Oxycel, 578
Oxycodone HCL (OxyContin), 293t, 688
  acetaminophen and, 299t
  aspirin and, 299t
OxyContin (oxycodone HCL), 293t, 688
Oxygel, 496
Oxygen therapy, 526, 543
Oxytocin, 409

P

Pacemaker cells, 561
Pacemakers, 335
Package inserts, 51, 52f, 53t, 61-62
Paclitaxel (Taxol), 378t
Pain
  acetaminophen for, 296
  acute and chronic, 290-91
  communicating levels of, 290b
  cultural attitudes toward, 303
  defined, 289, 624
  emotional responses and, 290
  fibromyalgia, 490-91
  headache, 399b, 639-41
  medications and, 290-91
  musculoskeletal conditions and, 491
  perception, 289
  severity, 289, 292
  threshold, 289
  tolerance, 289
Palliative drugs, 38t, 369, 497
Palonosetron HCL (Aloxi), 370t
Pamelor (nortriptyline), 300t
P-aminosalicylic acid (PAS), 351t
Panax ginseng, 396, 397t
Pancreas, 418, 432
  enzyme replacement, 506, 520
Pancrease MT (pancrelipase), 506
Pancreatin, 506
Pancrelipase (Cotazym, Pancrease MT), 506
Panmycin (tetracycline), 344t
Pantothenic acid, 389
Papules, 460f, 463
ParaGard (IUD), 610
Paraplatin (carboplatin), 374t
Parasites, intestinal, 333, 518
Parasympathetic nervous system, 623, 645-48
Parathyroid glands, 414, 478
Paregoric (camphorated opium tincture), 293t, 516
Parenteral route
  administering injectable medications, 274, 284t
  advantages, 262

Parenteral route (Continued)
  disadvantages, 262
  dosage calculations
    metric system, 194-95
    in units, 196-98
  equipment, 263-67
  forms, 190
  injectable, 60
  oil-based, 60
  preparation of medications for, 271-73, 274p
  psychosis treatment, 666-67
  reading syringes for administration of, 191-93
  routes of administration, 35t, 234-35, 274-81, 282-83p
  special precautions with, 262-63
  water-based, 58, 60
Parkinson's disease, 636-38, 653
Parlodel (bromocriptine), 614, 638
Paroxetine (Paxil), 662
Parsley, 398t, 399t
Partial seizures, 632
PAS (p-aminosalicylic acid), 351t
Passive immunity, 306, 307t, 309-11, 322, 324, 326t
Pastes, 59t, 249
Patches, transdermal, 249-51
  insulin, 428
Pathology, 3
Patients
  confidentiality, 89
  contact with allied health professionals, 6-8
  cultural differences among, 75-77
  drug abuse, 694-95
  education for medication safety, 8-10
  factors in choice of antibiotics, 335-36
  information, 64-65
  non-English speaking, 77
  teaching on over-the-counter drugs, 226-27
Paxil (paroxetine), 662
PCP (phencyclidine), 693
Pediarix, 321t
Pediatric patients. See Children
Pediazole (erythromycin-sulfisoxazole), 349t
Pediculosis, 472
Pellagra, 384
Pellets, 61
Penetrex (enoxacin), 346t
Penicillamine (Cuprimine, Depen), 486
Penicillins, 332, 333, 338-40
  antistaphylococcal, 338, 339t
  broad-spectrum, 338, 339t
  extended-spectrum, 339t, 340

Penicillins (Continued)
  narrow-spectrum, 338, 339t
  side effects, 339t
  for urinary tract infections, 588
Pens, insulin, 423, 428f
Pentavac, 318
Pentazocine (Talwin NX), 293t, 294, 302
Pentobarbital (Nembutal), 627
Pentoxifylline (Trental), 572
Peptic ulcers, 500, 501-5, 520
Pepto Bismol (bismuth salts), 504
Percents
  conversion to decimals, 116-17
  decimals conversion to, 117-18
  dividing, 118
  multiplying, 117-18
  using equations to figure, 120
  using fractions to figure, 118-20
Perception, pain, 289
Percocet (acetaminophen and oxycodone), 299t, 688
Percodan (aspirin and oxycodone), 299t, 688
Percutaneous medications, 35t, 58, 59t, 60b
  route of administration, 234, 235, 247-48
Pergolide (Permax), 496, 638
Pergonal (menotropin), 614
Periactin, 50
Peridex (hydrogen peroxide), 496
Peripherally acting adrenergic inhibitors, 568, 570t
Peripheral neuropathy, 314
Peripheral resistance in blood vessels, 562
Peripheral vascular diseases, 572, 573t
Peristalsis, 495
Periwinkle, 399t
Permax (pergolide), 496, 638
Permethrin (Nix, Elimite), 472
Peroxyl (hydrogen peroxide), 496
Persantine (dipyridamole), 576, 652
PH, drug, 34
Pharmacists
  duties in the medication pathway, 6-8
  ethics, 25-27
  legal implications for, 9
Pharmacodynamics, 36-37
Pharmacognosy, 31-32
Pharmacokinetics, 32-36
  absorption in, 33-34, 34t, 35t
  distribution, 34-36
  excretion/elimination in, 36
  factors that affect, 32, 33b
  metabolism in, 36

Pharmacology
  alternative medicine and, 394-400
  basic terms, 4b
  defined, 3-4, 4b
  drug receptor sites, 41-42
  ethics in, 25-27
  five basic categories of, 30-41
  history of, 4-6
  Internet, 5
  pharmacodynamics in, 36-37
  pharmacognosy in, 31-32
  pharmacokinetics in, 32-36
  pharmacotherapeutics in, 38
  reasons for studying, 6-8
  toxicology, 39-41
  undesirable effects of drugs, 41
Pharmacotherapeutics, 38
Phazyme, 510
Phenazopyridine (Pyridium), 590
Phencyclidine (PCP), 693
Phenelzine (Nardil), 641, 671
Phenergan (promethazine), 507, 617
Phenobarbital (Luminal), 627
Phenothiazines, 663t
Phenytoin Na (Dilantin), 300t, 558, 633
Phlebitis, 208
Phos-Ex, 392t
Phos-Lo, 392t
Phosphonated carbohydrate solution, 507
Phosphorus, 391, 392t, 393
Photosensitivity, 470
Physicians
  controlled substances in offices of, 20, 21t
  duties in the medication pathway, 6-8
  legal implications for, 9
Physicians' Desk Reference (PDR), 51, 53
Physiology and intravenous therapy, 206-7
Pilocarpine (Ocusert), 59t
Pin X (pyrantel), 518
Piperacillin (Pipracil), 339t
Pipracil (piperacillin), 339t
Pituitary gland hormones, 408-9, 432
Placebos, 16
Plague, 327t
Plant alkaloids, 372
Plaque, skin, 460f
Plaquenil (hydroxychloroquine), 358t, 486
Plasma protein binding, 36
Plasters, 59t
Platelets, aggregation of, 576
Platinol (cisplatin), 374t
Plavix (clopidogrel), 576

Plax, 496
Plendil (felodipine), 555
Pletal (cilostazol), 572
Pneumococcal vaccine, 317, 320t, 323t, 324
Pneumovax, 320t
Pnu-Immune, 320t
Point of maximum impulse, 548
Poisoning Prevention Packaging Act, 15
Poliomyelitis vaccines, 316, 319t, 323t
Palonosetron HCL (Aloxi), 370t
Polycarbophil (Fiber-Con), 512
Polycillin (amoxicillin), 339t
Polydipsia, 419
Polymox (amoxicillin), 339t
Polymyxin B (Polysporin), 347
Polyphagia, 419
Polypharmacy and the elderly, 73-74
Polysporin (polymyxin B), 347
Polyuria, 419
Portable insulin pumps, 423
Posaconazole (Noxafil), 353t
Postcoital contraception, 611-12
Posterior pituitary gland, 409
Potassium, 393-94, 393t
  loss, 586
  -sparing diuretics, 566t, 567
Potency, drug, 16
Potentiation, 42
Powder
  medications, 248
  reconstitution, 58, 175, 177t, 271, 272p, 283
Pramipexole (Mirapex), 638, 639
Prandin (repaglinide), 429
Praziquantel (Biltricide), 518
Precautions
  in handling antineoplastic agents, 379-80
  opioid and opiate analgesics, 294
  with parenteral medications, 262-63
  with special populations, 68-74
Precef (ceforanide), 342t
Prednisone (Deltasone), 300t
Prefilled syringes, 269, 283
Pregabalin (Lyrica), 296t
Pregnancy and lactation
  Accutane use during, 463
  antibiotic use during, 336
  herbal supplement use during, 397t, 400
  immunosuppression and, 329
  MMR vaccine and, 69, 311-12
  precautions and contraindications during, 68-69, 70b, 71b

Pregnancy and lactation (Continued)
  stimulant laxative use during, 512
  thyroid replacement during, 412
  vitamins and, 386
Premeasured cartridges, 58
Premenstrual syndrome, 399b, 613-14
Preparation of medications, for injections, 271-73, 274p
Presbyopia, 437
Prescriptions
  defined, 87
  parts of, 87-89
  preparation, 87
  refills, 89-90
  safeguarding pads used for, 90-91
Prevacid (lansoprazole), 503
Preventive/prophylactic drugs, 38t
Prevnar, 320t
Priapism, 616-17
Prilosec (omeprazole), 502
Primaquine, 358t
Primary hypertension, 562
Primatene mist aerosol, 59t, 537
Primidone (Mysoline), 635
Principen (ampicillin), 339t
Probenecid (Benemid), 487
Procainamide (Pronestyl, Procan-SR), 558
Procaine (Novocain), 627
Procan-SR (procainamide), 558
Procarbazine (Matulane), 378t
Prochlorperazine (Compazine), 370t
Progestasert (IUD), 610
Progesterone, 603-5
Progestins, 376t, 602, 605t, 618
Prograf (tacrolimus), 377t
Prokinetic agents, 505
Prolactin, 409
Proleukin (interleukin-2), 328
Promethazine (Phenergan), 507, 617
Pronestyl (procainamide), 558
Propecia (finasteride), 473
Proper fractions, 101
Prophylactic agents, 4b, 336-37
  asthmatic, 541t
  topical, 470-72
Proportions and ratios. See Ratios and proportions
Propoxyphene/acetaminophen (Darvocet N), 299t
Propoxyphene (Darvon), 294, 302, 688
Propranolol (Inderal), 552, 555, 558, 561, 568, 617
Proprietary drugs. See Brand-name drugs
ProQuad, 321t
Proscar (finasteride), 600

Prostaglandin agonists, 439
Prostate health, 399b, 600, 601t
Prosthetic joints, 335
Prostigmin (neostigmine), 490, 646
Proteolytic enzymes, 469
Proteus, 590
Proton pump inhibitors, 502-3
Protozoa, classification of, 333
Prozac (fluoxetine), 613, 659, 672-73
Psilocybin, 693
Psoriasis, 461, 473
Psychedelic drugs, 692-93
Psychomimetic drugs, 692-93
Psychoses, 659-60, 662-68
Psychotherapy, 658
Psyllium hydrophilic (Effersyllium, Perdiem, Metamucil, Serutan), 513t, 520
Pumps
  infusion, 214-15
  insulin, 423, 427, 428f
Pure Food and Drug Act of 1906, 14, 17b
Purinethol (mercaptopurine), 375t
Purity, drug, 16
Pustules, 460f, 463
Pyrantel (Antiminth, Pin X), 518
Pyrazinamide (PZA), 351, 351t
Pyridium (phenazopyridine), 590
Pyridostigmine (Mestinon, Regonol), 490
Pyridoxine, 384t, 387, 388t
Pyrimethamine (Daraprim), 358t
Pyrimethamine with sulfadoxine (Fansidar), 358t
Pyuria, 588
PZA (pyrazinamide), 351, 351t

Q

Quality assurance, drug, 16, 227
  medication delivery, 229-30
Questran (cholestyramine), 575
Quinethazone (Hydromox), 567
Quinidine, 558
Quinine, 356, 358t
Quinolone antimicrobials, 344-45, 346t

R

Rabeprazole (AcipHex), 503
Rabies vaccine, 321, 326t, 327t
Radiation therapy, 373
Radioactive iodine, 412
Radioisotopes, 373
Raloxifene (Evista), 376t, 478
Ranitidine (Zantac), 502, 617
Rapamune (sirolimus), 328t
RapidMist, 427
Rashes, 399b

Ratios and proportions
  converting between measurement systems using, 150-51
  figuring percents using, 122-23
  nonparenteral medications dosage calculations using, 168-69
  parenteral medications dosage calculations using, 194
  practical applications, 124-25
  solving for *x*, 121-22
Reach with fluoride, 496
Reality (female condom), 610-11
Rebound congestion, 531
Receptor sites, drug, 41-42
Recombinant DNA technology, 32
Recombivax HB, 320t
Reconstitution
  labeling, 83
  of powders, 58, 175, 177t, 271, 272p, 283
Record keeping, 22f, 23
Rectal medications, 241-45
  analgesic, 301t
Rectus femoris site for intramuscular injections, 281, 283p
Refills, prescription, 89-90
Reglan (metoclopramide), 370t, 505, 639
Regulation of medication
  herbal medicines, 396
  international, federal, and state statutes for, 13-16
Regurgitation, 370, 506-10, 510b, 521
Relaxation, 639
Relenza Rotadisk (zanamivir), 357t, 543
Relpax (eletriptan), 639
Rembrandt Blocking Gel, 497
Remeron (mirtazapine), 669
Remicade (infliximab), 486
Reminyl (galantamine), 675
Renova (tretinoin), 388t, 466
Repaglinide (Prandin), 429
Replacement therapy, 38t, 207-8, 407
Reproductive system, the
  anabolic steroids and, 598-600
  contraception and, 59t, 466, 606-13
  female, 595, 595f, 597f
    endometriosis and, 615-16
    estrogen and, 59t, 376t, 601-3, 604t
    menopause and, 596, 601-2
    premenstrual syndrome and dysmenorrhea, 613-14
    progesterone and, 603-5

Reproductive system, the
  (Continued)
  hormone replacement and, 59t, 598, 601-3
  infertility and, 614-15
  libido and, 617
  male, 595-600, 601t
    anabolic steroids and, 598-600, 618
    benign prostatic hypertrophy and, 600, 601t
    erectile dysfunction and, 616-17, 618
  sexually transmitted diseases and, 610
Requip (ropinirole), 638
Rescriptor (delavirdine), 357t
Reserpine (Serpasil), 568
Respiratory system, the
  anatomy and functions, 524-26
  antihistamines and, 300t, 527-29, 543
  asthma and, 537-42
  chronic obstructive pulmonary disease (COPD), 526, 529, 537-40, 543
  cough medications and, 533-35, 543
  cromolyn sodium and, 531
  decongestants and, 59t, 447, 529-30
  glucocorticoids and, 531
  herbal supplements for, 399b
  influenza virus and, 542-43
  lower, 526, 529, 535-42
  over-the-counter preparations for, 531-33
  oxygen therapy, 526, 543
  upper, 427, 531-35
  vaccines, 317
Respondeat superior, 24
Restasis (cyclosporine), 442
Restless legs syndrome (RLS), 638-39
Restoration therapy, 207
Retavase (reteplase), 576
Reteplase (Retavase), 576
Retina, 437
Retin A (tretinoin), 388t, 466
Retinol, 384t, 385-86, 388t
Retrovir (zidovudine), 358t
Revia (naltrexone), 686
Reye's syndrome, 296, 300, 317
Rheumatoid arthritis, 480, 481f
Rheumatrex (methotrexate), 375t, 486
Rhinitis, 427, 534t
Ribavirin (Virazole), 357t
Riboflavin, 384t, 387
Rickets, 384

Rifadin (rifampin), 351t
Rifamate (rifampin-isoniazid), 351t
Rifampin-isoniazid (Rifamate), 351t
Rifampin (Rimactane, Rifadin), 351t
Rimactane (rifampin), 351t
Rimantadine (Flumadine), 357t, 542
Ringer's solutions, 209
Risedronate (Actonel), 477-78
Ritalin (methylphenidate), 676
Ritonavir (Norvir), 357t
Rizatriptan (Maxalt), 639
Robaxin (methocarbamol), 488
Rocaltrol, 388t
Rocephin (ceftriaxone), 342t
Roferon-A (alpha-interferon), 328t, 377t
Rogaine (minoxidil), 50, 472-73
Ropinirole (Requip), 638
Rose hips, 398t
Rosiglitazone (Avandia), 429
Rotavirus vaccine, 318
Rounding decimals, 111-12
Route of administration
   anesthesia, 626-27
   immunization, 324
   injectable, 274-81, 282-83p
   labeling, 81, 83
   oral, 238, 239-41p, 242b
   percutaneous, 247-59
   rate of drug absorption and, 34t, 35t, 67
   rectal, 241-45
   types of, 34t, 35t, 67, 234-35
Rowasa (mesalamine), 517
Rubramin PC, 389t
Rubs, skin, 459
Ru-486 (mifepristone), 612-13

S
S. aureus, 590
Safe drugs, 30
Safety
   active immunization agents, 321-22
   antimicrobials, 362
   education, medication, 8-10, 226-27
   herbal supplements, 396, 400
   medication administration, 227, 228b, 230-31
   OSHA standards, 228-29
   over-the-counter medications, 226-27
   quality assurance and, 229-30
   self-medication, 227
Salicylate analgesics, 295-96, 297t
   for arthritis, 481-85
   combinations, 298, 299t
Salicylic acid (Compound W, Wart-Off, Mediplast, Sal-Plast), 59t

Salicylic acid spots, 59t
Saline, 58, 392t
   intravenous therapy and, 208
   osmotic, 511
Salinex, 392t
Salivart, 497
Saliva substitutes, 497, 520
Salmeterol (Serevent), 539
Sal-Plast (salicylic acid), 59t
Salts, 390
Samples, drug, 26
Sanctura (trospium), 590
Sandimmune (cyclosporine), 327, 328t, 329
Sandostatin (octreotide), 409
Sansert (methysergide), 640
Saquinavir (Invirase), 357t
Saw palmetto, 396, 397t
Scabies, 472
Scales, skin, 460f
Scalp needles, 213
Scars, 460f
Schizophrenia, 658, 659, 662, 664, 667
Scientific-biomedical beliefs on health and illness, 76
Sclera, 436-37
Scope mouthwash, 496
Scopolamine (Isopto Hyoscine Solution), 445t, 507, 647
Screening, intravenous, 220-21
Scurvy, 384
Seborrheic dermatitis, 468
Sedatives
   abuse, 690-92
   conscious sedation, 626
   sleep disorders and, 627-32
Seizures, 623, 632-36, 653
Selective norepinephrine reuptake inhibitors (SNRIs), 673
Selective serotonin reuptake inhibitors (SSRIs)
   for anxiety, 659
   for depression, 670-71t, 672-73
   for premenstrual syndome, 613
Selegiline (Eldepryl, Cortex), 638
Sensitivity, drug, 335
Septra (trimethoprim sulfamethoxazole), 349t, 588
Sera, 310
Serentil (mesoridazine), 664
Serevent (salmeterol), 539
Seromycin (cycloserine), 351t
Serotonin antagonists, 507
Serpasil (reserpine), 568
Sertaconazole (Ertaczo), 354t
Sertraline (Zoloft), 613, 659
Serums, 326t
Serzone (nefazodone), 669
Severity, pain, 289, 292

Sexually transmitted diseases, 610
Shape of microorganisms, 333
Shingles, 318, 324
Siberian ginseng, 397t
Side effects, 37, 39
   adrenergic agonists, 649t
   adrenergic antagonists, 601t, 651t
   adrenergic-inhibiting agents, 569-70t
   aminoglycosides, 345t
   anabolic steroids, 599t
   androgens, 599t
   anticholinergics, 539t, 647t
   antidepressants, 670-71t
   antihistamines, 528t
   antimalarials, 358t
   antineoplastic agents, 369-71
   antipsychotics, 665-66
   antiseizure medications, 634t, 635t
   antituberculosis drugs, 351t
   antiulcer drugs, 503-4t
   antivirals, 357t
   anxiolytics, 661t
   barbiturates, 629t
   benzodiazepines, 630t
   beta-adrenergic agents, 538t, 569t
   bronchodilators, 539t
   cephalosporins, 342t
   chemotherapy, 369-71, 507b
   chloramphenicol, 347t
   cholinergic agents, 646t
   decongestants, 530t
   dopamine agonists, 637t
   erythromycins, 343t
   estrogens, 604t
   fluoroquinolones, 346t
   glucocorticoids, 532t, 540t
   HIV antivirals, 358t
   hypolipidemics, 574t
   ketolides, 343t
   libido, 617
   lyncomycins, 347t
   methylxanthines, 539t
   mucolytics/expectorants, 536t
   nonopioids, 640t
   ophthalmic drugs, 438
   oral contraceptives, 609t
   penicillins, 339t
   phenothiazines, 663t
   progestins, 605t
   scabicides/pediculicides, 472
   spermicides, 611t
   sulfonamides, 349t
   systemic drugs, 353t
   tetracyclines, 344t
   topical antifungals, 354t
   urinary tract treatment, 350t, 589t
Sildenafil (Viagra), 616

Silvadene Cream (silver sulfadiazine), 349t
Silver nitrate, 360, 439
Silver preparations, 360
Silver sulfadiazine (Silvadene Cream), 349t
Simethicone, 510
Simplifying fractions, 102
Simvastatin (Zocor), 575
Sinequan (doxepin), 300t
Singulair (montelukast), 541
Sinoatrial (SA) nodes, 561
Sirolimus (Rapamune), 328t
Sitagliptin (Januvia), 430
Skin
  acne preparations, 463, 466-68
  cleansers, 458
  functions, 456
  layers, 456, 457f
  lesions, 460f, 473
  types of preparations for, 458-59
  See also Topical medications
Sleep disorders, 399b, 627-32, 653
Slo-Phyllin (theophylline/aminophylline), 540
Slow Fe, 392t
Slow-K, 393t
Slow Mag, 392t
Smoking, 683
  cessation products, 683-84
  and pregnancy, 69
Soaks, 248
Soaps, 458
Social anxiety disorder, 659
Sodium bicarbonate, 500
Sodium chloride, 392t, 393
Sodium hypochlorite, 360
Sodium loss, 586
Solarcaine (benzocaine), 59t
Solid oral preparations, 55, 56t, 239p
Solubility, drug, 33, 35
Solutions, 57
  intravenous therapy, 208-9
Solvents and solutes, body, 206, 391, 584-85
Soma (carisoprodol), 488
Sominex (diphenhydramine), 632
Sotalol (Betapace), 561
Sources
  drug, 31-32
  medication errors, 234
Spasticity, muscle, 488, 490, 491, 641, 642t
Special populations
  children, 70-72
  compliance assistance for, 74-75
  cultural differences and, 75-77
  drug dosing for, 65-68
  elderly, 72-74
  immunizations for, 312-13, 321

Special populations (Continued)
  precautions and contraindications to medication use in, 68-74
  pregnant and lactating, 68-69, 70b, 71b
Spectinomycin, 345
Spectrobid (bacampicillin), 339t
Spermicides, 610, 611t
Spikes, infusion therapy, 213
Spironolactone (Aldactone), 567, 617
Sporanox (itraconazole), 353t
Spotted cowbane, 399t
Sprays, 59t, 251
Sputum, 536
St. Bennett's herb, 399t
St. John's wort, 396, 398t
Stadol (butorphanol nasal spray), 639
Staining agents, ophthalmic, 447, 449t
Standardization of medications, 13
Standards and safety, drug, definitions, 16
Standing orders, 86
Staphcillin (methicillin), 339t
Statins, 574t, 575
Stavudine (Zerit), 357t
Steclin (tetracycline), 344t
Sterilization using disinfectants, 360
Steroids
  administration of, 414-18
  anabolic, 598-600, 618, 694
  drugs used as, 416-17t
  hormones, 406, 414
Stilphostrol (diethylstilbestrol), 376t
Stimulant drugs, 37t
Stimulant laxatives, 512
Stomach ulcers, 500
Stomatitis
  causes of, 496, 537
  chemotherapy and, 370
Stool softeners/moistening agents, 515
Storage, vaccine, 324
Strattera (atomoxetine), 676
Strength of drugs, 13, 14, 18, 50-51
  labeling on, 81
Streptase (streptokinase), 576
Streptokinase (Streptase), 576
Streptomycin (neomycin), 345t, 351t
Stress, 399b, 414
Stroke prevention drugs, 576, 652
Subcutaneous injections, 275, 276-77p, 278-79p, 279f
Sublimaze (fentanyl), 293t
Sublingual medications, 252
Sublingual nitroglycerin, 552

Subtraction
  decimals, 113-14
  fractions, 105-6
Succinimides, 634t
Sucralfate (Carafate), 501
Sulamyd (sulfacetamide ophthalmic ointment/solution), 349t
Sulfacetamide ophthalmic ointment/solution (Sulamyd), 349t
Sulfadiazine (Microsulfon), 588
Sulfamethoxazole (Gantanol), 349t
Sulfasalazine (Azulfidine), 349t, 486, 517
Sulfinpyrazone (Anturane), 487
Sulfisoxazole (Gantrisin), 349t, 588
Sulfonamides, 332, 348, 349t, 362, 589t
  for burns, 468
  for urinary tract infections, 588
Sulfonylureas, 428-29
Sumatriptan (Imitrex), 639
Summation, 43
Sumycin (tetracycline), 344t
Sunscreens, 59t, 470-71
Superinfections, 336
Supershots, 318, 321t
Supplemental drugs, 38t
Supportive drugs, 38t
Suppositories, 59t, 242, 243p, 244p, 515
Suprax (cefixime), 342t
Surgicel, 578
Surveillance, drug, 18, 20t
Suspensions, 57, 59t
Symbols and abbreviations in measurement systems, 141, 142t
Symmetrel (amantadine), 357t, 636
Sympathetic nervous system, 623, 645-48, 653-54
Sympathomimetic agents, 439
Synarel (nafarelin), 615
Synergism, 42
Synovitis, 480
Synthetic drugs, 32
  opioids, 516-17
Synthetic human amylin, 430
Syringes
  disposal, 228-29
  oral, 241p
  for parenteral drug administration, 191-93
  prefilled, 269, 283
  selection, 263-65
  types and sizes, 263, 283
Systemic effects, 37

T

Tablets, 55, 56t
Tacrine (Cognex), 674
Tacrolimus (Prograf), 377t

Tadalafil (Cialis), 616
Tagamet (cimetidine), 502, 617
Talwin NX (pentazocine), 293t, 294, 302
Tamiflu (oseltamivir), 542-43
Tamoxifen (Nolvadex), 376t
Tampons, 61
Tamsulosin (Flomax), 600
Tarceva (erlotinib), 378t
Tardive dyskinesia, 665, 667
Tasmar (tolcapone), 636
Taxol (paclitaxel), 378t
Taxotere (docetaxel), 378t
Tazarotene (Tazorac), 466
Tazidime (ceftazidime), 342t
Tazorac (tazarotene), 466
T-cells, 308, 328
Td. See Diphtheria, tetanus, and pertussis vaccine
Tdap. See Diphtheria, tetanus, and pertussis vaccine
Tears, 438
   artificial, 442
Tea tree oil, 398t
Teeth whitening, 497
Tegopen (cloxacillin), 339t
Tegretol (carbamazepine), 300t, 633, 635, 673
Telithromycin (Ketek), 343t
Temodar (temozolomide), 374t
Temozolomide (Temodar), 374t
Temperature, measurements, 147-50
Tempra (acetaminophen), 297t
Tenex (guanfacine), 617
Tenormin (atenolol), 686
Tension headaches, 641
Tenuate (diethylpropion), 520
Tequin (gatifloxacin), 346t
Teratogenic substances, 379
Terazol (terconazole), 354t
Terazosin (Hytrin), 600
Terbinafine (Lamisil), 353t
Terconazole (Terazol), 354t
Teriparatide (Forteo), 478
Teslac (androgen), 376t
Tessalon (benzonatate), 535
Testoderm, 598
Testolactone (Teslac), 376t
Testosterone, 597, 598
Tetanus
   antitoxin, 326t
   toxoid, 315, 319t, 320t
Tetany, 386
Tetracyclines, 69, 72, 342-44, 344t
   for acne, 463
   for peptic ulcers, 504
   for urinary tract infections, 588
Tetramune, 319t
Thalidomide (Thalomid), 15, 328t

Theophylline/aminophylline (Slo-Phyllin, Elixophyllin), 540
TheraCys (BCG vaccine), 317, 320t, 377t
Therapeutics, 4b, 38t
Thiabendazole (Mintezol), 518
Thiamine, 384t, 387
Thiazide diuretics, 565, 566t, 567, 617
Thiazolidinediones, 429
Thienobenzodiazepines, 663t
Thiothixene (Navane), 666
Thioxanthenes, 663t
Thorazine (chlorpromazine), 664, 665-66
Threshold, pain, 289
Thrombi, 220, 576, 577f
Thrombin, 578
Thrombinar, 578
Thromboembolisms, 576
Thrombolytic medications, 576
Thrombostat, 578
Thyroid hormone, 37, 409, 411-14, 432
Thyroid-stimulating hormone, 409
Thyrotropin (TSH), 409
Tiagabine (Gabitril), 635
Ticlid (ticlopidine), 576
Ticlopidine (Ticlid), 576
Tigan (trimethobenzamide), 370t, 507
Tilade (nedocromil), 541
Time
   of administration, 67
   conversions, 146-47
   infusion, 217-18
Tinactin (tolnaftate), 248
Tinctures, 59t, 293t, 359-60
Tinnitus, 450, 482
Tioconazole (Vagistat), 354t
Titer, antibody, 313
Titralac, 392t
Tizanidine (Zanaflex), 488
Tobacco, 399t, 683-85
Tobramycin (Nebcin, Tobrex), 345t
Tobrex (tobramycin), 345t
Tocainide (Tonocard), 558
Tofranil (imipramine), 300t, 591
Tolcapone (Tasmar), 636
Tolerance
   drug, 42
   pain, 289
Tolnaftate (Tinactin, Absorbine, Aftate), 248
Tolterodine (Detrol-LA), 590
Tonocard (tocainide), 558
Tonometry, 442
Toothpaste, 59t
Topamax (topiramate), 300t, 635

Topical medications, 34, 58, 247
   absorption, 457-58
   acne, 463, 466-68
   anesthetics, 59t, 468, 496-500, 627
   antibiotic, 459
   antifungal, 353-54t, 453, 464-65t
   antiinfective/antiinflammatory, 459, 461-63
   antipruritics, 468
   antiviral, 459, 461
   for burns, 468-70
   classification of, 456-57
   corticosteroids, 461-63
   for geriatric patients, 251
   hemostatics, 576, 578
   keratolytic agents, 466, 468
   nitroglycerin, 552
   prophylactic, 470-72
   scabies and pediculosis, 472
   seborrheic dermatitis, 468
   sulfonamide, 332, 349t
   types of, 248-52, 458-59
Topiramate (Topamax), 300t, 635
Tourette's syndrome, 666
Toxicology, 39-41
Toxoids, 312, 315
Tracheobronchial tree, 525
Trade names, 81
Tramadol (Ultram), 296t
   acetaminophen and, 299
Tranquilizers
   for alcoholism, 686
   major, 662-68
   minor, 660-62
Transdermal medications, 58, 59t, 61f, 252
   contraceptive, 607, 609-10
   nitroglycerin, 552
   opioids, 301t
   route of administration, 234, 247
   testosterone, 598
   types of, 249-51
Transplantation and immunosuppressants, 325, 327
Travel and vaccinations, 325
Trazodone (Desyrel), 662, 669
Tremors, 660
Trental (pentoxifylline), 572
Tretinoin (Retin A, Renova, Antragen), 377t, 388t, 466
Trexall (methotrexate), 377t
Triacetin (Fungoid, Ony-Clear Nails), 354t
Triamcinolone (Aristocort, Kenacort), 485
Tricyclic antidepressants, 300t, 659, 669, 670t
Trifluridine (Viroptic), 357t
Triglycerides, 572-75
Tri-Immunol, 319t

Trileptal (oxcarbazepine), 635
Trimethobenzamide (Tigan), 370t, 507
Trimethoprim sulfamethoxazole (Bactrim, Septra, Cotrim), 349t, 588
Trimox (amoxicillin), 339t
Triple Antibiotic Cream, 248
Triple Sulfa (trisulfapyrimidines), 349t
Trisulfapyrimidines (Triple Sulfa), 349t
Troches, 55
Tropic hormones, 408
Trospium (Sanctura), 590
Tuberculosis, 332
  drugs to treat, 350-52
  vaccine, 317
Tubing, infusion, 212f, 213
Tumors, skin, 460f
Tums, 392t, 477
Twinrix, 320t
Tylenol (acetaminophen), 297t
Tylox (acetaminophen and oxycodone), 299t
Tympanic membrane, 449
Typhoid, 327t

U
Ulcers
  peptic, 50, 501-5, 520
  skin, 460f, 473
Ultracet (acetaminophen and tramadol), 299
Ultralente insulin, 422
Ultram (tramadol), 296t
Unbound drugs, 34
Undecylenic acid (Desenex, Cruex, Caldesene, Fungoid), 354t
Undesirable effects, identification of, 41
Unipen (nafcillin), 339t
Unisom (doxylamine), 632
United States Pharmacopoeia (USP), 14, 50, 51, 65, 379
Units, measurement, 140-41, 196-97
Unstable angina, 551
Upper respiratory tract, 427, 531-35
Uracil mustard ifosfamide (Ifex), 374t
Urecholine (bethanechol), 645
Urinary system, the
  diuretics and, 584
  enuresis and, 589t, 590-91
  fluid and electrolyte balance and, 392t, 584-85
  fluid replacement therapy, 585-87
  infections, 350, 399b, 587-90
Urinary tract infections, 350, 399b, 587-90

Urispas (flavoxate), 590
Urofollitropin (Metrodin), 614
Urokinase (Abbokinase), 576
Ursodiol (Actigall), 506
U.S. Customary System of Measurement, 138-40
  length measurements, 159-61
  volume measurements, 152-54
  weight measurements, 154-59
U.S. Department of Agriculture, 396
Uveitis, 438

V
Vaccinations, 306, 307f, 309
  adverse reactions to, 314
  BCG (TheraCys), 317, 320t, 377t
  chickenpox, 316-17, 320t, 321t, 323t
  diphtheria, tetanus, and pertussis, 315, 319t, 321t, 323t
  documentation, 314-15
  Haemophilus influenzae, 316, 319t, 323t
  hepatitis, 316, 320t, 323t
  human papillomavirus, 318, 320t, 324
  indications for, 313
  influenza, 317, 320t, 323t
  lyme, 320t, 321
  measles, mumps, and rubella, 69, 311-12, 315-16, 319t, 321t, 323t
  meningococcal, 318, 320t, 321t, 323t
  nicotine deterrent, 684
  patient education, 324-25
  pneumococcal, 317, 320t, 323t, 324
  poliomyelitis, 316, 319t, 323t
  rabies, 321, 327t
  for respiratory conditions, 317
  rotavirus, 318
  safety, 321-22
  schedule, 323t
  for specific populations, 321
  storage, 324
  supershot, 318, 321t
  travel and, 325
  types, 311-12
  zoster, 318
Vaccine Adverse Event Reporting System (VAERS), 314
Vaccine Information Statements (VIS), 314
Vaginal medications, 59t, 256-57
  estrogen, 602-3
Vagistat (tioconazole), 354t
Valacyclovir (Valtrex), 357t
Valerian, 396, 398t, 632
Valium (diazepam), 50, 489, 507
  for anxiety, 659
  libido and, 617

Valium (diazepam) *(Continued)*
  for seizures, 633
  for spasticity, 641
Valproate (Depakote), 635, 673
Valproic acid (Depakene), 635, 640, 641
Valtrex (valacyclovir), 357t
Vancocin (vancomycin), 345, 347t
Vancomycin (Vancocin), 345, 347t
Vantin (cefpodoxime), 342t
Vardenafil (Levitra), 616
Varenicline (Chantix), 684
Variant angina, 551
Varicella virus vaccine, 316-17, 320t, 321t, 323t
Varivax vaccine, 316-17, 320t
Vasocon (Bepridil), 59t, 555
Vasocongestion, 442
Vasodilan (isoxsuprine), 572
Vasodilators, 550, 556, 561, 568, 571t, 580
Vasospastic angina, 551
Vasotec (enalapril), 568
Vastus lateralis site for intramuscular injections, 281, 283p
Velban (vinblastine), 375t
Velosef (cephradine), 342t
Velsar (vinblastine), 375t
Venlafaxine (Effexor), 659, 662
Venofer, 392t
Ventolin (albuterol), 59t, 537
Ventrogluteal site for intramuscular injections, 281
Verapamil (Calan, Isoptin), 555, 561, 641
Verbal medication orders, 86
Vermox (mebendazole), 518
Versed (midazolam), 626
Vertigo, 449, 453t
Vesicles, skin, 460f
Viactiv, 392t, 477
Viagra, 50
Viagra (sildenafil), 616
Vials, 58, 61f, 263, 267, 269-70p, 283
  mixing medications in, 273-74p, 284
Vibramycin (doxycycline), 344t, 358t
Vicoprofen (ibuprofen and hydrocodone), 299t
Vidarabine (Vira-A), 357t
Videx, ddI (didanosine), 357t
Vinblastine (Velban, Velsar), 375t
Vinca, 399t
Vincristine (Oncovin), 375t
Vinorelbine (Navelbine), 375t
Vioform (clioquinol), 354t
Vira-A (vidarabine), 357t
Viracept (nelfinavir), 357t

Viral infections, drugs used to treat, 355-56, 357t
Viramune (nevirapine), 357t
Virazole (ribavirin), 357t
Viroptic solution, 357t
Viruses, classification of, 333
Vistaril (hydroxyzine), 300t, 662
Vistide (cidofovir), 357t
Vitamins
    A, 384t, 385-86, 388t
    B, 384t, 387-89
    C, 389-90, 389t
    D, 384t, 386-87, 388t
    deficiency, 384-85
    E, 384t, 387, 388t
    for the elderly, 390
    fat-soluble, 384t, 385-87, 388t, 400
    functions of, 383-84
    H, 389
    indications for, 400
    K, 384t, 387, 388t
    lifestyle choices and, 390, 390t
    sources of, 385, 386t
    water-soluble, 384t, 387-90, 388t, 400
Vite E cream, 388t
Vitreous humor, 437
Vivotif Berna vaccine, 327t
Volume measurement and conversion in metric system, 134-36, 152-54
Vomiting, 370, 506-10, 510b, 521
Vyvanse (lisdexamfetamine), 676

W

Warfarin (Coumadin), 576
Wart-Off (salicylic acid), 59t
Water-based parenteral medications, 58, 60

Water-soluble vitamins, 384t, 387-90, 388t, 400
Weight
    appetite suppressants and, 518-20
    drug dosing and, 65-66, 178-82
    loss and chemotherapy, 370
    measurement and conversion in metric system, 136-39, 154-59
Wellbutrin (bupropion), 669, 673
Wellcovorin (leucovorin), 375t
Wheals, 460f
Whitening agents, tooth, 497
Wild tobacco, 399t
Winged-infusion needles, 213
Wolfsbane, 399t
World Health Organization, 292
Worms, parasitic, 518
Wormwood, 399t
Wounds, cleansing of, 359
Wytensin (guanabenz), 617

X

Xanax (alprazolam), 613
Xanthine derivatives, 540
Xeloda (capecitabine), 375t
Xerostomia, 497
Xopenex (levalbuterol), 59t

Y

Yin and yang, 396

Z

Zafirlukast (Accolate), 541
Zalcitabine (Hivid), 357t
Zanaflex (tizanidine), 488
Zanamivir (Relenza Rotadisk), 357t, 543

Zantac (ranitidine), 502, 617
Zaroxolyn (metolazone), 567
Zephiran (benzalkonium chloride), 359
Zerit (stavudine), 357t
Ziagen (abacavir), 357t
Zicam, 533
Zidovudine (Retrovir), 358t
Zileuton (Zyflo), 541
Zinc, 393t, 394
    based decongestants, 530t, 533
    insulin and, 421
    oxide, 249
Ziprasidone (Geodon), 666
Zithromax, 175, 176f, 177t, 341, 343t
Zocor (simvastatin), 575
Zofran (ondansetron), 370t, 507
Zoladex (goserelin), 376t, 615
Zolmitriptan (Zomig), 639
Zoloft (sertraline), 613, 659
Zolpidem (Ambien), 631
Zomig (zolmitriptan), 639
Zonegran (zonisamide), 635
Zonisamide (Zonegran), 635
Zostavax, 318
Zoster vaccine, 318
Zovirax (acyclovir), 357t, 497
Z-track, 507
Zyban (bupropion), 669, 684
Zyflo (zileuton), 541
Zyloprim (allopurinol), 487
Zyprexa (olanzapine), 666